Temperature

0° C (Centigrade) = 32° F (Fahrenheit) = 273° K (Kelvin)
100° C = 212° F

Pressure

1 Atmosphere = 760 mmHg (at 0° C) = 760 torr = 29.0213 inch
H_2O (at 32° F)

Volume

1 liter (L) = 1000 milliliters (mL)
1 L = 1.057 quarts (qt)
1 qt = 0.9463 L = 946.3 mL = 32 ounces (oz)
1 gallon (gal) = 4 qt = 128 oz = 3.785 L
1 pint (pt) = 16 oz = 2 cups (c)

SI Units (Systeme International)

Physical quantity	Unit	Symbol
Mass	kilogram	kg
Distance	meter	m
Time	second	sec
Amount of substance	mole	mol
Force	newton	N
Work	joule	J
Power	watt	W
Pressure	pascal	Pa
Velocity	meters per sec	$m \cdot sec^{-1}$
Torque	newton-meter	N-m
Angle	radian	rad
Angular Velocity	radians per second	$rad \cdot sec^{-1}$
Acceleration	meters per second^2	$m \cdot sec^{-2}$
Volume	liter	L

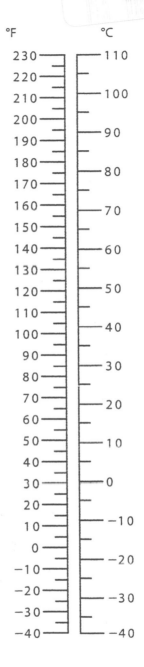

Fahrenheit
Temperature

To convert temperature scales:

Fahrenheit to Celsius $°C = 0.555(°F - 32)$

Celsius to Fahrenheit $°F = 1.8(°C) + 32$

Traditionally, in the United States, English units of measurement have been used, and we have presented equivalents for various units. However, practitioners and researchers are encouraged to use the SI units. (Knuttgen, H. G., and Komi, P. V.: *Basic definitions for exercise.* In Komi, P. V. (ed.): *Strength and Power in Sports.* Oxford, Blackwell Scientific Publications, 1992, pp. 3–6).

Fox's
Physiological Basis
for Exercise and Sport

sixth edition

Fox's
Physiological Basis
for Exercise and Sport

Merle L. Foss
University of Michigan

Steven J. Keteyian
Henry Ford Heart & Vascular Institute

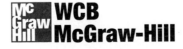

Boston, Massachusetts   Burr Ridge, Illinois   Dubuque, Iowa
Madison, Wisconsin   New York, New York   San Francisco, California   St. Louis, Missouri

WCB/McGraw-Hill
A Division of the McGraw-Hill Companies

Fox's Physiological Basis for Exercise and Sport

 This book is printed on recycled, acid-free paper containing 10% postconsumer waste.

1 2 3 4 5 6 7 8 9 0 QPD/KPH 9 0 9 8 7

ISBN 0-697-25904-8

Publisher: *Edward E. Bartell*
Sponsoring Editor: *Theresa Grutz*
Developmental Editor: *Patricia A. Schissel*
Marketing Manager: *Pamela S. Cooper*
Project Manager: *Donna Nemmers*
Production Supervisor: *Laura Fuller*
Designer: *Katherine Farmer*
Cover Designer: *Elise Lansdon*
Photo Research Coordinator: *John C. Leland*
Art Editor: *Joyce Watters*
Compositor: *York Graphic Services, Inc.*
Typeface: *10/12 Times*
Printer: *Quebecor Printing Book Group/Dubuque*

The Credits section of this book appears on page 611, and is considered an extension of the copyright page.

Library of Congress Cataloging-in-Publication Data
Foss, Merle L., 1936–
    Fox's physiological basis for exercise and sport. —6th ed./
Merle L. Foss, Steven J. Keteyian.
        p. cm.
    Rev. ed. of: The physiological basis for exercise and sport/
Edward L. Fox, Richard W. Bowers, Merle L. Foss. 5th ed. ©1993.
    First through 4th eds. published under title: The physiological
basis of physical education and athletics.
    Includes bibliographical references and indexes.
    ISBN 0-697-25904-8
    1. Sports—Physiological aspects. 2. Exercise—Physiological
aspects. I. Keteyian, Steven J. II. Fox, Edward L. Physiological
basis for exercise and sport. III. Fox, Edward L. Physiological
basis of physical education and athletics. IV. Title. V. Title:
Physiological basis for exercise and sport.
    [DNLM: 1. Sports. 2. Sports Medicine. 3. Physical Education and
Training. 4. Exercise. QT 260 F75lf 1998]
RC1235.F65 1998
612'.044—DC21
DNLM/DLC
for Library of Congress

www.mhhe.com

To my loving wife, Peggy Meister Foss, who
encourages me in my work, and to my mother,
Gladys Campbell Foss, who, perhaps unknowingly,
taught me to write.
—M.L.F.

Work without the love and interest of others
represents "hard labor." This work is dedicated to
three people who turned my toils into joy:
Lynette Karyl Laidler-Keteyian,
"Princess" Stephanie Rose Keteyian,
and in loving memory of
Virginia Keteyian (1923–1996)
—S.J.K.

Brief Contents

Contents

Section Two
Neuromuscular Concepts 105

Chapter 5
Nervous Control of Muscular Movement 105

Chapter 6
Skeletal Muscle: Structure and Function 130

Section Three
Cardiorespiratory Considerations 169

Chapter 7
Pulmonary Ventilation and Mechanics 170

Chapter 8
Gas Exchange and Transport 194

Chapter 9
Cardiovascular System: Function and Exercise Responses 214

Chapter 10
Cardiorespiratory Control 248

Section Four
Physical Training 267

Chapter 11
Methods for Anaerobic Training and Physiologic Responses 268

Chapter 12

Methods for Aerobic Training and Physiologic Responses 294

Chapter 13

Development of Muscular Strength, Endurance, and Flexibility 338

Chapter 14

Physical Activity and Health 374

Section Five

Nutrition and Body Weight Control 409

Chapter 15

Nutrition and Exercise Performance 410

Chapter 16

Exercise, Body Composition, and Weight Control   438

Section Six

Humoral Responses and Performance Aids   469

Chapter 17

Exercise and the Endocrine System   470

Chapter 18

Drugs and Ergogenic Aids   492

Section Seven

The Environment   509

Chapter 19

Temperature Regulation: Exercise in the Heat and Cold   510

Chapter 20

Performance Underwater, at High Altitude, and during and after Microgravity 540

Feature Boxes

Foreword

The sixth edition of this text carries within its title the name of its original author, the late Dr. Edward L. Fox. As professional colleagues and personal friends of Ed Fox at The Ohio State University during the years he developed the original versions of this text with Dr. Donald Mathews, we are well aware of his vision for this text and of his genuine concern for students in this discipline.

Ed Fox was a native of Dayton, Ohio. He received his B.S. and M.A. degrees in physical education and his Ph.D. degree in physiology, all from The Ohio State University. He then went on to Indiana University to do post-doctoral study with Dr. Sid Robinson. Returning to Ohio State to begin a career of teaching and research, he had widely varied research interests within the field of exercise physiology, spanning the range from gifted young athletes to the elderly. He was a long-time member of the American College of Sports Medicine and at one time ran for the office of president of that organization. He was liked and admired by his students, not only for his expertise, but for his sense of humor and for the deep care he showed the students whom he felt were trusting him to educate them and to guide them in their careers. He was a gifted writer with a knack for clarifying difficult concepts. His untimely passing in 1983 ended an all-too-brief career that included many scientific publications and texts in the area of exercise physiology.

This text, in its early form, represented the single effort of which Ed Fox was most proud. He felt that this text should help students and others who were going to guide people engaging in exercise programs under a wide variety of circumstances. He also believed that those who conduct such programs have an obligation to understand the physiological effects of activity through which they are directing the individual. This is the essence of exercise physiology. In this book he provided a carefully researched, comprehensive view of the physiological basis for exercise and sport—done in a format that enabled students to understand difficult and important concepts with minimal scientific prerequisite. The name Fox has become synonymous with well-written, easily understood exercise physiology.

This text has had a strong and continuing influence in the field, due largely to the efforts of Ann Fox Day, who worked tirelessly to ensure that Ed's vision for this text and its high quality be maintained. Her goals were accomplished in conjunction with the writing skill and knowledge of the field of previous co-authors. This sixth edition of Fox's original text remains true to the goals that Ed Fox had established. It remains well-written and easily understood, thanks to the efforts of Drs. Foss and Keteyian and the editorial staff at WCB/McGraw-Hill Publishers. Material and figures throughout help to clarify sometimes difficult concepts and to highlight important facts. Most importantly, the text includes the latest research-based information in all the areas covered. This edition, containing updated research information, continues to fulfill Ed Fox's vision to be comprehensive, and expands on these areas to include timely material, particularly in the areas that have been updated by the current authors. Some of these concern training methods, exercise prescription, and physical activity and health. Former colleagues, students, and friends (of which there are very many) will be pleased to see that this edition continues to carry the goals and visions of Ed Fox into the future. We feel that he would be as proud of this effort as he was of the early editions.

Dr. Robert L. Bartels
Dr. Timothy E. Kirby

Preface

Ever since 1927 when the "roots" of exercise physiology first took hold in the United States at the Harvard Fatigue Laboratory, our field has grown in both depth and stature. Within the past five years alone, the role of physical activity in health maintenance and health improvement has risen to one of national importance. More than ever, students are seeking careers that require formal instruction in what we believe is a stimulating and dynamic field.

This textbook is no longer written for just the physical education teacher or coach. As a result, it is no longer used only in physical education and kinesiology departments. Instead, exercise physiology courses are now being taught in departments of physical therapy, occupational therapy, allied health, public health, and physiology. We take great pleasure in knowing that, for many students, their ability to advance a profession and contribute to society in the future will be partly influenced by our efforts.

New to this Edition

This book was written with the intention of being a comprehensive text used in an upper-level undergraduate or lower-level graduate course of study. The breadth of the material found between its covers far exceeds what can be covered in one semester, giving rise to its value as a resource for many years in the future.

Without question, this text has undergone numerous organizational and content changes—more so now than at any other time in its more than 25 year history. The number of chapters have been reduced to 20, and material formerly covered in a separate chapter devoted to female issues has been integrated where appropriate. These decisions were made because of our belief that a female's participation in exercise and sport should no longer be viewed as if it were unexpected or unique. We acknowledge that areas do exist where females and males differ in terms of basic physiology or physiologic response to exercise, and these issues are now integrated into each chapter as indicated.

We also take great joy in pointing out that not just two or three, but 12 of the 20 chapters have undergone *major* revision. In doing so we have brought to students the most up-to-date science and information that can be applied in the classroom setting. Some highlights and other features or changes include:

- Inclusion of more clinical discussion and examples to aid those students entering such professions in the future.

- Addition of feature boxes that highlight unique aspects of coaching, advanced study, or clinical practice.

- Chapter 1 has been expanded to include the rich history that preceded those of us now practicing in the field.

- Chapter 9 now includes a more comprehensive presentation of the major determinants of cardiac function at rest and of how these factors are altered during an acute bout of exercise.

- Chapter 10 provides a much stronger presentation of the roles of central command and the body's receptors in regulating cardiorespiratory adaptations before, during and after exercise, reflecting much of what we have learned in just the past several years.

- Our approach to training principles and chronic adaptations to training has been completely reworked. Chapter 11 covers training principles and chronic adaptations to sprint/power- or anaerobic-type sports, whereas chapter 12 does the same for endurance- or aerobic-type sports.

- Chapter 13 has been revised to emphasize some of the side benefits to progressive resistance training and its use by older people.

- Chapter 14 is fully revised and addresses what continues to be a rapidly growing subspecialty within the discipline of exercise physiology: public health. To facilitate our efforts, we highlight the Surgeon General's first report on *Physical Activity and Health*.

- Chapter 18 now includes a summary of "contemporary" ergogenic aids, with an index of their efficacy and risks.

- Chapter 20 has extended its coverage of the environment to include humankind's adaptations and responses to microgravity (i.e., space).

- Finally, we hope the larger page size with full-color format enhances this edition's role as a teaching and learning tool.

Walk Through

Contents and Organization

To correctly revise and generate the sixth edition of this text, we literally started where all scientists begin when striving to solve as yet unanswered questions: in the literature. Evidence of our efforts is clear if you scan through the reference lists found at the end of each chapter. When doing so you will notice that extensive, current additions have been made. We are confident in saying this text is up-to-date.

Following an introduction (chapter 1), we have divided our efforts into seven distinct sections. These include:

- Bioenergetics
- Neuromuscular Concepts
- Cardiorespiratory Considerations
- Physical Training
- Nutrition and Body Weight Control
- Humoral Responses and Performance Aids
- The Environment

As highlighted in the table of contents, each section is compartmentalized using two or more chapters, allowing the instructor and the student to choose those topics they feel are most relevant for study during a particular course. Although information in one chapter may depend upon that given in another, much cross-referencing by page number is given for easy identification.

Whenever possible, we have tried to integrate our teachings across various populations and among persons who are healthy and those with specific diseases. As has been the case throughout history, much is learned about normal human physiology when comparing those who are healthy to those with clinically manifest disease. However, we have taken the next step and often compare these same two groups relative to their acute and chronic responses to exercise. Doing so only expands that much more our ability to learn and teach.

Pedagogical Aids

Chapter Opening Features

- Chapter Introduction: Each chapter begins with an overview of the chapter content. In addition to preparing students for the key ideas to be explored, the introduction ties the chapter to other relevant material in the textbook.

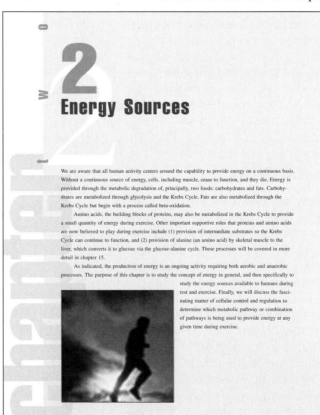

2
Energy Sources

We are aware that all human activity centers around the capability to provide energy on a continuous basis. Without a continuous source of energy, cells, including muscle, cease to function, and they die. Energy is provided through the metabolic degradation of, principally, two foods: carbohydrates and fats. Carbohydrates are metabolized through glycolysis and the Krebs Cycle. Fats are also metabolized through the Krebs Cycle but begin with a process called beta-oxidation.

Amino acids, the building blocks of proteins, may also be metabolized in the Krebs Cycle to provide a small quantity of energy during exercise. Other important supportive roles that proteins and amino acids are now believed to play during exercise include (1) provision of intermediate substrates so the Krebs Cycle can continue to function, and (2) provision of alanine (an amino acid) by skeletal muscle to the liver, which converts it to glucose via the glucose-alanine cycle. These processes will be covered in more detail in chapter 15.

As indicated, the production of energy is an ongoing activity requiring both aerobic and anaerobic processes. The purpose of this chapter is to study the concept of energy in general, and then specifically to study the energy sources available to humans during rest and exercise. Finally, we will discuss the fascinating matter of cellular control and regulation to determine which metabolic pathway or combination of pathways is being used to provide energy at any given time during exercise.

- Outline of Topics: The outline provides a concise "map" of the content to be covered and a framework for students to use as they mentally organize the material.

- Major Concepts: The key learning objectives can be used to help students focus on the most important material in each chapter; they also provide an excellent starting point for reviewing the material before quizzes and exams.

- Key Terms: Students see all of the important terms up front, alerting them to terms they should know. After completing the chapter, this material can be used to test understanding of the key terms.

Featured Box Readings

The feature boxes allow us to stray a bit from the main body of the text, drawing students into a specific point of study.

- **Clinic Note:** Over the past decade many students graduating with their major field of study in kinesiology, exercise science, or exercise physiology have entered careers in cardiac rehabilitation, occupational therapy, nursing, and physical therapy. Our Clinic Notes make the connection between academics and clinical practice. For all students this feature provides first-hand, real-life clinical applications of what is learned in the classroom.

- **Coaches' Corner:** This feature represents our initiative to bring together what is observed in the exercise physiology laboratory with what happens on the field. We touch on a wide variety of issues, such as "new wave" training methods, special safety concerns, and performance-enhancing techniques.

  - **Advanced Study:** With this feature students have the opportunity to explore topics in greater depth, and instructors can use this material when teaching challenging concepts.

New Illustration Program

- Full-color illustrations: Detail, clarity, and consistency characterize the new full-color illustration program. Students will be able to better visualize structures and processes and to clearly see complex ideas.

- Enhanced photograph program: This edition is enlivened by more photographs in full color that show students up-to-date practices and procedures in exercise physiology.

End-of-Chapter Features

- Summary: Each chapter ends with a review summary to help students effectively internalize the important concepts.

- Questions: Interesting questions at the end of each chapter give students the opportunity to think critically about the content and to assess their mastery of the concepts.

- References: Thoroughly updated references support the presentation in each chapter.

- Selected Readings: Students and instructors seeking additional information on topics presented in any of the chapters can turn to additional resources found at the end of each chapter.

Sample page: Clinic Note

120   Section 2 • Neuromuscular Concepts

Clinic Note

Stretch Reflexes

You can test your neuromuscular stretch reflexes by exerting a quick forceful tap with a rubber reflex hammer to the tendon. Three such examples are given as follows.

Biceps Reflex

Flex your forearm 90 degrees and have a partner support it; have the partner place his or her thumb over the tendon of insertion of the biceps (tubercle of radius). Now strike the thumb with the hammer; the force is transferred to your biceps tendon. The biceps muscle will contract, flexing the forearm. (Note: spinal cord segment servicing the muscle biceps brachii is C5–C6 [i.e., fifth and sixth cervical vertebrae].)

Triceps Reflex

Support your arm in a similar fashion as in the biceps reflex. When the triceps tendon of insertion (olecranon process of ulna) is struck directly with the hammer, the triceps will contract, extending the forearm. (Note: spinal cord segment servicing the muscle triceps brachii is C6–C7 [i.e., sixth and seventh cervical vertebrae].)

Patellar Reflex

Sit comfortably on the edge of a table, with your legs dangling and relaxed. Strike the patellar tendon with a sharp blow. The quadriceps femoris muscles will contract, causing extension of the leg (see figure 5.15). (Note: spinal cord segment servicing the four quadricep muscles is L2, L3, L4 [i.e., second, third, and fourth lumbar vertebrae].)

In each reflex, stimulation of the muscle spindles by rapping the tendon with a sharp, firm blow conveys information to the CNS, where motor stimuli are relayed to the appropriate muscle and contraction of the muscle is initiated. A positive response (i.e., lack of contraction for the specified muscle) is indicative of a malfunction or lesion at the level of the spinal cord servicing that particular muscle (e.g., biceps brachii—fifth or sixth cervical vertebrae). Likewise, the absence of limb reflexes might indicate a disruption of a normal function in the sensory afferent or motor efferent nerve systems due to injury or disease. Team physicians and trainers frequently conduct basic reflex tests to determine whether an injured athlete has experienced nerve damage. Similar reflex testing can be used to check for CNS hyperexcitability or depression caused by the possible presence of drugs and medications in the body.

Sample page: Figure 8.5

muscles supplied with these motor fibers. Severing the nerve results in total paralysis.

Voluntary Control of Motor Functions

136   Section 2 • Neuromuscular Concepts

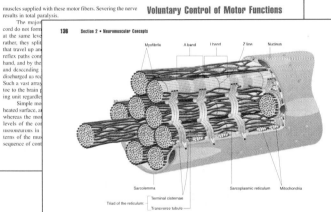

Figure 8.5

The sarcoplasmic reticulum and transverse tubules form a netlike system of tubules and vesicles surrounding the myofibrils. The outer vesicles store large quantities of calcium ions (Ca^{++}), one of the ingredients required for the contractile process. The transverse tubules are concerned with conduction of the nervous impulses deep into the myofibrils. The two outer vesicles (terminal cisternae) and the transverse tubule separating them are known as a triad.

(Labels: Myofibrile, A band, I band, Z line, Nucleus, Sarcolemma, Terminal cisternae, Triad of the reticulum, Transverse tubule, Sarcoplasmic reticulum, Mitochondria)

Sample page: Chapter 16

Chapter 16 • Exercise, Body Composition, and Weight Control   463

expenditure of elderly persons ought to be rather than to spend more time in assessing what they currently are. He suggests that we should "actively" encourage physical activity in the elderly, which, in turn, will be accompanied by an increase in their energy expenditure and a decrease in fatness, and at the same time promote the need to ingest adequate amounts of essential dietary nutrients. In essence, the elderly should strive for an activity-driven metabolic system that is truly in a harmonious balance.

Numerous studies have emphasized the capacity of older men and women to adapt to regularly performed "aerobic" exercise with consistent improvements in functional capacity.[33] Other studies indicate that progressive resistance training produces improvements in strength, muscle size, and skeletal muscular function and reduces the losses of muscle mass associated with sarcopenia.[35] Evans[34] suggests that the positive changes in body composition that occur with exercise, and especially with resistance training, may not only prevent sarcopenia but also a wide array of associated abnormalities. Further, there is no pharmacological intervention that holds a greater promise of improving health and promoting independence in the elderly than exercise. Poehlman[94] cautions that aerobic exercise might be counterproductive to stimulating fat loss if older subjects become less active during the remainder of the day. This may make resistance training the exercise of choice since it helps to both preserve fat-free mass and raise resting metabolic rate. This combination of adaptations results in a more predictable oxidation of whole body fat.

Summary

Endomorph, mesomorph, and ectomorph are the terms employed in describing the somatotype or body type of a person. Endomorph refers to fat; mesomorph to muscle; and ectomorph to a body that is lean. Each of us has a degree of all three body-type components. Athletes and other active people tend to have higher mesomorphic and ectomorphic components than do nonathletes or sedentary individuals.

Fat content of the body is significantly associated with physical activity. Athletes and other active people are less obese than sedentary individuals. Lack of exercise with overeating is the prime cause of obesity in all age groups. Obesity refers to the above-average amount of fat contained in the body, which in turn is dependent on the lipid (fat) content of each adipocyte (fat cell) and on the total number of fat cells. The prevention of obesity through regular exercises and proper diet is more successful than is the treatment for it.

Two methods are commonly employed in estimating fat content of the body: (1) measuring the density of the person and (2) measuring skinfolds to estimate body density. The density of the body can be measured by hydrostatic (underwater) weighing. This is the most accurate, readily available method for estimating body density, but it is also difficult from a technical standpoint. Estimates of body density from skinfold measures are less accurate and more specific than underwater weighing but are a less difficult and more practical method. Body fat can be estimated from body density measures using one of two equations: (1) Brozek, percent fat = (457/body density) − 414.2, or (2) Siri, percent body fat = (495/body density) − 450.

Energy balance means consuming the same amount of energy through food intake as is being expended by activity. When more energy is consumed than expended, the person is said to be in a positive energy balance and body weight is gained. When less energy is consumed than expended, the person is said to be in a negative energy balance and body weight is lost. The weight gained may be in the form of fat or fat-free (lean or muscle) weight. The latter is possible when a person is in a positive energy balance while participating in an exercise program.

Considerable attention is being given to the serious malpractices associated with "making weight" in wrestling. This is particularly true for high-school wrestlers. Various methods are available that give a reasonable estimate for minimum weight for the young wrestler. Women gymnasts also represent a special challenge in body weight control and nutrition education.

Questions

1. Define endomorphy, mesomorphy, and ectomorphy.
2. According to Sheldon's rating form, what would be the somatotype of an extreme endomorph?
3. How do the somatotypes of marathon runners compare with those of football players, according to Carter?
4. Would you consider that female and male somatotypes in comparable sport events are similar?
5. Explain how the difference in track performance between men and women might be partially attributed to the body's fat content.
6. Illustrate how density determinations are used to compute body fat.
7. Calculate the body density (JPW equation) of a 21-year-old female who has the following skinfold measurements: triceps = 13mm, iliac crest = 19mm, midthigh = 29mm. (Answer below.*)
8. Compute the percentage of fat, using both the Brozek and Siri formulas, of a person whose body density equals 1.0456 g/cm³.
9. Explain and give an example of a person in a positive energy balance.

*Answer: About 20.6%.

End-of-Book Features

Consistent with our desire to provide a thorough revision of the entire text, each appendix has been critically reviewed and revised as needed. As a result, dated material has been dropped and newer material added. To aid those students who sometimes have difficulty recalling mathematical equations, a new appendix includes six key equations often used in exercise physiology.

The glossary again provides a concise definition of words and terms that are **boldfaced** throughout the text. The two pages inside the front cover provide valuable information meant to assist students with units of measure and conversions, contributing further to the important role this text plays as a life-long resource.

Ancillary Material

Valuable supplements are available from McGraw-Hill publishers to qualified adopters of *Fox's Physiological Basis for Exercise and Sport,* sixth edition:

- Course Bits: Qualifying adopters now can have access to valuable electronic tools on our website—download software, images, and more!

- Instructor's Manual and Test Bank, by Merle L. Foss, Steven J. Keteyian, Jacquelyn La New, and Clinton A. Brawner: This manual provides a chapter-by-chapter overview of key concepts and a test bank tied to the computerized testing software.

- MicroTest computerized testing software for IBM-compatible and Macintosh computers eases the task of preparing tests: the test items can be edited, deleted, ordered, and your own test items can be imported into the program to customize the testing software to fit your needs.

- Instructor's Presentation Software Program (CD-ROM): enhance your classroom presentations with this new, illustrated Power Point program developed specifically for the sixth edition by Susan Muller with digital graphics by Dan Clark. The Power Point files also include detailed notes for your presentations.

- Exercise Physiology Transparencies: The color acetates have been revised and expanded to complement this edition.

- Exercise Physiology Videolabs: This series of *thirteen* videotapes shows clear and complete demonstrations of common lab experiments. Students with limited lab access can still become familiar with standard exercise physiology lab activities. Also included is an Instructor's Manual that provides guidance on using the videolabs.

  - Student Videolab Manual to accompany the Exercise Physiology Videolabs: This convenient manual actively involves students in the videolab presentations and reinforces concepts through worksheets and activities. This manual is available for student purchase and can be packaged with the sixth edition of *Fox's Physiological Basis for Exercise and Sport.**

- Student Study Guide: This student learning tool includes summaries of all key concepts, terms, and study questions for each chapter. The guide is available at a special price when packaged with *Fox's Physiological Basis for Exercise and Sport,* sixth edition.*

- Exercise Physiology Lab Manual: The new Exercise Physiology Lab Manual by Gene Adams can be customized to fit your course. This lab manual is available packaged with *Fox's Physiological Basis for Exercise and Sport,* sixth edition, at a savings to your students.*

Acknowledgments

Let there be no mistake, by no means does this text represent the work of just two people. It is with great appreciation that we recognize the many people who helped us

---

*Ask your bookstore manager to order any of these special packages from McGraw-Hill Publishers.

---

glossary

A

A Band That area located in the center of the sarcomere containing both actin and myosin.

Acceleration Sprint A training method in which running speed is gradually increased from jogging to striding and finally to sprinting.

Acclimation Short-term or acute changes that occur in the body to lessen the physiological strain that develops in response to changes in climatic factors.

Acclimatization Pertaining to certain physiological adjustments brought about through continued exposure to a different climate, for example, changes in altitude and heat.

Accommodating Resistance A feature unique to isokinetic testing or training apparatus where a counterforce is provided so that the speed of contraction is controlled.

Acetylcholine (ACh) A chemical substance involved in several important physiological functions such as transmission of an impulse from one nerve fiber to another across a synapse.

Acid A chemical compound that gives up hydrogen ions (H^+) in solution.

Acidosis A condition of reduced alkali reserve (bicarbonate) of the blood and other body fluids; usually, but not always, associated with an increase in H-ion concentration and a fall below normal in pH.

Actin A protein involved in muscular contraction.

Action Potential The electrical activity developed in a muscle or nerve cell during activity or depolarization.

Active Transport The movement of substances or materials against their concentration gradients by the expenditure of metabolic energy.

Actomyosin A protein complex formed from actin and myosin when myosin cross-bridges form a chemical bond with selected sites on actin filaments.

Acute Muscular Soreness Pain that occurs during or immediately after performance of relatively high-intensity exercise; associated with inadequate blood flow.

Adenine An aromatic base that when linked to ribose forms adenosine, the molecular foundation for ATP, ADP, and AMP.

Adenohypophysis The anterior lobe of the pituitary gland; *aden* means "in relationship to a gland," in this case the hypophysis (pituitary); secretes six major hormones.

Adenosine The molecular foundation for ATP, ADP, and AMP, comprised of a five-carbon sugar (ribose) linked to an aromatic base (adenine).

Adenosine Diphosphate (ADP) A complex chemical compound which, when combined within organic phosphate (Pi), forms ATP.

Adenosine Triphosphate (ATP) A complex chemical compound formed with the energy released from food and stored in all cells, particularly muscles. Only from the energy released by the breakdown of this compound can the cell perform work.

Adipocyte A fat cell; a cell that stores fat.

Adipose Tissue Fat tissue.

Adrenal Cortex Outer portion of the adrenal gland; secretes some forty different hormones known as steroids, which can be categorized as mineralocorticoids, glucocorticoids, and androgens.

Adrenal Medulla Inner portion of the adrenal gland; often viewed as a direct extension of the sympathetic nervous system; secretes epinephrine and norepinephrine.

Adrenocorticotropic Hormone (ACTH; or Corticotropin) A hormone secreted by the anterior lobe of the pituitary gland that stimulates the production and release of the glucocorticoid hormones from the adrenal cortex.

Aerobic In the presence of oxygen.

Aerobic Glycolysis See *Glycolysis.*

Aerobic Power Maximal rate at which an individual can consume oxygen during the performance of all-out, exhaustive exercise; "best" index of cardiorespiratory fitness.

Aerotitis Inflammation or disease of the ear.

Afferent Nerve A neuron that conveys sensory impulses from a receptor to the central nervous system.

Alactacid Oxygen Debt That portion of the recovery oxygen used to resynthesize and restore ATP + PC in muscle following exercise. The rapid recovery phase.

Aldosterone A mineralocorticoid.

Alkali Reserve The amount of bicarbonate (base) available in the body for buffering.

¹Definitions followed by an asterisk (*) are from the Publications Advisory Committee, IOC Medical Commission, and personal communication with H. G. Knutgen.

595

throughout our journey of preparing and completing a contemporary edition of this classic classroom text. Special recognition is extended to both the University of Michigan and Henry Ford Health System for their support of our efforts, as well as of those who influenced our thinking through both their teachings and their appreciation of the "art of science." This includes Drs. Robert S. Shepard, Sidney Goldstein, Betty Gates, Louis E. Alley, Charles M. Tipton, and the late Donald Magilligan. Without question, great thanks are also due to those who helped write or review various chapters of this or earlier editions of the text. Their efforts, although hidden within our words, remain forever meaningful.

John Davis
Alma College
Carlos J. Crespo
National Heart, Lung, and Blood Institute
Jonathan K. Ehrman
Eastern Michigan University
Carl Foster
Sinai Samaritan Medical Center
Paul M. Gordon
West Virginia University
Paul S. Visich
Central Michigan University
Randy L. Wilber
U.S. Olympic Committee, Sport Science and Technology
Robert E. Neeves
University of Delaware
Gregory A. Kenney
SUNY College at Brockport
L. Jerome Brandon
Georgia State University
Frederick F. Andres
University of Toledo
Tom Ball
Northern Illinois University
Bethany Anne Ledford
Henry Ford Health System
Dennis Jacobsen
University of Nebraska–Kearney
Luke E. Thomas
Northeast Louisiana University
Richard Latin
University of Nebraska
Loren Cordain
Colorado State University
Steven P. Hooker
University of Northern Colorado
Eric W. Banister
Simon Fraser University
Matthew D. Vukovich
Wichita State University

Robert Bartels
Emeritus, The Ohio State University
Josh Palgi
Kean College of New Jersey
Wayne H. Osness
University of Kansas
Steven Loy
California State University–Northridge
Jacalyn J. Robert
Texas Tech University
Charles Marks
Oakland University
Melvin H. Williams
Old Dominion University
Priscilla M. Clarkson
University of Massachusetts, Amherst
William Floyd
University of Wisconsin–LaCrosse
Roberta Pohlman
Wright State University
Sandra Kay Burrus
Indiana University
Thomas Balon
University of Iowa
Stewart Petersen
University of Alberta
Edward Zambraski
Nelson Laboratory

Our deepest thanks to Theresa Grutz, Donna Nemmers, and McGraw-Hill for their support, timeliness, and willingness to publish yet another edition of this book. We also offer a special note of thanks to Mr. Clinton Brawner who served as technical editor, and Mr. Mark Perkins, a special assistant. Great things lie ahead for these young men.

Finally, as Drs. Bartels and Kirby so elegantly state in their Foreword to this text, we remain conscious and ever-thankful of the legacy and efforts of the late Dr. Edward L. Fox. We have again tried to meaningfully translate difficult physiological concepts to the open-minded student, a skill at which Dr. Fox was truly a master. We are so very pleased that his name now leads the title of this—and of all subsequent editions of our textbook.

—Merle L. Foss, Ph.D., FACSM
Division of Kinesiology
University of Michigan
Ann Arbor, Michigan

—Steven J. Keteyian, Ph.D., FACSM
Heart & Vascular Institute
Henry Ford Health System
Detroit, Michigan

Fox's
Physiological Basis
for Exercise and Sport

1

Introduction to Exercise Physiology, Sports Medicine, and Kinesiology

Today, more than ever before, it is necessary for physical educators, therapists, coaches, trainers, fitness instructors, and kinesiologists to recognize the vital part science plays in the successful conduct of physical education, athletic rehabilitation, and activity programs. Toward this objective, all such exercise professionals must have a solid understanding of basic **exercise physiology.** This essential knowledge will provide the foundation for many decisions they will make on a daily basis in the performance of their jobs. These decisions could be in any number of areas related to performance, safety, nutrition, use of ergogenic aids, fatigue, heat intolerance, and so on, but will invariably come down to the application of a concept or principle learned in exercise physiology class. This rapidly developing field provides some real challenges for everyone to keep up with. Let's explore this rapid change.

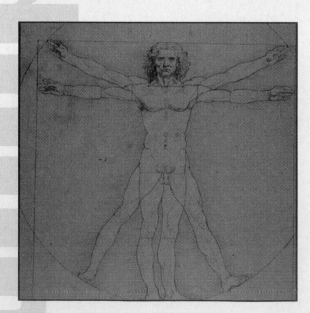

A Brief History of Exercise Physiology

What Are Sports Medicine and Kinesiology?

The Body as a "Machine"—Systems and Molecules

Overview of the Text

The major concepts to be learned from this chapter are as follows:

- Comprehension of exercise physiology and its underlying scientific principles and concepts is important for physical educators, clinicians, coaches, trainers, and fitness instructors.
- Several professional societies are open to student membership and some offer certification programs that require examination of both "textbook" knowledge and hands-on practical expertise.
- The rich history of exercise physiology includes the contributions of both early researchers, who conducted classical laboratory studies, and of physical educators who also researched and interpreted scientific findings.
- Because of recent research and an upsurge of interest in physical fitness, health, and wellness, today's young professionals are faced with increased learning challenges and career opportunities.
- *Sports medicine* is an umbrella term that refers to all aspects of sport and exercise science, including kinesiology, cardiac rehabilitation, adult fitness, athletic medicine, and anthropometry.
- *Kinesiology* is defined as the scientific study of human movement. This includes such aspects of study as exercise physiology, motor learning/control, and biomechanics.
- *Exercise physiology* is an aspect of kinesiology and sports medicine that involves the study of how the body—from a functional standpoint—responds, adjusts, and adapts to exercise and training.
- There are reasons to be in awe of the performance capabilities of the human body when viewed as a working "machine."
- Both the older *systems approach* and the more recent emphasis on *cellular and molecular biology* are important to better understanding the body's functions and limitations. This is the challenge of the future.

Over the past 35 years, the number of exercise physiology laboratories has increased tremendously. As a result, much new knowledge dealing with how best to train for recreational or competitive athletics and to develop fitness for health and disease prevention has appeared in the scientific literature. Likewise, the field itself has expanded beyond the physical education classroom and the sports arenas to include programs founded in communities, hospitals, worksites, and governments as well as an emphasis on groups such as children, the elderly, and persons with chronic diseases. Also, within exercise physiology itself, there has been a shift toward research in the areas of biochemistry of exercise, clinical applications, endocrinology, molecular biology, and aging, to name a few. One has only to review the abstracts for upcoming society meetings where exercise physiologists present their most recent research findings to gain a sense of rapid movement and change. The use of terms like antioxidants, gene expression, killer cells, heart transplants, and magnetic resonance imagery (MRI) are the tip-offs—at least for the moment!

Further evidence of advancement in the science of physical education and athletics was the formation of the American College of Sports Medicine (ACSM) in 1954. Our intent here is to describe the ACSM and other professional organizations that students may choose to join so they become involved at the earliest possible time. The ACSM "college" membership is made up of physical educators, athletic trainers, biochemists, coaches, exercise physiologists, physicians, nutritionists, and numerous other related professional groups. Membership in the college rose to 3000 from 1954 to 1975, and then doubled to more than 6000 between 1975 and 1978. Now with more than 16,000 members, the American College of Sports Medicine is the largest and most influential sports medicine group in the world.

In 1984 the ACSM National Center was moved from Madison, Wisconsin, to Indianapolis, Indiana. There also are twelve regional chapters located throughout the United States (figure 1.1). The national ACSM organization meets once a year, at which time research papers covering all aspects of the science of sports and exercise are presented. *Medicine and Science in Sports and Exercise,* published monthly by the College, is an international journal containing research articles dealing with all facets of sports medicine. The ACSM also publishes position stands and opinion statements on specific topics and public issues and offers an educational program for lay subscribers called "ACSM Fit Society." This program was started in 1992, currently has 1000 members, and is targeted for much future growth.

Another service provided by ACSM is their exercise-related certification programs, which are recognized for their quality and comprehensiveness. The establishment of these programs was an important step for our profession because they put in place, for the first time, standard "quality assurance" measures, as evidenced by applicants passing written tests of knowledge and practical exams of hands-on skills. These programs offer certification in two different tracks: the clinical track and the health and fitness track. Under the clinical track, a person can become certified as a program director, an exercise specialist, or an exercise test technologist. Under the health and fitness track, one can obtain certification as a health/fitness director, a health/fitness instructor, or an exercise leader. Students should keep in mind that they can seek certification in any of the categories for which they otherwise qualify and that such credentials may help them compete for available jobs in the future. Ask your instructor about how this works!

Another outgrowth of the ever-increasing interest in sports medicine was the formation, in 1959, of the Committee on the Medical Aspects of Sports, an organization of the American Medical Association. This group does an excellent job disseminating literature concerned with protecting the health of the athlete as well as holding seminars for coaches, trainers, and physicians. Similarly, the Association for Worksite Health Promotion (AWHP), initially called the American Association of Fitness Directors in Business and Industry (AAFDBI) and later the Association for Fitness in Business (AFB), was organized in 1974. This organization was established to meet the growing need of a variety of professionals and their support staffs who began to develop worksite fitness and health promotion programs. The AWHP holds a national conference each year and also has developed a network of ten regional chapters and international affiliates to disseminate information regarding the promotion and management of wellness programs in corporate, hospital, private, and community settings.

Still other organizations of which the informed student should be aware are the American Alliance for Health, Physical Education, Recreation, and Dance (AAHPERD); the United States Olympic Committee (USOC); the President's Council on Physical Fitness and Sports (President's Council); Federation Internationale Medico Sportive (FIMS); the National Athletic Trainers Association (NATA); and the American Association of Cardiovascular and Pulmonary Rehabilitation (AACVPR). AAHPERD grew out of the former American Physical Education Association (APEA), which we will discuss later in this chapter, along with the origins of the President's Council, FIMS, and NATA. College student membership is available in ACSM, AWHP, AAHPERD, NATA, and AACVPR, whereas appointment to the other groups is necessary for direct involvement. AWHP and NATA also offer certification testing programs.

As mentioned earlier, for you to contribute to the best of your ability to all aspects of physical education, athletics, and fitness leadership, you will need a good understanding of the available scientific knowledge. Such understanding will not only result in better teams and better programs of activities but will also enable you to guard the

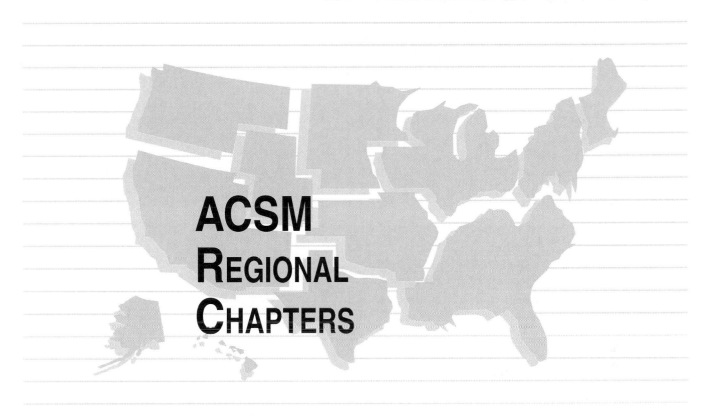

Figure 1.1
Map of U.S. showing 12 ACSM regional chapters.

health of your students, athletes, patients, and clients, which is one of your primary responsibilities. Additionally, knowing the reasons why you select a particular approach for accomplishing a specific task immediately establishes you as a professional rather than a technician. Sometimes "why" is the most difficult of all questions because your response reflects the depth of your knowledge base. You might reflect on this as you evaluate the answers you have received from respected professionals lately. Were you favorably impressed?

The recent and rapid expansion of knowledge and interest in sports medicine requires that you learn much more factual and technical information than did your predecessors. At the same time, you are favored by having a greater number of career opportunities open to you. In fact, there are few career tracks today that offer more variety, personal challenge, and opportunity for service than those related to the educational, scientific, and clinical aspects of sports medicine and contemporary physical education. The shift that physical education has made toward an emphasis on teaching concepts related to heath and well-being is a welcomed one, as evidenced in a 1995 special issue of the *Research Quarterly for Exercise and Sport,* which contained the proceedings of the International Scientific Consensus Conference on "Physical Activity, Health, and

Well-Being." The article predicts that this shift will stimulate many young professionals to once again pursue teaching as their undergraduate major and to go on to work in this most important career track. As we shall see, physical educators have played a crucial role in the development of exercise physiology as we now study it.

A Brief History of Exercise Physiology

In all of human endeavor, maintaining a sense of history is of vital importance. This holds true as well for academic disciplines where it is important for current scholars, including both students and faculty, to have some clear idea of their foundation and "roots." The history-related questions often asked in professional settings are what were the major events and who were the key players that led to the development of the course of study we now call exercise physiology? Since you have now chosen to study this discipline, these also are questions about which you would naturally become inquisitive. This sense of curiosity is an indication that you are beginning to feel connected to a myriad of important events that have unfolded prior to your

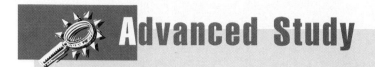

Advanced Study

Historical Highlights

- **1789 Lavoisier** (France) Conducts first quantitative exercise physiology study

- **1847 von Helmholtz** (Germany) Elucidates the Law of Conservation of Energy

- **1850–1890 Golden Era** (Germany) Research on the energy cost of various activities

- **1894 Rubner** (Germany) Uses calorimeter to measure energy metabolism in dogs

- **1913 Benedict & Cathcart** (United States) Publish classic study of "Human Body as a Machine"

- **1923 A. V. Hill** (England) Begins as professor of physiology at University College in London

- **1927 L. J. Henderson** (United States) Starts the Harvard Fatigue Laboratory with D. B. Dill as director until it closed in 1947

- **1930s** (circa) **Nobel Prizes** Awarded to **A. V. Hill** (England), **August Krogh** (Denmark), and **Otto Meyerhof** (Germany)

- **1940s** (circa) **World War II** Research emphasis shifts to physical fitness and strength as related to combat

- **1953 Kraus & Hirschland** (United States) Report that American kids are less fit than European kids

- **1954 ACSM** (United States) Unique organization formed by physicians, researchers, and educators

- **1968 Kenneth Cooper** (United States) Publishes paperback book **Aerobics** to start interest in jogging

- **1970s Era of Rapid Expansion** Significant increase in number of labs and research production in the US and Scandinavia

- **1980s Athletes and rehabilitation** Emphasis placed on muscle fibers, nutrition, CR training and how best to rehabilitate from injuries and diseases

- **1990s Applications to Health** Shift toward "Healthy People 2000: National Health Promotion and Disease Prevention Objectives" (USDHHS)

- **1996 US Surgeon General** Issued a report emphasizing the importance and benefits of a physically active lifestyle

- **1996 ASCM and NCPPA** (United States) More than 100 organizations join The National Coalition for Promoting Physical Activity, led by ACSM

---

involvement. Each new participant is bound to reflect on his or her own possible future involvement in contributing to the overall mosaic of the field as it undergoes continual growth and modification. What small or larger piece might you personally contribute? A most exciting question to ponder!

Brief histories are difficult to write because many important events and people must be left out (i.e., the writer is forced to be selective). We are fortunate to have some earlier and some more recent works to review that contain many important details and allow us to make some generalized statements regarding the origins of exercise physiology as an academic discipline. In this regard, we relied heavily on Chapman and Mitchell's 1965 article "The Physiology of Exercise"[4] and Dill's 1967 article "The Harvard Fatigue Laboratory: Its Development, Contributions and Demise"[6]. Later references include Johnson and Buskirk's 1974 book, *Science and Medicine of Exercise and Sports*[7] and Buskirk's 1981 article "The Emergence of Exercise Physiology"[3]. Our most recent resources were

Brook's 1987 article "The Exercise Physiology Paradigm in Contemporary Biology"[2] and Berryman's excellent 1995 history of the American College of Sports Medicine, *Out of Many, One*[1]. As always, the interested reader is encouraged to review these resources in detail for insights that go far beyond this brief history.

With this background to work from, we will outline the origins of exercise physiology in terms of the early scientists who did classical studies in the 1700s, 1800s, and early 1900s. This will allow a later break to identify key physical educators and physicians who served in the important roles of interpreters and applicators. Dill[7] indicates that the first exercise physiology experiment, which was conducted in France by Lavoisier and Sequin in 1789, pertained to the measurement of oxygen uptake in a young man at rest, after eating a meal, and during the performance of exercise (figure 1.2). Dill then mentions von Helmholtz of Germany for his work in clarifying the law of conservation of energy in 1847, and Rubner (1894), also of Germany, for his precise experiments using an indirect calorimeter to

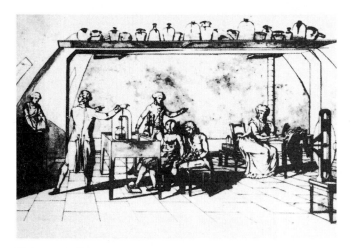

Figure 1.2

A plate showing the first exercise physiology experiment conducted by Lavoisier in France around 1789.

measure the intake and output of energy in dogs as predicted by the conservation of energy law. This work, along with that of Atwater and Benedict in the United States in the early 1900s, established that metabolic rates could be estimated in man by measuring the volume and composition of expired air. All this helped to establish the caloric values of carbohydrates, fats, and proteins and provided a basis for calculating the percentage of fat and carbohydrates used in steady-state exercise. It should be noted that many of these same terms and concepts will be frequently used throughout our text so you sense the connection between the historical and present-day terminologies.

Dill[7] points out two names related to respiratory physiology: Hutchinson, who described the spirometer for measuring vital capacity in 1844, and Tissot, who 60 years later described a tank for measuring expired air volumes and recording respiration rates. This is the well known "Tissot tank" that could be found in nearly every exercise physiology lab from the period 1910–1970. Around 1897–1898, Haldane of England was developing apparatus that made the analysis of expired air samples easier and more precise. Other equipment was being developed, and Benedict and Cathcart used the first treadmill in the United States at the Carnegie Nutrition Laboratory in Boston (circa 1913). Very early methods for monitoring heart rate during exercise with a string galvanometer and chest electrodes were also used during the first two decades of the 1900s.

This brings us to an important time in our history, around 1923, when A. V. Hill became a professor of physiology at University College in London, England. Hill and his students are recognized for conducting the first studies on strenuous, anaerobic exercise in man as opposed to mostly steady-state activity, which was being studied in Germany and the United States. Hill is recognized as a real giant in our field; he and Krogh of Denmark and Meyerhof of Germany all received Nobel prizes for their work related

to muscle or muscular exercise[4]. Just a bit later (1927) the Harvard Fatigue Laboratory was started, and it became a "world center" for the study of muscular exercise. This laboratory with the unusual name of "fatigue" was started by L. J. Henderson. D. B. Dill distinguished himself through his work there and finally wrote a history regarding its development, contributions, and demise[6]. In some ways it was an end to an important era, but it also bore great fruit in the form of spin-off laboratories as noted researchers spread out across the United States and the world to continue their exercise science work.

Clearly, much of what we now call exercise physiology as a course of study had its beginnings in the field of physical education in the United States and can be traced back to the second half of the nineteenth and first half of the twentieth centuries. During the latter part of the 1800s, an influx of European immigrants brought along their systems for calisthenics exercise—for instance, Swedish Gymnastics and the German Turnverein—and these were taught as part of the physical education curriculum. Emphasis then shifted to games and sports during the early part of the 1900s as the physical education profession sought to gain greater recognition and acceptance. There was not as much emphasis on the health and fitness aspects of being a physically well-educated person as there is today.

The onset of World War I spurred interest in research related to the measurement of physical fitness and how best to train military personnel so they were ready for combat. A greater emphasis also was placed on research related to physical rehabilitation methods for wounded soldiers, energy cost of performing work tasks, heat tolerance, dietary modification, and environmental factors—all topics that are common in exercise physiology today. This research was conducted by physical educators, physicians, physiologists, and related scientists coalesced to form the foundation of our current profession. Without question, the First World War (1914–1918) had a significant impact on our field of study.

Other professional groups that helped to form the foundation for exercise physiology as we now know it were the team physicians and athletic trainers of the early 1900s. Sports were very popular in the United States and Europe and this stimulated a need for "how best research"—i.e., how best to train athletes for superior performance and how best to treat their many injuries. A strong need to share information led to the formation of professional societies such as the American Physical Education Association (APEA) in 1896, the Federation Internationale Medico Sportive (FIMS) in 1928, the National Athletic Trainers Association (NATA) in 1938, and the American College of Sports Medicine (ACSM) in 1954. These organizations began to publish scientific research journals (these are different than magazines), which greatly aided in making exercise physiology a recognized and respected field of study.

As always, many forces have come together to shape this history. Numerous other events and the efforts of many outstanding people have influenced the body of knowledge we currently call exercise physiology. World War II (1941–1945) was one influence, with its renewing focus on physical fitness and strength development for combat and an accompanying emphasis on drills and calisthenics in school physical education classes. Additionally, the 1953 research report by Kraus and Hirschland that nearly 60% of American school children had failed to meet even a minimum standard of strength required for health compared to only an 8% failure rate for European children[8]. This report prompted President Dwight D. Eisenhower to establish the President's Council on Youth Fitness a few years later and to establish the President's Citizens Advisory Committee on Fitness.

Then, in 1968 a $1 paperback book was written by Dr. Kenneth Cooper, a major in the United States Air Force Medical Corps[5]. It was simply titled *Aerobics*, but the Foreword described it as "a scientific program of exercise aimed at the overall fitness and health of your body, with a unique point system for measuring your progress toward maximal health." Note here the use of the words *your fitness, health,* and *progress.* This popular best seller did much to sensitize both the lay reader and scientist to the fast approaching emphasis that would be placed on what many began to call "heart, lungs, and legs" fitness. The aerobics craze had begun and would express itself in ways such as jogging, marathon runs, aerobics dance, aqua-aerobics, senior aerobics, century bike rides, triathlons, orienteering, cardiac rehabilitation, and so on.

Of course, all of these special outgrowths were of interest to the researcher in exercise physiology. A most important legacy from this latter period in our history was a renewed emphasis on research related to maintaining the health and wellness of all citizens—i.e., a return to prevention of disease and ill-health. Likewise, an increased emphasis was put on the role of exercise in the rehabilitation of special populations such as the obese, diabetics, cardiac patients, the elderly, and those with physical impairments. Importantly, much emphasis was also placed on the exercise physiology of girls and women who were finally gaining their rightful place in the world of physical activity and sports.

Some others who have been recognized as founders of modern day exercise physiology and sports medicine merit identification. Arguably, many other notable figures will inevitably be passed over in this brief overview of our history. We will rely heavily here on the 1995 history of the American College of Sports Medicine as written by Berryman[1]. We have selected six leaders because of the important educational roles that they played and the contributions they made to the interwoven fabric we call exercise physiology.

R. Tait McKenzie (figure 1.3), noted physician and physical educator, made numerous contributions in many areas of exercise physiology, preventive medicine, rehabilitative medicine, and sculpture. His professional life spanned the years 1904–1938, and he is identified as the person who planted the philosophical seed that grew into the formation of the ACSM. Next consider Arthur H.

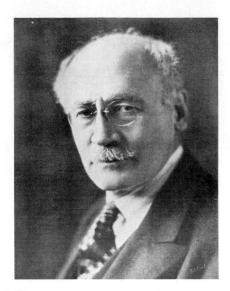

Figure 1.3

R. Tait McKenzie, noted physician and educator whose philosophy and efforts grew into the ACSM.

Steinhaus, a renowned physical educator and widely known and respected lecturer; he published papers in the early volumes (circa 1930) of the *Journal of Health and Physical Education,* with titles like "Physiology at the Service of Physical Education." Steinhaus became dean of the program at George Williams College in Illinois, which, along with Springfield College in Massachusetts, laid the groundwork to prepare personnel for the YMCA. He also was one of eleven founders, eight physical educators, and three physicians of the ACSM in 1954.

Two other founders of the ACSM were Peter V. Karpovich and his wife, Josephine L. Rathbone. Karpovich was a physician and professor of physiology at Springfield College, while Rathbone was a physical educator with appointments as technical director of training courses in physical therapy at Columbia University. She was best known for her contributions to corrective physical education and relaxation therapy from 1934–1945. Karpovich was one of three Springfield College faculty who was thrust into the limelight by the 1941 publication of an article called "Physical Fitness" in a special issue of the *Research Quarterly.* The other two were ACSM founder Leonard A. Larson and ACSM charter member Thomas K. Cureton. Larson later chaired departments of physical education at New York University and the University of Wisconsin-Madison and served the ACSM as its president. All three of these people conducted research in the area of exercise physiology and had been publishing articles in the scientific journals as early as the 1930s. Physical fitness was then the hot topic of the day, and Cureton was hired at the University of Illinois in 1941 to later become director of its Research Laboratory for Physical Fitness in 1945.

This brief history lesson should help you feel more informed of and connected to your exercise physiology

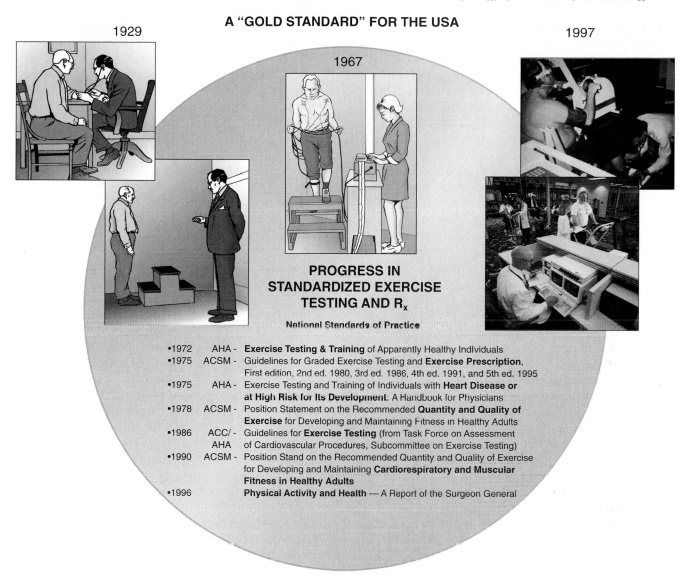

A "GOLD STANDARD" FOR THE USA

1929

1967

1997

PROGRESS IN
STANDARDIZED EXERCISE
TESTING AND R$_x$

National Standards of Practice

- •1972 AHA - **Exercise Testing & Training** of Apparently Healthy Individuals
- •1975 ACSM - Guidelines for Graded Exercise Testing and **Exercise Prescription**,
    First edition, 2nd ed. 1980, 3rd ed. 1986, 4th ed. 1991, and 5th ed. 1995
- •1975 AHA - Exercise Testing and Training of Individuals with **Heart Disease or
    at High Risk for Its Development**: A Handbook for Physicians
- •1978 ACSM - Position Statement on the Recommended **Quantity and Quality of
    Exercise** for Developing and Maintaining Fitness in Healthy Adults
- •1986 ACC/ - Guidelines for **Exercise Testing** (from Task Force on Assessment
    AHA of Cardiovascular Procedures, Subcommittee on Exercise Testing)
- •1990 ACSM - Position Stand on the Recommended Quantity and Quality of Exercise
    for Developing and Maintaining **Cardiorespiratory and Muscular
    Fitness in Healthy Adults**
- •1996 **Physical Activity and Health** — A Report of the Surgeon General

roots. Seeing the common linkage or lineage that runs through the earlier classical laboratory studies and the efforts of the physical educators is not difficult. Buskirk[3] rightly points out that the research has contributed to human well-being, largely through the interpretation of such research by those involved with physical education. It would be easy to trace many other equally important strands that have helped to bind the fabric together. We feel pleased to have introduced you to a few selected key players to go along with the major events that have guided our history. Among physical educators, names like McKenzie, Steinhaus, Larson, Karpovich, Rathbone, and Cureton will ring on forever as the early founders of what we call classroom exercise physiology. Likewise, words like immigrants, gymnastics, calisthenics, sports emphasis, wars, physical training, rehabilitation, fitness, aerobics, health, and wellness will remind us of events that have helped to shape exercise physiology as an academic discipline or area of study. Welcome to your newly found family tree!

What Are Sports Medicine and Kinesiology?

In the preceding discussion, the terms *exercise physiology* and *sports medicine* were mentioned several times but **kinesiology** was not. The reason for this disproportional usage will be made clearer as we go. Since these terms may have different meanings to different people, let's define them here. In the United States, sports medicine is an all-encompassing term that refers to all aspects, not just medical, of sport and exercise. Examples of such aspects would be (1) athletic medicine, (2) biomechanics, (3) clinical medicine, (4) growth and development, (5) psychology and sociology, (6) nutrition, (7) motor control, and (8) physiology. This latter term refers to exercise physiology or the physiology of exercise.

As the terms imply, this physiological side of sports medicine involves the study of how the body, from a functional standpoint, responds, adjusts, and adapts to exercise. This includes acute exercise (i.e., single bouts of exercise) as well as chronic or prolonged exercise, as is the case with exercise training. The term *adaptation* is important here since it emphasizes that somewhat permanent changes occur in a variety of body systems and within cells when whole body organisms are systematically and progressively "trained." In other words, exercise physiology provides the physiological basis or functional foundation of physical education, fitness, athletic, and rehabilitation programs. For brevity, we have chosen to use as our textbook title *Fox's Physiological Basis for Exercise and Sport.*

The term *kinesiology* has undergone some changes in usage and deserves some clarification of its current definition. Its root meaning is from the Greek word *kinein* (to move), and it is combined with *-logy* from the Greek word *-logia,* which means a science, doctrine, or theory of some topic. For our common use, kinesiology means the scientific study of human movement. Kinesiology, at one time, was taught as a single course within most college and university physical education curriculums and included material now covered in biomechanics classes. In addition to biomechanics, current kinesiology curricula include the study of exercise physiology and motor learning/control. Another change in the use of the term *kinesiology* is more widespread. During the late 1980s, many physical education units at institutions of higher learning in the United States and Canada changed their names to kinesiology or some derivation thereof. This elevated the term to a higher level of usage and denoted a broader definition. It also placed a large burden on physical education practitioners to be certain that the ever-important traditional aspects of the physical education curriculum were not lost in the transition process.

The Body as a "Machine"— Systems and Molecules

Although humanists might take issue with an engineering approach that views the body as a "working machine," doing so has a number of advantages and justifications. First, the learner can relate physiological functions to the workings of other devices that they may have experienced in the more observable world of machines. For example, a basic understanding of how fluids are circulated under pressure in the closed cooling system of a car provides for an easier appreciation of how the body adjusts to remain cool during the performance of work. Likewise, a basic knowledge of cellular metabolic functions allows for a better understanding of the production sites and of quantities of useful as well as bothersome heat produced during exercise. A combination of these thought processes allows the well-informed analyst to diagnose and reasonably predict the effects of any compromised function by parts analogous to both machines. By way

of example, wouldn't covering both an outdoor worker and the radiator of a car with blankets on a hot day have a similar effect on internal temperature if their "motors" were kept running? The temperatures of both "machines" would increase primarily because of the continued production and circulation of nonusable heat in a setting that drastically limits heat dissipation.

The foregoing analogy makes the point that a knowledge of both systems physiology and cellular biology are important to our contemporary understanding of how the body works. Since most of the systems aspects have been worked out and are reasonably well understood, many professionals believe that the future of exercise physiology, as an academic discipline, resides more in our understanding of cellular and subcellular *mechanisms* (note this choice of words which is used throughout biology). For this reason, students are encouraged to think on both levels but to ever increase their depth of knowledge about cellular processes. For more on this, refer to the treatise by Brooks, whose subtitle is, "To Molbiol or Not to Molbiol—That is the Question"[2]. He concludes that while molecular biology will become an important tool in the repertoire of the exercise physiologist, there will always be room for physical educators to contribute through more traditional "organs and systems" research. In other words, an understanding of both systems mechanisms and molecular mechanisms are viewed as important to our future.

With this in mind, and returning to the discussion of the human body as a machine, there may be little wonder why many exercise scientists are awed by the human body's potential performance capabilities. World records substantiate that the body is capable of both impressive sprint (100 meters in about 10 seconds) and long-distance running performances (26.2 miles on foot and 85 kilometers on skis, each in about 4 hours). It also allows for awesome feats of muscular strength (ability to lift two to three times one's body weight) and hypertrophy of muscle tissue (from 12-inch circumference biceps to over 24 inches) when it is subjected to specific overload training regimens. At the same time, differences in its makeup may give women athletes an advantage in selected competitions (channel swimming, ultramarathons, gymnastics). What examples can you think of for other individuals, events, or groups where the performances are nothing short of phenomenal? Be prepared to offer these in class as part of the opening discussions.

All of the above examples are performed by extraordinary human machines—machines that can increase their rate of whole-body energy "combustion" twenty times, increase their intake of air into "carburetor-like" lungs thirty times, and electrically signal their heart "fuel/oxygen/exhaust" pump to rapidly increase its "firing rate" some three or four times above its "idling" rate. These processes are controlled and regulated through complex neurohumoral "circuits," with data integration and memory capabilities that exceed the most sophisticated computers. Finally, add

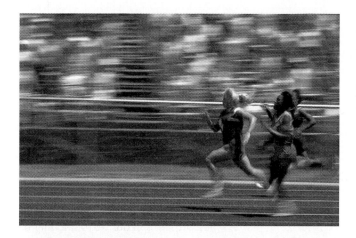

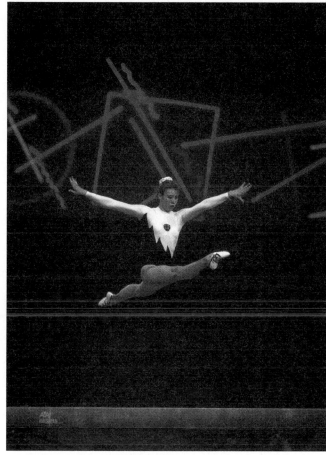

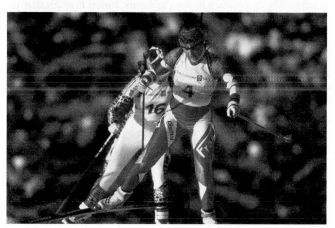

the internal autonomous ability to repair "damaged component" cells (which are likely no longer under warranty!), to reduce "sludge-like" cholesterol deposits, to neutralize "corrosive acids," to filter out "airborne particles" that are toxic in nature, and to restore reserve "fuel supplies" through adequate rest and nutrient intake. All things considered, wouldn't you agree that the human body has the potential to be an awesome working machine? And consider the age-old question of whether most human machines wear out or rust out? An important question for our profession is, What effect does participation in a regular exercise program have on the process of wearing out or rusting out? You should be much better prepared to answer these questions after reading this text and completing this course.

You may find it helpful to begin to think more like an engineer. For example, after you have mastered the major concepts of the circulatory system, continue to probe with "what if" thoughts and questions. What if parts of the circulatory system became partially or completely clogged with plaque? What if a vessel becomes completely blocked? The answer is that pressure in the system would increase and flow would progressively decrease until it stops. You know this not only because of equations and principles you have learned but also because of your past experience in

kinking a garden hose. Water flow is reduced when you gradually kink the hose to take a drink, and it may be completely stopped if the hose twists when you move the lawn sprinkler. Furthermore, an increase in pressure within the hose is apparent back at the faucet because more water squirts out around the connection. These are events that we all have seen and experienced in the practical world of applied mechanics. What do you think would happen to the pressure and flow within the hose if the connection at the faucet was loosened even more? Might this be similar to severing a major artery in the body? What does your new line of thinking tell you?

Overview of the Text

This textbook focuses exclusively on exercise physiology. Therefore, to further define and understand what exercise physiology is all about, an overview of the text is appropriate at this time. In writing the chapters that follow, we have made a concerted effort to eliminate those aspects of physiology that, from your standpoint, might be of academic interest only. Our concern has been to cover materials you will be able to put to immediate use in the school gymnasium, in the exercise center, in the laboratory, and on the athletic field. In other words, we have kept you, the student, in mind, rather than your professor. This book is divide into seven sections: Bioenergetics, Neuromuscular Concepts, Cardiorespiratory Considerations, Physical Training, Nutrition and Body Weight Control, Humoral Responses and Performance Aids, and the Environment.

Bioenergetics

If you were asked to select a term that might be considered a common denominator for all aspects of physical education, exercise, and athletics, what would it be? After a little deliberation, we hope you would agree that *energy* is the term most appropriate. The material of chapters 2, 3, and 4 are the foundation for this text, and it is important that you master the concepts contained therein. The term *energy* appears in every chapter of this book because it truly is what you deal with in the fields of physical education, physical fitness, clinical exercise physiology, and sport. For that matter, energy is essential to life. Muscles can contract only if there is an adequate source of energy; foods are selected on the basis of their energy content; fatigue occurs in the absence of energy; special training and dietary approaches can result in improved energy storage. Furthermore, a knowledge of energy recovery rates and how to measure and express work performance is basic to intelligently designing appropriate training and fitness programs for athletes, apparently healthy persons, and patients with chronic diseases alike. For these reasons, metabolic pathways, adenosine triphosphate (ATP), lactic acid, and maximal oxygen uptake are emphasized in this section.

Neuromuscular Concepts

An understanding of the nervous control of muscular movement in terms of motor unit recruitment and how reflexes can be used to enhance performance is invaluable to the well-informed exercise science professional (chapter 5). Likewise, clinicians and trainers need a knowledge of basic neural function to evaluate injuries involving nerve damage and to diagnose muscular weaknesses. All movement clearly depends on muscular contractions. Therefore, performance levels can be better enhanced if the exercise professional more completely understands the structure and function of skeletal muscle in terms of different fiber types, the fuels they use, and how quickly they fatigue (chapter 6). Furthermore, teachers and coaches have a better understanding of the genetic limitations of performers and why some are good at power events like jumping and sprinting, while others excel in activities that require more prolonged endurance. It is especially for these reasons that section 2 helps the instructor as well as the participant to better understand the fundamental neuromuscular processes involved in the improvement of motor skills.

Cardiorespiratory Considerations

Understanding the functions of the respiratory and circulatory systems is important to the exercise professional, perhaps more so today than ever before. For example, adult fitness programs for presumably healthy individuals, as well as for patients with chronic lung or heart disease, are centered on increasing the functional capacity of the cardiorespiratory system and on preventing future illness. Such programs are fast becoming major responsibilities of persons with academic training in exercise physiology. While pulmonary ventilation (moving air in and out of the lungs) may only be 5 or 6 liters per minute at rest, it may reach as high as 170 liters per minute during all-out exercise (chapter 7). In chapter 8, appropriately titled Gas Exchange and Transport, we describe the influence of gas partial pressures on the diffusion and loading/unloading of oxygen and carbon dioxide onto and off of hemoglobin. Chapter 9 emphasizes how the heart and circulatory system respond and adapt to ensure that adequate blood flow is maintained to both resting and active regions of the body during exercise. Finally, chapter 10 covers the brain's regulatory control of the cardiorespiratory systems, given the help of sensory information provided by a variety of other bodily sources.

Physical Training

The concept of "specificity of training" indicates that not all individuals should be trained the same but that their training programs should be custom-tailored to best meet their needs. That is to say that the outcomes of training can be specifically related to the input. Yet there are some general principles of training that broadly apply to most any program and some training methods that would be appropriate for only a certain category of performers such as sprinters versus endurance runners. The trick is to know the difference and when to incorporate each into a program specifically designed to improve anaerobic (chapter 11) or aerobic (chapter 12) performance. It also is important to have a good idea of expected outcomes of training to know if a program is producing reasonable results and which variables can be manipulated in an effort to better influence the outcomes. Such outcomes are detailed for anaerobic and aerobic activities in chapters 11 and 12, respectively. Chapter 13 addresses training questions such as What is the best way to develop strength? Which equipment is best? Are isometric exercises better than isotonic exercises? What is an isokinetic contraction? How can flexibility be improved? This section concludes with physical activity and health (chapter 14), which includes how to safely prescribe exercise programs for adults and the beneficial effects of these prescriptions on overall health status. This material is arguably among the more important things you will learn in your course of study!

Nutrition and Body Weight Control

To perform at peak efficiency, an athlete (or anyone for that matter) must be well nourished—i.e., following a diet that is well balanced and providing adequate nutrients. But proper nourishment goes beyond mere "energy" nutrients, such as the kilocalories of carbohydrates, fats, and proteins, and includes "non-energy" nutrients like the equally important vitamins, minerals, and water. The material in chapter 15 not only helps you to teach and apply proper dietary practices, but also includes suggestions for good nutrition before, during, and following exercise. Additionally, you will find a suggested dietary regimen to increase intramuscular glycogen stores for improving endurance performance, commonly called carbohydrate loading. The subject of obesity—its definition and suggestions for contending with this problem which is of epidemic proportions in the United States today—is contained in chapter 16. We also include instructions for determining certain skinfolds and anthropometric measures as well as many newer methods for estimating both percentage of body fat and lean body mass. This all leads to the use of equations to predict minimal weights for high-school and college wrestlers, which are presented in this chapter—a good example of applied exercise science.

Humoral Responses and Performance Aids

The special considerations presented in this section include other regulatory systems in the body and athletic practices that are very much in the news these days. Interestingly, these practices also have elements of morbidity and mortality associated with them—for example, attempts to modify circulating levels of endocrine hormones like testosterone and growth hormone (chapter 17) or to take work-enhancement substances (ergogenic aids) such as anabolic steroids, amphetamines, or other drugs (chapter 18). We review both the physiological and ethical aspects of these hazardous, illegal, and unwarranted practices. These chapters include an overview of mechanisms related to the specific actions of hormones and drugs, as well as the concepts of dose-response, LD-50, toxicity, safety factors, dangerous or untoward side effects, and so on. The main emphasis is on the effects of hormones and so-called ergogenic aids on exercise responses, training adaptations, and safety considerations. This knowledge should prepare students to intelligently speak out against potentially harmful and unsafe practices.

The Environment

In a similar vein, not too long ago, lack of knowledge concerning the inherent risks of athletes exercising in hot, humid environments was responsible for many unnecessary football fatalities. In chapter 19 you will learn about the principal mechanisms for body temperature regulation in response to both hot and cold environments, how workers can *acclimatize* to these conditions, and how safety can be enhanced. We emphasize practical suggestions for intelligently managing these environmental stressors in terms that can be applied to the administration of late summer marathon runs, winter cross-country ski competitions, and other common sports events. In chapter 20, our emphasis will be on exercise performance in other environments, which can be harmful or even life-threatening if certain "governing laws" are violated—namely, while underwater, at higher altitude, or while exploring microgravity (space). Although most of us may never probe the limitations to performance imposed by these environments, we hope that the informed student may caution others about certain inherent risks, all in the name of managing risks and promoting safety.

Finally, we include a glossary plus eight appendixes. You are strongly encouraged to improve your professional word power, as this is an important indication of learning; consider how well and how correctly you can use these words. Obviously, it is difficult, if not impossible, to use them correctly if you don't know their meaning or can't pronounce and spell them. Be sure to practice this by using the key words at the beginning of each chapter and by checking the glossary for quick working definitions. Appendix A includes a list of common symbols, abbreviations, and norms used by most exercise physiologists in this country and elsewhere. Appendix B is a basic review of the cell and the driving forces that result in movement of substances across cell membranes. Appendix C is a comprehensive discussion of gas laws and their application to exercise physiology. Appendix D gives the formulas for the calculation of oxygen consumption and carbon dioxide production. Appendix E provides nomograms for calculating body surface area and body mass index, and for the conversion of body mass in pounds to kilograms. Appendix F contains tests of anaerobic and aerobic power. Appendix G contains equations for computing work efficiency. Appendix H details six key equations commonly used in exercise physiology.

References

1. Berryman, J. W. 1995. *Out of Many, One: A History of the American College of Sports Medicine*. Champaign, Human Kinetics Publishers.
2. Brooks, G. 1987. The exercise physiology paradigm in contemporary biology: To molbiol or not to molbiol—That is the Question. *Quest*, 39:231–242.
3. Buskirk, E. R. 1981. The emergence of exercise physiology. In Brooks, G. (ed.), *Perspectives on the Academic Discipline of Physical Education*. Champaign, Human Kinetics Publishers. 55–74.
4. Chapman, C. B., and J. H. Mitchell. 1965. The physiology of exercise. *Scientific American*. 212:88–96.

5. Cooper, K. H. 1968. *Aerobics*. New York, Bantam Books.
6. Dill, D. B. 1967. The Harvard Fatigue Laboratory: Its development, contributions and demise. In Chapman, C. B. (ed.), *Physiology of Muscular Exercise*. New York, American Heart Association. 161–170.
7. Dill, D. B. 1974. Historical review of exercise physiology science. In Johnson, W. R., and E. R. Buskirk, *Science and Medicine of Exercise and Sports*. New York, Harper and Row, 37–41.
8. Kraus, H., and R. P. Hirschland. 1953. Muscular fitness and health. *Journal of Health, Physical Education, and Recreation*. 24:17–19.

Selected Readings

Periodicals dealing predominantly with the science of exercise physiology, physical education, and athletics:

Acta Physiologica Scandinavica *(Acta Physiol Scand)*

American Journal of Sports Medicine *(Am J Sports Med)*

British Journal of Sports Medicine *(Br J Sports Med)*

Canadian Journal of Applied Sports Sciences *(Can J Appl Sports Sci)*

Ergonomics *(Ergonomics)*

The European Journal of Applied Physiology *(Eur J Appl Physiol)*, formerly Arbeitsphysiologie *(Arbeitsphysiol)*, and Internationale Zeitschrift fur Angewandte Physiologie Einschlesslich Arbeitsphysiologie *(Int Z Angew Physiol)*

International Journal of Sports Medicine *(Int J Sports Med)*

International Journal of Sports Nutrition *(Int J Sports Nutri)*

Journal of Applied Physiology *(J Appl Physiol)* or Journal of Applied Physiology: Respiratory, Environmental and Exercise Physiology *(J Appl Physiol: Respirat Environ Exerc Physiol)*

Journal of Cardiopulmonary Rehabilitation *(J Cardiopulmonary Rehabil)*

Journal of Sports Medicine and Physical Fitness *(J Sports Med Phys Fitness)*

Medicine and Science in Sports *(Med Sci Sports)* or Medicine and Science in Sports and Exercise *(Med Sci Sports Exerc)*

The Physician and Sportsmedicine *(Phys Sportsmed)*

Research Quarterly *(Res Q)* or Research Quarterly for Exercise and Sport *(Res Q Exerc Sport)*

Sports Medicine *(Sports Med)*

Books dealing with the physiology of exercise and human performance:

American College of Sports Medicine. 1971. *Encyclopedia of Sport Sciences and Medicine*. New York: Macmillan.

American College of Sports Medicine. *Exercise and Sport Sciences Reviews*. Vols. 1–3, Orlando: Academic Press, Inc., 1973–1975. Vols. 4 & 5, Santa Barbara: Journal Publishing Affiliates, 1976 & 1977. Vols. 6–17, New York: Macmillan, 1978–1989. Vols. 18–24, Baltimore: Williams & Wilkins, 1990–1996.

Astrand, P.-O., and K. Rodahl. 1986. *Textbook of Work Physiology*, 3rd ed. New York: McGraw-Hill.

Bouchard, C., B. D. McPherson, R. J. Shepherd, T. Stephens, and J. R. Sutton (eds.). 1990. *Exercise, Fitness and Health—A Consensus of Current Knowledge*. Champaign: Human Kinetics Publishers.

Bowers, R. W., and E. L. Fox. 1992. *Sports Physiology*. Dubuque: Wm. C. Brown.

Brooks, G., and T. Fahey. 1995. *Exercise Physiology: Human Bioenergetics and Its Applications*. 2d ed. Mt. View, CA: Mayfield.

deVries, H., and T. J. Housh. 1993. *Physiology of Exercise for Physical Education, Athletics and Exercise Science*, 5th ed. Dubuque, Brown & Benchmark.

Falls, H. B. 1980. *Essentials of Fitness*. Dubuque: Wm. C. Brown.

Hickson, J. F., Jr., and I. Wolinsky (eds.). 1989. *Nutrition in Exercise and Sports*. Boca Raton: CRC Press.

Horton, E. S., and R. L. Terjung. 1988. *Exercise, Nutrition and Energy Metabolism*. New York: Macmillan.

Larson, L. (ed.). 1974. *Fitness, Health, and Work Capacity: International Standards for Assessment*. New York: Macmillan.

McArdle, W. D., F. I. Katch, and V. L. Katch. 1996. *Exercise Physiology: Energy, Nutrition and Human Performance*, 4th ed. Baltimore: Williams & Wilkins.

Noble, B. J. 1991. *Physiology of Exercise and Sport*, 2d ed. St Louis: Times Mirror/Mosby College.

Pollock, M. L., and J. H. Wilmore. 1990. *Exercise in Health and Disease: Evaluation and Prescription for Prevention and Rehabilitation*, 2d ed. Philadelphia: W. B. Saunders.

Poortmans, J. R. (ed.). 1988. *Principles of Exercise Biochemistry*. (Medicine and Sport Science Series, Vol. 27). New York: S. Karger.

Powers, S. K., and E. T. Howley. 1997. *Exercise Physiology: Theory and Application to Fitness and Performance*. 3rd ed. Dubuque: Brown & Benchmark.

Rarick, G. (ed.). 1973. *Physical Activity: Human Growth and Development*. New York: Academic Press.

Robergs, R. A., and S. O. Roberts. 1997. *Exercise Physiology: Exercise, Performance, and Clinical Applications*. St. Louis: Mosby-Year Book, Inc.

Ryan, A. J., and F. L. Allman, Jr. (eds.). 1989. *Sports Medicine*, 2d ed. New York: Academic Press.

Shephard, R. J. 1984. *Biochemistry of Physical Activity*. Springfield: Charles C Thomas.

Strauss, R. H. (ed.). 1990. *Sports Medicine*, 2d ed. Philadelphia: W. B. Saunders.

Strauss, R. H. 1987. *Drugs and Performance in Sports*. Philadelphia: W. B. Saunders.

Wilmore, J. H., and D. L. Costill. 1988. *Training for Sport & Activity: The Physiological Basis of the Conditioning Process*. 3rd ed. Champaign: Human Kinetics Publishers.

Wilmore, J. H., and D. L. Costill. 1994. *Physiology of Sport & Exercise*. Champaign: Human Kinetics Publishers.

1

Bioenergetics

The main theme of this section is energy—what it is, where it comes from, how it is measured, and how it is produced and used by the human body at rest and during exercise. The objective is to enable you to apply in the gymnasium, on the athletic field, in the classroom, or in a clinical setting the knowledge gained from understanding energy. For example, you will learn that the body can store energy in small quantities and can "turn on" metabolic pathways within cells to provide "back up" energy for continued physical activity. Later, you will be shown how the scientific basis for the development of physical fitness and enhanced athletic performance is closely tied to conditioning programs that enhance the rate of energy utilization.

Has the thought ever occurred to you that there is an important physiological reason why the sprinter should be trained differently from the distance runner? Or, even more fundamentally, why some individuals are sprinters and others are better at endurance activities? Have you ever thought about what enables muscles to contract or what fatigue is and how its onset may be delayed by certain activities? Or during exercise, how the body regulates the types of fuels that are being "burned" to produce energy? Finally said, all of these considerations relate in some way to the storage and use of energy by actively contracting muscle cells or by the cells of important support organs/systems, such as the lungs, liver, heart, kidneys, nervous system, endocrine glands, and so on. A very complex interaction to say the least, but one with a common basis: energy.

The materials contained in this section will also provide the physiological basis, foundation if you like, for you to better understand the important concepts of "training specificity" and the interrelationships of nutrition, performance, and body weight regulation. Finally, you will learn that the energy concept pervades *all* phases of physical activity, from athletics to clinical practice. For these reasons we, once again, encourage you to master the material of these early chapters. This will set the stage for a better overall learning experience when the more applied topics are introduced in later chapters. Our discussion of energy starts with the energy sources available to the human body and how they are used during rest and exercise (chapter 2). Next, we proceed to the replenishment of these sources during recovery from exercise (chapter 3). We end the section with a discussion of the measurement of energy production and the efficiency of the human body during performance of various kinds of exercise (chapter 4). Enough talk; let's get started with this exciting venture!

Energy Sources

We are aware that all human activity centers around the capability to provide energy on a continuous basis. Without a continuous source of energy, cells, including muscle, cease to function, and they die. Energy is provided through the metabolic degradation of, principally, two foods: carbohydrates and fats. Carbohydrates are metabolized through glycolysis and the Krebs Cycle. Fats are also metabolized through the Krebs Cycle but begin with a process called beta-oxidation.

Amino acids, the building blocks of proteins, may also be metabolized in the Krebs Cycle to provide a small quantity of energy during exercise. Other important supportive roles that proteins and amino acids are now believed to play during exercise include (1) provision of intermediate substrates so the Krebs Cycle can continue to function, and (2) provision of alanine (an amino acid) by skeletal muscle to the liver, which converts it to glucose via the glucose-alanine cycle. These processes will be covered in more detail in chapter 15.

As indicated, the production of energy is an ongoing activity requiring both aerobic and anaerobic processes. The purpose of this chapter is to study the concept of energy in general, and then specifically to

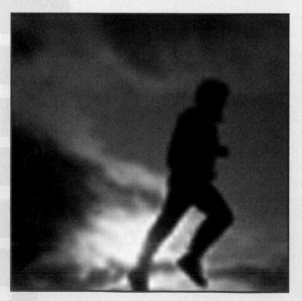

study the energy sources available to humans during rest and exercise. Finally, we will discuss the fascinating matter of cellular control and regulation to determine which metabolic pathway or combination of pathways is being used to provide energy at any given time during exercise.

Energy Defined

The Biological Energy Cycle

Adenosine Triphosphate—ATP

Control and Regulation of Metabolic Pathways

Summary

The major concepts to be learned from this chapter are as follows:

- All energy used by the biological world is ultimately derived from the sun.
- The immediate energy source for all activity in humans, as well as in most other biological systems, comes from the breakdown of a single chemical compound—adenosine triphosphate, or ATP.

- The metabolic production of ATP by muscle and other cells comes from the energy released through the breakdown of foods and other high-energy compounds and involves both an anaerobic (without oxygen) and aerobic (with oxygen) series of chemical reactions.
- Three basic metabolic systems—the phosphagens, anaerobic glycolysis, and aerobic systems—work together to provide needed ATP during exercise.
- Fats (fatty acids), carbohydrates (glucose and glycogen) and to a much lesser extent, proteins (amino acids), provide fuel for energy at rest and during exercise.
- Carbohydrates can be "burned" in the absence of oxygen, whereas fats are "always burned in the flame of carbohydrate" and in the presence of oxygen—i.e., metabolism of both substrates occurs simultaneously.
- Whether ATP is predominantly supplied to the working muscles by way of anaerobic or aerobic metabolic pathways depends on the intensity and duration of the activity performed.
- Lactate is present in the bloodstream even at rest because of lactate dehydrogenase (LDH) activity but increases greatly during anaerobic exercise when the rate of ATP use exceeds ATP resynthesis via oxidative-phosphorylation.
- A depletion of energy substrates (phosphagens, blood glucose, muscle glycogen) or an accumulation of intracellular and blood lactate leads to muscle cell fatigue and forces the performer to slow down or stop activity.
- Muscle cell metabolism during exercise is regulated among pathways depending on the energy state of the cell, required rate of energy production, its mitochondrial capacity, and oxygen availability.
- Immediate regulation and control starts with ADP production at the beginning of muscle contractions, continues through hormone "amplification" via c-AMP, and ends with oxygen—all of which tend to activate or inhibit key rate-limiting enzymes.
- Sports can be categorized along a continuum going from mostly aerobic (long distance), through a mixture of aerobic and anaerobic (middle distances), and on to mostly anaerobic (short sprint) activities.
- A working knowledge of this continuum and how the three metabolic systems cooperate to provide ATP energy is basic to sound athletic coaching, training, and exercise prescription.
- Although, generally speaking, females have lower anaerobic energy capacities (ATP, CP, and glycolysis) and lower aerobic powers (max $\dot{V}O_2$) than males at the same status of training, there is much overlap when trained and untrained populations are compared.
- Trained female athletes exceed untrained females on all energy measures and more closely approximate trained male athletes when differences in body size, weight, body fat, and active muscle mass are factored out by using relative units of expression.

Energy Defined

Before much meaning can be given to a discussion of energy sources, we need to define energy. Probably all of us have some idea of the nature of energy. Such common words as *force, power, strength, vigor, movement, life,* and even *spirit* more or less suggest the idea of energy. These terms, however, do not give us a satisfactory description of the exact meaning of energy. Furthermore, they do not lend themselves to scientific quantitation. Scientists, therefore, define **energy** as the *capacity or ability to perform work.* **Work** we define as the application of a force through a distance. As a result, energy and work are inseparable. We will explore the relationships between energy and work in chapter 4. Right now, let us continue with our discussion of energy.

There are six forms of energy: (1) chemical, (2) mechanical, (3) heat, (4) light, (5) electrical, and (6) nuclear. Each can be converted from one form to another. This "transformation of energy" is a fascinating and exciting story, particularly as applied to the biological world. Specifically, we are interested in the transformation of chemical energy into mechanical energy. Mechanical energy is manifested in human movement, the source of which comes from converting food to chemical energy within our body.

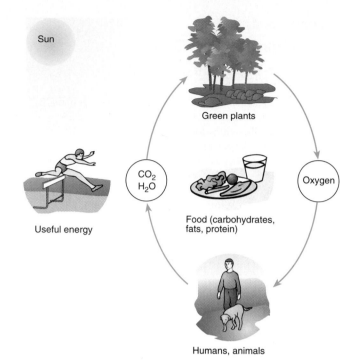

Figure 2.1

The biological energy cycle. Energy from sunlight is used by plants to build food molecules from CO_2 and H_2O, with oxygen being given off. Both plants and animals, including humans, in turn, use oxygen to break down foods for the energy they need to live.

The Biological Energy Cycle

All energy in our solar system originates in the sun. Where does this energy, called *solar energy,* come from? Solar energy actually arises from nuclear energy. Some of this nuclear energy reaches the earth as sunlight or light energy. The millions of green plants that populate our earth store a portion of this energy from the sunlight in still another form—chemical energy. In turn, this chemical energy is used by green plants to build food molecules such as glucose, cellulose, proteins, and lipids from carbon dioxide (CO_2) and water (H_2O). This process, whereby green plants manufacture their own food, is called **photosynthesis.** We, on the other hand, are not capable of doing this; we must eat plants and other animals for our food supplies. We are, therefore, directly dependent on plant life and, ultimately, on the sun for our energy.

Food in the presence of O_2 is broken down to CO_2 and H_2O with the liberation of chemical energy by a metabolic process called respiration. The sole purpose of metabolic respiration is to supply the energy we need to carry out such biological processes as the chemical work of growth and the mechanical work of muscular contraction. The entire process is called the biological energy cycle (figure 2.1).

Adenosine Triphosphate— ATP

We now know what energy is, where it originates, and that it is supplied to us by the foods we eat. Our next problem is to understand how this energy is used to perform physiological work, particularly the mechanical work of muscular contraction. The energy liberated during the breakdown of food is *not directly* used to do work. Rather, it is employed to manufacture another chemical compound called **adenosine triphosphate,** or, more simply, **ATP,** which is stored in all muscle cells. *Only from the energy released by the breakdown of ATP can the cell perform its specialized work.*[20]

The structure of ATP* consists of one very complex component, adenosine, and three less complicated parts called phosphate groups. For our purposes, its chemical importance lies in the phosphate groups. In figure 2.2*A,* a simplified structure of ATP is shown. The bonds between the two terminal phosphate groups represent so-called high-energy bonds. When 1 mole (a unit defined later) of these

---

*For a detailed discussion of the structure of ATP, refer to McGilvery (1975).

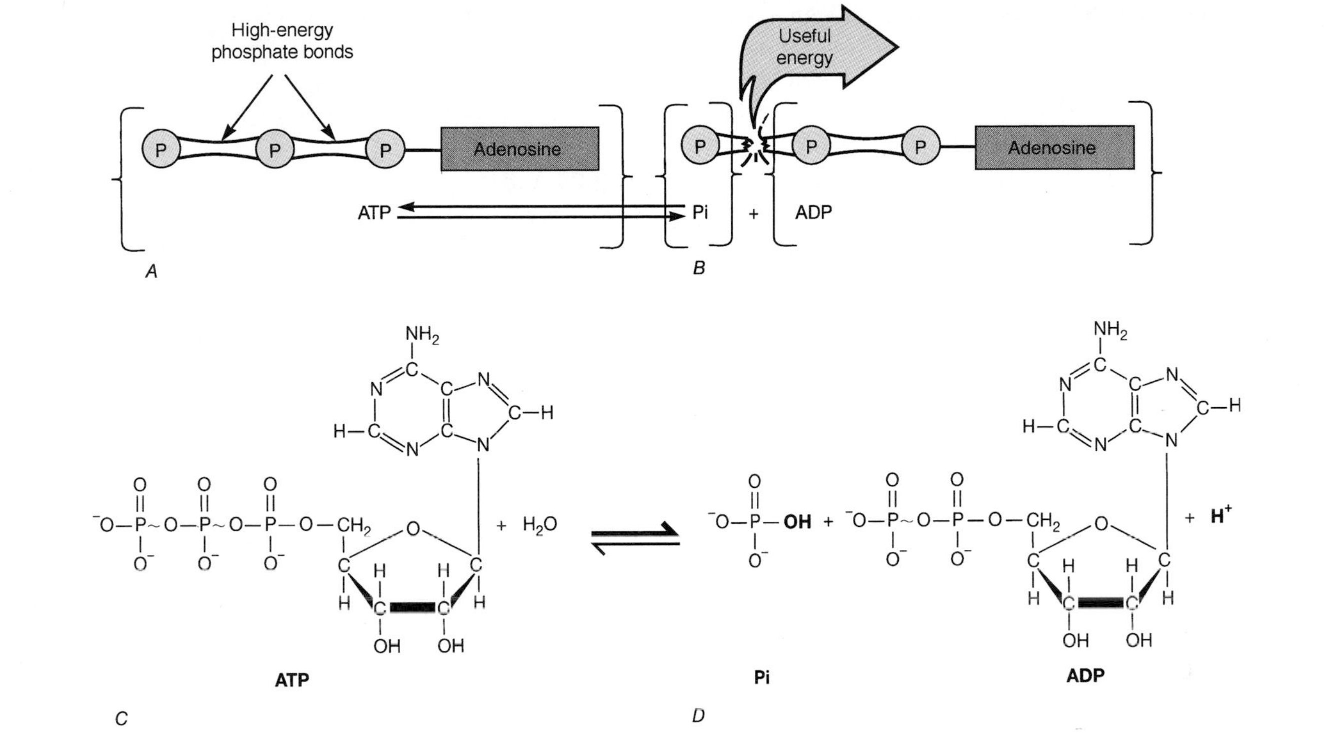

Figure 2.2

A. Simplified structure of ATP, showing high-energy phosphate bonds. *B.* Breakdown of ATP to ADP and inorganic phosphate (Pi), with the release of useful energy. The breakdown of 1 mole of ATP yields between 7 and 12 kilocalories (kcal) of energy. *C.* The molecular structure of adenosine triphosphate (ATP) showing two unstable energy-rich anhydride bonds (~). *D.* Hydrolysis reaction to the right with the splitting off of inorganic phosphate (Pi) and production of adenosine diphosphate (ADP). The thinner arrow to the left shows that reformation of ATP is possible.

phosphate bonds is broken off (i.e., removed from the rest of the molecules), 7 to 12 **kilocalories**[†] of energy are liberated, and **adenosine diphosphate (ADP)** plus **inorganic phosphate (Pi)** are formed (figure 2.2*B*). *This energy released during the breakdown of ATP represents the immediate source of energy that can be used by the muscle cell to perform its work.*

Figure 2.2*C* shows ATP in its chemical form. The aromatic base, **adenine,** is at the top and is linked to a five-carbon sugar, **ribose,** to form **adenosine.** The ~ indicate the energy-rich but unstable anhydride bonds that link the last two phosphate groups to the molecule. These bonds can be broken in the presence of water (called hydrolysis) as shown by the reaction going to the right in the direction of the heavy arrow. Note the location of the oxygen and the two hydrogens from H_2O as they are involved in the reaction (figure 2.2*D*). Note also the formation of the hydrogen ion in its free form (H^+), which you will learn represents the first expression of acidity with which the cell must deal.

The reaction can be immediately reversed to form ATP (see light arrow in figure 2.2*D* to *C*), but this requires the presence of a similar high-energy source, which is stored **phosphocreatine (PC).** The reaction also can be reversed at a few selected points in the cellular metabolic pathways where the "drop" in stored energy is enough to allow the reaction to proceed. But you will learn that these reactions are more complex and slower to occur. Look for these latter reactions by their names of **oxidation-reduction** and **oxidative phosphorylation.** At this juncture you might begin to associate the names for the above reactions with the involvement of oxygen, hydrogen, and phosphorus.

Sources of ATP

Because the hydrolysis (breakdown) of ATP releases energy for muscular contraction, the question is raised: How is this important compound supplied to each muscle cell? First, it must be realized that (1) at any one moment there is only a limited quantity of ATP in a muscle cell and that (2) ATP is constantly being used and regenerated. Regeneration of ATP requires energy. There are three common energy-yielding processes for the production of

---

[†]A kilocalorie (kcal) is the amount of heat energy required to raise 1 kilogram (kg) of water 1° Celsius (°C). A calorie (cal) is the amount of heat required to raise 1 gram (g) of water 1°C. One thousand cal equals 1 kcal. The kcal is the calorie term used most often in this text.

ATP: (1) the **ATP-PC system** (or **phosphagen system**), the system in which the energy for resynthesis of ATP comes from only one compound, phosphocreatine (PC); (2) **anaerobic glycolysis,** the system that generates lactic acid but provides some ATP from the partial degradation of glucose or glycogen in the absence of oxygen; and (3) the **aerobic system,** which involves the use of oxygen and really has two parts: part A involves the completion of the oxidation of the carbohydrates, and part B involves the oxidation of fatty acids and some amino acids. Both parts of the aerobic system have the Krebs Cycle as their final route of oxidation. Because some protein can also be oxidized through the Krebs Cycle, it is appropriately called the final common pathway.

All three suppliers of energy for ATP resynthesis operate in the same general manner. The energy liberated from the breakdown of foodstuffs and the energy released when PC is broken down are used to put the ATP molecule back together again; in other words, the energy is used to "drive" the reaction shown in figure 2.2 from right (*B*) to left (*A*). The energy released from the breakdown of foods and PC is functionally linked or coupled to the energy needs of resynthesizing ATP from ADP and Pi (figure 2.3). The functional coupling of energy from one series of reactions to another is referred to biochemically as **coupled reactions** and is the fundamental principle involved in the metabolic production of ATP.

Anaerobic Sources of ATP— Anaerobic Metabolism

Two of the three metabolic systems involved in ATP resynthesis mentioned previously, the ATP-PC (phosphagen) system and anaerobic glycolysis, are **anaerobic.** Anaerobic means without oxygen, and metabolism refers to the various series of chemical reactions that take place within the body (e.g., the muscle cell), including those just mentioned. Thus *anaerobic metabolism,* or the anaerobic generation of ATP, refers to the resynthesis of ATP through chemical reactions that do not require the presence of the oxygen we breathe.

The ATP-PC (Phosphagen) System

Because this anaerobic system is least complicated (but in no way least important), we will discuss it first. Phosphocreatine, like ATP, is stored in muscle cells. Because both ATP and PC contain phosphate groups, they are collectively referred to as **high-energy phosphagens** (hence the name "phosphagen system"). PC is also similar to ATP in that when its phosphate group is removed, a large amount of energy is liberated (figure 2.4*A* & *B*). The end products of this breakdown reaction are creatine (C) and inorganic phosphate (Pi). The molecular structure of PC with its bonded high-energy phosphate group (~) is shown in figure 2.4*C*. As previously discussed, the energy is immediately avail-

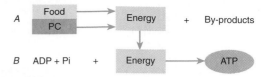

Figure 2.3

The principle of coupled reactions. The energy released from the breakdown of foods and phosphocreatine (PC) is functionally linked or coupled to the energy needs of resynthesizing ATP from ADP (adenosine diphosphate) and Pi (inorganic phosphate).

able and is biochemically coupled to the resynthesis of ATP. For example, as rapidly as ATP is broken down during muscular contraction, it is continuously re-formed from ADP and Pi by the energy liberated during the breakdown of the stored PC. These coupled reactions can be summarized as follows:

$$PC \longrightarrow Pi + C + \textbf{Energy}$$
$$\textbf{Energy} + ADP + Pi \longrightarrow ATP$$

The preceding equations are overly simplified. In the body, they are more complicated and require the presence of **enzymes,** which are protein compounds that accelerate the speed of the individual reactions. Actually, all metabolic reactions occurring in the body require the presence of enzymes, including the breakdown of ATP. The enzyme that catalyzes (speeds) the breakdown of PC with the resultant formation of ATP is appropriately named *creatine kinase.* Note here that any enzymes that regulate phosphorylation-dephosphorylation reactions (i.e., transfer of high-energy phosphate) all end in -kinase. This reaction can be shown as $PC + ADP \xrightarrow{\text{creatine kinase}} ATP + C$. It is also possible for ADP to react to form ATP, because ADP still has one high-energy phosphate bond intact. This reaction, referred to as the myokinase reaction, occurs in muscle cells, is catalyzed by the enzyme *myokinase,* and results in the production of one ATP from two ADP. It can be written $ADP + ADP \xrightarrow{\text{myokinase}} ATP + AMP$. Note the production of a new by-product of the reaction, namely, adenosine monophosphate (AMP). But that is as far as the breakdown occurs. The last phosphate group that remains on AMP is tightly bonded and therefore is not available as an energy source. It remains as AMP or is broken down (degraded) to its basic parts. When this happens, AMP is lost from the potential phosphagen pool.

Ironically, the only means by which PC can be reformed from Pi and C is from the energy released by the breakdown of ATP. This occurs *during recovery* from exercise, with the primary source of ATP coming from that obtained through the breakdown of foodstuffs. *Thus, when PC stores are depleted in the ultra high-intensity activity of sprinting, they cannot effectively be replenished until recovery has started.* We will discuss this and other recovery processes in more detail in the next chapter.

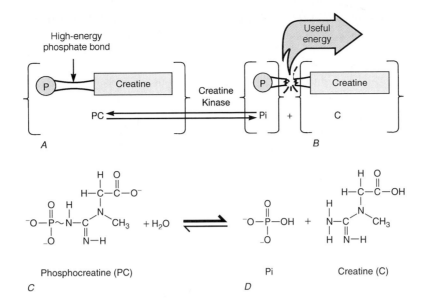

Figure 2.4

A. Simplified structure of phosphocreatine (PC) showing its high-energy phosphate bond. *B.* Breakdown of PC to creatine (C) and inorganic phosphate (Pi), with the release of energy used to resynthesize ATP. *C.* The chemical structure of phosphocreatine showing its high-energy bond (∼). *D.* Splitting of phosphocreatine into inorganic phosphate (Pi) and creatine. The thinner arrow to the left shows that reformation of PC is possible.

2.1

Estimation of the energy available in the body through the phosphagen (ATP-PC) system

	ATP	PC	Total phosphagen (ATP + PC)
1. Muscular concentration			
a. mmol · kg muscle^{-1}*	4–6	15–17	19–23
b. mmol total muscle mass†	120–180	450–510	570–690
2. Useful energy‡			
a. kcal · kg muscle^{-1}	0.04–0.06	0.15–0.17	0.19–0.23
b. kcal total muscle mass	1.2–1.8	4.5–5.1	5.7–6.9

*Based on data from Hultman[14] and Karlsson[18]
†Assuming 30 kg of muscle in a 70 kg man.
‡Assuming 10 kcal per mole ATP.

How much ATP energy is available from the phosphagen system? The answer to this question is contained in table 2.1. Several points in the table are worth highlighting. First, notice that storage of PC in the muscle is about three times that of stored ATP. This makes sense, because the function of stored PC is to provide "backup" energy for ATP resynthesis. Second, the abbreviation mmol refers to **millimoles,** a unit of measure used in quantifying amounts of chemical compounds. A **mole** is a given amount of a chemical compound by weight, the weight being dependent on the quantities of each kind of atom making up the compound. Since the weight of a mole is always expressed in grams (g), a mole of any substance is commonly referred to as its gram molecular weight. A millimole of any substance would be 1/1000 of a mole since 1000 millimoles = 1 mole. Note that conversion from millimoles to moles requires a decimal shift of three positions to the left (dividing by 1000). Of course, the decimal shift is three positions to the right if you are converting from moles to millimoles (multiplying by 1000). For example, 120 to 180 mmol of

ATP in the total muscle mass as shown in table 2.1 could be expressed as .120 to .180 moles. Practice this if you are rusty!

To better understand the concept of moles and millimoles, let's consider what a mole of glucose and a mole of lactic acid crystals would weigh and look like. It is probably easier to picture glucose crystals, because we have all seen table sugar, which is very similar in its makeup. Glucose has the molecular formula $C_6H_{12}O_6$. The weight of a mole of glucose is determined by first multiplying the quantities of each kind of atom by its atomic mass unit (amu), which can be found in a periodic table for the elements. Therefore, (6 C × 12 amu = 72 amu) + (12 H × 1 amu = 12 amu) + (6 O × 16 amu = 96 amu) for a total of 180 amu. Expressed in grams (g), a mole of glucose weighs 180 g or about 6 ounces and would nearly fill both of your hands if they were cupped to form a "bowl." The formula for lactic acid is $C_3H_6O_3$ for a total of 90 amu and therefore 90 g · mole^{-1}. Note that a mole of lactic acid is one-half the weight and size of a mole of glucose and could likely be held in one cupped hand if the crystals were carefully poured to form a pile in the center of the palm. For some additional practice on this, refer back to figures 2.2 and 2.4 and calculate how much a mole of ATP and a mole of PC would each weigh. Use 14 for the amu of nitrogen and 31 for the amu of phosphorus. Did you get 503 g for a mole of ATP and 236 g for a mole of PC? Comparatively speaking, ATP is quite a large and heavy molecule, isn't it?

Let's return now to table 2.1. Remember that when 1 mole of ATP is broken down, between 7 and 12 kcal of usable energy are released. An average of 10 kcal per mole of ATP is assumed. Also, notice that only 19 to 23 mmol of total phosphagen (ATP + PC) are stored in each kilogram (1 kg = 2.2 lbs) of muscle. When multiplied by 30 to determine mmol per total muscle mass (note the assumption of 30 kg of muscle in a 70 kg "anatomical man") the amount is 570 to 690 mmol of stored phosphagen for the entire body. This could also be written as .570 to .690 moles of phosphagen. When multiplied by 10 kcal · mole^{-1}, this is equivalent to between 5.7 and 6.9 kcal of ATP energy, which does not represent very much energy for use during exercise. For example, the phosphagen stores in the working muscles would be exhausted after only the first three to five seconds of all-out exercise, such as sprinting 100 meters. The total amount of ATP energy available from the phosphagen system is, indeed, very limited!

The importance of the phosphagen system to physical performance and athleticism is exemplified by the powerful, quick starts of sprinters, football players, high jumpers, and shot-putters. Without this system, fast, powerful movements could not be performed, because such activities demand a rapidly available supply rather than a large amount of ATP energy. The phosphagen system *represents the most rapidly available source of ATP for use by the muscle.* Some of the reasons for this are:

1. Both ATP and PC are stored directly within the contractile mechanism of the muscles,
2. It does not depend on a long series of chemical reactions, and
3. It does not depend on transporting the oxygen we breathe to the working muscles.

Anaerobic Glycolysis System*

The other anaerobic system in which ATP is resynthesized within the muscle, anaerobic glycolysis, involves an incomplete breakdown of one of the foodstuffs, **carbohydrate** (sugar), to **lactic acid.** In the body, all carbohydrates are converted to the simple sugar **glucose,** which can either be immediately used in that form or stored in the liver and muscle as **glycogen** for later use. Stored glycogen consists simply of numerous glucose molecules that are linked together in branched chains by special oxygen bonds called glycosidic bonds. We will see later that these bonds can be broken, called glycogenolysis, to release glucose from the liver into the blood stream for delivery to active muscles or can be broken within muscle cells themselves for a more direct use of stored glucose.[14] In either case, the glucose is only partially metabolized through the process of anaerobic glycolysis, which occurs in the cytosol (intracellular fluid) of the muscle cell without any need for oxygen. Therefore, for our purposes, carbohydrates, sugar, glucose, and glycogen have equivalent meanings with respect to metabolism. It is important to reemphasize here that lactic acid results from anaerobic glycolysis.

From a chemical standpoint, anaerobic glycolysis is more complicated than the phosphagen system in that it requires twelve separate but sequential chemical reactions for completion. This series of reactions was discovered in the 1930s by Gustav Embden and Otto Meyerhof, two German scientists. For this reason, anaerobic glycolysis is sometimes referred to as the Embden-Meyerhof pathway, but more commonly it is referred to simply as glycolysis.

How are glucose and glycogen used for resythesizing ATP? As just indicated, glucose itself or glucose from glycogen is chemically broken down into lactic acid by a series of reactions. During this breakdown, energy is released and, through coupled reactions, is used to resynthesize ATP. This process is shown schematically in figure 2.5. Again, the reactions are overly simplified and the twelve individual reactions known to be involved in glycolysis are collectively shown in the box labeled "glycolytic sequence." In addition, each of the reactions requires the presence of a specific enzyme for the reactions to occur at a sufficient speed. As you know, enzymes are special proteins that make biochemical reactions "go"

---

*Glycolysis literally means the splitting of glucose (McGilvery, 1983, p. 484). Anaerobic glycolysis then refers to the partial breakdown of glucose in the absence of oxygen.

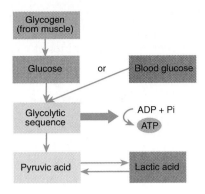

Figure 2.5

Anaerobic glycolysis. Glycogen is chemically broken down by a series of reactions into lactic acid. During this breakdown, energy is released and, through coupled reactions, is used to resynthesize ATP.

without being consumed themselves in the process—i.e., they are reusable. There will be much more on the metabolic control and regulatory function of enzymes later in this chapter.

Only a few moles of ATP can be resynthesized from glucose or glycogen during anaerobic glycolysis as compared with the yield possible when conditions are more conducive to their complete oxidation. For example, during anaerobic glycolysis only 2 or 3 moles of ATP can be resynthesized from the breakdown of 1 mole, or 180 grams (about 6 ounces), of glucose or glycogen, respectively. As we will soon see, at a lower rate of ATP energy demand and in the presence of sufficient oxygen, the complete breakdown of the same amount of glucose and glycogen yields 38 and 39 moles of ATP respectively—roughly a 16 times higher yield from the same energy substrate. If you had your choice, which route of ATP resynthesis would you rather have working for you? During the performance of competitive athletics, do you always have a choice if you want to win? What about a life-threatening or survival situation?

The summary equations of the coupled reactions for ATP resynthesis from anaerobic glycolysis when glycogen is the fuel substrate are as follows (**n** indicates numerous linked molecules, unspecified in number):

$$(C_6H_{12}O_6)_n \longrightarrow 2C_3H_6O_3 + \textbf{Energy}$$
$$\text{(glycogen)} \qquad \text{(lactic acid)}$$
$$\textbf{Energy} + 3 \text{ ADP} + 3 \text{ Pi} \longrightarrow 3 \text{ ATP}$$

During exercise, the useful ATP production from anaerobic glycolysis is actually less than the 3 moles of ATP (3 ATP) shown in the preceding equations. The reason for this is that during exhaustive exercise, the muscles and blood can tolerate the accumulation of only about 60 to 70 grams of lactic acid before fatigue sets in. This amount of lactic acid is shown in table 2.2. When spread throughout 30 kg of muscle (assumed for a 70 kg man) it represents a concentration of 2.0 to 2.3 grams per kg. The main point is,

if all 180 grams of glycogen were broken down anaerobically during exercise, 180 grams of lactic acid (represented at $2C_3H_6O_3$ in the above equation) would be formed and this would be intolerable. Therefore, from a practical viewpoint, only between 1 and 1.2 moles of ATP can be totally resynthesized from anaerobic glycolysis during heavy exercise before lactic acid in blood and muscles reaches exhausting levels.*

Holloszy agrees that there appears to be an upper limit to the amount of lactic acid that can accumulate before a performer must stop with severe muscular fatigue.[13] One possible explanation for this limitation is that intracellular concentration of hydrogen ions increases (pH drops) as lactic acid accumulates in muscle, resulting in inhibition of the **rate-limiting enzyme** phosphofructokinase (PFK) in the anaerobic glycolysis pathway.[25,28] The significance of this "down regulation" of a rate-limiting enzyme is the creation of a bottleneck in the pathway, which holds back all of the sequential reactions on either side of the "obstruction." One of the most important enzymes in this respect is PFK, but you will be introduced to other key regulatory enzymes of anaerobic glycolysis with names like phosphorylase, hexokinase, pyruvate kinase, and lactate dehydrogenase.[2,23]

Anaerobic glycolysis, like the phosphagen system, is extremely important to us during exercise primarily because it also provides a relatively rapid supply of ATP. For example, exercises that can be performed at a maximal rate for between 1 and 3 minutes (such as sprinting 400 and 800 meters) depend heavily on the phosphagen system and anaerobic glycolysis for ATP formation.

The total ATP energy available in the body through anaerobic glycolysis is estimated in table 2.2. As mentioned before, if the muscles can tolerate 2.0 to 2.3 grams of lactic acid per kilogram of muscle, or 60 to 70 grams for the total muscle mass, then the maximal amount of ATP manufactured by glycolysis would be between 1.0 and 1.2 moles (1000 to 1200 millimoles). As before, multiplying by 10 kcal $\cdot$ mole^{-1} of ATP yields a total of 10 to 12 kcal of useful energy. Given these assumptions and conditions, notice that this is about twice as much ATP as that which is obtainable from the ATP-PC system. It is still only a relatively small amount of energy considering that approximately 125 kcal are required to run a mile. Clearly, the additional energy will have to come from a different source to avoid a buildup of lactic acid. This is accomplished in cooperation with the aerobic system—i.e., oxygen begins to enter the metabolic scene.

---

*The complete breakdown of 1 mole of glycogen to 180 grams of lactic acid yields enough energy for the resynthesis of 3 moles of ATP. Therefore, the partial breakdown of a mole of glycogen to only 60 or 70 grams of lactic acid yields enough energy for the resynthesis of $180/3 \times 60/X = 1$ mole of ATP or $180/3 \times 70/X = 1.16$ ($\sim$1.2) moles of ATP.

2.2

table

Estimation of the energy available in the body through anaerobic glycolysis*

	Per kg muscle	Total muscle mass
1. Maximal lactic acid tolerance (grams)[†]	2.0–2.3	60–70
2. ATP formation (millimoles)	33–38	1000–1200[‡]
3. Useful energy (kilocalories)	0.33–0.38	10.0–12.0

*Assumptions same as in table 2.1.
[†]Based on data from Karlsson.[18]
[‡]1.0–1.2 moles from previous calculations.

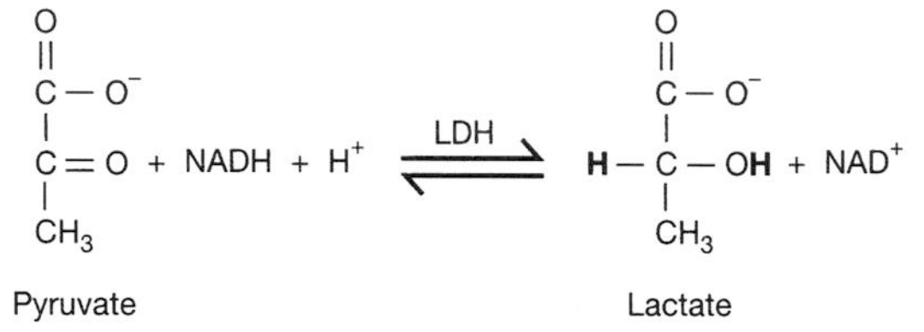

Before we leave this area of anaerobic glycolysis, let's take a closer look at some things about lactic acid. Pyruvic acid, which was shown in figure 2.5, is a precursor to lactic acid. The molecular structure of pyruvic acid and lactic acid are shown in figure 2.6; a double arrow for the reactions indicates that these acids can be converted back and forth. Note the use of the terms *pyruvate* and *lactate,* which mean that these acids are in ionized form; in other words, they both have given off (dissociated) hydrogen ions (H^+) into intracellular or extracellular fluids (like blood). Note the oxygen with its negative charge (O^-) on each of the molecules. These are the sites where the hydrogen was previously bonded. At physiological pH this dissociation is complete, so the buildup of lactic acid during anaerobic glycolysis and resultant dissociation of H^+ makes the intracellular fluids more acidic. As indicated earlier, H^+ can severely impair function and cause fatigue in working muscle cells.[18] Now you see where the acidity is coming from.

Note also in figure 2.6 that the reaction for the conversion of pyruvate to lactate is catalyzed by lactate dehydrogenase (LDH) and can proceed in either direction. During anaerobic glycolysis, when large increases in lactic acid occur, factors drive the reaction to the right. It will become clearer that the principal factors are high power outputs that require rates of ATP resynthesis that exceed the cell's oxidative capabilities. This may be due to a relative lack of adequate oxygen delivery to the cells during such intense exercise. Because of the two-way direction of this reaction, the lactate can be converted back to pyruvate when conditions are more favorable in terms of oxygen delivery relative to oxygen demands. This process will occur when the intensity of activity is reduced or the worker stops altogether.

Yet another interesting part of the pyruvate-lactate reaction in figure 2.6 is the role played by another molecule that contains adenine. This is **nicotinamide adenine dinucleotide (NAD),** whose nicotinamide group is derived from a B vitamin. People who are deficient in B vitamins are known to suffer from low energy levels. This makes sense because NAD is an important carrier of H, which will be described in more detail later in this chapter. In the reaction,

Figure 2.6

Reaction of pyruvate with $NADH + H^+$ to yield a reduced form of pyruvate, which is lactate, and the freeing up of NAD in oxidized form, NAD^+. Lactate dehydrogenase (LDH) is the enzyme that speeds the reaction in either direction depending primarily on oxygen availability (note the double arrow). Note also the location of the hydrogens that are taken on.

$NADH + H^+$ gives off two hydrogen to pyruvate in order to form lactate. The two locations where hydrogen is incorporated into the lactate molecule are known (see bold **H**'s in figure 2.6). This frees up NAD^+, which is an important event because NAD^+ is required for earlier reactions in the anaerobic glycolysis pathway to continue.

In a sense, lactic acid is produced and tolerated so that a precious few additional ATP can be generated. Albeit, not many, but a few more until the cells become so acidic that they cannot effectively function. This ability to continue to generate some ATP and tolerate the buildup of lactic acid and compromised muscle function may have important implications for survival in life-threatening situations, such as asphyxiation due to drowning or strangulation. It also has important implications during all-out sprint efforts to avoid harmful injury or when struggling to flee an oxygen-deficient environment. In fact, in these situations, the accumulation of lactic acid should be viewed as a most helpful and welcome ally by providing a few more ATP to support final efforts for survival.

In summary, anaerobic glycolysis (1) results in the formation of lactic acid, which is related to muscular fatigue; (2) does not require the presence of oxygen; (3) uses *only* carbohydrates (glucose and glycogen) as its food fuel; and (4) releases enough energy for the resynthesis of only a very

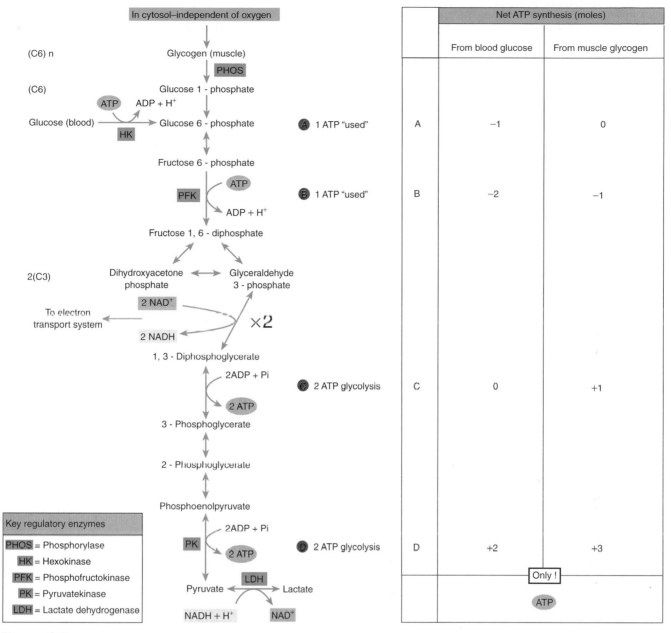

Figure 2.7

Sources of ATP from the anaerobic glycolysis of carbohydrate in the form of either 6 carbon blood glucose or muscle glycogen to 3 carbon pyruvate or lactate. Note the key regulatory enzymes.

few moles of ATP. Now let's closely review figure 2.7 and look for some of these outcomes. This figure names the intermediate products of the reactions and identifies five key regulatory enzymes that control the speed with which these reactions proceed. Instructors commonly require students to learn this series of reactions so well that they can be written out from memory. A very reasonable assignment.

First, note that the anaerobic glycolysis reactions are all occurring in the cytoplasm (intracellular fluid) and are independent of the presence of oxygen. Our objective here is to do a "bottom line" accounting for ATP, taking into con-

sideration places where ATP is used as well as where ATP is resynthesized. The *net* yield of ATP is our primary concern. In this regard it makes a difference whether glycogen that is already inside the muscle cell is used as the fuel substrate or whether glucose must be brought in at a cost of 1 ATP (see reaction A). Said differently, using muscle glycogen saves 1 ATP. Two regulatory enzymes are involved here, phosphorylase (PHOS), which speeds the breakdown of muscle glycogen to Glucose 1-phosphate, and hexokinase (HK), which speeds the conversion of Glucose to Glucose 6-phosphate. Note also that one additional ATP is used in the reaction when Fructose 6-phosphate is converted to Fructose 1, 6-diphosphate (see reaction B). Here we see the presence of the rate-limiting enzyme phosphofructokinase (PFK), which can control the flux of precursors through the entire glycolysis pathway. You might say that PFK is the glycolysis "gatekeeper."

At this point the 6-carbon sugar has been split into two 3-carbon compounds so all events are doubled downstream (see the **×2** signal). This means that 2 NADH are formed from 2 NAD^+ to go on to the electron transport system of the mitochondrion, if and when conditions are favorable for their oxidation—namely when adequate oxygen is present. Combining H to NAD is an important event that won't occur unless NAD is in its oxidized form of NAD^+. Let's not forget that these 2 NADH have been generated but are not yet included in our ATP accounting efforts. The H still have to enter the mitochondria, and NAD plays an important role as their carrier across the mitochondrial membrane. Let's also remember to look for ways that NAD^+ can readily be made available. Otherwise, the downstream reactions will not occur, and we will be left with using up one or two ATP and not resynthesizing any new ones. Not a very happy state in terms of cellular energy production.

On the other hand, if the reactions can proceed unhindered, 2 ATP will be resynthesized at reaction C and 2 more at reaction D. This all matches up with the earlier summary equations that indicated a net synthesis of either 2 or 3 ATP as a result of anaerobic glycolysis. Since we are near the end of the reaction sequence, note the presence of pyruvatekinase (PK) and lactate dehydrogenase (LDH), the last of the regulatory enzymes. Also note the important role that the formation of lactate plays in freeing up NAD^+ so it is available to be used in the earlier reaction at X2. Lactic acid often gets a bad reputation but really it can be viewed as a hero that allows glycolysis to continue to at least yield a few ATP in the face of inadequate or no oxygen within the cell. In summary, pyruvate is reduced (takes on hydrogens) to form lactate, while NADH is oxidized (hydrogens removed) to free up NAD^+. Lactate may be viewed as a "dead end" product, but it often does much to win races or sustain life. In the absence of oxygen, 2 or 3 ATP are better than none!

Aerobic Sources of ATP— Aerobic Metabolism

Before describing the reactions of the aerobic system, it is important to introduce a number of biochemical terms: acetyl group, acetyl-CoA, NAD^+, NADH, FAD^+, and $FADH_2$. An acetyl group, for our purposes, can be simply defined as a two-carbon molecule. For example, **pyruvic acid** (a three-carbon molecule) loses CO_2 to become an acetyl group, which combines with co-enzyme A to form acetyl-CoA before entering the Krebs Cycle. Likewise, in fatty acid metabolism, two-carbon acetyl groups are

"chunked off" in the process of β-oxidation and go on to enter the Krebs Cycle. The metabolism of protein (amino acids) is more complex because only some of them enter the Krebs Cycle as acetyl groups.

NAD^+ (nicotinamide adenine dinucleotide) and **FAD^+ (flavin adenine dinucleotide)** serve as hydrogen acceptors and carriers. H^+ are cleaved from carbohydrates during glycolysis and Krebs Cycle activity. The removal of H^+ ions from a compound is one form of **oxidation.** When a compound "accepts" a H^+, it is said to be reduced or to have undergone reduction. Thus, NADH and $FADH_2$ are the reduced forms of NAD^+ and FAD^+. The function of both NADH and $FADH_2$ is to carry electrons through the electron transport system (see p. 30).[*] See figures 2.8 and 2.9 for the molecular structures of NAD and FAD as well as the locations where hydrogen are carried.

In the presence of oxygen, 1 mole of glucose is completely broken down to carbon dioxide (CO_2) and water (H_2O), releasing sufficient energy to resynthesize 38 or 39 moles of ATP. This is by far the largest yield of ATP energy. Such a yield, as you might guess, requires many reactions and enzyme systems, all of which are much more complex than in the two anaerobic systems just discussed. Like the anaerobic systems, the reactions of the oxygen system occur within the muscle cell but, unlike the former, are confined to specialized, subcellular organelles called **mitochondria** (singular = **mitochondrion**). These compartments contain an elaborate membrane system consisting of a series of inward folds and convolutions called **cristae,** as shown in figure 2.10. Cristae are thought to contain most, if not all, of the enzyme systems required for aerobic metabolism. Skeletal muscle is proliferated with mitochondria (see figure 2.10A). Although only a single isolated mitochondrion is shown in the sketch (figure 2.10B), the mitochondria dispersed throughout muscle are connected through a network of fine membranes. This network is similar to the sarcoplasmic reticulum discussed in chapter 6.

The many reactions of the aerobic system can be divided into three main series: (1) **aerobic glycolysis,** (2) the **Krebs Cycle,** and (3) the **electron transport system (ETS).**

Aerobic Glycolysis

The first series of reactions involved in the aerobic breakdown of glycogen to CO_2 and H_2O is glycolysis. This may come as a surprise, since it was just said that glycolysis is an anaerobic pathway. Actually, there is only one difference between the anaerobic glycolysis discussed earlier and the aerobic glycolysis that occurs when there is a sufficient supply of oxygen: *lactic acid does not accumulate.* In other words, the presence of oxygen inhibits the accumulation of lactic acid but *not* the resynthesis of ATP. This is accom-

---

[*]For further explanation refer to McGilvery (1983) and West (1991).

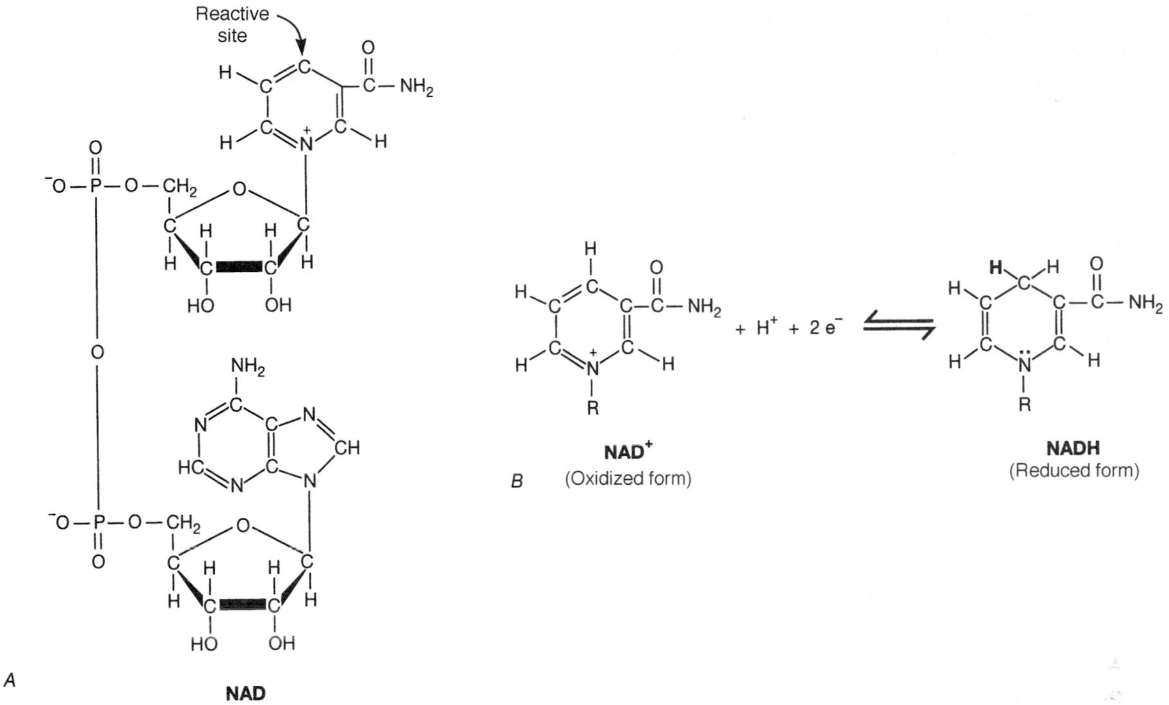

Figure 2.8

A. Nicotinamide adenine dinucleotide (NAD) showing reactive site. *B.* Structure of the oxidized form of nicotinamide adenine dinucleotide (NAD⁺) and the reduced form (NADH). R represents the remainder of the molecule which is unchanged. Note that a H^+ and two electrons (e^-) are incorporated into the molecule when it is reduced.

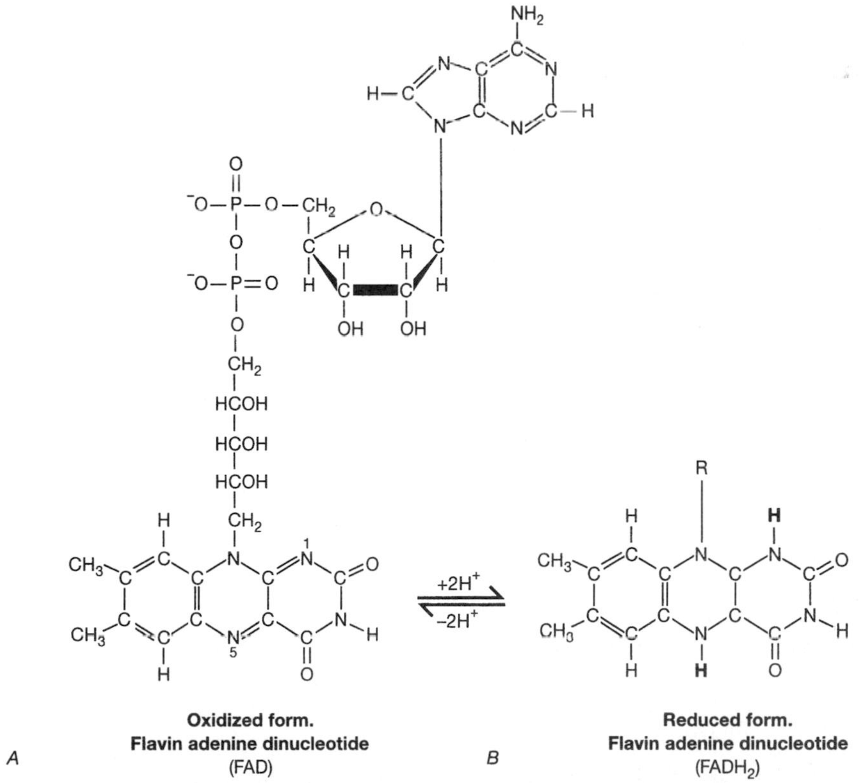

Figure 2.9

A. Oxidized form of FAD indicating the two sites (see 1 and 5) where hydrogen bonds to this coenzyme carrier. *B.* Reduced form of FAD showing the isoalloxazine ring, which is the reactive part of the molecule. R means the remainder of the molecule, which is unchanged. Note the bonding of 2 H^+ to nitrogens and the loss of associated double bonds.

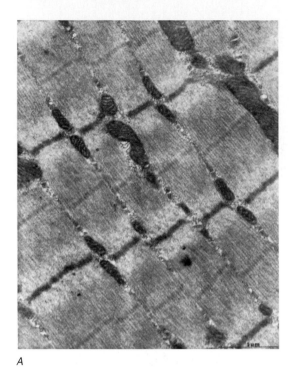

A

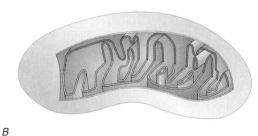

B

Figure 2.10

Mitochondria. *A.* An electron micrograph of a longitudinal section of rat skeletal muscle, showing several mitochondria. *B.* A schematic illustration of a mitochondrion showing its extensive membrane system and cristae, the latter of which contain the enzyme systems for aerobic metabolism. The cristae are also visible in the mitochondria shown in the electron micrograph.

(Electron micrograph courtesy Dr. James Cirrito, The Ohio State University, Columbus, Ohio.)

plished by diverting the majority of the lactic acid precursor pyruvic acid, into the aerobic system *after* the ATP is resynthesized (figure 2.11). Thus, during aerobic glycolysis, 1 mole of glycogen is broken down into 2 moles of pyruvic acid, releasing enough energy for resynthesizing 3 moles of ATP. These coupled reactions can be summarized as follows:

$$(C_6H_{12}O_6)_n \longrightarrow 2C_3H_4O_3 + \textbf{Energy}$$
$$\text{(glycogen)} \quad \text{(pyruvic acid)}$$
$$\textbf{Energy} + 3ADP + 3Pi \longrightarrow 3ATP$$

Additionally, 2 NAD^+ are reduced to 2 NADH, which are diverted to the electron transport system of the mitochondria where 6 more ATPs are generated (3 for each NADH).

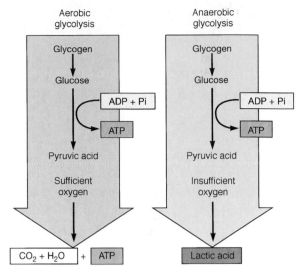

Figure 2.11

Aerobic and anaerobic glycolysis. The breakdown of glycogen to pyruvic acid with ATP resynthesis does not require oxygen. With oxygen present (aerobic glycolysis), pyruvic acid is further broken down to CO_2 and H_2O with more ATP resynthesized. Without oxygen (anaerobic glycolysis), pyruvic acid is converted to lactic acid with no further ATP resynthesized.

Let's look for these later when we review some of the reactions leading to the Krebs Cycle and the ETS (figure 2.12).

The Krebs Cycle

Next, the pyruvic acid formed during aerobic glycolysis passes into the mitochondria and continues to be broken down in a series of reactions called the *Krebs Cycle* after its discoverer, Sir Hans Krebs. For this important discovery, he won the Nobel Prize in physiology and medicine in 1953. This cycle may also be referred to as the *tricarboxylic acid (TCA) cycle* or the *citric acid cycle*, after some of the chemical compounds found in the cycle. A number of significant events occur during the Krebs Cycle in which we have an interest: (1) carbon dioxide is produced, (2) oxidation (and reduction) occur, and (3) ATP is produced through the conversion of a closely related compound, guanosine triphosphate (GTP).

Immediately, CO_2 is removed from pyruvic acid transforming it from a three-carbon compound to a two-carbon compound (an acetyl group). This acetyl group combines with co-enzyme A to form acetyl co-enzyme A. CO_2 is also formed in the Krebs Cycle. All CO_2 produced diffuses into the blood and is carried to the lungs where it is eliminated from the body.

Remembering that oxidation is the removal of electrons from a chemical compound, electrons are removed in the form of hydrogen atoms from the carbon atoms of what was formerly pyruvic acid and before that, glycogen. The

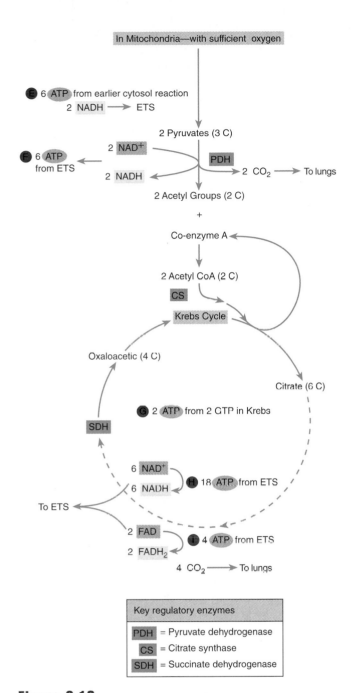

Net ATP synthesis (moles)		
	From blood glucose (+2)	From muscle glycogen (+3)
E	+8	+9
F	+14	+15
G	+16	+17
H	+34	+35
I	+38	+39

13 to 19 × more!

Figure 2.12

Sources of ATP from the complete oxidation (Aerobic Glycolysis) of pyruvate through the Krebs Cycle and Electron Transport System (ETS). The dashed lines indicate that several reactions have been omitted. Note the key regulation enzymes.

hydrogen atom, you may recall, contains a positively charged particle called a proton (referred to here as a free hydrogen ion) and a negatively charged particle called an electron. In other words:

$$H \longrightarrow H^+ + e^-$$
(hydrogen atom) (hydrogen ion) (electron)

Thus, when hydrogen atoms are removed from a compound, that compound is said to have been oxidized.

The production of CO_2 and the removal of electrons in the Krebs Cycle are related as follows: pyruvic acid (in its modified form) contains carbon (C), hydrogen (H), and oxygen (O); when H is removed, only C and O (i.e., the chemical components of carbon dioxide) remain. Thus in the Krebs Cycle, pyruvic acid is oxidized resulting in the production of CO_2. The Krebs Cycle is shown schematically in figure 2.13. In the Krebs Cycle itself, only 2 moles of ATP (via GTP) are formed for each mole of glycogen

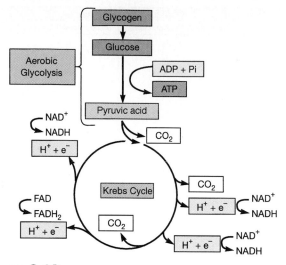

Figure 2.13

The Krebs Cycle. Pyruvic acid, the end product of aerobic glycolysis, enters the Krebs Cycle after a slight chemical alteration. Once in the cycle, two further chemical events take place: (1) the release of CO_2, which eventually is eliminated from the body by the lungs; and (2) oxidation, i.e., the removal of hydrogen ions (H^+) and electrons (e^-), which ultimately enter the electron transport system for further chemical alterations.

metabolized. At four different sites in the Krebs Cycle, H^+ are removed and passed through the electron transport system where the end result is the formation of water and ATP units.

The Electron Transport System (ETS)

Continuing in the breakdown of glycogen, the end product, H_2O, is formed from the H^+ and electrons that are removed in the Krebs Cycle and the *oxygen* we breathe. The specific series of reactions in which H_2O is formed is called the *electron transport system* (ETS) or the *respiratory chain.* Essentially what happens is that the hydrogen ions and electrons enter the ETS via $FADH_2$ and NADH and are "transported" to oxygen by "electron carriers" in a series of enzymatic reactions, the end product of which is water. In other words:

$$4H^+ + 4e^- + O_2 \longrightarrow 2H_2O$$

that is, 4 hydrogen ions ($4H^+$) plus 4 electrons ($4e^-$) plus 1 mole of oxygen (O_2) yield 2 moles of water ($2H_2O$). The electron carriers are often referred to as the **cytochromes,** which have **iron (Fe)** as an important part of their structure. The hydrogens and electrons are passed downward from a level of higher energy to a level of lower energy through reversible changes in the state of iron between Fe^{++} and Fe^{+++}. It is this energy, which is given up in a series of small release steps, that eventually is used to resynthesize ADP and Pi back to ATP. This ATP resynthesis process is called **oxidative phosphorylation.** Because iron

is so critical to this process of electron transport leading to ATP resynthesis there is small wonder why people with iron deficiencies have little energy and are lethargic. As the electrons are carried down the respiratory chain, energy is released, and ATP is resynthesized in coupled reactions. NADH enters the ETS at a slightly higher level than $FADH_2$ and thus "yields" 3 ATP per pass, whereas $FADH_2$ yields only 2 ATP per pass. This is shown in figure 2.14. Overall, twelve pairs of electrons are removed from 1 mole of glycogen and are carried as NADH or $FADH_2$ (see reactions E, F, H, I in figure 2.12). Thus 36 moles of ATP are generated. Therefore, during aerobic metabolism, most of the total of 38 or 39 moles of ATP for glucose and glycogen, respectively, are resynthesized in the electron transport system at the same time water is formed.

Summary Equations for Aerobic Metabolism

A summary of the coupled reactions involved in the aerobic breakdown of 1 mole of glycogen is as follows:

$$(C_6H_{12}O_6)_n + 6O_2 \longrightarrow 6CO_2 + 6H_2O + \textbf{Energy}$$
(glycogen)

$$\textbf{Energy} + 39ADP + 39Pi \longrightarrow 39ATP$$

Note that 39 moles of ATP are resynthesized: 3 ATP from aerobic glycolysis, 30 ATP from the passage of NADH into the ETS, 4 ATP from the passage of $FADH_2$ into the ETS, and 2 ATP (via GTP) from the Krebs Cycle itself. Also note that when blood glucose is the source of carbohydrate fuel, one additional ATP is "consumed" in converting glucose to glucose 1-phosphate (see figure 2.7). It should be further noted that it requires 6 moles of oxygen ($6O_2$) to break down 180 grams (1 mole) of glycogen. Because 1 mole of any gas (in our case, oxygen) occupies 22.4 liters at standard temperature and pressure, 6 moles of $O_2 = 6 \times 22.4 = 134.4$ liters. Therefore, 134.4 liters of O_2 are required to resynthesize 39 moles of ATP or $134.4 \div 39 = 3.45$ liters of O_2 required per mole of ATP resynthesized. In other words, any time 3.45 liters of O_2 are consumed by the body, 1 mole of ATP is aerobically synthesized. At rest, this would take between 10 and 15 minutes. During maximal exercise, however, it would take most of us only about 1 minute.

The most important advantage to aerobic metabolism is that H^+ picked up by NAD^+ from glycolytic reactions and from lactate to pyruvate conversion can now be oxidized to yield ATP energy. Before they simply accumulated as a NADH or lactate byproduct of anaerobic glycolytic metabolism. Note reaction E (figure 2.12) and the gain of 6 moles of ATP in our continued accounting for ATP energy sources. Also note that 6 more moles of ATP are resynthesized at reaction F, which, like before, is dependent on NAD^+. This reaction is an important one regulated by pyruvate dehydrogenase (PDH) in that carbon dioxide is produced for the first time as 3 carbon pyruvates are converted to 2 carbon acetyl groups.

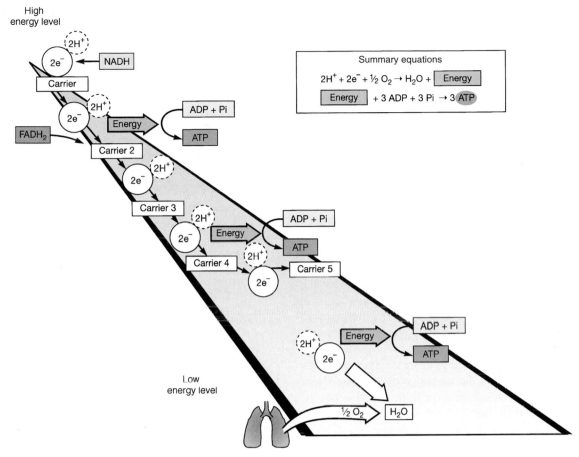

Figure 2.14

The electron transport system. The hydrogen ions (H$^+$) and electrons (e$^-$) removed in the Krebs Cycle have a high energy level as they enter the electron transport system. Here two major chemical events take place. First, the hydrogen ions and electrons are "transported" by electron carriers to the oxygen we breathe to form water (H$_2$O) through a series of enzymatic reactions; and second, at the same time, ATP is resynthesized in coupled reactions from the energy released. For every pair of electrons transported, an average of 3 moles of ATP is resynthesized.

In turn, the acetyl groups can combine with co-enzyme A to form acetyl CoA, which can then enter the Krebs Cycle. The 2 carbon acetyl CoA combines with 4 carbon oxaloacetate to form 6 carbon citrate and co-enzyme A is freed up to be reused (note arrow returning to co-enzyme A pool in figure 2.12). The "gatekeeper" enzyme here is citrate synthase (CS). Citrate undergoes a series of biochemical degradations in the Krebs Cycle, as shown by the dashed line. These reactions proceed only in the direction of the arrows so it is a true cycle. A key regulatory enzyme in this series of reactions is succinate dehydrogenase (SDH). In fact, this ends our summary of key regulatory enzymes, which started with phosphorylase and now numbers as many as eight. We will return to these in our upcoming discussion of control and regulation of cellular metabolism.

This also completes our ATP accounting business. Two more moles of ATP (reaction G) are indirectly resynthesized in the Krebs Cycle via guanosine triphosphate (GTP) in the coupled reaction 2 ADP + 2 GTP→

2 GDP + 2 ATP. GTP is actually formed but since its energy is the same as ATP, the reaction proceeds unhindered. Finally, 6 NADH (reaction H) and 2 FADH$_2$ (reaction I) are produced in the Krebs Cycle to go on to the ETS. Happily, this results in the resynthesis of 18 (3 for each NADH) and 4 (2 for each FADH$_2$) more moles of ATP to bring the final accounting to 38 or 39 moles as anticipated. Finally, note the important roles that NAD and FAD in their oxidized forms played in this process and the additional 4 moles of CO$_2$ that are given off in the Krebs Cycle. This accounts for all 6 of the CO$_2$ shown in earlier outlines of the overall reactions (recall C$_6$H$_{12}$O$_6$ + 6 O$_2$ → **6 CO$_2$** + 6 H$_2$O + 38 or 39 ATP).

It is clear that NAD$^+$ and FAD$^+$ must be continually freed up so that they can participate in the processes of oxidation-reduction of precursor energy substrates and in the transportation of hydrogens to the ETS. For only then can the oxidative-phosphorylation process be taken to completion with the formation of metabolic water and much ATP energy. This entire process moves freely when there is adequate oxygen at the terminal endpoint of the ETS but becomes bogged down when oxygen is either marginal or inadequate in quantity. A high energy state of the cell then is when there is a high ratio of NAD^+:NADH and FAD:$FADH_2$. A low energy state is present when the ratios are reversed—i.e., too much NADH and $FADH_2$ have accumulated.

These terms of low- and high-energy states will show up again in the next section as we discuss metabolic control and regulation. At this point, thinking mechanistically, how would you respond to this question: why do NADH and $FADH_2$ sometimes accumulate in the cytosol and mitochondria of muscle cells? Might you answer that they are produced faster than they can be carried away and/or that there is too little oxygen available to rapidly oxidize the hydrogens they are carrying? These are good answers. In either case, the real bottom line is that the resynthesis of ATP will be compromised. This means that the force and tension outputs of muscle cells will be diminished because less energy is available. And this means that the performer will have to slow down or stop altogether. Fatigue, then, can be related to the combined effects of lactate buildup but also to the oxygenation state of the cells. As we will see, these effects ultimately relate to the intensity of exercise (low, medium, high power output) relative to the **aerobic power ($\dot{V}O_2$ max)** of the performer.

The Aerobic System and Fat Metabolism

So far, we have discussed the aerobic breakdown only of glycogen, a carbohydrate. The other two foodstuffs, **fat** and **protein,** can also be aerobically broken down to CO_2 and H_2O, releasing energy for ATP resynthesis. One key difference in substrates is that while carbohydrates can be metabolized in either the absence or presence of oxygen, fat and protein can *only* be metabolized in the presence of oxygen. Fats (usually 16- or 18-carbon chains) in the form of triglycerides are broken down into two-carbon compounds (acyl groups) by a series of reactions called **beta-oxidation** for entry into the Krebs Cycle and ETS (see figure 2.15).

Fatty acids must be "activated" for beta-oxidation (β-oxidation) at the expense of 1 ATP. Then in the process of β-oxidation, one $FADH_2$ and one NADH are generated, which pass through the ETS. A total of 5 ATP will be generated in this initial process (3 ATP from NADH and 2 ATP from $FADH_2$). Just as with the acyl groups from pyruvic acid, 1 ATP (via GTP), 3 NADH, and 1 $FADH_2$ are produced in the Krebs Cycle for each acyl group. Remembering that for each NADH 3 ATP are resynthesized and for each $FADH_2$ 2 ATP are resynthesized, a total of 12 ATP are produced in the Krebs Cycle and ETS. The net production of ATP with activation of fatty acids, β-oxidation, and first passage through the Krebs Cycle is 16 ATP (17–1).

On subsequent passes of acyl groups through β-oxidation and the Krebs Cycle, a full 17 ATP will be resynthesized as there is no need for additional activation. On the

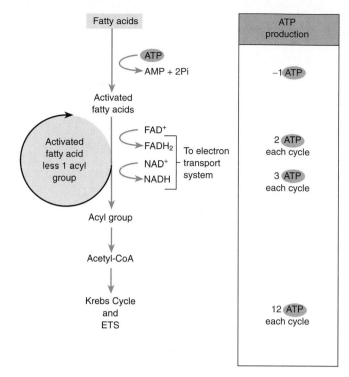

Figure 2.15

Summary of fatty acid metabolism (aerobic). Fatty acids are "activated" for beta-oxidation, then in a series of cyclic events, 2-carbon units (acyl groups) are separated and enter the Krebs Cycle as acetyl-CoA. The total number of moles of ATP produced depends on the specific fatty acid and the number of carbons in the fatty acid.

last passage, involving a four-carbon chain, there will be 17 and 12 ATP resynthesized (the last acyl group does not go through β-oxidation). Different fatty acids will result in varying amounts of ATP resynthesized. For two typical fatty acids, stearic acid (an 18-carbon molecule) and palmitic acid (a 16-carbon molecule) there would be 147 and 130 ATP produced, respectively. Table 2.3 summarizes these observations. See figure 15.2 for the chemical structure of palmitic acid. Stearic acid would look the same as palmitic acid but with two more carbons and two more hydrogens in its structural backbone.

Note that 1 mole of palmitic acid (a little over half of a pound) releases enough energy to resynthesize 130 moles of ATP, substantially more than from 1 mole of glycogen. However, 23 moles of oxygen are required to completely oxidize this fatty acid. This means that 23 moles × 22.4 liters of O_2 per mole = 515.2 liters of O_2 are required. Therefore, 3.96 liters of O_2 are required per mole of ATP resynthesized (515.2 ÷ 130 = 3.96). This is 15% more than the 3.45 L · $mole^{-1}$ of ATP calculated for glycogen. It clearly makes the point that it requires more oxygen to completely oxidize fats than it does for carbohydrates. But given that there is plenty of oxygen available, fats represent highly concentrated, relatively light weight, and very large reserves

2.3

Net production of ATP from two typical fatty acids

	Stearic acid (18-carbon chain)	Palmitic acid (16-carbon chain)
Activation and first pass (17 − 1):	16 ATP	16 ATP
Next 6 passes (6 × 17)	102 ATP	——
Next 5 passes (5 × 17)	——	85 ATP
Last pass (17) plus (12)	29 ATP	29 ATP
TOTAL ATP PRODUCTION	147 ATP	130 ATP

2.4

Estimation of the energy available from muscle glycogen through the aerobic (oxygen) system*

	Muscle glycogen	
	Per kg muscle	**Total muscle mass**
1. Muscular concentration (grams)	13–15[†]	400 450
2. ATP formation (moles)	2.8–3.2	87–98
3. Useful energy (kcal)	28–32	870–980

*Assumptions the same as in table 2.1.
[†]Based on data from Hultman.[14]

of stored energy that can be tapped for the performance of exercise. This would be the case for lower-intensity, long-duration activities like walking, jogging, in-line skating, marathon runs, channel swims, and the like.

Role of Protein in Aerobic Metabolism

Thus far we have discussed the fate of carbohydrates and fats in the metabolic scheme. What of protein? Protein is indeed a source of ATP but it plays only a very minor role during rest. Also, under most conditions of exercise the contribution of proteins to the overall energy supply will not exceed 5% to 10%, and in some cases there will be no measurable contribution at all. However, in cases of starvation or semi-starvation, conditions of carbohydrate deprivation, and feats of unusual endurance (6-day races), protein catabolism has been shown to significantly contribute to the overall energy provision.[3,21,22] Likewise, Felig* and coworkers have suggested that amino acids from proteins play a supportive role in providing energy during the performance of prolonged exercise that leads to exhaustion in human subjects. The energy is provided partly through the **glucose-alanine cycle** described in chapter 15. Because protein is not a major source of energy during most types of exercise it will not be further emphasized here. That is to say, carbohydrates and fats remain as the primary sources of fuel for ATP production during aerobic glycolysis. However, we will include discussion of protein metabolism in other chapters as it relates to special nutritional considerations and training conditions.

Total Aerobic Energy in Muscle

The total muscular energy that can be manufactured through the aerobic system is difficult to estimate, because all three foodstuffs are used in varying amounts. However, as a basis for comparison with the anaerobic systems, the total aerobic energy available in the muscles from glycogen alone is given in table 2.4. The aerobic system has by far the greatest capacity with respect to ATP production (compare with tables 2.1 and 2.2). For example, the amount of ATP available from the aerobic breakdown of all the glycogen in the

*Felig, P. and Wahren, J. Amino acid metabolism in exercising man. *J. Clin. Invest.* 50:2703, 1971.

2.5
General characteristics of the three systems by which ATP is formed

System	Food or chemical fuel	O_2 required	Speed	Relative ATP production
Anaerobic				
ATP-PC system	Phosphocreatine	No	Fastest	Few; limited
Glycolysis system	Glycogen (glucose)	No	Fast	Few; limited
Aerobic				
Oxygen system	Glycogen, fats, proteins	Yes	Slow	Many; unlimited

muscles is between 87 and 98 moles! This is nearly 50 times more than that made available by the two anaerobic systems combined. Additionally, another 80 to 100 grams of glycogen are stored in the liver,[16] and if all were used for aerobic metabolism, another 17 to 22 moles of ATP would be generated. All combined this would provide about 120 moles of ATP and at 10 kcal $\cdot$ mole^{-1} would yield about 1200 kcal of energy. Enough to jog 10 miles at an expenditure of 120 kcal per mile. That's a significant quantity of stored energy. Keep in mind that this is simply for stored muscle and liver glycogen and doesn't consider the energy reserves in body fat and proteins. Impressive, huh?

We have seen that the aerobic system is capable of utilizing both fats and glycogen for resynthesizing large amounts of ATP without simultaneously generating fatiguing by-products. For this reason, it is the preferred system under resting conditions. With respect to exercise for health and sports participation, the aerobic system is particularly suited for manufacturing ATP during prolonged endurance-type activities. For example, during marathon running (42.2 kilometers, or 26.2 miles) we estimate that a total of about 140 moles of ATP (approximately 1 mole of ATP every minute) are required.[5,10] Such a large, sustained output of ATP energy is possible because large amounts of glycogen, fats, and oxygen are readily available to the working skeletal muscles. A summary of the complete aerobic system is shown in figure 2.16.

Comparing the Energy Systems

As a final consideration, let us compare the three energy systems. First, in their general characteristics (table 2.5), and second, in their maximal **energy capacity** and **power** with respect to ATP production. Capacity refers to an amount independent of time, whereas power refers to rate (i.e., an amount in a given time). From what has already been said concerning the energy systems, you should be able to rank them with respect to both their relative capacities and powers. The aerobic system, by far, has the largest capacity

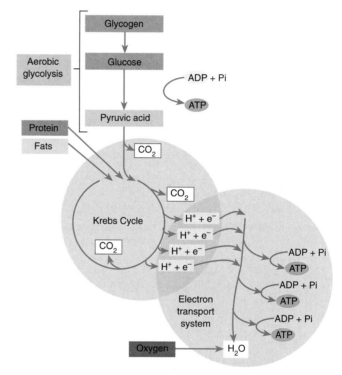

Figure 2.16
Summary of the aerobic (oxygen) system. Glycogen is oxidized in three major series of chemical reactions: aerobic glycolysis in which pyruvic acid is formed and some ATP resynthesized; the Krebs Cycle in which CO_2 is produced, and H^+ and e^- are removed; and the electron transport system in which H_2O is formed from H^+, e^-, and oxygen, and more ATP is resynthesized. Fats and proteins, when used as fuels for ATP resynthesis, also go through the Krebs Cycle and the electron transport system.

whereas the phosphagens have the largest power, right? To check your answers, consult table 2.6. Notice that anaerobic glycolysis contributes relatively more to maximal power and very little to the maximal capacity of the three combined energy systems.

2.6 table

Maximal capacity and power of the three energy systems

System	Maximal power (moles of ATP per minute)	Maximal capacity (total moles of ATP available)
Phosphagen (ATP-PC)	3.6	0.7
Anaerobic glycolysis	1.6	1.2
Aerobic or oxygen (from glycogen only)	1.0	90.0

The Aerobic and Anaerobic Systems during Rest and Exercise

There are at least three important features of the anaerobic and aerobic systems under conditions of rest and exercise that need further consideration: (1) the types of foodstuffs being metabolized, (2) the relative roles played by each system, and (3) the presence and accumulation of lactic acid in the blood.

Rest

From figure 2.17*A* we see that under resting conditions about two-thirds of the food fuel is contributed by fats and the other one-third by carbohydrates (glycogen and glucose). Protein is not shown in the diagram because, as pointed out earlier, its contribution as a food fuel is negligible. Also, as is indicated, the aerobic system is the principal energy system in operation. This is true because our oxygen transport system (heart and lungs) is capable of supplying each cell with sufficient oxygen and, therefore, with adequate ATP to satisfy all the energy requirements of the resting state (figure 2.17*B*). The molecules of ATP shown coming from the anaerobic system are considered as part of the aerobic yield, because, as we indicated earlier, they are likewise formed in the presence of oxygen.

Although the aerobic system is the primary one in operation, perhaps you have noticed (figure 2.17*B*) that there is a small but constant amount of lactic acid present in the blood (about 10 mg for every 100 mL of blood).* The reason for this relates to the abundance and effectiveness of LDH (lactate dehydrogenase), the enzyme that catalyzes the reaction of pyruvic acid to lactic acid. LDH is always converting some pyruvate to lactate. The fact that the lactic acid level remains constant and does not accumulate tells us that

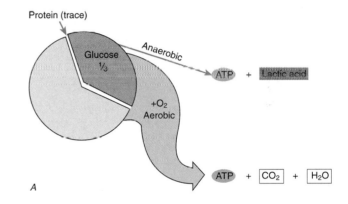

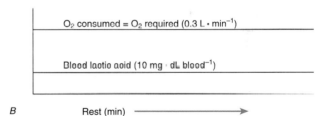

Figure 2.17

A. The aerobic system supplies all the ATP required in the resting state. *B.* During rest, oxygen consumption (0.3 L · min⁻¹) remains constant and is adequate to supply the required ATP; as a consequence, the blood lactic acid level remains within the normal range (10 mg · dL blood⁻¹). The combination of these factors indicates that metabolism is aerobic.

anaerobic glycolysis is not operating at any significant level. We see, then, that at rest the foodstuffs utilized are fats and carbohydrates, and the necessary ATP is supplied primarily by the aerobic system.

Exercise

Both anaerobic and aerobic systems contribute ATP during exercise; however, their relative roles depend on (1) the intensity of exercises performed, (2) the state of training, and

*Ten milligrams (mg) in 100 milliliters (mL) of blood is usually expressed as milligrams percent (mg %) or mg per deciliter (mg · dL⁻¹). Another example: 15 g of hemoglobin in 100 mL of blood would be read as 15 g %.

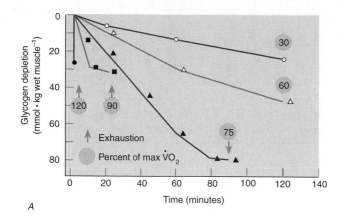

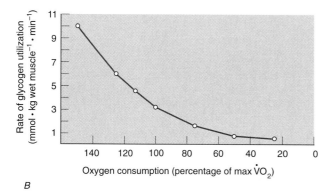

Figure 2.18

Glycogen depletion patterns during exhaustive work on the cycle ergometer. Both absolute (*A*) and relative (*B*) glycogen depletion are related to the intensity of work. Note that in graph *A,* exhaustion was not achieved during the 30% and 60% rides.

Source for (A): Data from B. Saltin and J. Karlsson, "Muscle Glycogen Utilization During Work of Different Intensities" in Muscle Metabolism During Exercise, 1971, Plenum Publishing Corporation, New York.

(3) the diet of the athlete. To begin our discussion, we can divide the many types of exercises into two categories: (1) exercises that can be performed for only short periods of time but which require maximal or near-maximal efforts, and (2) exercises that can be performed for relatively long periods of time but which require submaximal effort. Later we will point out the interaction and significance of the roles played by the three energy systems in exercises that do not easily fit into one or the other of these categories. The understanding of this concept is vitally important to you in planning training programs that specifically emphasize the development of one or more of these energy pathways.

Saltin and Karlsson[27] have described glycogen depletion patterns with activities requiring from 30% to 120% of maximal oxygen consumption (see figure 2.18*A*). Along with other observations to be made in the following paragraphs, we can begin to comprehend some of the limiting factors in exercise. With activities requiring less than 60% or more than 90% of aerobic capacity, glycogen stores are

not significantly depleted. The muscle glycogen depletion for these work intensities is only one-half to one-fourth of the depletion shown for work at 75% of max $\dot{V}O_2$. In figure 2.18*B* the rate of glycogen utilization can be seen to be related to the relative work load. The rate of glycogen utilization increases sharply with increasing work loads. At very high work loads, where exhaustion occurs very rapidly, there is still about 70% of the initial glycogen stores remaining. As shown in figure 2.18*A*, at a work load requiring 75% of the subject's aerobic capacity, exhaustion was highly related to a glycogen level approaching zero.

Saltin and Karlsson have reported glycogen utilization rates of 0.3, 0.7, 1.4, 3.4, and 10 mmol glucose units per kg of wet muscle per minute for work loads of 25%, 50%, 75%, 100%, and 150% of the aerobic capacity, respectively.[27] Figure 2.18*B* illustrates these observations.

Exercises of Short Duration

Exercises in this category include sprinting events such as the 100-, 200-, and 400-meter dashes, the 800-meter run, and other events in which the required rate of work can be maintained for up to only 2 or possibly 3 minutes.

Figure 2.19*A* shows the relative roles of the energy systems when performing these types of exercises. Here we see that the major food fuel is carbohydrates, with fats minor and proteins—once again—negligible contributors. We also see that the predominant system is anaerobic. This does not mean to imply, however, that it is the *only* system operating. It merely indicates that the energy or ATP required for these types of exercises cannot be supplied via the aerobic system alone. As a consequence, most of the ATP must be supplied anaerobically by the phosphagen system and anaerobic glycolysis. Phosphocreatine (PC) levels, with short, very high-intensity work will quickly drop to very low levels and remain there until the exercise stops. Likewise, PC is rapidly replenished (within minutes) during recovery.

The aerobic system is limited in supplying adequate ATP during the performance of any exercise for two reasons: (1) each of us has a ceiling for his or her aerobic power or the maximum rate at which we can consume oxygen; and (2) it takes at least 2 or 3 minutes for oxygen consumption to increase to a new, higher level. For example, well-trained female[7] and male[26] athletes have maximal aerobic powers that range between 3.0 and 5.0 liters of O_2 per minute; maximum for the untrained female[8] is around 2.2 liters per minute and for the untrained male,[9] 3.2 liters per minute. These levels of O_2 consumption are not nearly enough in either case to supply all the ATP needed for such an effort as the 100-meter dash, which would theoretically require in excess of 45 liters per minute (about 8 liters of O_2 per 100 meters or per 10 seconds).

Even if it were possible to consume oxygen at a rate that would alone meet the energy or ATP requirement, it would take the first 2 or 3 minutes of exercise to accelerate the oxygen consumption to the required level. This is because

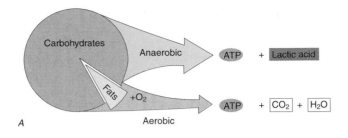

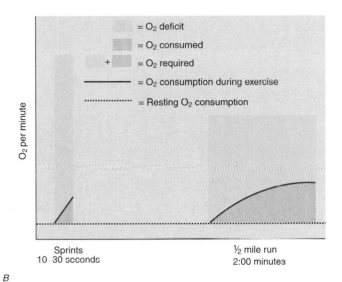

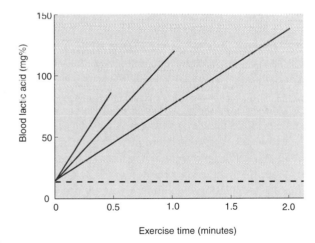

Figure 2.19

A. During all-out exercises of short duration the anaerobic systems, anaerobic glycolysis, and the phosphagen system (not shown) supply most of the required ATP. *B.* Relationships among the oxygen deficit, oxygen consumption, and oxygen requirement during exercises of short duration. *C.* Accumulation of lactic acid in the blood during exhausting exercises lasting from 30 seconds to 2 minutes.

of the time it takes for adequate biochemical and physiological adjustments to become manifest. This holds true during the transition from rest to an exercise of any

intensity and from an exercise of lower intensity to one of higher intensity. The period during which the level of oxygen consumption is below that necessary to supply all the ATP required of any exercise is called the **oxygen deficit** (figure 2.19*B*). It is during this oxygen deficit period that the phosphagen system and anaerobic glycolysis are called on to supply most of the ATP required for the exercise. This means that during short-term but high-intensity exercises, such as those mentioned before, there will always be an oxygen deficit throughout the duration of the exercise, with the major source of ATP being the two anaerobic systems.

From figure 2.19*C* we see that the rapid acceleration in anaerobic glycolysis is accompanied by an equally rapid accumulation of lactic acid. However, accumulated lactic acid assumes a significant role in activities lasting from about 2 minutes to 10 minutes. PC depletion and the rate of ATP resynthesis are very important in activities lasting less than 3 minutes. To give relief to the intense work stress, exercise must either be stopped or continued at a much lower intensity. Blood lactate levels as high as 200 mg % have been recorded during competitive sprinting events in track and in swimming.[24] Such high levels are some twenty times greater than those normally found under resting conditions (10 mg %).

The level of blood lactate, then, is an excellent indicator of which energy system is predominantly used during exercise. If the level is high, the primary system used must have been anaerobic glycolysis; if the level is low, the aerobic system predominated. For this reason, coaches and trainers have used blood lactate levels to indicate shifts in the sources of energy provision during the course of a training program—i.e., another index of training status. This approach is sensible and has been applied to both human athletes (chapter 11) as well as race horses and dogs.

Prolonged Exercises

Any exercise that can be maintained for relatively long periods of time should be included under this category. By relatively long periods of time, we mean 10 minutes or longer. In such cases, the major foodstuffs are again carbohydrates and fats (figure 2.20*A*). For activities lasting up to 20 minutes (e.g., continuous running) carbohydrates generally are the dominant fuel source for resynthesis of ATP, with fats playing a relatively minor but supportive role. Higher, but not maximal, levels of lactic acid will appear in the blood. As the time of performance proceeds past an hour, glycogen stores begin to show significant decreases in concentration and fats become more important as a source for ATP resynthesis. The "mix" of glycogen and fat utilization will vary with different athletes for a variety of reasons including state of training, proportions of Type I and Type II muscle fibers (see chapter 6), and initial glycogen stores.

In these types of exercises, the major source of ATP is supplied by the aerobic system. The anaerobic glycolysis and ATP-PC systems also contribute, but only at the

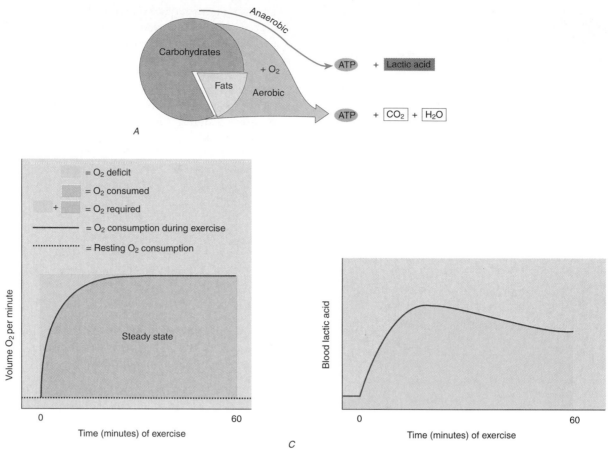

Figure 2.20

A. During prolonged submaximal exercises, the major source of ATP is through the aerobic system. *B.* Anaerobic glycolysis and the phosphagen system also contribute ATP but only at the beginning of submaximal exercise (O_2 deficit), before oxygen consumption reaches a constant level (steady-state). *C.* Once a steady-state oxygen consumption is reached, the small amount of lactic acid accumulated during the O_2 deficit period remains relatively constant until the end of exercise.

beginning of the exercise, before oxygen consumption reaches a new steady-state level; during this time an oxygen deficit is incurred. Once oxygen consumption reaches a new steady-state level (in about 2 or 3 minutes) it is sufficient to supply all of the ATP energy required for the exercise (figure 2.20*B*). For this reason, blood lactic acid does not accumulate to very high levels during exercise lasting more than an hour. Anaerobic glycolysis is diminished once steady-state oxygen consumption is reached, and the small amount of lactic acid accumulated prior to this time remains relatively constant until the end of the exercise or may actually diminish somewhat (see figure 2.20*C*).

Understandably, the anaerobic systems might be re-engaged during "kick" efforts to win a long-distance race, thereby raising blood lactate levels at the end. In other runners the event might be ended with an aerobic steady-state effort. A good example of this is during marathon running.[5,10] These athletes run 42.2 kilometers (26.2 miles) in about 2.5 hours, but at the end of the race their blood lactic acid levels are only about two to three times those found at rest.[5] The fatigue experienced by these runners at the end of

a race is, therefore, due to factors other than high blood lactic acid levels. Some of the more important factors leading to this type of fatigue are: (1) low blood glucose levels from depletion of liver glycogen stores; (2) local muscular fatigue from depletion of muscle glycogen stores; (3) loss of water (dehydration) and electrolytes, which leads to high body temperature; (4) boredom; and (5) the general physical beating that the body has sustained.[4]

In prolonged activities of very low intensity such as walking, playing golf, and certain industrial tasks, lactate does not accumulate in the blood above the normal resting level. This is so because the phosphagen system alone is sufficient to supply the additional ATP energy needed prior to reaching a steady state of oxygen consumption. In these cases, fatigue can be delayed up to 6 hours or more. When fatigue does occur, its cause is not clear but might relate most to the prolonged strain on muscles, tendons, and joints from the overload stresses that are experienced.

The preceding information can be extremely useful to you as a coach or trainer of athletes. For example, one of the most important aspects of competitive middle-distance

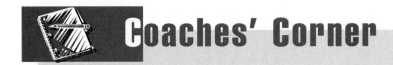

Coaches' Corner

- The muscular concentrations of ATP and PC in females are the **same** as in males (i.e., about 4 $mM \cdot kg^{-1}$ muscle for ATP and 16 $mM \cdot kg^{-1}$ muscle for PC).[15]

- Because of the smaller total skeletal muscle mass in the female, there is **less total phosphagen** available for use during exercise.

- Comparisons of the functional capacities of the ATP-PC system between males and females can be made in four ways, all of which work **equally well** for both genders.

- These **methods include** (1) measurement of oxygen during immediate recovery, (2) the Margaria Anaerobic Power Test, (3) the Wingate Peak Power Test and (4) performance ratios.

- Highly trained oarswomen on the US national team have maximal fast-component O_2 recovery values equal to untrained men but only about **60%** of the level of male oarsmen.[12]

- The results of the Margaria-Kalamen stair-climbing test for the rapid utilization of stored ATP and PC in leg muscles indicates **no difference** between females and males over an age range from 6 to 25 years.[6]

- The maximal anaerobic peak power capability of the whole body is approximately **2.1 horsepower** (HP) for the average male and **1.7 HP** for the average female.

- The maximal anaerobic power of both men and women **decreases** after the age of 25 years, likely accounting for the dramatic drop off in vertical jumping ability.

- When male-to-female performance ratios for running events are contrasted, the **best events** for females are the 100- and 200-meter sprints, which rely heavily on muscular stores of ATP and PC for their source of energy.

- Females tend to have **lower levels of lactic acid** in their blood following maximal exercise than do males, strongly suggesting that the capacity of their anaerobic glycolysis system also is lower.

- The lower capacity of the **anaerobic glycolysis system** in females puts them at a slight disadvantage when competing in events lasting 1 to 4 minutes because these events involve anaerobic glycolysis to a large extent.

- The maximal aerobic power (**max $\dot{V}O_2$**) of females is also **smaller by 15–25%** than that of males, mainly because of body size factors, including less hemoglobin and blood volume and a smaller heart size.

- The differences in max $\dot{V}O_2$ between males and females is **negligible prior to puberty,** when body size and composition differences are minimal, and greatest during the adult, middle-age years.

- Differences in absolute max $\dot{V}O_2$ ($L \cdot min^{-1}$) between the genders are smaller when this measure is expressed **relative to a body size** dimension such as body weight ($mL \cdot kg^{-1} \cdot min^{-1}$).

- Because the metabolism of the working skeletal muscles dictates the size of the max $\dot{V}O_2$, differences between male and female are minimal when **lean body mass** is used, and to an even lesser extent when **active muscle mass** is used for relative expressions.

- Likewise, such relative expressions **tend to cancel out** many of the differences in phosphagen and anaerobic glycolytic function, which are mainly related to a larger body size and total muscle mass in males. Recognition of *energy equity* is encouraged here.

and distance running is pacing. If an athlete starts an endurance race too fast or begins his or her final sprint too soon, lactic acid will accumulate to very high levels and cause race-limiting fatigue. As you will recall, this is true because as the intensity of the exercise increases, so does the amount of energy required from the anaerobic systems. Consequently, the race may be lost, owing to this early onset of fatigue. Well-informed coaches, or athletes for that matter, would never let this happen. Instead, from a physiological standpoint, they would advocate that the runner maintain a steady, but sufficient, pace throughout most of the race, then finish with an all-out effort. In other words, the onset of fatigue due to lactic acid accumulation should be delayed until the end of the race.

To a lesser degree, these same principles would be applied by someone who works in a clinical position and is involved in the rehabilitation of previously sedentary patients. The main difference being that they might be walking, jogging, or exercising at a slower speed for their workouts, but they, and you, must pay heed to the importance of sensible pacing.

Having made these generalized observations, we must also recognize that in the special case of middle-distance runners there are a variety of racing strategies. In one instance, a particular runner always seems to come from behind and "out sprint" the field during the last 200 meters whereas another runner has to "break on top and improve his or her position." Each elite runner has found a strategy that works best for him or her physiologically. The "sprinter" perhaps has a higher percentage of Type II (fast-twitch, glycolytic) fibers whereas the "front runner" may have more Type I (slow-twitch, oxidative) fibers.

Just as an anaerobic capacity is important in the performance of exercises of short duration, the **maximal oxygen consumption** or **aerobic power** is a significant factor in the performance of prolonged activities. This stems from the fact that the aerobic system supplies the majority of energy required for these types of exercises. Maximal aerobic power (abbreviated **max $\dot{V}O_2$, or $\dot{V}O_2$ max**)* is defined as the maximal rate at which oxygen can be consumed. *The higher an athlete's maximal aerobic power, the more successfully he or she will likely perform in endurance events, provided all other factors that contribute to a championship performance are present* (figure 2.21). The best runners in this study had $\dot{V}O_2$ maxes as high as 75 mL $\cdot$ kg^{-1} $\cdot$ min^{-1}. Sedentary, nontrained people may only have values in the range of 25 to 40 mL $\cdot$ kg^{-1} $\cdot$ min^{-1}.

Interaction of Aerobic and Anaerobic Energy Sources during Exercise

Thus far, we have discussed the energy systems during exercises that have either been short-term, high-intensity efforts (anaerobic) or long-term, low-intensity efforts (aerobic). What about those exercise activities that fall in between these categories? Are they anaerobic or aerobic activities? As illustrated in figure 2.22, it is not possible to classify such activities as strictly either anaerobic or aerobic. Rather, they require a blend of both anaerobic or aerobic metabolism. Take, for example, the 1500-meter and 2-mile runs. In these activities, the anaerobic systems supply the major portion of ATP during the sprint at both the start and finish of the race, with the aerobic system predominating during the middle, or steady-state, period of the run. Overall, these runs demand about half of the required ATP from anaerobic sources and half from aerobic sources.

The illustration in figure 2.22 represents what we can call an energy continuum for track events. In other words,

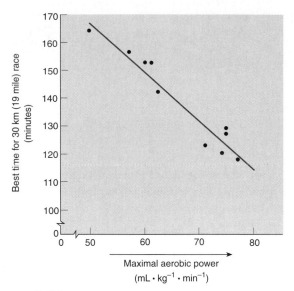

Figure 2.21

The higher an athlete's maximal aerobic power, the more successfully he or she will perform in endurance events, provided all other factors contributing to a championship performance are present. (Based on data from Karlsson and Saltin.[19])

those events to the left, such as the 100-meter dash, are almost 100% anaerobic, whereas those far to the right, such as the marathon, are clearly aerobic. In between these two extremes are the so-called gray zones, in which various mixtures of anaerobic and aerobic metabolism are required during performance. These latter activities are often the most difficult for the athlete to perform because all the energy systems are involved to a large extent. Also, these activities are often most difficult to prepare an athlete for, because he or she must spend time during training developing both anaerobic and aerobic systems. The energy continuum concept applies to all activities, not just track events. It will be useful to us during our discussions of training programs in chapters 11 and 12.

Control and Regulation of Metabolic Pathways

Earlier we indicated that the types of energy sources and food fuels used during the performance of exercise were related to the intensity and duration of the activity. But how do cells "know" when to switch from high energy phosphagens, to anaerobic glycolysis of carbohydrates, to oxidation of a combination of fats and carbohydrates, and so on? This is what control and regulation of metabolic pathways is all about: matching the provision of energy to the rate at which it is being used so that the performer does not experience early or undue fatigue. In this discussion we will

---

*The V stands for volume, O$_2$ for oxygen, and the dot over the V ($\dot{V}$) stands for per unit of time, usually 1 minute. Thus max $\dot{V}O_2$ or $\dot{V}O_2$ max, = maximal oxygen consumption = maximal aerobic power.

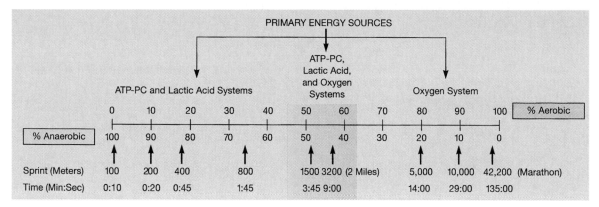

Figure 2.22

The approximate percentage of contribution of aerobic and anaerobic energy sources in selected track events. Nonshaded areas represent predominance of either anaerobic (left) or aerobic (right) metabolism. The shaded area represents events in which anaerobic and aerobic systems are of nearly equal importance.

table 2.7

List of key factors in control and regulation of metabolic pathways

1. High vs. low energy state of the cell
2. Circulating levels of hormones
3. "Amplification" of hormone effect via c-AMP
4. Activation or inhibition of key rate-limiting enzymes
5. Power output level relative to aerobic power
6. Adequacy of oxygen supplied to the cell
7. Competition for ADP substrate by CPK isoforms

refer to the eight key enzymes that regulate glycolysis as well as to other enzymes, hormones, and substrates that interact to regulate fat and protein metabolism. You will find that there are several key players in this fascinating story, so let's start by reviewing them in table 2.7.

Next, it would be well to review figure 2.23, which summarizes much of what is known about the enzyme and hormonal regulation of substrate choice and metabolic pathways during exercise. The notations are intended to give some additional insight into what appears on the surface to be a rather complex matter. Actually, the story is quite consistent with what we know intuitively and with what we now know about this aspect of exercise physiology. Our first emphasis is that there are two major methods of control and regulation, one that operates *within* the muscle cells and the other that influences the cells from the *outside.* Both of these methods act to either *activate or inhibit* the key regulatory hormones that we reviewed in figures 2.7 and 2.12. You may want to go back and review those now. Also, as you study the upcoming figures 2.23 and 2.24, look for the terms that are emphasized in **bold type.** By "working" them back and forth, you will come to a better understanding of the complexity of metabolic control and regulation.

Energy State Regulation

Intracellular regulation is partially accomplished by the activation of key enzymes when the cellular energy is at a lower level, such as would occur during exercise. Note that ADP, which is immediately produced when ATP is split, often serves as the factor that activates the regulatory enzymes. Conversely, these enzymes would be inhibited when the intracellular energy is at a higher level—i.e., there is plenty of ATP around. This method of control, which we might call **energy state regulation,** is very quick in its response and is tightly linked to the rate of energy expenditure during exercise. We will return to ADP as a key player in control and regulation when we discuss a theoretical model that considers several factors acting together during exercise.

Hormone Amplification

The second major method of control and regulation is of equal importance but is slower in its response. It operates through **hormones** that cause increases in cyclic adenosine monophosphate (c-AMP) to be formed on the inside sur-

Enzymes / Substrate   Notation

Activated by	Enzyme/Substrate	Inhibited by	Notation
Lower energy state		Higher energy state	The general principle of "intra" cellular regulation; lower energy during exercise "drives" system
↑ Hormone→↑[c-AMP]		↓ Hormone→↓[c-AMP]	Equally important; slower but widespread and persistent "amplification" drive to system

Carbohydrates

Activated by	Enzyme/Substrate	Inhibited by	Notation
$ATP \rightarrow ADP + H^+$	↑[ADP]	$CP + ADP \rightarrow ATP + C$	Immediate and much ↑ [ADP] with exercise; competed for by CPKc and CPKm isoforms (see figure 2.24)
↑ [AMP],↑ [CA^{++}] ↑ EPI & Glucagon	PHOS b → a	[ATP], Glucose 6-P ↑ Insulin,↑ Cortisol	Immediate increase in muscle and liver glycogenolysis to provide more glucose for glycolysis
↑ Glucose	HK	↑ [ATP], Glucose 6-P	First of 3 key glycolytic regulatory enzymes which is mainly "turned on" by ↑ glucose levels
↑ [ADP],↑ [AMP] ↑ F 2, 6 di P,↑ [NH4$^+$]	PFK	↑ [ATP], ↑ [Citrate] ↑ Glucagon——→ Protein kinase	PFK is the most important "rate limiter" of substrate flux; activators are all by-products of metabolism that stimulate continued glycolytic energy production. Inhibitors signal "plenty" of energy in cell
↑ ADP,↑ F 1, 6 di-P	PK	↑ Glucagon——→ Protein kinase	Third enzyme that regulates glycolysis during exercise
↑ NADH or ↑ $\frac{NADH}{NAD^+}$	LDH		If cytosolic NADH production from glycolysis exceeds oxidation capacity of ETS more lactate and NAD$^+$ is formed so glycolysis can continue
↑ Pyruvate	PDH		A powerful enzymatic control just before Krebs Cycle that regulates an irreversible reaction called oxidative carboxylation where CO_2 is released, and NADH and acetyl CoA are produced to go on
↑ ADP	CS	↑ ATP, ↑ NADH, ↑ Acetyl–CoA, ↑ Citrate ↑ Oxaloacetic ↑ Succinyl–CoA, ↑ Acyl-CoA	Key regulatory enzyme in the Krebs (citric acid) Cycle since the whole cycle must "turn" at the same rate as this first important step. Note that derivatives from fatty acid metabolism inhibit citrate synthase activity
Exercise training	SDH	↑ Malonate	Krebs Cycle enzyme that responds to training by an enhanced specific activity so FADH$_2$ is more readily produced
O$_2$ available ↑ ADP	cyta + a3 (CO)	O$_2$ deprivation	Also called cytochrome oxidase (CO); operates "closest" to O$_2$ in ETS; key to its activation is readily available O$_2$ whereas it is inhibited by low O$_2$

Fats

Activated by	Enzyme/Substrate	Inhibited by	Notation
↑ EPI & Glucagon→ c-AMP dependent protein kinase	TG lipase (HSL)	↑ Glucose ↑ Insulin	Also called hormone sensitive lipase (HSL), which starts the breakdown of stored triglycerides to glycerol and fatty acids; fatty acids are circulated to or are oxidized directly by muscle cells to synthesize ATP
↑ EPI & Glucagon→ c-AMP dependent protein kinase	LPL	↑ Glucose ↑ Insulin	Lipoprotein lipase (LPL) acts like TG lipase only on bloodborne TG which is carried in combination with lipoproteins, i.e., glycerol and fatty acids are freed up for further conversion (glycerol in liver) or oxidation (fatty acids in muscle)
↑ Acyl CoA	CAT	↑ Malonyl CoA	Fatty acids are converted to fatty acyl CoA, which activates carnitine acyltransferase (CAT) to increase its transport across the mitochondrial inner membrane so it can enter the process of β-oxidation. When cellular energy is high, surplus acetyl CoA is diverted from the Krebs Cycle toward FA synthesis and this "carnitine shuttle" is inhibited by malonyl CoA (a fatty acid precursor)
Hydroxylacyl CoA	3HAD		3HAD (L-3 hydroxyacyl CoA dehydrogenase) is a key rate-limiting enzyme in β-oxidation where fatty acyl CoA is converted to acetyl CoA; it is activated by hydroxyacyl CoA, a substrate precursor that is provided when fatty acids are broken down

Proteins

Activated by	Enzyme/Substrate	Inhibited by	Notation
Low energy ↑ EPI & Glucagon→ c-AMP dependent protein kinase ↑ Cortisol	3 Compartments Blood Liver Muscle	High energy	When level of cellular energy is low, amino acids are broken down to support energy demands of exercise via the glucose-alanine cycle (see figure 15.4). If the energy state of the cell is high, amino acids can be converted to acetyl CoA and subsequently stored as fat. Epinephrine, glucagon, and cortisol stimulate gluconeogenesis in the liver so additional amino acids are converted to glucose and released to the blood as circulating energy

faces of target cell membranes. c-AMP is formed from ATP, so energy is directly involved. The reaction is sped up by the enzyme adenyl cyclase as is shown in detail in chapter 17. Although this control method is slower, it is also more widespread and persistent. This is because the effects of c-AMP are greater than would simply be caused by a direct link between a hormone and its effect—i.e., there is an on-going amplification drive to the system, which we will call **c-AMP amplification.**[11,17]

A review of figure 2.23 indicates three enzymes that are **activated** by the hormones **epinephrine (EPI)** and **glucagon** at a time when the cell would be experiencing a lowered energy state. Note that phosphorylase "b" is converted to "a" (the active form) so that more glycogen will be broken down to provide glucose for the glycolysis pathway. At the same time, triglycerides (TG) lipase or hormone sensitive lipase (HSL) and lipoprotein lipase (LPL) are activated to begin the breakdown of stored and blood-borne triglycerides so that fats can be metabolized through the Krebs Cycle. These same hormones act, along with **cortisol,** to stimulate the liver to convert amino acids to glucose as an additional source of energy if cellular energy is low during prolonged periods of exercise. Note that some other hormones like **insulin,** and glucose itself, have an inhibitory effect on these same enzymes. This makes sense because if there is plenty of glucose present during a high energy state of the cell, there is little need to generate more through the breakdown of stored carbohydrates, fats, or proteins. Some call it the "wisdom of the body."

Substrate/Enzyme Regulation

Another method of control that is less immediate but very powerful in its effects relates to substrates that are produced or used during reactions that, in turn, activate or inhibit specific enzymes. For example, if NADH builds up in the cytosol, it will activate lactate dehydrogenase (LDH) to convert more pyruvate to lactate and free up NAD^+. This would happen when energy demands are very high, glycolysis is "turned on" and the oxidation capacity of the ETS to process NADH is exceeded. Likewise, an increase in pyruvate would occur with a high level of glycolysis. This increase in pyruvate activates pyruvate dehydrogenase (PDH), which is a powerful enzymatic control just before the Krebs Cycle. PDH regulates an irreversible reaction called oxidative carboxylation, during which CO_2 is produced and both NADH and acetyl CoA are produced to go forward—forward toward oxygen, that is, which brings us to our final consideration of individual substrate control.

Oxidative State Regulation

Actually, the availability of oxygen or its relative state of deprivation was, at one time, considered to be the main controller of metabolic pathway selection. This **oxidative state regulation** is still considered to be very important, but we now recognize other controlling influences. When oxygen is readily available, along with ADP, it activates the enzyme that is closest to it in the ETS, cytochrome oxidase (CO). This might be viewed as "terminal position" control, which can have widespread effects on speeding up or slowing down the rate at which hydrogen is eventually combined with O_2 to form metabolic H_2O. The main consideration in this is that NAD^+ and FAD are freed up, and a major portion of all ATP are formed via oxidative phosphorylation. If oxygen is in low supply, for whatever reason during exercise, CO is inhibited with a backup of NADH, $FADH_2$, and ADP. These serve as clear signals that anaerobic glycolysis will have to step up its efforts to carry the load in terms of providing needed ATP—at least until the oxidative mechanisms of the ETS that rely on the chief of all oxidizers, oxygen, have a chance to catch up. The key determining factor in this regulatory process is **exercise intensity.**

A theoretical model[1,23] to explain how exercise intensity determines which metabolic pathway will be most used for ATP production is shown in figure 2.24. Three exercise conditions are defined at the top of the model in terms of $\dot{V}O_2$ max, power output, and adequacy of oxygen. These might simply be viewed as low-, medium-, and high-intensity exercise. These conditions are matched at the bottom of the model to expected fatigue outcomes and metabolic pathways. For example, for the low-intensity condition, a slow rate of fatigue with mainly fat and some carbohydrate oxidation in the presence of adequate oxygen is shown. Conversely, the high intensity condition shows a rapid rate of fatigue related to the rapid depletion of ATP and PC in the face of inadequate oxygen. For both of these conditions, cytosolic creatine phosphokinase (CPKc) can outcompete any other enzymes for available ADP and phosphorylate it to ATP at the expense of PC. This occurs without any appreciable build-up of ADP or creatine (see small ADP and C). The relatively small increases in ADP for the high intensity condition are believed due to rapid fatigue before ADP levels can build up. This is not the case for the more prolonged medium-intensity exercise condition, however, where ADP and C do build up. See the large ADP and C in the center of the model (medium-exercise condition).

The build-up of ADP and C during the performance of medium intensity exercise relates to the use of more ATP to meet the higher power outputs (note 50% to 70% of

Figure 2.23 (opposite page)

Summary of enzyme and hormonal regulation of substrate choice and metabolic pathways during exercise. See figures 2.7 and 2.12 for explanation of abbreviations used for carbohydrate enzymes.

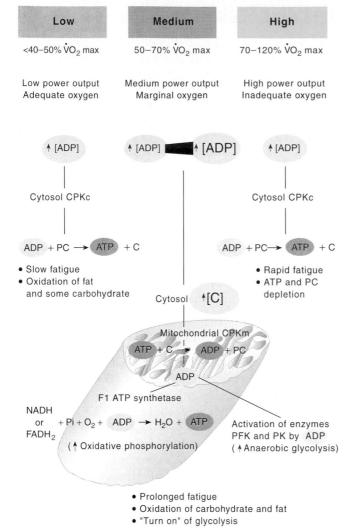

Low	Medium	High
<40–50% $\dot{V}O_2$ max	50–70% $\dot{V}O_2$ max	70–120% $\dot{V}O_2$ max
Low power output	Medium power output	High power output
Adequate oxygen	Marginal oxygen	Inadequate oxygen

Figure 2.24

Regulation of metabolism during low, medium, and high intensity exercise via ADP (direct) and ADP shuttle (indirect).

$\dot{V}O_2$ max). At first, these extra ATP can be provided by the oxidation of additional carbohydrates and fat, but at about 70% of $\dot{V}O_2$ anaerobic glycolysis must also be "turned on." With both systems now producing ATP, there is a prolongation of fatigue, as shown in the model. A key signal in this model is the build-up of C in the cytosol, which activates an ADP shuttle. Once the ADP shuttle is activated, the F1 ATP synthetase will outcompete the cytsolic CPKc for the available ADP. Note the role of the mitochondrial creatine phosphokinase (CPKm), which rephosphorylates C and provides ADP to the F1 ATP synthetases. The impact of additional ADP in the mitochondrion is twofold. If there is adequate oxygen, it can be used in oxidative phosphorylation to produce ATP. If oxygen becomes limited, then the CPKc once again becomes the strongest competitor for ADP, and it diffuses back to the cytosol. In this case PC would provide the energy needed for ATP resynthesis.

ADP in the cytosol would also serve to activate the phosphofructokinase (PFK) and pyruvatekinase (PK) enzymes so there is a continued high drive for anaerobic glycolysis. And so we see that the relative concentration (low vs. high) and location (cytosol vs. mitochondrion) of ADP plays a most important role in matching cellular metabolic systems to exercise intensity.

Miller has written an excellent review[23] of how this biochemical model explains the connection between exercise intensity and the metabolic system "selected" by the cell for ATP production. He has summarized it as follows: "Therefore, under conditions of very high intensity or low intensity exercise, small changes in [ADP] will activate the appropriate metabolic pathway, depending on oxygen availability and power output demand. Both of these conditions preclude any contribution from glycolysis. When the exercise intensity is too high for oxidative phosphorylation and the exercise duration is beyond that of the PC system, [PC] decreases with a concomitant increase in [ADP]. This elevation in [ADP] is greater than that seen during either very low or very high intensity work. The significance is that large changes in [ADP] will activate the PFK and PK enzymes of glycolysis, whereas small changes in [ADP] will activate either the PC pathway or oxidative phosphorylation." Although this is a theoretical model, it does predict many of the events that are known to occur during various intensities of exercise. It also serves as a model for future research, and you will likely learn more about it as you continue your studies.

Summary

The primary concern of this chapter is energy. The sun is the ultimate source of all energy on earth, for it is through solar radiation that carbohydrates are formed in plants. Humans and animals eat plants and other animals for food. In the human body, food energy is used to manufacture adenosine triphosphate, or ATP—the chemical compound that, when broken down, supplies energy for muscular contraction and other biological processes.

The production of ATP involves both anaerobic (without oxygen) and aerobic (with oxygen) metabolism (chemical reactions). There are two anaerobic systems: (1) the phosphagen, or ATP-PC system; and (2) anaerobic glycolysis, the lactic acid producing system.

The phosphagens (ATP + PC, a chemical compound similar to ATP) are stored within the contractile mechanisms of muscle and provide the most rapidly available source of ATP for use by the muscle. This energy system is the major one used for ATP production during high-intensity, short-duration exercises, such as sprinting 100 meters.

Anaerobic glycolysis releases energy for ATP synthesis through the partial breakdown of carbohydrates (glycogen and glucose) to lactic acid. Lactic acid (called lactate in its dissociated form) causes muscular fatigue when it accumulates in the blood and muscles. Anaerobic glycolysis is also a major supplier of ATP during high-intensity, short-duration activities, such as sprinting 400 and 800 meters. Activities that depend heavily on the phosphagen system and anaerobic glycolysis are called anaerobic activities.

The aerobic, or oxygen utilizing system releases energy for ATP production from the breakdown mainly of carbohydrates and fats, and sometimes of protein, to carbon dioxide and water. Although the aerobic system yields by far the most ATP, it requires several series of complex chemical reactions. With carbohydrates, in the first series of reactions, called aerobic glycolysis, glycogen is broken down to pyruvic acid; then in the Krebs Cycle, carbon dioxide is produced and electrons, in the form of hydrogen atoms, are removed. In the final series of reactions, hydrogen atoms (electrons) are "transported" to the mitochondria, where they combine with the oxygen we breathe; water is formed, and ATP is synthesized. With fats as the fuel, the reactions are the same with the exception of the first series, which is called beta-oxidation and prepares 2-carbon acyl groups to enter the Krebs Cycle. The oxygen system is used during rest and predominates during low intensity, long-duration exercises, such as the marathon. Such activities are called aerobic exercises.

Many exercise activities require a blend of both anaerobic and aerobic metabolism. For example, in the 1500-meter run, the anaerobic systems supply the major portion of ATP during the sprint at both the start and finish of the race, with the oxygen systems predominating during the middle, or steady-state, period of the run. This information is useful when developing training programs.

Females have the same concentrations of muscular ATP + PC as males, but because of their lesser total muscle mass, the total stores of these phosphagens are smaller. However, female performances in the shortest events (running 100 meters), in which ATP + PC are important sources of energy, are closest to male performances.

Females tend to have lower levels of lactate in their blood following maximal exercise than males (same training status). This indicates a limitation to the anaerobic glycolysis system, which makes it comparatively more difficult for them to perform events lasting around one to four minutes.

Likewise, males have larger aerobic power measures in absolute units (max $\dot{V}O_2$, L · min^{-1}), but differences between the genders become progressively smaller when O_2 uptake is expressed relative to body weight (mL · kg^{-1} · min^{-1}), lean body mass (mL · kg LBM^{-1} · min^{-1}) or active muscle volume. In fact, max $\dot{V}O_2$ measures have been shown to be the same for males and females when expressed relative to active muscle volume.

However, in the real world of athletic performance, the only meaningful relationship is between max $\dot{V}O_2$ and total body weight. Female performances are relatively good in distance events, especially in swimming, where water partially supports body weight. By contrast, in distance running, where movement of the total body weight comprises the largest part of the work load, females are clearly at a disadvantage because of their smaller max $\dot{V}O_2$.

Control and regulation of metabolic pathways during exercise are dependent on several factors operating at the same time. Two major influences are the energy state of the cell (intracellular control) and the hormone-amplification drive from outside the cell. These influence the activation or inhibition of regulatory enzymes at key positions (some of them rate limiting) in metabolic pathways so metabolism can be speeded up or slowed down. Use of food fuel substrates goes hand-in-hand with metabolic pathway selection.

A biochemical model of how exercise intensity determines which metabolic pathway will be utilized for ATP production has been suggested. In this model, a build-up of ADP and the adequacy of oxygen are two key determinants of pathway choice during the performance of low-, medium-, and high-intensity activities.

Questions

1. How is energy defined?
2. Name the six forms of energy.
3. Diagram the biological energy cycle.
4. What is the immediate source of energy for muscular contraction?
5. What are coupled reactions and what biochemical purpose do they serve?
6. Define anaerobic and aerobic metabolism.
7. Describe each of the three ways by which ATP is resynthesized.
8. How is lactic acid formed?
9. Distinguish between aerobic and anaerobic glycolysis.
10. What are the functions of the Krebs Cycle and the electron transport system?
11. How is fat used to synthesize ATP?
12. What are the capacities and powers of the three energy systems?
13. Under conditions of either rest or submaximal exercise, what are the three important features of the anaerobic and aerobic pathways that we must consider?
14. Discuss the considerations in question 13 as they would apply during all-out exercise.
15. Identify the predominant energy systems (phosphagen, anaerobic glycolysis, or oxygen system) used during the following activities: (a) 100-meter

dash, (b) 400-meter dash, (c) 1500-meter run, and (d) marathon.

16. What known gender differences exist for the energy systems identified in question 15?

17. What are the primary factors that account for these gender differences?

18. Which relative expression of max $\dot{V}O_2$ appears "fairest" for gender comparisons? Which is most practical?

19. Which of the running events listed in question 15 would females be expected to perform most like males? Why might they do even better at distance swimming events?

20. What categories of mechanisms control and regulate cellular energy systems during exercise?

21. Outline the biochemical model involving ADP that explains matching of energy systems and substrates to exercise intensity.

References

1. Booth, F. W., and D. B. Thomason. 1991. Molecular and cellular adaptations of muscle in response to exercise: perspectives of various models. *Physiol Rev.* 71(2):541–585.

2. Brooks, G. A., and T. D. Fahey. 1984. *Exercise Physiology: Human Bioenergetics and Its Applications.* New York: John Wiley, p. 82.

3. Cahill, G. F., Jr. 1971. Metabolic role of muscle. In Pernow, B., and B. Saltin (eds.), *Muscle Metabolism during Exercise.* New York: Plenum Press, pp. 103–109.

4. Costill, D. L. 1974. Muscular exhaustion during distance running. *Phys Sportsmed.* 2(10):36–41.

5. Costill, D. L., and E. L. Fox. 1969. Energetics of marathon running. *Med Sci Sports.* 1:81–86.

6. De Souza, M. J., M. S. Maguire, K. R. Rubin, and C. M. Maresh. 1990. Effects of menstrual phase and amenorrhea on exercise performance in runners. *Med Sci Sports Exerc.* 22(5):575–580.

7. Drinkwater, B. L. 1973. Physiological responses of women to exercise. In Wilmore, J. L. (ed.), *Exercise and Sport Sciences Reviews,* vol. 1. New York: Academic Press, pp. 125–153.

8. Drinkwater, B. L., S. M. Horvath, and C. L. Wells. 1975. Aerobic power of females, ages 10 to 68. *J Gerontol.* 30(4):385–394.

9. Fox, E. L., C. E. Billings, R. L. Bartels, R. Bason, and D. K. Mathews. 1973. Fitness standards for male college students. *Int Z Angew Physiol.* 31:231–236.

10. Fox, E. L., and D. L. Costill. 1972. Estimated cardiorespiratory responses during marathon running. *Arch Environ Health.* 24:315–324.

11. Goldfarb, A. H., J. F. Bruno, P. J. Buckenmeyer. 1989. Intensity and duration of exercise effects on skeletal muscle cAMP, phosphorylase, and glycogen. *J Appl Physiol.* 66(1):190–194.

12. Hagerman, F., E. Fox, M. Connors, and J. Pompei. 1974. Metabolic responses of women rowers during ergometric rowing. *Med Sci Sports.* 6(1):87.

13. Holloszy, J. O. 1982. Muscle metabolism during exercise. *Arch Physical Med Rehab.* 63:231–234.

14. Hultman, E. 1967. Studies on muscle metabolism of glycogen and active phosphate in man with special reference to exercise and diet. *Scand J Clin Lab Invest* (Suppl 94). 19:1–63.

15. Hultman, E., J. Bergstrom, and N. McClennan-Anderson. 1967. Breakdown and resynthesis of phosphocreatine and adenosine triphosphate in connection with muscular work in man. *Scand J Clin Invest.* 19:56–66.

16. Hultman, E., and L. H. Nilsson. 1971. Liver glycogen in man. Effect of different diets and muscular exercise. In Pernow, B., and B. Saltin (eds.), *Muscle Metabolism during Exercise.* New York: Plenum Press, pp. 143–151.

17. Kalinski, M. I., A. Y. Antipenko, C. C. Dunbar, and D. W. Michielli. 1995. *Exercise and Intracellular Regulation of Cardiac and Skeletal Muscle.* Champaign: Human Kinetics.

18. Karlsson, J. 1971. Lactate and phosphagen concentrations in working muscle of man. *Acta Physiol Scand* (Suppl). 358:1–72.

19. Karlsson, J., and B. Saltin. 1971. Diet, muscle glycogen and endurance performance. *J Appl Physiol.* 31(2): 203–206.

20. Lehninger, A. L. 1971. *Bioenergetics,* 2d ed. New York: W. A. Benjamin, p. 100.

21. Lemon, P. W. R. 1980. Effect of initial muscle glycogen levels on protein catabolism during exercise. *J Appl Physiol.* 48: 624–629.

22. Lemon, P. W. R., and F. J. Nagle. 1981. Effects of exercise on protein and amino acid metabolism. *Med Sci Sports Exerc.* 13:141–149.

23. Miller, W. C. 1992. *The Biochemistry of Exercise and Metabolic Adaptation.* Dubuque: Brown & Benchmark.

24. Robinson, S. 1974. Physiology of muscular exercises. In Mountcastle, V. B. (ed.), *Medical Physiology,* 13th ed., vol. 2. St. Louis: C. V. Mosby, p. 1279.

25. Sahlin, K. 1978. Intracellular pH and energy metabolism in skeletal muscle in man. *Acta Physiol Scand* (Suppl 455). 1–56.

26. Saltin, B., and P.-O. Astrand. 1967. Maximal oxygen uptake in athletes. *J Appl Physiol.* 23:353–358.

27. Saltin, B., and J. Karlsson. 1971. Muscle glycogen utilization during work of different intensities. In Pernow, B., and B. Saltin (eds.), *Muscle Metabolism during Exercise.* New York: Plenum Press, pp. 289–299.

28. Triveldi, B., and W. H. Danforth. 1966. Effect of pH on kinetics of frog muscle phosphofructokinase. *J Biol Chem.* 241:4110–4112.

Selected Readings

Bowers, R. W., and E. L. Fox. 1992. *Sports Physiology.* Dubuque: Wm. C. Brown.

Coggan, A. R., and E. F. Coyle. 1991. Carbohydrate ingestion during prolonged exercise: effects on metabolism and performance. *Exercise and Sports Sciences Reviews.* 19:1–40.

Gladden, L. B. 1989. Lactate uptake by skeletal muscle. *Exercise and Sports Sciences Reviews.* 17:115–155.

Gollnick, P. D., and L. Hermansen. 1973. Biochemical adaptations to exercise: anaerobic metabolism. In Wilmore, J. H. (ed.), *Exercise and Sport Sciences Reviews,* vol. 1. New York: Academic Press, pp. 1–43.

Gollnick, P. D., and D. W. King. 1969. Energy release in the muscle cell. *Med Sci Sports.* 1:23–31.

Hermansen, L. 1969. Anaerobic energy release. *Med Sci Sports.* 1:32–38.

Holloszy, J. O. 1973. Biochemical adaptations to exercise: aerobic metabolism. In Wilmore, J. H. (ed.), *Exercise and Sport Sciences Reviews,* vol. 1. New York: Academic Press, pp. 45–71.

Howald, H., and J. R. Poortmans (eds.). *Metabolic Adaptations to Prolonged Physical Exercise.* Basel, Switzerland: Birkhauser-Verlag.

Katz, A., and K. Sahlin. 1990. Role of oxygen in regulation of glycolysis and lactate production in human skeletal muscle. *Exercise and Sports Sciences Reviews.* 18:1–28.

Keul, J., E. Doll, and D. Keppler. 1972. *Energy Metabolism of Human Muscle* (trans. J. S. Skinner). Baltimore: University Park Press.

Lehninger, A. L. 1971. *Bioenergetics,* 2d ed. New York: W. A. Benjamin.

Maclaren, D. P. M., H. Gibson, M. Parry-Billings, and R. H. T. Edwards.

1989. A review of metabolic and physiological factors in fatigue. *Exercise and Sports Sciences Reviews.* 17:29–66.

Margaria, R. 1976. *Biomechanics and Energetics of Muscular Exercise.* Oxford: Oxford University Press, pp. 1–58.

McGilvery, R. W. 1975. The use of fuels for muscular work. In Howald, H., and J. R. Poortmans (eds.), *Metabolic Adaptations to Prolonged Physical Exercise.* Basel, Switzerland: Birkhauser-Verlag, pp. 12–30.

McGilvery, R. W. 1983. *Biochemistry: A Functional Approach.* Philadelphia: W. B. Saunders.

Milvey, P. (ed.). 1977. Metabolism in prolonged exercise. *Ann NY Acad Sci.* 301(1):3–97.

Pernow, B., and B. Saltin (eds.). 1971. *Muscle Metabolism during Exercise.* New York: Plenum Press.

Poortmans, J. R. (ed.). 1968. *Biochemistry of Exercise.* Baltimore: University Park Press.

Sahlin, K., G. Palmskog, and E. Hultman. 1978. Adenine nucleotide and IMP contents of the quadriceps muscle in man after exercise. *Pflugers Arch.* 374:193–198.

Stainsby, W. N., and G. A. Brooks. 1990. Control of lactic acid metabolism in contracting muscles and during exercise. *Exercise and Sports Sciences Reviews.* 18:29–63.

Tullson, P. C., and R. L. Terjung. 1991. Adenine nucleotide metabolism in contracting skeletal muscle. *Exercise and Sports Sciences Reviews.* 19:507–537.

West, J. B. 1991. (*Best and Taylors*) *Physiological Basis of Medical Practice.* Baltimore: Williams and Wilkins.

3 Recovery from Exercise

Devlin and Horton[46] have nicely summarized the need for a recovery period after exercise. The post-exercise recovery period is characterized by a transition from the acutely catabolic (breaking down) phase that occurs during exercise to an anabolic (building up) phase. For example, muscle glycogen stores are replenished after exercise even in the absence of refeeding. Therefore lactate, rather than being viewed simply as a "waste product" of metabolism, should be thought of as a fuel source for muscle and as a source for the partial regeneration of liver and muscle glycogen. This works best if lactate is "utilized" properly. Also, the increase in net protein degradation that occurs during exercise at even low-to-moderate workloads is replaced by net protein resynthesis as soon as exercise is stopped. These anabolic responses are essential for physical training to result in increased glycogen stores and lean body mass.

Therefore, in addition to understanding the different roles played by the metabolic energy systems during rest and exercise, we need to understand how the energy systems respond during the recovery process. Any form of exercise represents an acute disturbance in the homeostasis of the resting athlete, patient, or subject. Recovery from exercise, then, represents the sum total of the processes that return the exerciser to the resting state. To address the complex processes of recovery, the following topics will be

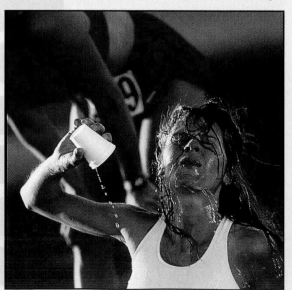

discussed: (1) excess postexercise oxygen consumption (formerly called oxygen debt), (2) replenishment of energy stores, (3) reduction of lactic acid in blood and muscle, (4) restoration of oxygen stores, (5) intensity- and activity-specific effects on the recovery process, and (6) practical guidelines for recovery. Prior to this discussion, we need to review the basic terminology associated with recovery from exercise.

Terminology

The major concepts to be learned from this chapter are as follows:

- The purpose of elevated oxygen consumption levels during recovery from exercise is to restore the muscles and the rest of the body to their pre-exercise condition.
- Restoration of the body during recovery includes replenishing the energy stores that were depleted and removing lactate that was accumulated during exercise; both processes require ATP energy.
- The oxygen consumed during the recovery period, in part, supplies the immediate ATP energy required during the recovery period.
- Restoration of the muscle phosphagen stores (ATP + PC) requires only a few minutes, whereas full restoration of the muscle and liver glycogen stores requires a day or more.
- The speed of the reduction of lactate in the circulation and muscle can be greatly increased by performing light exercise rather than by resting during the recovery period.
- Small amounts of oxygen, stored in muscle in chemical combination with myoglobin, are important during the performance of intermittent exercise because they are used during the work intervals and are quickly restored during the recovery intervals.

Terminology

The concept of **oxygen debt,** introduced in 1922 and 1923 by A. V. Hill* and H. Lupton,[80,81] states that most of the lactate formed during exercise is converted to glycogen immediately after stopping activity, and the remaining lactate is oxidized to CO_2 and H_2O. The proportions allocated to these processes were 80% of the lactate converted to glycogen and the remaining 20% to oxidation. Later, Margaria, Edwards, and Dill[112] introduced the concept of alactacid and lactacid oxygen debt components. They observed that the decline in blood lactate did not occur immediately after exercise but appeared to follow two separate rate curves. They further concluded that the initial rapid decline in the rate of oxygen consumption was alactacid in origin (the prefix "a" denoting "not due to" lactic acid formation in muscle) and suggested that this portion was a result of the replacement of phosphagens (ATP and PC) in muscle. They also observed that the lactacid portion was characterized by a similar decay time in lactate concentration and by the slow component of recovery oxygen consumption.[112] Gaesser and Brooks[59] have published a review of the pertinent literature that elucidates this controversial matter; it brings into serious question the original lactate clearance concept and, thus, the terminology related to oxygen debt.

For a number of years we have known that the elevated oxygen consumption during recovery is reflective of more than merely replacing oxygen that was "borrowed" during exercise or converting lactate to pyruvate or replenishing glycogen stores immediately after exercise. For this reason, a number of authors[29,30,58,59,60,101,137] have suggested names that might more appropriately describe events that occur during recovery. Such terms as *recovery oxygen*[137] and *excess post-exercise oxygen consumption*[29,30,58,59,60] have been proposed. Further, the oxygen consumption pattern in recovery clearly shows two major components typical of an exponential decline: a faster component, previously identified as the alactacid oxygen debt; and a slower component, previously called the lactacid oxygen debt. Knuttgen,[98] in 1970, declared that "the alactacid portion of the total debt could very well be considered as the fast component." In this same reference,[98] he also referred to the slow component. Additionally, prolonged elevation of post-exercise oxygen consumption has been characterized as an "ultra-slow component."[118,119]

Although there is not universal agreement on terminology, *excess post-exercise oxygen consumption,*[110,118] or EPOC, and *recovery oxygen*[137] have been suggested as contemporary terms for the classic oxygen debt. In this text we will use **recovery oxygen,** or merely *recovery,* to describe oxygen consumption during the recovery process. Further we will refer to the **fast component** and **slow component** in reference to what formerly was identified as the *alactacid*

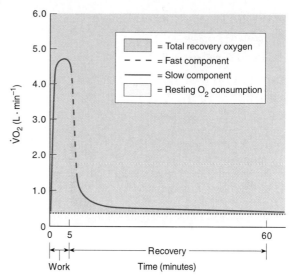

Figure 3.1

Recovery oxygen. The amount of oxygen consumed during recovery above that which would have been consumed at rest in the same time period is called the recovery oxygen. Recovery oxygen consumption consists of a fast component and a slow component.

(Based on data from Fox et al.[56])

oxygen debt and *lactacid oxygen debt,* respectively. The components of oxygen consumption during recovery are shown schematically in figure 3.1. Table 3.1 is a summary of the classic and suggested terminology. Again, there is not universal agreement on terminology and in the literature, any of the above terms, as well as several others, will be found.

Recovery Oxygen

Recovery oxygen may be defined as the net amount of oxygen consumed during recovery from exercise, or as the amount of oxygen consumed during recovery in excess of that which would have ordinarily been consumed at rest in the same amount of time. To calculate the net recovery oxygen, we need to know the pre-exercise resting oxygen consumption rate and the total recovery time.

Net recovery O_2 = (Total $\dot{V}O_2$ rec) − (T) ($\dot{V}O_2$ rest)

Where

Total $\dot{V}O_2$ rec = the gross oxygen consumption during recovery in liters (L)

T = the time, in minutes, required for oxygen consumption to return to pre-exercise level

$\dot{V}O_2$ rest = measured pre-exercise resting oxygen consumption in liters per minute $(L \cdot min^{-1})$

During recovery from exercise the energy demand is considerably less because exercising has ceased. However,

---

*A. V. Hill and O. Meyerhof received the Nobel Prize for physiology and medicine in 1922.

3.1
table

Classic and contemporary expressions for oxygen consumption during recovery from exercise

Classic	Contemporary	Volumes
Oxygen debt	Recovery oxygen Excess post-exercise oxygen consumption (EPOC)	5 to 18 liters
Alactacid oxygen debt	Fast component Rapid recovery Rapid phase	0.5 to 4 liters (rarely, up to 6 liters)
Lactacid oxygen debt	Slow component Slow recovery Slow phase	5 to 14 liters
	Ultra-slow component	Not well established

oxygen consumption continues at a relatively high level for a period of time—the length of which depends on the intensity and, to a lesser degree, the duration of exercise.[64] For example, the energy expenditure following either a 3.2 km walk or run at a steady-state rate between 18% and 68% of peak $\dot{V}O_2$ ranges between 13 to 71 kJ (3 to 17 kcal).[23] Training status also effects the size of the recovery O_2 volume. Endurance-trained people undergo adaptation that enables them to adjust more quickly to the energy requirements of constant load submaximal work. They, therefore, develop a smaller O_2 deficit, and their rate of recovery on cessation of exercise is more rapid, so the magnitude of their recovery O_2 volume is smaller.[66]

The concept of oxygen debt, as originally developed by Hill, meant that the oxygen consumed during recovery was used primarily in restoring the body to its pre-exercise condition, including replenishing the energy stores that were depleted and removing any lactic acid that was accumulated during exercise. Many erroneously interpret the classical term *oxygen debt* to mean that extra oxygen consumed during recovery is being used to replace oxygen that was "borrowed" from somewhere within the body during exercise. Actually, during maximal exercise, depletion of the oxygen stored in muscle itself (in combination with myoglobin) and in venous blood would amount to only about 0.6 liters. The recovery oxygen level, on the other hand, is probably thirty times larger than this in an athlete following maximal exercise. It is also higher in physically active lean men than in active women.[14]

Fast and Slow Components

In figure 3.1, the time course of oxygen consumption following exhaustive exercise decreases exponentially. That is to say, the rate at which oxygen is consumed is not constant throughout the recovery period. During the first two or three minutes of recovery, oxygen consumption declines very rapidly, then more slowly until a constant rate, equivalent to resting level, is reached. The initial rapid portion of recovery is now identified as the fast component,[101] whereas the slower phase is now referred to as the slow component (see p. 61).[81,101,112] Again, the slow component was formerly identified as the *lactacid* component, because it was observed that the oxygen consumed during this phase of recovery was quantitatively related to the removal of the lactic acid accumulated in the blood and muscles during exercise. The term *alactacid* was used because the oxygen consumed during the fast component of recovery was thought to be independent of the removal of lactic acid during recovery. At one time, it was thought that the entire recovery oxygen was lactacid in nature (i.e., that it resulted from the removal of the lactic acid accumulated during exercise).[79] When first proven in 1933 that an elevated recovery oxygen consumption could be incurred in the absence of lactic acid accumulation, the term *alactacid oxygen debt* was used.[112]

The elevated oxygen consumption during the fast component of recovery includes oxygen fueling the post exercise energetic need of: (1) resaturation of myoglobin with oxygen, (2) restoration of blood levels of oxygen (see chapter 8), (3) the energy cost of elevated ventilation (see chapter 7), (4) elevated heart activity (see chapter 9), and probably most significantly, (5) the replenishment of phosphagens (ATP and PC).[101] The volume of the fast component of O_2 recovery is calculated from the area under the curve for O_2 uptake rates, in $L \cdot min^{-1}$, plotted against time in min. The magnitude of the fast component volume is related to the submaximal exercise intensity (50% to 80% of $\dot{V}O_2$ max) but not to the duration of exercise.[67] Likewise, measures of minute ventilation ($\dot{V}_E$), carbon dioxide production ($\dot{V}CO_2$) and oxygen uptake ($\dot{V}O_2$) are elevated after the performance of the "same" exercise at a higher intensity.[148] There appears to be a limit to the effect exercise intensity has on increasing the fast component of O_2 recovery;

however, since the fast component following short duration (1 min), supramaximal cycling work (maximal speed against 5.5 kg resistance) is similar to that of other work intensities.[93]

The elevated oxygen consumption during the slow component of recovery is known to be associated with a number of physiological events including: (1) an elevated body temperature[2,67] involving the **Q_{10} effect;**[*] (2) the oxygen cost of ventilation; (3) the oxygen cost of increased myocardial activity; (4) an increase in sodium and potassium pump activities (ion redistribution); (5) glycogen resynthesis; (6) the calorigenic effect of catecholamines;[10,11] and (7) oxidation of lactic acid (i.e., conversion to CO_2 and H_2O), among other factors.[60,137] Hagberg et al. state that the greater part (60% to 70%) of the slow component oxygen consumption can be accounted for simply by the effect of temperature on metabolism.[67]

The effects of exercise intensity and duration on the magnitude of the slow component of recovery warrants our consideration. Metabolic system measures such as $\dot{V}_E$, $\dot{V}CO_2$, and $\dot{V}O_2$ made during the slow component are not affected following performance of the "same" work at a higher intensity.[148] Similarly, performing submaximal (50% to 80% $\dot{V}O_2$ max) cycling exercise for a longer duration (20 vs. 5 min) has no effect on the slow component of O_2 recovery.[67] However, a combination of the highest intensity (80% $\dot{V}O_2$ max) and longest duration (20 min) increases the slow component 5 times above that measured after a shorter duration (5 min) at the same intensity. In summary, the slow component is relatively unaffected by a change in exercise intensity or duration until a threshold of a combined intensity × duration stimulus is presented. Then it increases.

Replenishment of Energy Stores during Recovery

There are two important questions to answer here: (1) what energy stores are depleted during exercise, and (2) how are they replenished during recovery? First, there are two sources of energy that are depleted to varying extents during exercise: (1) the phosphagens, or ATP and PC, stored in the muscle cells; and (2) glycogen stored in large quantities in both muscle and liver, which serves as an important dual source of fuel during most exercise activity. If you are wondering why fats have not been included in our list, it's because they are not directly replenished during recovery but instead are rebuilt indirectly through the replenishment of carbohydrates (glucose and glycogen). We will not concern ourselves too much with this latter point but will, in answering the second question, concentrate on the replenishment of the other two energy sources: ATP-PC and glycogen.

Restoration of ATP + PC and the Fast Component of Recovery

Direct measurement of the phosphagen stores in human skeletal muscle is rather difficult. It requires the removal of a small sample of muscle tissue using biopsy techniques under sterile surgical conditions (see figure 6.13) and a well-equipped laboratory for analysis. A newer method uses a radioactive isotope of phosphorus (31P) combined with magnetic resonance spectroscopy called 31P MRS. The latter method allows measurements to be made every few seconds so more detailed response curves can be plotted. Sullivan[140] reports no differences in ATP or pH measurements between the two techniques at rest, during peak exercise, or in recovery. We will review a combination of studies that have used these methods to provide a clear picture of the change that occurs in ATP + PC during exercise and during the fast component of recovery. Several of these studies have demonstrated a linear relationship between work intensity and in the net change in the concentration of high energy phosphates. A linear relationship between these variables would mean that for a given change in the work intensity, the degree to which the phosphate stores are depleted is constant. There is also evidence, however, that the metabolic system does not behave as a linear system.[106]

Kemp used 31P MRS to estimate normal muscle ATP production rates to be as high as 20 to 25 mmol $\cdot$ L^{-1} $\cdot$ min^{-1} during exercise when glycogen was being used as a fuel. A similar rate of ATP production was found during the oxidative metabolism of all fuel substrates, including carbohydrates, fatty acids, and amino acids.[96] He has also suggested that the rate of PC recovery after exercise is a useful estimate of net oxidative ATP synthesis.[95] This gives an impression of the very rapid rate of ATP production during exercise. But how low do ATP and PC concentrations go? Intramuscular PC is reduced to approximately 20% of resting concentration at the end of a 30 sec all-out maximal sprint on a cycle ergometer, whereas ATP is reduced to a lesser degree, remaining at about 70% of resting level.[17] A somewhat lower post-exercise PC concentration (15% of resting level) has been reported at the end of both exhaustive dynamic exercise and isometric contractions sustained to fatigue.[71] PC reaches its minimal value at the time of muscle exhaustion and begins to return toward pre-exercise level immediately upon cessation of exercise.[149] A fast phase of PC recovery with a half-time (time required for a concentration to return to 50% of its peak point above a baseline level) of 21 to 22 sec has been shown to be followed by a slower phase with a half-time greater than 3 min.[71]

Several studies have shown that most of the ATP and PC depleted in the muscle during exercise is restored very rapidly (i.e., within a few minutes following exercise).[71,86,91,92,122,123] The results of one of the first studies[60] of this kind are shown in figure 3.2. In this experiment,

---

[*]The metabolic activity of a cell doubles for every 10° C increase in temperature.

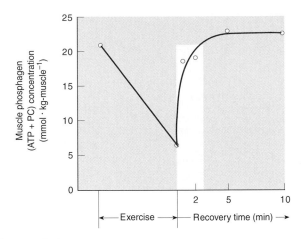

Figure 3.2

The muscular stores of ATP + PC that were depleted during exercise are restored within a few minutes following exercise. Notice that the phosphagen restoration is 70% completed in 30 seconds and is essentially 100% completed within about 3 to 5 minutes.

(Based on data from Hultman et al.[86])

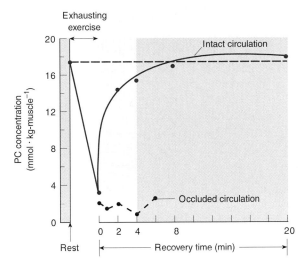

Figure 3.3

Restoration of PC during recovery from exhausting exercise. Two recoveries were used: (1) when the muscles had a normal blood flow (intact circulation) and (2) when the blood flow to the muscles was occluded (occluded circulation). With an intact circulation, the majority (90%) of PC was restored to the muscles within four minutes of recovery. No restoration of PC took place when the blood flow was occluded, indicating that oxygen is required for this process.

(Based on data from Harris et al.[71])

the subjects rode a cycle ergometer (stationary bicycle) for 10 minutes. Muscle tissue samples were taken from the vastus lateralis (one of the quadriceps muscles) by needle biopsy before exercise and at various times during recovery. The samples were subsequently analyzed for ATP and PC concentrations. Notice from the figure that the phosphagen restoration is very rapid at first (shaded area), then somewhat slower, being 70% completed within 30 seconds and 100% completed within 3 to 5 minutes. Under very heavy exercise conditions, Knuttgen and Saltin[100] have observed that ATP and PC levels have been reestablished within six minutes.

In this study, ATP and PC recovery were assessed together. The restoration, specifically of muscle phosphocreatine (PC), has also been examined, again in the vastus lateralis, during recovery from exhausting cycle exercise.[71] In these experiments, PC restoration was examined under two different recovery conditions: (1) when the muscles under study had a normal blood flow (intact circulation) and (2) when the blood flow to the muscles was occluded (occluded circulation) to produce **ischemia.** The results are shown in figure 3.3. With an intact circulation, restoration of PC was very rapid at first (shaded area), then much slower. For example, after two minutes of recovery, 84% of the PC depleted during exercise was restored, with 89% restored after four minutes. By eight minutes, 97% of the PC was restored to the muscles. Although the complete restoration of PC was somewhat longer in this latter experiment, the findings essentially confirm the earlier studies in that the majority of the muscular stores of ATP and PC depleted during exercise are restored within a few minutes of recovery.

The above studies clearly indicate the important role that adequate blood flow and the delivery of oxygen to muscles play during recovery from exercise. This has been verified in a number of other studies where blood flow has been partially occluded during sustained-grip exercise[94] and isometric contractions to fatigue,[71] or totally occluded following steady-state cycling exercise.[88] In all cases, the rate of recovery was impaired when blood flow was compromised. In keeping with this, Tesch[141] has found that both the amount of fatigue and the rate of muscle force recovery correlate with muscle capillary density—i.e., provision of potentially more blood flow.

In addition, the results from studies in which the muscle phosphagens have been directly measured agree with other studies that have indirectly or theoretically dealt with phosphagen restoration.[47,110,111] Brooks et al. have estimated the amount of oxygen necessary for rephosphorylation of ATP and PC to be about 1.5 liters.[29]

Energetics of Phosphagen Restoration

The ATP energy required for phosphagen restoration is provided mainly by the aerobic system through the oxygen consumed during the fast component of the recovery oxygen period.[49,122,123] The fact that oxygen is required for this process is clearly shown in figure 3.3. When the blood flow

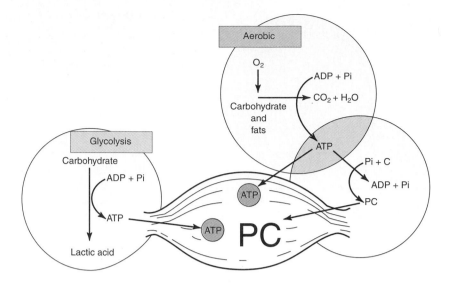

Figure 3.4

The oxygen consumed during the fast component of recovery provides the majority of energy necessary to replenish ATP and PC stores in muscle that were depleted during exercise. Some of the ATP resynthesized is directly stored in muscle, and some is broken down immediately to resynthesize PC, which is then stored in the muscle. Anaerobic glycolysis may also provide some energy (ATP) for phosphagen restoration.

(From Bowers and Fox.[22])

(circulation), and thus the oxygen supply, to muscle was occluded during recovery, little or no resynthesis of PC took place. Nevertheless, a small part of the energy required for phosphagen restoration may also be derived without oxygen through anaerobic glycolysis.[35,50]

As shown in figure 3.4, the aerobic energy made available for phosphagen replenishment comes about from the breakdown of carbohydrate and fats (and perhaps a small amount of lactic acid) to CO_2 and H_2O via the Krebs Cycle and the electron transport system. Some of the resynthesized ATP is stored directly in muscle, whereas some is broken down immediately, to resynthesize the PC that is stored in the muscle. PC can only be resynthesized in coupled reactions from the energy released when ATP is broken down (see chapter 2). In other words, ATP, but not PC, is directly resynthesized from the energy released from the breakdown of foods.

Most of the energy for phosphagen restoration arises from metabolic activity occurring during the period of the fast component of recovery. The fast component declines very rapidly and is complete in three to six minutes (usually less than four minutes) (figure 3.1). Its decline can be estimated from analysis of the oxygen consumption curve during the first few minutes of recovery. When estimated in this manner, the **half-reaction time** of replenishment is 30 seconds or less.[67,109] This means that in 30 seconds, $1/2$ of the total fast component of recovery is complete; in 1 minute, $3/4$; in $1 1/2$ minutes, $7/8$; and in 3 minutes, $63/64$. However, as just pointed out, the actual rate at which the ATP and PC stores are replenished is some-

what faster (i.e., with 70% rather than 50% restored in 30 seconds).*

The reason for this discrepancy is that the amount of oxygen consumed during recovery includes not only the amount of oxygen required to oxidize substrate sufficient to replenish the ATP and PC stores, but also (1) a certain amount of extra oxygen needed to replace the depleted oxygen stores (about 0.6 L of oxygen with maximal exercise), (2) about 50 mL of extra oxygen required for the still-activated heart and respiratory muscles,[48,146] and (3) a certain amount of extra oxygen required by the body because of increased tissue temperature[28,29,30] and catecholamine (norepinephrine).[62] With these corrections, the half-reaction time is approximately 20 seconds, which is in close agreement with the actual phosphagen restoration rate as determined from muscle sample analysis.[49,111,112]

The greater the phosphagen depletion during exercise, the greater the oxygen required for the restoration during recovery. Thus, these two quantities—phosphagen restoration and the fast component oxygen consumption—should be related. Knuttgen and Saltin[99,100] have demonstrated under a variety of conditions that there is a high degree of relationship between phosphagen depletion and the fast component oxygen volumes. Figure 3.5 demonstrates this relationship. A small volume of oxygen calculated for the fast component (low-intensity exercise), demonstrates there is little deple-

---

*Both Knuttgen[98] and Hagberg et al.[67] have presented an equation for calculating the slow component of recovery oxygen.

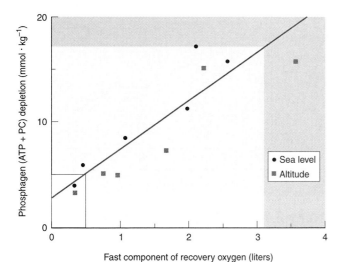

Figure 3.5

Phosphagen depletion and the fast component of recovery oxygen consumption. The greater the phosphagen depletion during exercise, whether at altitude or sea level, the greater the amount of oxygen required during recovery for restoration.[98,99] This relationship between the fast component of recovery oxygen and phosphagen restoration in muscle is based on the fact that 3.45 liters of oxygen are required in the oxidative process to produce 1 mole of ATP. Typical values of phosphagen stores depletion and fast component oxygen volumes are illustrated by the shaded areas.

tion of the ATP and PC concentrations in muscle. On the other hand, as the fast component volumes (associated with exercise levels above 60% to 70% of the aerobic capacity) become greater, the depletion of the phosphagen stores (ATP and PC) is greater.[99,100] The relationship is based on the fact that it requires 3.45 liters of oxygen to manufacture 1 mole of ATP. This relationship has been used indirectly to evaluate the maximal phosphagen capacity in males[55] and females.[70] Typical values for both the depletion of phosphagen stores and the fast component are indicated in figure 3.5.

The maximum size of fast component post-exercise oxygen use ranges between 2 and 3 liters in untrained males;[126] a higher value is associated with well-trained athletes. For example, a level of 6 liters has been recorded in male competitive rowers.[69] As shown by the relationship in figure 3.5, such a large fast component for recovery can be interpreted to mean that a large amount of phosphagen was depleted during exercise and would need to be restored during recovery. Reciprocally, a large quantity of phosphagen was available for use during exercise. This has important applications in human performance because the sprinter who can develop, through training, a greater capacity of the fast oxygen component will be more successful than one who has a smaller level. As indicated in chapter 2, the amount of ATP + PC available (capacity) and its rate of utilization (power) are directly related to an athlete's ability to generate and sustain power in an activity such as sprinting. Through a properly designed training program, the phos-

phagen system, and hence performance, in such activities may be improved. In chapter 4 and Appendix F we describe practical ways to indirectly measure the power capability of the phosphagen system of an athlete.

Muscle Glycogen Resynthesis

For nearly 50 years scientists believed that the muscular store of glycogen depleted during exercise was resynthesized from lactic acid during the immediate recovery period (one to two hours) following exercise. We now know this is not true.[26,77,85,108,117,121] The full repletion of the muscle glycogen following exercise requires several days and depends on two major factors: (1) the type of exercise performed that caused the glycogen depletion, and (2) the amount of dietary carbohydrate consumed during the recovery period. Two different types of exercises have been used to study muscle glycogen depletion and repletion: (1) *continuous endurance-like activities* (i.e., low-intensity, long-duration exercises); and (2) *intermittent, exhaustive activities* (i.e., high-intensity, short-duration exercises). The following discussion centers on these two types of exercise and considers the influence of the dietary intake of carbohydrates.

1. *Muscle Glycogen Depletion and Repletion—Continuous-Endurance Exercise.* Figure 3.6 shows the pattern of muscle glycogen depletion-repletion during and following endurance exercise. The exercise in these studies consisted of one hour of endurance activity (e.g., swimming, running, or bicycling) and one hour of heavier, exhausting exercise. From this figure, we can observe that:
   a. Only an insignificant amount of muscle glycogen is resynthesized within the immediate recovery period (one to two hours) following endurance exercise. However, Maehlum[109] has reported some measurable muscle glycogen repletion during the first four hours of recovery from prolonged exercise (70% $\dot{V}O_2$ max) to exhaustion even if the subjects were fasted. This process does not continue during the last 8 hours of a 12-hour fasted recovery period.
   b. The complete resynthesis of muscle glycogen following endurance exercise requires a high dietary intake of carbohydrates during a two-day (~ 46 hours) recovery period.
   c. Without a high carbohydrate intake, only a small amount of glycogen is resynthesized even during a five-day period.
   d. Replenishment of muscle glycogen following a high-carbohydrate diet is most rapid during the first several hours of recovery from endurance exercise, being 60% completed in 10 hours.
   e. There appears to be no difference in glycogen resynthesis whether simple sugars (sucrose,

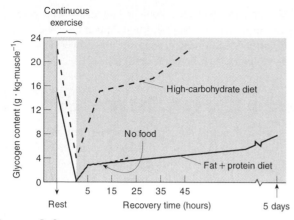

Figure 3.6

Only an insignificant amount of muscle glycogen is resynthesized within the immediate recovery period following continuous, prolonged exercise. The complete resynthesis of muscle glycogen following this kind of exercise requires a high dietary intake of carbohydrate during at least a two-day (46-hour) period. Without carbohydrate intake, only a small amount of glycogen is resynthesized even during a five-day period.

(Based on data from Hultman and Bergstrom[85] and Piehl.[121])

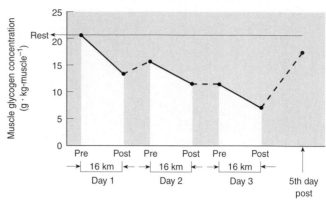

Figure 3.7

Muscle glycogen is progressively depleted during a three-day period when 16 kilometers (10 miles) are run each day.

(Based on data from Costill et al.[41])

glucose) or complex sugars (starches) are consumed during the first 24 hours following exhaustive work. However, during the next 24 hours, greater glycogen storage occurred with complex carbohydrates as the food source.[42]

f. It is interesting to note that muscle glycogen synthesis during recovery from prolonged exercise is similar for juvenile diabetics and non-diabetics.[73] This means that diabetics can recover from strenuous daily physical activity just as non-diabetics if their carbohydrate intake is carefully managed.

g. Finally, prior exercise—in the form of four hours of low-intensity swimming—primarily promotes the local incorporation of recycled glucose within the muscle itself.[129]

From a practical viewpoint, such information is important to the coach and athlete because of the importance muscle glycogen has as a metabolic fuel during heavy and prolonged exercise activity. As described in chapter 2, glycogen represents the only metabolic fuel for glycolysis and is a major fuel for the aerobic system during various types of endurance activity. There is also some evidence that when the glycogen stores in muscle are low or depleted, muscle fatigues, even though fat is still available as a fuel.[15,74] Thus, an adequate concentration of muscle glycogen should be maintained at all times. This is not always easy, given the severe endurance demand of training, such as running several miles every day, and the time necessary to adequately replenish muscle glycogen. Figure 3.7 shows progressive depletion of muscle glycogen stores during a three-day

period when 16 kilometers (10 miles) were run each day.[41] This occurred in spite of the fact that the runners consumed normal amounts of carbohydrates during this time.

2. *Muscle Glycogen Depletion and Repletion—Intermittent, Short-Duration Exercise.* Several studies[77,107] have examined muscle glycogen replenishment following intermittent, short-duration exercise; the results of these studies are shown in figure 3.8*A* and *B*. In *A*, the exercise consisted of riding a cycle ergometer at very heavy work rate for one-minute intervals with three minutes of rest between bouts. This pattern was continued until a subject was exhausted and could no longer maintain at least 30 seconds of work during one of the exercise bouts. During a 24-hour recovery period, either a normal mixed diet or a high-carbohydrate diet was consumed. In *B*, the subjects performed three exhausting one-minute exercise bouts, again on a cycle ergometer, with four minutes of rest allowed between bouts. Their recovery was monitored for only 30 minutes, during which time no food was consumed by the subjects. The following conclusions were made:

a. A significant amount of muscle glycogen can be resynthesized within 30 minutes to two hours of recovery, even in the absence of food (carbohydrate) intake.

b. The complete resynthesis of muscle glycogen does *not* require a greater-than-normal intake of carbohydrate.

c. Complete resynthesis of muscle glycogen required a 24-hour recovery period when a normal or high-carbohydrate diet is consumed.

d. Muscle glycogen resynthesis is most rapid during the first several hours of recovery, being 39% completed in two hours and 53% completed in five hours.

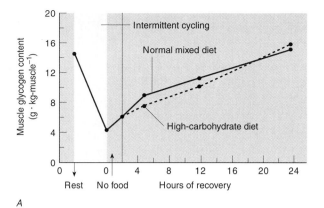

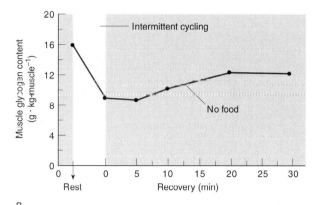

Figure 3.8

Muscle glycogen resynthesis following intermittent exercise to exhaustion. *A,* a significant amount of glycogen is resynthesized during the first 2 hours of recovery, even in the absence of food intake. *B,* resynthesis also occurs during the first 30 minutes of recovery under no-food conditions. A complete resynthesis of muscle glycogen following this kind of exercise requires 24 hours.

(Data in A from MacDougall et al.,[107] data in B from Hermansen and Vaage.[77])

It is important for coaches and trainers to know that significant amounts of muscle glycogen can be resynthesized within two hours of recovery from intermittent, short-duration exercise without food intake; likewise, these facts have application to nonendurance athletes who often must compete several times in one day (e.g., heats in track and swimming events; and gymnastics, wrestling, and basketball tournaments). A similar pattern of muscle glycogen replenishment has been reported by Bangsbo[8] for three minutes of intense one-legged knee extension contractions leading to exhaustion. Muscle glycogen increased from 94 mmol · kg wet wt^{-1} at the end of exercise to 109 mmol after one hour of recovery. This partial restoration of muscle glycogen after short-term, intense, exhaustive exercise occurred without refeeding and would be representative of those athletic efforts we commonly refer to as "all out." Interestingly, the total net recovery oxygen for the exercised leg was calculated to be 1.5 L, of which only one-third could be accounted for by the combined resynthesis of ATP,

PC, and glycogen plus the reloading of hemoglobin and myoglobin.

Physiological Factors Related to Differences in Muscle Glycogen Resynthesis

Why is muscle glycogen resynthesis different following continuous versus intermittent exercise? The answer to this question is not entirely known. However, several factors may be involved. One could be related to the overall amount of glycogen depleted during exercise. For example, with continuous exercise, about twice the amount of glycogen is depleted as with intermittent exercise (compare figures 3.7 and 3.8). Thus, with less overall glycogen to resynthesize, less time is needed. This idea is supported by the fact that in the first 24 hours of recovery, about the same total amount of glycogen was resynthesized regardless of whether the preceding exercise was continuous or intermittent.

Another factor that may be important is the availability of *glycogen precursors.* To synthesize glycogen (as well as any compound), an adequate amount of its constituents (precursors) must also be available.[45] Common precursors of glycogen are lactate, pyruvate, and glucose. These must be available to the liver and muscle, where most of the resynthesis begins. Following prolonged continuous exercise, most of these precursors are found in limited amount,[4] whereas following intermittent exercise, they are usually found in normal or even in above-normal circulating amounts. For example, there is a rapid and large increase in glucose production when subjects exercise to exhaustion on a cycle ergometer at approximately 100% $\dot{V}O_2$ max.[113] Turnover of this excess glucose (called post-exercise hyperglycemia) follows a biphasic response pattern during the first 30 minutes of recovery.[31] Glucose production exceeds utilization during the first five minutes, then reverses during the next 10 to 30 minutes of recovery. Following intermittent exercise, glycogen synthesis starts sooner and has more readily available glycogen precursors for glycogen synthesis. Dietary intake of carbohydrate following continuous exercise facilitates glycogen repletion—but does not do so following intermittent exercise—which is why a greater-than-normal intake of carbohydrate does not improve glycogen resynthesis following intermittent exercise.

A final factor that may explain differences in glycogen resynthesis following intermittent and continuous activity is the different types of fibers found in mixed skeletal muscle (see chapter 6). Most human muscles contain two basic fiber types: a Type II (*fast, glycolytic*) fiber, which is preferentially recruited during the performance of short-duration, high-intensity work (such as the intermittent exercises discussed here), and a Type I (*slow, oxidative*) fiber, which is used preferentially during prolonged, continuous exercise. There is evidence that glycogen resynthesis in Type II fibers is faster than in Type I fibers.[121] Glycogen resynthesis is therefore faster following intermittent exercise because the Type II fiber is used to a greater extent in this kind of activity than in endurance exercise.

Energetics of Muscle Glycogen Resynthesis

The resynthesis of glycogen involves a series of complicated chemical reactions, each requiring specific enzymes.[100] These reactions were outlined in chapter 2 and were summarized in figure 2.13. We encourage you to review the relevant reactions and note that this process requires energy. For the most part, this energy is provided from ATP generated aerobically. Part of this energy requirement might be met through the oxygen consumed during the slow component of recovery. However, this would be true only for the glycogen resynthesized during the immediate post-exercise recovery period (one to two hours) because the slow-recovery component is generally completed within this time. Also, a quantitative relationship between glycogen resynthesis during recovery and the ATP energy provided during the slow component of recovery has not been experimentally determined.

Muscle Glycogen Supercompensation

The amount and rate of glycogen resynthesis in skeletal muscle during recovery from exercise may be increased to a much higher concentration than normal (supercompensated) by following a special exercise/diet procedure. This information has proved useful to athletes, for such a procedure has been shown to significantly improve endurance performance. More detailed information concerning muscle glycogen supercompensation procedures appears in chapter 15. It is noteworthy that nearly the same amount of carbohydrate loading can be obtained by simply ingesting greater amounts of carbohydrate as contrasted to the more complicated exercise/dietary regimens advocated in years past.

Liver Glycogen Replenishment

As mentioned in chapter 2, liver glycogen represents a sizable energy store. Unfortunately, not many studies in humans have been conducted in which the liver glycogen stores were examined. However, the results of one such study[87] are shown in figure 3.9. Liver glycogen concentration was determined at rest (by removing small pieces of tissue from the liver with a special biopsy needle) following one hour of heavy cycle exercise (figure 3.9A) and on several days of carbohydrate starvation followed by a high-carbohydrate diet (figure 3.9B). Liver glycogen was considerably reduced following exercise and was further reduced during several days of carbohydrate starvation. An overshoot, or supercompensation, takes place within one day after carbohydrate refeeding.

In dogs, the liver has been shown to be a valuable supply source of glucose during 150 minutes of moderate intensity treadmill running. Net hepatic glucose output rose

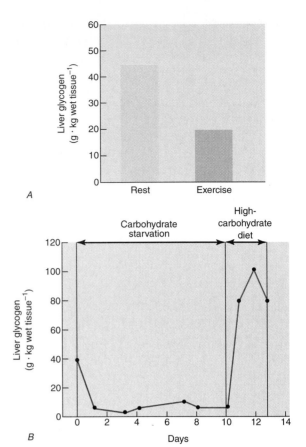

Figure 3.9

A. Liver glycogen is considerably reduced following exercise, *B.* with a further reduction during several days of carbohydrate starvation. Note the overshoot, or supercompensation, one day after carbohydrate refeeding.

(Based on data from Hultman and Nilsson.[87])

gradually from 2.6 mg · kg^{-1} · min^{-1} at rest to 8.9 units after 60 minutes of exercise and then remained essentially unchanged until exercise was stopped.[143] Interestingly, hepatic glucose uptake did not change from resting levels of 1.4 mg · kg^{-1} · min^{-1} either during exercise or during 90 minutes of recovery. In rats[26] studies show that no resynthesis of liver glycogen occurs during 24 hours of recovery from exercise when no food is consumed. Although comparable studies on humans have not been conducted, it is reasonable to assume that a similar result would be found. As with muscle glycogen resynthesis, the energy requirement for liver glycogen resynthesis is provided from ATP generated aerobically. This resynthesis process is also called **glyconeogenesis.**

Reduction of Lactate in Blood and Muscle

When lactic acid, the product of glycolysis (the anaerobic phase of carbohydrate metabolism), reaches a high concentration in blood and muscle, fatigue sets in. At this point we will switch from the use of the term *lactic acid* to *lactate*. This is appropriate since, at a blood or intracellular fluid pH of 6.5, fully 99.8% of lactic acid exists in its ionized form of $C_3H_5O_3^-$ and H^+—i.e. lactate and its disassociated hydrogen ion. Therefore, full recovery from exercises in which a maximal concentration of lactate has been reached involves the reduction of lactate from both blood and skeletal muscle that was active during the preceding exercise period. Just how large is the blood lactate increase and how does the immediate post-exercise blood lactate concentration relate to the intensity and duration of activity?

Blood lactate and pyruvate levels have been directly related to exercise intensity but there is only a slight increase in blood lactate at a low level of exercise intensity and no change in lactate-to-pyruvate ratios until a threshold work rate is reached.[145] At this threshold, lactate abruptly increases without an associated increase in pyruvate. For example, the blood lactate concentration increases only tenfold after a 800 m submaximal swim but a full 15-fold after a 100 m maximal effort swim.[63] The blood lactate concentrations also have been studied immediately after subjects have pedaled a cycle ergometer at various combinations of submaximal intensity (50%, 65%, and 80% of $\dot{V}O_2$ max) and duration (5 or 20 minutes). The lowest post-exercise blood lactate concentration occurred with a combination of low-intensity and short-duration (50% $\dot{V}O_2$ max, 5 minutes) whereas a combination of high-intensity and long-duration (80% $\dot{V}O_2$ max, 20 minutes) produced the highest concentration.[67] Other intermediate combinations produced an intermediate increase in blood lactate concentration. In summary, we may conclude that immediate post-exercise blood lactate concentration generally relates to exercise intensity but also is influenced by exercise duration.

The variation in blood lactate concentration also depends on the number of repeat bouts of short-duration, high-intensity exercise that is performed and on the length of the rest period taken between bouts. For example, a peak whole-blood lactate concentration of 15.3 meq $\cdot$ L^{-1} (arterial) and 16.7 meq $\cdot$ L^{-1} (femoral vein) were found at the end of the fourth and last bout of 30-sec maximal isokinetic cycling exercise.[104] Balsom[7] studied sprinters who performed 15 repeat 40-m sprints with either a 120-, 60-, or 30-sec rest between each sprint. The sprinters who were allowed the shortest rest period showed the greatest accumulation of blood lactate. This indicates the importance of adequate rest time for the removal of large quantities of blood lactate that build up during repeat bouts of all-out exercise. Surprisingly, after six sprints there was no significant difference in blood lactate concentration due to further bouts of sprinting, regardless of the length of the rest period.

We can pose several important questions about this process of lactate removal during recovery from exercise. For example, how long does it take to remove the accumulated lactate? What factors influence the speed of lactate reduction? What happens to the lactate? What is the relationship between the removal of lactate during recovery and the slow-recovery phase?

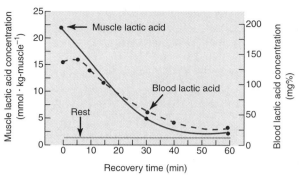

Figure 3.10

Lactic acid is removed from the blood and muscles, during recovery from exhausting exercise. In general, 25 minutes of rest-recovery are required to remove half of the accumulated lactic acid.

(Based on data from Karlsson and Saltin.[92])

Speed of Lactate Removal

The time course of the removal of lactate from blood and muscle is shown in figure 3.10. Exercise consisted of five one-minute bouts of pedaling on a cycle ergometer.[92] Five-minute rest periods were allowed between work bouts. During the recovery period, the subjects (all males) rested while seated on the cycle (rest-recovery). At least one hour of recovery was required to remove most of the accumulated lactate. The same amount of time was also required following running to exhaustion on a treadmill.[98] In general, 25 minutes of rest-recovery are required following maximal exercise to remove half of the accumulated lactate.[75] This means that about 95% of the lactate will be removed in 1 hour and 15 minutes of rest-recovery from maximal exercise.

The lactate concentration shown in figure 3.10 represents average maximal values for both muscle and blood. During submaximal, but heavy, exercise—in which the accumulation of lactate is not as great—less time is required for its removal during recovery. A shorter (three-minute) period of intense one-leg knee extensions leading to exhaustion produced even higher (27 mmol $\cdot$ kg wet $wt^{-1} \cdot min^{-1}$) muscle lactate concentration but showed a faster rate of initial recovery than is shown in figure 3.10.[8] We can estimate that more than two-thirds of the lactate that accumulated in muscle during intense exercise is released to the blood. Muscle lactate concentration in mmol $\cdot$ kg wet $wt^{-1} \cdot min^{-1}$ decreased during recovery to 14.5 (3 minutes), 6.7 (10 minutes), and 3.0 (60 minutes).

Effects of Exercise during Recovery on the Speed of Lactate Removal

The terms **passive** or **resting-recovery** mean that a subject has rested throughout the duration of the recovery period. However, following heavy to maximal exercise, lactate is

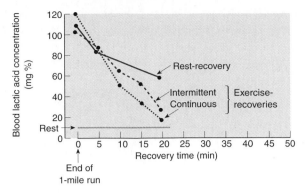

Figure 3.11

Lactic acid can be removed from blood and muscle more rapidly following heavy to maximal exercise by performing light exercise during recovery (exercise-recovery) rather than by resting throughout the recovery period (rest-recovery).

(Based on data from Bonen and Belcastro.[18])

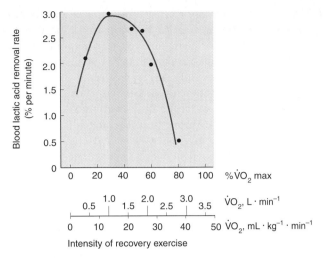

Figure 3.12

For untrained subjects, the recovery exercise that produces the fastest or optimal rate of removal of blood lactic acid is one in which the oxygen consumption ($\dot{V}O_2$) is between 30% and 45% $\dot{V}O_2$ max, or 30% to 45% of $\dot{V}O_2$ max (shaded area).

(Based on data from Belcastro and Bonen.[13])

cleared from blood and muscle more rapidly when light exercise is performed during recovery versus during rest-recovery.[13,18,19,20,61,75,76] Such a recovery is referred to as **exercise recovery,** or active recovery, and is similar to the cool-down procedures that most athletes have practiced for many years. An example of the effects of exercise-recovery on lactate removal is shown in figure 3.11. In these experiments,[18] the subjects ran one mile on three separate days. Three different recovery periods were used: (1) rest, (2) continuous exercise consisting of jogging at a self-selected pace, and (3) intermittent exercise of the kind normally practiced by athletes. Both exercise recoveries resulted in substantial increases in the rate of lactate removed from the blood. The removal rate was fastest during the continuous jogging recovery. This information suggests that athletes should exercise continuously throughout the recovery period rather than intermittently, which is their normal practice.

The early work of Royce[128] indicates that there may be some limitation to the use of an active-recovery procedure. Subjects displayed a slower slow component of O_2 recovery from a maximal cycle ergometer test when they continually pedaled at the same RPM against minimal resistance. This finding for low-intensity active recovery prompted the following question: what intensity of exercise should be performed during recovery to promote optimal lactate removal? The answer can be found in figure 3.12. The rate of blood lactate removal (*y,* vertical axis) is shown plotted against the intensity of the exercise performed during recovery (*x,* horizontal axis). The latter is expressed in three different units: (1) the amount of oxygen consumed during exercise as a percentage of the subject's maximal aerobic power (% $\dot{V}O_2$ max),* (2) as the amount of oxygen consumed

during exercise in liters per minute ($L \cdot min^{-1}$), and (3) as milliliters of oxygen consumed by each kilogram of body weight per minute of exercise ($mL \cdot kg^{-1} \cdot min^{-1}$) The recovery exercise intensity that produces the fastest or optimal rate of removal of blood lactate has been calculated to be between 30% and 45% $\dot{V}O_2$ max.[43] This corresponds to oxygen consumptions of 1.0 to 1.5 $L \cdot min^{-1}$, or of 15 to 20 $mL \cdot kg^{-1} \cdot min^{-1}$ (shaded area in figure 3.12).

These figures, however, were calculated for exercise recovery performed on a cycle ergometer with untrained subjects. With trained subjects whose recovery exercise consisted of running or walking, studies show that lactate removal is optimal at an intensity between 50% and 65% $\dot{V}O_2$ max.[61,76] The major reason for this difference is likely related more to the subject's state of training than to the difference in exercise mode (running or walking versus cycling). In other words, the higher the fitness level (with greater mitochondrial density, blood perfusion, and enzyme capacity), the higher the recovery exercise intensity may need to be for optimal lactate removal. Koutedakis[102] has reported that competitive rowers have the fastest rate of lactate removal when they continue to row at 40% rather than at 60% of their maximal rowing speed.

Note that an optimal active-recovery exercise intensity recommendation is more precise when it is "activity specific"—i.e. the same mode of exercise is used in the criterion test as in the activity itself and the unit of measurement is relevant to exercise performed. Such "specificity" has been shown for active recovery after two minutes of exercise (90% $\dot{V}O_2$ max) on a swimming ergometer.[133] A 15-minute period of free swimming was more effective in reducing blood lactate during recovery than a 15-minute period of walking. By contrast, studies have shown low-intensity leg exercise to be more effective in promoting

---

*For example, if a subject's $\dot{V}O_2$ max is 50 milliliters of oxygen per kg BW per minute ($mL \cdot kg^{-1} \cdot min^{-1}$), or 3.5 liters of oxygen per minute ($L \cdot min^{-1}$), then an exercise load requiring 25 $mL \cdot kg^{-1} \cdot min^{-1}$, or 1.75 $L \cdot min^{-1}$, would represent 50% $\dot{V}O_2$ max (25/50 or 1.75/3.5 × 100 = 50%).

lactate clearance during a 30-minute recovery period after exhaustive arm exercise (canoeing ergometer) than either passive-recovery or low-intensity arm exercise.[6]

Other studies indicate that 10 minutes of active recovery after a maximal oxygen uptake treadmill run increases blood lactate elimination in physically trained prepubescent boys.[115] Also, low intensity cycling (10 W) with one leg resulted in a lowered blood and muscle lactate concentration during the first 10 minutes of recovery from an exhaustive bout of high-intensity exercise (61 $\pm$ 5 W, lasting 3.5 minutes).[9] Adding a hot environment (35 degrees C, 30% RH) did not improve on the superior effectiveness of the active recovery procedure in enhancing blood lactate reduction in subjects recovering from six one-minute bouts of exercise at 100% $\dot{V}O_2$ peak on a cycle ergometer, with one minute rest between bouts.[53] Blood lactate concentration returned more rapidly to a pre-exercise concentration when subjects continued cycling with one leg for 45 minutes and rested for 45 minutes (partial active recovery) as opposed to resting for 90 minutes following high-intensity intermittent cycle exercise.[120] A 20-minute swim at a self-selected pace was an effective form of active recovery to lower blood lactate concentration after a maximal 100-m freestyle sprint performed by male competitive masters swimmers.[125] Active recovery (pedaling at 60 rpm against a 1 kg resistance) is beneficial for the performance of a very short duration (six seconds), high-intensity power test, where only a brief (30-second) recovery interval is allowed.[134]

Contrary findings have shown little profit to the above type of activity in improving recovery from exercise stress. For example, performing an active leg recovery procedure caused further elevation in heart rate and arterial hypotension following repeat six-minute bouts of anaerobic arm crank exercise.[78] Cerretelli[35] designed a unique experiment to study the effect of three minutes of "very active" recovery on blood lactate concentration. A subject who has just completed a 20-second bout of supramaximal exercise (2.5 times $\dot{V}O_2$ max) agreed to perform three additional minutes of anaerobic exercise (at $\dot{V}O_2$ max). The very active "recovery" period was so intense that an even higher blood lactate concentration resulted. A final study addresses muscle glycogen resynthesis after 60 minutes of passive recovery compared with a combination of 30 minutes active (cycling at 40% to 50% $\dot{V}O_2$ max) and 30 minutes passive recovery.[39] Subjects were recovering from three one-minute cycling bouts (130% $\dot{V}O_2$ max) with four minutes of rest between bouts. In this case, mean muscle glycogen after 60 minutes of passive recovery increased 15 mmol $\cdot$ kg wet wt^{-1}, whereas it actually decreased 6.3 units following the 60-minute active recovery protocol. This suggests that passive recovery following intense exercise results in a greater amount of muscle glycogen resynthesis than active recovery of the same duration.

As shown in figure 3.12, when the intensity of the recovery exercise is either below or above the optimal limit (shaded area), lactate is metabolized/degraded more slowly. In fact, when the intensity of the recovery exercise is greater than 60% $\dot{V}O_2$ max, the degradation rate of lactate is actually less than that during rest recovery. The obvious reason is that during the recovery exercise itself, more lactate is being produced than is being removed. One investigator suggested that active recovery should be nearer to 70% of $\dot{V}O_2$ max for the first few minutes, then about 40% of $\dot{V}O_2$ max for the later recovery period.[137] Intuitively, the elite, middle-distance athlete often appears to follow this procedure after a race—a brief period of standing or walking recovery followed by running at a fairly rapid pace and then a slower pace. Dodd et al.,[51] however, has studied this matter in subjects recovering from shorter, (50 seconds) maximal intensity work with a different outcome. The performance of continuous submaximal exercise (35% $\dot{V}O_2$ max for 40 minutes) was more effective than a combination of intensities (65% $\dot{V}O_2$ max for 7 minutes followed by 35% $\dot{V}O_2$ max for 33 minutes) in lowering blood lactate concentration.

Fate of Lactate—Physiology of Lactate Removal

So far we have learned that blood lactate concentration returns toward its resting concentration during recovery from exercise, and that it is removed faster during controlled exercise recovery than during rest-recovery. But what actually happens to the lactate and how is it removed faster during exercise recovery?

Lactate as a fuel in the aerobic pathway accounts for the majority of the lactate removed during recovery from exercise. Although this holds true for both rest- and exercise-recovery procedures, oxidation accounts for more lactate removal in the latter than in the former. Several organs are capable of oxidizing lactate. However, there is consensus that skeletal muscle is the major organ involved in the process.[26,60,75,76,83] Most of the lactate oxidized by muscle occurs within Type I rather than Type II fibers.[18,19,20] This is a major reason why lactate removal is faster during exercise recovery than during rest-recovery. In the former, both the blood flow carrying lactate to the muscles and the metabolic rate of the active muscles is greatly increased. In addition, the type of exercise selected during most exercise-recovery procedures preferentially recruit Type I fibers to perform the work.

A summary of the fate of the lactate removed from blood and muscle during rest-recovery is shown in figure 3.13. The percentages given in the figure were determined from experiments performed on rats after four hours of recovery.[60]

Lactate Removal and the Slow Component of Recovery

For years we assumed that the oxygen consumed during the slow component of recovery was quantitatively related to the removal of lactate during the immediate recovery period

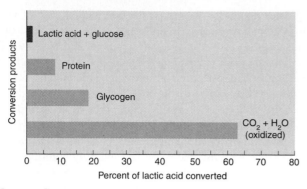

Figure 3.13

The fate of lactic acid. Lactic acid removed from blood and muscle during recovery is metabolically converted to glucose, protein, glycogen, CO_2 and H_2O (oxidized). The last two conversions are the major fates.

(Based on data from Gaesser and Brooks.[60])

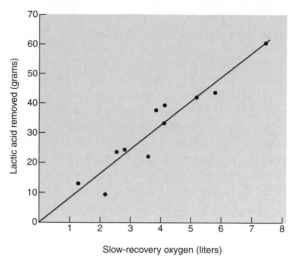

Figure 3.14

A relationship exists between the oxygen consumed during the slow component of recovery and the removal of lactic acid from the blood;[56] however, the exact amount of oxygen required to remove a given quantity of lactic acid varies considerably.[61,127]

from exercise. In fact, figure 3.14 shows a good relationship between the slow recovery component and the removal of lactate from the blood. However, the exact amount of oxygen required to metabolize a given quantity of lactate varies considerably,[61,127] and it is difficult to account for all of the lactate.[84] Such a poor quantitative relationship is not surprising, since there are many possible fates for lactate, each of which requires varying amounts of free energy to be completed. Nevertheless, at least part of the oxygen and ATP energy requirement associated with lactate removal may be met by the oxygen consumed during the slow component of recovery phase.

The magnitude of the slow component of recovery is not greatly affected by the intensity of work below 65% of $\dot{V}O_2$ max. However, for exercise above 65% $\dot{V}O_2$ max and lasting longer than five minutes, the slow-recovery phase has a greater magnitude.[67] The maximum cumulative volume of oxygen during the time course of the slow-component oxygen recovery curve ranges between 5 and 10 liters.[56] It is usually larger in athletes, particularly in those who train for and participate in activities such as the long sprints and 800 meters.

The slow recovery period occupies five time constants with a decay time constant equal to 21.6 minutes—i.e. 30 times slower than that of the fast component.[111] This means that after one hour and 48 minutes of rest recovery, slow recovery is generally completed. During exercise recovery, the slow component is not only smaller by about 1 to 2 liters, but is reduced more quickly.[61]

Restoration of Oxygen Stores

Although the body oxygen stores are small, they are of importance during exercise, particularly during intermittent exercise, because they are used during each work period and replenished during each rest period.

O_2-Myoglobin Stores

Oxygen is stored mainly in the muscle in chemical combination with **myoglobin,** a complex protein compound similar to **hemoglobin** found in the blood. In fact, myoglobin is sometimes referred to as muscle hemoglobin. Although myoglobin acts as a store for oxygen, it is also involved functionally in the actual transfer of oxygen from inside the cellular membrane to the mitochondria within the muscle cell. Thus, myoglobin has a dual role: storage of oxygen and facilitation of the diffusion of oxygen from blood to the mitochondria.

Size and Importance of O_2-Myoglobin Stores

The O_2-myoglobin stores are small. For example, estimates are that only 11.2 milliliters (mL) of oxygen are stored in myoglobin per kilogram (kg) of muscle mass.[72] Assuming a total of 30 kg (66 pounds) of muscle mass in a person weighing 70 kg (154 pounds), this amounts to 336 mL of oxygen ($30 \times 11.2 = 336$ mL O_2). In athletes, who generally have a larger muscle mass, the total O_2-myoglobin stores, although larger, may still be only 500 mL.* However, the O_2-myoglobin stores are important during intermittent exercise—not because of their size, but because of their rapid restoration during a recovery period. This allows them to be used repeatedly during intermittent exercise. An

---

*Assuming that the stored oxygen is used in breaking down carbohydrate, 500 mL of oxygen would resynthesize 145 millimoles, or 0.145 moles, of ATP—enough to meet the energy requirements for about two minutes of resting metabolism.

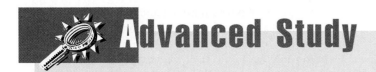

Advanced Study

Lactate in Recovery

There are four possible fates of lactate.

1. *Excretion in urine and sweat.* Lactate is known to be excreted in the urine[90] and sweat.[3] However, the amount of lactate removed in this manner during recovery from exercise is negligible.

2. *Conversion to glucose and/or glycogen.* Because lactate is a byproduct of carbohydrate metabolism (glucose and glycogen) during anaerobic work, it can be reconverted to these compounds in the liver (glycogen and glucose) and in muscle (glycogen) if the required ATP energy is supplied. However, as previously mentioned, glycogen resynthesis in muscle and liver is extremely slow compared with lactate degradation/removal. In addition, the magnitude of the change in the blood glucose concentration during recovery is also minimal. Therefore, conversion of lactate to glucose and glycogen accounts for only a small portion of the total lactate removed.[26,27,44,60] Wasserman et al.[143] have shown that the increase in net hepatic lactate concentration is eight times above rest in catheterized dogs at completion of 10 minutes of moderate-intensity running on a treadmill. The net concentration then decreased so that the liver became an overall net lactate consumer by the end of 150 minutes of exercise and throughout 90 minutes of recovery. Other studies where electrical stimulation was used to elicit maximal exercise indicate that only a small portion (10%) of the lactate formed during exercise is taken up by the liver during an immediate period of recovery.[84] A higher accumulation of lactate, however, tends to stimulate the conversion of circulating lactate to muscle glycogen.[129]

3. *Conversion to protein.* Carbohydrates, including lactate, are converted to protein in the body. However, only a relatively small amount of lactate is converted to protein during the immediate recovery period following exercise.[60]

4. *Oxidation/conversion to CO_2 and H_2O.* Lactate is also a metabolic fuel, principally for skeletal muscle,[26,59,60,75,76,83] but heart muscle,[136] brain,[117] liver,[121] and kidney[151] tissues are also capable of this function. In the presence of oxygen, lactate is first converted to pyruvate[54] and then to CO_2 and H_2O in the Krebs Cycle and the electron transport system, respectively. ATP is resynthesized in coupled reactions in the electron transport system.

---

example of this effect is shown in figure 3.15. The intermittent work performed in these experiments consisted of alternating 15 seconds of work on a cycle ergometer with 15 seconds of rest recovery for one hour. The O_2-myoglobin stores may be calculated to contribute 20% of the total ATP energy required during this time.[52] This is more than from either the stored phosphagens or anaerobic glycolysis.

The importance of the oxygen stores is emphasized in the following:

1. Assuming that the total muscle mass involved during the intermittent work performed in the preceding experiments was 15 kg, then the total O_2-myoglobin stores involved was 168 mL of oxygen (15 × 11.2 = 168 mL).

2. Alternating 15 seconds of work with 15 seconds of rest recovery during a period of one hour means that there were two rest-recovery periods each minute, or 120 during the hour. Assuming that only half of the stores were replenished during each of the rest-recovery periods, then 84 mL of oxygen (168 ÷ 2 = 84 mL) were restored per rest period, or 10 liters of oxygen over the hour (84 × 120 = 10,080 mL). This represents a substantial amount of oxygen for use during the work periods (e.g., enough to generate 3 moles of ATP aerobically).

Mechanism of Replenishment of the O_2-Myoglobin Stores

Because oxygen is bound to myoglobin in chemical combination, the restoration of the O_2-myoglobin stores depends mainly on the availability of oxygen. In turn, the availability of oxygen depends on its *partial pressure*. For a discussion on the concept of partial pressure, refer to chapter 8. For our present purposes, we need only remember that during exercise, particularly during heavy exercise, the demand for oxygen is high. Consequently, the oxygen that was combined with myoglobin is readily given up to the mitochondria. Just the opposite is true during recovery from exercise. Here the availability of oxygen is greatly increased, causing a recharging of myoglobin with oxygen, a process requiring only a few seconds to complete.[29] Oxygen consumed

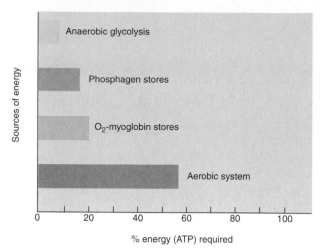

Figure 3.15

The O_2-myoglobin stores are important during intermittent exercise because they are used during the work intervals and are quickly restored during the recovery intervals. As shown here, 20% of the total energy required during 1 hour of work, consisting of 15 seconds of work alternated with 15 seconds of recovery, was derived from the O_2-myoglobin stores.

(Based on data from Essen et al.[52])

during the fast component of recovery supplies the necessary oxygen for restoration of the O_2-myoglobin stores. The recovery time for the hemoglobin-to-myoglobin ratio in the quadriceps capillary bed of elite male and female rowers following near-maximal voluntary contraction ranges from 10 to 80 seconds.[36]

Other Recovery Considerations

The following section indicates some elements measured in blood and muscle that signal the disruptive effect of exercise that necessitates post-exercise rest and recovery. They are considered under the headings of lipid and amino acid metabolism and H^+, Pi, and K^+ concentrations, respectively. Some of these factors have only been implicated recently in the search for a comprehensive explanation for the alteration of events during the fast and slow components of recovery.

Lipid Metabolism

Up to this point our emphasis has been on changes related to the restoration of high-energy phosphagens, blood glucose, muscle and liver glycogen, and the degradation of lactate during recovery from exercise. This is primarily a consideration of how best to return these substances back to their resting concentration as quickly and as completely as possible. Let's now ask what the role of lipid metabolism

is. Fats are metabolized during exercise, so it is reasonable to assume that their metabolism continues during recovery. Hagenfeldt[68] used continuous infusion of 14C-labeled oleic acid to study the turnover of free fatty acids (FFA) following exercise. Arterial FFA reached a maximum of twice the exercise value after six minutes of recovery and remained 75% above the basal concentration for 20 minutes. The post-exercise rise in circulating FFA concentration during the early stage of recovery may be due to the removal of sympathetic vasoconstrictor tone. This leads to an increase in the release of FFA into the plasma pool above the level observed during exercise. The final result is an increase in the rate of removal of FFA at the end of exercise that remains above basal level during recovery for as long as the arterial concentration is elevated. Plasma FFA and glycerol concentration are both related to the intensity and duration of exercise and may remain elevated for at least 12 hours after exhaustive exercise.[16] This represents a large energy flux from lipid metabolism, with the ATP generated used to restore the other depleted energy sources.[4]

The response to a 100-g oral glucose tolerance test administered after an overnight fasted rest is dramatically influenced by previously performing three hours of treadmill exercise at 50% of $\dot{V}O_2$ max[103] in that there is a significant increase in lipid oxidation compared with rest. Carlin[32] reported no net loss of muscle carnitine after 90 minutes of cycle ergometer exercise, indicating that this important lipid metabolite remains fully in place. Lipid metabolism in the heart of rats after two hours of continuous swimming display an elevated lipolytic activity (26% above the control animals) after one hour of recovery, which does not return to the resting concentration until four hours later.[124] Cardiac triglyceride (TG) concentration returned to normal in the same animals after only two hours of recovery, meaning that the rate of TG synthesis during recovery is in excess of its hydrolysis.

There appears to be a time constraint to the degree of exercise-induced increase in lipid metabolism during recovery. Maron[114] reported no prolonged alteration in FFA, glycerol, or TG after one, two, and three days of recovery from running a competitive marathon. Finally, studies have suggested that two-thirds of the total net recovery oxygen following one-legged short-term, intense, exhaustive exercise may be linked to the metabolic use of intramuscular triacyglycerol, a byproduct of TG breakdown.[8] In summary, it appears that an elevated lipid metabolism continues into recovery and is a more important source of O_2 utilization and ATP production than previously believed.

Amino Acid Conversion

Although the contribution of amino acid's metabolism to ATP production is limited during exercise, it is important to long-duration activity and the subsequent recovery from it. Brooks[21] found that amino acids may provide up to 10% of the total energy for sustained exercise, therefore affecting muscle glycogen use. If less muscle glycogen is used, there is an increased potential for prolonged exercise at a high metabolic rate. Alanine, lactate, and pyruvate are major metabolites in **gluconeogenesis.** Since several other amino acids can be converted to alanine following conversion to glutamate, they provide a carbon source to assist in maintaining blood glucose concentration during exercise and to glycogen restoration during recovery. A marked increase in liver gluconeogenesis has been shown in dogs after 150 minutes of treadmill running.[144] The increase primarily results from an increase in the fractional extraction of alanine from the circulation by the liver, where it is effectively channeled into glucose. Gluconeogenesis via alanine increases during recovery as the delivery of alanine to the liver increases above the rate observed during exercise.[144] Prolonged aerobic exercise (four hours at 40% $\dot{V}O_2$ max) stimulates muscle protein breakdown, which does not result in a significant depletion of muscle mass because muscle protein synthesis is stimulated throughout four hours of recovery.[34] A high intake ($2.0 \ g \cdot kg^{-1} \cdot d^{-1}$) of protein facilitates this response, when compared to the recommended daily intake ($0.9 \ g \cdot kg^{-1} \cdot d^{-1}$) of protein.[33] As for lipids, it appears that amino acid conversion and metabolism plays a larger role during recovery from exercise than previously believed.

Concentrations of H^+, Pi and K^+

With the application of 31P magnetic resonance spectroscopy (MRS), magnetic resonance imagery (MRI), and nuclear magnetic resonance (NMR) techniques, it has been possible to follow the time course of change in the intramuscular concentrations of H^+, Pi, and K^+, as well as muscle proton transverse relaxation times during exercise and recovery.[37,97,149] This has provided new insight into the dynamics of change at the molecular level in ion exchange and has brought some challenges to traditional ideas. The rate of return of arterial pH (hydrogen ion concentration, H^+) in normal subjects during passive recovery depends on the intensity of the work rate.[139] There is a rapid return to a pre-exercise value after moderate work, but a further decrease during the first two minutes of recovery for both heavy intensity and very heavy intensity work—then a slower return toward a resting value for all work intensities. Intramuscular pH declined from 7.1 to 6.4 in the adductor pollicis muscle of humans at the point of fatigue and returned to normal within 20 minutes.[116] A similar pattern was produced by exhaustive dynamic leg extension exercise[65] and by exhaustive cycle ergometer exercise. Intramuscular pH decreased from 7.0 at rest to 6.4 at the point of exhaustion and returned to resting level after 20 minutes of recovery.[130] By contrast, subjects who sprinted for 30 seconds still showed a decreased pH after 30 minutes of passive recovery.[1] The proton flux from lactic acid is buffered passively during

exercise,[97] but pH may continue to decrease during the first two minutes of recovery.[149]

Generally, it is believed that the reduction in intramuscular pH is accompanied by reduction in indexes of work performance resulting from the increase in blood lactate concentration. pH measured by the 31P MRS technique is closely correlated ($r = -0.84$) with muscle lactate accumulation.[140] However, recovery from repeated 30-second maximal sprints on a cycle ergometer takes place despite the fact that muscle pH remains very low[17] and that there is evidence for nonlinearity in the oxidative recovery process.[106] Boska[21] has reported an approximate linear relationship between the decline in maximal voluntary contraction (MVC) during a four minute sustained contraction and the accumulation of H^+ and Pi during both fatigue and recovery. Since MVC correlated best with the change in Pi, it was felt that this metabolite is an important factor in muscle fatigue and recovery. Pi reaches its maximal concentration at the time of exhaustion and begins to return toward a pre-exercise concentration immediately on cessation of dynamic exercise.[149] Pi correlates closely to ATP production from glycogen breakdown during the start of aerobic exercise and throughout exercise performed under ischemic conditions,[96] and it maintains an approximate linear relationship to PC resynthesis during the recovery process.[95] Pi concentration has been used as an indication of metabolic restoration after the production of moderate fatigue in a relatively short (2 minutes) versus a longer (15 to 20 minutes) exercise period.[5] Fatigue closely correlated with increased Pi, but both measures had recovered within 5 minutes after exercise was stopped.

Lindener indicates that several studies have shown that exercise results in a release of K^+ ions from contracting muscles, which produces a decrease in the intracellular K^+ concentration and an increase in plasma K^+ concentration.[104,105] The response of muscle to the loss of intracellular K^+ has been cited as a contributing factor to muscle fatigue due to the concomitant increase in intracellular Na^+ concentration that disrupts normal sarcolemma membrane potential and cell excitability. During exercise there is an ongoing attempt to regulate cellular and whole body K^+ homeostasis via an increased uptake of K^+ by contracting muscles and inactive tissues. These efforts are made through activation of the Na^+-K^+ pump to restore the active muscle intracellular K^+ concentration to a pre-contraction level and to prevent plasma K^+ concentration from rising to a toxic level. Following exercise, plasma K^+ concentration $[K^+]$ rapidly returns to resting level, a change that is associated with improvements in muscle contraction. The change in both arterial and femoral venous $[K^+]$ is more rapid during exercise (30 second bouts of maximal isokinetic cycling) and recovery than is the change in lactate.[104] Plasma $[K^+]$ increases immediately upon completion of a 100 m maximal swim effort, then decreases significantly at the 2.5- and 5-minute post-exercise points, respectively, and returning to a near baseline concentration after 30 minutes of recovery.

Performance Recovery

Some recent studies have addressed the matter of performance recovery—i.e., how quickly do subjects recover a given measure of performance like force, power, or isometric tension? For example, Sherman[132] has emphasized that although muscle and liver glycogen levels may be normalized 24 hours after exercise, muscle function and performance measures may not be fully recovered. Does this pattern hold true for different types, intensities and durations of exercise—i.e., is there any generalizable pattern of performance recovery? The 48-hour recovery pattern was similar for subjects who performed 60 minutes of either level jogging, downhill jogging on a −5% grade, or stationary cycling, all at 60% of $\dot{V}O_2$ max.[142] Energy expenditure levels were still elevated and recovery was not complete after nine hours of "regulated" recovery. This indicates that the type of aerobic exercise may not be a strong influence on the recovery pattern provided that the intensity and duration are similar.

The type of exercise may have a stronger influence on the length of the performance recovery period. For example, recovery of isometric handgrip endurance capacity after complete fatigue is very rapid at first, much slower after 10 minutes, but is still 85 to 90% complete after 40 minutes.[57] This finding matches well with a 60-minute period that was needed to attain full recovery of isometric endurance time following voluntary contractions to fatigue.[40] It is of interest that the amplitude of the EMG had still not returned to pre-fatigue levels after four hours of recovery. The time course of recovery is somewhat faster for dynamic muscular contractions performed to failure; progressing very rapidly at first, reaching 50% at 2.25 minutes and being 90% complete at 20 minutes.[150] Recovery from maximal effort isokinetic cycling to fatigue was even faster with full recovery of peak voluntary or peak stimulated (percutaneous electrical) pedalling force in about three minutes.[12]

The intensity of prior exercise may also present a strong influence on performance measures during recovery. For example, dynamic exercise on a cycle ergometer influences the speed of recovery of short term power output. Subjects who pedalled at 60% and 80% of $\dot{V}O_2$ max were fully recovered in one minute, whereas full recovery from 100% $\dot{V}O_2$ max effort required 4 min, and only 90% recovery from supramax efforts (120% $\dot{V}O_2$ max) had occurred after 8 min of recovery.[82] The importance of a solid aerobic foundation—i.e., relatively high $\dot{V}O_2$ max—on the rate of recovery from short-term, high-intensity exercise has been demonstrated. Sinacore[135] reports a high, negative correlation ($r = -.84$) between the percentage of reduction in torque after 30 seconds of recovery from a 60-second isokinetic exercise test and a subject's $\dot{V}O_2$ max. This means that those with the highest maximal oxygen uptake capabilities showed the least amount of residual fatigue after 30 seconds of recovery. Said differently, those with a higher "aerobic base" recovered their muscle function faster. Many

of the metabolic changes during recovery including ATP, CP, and ADP restoration toward normal correlate with the aerobic-oxidative potential of skeletal muscle and this is a most important determinant of recovery rates.[89]

It is of interest to note that there can be mismatches between commonly expected metabolic markers of recovery status and performance measures. For example, elevated blood lactate levels at the end of 20 minutes of recovery did not adversely effect the work output of subjects who repeated a 5-min all out effort on a stationary cycle ergometer.[147]

Some Practical Recovery Guidelines

From the previous discussion, you should now be able to draw some conclusions about the relative time required for adequate recovery from various exhausting exercise performances. Table 3.2 presents some suggestions.

Summary

The process of recovery from exercise involves restoration of the muscle and the rest of the body to their pre-exercise condition. During recovery from exercise, oxygen consumption remains elevated above the resting level for varying lengths of time. The additional oxygen consumed above rest is termed the recovery oxygen. During the first two or three minutes of recovery, there is a high rate of oxygen consumption followed by a gradual decline to near-resting level. The initial three to six minutes of recovery has been named the fast component, whereas the slower phase has been named the slow component of recovery. In contemporary literature, the terminology of recovery events is in an evolutionary stage, and some sources continue to use the expression *oxygen debt* for recovery oxygen.

Much of the muscular ATP and PC store that is depleted during exercise is rapidly restored during the first three to five minutes of the recovery period. The ATP energy required for this process is supplied mainly by the aerobic system through the oxygen consumed during the fast component of recovery. The reduction of the fast component is completed in only a few minutes. The maximum size of the fast component ranges between 2 and 3 liters of oxygen, although a much higher value has been recorded in trained athletes.

Lactate, as a metabolic product of glycolysis during exercise, has, as a principal fate, oxidation to CO_2 and H_2O. The concentration of lactate found in the blood at any time during either rest or activity is a function of the rate of production and the rate of degradation of this important metabolite.

3.2

Suggested minimum and maximum recovery times following exhaustive exercise

Recovery process	Suggested recovery time	
	Minimum	**Maximum**
Restoration of muscle phosphagen stores (ATP + PC)	2 minutes	5 minutes
Disappearance of the fast component of recovery O_2	3 minutes	6 minutes
Muscle glycogen replenishment	10 hours (after continuous exercise)	46 hours
	5 hours (after intermittent exercise)	24 hours
Liver glycogen replenishment	unknown	12–24 hours
Reduction of lactic acid in blood and muscle	30 minutes (with exercise-recovery)	1 hour
	1 hour (with rest-recovery)	2 hours
Reduction of the slow component of the recovery O_2	30 minutes	1 hour
Restoration of O_2 stores (plasma, myoglobin)	10–15 seconds	1 minute

Although not discussed directly in the chapter, an understanding of the importance of lactate in metabolism—its fate, its role in muscle fatigue, and its production and removal—has undergone a significant change. The reviews by Katz and Sahlin (1990) and Stainsby and Brooks (1990) present a concise exposition of the role of this important metabolite in exercise and recovery.

Restoration of the muscle and liver glycogen stores depleted during exercise depends on the type of exercise performed (continuous versus intermittent) and may require several days for completion, during which time dietary intake of carbohydrate is necessary. Following continuous, exhausting exercise, muscle glycogen restoration is 60% completed in 10 hours of recovery and is fully completed within 46 hours. Following intermittent, exhausting exercise, restoration of muscle glycogen is 53% completed in five hours and is fully completed in 24 hours. Only small amounts of muscle and liver glycogen are restored within the immediate (one to two hours) recovery period following maximal exercise of either type. The ATP energy for muscle and liver glycogen restoration comes from the aerobic system, but does not involve the oxygen consumed during the slow component of recovery to a great extent.

The lactate accumulated in blood and muscle during exercise is removed during the recovery period. The speed of lactate removal depends on whether a subject rests during recovery (rest-recovery) or performs light exercise (30% to 65% $\dot{V}O_2$ max) during recovery (exercise recovery). Lactate is removed faster during exercise recovery. Blood lactate is degraded by (1) conversion to glucose and/or glycogen, (2) conversion to protein, and (3) oxidation to CO_2 and H_2O by the aerobic system. The blood lactate's major fate is oxidation to CO_2 and water, which occurs mainly in skeletal muscle, but also occurs in heart, kidney, liver, and brain tissues. Although at least part of the oxygen and ATP energy required for lactate removal probably comes from the slow component of recovery, no quantitative relationship between the two has thus far been determined. The maximal size of the slow component is usually between 5 and 10 liters of oxygen.

Oxygen is stored in skeletal muscle in chemical combination with myoglobin. Although the stores are small, they are of importance during intermittent exercise because they are used during the work periods and are restored during the rest periods. Restoration of the O_2-myoglobin stores during recovery is rapid, requiring only a few seconds, and depends on the availability (partial pressure) of oxygen. The oxygen is part of the fast component of recovery.

Questions

1. Describe the revision of post-exercise oxygen-consumption terminology.
2. Define recovery oxygen and its components.
3. How rapidly are the phosphagen stores (ATP + PC) replenished during recovery?
4. What is the relationship between restoration of the ATP and PC stores in the muscle and the fast component of recovery?
5. How large is the fast component of recovery and what is the significance of its size?

6. Discuss the restoration of the muscle glycogen stores with respect to: (a) the type (continuous versus intermittent) of previous exercise performed, (b) the presence or absence of food intake during recovery, (c) the physiological factors related to the different rates of glycogen restoration, and (d) the energetics of glycogen replenishment.

7. What are the effects of exercise, diet, and recovery from exercise on liver glycogen stores?

8. What is meant by rest recovery and exercise recovery, and how do they influence the rate of lactate removed?

9. Discuss the fate of lactate removed during recovery. What organs and tissues are involved in this process?

10. What is the relationship between lactate removal and the fast component of recovery?

11. Explain the importance of the oxygen stores during intermittent exercise.

12. Suppose an athlete were to compete first in the 800-meter run, then about an hour or so later in the 1500-meter run. What would you, as a coach, tell the athlete concerning the fastest way to recover between events?

References

1. Allsop, P., M. Cheetham, S. Brooks, G. M. Hall, and C. Williams. 1990. Continuous intramuscular pH measurement during the recovery from brief, maximal exercise in man. *Eur J Appl Physiol.* 59(6):465–470.

2. Altman, P. L., and D. S. Dittmer (eds). 1966. Environmental Biology. *Fed of Amer Soc for Exper Biol.*, pp. 4–5.

3. Åstrand, I. 1963. Lactate content in sweat. *Acta Physiol Scand.* 58:359–367.

4. Bahr, R., A. T. Hostmark, E. A. Newsholme, O. Gronnerod, and O. M. Sejersted. 1991. Effect of exercise on recovery changes in plasma levels of FFA, glycerol, glucose and catecholamines. *Acta Physiol Scand.* 143:105–115.

5. Baker, A. J., K. G. Kostov, R. G. Miller, and M. W. Weiner. 1993. Slow force recovery after long-duration exercise: Metabolic and activation factors in muscle fatigue. *J Appl Physiol.* 74(5):2294–2300.

6. Baker, S. J., and N. King. 1991. Lactic acid recovery profiles following exhaustive arm exercise on a canoeing ergometer. *Br J Sports Med.* 25(3):165–167.

7. Balsom, P. D., J. Y. Seger, B. Sjodin, and B. Ekblom. 1992. Maximal-intensity intermittent exercise: Effect of recovery duration. *Int J Sports Med.* 13(7):528–533.

8. Bangsbo, J., P. D. Gollnick, T. E. Graham, and B. Saltin. 1991. Substrates for muscle glycogen synthesis in recovery from intense exercise in man. *J Physiol.* (London) 434:423–440.

9. Bangsbo, J., T. Graham, L. Johansen, and B. Saltin. 1994. Muscle lactate metabolism in recovery from intense exhaustive exercise: impact of light exercise. *J Appl Physiol.* 77(4):1890–1895.

10. Barnard, R. J., and M. L. Foss. 1969. Oxygen debt: effect of beta-adrenergic blockade on the lactacid and alactacid components. *J Appl Physiol.* 27:813–816.

11. Barnard, R. J., C. M. Tipton, and M. L. Foss. 1970. Oxygen debt: Involvement of the Cori cycle. *Int Z Angew Physiol.* 28:105–119.

12. Beelen, A., A. J. Sargeant, D. A. Jones, and C. J. de Ruiter 1995. Fatigue and recovery of voluntary and electrically elicited dynamic force in humans. *J Physiol* (London) 484:227–235.

13. Belcastro, A. N., and A. Bonen. 1975. Lactic acid removal rates during controlled and uncontrolled recovery exercise. *J Appl Physiol.* 39(6):932–936.

14. Berg, K. E. 1991. Comparison of energy expenditure in men and women at rest and during exercise recovery. *J Sports Med Phys Fitness* 31(3):351–356.

15. Bergstrom, J., L. Hermansen, E. Hultman, and B. Saltin. 1967. Diet, muscle glycogen and physical performance. *Acta Physiol Scand.* 71:140–150.

16. Bielinski, R., Y. Schutz, and E. Jequier. 1985. Energy metabolism during the postexercise recovery in man. *Am J Clin Nutr.* 42(1):69–82.

17. Bogdanis, G. C., M. E. Nevill, L. H. Boobis, H. K. Lakomy, and A. M. Nevill. 1995. Recovery of power output and muscle metabolites following 30 s of maximal sprint cycling in man. *J Physiol.* (London) 482:467–480.

18. Bonen, A., and A. N. Belcastro. 1976. Comparison of self-selected recovery methods on lactic acid removal rates. *Med Sci Sports.* 8(3):176–178.

19. Bonen, A., C. J. Campbell, R. L. Kirby, and A. N. Belcastro. 1979. A multiple regression model for blood lactate removal in man. *Pflugers Arch.* 380:205–210.

20. ———. 1978. Relationship between slow-twitch muscle fibers and lactic removal. *Can J Appl Sport Sci.* 3:160–162.

21. Boska, M. D., R. S. Moussavi, P. J. Carson, M. W. Weiner, and R. G. Miller. 1990. The metabolic basis of recovery after fatiguing exercise of human muscle. *Neurology* 40(2):240–244.

22. Bowers, R. W., and E. L. Fox. 1992. *Sports Physiology.* Dubuque, IA: Wm. C. Brown.

23. Brehm, B. A., and B. Gutin. 1986. Recovery energy expenditure for steady state exercise in runners and nonexercisers. *Med Sci Sports Exerc.* 18(2):205–210.

24. Brooks, G. A. 1987. Amino acid and protein metabolism during exercise and recovery. *Med Sci Sports Exerc.* 19(5 Suppl.): S150–156.

25. Brooks, G. A. 1986. The lactate shuttle during exercise and recovery. *Med Sci Sports Exerc.* 18(3):360–368.

26. Brooks, G. A., K. E. Brauner, and R. G. Cassens. 1973. Glycogen synthesis and metabolism of lactic acid after exercise. *Am J Physiol.* 224:1162–1166.

27. Brooks, G. A., and G. A. Gaesser. 1980. End points of lactate and glucose metabolism after exhausting work. *J Appl Physiol.* 49:1057–1069.

28. Brooks, G. A., K. J. Hittelman, J. A. Faulkner, and R. E. Beyer. 1971. Temperature, liver mitochondrial respiratory functions, and oxygen debt. *Med Sci Sports.* 3(2):72–74.

29. ———. 1971. Temperature, skeletal muscle mitochondrial functions, and oxygen debt. *Am J Physiol.* 220(4):1053–1059.

30. ———. 1971. Tissue temperatures and whole-animal oxygen consumption after exercise. *Am J Physiol.* 221(2):427–431.

31. Calles, J., J. J. Cunningham, L. Nelson, N. Brown, E. Nadel, R. S. Sherwin, and P. Felig. 1983. Glucose turnover during recovery from intense exercise. *Diabetes.* 32:734–738.

32. Carlin, J. I., W. G. Reddan, M. Sanjak, and R. Hodach. 1986. Carnitine metabolism during prolonged exercise and recovery in humans. *J Appl Physiol.* 61(4):1275–1278.

33. Carraro, F., W. H. Hartl, C. A. Stuart, D. K. Layman, F. Jahoor, and R. R. Wolfe. 1990. Whole body and plasma protein synthesis in exercise and recovery in human subjects. *Am J Physiol.* 258(5 Pt 1):E821–831.

34. Carraro, F., C. A. Stuart, W. H. Hartl, J. Rosenblatt, and R. R. Wolfe. 1990. Effect of exercise and recovery on muscle protein synthesis in human subjects. *Am J Physiol.* 259(4 Pt 1):E470–476.

35. Cerretelli, P., G. Ambrosoli, and M. Fumagalli. 1975. Anaerobic recovery in man. *Eur J Appl Physiol.* 34:141–148.

36. Chance, B., M. T. Dait, C. Zhang, T. Hamoaka, and F. Hagerman. 1992. Recovery from exercise-induced desaturation in the quadriceps muscles of elite competitive rowers. *Am J Physiol.* 262(3 Pt 1):C766–775.

37. Cheng, H. A., R. A. Robergs, J. P. Letellier, A. Caprihan, M. V. Icenogle, and L. J. Haseler. 1995. Changes in muscle proton transverse relaxation times and acidosis during exercise and recovery. *J Appl Physiol.* 79(4):1370–1378.

38. Chick, T. W., T. G. Cagle, F. A. Vegas, J. K. Poliner, and G. H. Murata. 1991. The effect of aging on submaximal exercise performance and recovery. *J Gerontol.* 46(1):B34–38.

39. Choi, D., K. J. Cole, B. H. Goodpaster, W. J. Fink, and D. L. Costill. 1994. Effect of passive and active recovery on the resynthesis of muscle glycogen. *Med Sci Sports Exerc.* 26(8):992–996.

40. Cornwall, M. W., L. P. Krock, and L. M. Wagner. 1994. Muscular fatigue and recovery following alternating isometric contractions at different levels of force. *Aviat Space Environ Med.* 65(4):309–314.

41. Costill, D. L., R. W. Bowers, G. Branam, and K. Sparks. 1971. Muscle glycogen utilization during prolonged exercise on successive days. *J Appl Physiol.* 31:834–838.

42. Costill, D. L., W. M. Sherman, W. J. Fink, C. Maresh, M. Witten, and J. M. Miller. 1982. The role of dietary carbohydrate in muscle glycogen resynthesis after strenuous running. *Am J Clin Nutri.* 34:1831–1836.

43. Davies, C. T., A. V. Knibbs, and J. Musgrove. 1970. The rate of lactic acid removal in relation to different baselines of recovery exercise. *Int Z Angew Physiol.* 28(3):155–161.

44. Depocas, F., Y. Minaire, and J. Charonnet. 1969. Rates of formation and oxidation of lactic acid in dogs at rest and during moderate exercise. *Can J Physiol Pharmacol.* 47:603–610.

45. Devlin, J. T., J. Barlow, and E. S. Horton. 1989. Whole body and regional fuel metabolism during early postexercise recovery. *Am J Physiol.* 256:E167–172.

46. Devlin, J. T., and E. S. Horton. 1989. Metabolic fuel utilization during postexercise recovery. *Am J Clin Nutr.* 49(5 Suppl.): 944–948.

47. DiPrampero, P. E. 1971. The alactacid oxygen debt: its power, capacity and efficiency. In Pernow, B., and B. Saltin (eds.), *Muscle Metabolism during Exercise.* New York: Plenum Press, pp. 371–382.

48. DiPrampero, P. E., and R. Margaria. 1969. Mechanical efficiency of phosphagen (ATP + PC) splitting and its speed of resynthesis. *Pflugers Arch.* 308:197–202.

49. ———. 1968. Relationship between O$_2$ consumption, high energy phosphates and the kinetics of the O$_2$ debt in exercise. *Pflugers Arch.* 304:11–19.

50. DiPrampero, P. E., L. Peeters, and R. Margaria. 1973. Alactic O$_2$ debt and lactic acid production after exhausting exercise in man. *J Appl Physiol.* 34:628–632.

51. Dodd, S., S. K. Powers, T. Callender, and E. Brooks. 1984. Blood lactate disappearance at various intensities of recovery exercise. *J Appl Physiol.* 57(5)1462–1465.

52. Essen, B., L. Hagenfeldt, and L. Kaijser. 1977. Utilization of blood-borne and intramuscular substrates during continuous and intermittent exercise in man. *J Physiol.* 265:480–506.

53. Falk, B., M. Einbinder, Y. Weinstein, S. Epstein, Y. Karni, Y. Yarom, and A. Rotstein. 1995. Blood lactate concentration following exercise: effects of heat exposure and of active recovery in heat-acclimatized subjects. *Int J Sports Med.* 16(1):7–12.

54. Freund, H., J. Marbach, C. Ott, J. Lonsdorfer, A. Heitz, P. Zouloumian, and P. Kehayoff. 1980. Blood pyruvate recovery curves after short heavy submaximal exercise in man. *Eur J Appl Physiol.* 43(1):83–91.

55. Fox, E. L. 1973. Measurement of the maximal alactic (phosphagen) capacity in man. *Med Sci Sports.* 5:66.

56. Fox, E. L., S. Robinson, and D. Wiegman. 1969. Metabolic energy sources during continuous and interval running. *J Appl Physiol.* 27:174–178.

57. Funderburk, C. F., S. G. Hipskind, R. C. Welton, and A. R. Lind. 1974. Development of and recovery from fatigue induced by static effort at various tensions. *J Appl Physiol* 37(3):392–396.

58. Gaesser, G. A., and G. A. Brooks. 1980. Glycogen repletion following continuous and intermittent exercise to exhaustion. *J Appl Physiol.* 49:722–728.

59. ———. 1984. Metabolic bases of excess post-exercise oxygen consumption: A review. *Med Sci Sports Exerc.* 16(1):29–43.

60. ———. 1979. Metabolism of lactate after prolonged exercise to exhaustion. Gaesser, G. A., and G. A. Brooks. (Abstract). *Med Sci Sports.* 11:76.

61. Gisolfi, C., S. Robinson, and E. S. Turrell. 1966. Effects of aerobic work performed during recovery from exhausting work. *J Appl Physiol.* 21:1767–1772.

62. Gladden, L. B., W. B. Stainsby, and B. R. McIntosh. 1982. Norepinephrine increased canine skeletal muscle $\dot{V}O_2$ during recovery. *Med Sci Sports Exerc.* 14:471–476.

63. Goodman, C., G. G. Rogers, H. Vermaak, and M. R. Goodman. 1985. Biochemical responses during recovery from maximal and submaximal swimming exercise. *Eur J Appl Physiol.* 54(4):436–441.

64. Gore, C. J., and R. T. Withers. 1990. The effect of exercise intensity and duration on the oxygen deficit and excess post-exercise oxygen consumption. *Eur J Appl Physiol.* 60:169–174.

65. Graham, T. E., J. Bangsbo, P. D. Gollnick, C. Juel, and B. Saltin. 1990. Ammonia metabolism during intense dynamic exercise and recovery in humans. *Am J Physiol.* 259:E170–176.

66. Hagberg, J. M., R. C. Hickson, A. A. Ehsani, and J. O. Holloszy. 1980. Faster adjustment to and recovery from submaximal exercise in the trained state. *J Appl Physiol.* 48(2):218–224.

67. Hagberg, J. M., J. P. Mullin, and F. P. Nagle. 1980. Effect of work intensity and duration on recovery O$_2$. *J Appl Physiol.* 48.540–544.

68. Hagenfeldt, L., and J. Wahren. 1975. Turnover of free fatty acids during recovery from exercise. *J Appl Physiol.* 39(2):247–250.

69. Hagerman, F. C., M. C. Conners, J. A. Gault, G. R. Hagerman, and W. J. Polinski. 1978. Energy expenditure during stimulated rowing. *J Appl Physiol.* 45(1):87–93.

70. Hagerman, F. C., E. L. Fox, M. Conners, and J. Pompei. 1974. Metabolic responses of women rowers during ergometric rowing. *Med Sci Sports.* 6(1):87.

71. Harris, R. C., R. H. T. Edwards, E. Hultman, L.-O. Nordesjo, B. Nylind, and K. Sahlin. 1976. The time course of phosphorylcreatine resynthesis during recovery of the quadriceps muscle in man. *Pflugers Arch.* 367:137–142.

72. Harris, R. C., E. Hultman, L. Kaijser, and L.-O. Nordesjo. 1975. The effect of circulatory occlusion on isometric exercise capacity and energy metabolism of the quadriceps muscle in man. *Scand J Clin Invest.* 35:87–95.

73. Hermansen, L. 1980. Resynthesis of muscle glycogen stores during recovery from prolonged exercise in non-diabetic and diabetic subjects. *Acta Paediatr Scand Suppl.* 283:33–38.

74. Hermansen, L., E. Hultman, and B. Saltin. 1967. Muscle glycogen during prolonged severe exercise. *Acta Physiol Scand.* 71:129–139.

75. Hermansen, L., S. Maehlum, E. D. R. Pruett, O. Vaage, H. Waldum, and T. Wesselman. 1975. Lactate removal at rest and during exercise. In Howald, H., and J. R. Poortmans (eds.), *Metabolic Adaptation to Prolonged Physical Exercise.* Basel, Switzerland: Birkhauser-Verlag, pp. 101–105.

76. Hermansen, L., and I. Stensvold. 1972. Production and removal of lactate during exercise in man. *Acta Physiol Scand.* 86:191–201.

77. Hermansen, L., and O. Vaage. 1977. Lactate disappearance and glycogen synthesis in human muscle after maximal exercise. *Am J Physiol.* 233(5):E422–E429.

78. Hildebrandt, W., H. Schutze, and J. Stegemann. 1992. Cardiovascular limitations of active recovery from strenuous exercise. *Eur J Appl Physiol.* 64(3):250–257.

79. Hill, A. V., C. N. H. Long, and H. Lupton. 1924. Muscular exercise, lactic acid and the supply and utilization of oxygen. *Proc Roy Soc.* (London). 96:438–475.

80. Hill, A. V., and H. Lupton. 1923. Muscular exercise, lactic acid and the supply and utilization of oxygen. *Q J Med.* 16:135–171.

81. ———. 1922. The oxygen consumption during running. *J Physiol.* 56:xxxii–xxxiii.

82. Hitchcock, H. C. 1989. Recovery of short-term power after dynamic exercise. *J Appl Physiol.* 67(2):677–681.

83. Hubbard, J. L. 1973. The effect of exercise on lactate metabolism. *J Physiol.* 231:1–18.

84. Hultman, E. H. 1986. Carbohydrate metabolism during hard exercise and in the recovery period after exercise. *Acta Physiol Scand Suppl.* 556:75–82.

85. Hultman, E., and J. Bergstrom. 1967. Muscle glycogen synthesis in relation to diet studied in normal subjects. *Acta Med Scand.* 182:109–117.

86. Hultman, E., J. Bergstrom, and N. McLennan-Anderson. 1967. Breakdown and resynthesis of phosphorylcreatine and adenosine triphosphate in connection with muscular work in man. *Scand J Clin Invest.* 19:56–66.

87. Hultman, E., and L. H. Nilsson. 1971. Liver glycogen in man: Effect of different diets and muscular exercise. In Pernow, B., and B. Saltin (eds.), *Muscle Metabolism during Exercise.* New York: Plenum Press, pp. 143–151.

88. Innes, J. A., I. Solarte, A. Huszczuk, E. Yeh, B. J. Whipp, and K. Wasserman. 1989. Respiration during recovery from exercise: effects of trapping and release of femoral blood flow. *J Appl Physiol.* 67(6):2608–2613.

89. Jansson, E., G. A. Dudley, B. Norman, and P. A. Tesch. 1990. Relationship of recovery from intensive exercise to the oxidative potential of skeletal muscle. *Acta Physiol Scand.* 139(1):147–152.

90. Johnson, R. E., and H. T. Edwards. 1937. Lactate and pyruvate in blood and urine after exercise. *J Biol Chem.* 118:427–432.

91. Karlsson, J., F. Bonde-Petersen, J. Hendriksson, and H. G. Knuttgen. 1975. Effects of previous exercise with arms or legs on metabolism and performance in exhaustive exercise. *J Appl Physiol.* 38:763–767.

92. Karlsson, J., and B. Saltin. 1971. Oxygen deficit and muscle metabolites in intermittent exercise. *Acta Physiol Scand.* 82:115–122.

93. Katch, V. L. 1973. Kinetics of oxygen uptake and recovery for supramaximal work of short duration. *Int Z Angew Physiol.* 31(3):197–207.

94. Kearney, J. T. 1973. Strength recovery following rhythmic or sustained exercise. *Am Correct Ther J.* 27(6):163–167.

95. Kemp, G. J., D. J. Taylor, and G. K. Radda. 1993. Control of phosphocreatine resynthesis during recovery from exercise in human skeletal muscle. *NMR Biomed.* 6(1):66–72.

96. Kemp G. J., D. J. Taylor, P. Styles, and G. K. Radda. 1993. The production, buffering and efflux of protons in human skeletal muscle during exercise and recovery. *NMR Biomed.* 6(1):73–83.

97. Kemp, G. J., C. H. Thompson, A. L. Sanderson, and G. K. Radda. 1994. pH control in rat skeletal muscle during exercise, recovery from exercise, and acute respiratory acidosis. *Magn Reson Med.* 31(2):103–109.

98. Knuttgen, H. G. 1970. Oxygen debt after submaximal physical exercise. *J Appl Physiol.* 29(5):651–657.

99. Knuttgen, H. G., and B. Saltin. 1972. Muscle metabolites and oxygen uptake in short-term submaximal exercise in man. *J Appl Physiol.* 32(5):690–694.

100. ———. 1973. Oxygen uptake, muscle high-energy phosphates, and lactate in exercise under acute hypoxic conditions in man. *Acta Physiol Scand.* 87:368–376.

101. Kochan, R. G., D. R. Lamb, S. A. Lutz, C. V. Perrell, E. M. Reiman, and R. R. Schlender. 1979. Glycogen synthetase activation in human skeletal muscle: Effect of diet and exercise. *Am J Physiol.* 235:E660–E666.

102. Koutedakis, Y., and N. C. Sharp. 1985. Lactic acid removal and heart rate frequencies during recovery after strenuous rowing exercise. *Br J Sports Med.* 19(4):199–202.

103. Krzentowski, G., F. Pirnay, A. S. Luyckx, N. Pallikarakis, M. Lacroix, F. Mosora, and P. J. Lefebvre. 1982. Metabolic adaptations in post-exercise recovery. *Clin Physiol.* 2(4):277–288.

104. Lindinger, M. I., G. J. Heigenhauser, R. S. McKelvie, and N. L. Jones. 1992. Blood ion regulation during repeated maximal exercise and recovery in humans. *Am J Physiol.* 262:R126–136.

105. Lindinger, M. I., and G. Sjogaard. 1991. Potassium regulation during exercise and recovery. *Sports Med.* 11(6):382–401.

106. McCann, D. J., P. A. Mole, and J. R. Caton. 1995. Phosphocreatine kinetics in humans during exercise and recovery. *Med Sci Sports Exerc.* 27:378–389.

107. MacDougall, J. D., G. R. Ward, D. G. Sale, and J. R. Sutton. 1977. Muscle glycogen repletion after high-intensity intermittent exercise. *J Appl Physiol.* 42:129–132.

108. Maehlum, S., P. Felig, and J. Wahren. 1978. Splanchnic glucose and muscle glycogen metabolism after glucose feeding during postexercise recovery. *Am J Physiol.* 235(3):E255–260.

109. Maehlum, S., and L. Hermansen. 1978. Muscle glycogen concentration during recovery after prolonged severe exercise in fasting subjects. *Scand J Clin Lab Invest.* 38(6):557–560.

110. Margaria, R., P. Cerretelli, P. E. diPrampero, C. Massari, and G. Torelli. 1963. Kinetics and mechanism of oxygen debt contraction in man. *J Appl Physiol.* 18:371–377.

111. Margaria, R., P. Cerretelli, and F. Mangile. 1964. Balance and kinetics of anaerobic energy release during strenuous exercise in man. *J Appl Physiol.* 19:623–628.

112. Margaria, R., H. T. Edwards, and D. B. Dill. 1933. The possible mechanism of contracting and paying the oxygen debt and the role of lactic acid in muscular contraction. *Am J Physiol.* 106:687–714.

113. Marliss, E. B., E. Simantirakis, P. D. Miles, R. Hunt, R. Gougeon, C. Purdon, J. B. Halter, and M. Vranic. 1992. Glucose turnover and its regulation during intense exercise and recovery in normal male subjects. *Clin Invest Med.* 15(5):406–419.

114. Maron, M. B., S. M. Horvath, and J. E. Wilkerson. 1977. Blood biochemical alterations during recovery from competitive marathon running. *Eur J Appl Physiol.* 36:231–238.

115. Mero, A. 1988. Blood lactate production and recovery from anaerobic exercise in trained and untrained boys. *Eur J Appl Physiol.* 57(6):660–666.

116. Miller, R. G., D. Giannini, H. S. Milner-Brown, R. B. Layzer, A. P. Koretsky, D. Hooper, and M. W. Weiner. 1987. Effects of fatiguing exercise on high-energy phosphates, force, and EMG: Evidence for three phases of recovery. *Muscle Nerve* 10(9):810–821.

117. Nemoto, E. M., J. T. Hoff, and J. W. Severinghaus. 1974. Lactate uptake and metabolism by brain during hyperlactacidemia and hypoglycemia. *Stroke.* 5:48–53.

118. Newsholme, E. A. 1978. Substrate cycles: their metabolic, energetic and thermic consequences in man. *Biochem Soc Symp.* 43:183–205.

119. Newsholme, E. A., and A. R. Leetch. 1983. *Biochemistry for the Medical Sciences.* New York: John Wiley.

120. Peters Futre, E. M., T. D. Noakes, R. I. Raine, and S. E. Terblanche. 1987. Muscle glycogen repletion during active postexercise recovery. *Am J Physiol.* 253(2 Pt 1):E305–311.

121. Piehl, K. 1974. Time course for refilling of glycogen stores in human muscle fibers following exercise-induced glycogen depletion. *Acta Physiol Scand.* 90:297–302.

122. Piiper, J., P. E. diPrampero, and P. Cerretelli. 1968. Oxygen debt and high-energy phosphates in gastrocnemius muscle of the dog. *Am J Physiol.* 215:523–531.

123. Piiper, J., and P. Spiller. 1970. Repayment of O$_2$ debt and resynthesis of high energy phosphates in gastrocnemius muscle of the dog. *J Appl Physiol.* 28:657–662.

124. Podbielski, B., and W. K. Palmer. 1989. Cardiac triacylglycerol content and lipase activity during recovery from exercise. *J Appl Physiol.* 66(3):1099–1103.

125. Reaburn, P. R., and L. T. Mackinnon. 1990. Blood lactate responses in older swimmers during active and passive recovery following maximal sprint swimming. *Eur J Appl Physiol.* 61(3–4):246–252.

126. Roberts, A. D., and A. R. Morton. 1978. Total and alactic oxygen debts after supramaximal work. *Eur J Appl Physiol.* 38:281–289.

127. Rowell, L. B., K. K. Kraning, T. O. Evans, J. W. Kennedy, J. R. Blackmon, and F. Kusumi. 1966. Splanchnic removal of lactate and pyruvate during prolonged exercise in man. *J Appl Physiol.* 21:1773–1783.

128. Royce, J. 1969. Active and passive recovery from maximal aerobic capacity work. *Int Z Angew Physiol.* 28(1):1–8.

129. Ryan, C., and J. Radziuk. 1995. Distinguishable substrate pools for muscle glyconeogenesis in lactate-supplemented recovery from exercise. *Am J Physiol.* 269:E538–550.

130. Sahlin, K., A. Alvestrand, R. Brandt, and E. Hultman. 1978. Intracellular pH and bicarbonate concentration in human muscle during recovery from exercise. *J Appl Physiol.* 45(3):474–480.

131. Sahlin, K., and J. Henricksonn. 1984. Lactate content and pH in muscle samples of trained and untrained men. *Acta Physiol Scand.* 122:331–339.

132. Sherman, W. M. 1992. Recovery from endurance exercise. *Med Sci Sports Exerc.* 24(9 Suppl.):S336–339.

133. Siebers, L. S., and R. G. McMurray. 1981. Effects of swimming and walking on exercise recovery and subsequent swim performance. *Res Q Exerc Sport.* 52(1):68–75.

134. Signorile, J. F., C. Ingalls, and L. M. Tremblay. 1993. The effects of active and passive recovery on short-term, high intensity power output. *Can J Appl Physiol.* 18(1):31–42.

135. Sinacore, D. R., E. F. Coyle, J. M. Haaberg, and J. O. Holloszy. 1993. Histochemical and physiological correlates of training- and detraining-induced changes in the recovery from a fatigue test. *Phys Ther.* 73(10):661–667.

136. Spitzer, J. J. 1974. Effect of lactate infusion on canine myocardial free fatty acid metabolism in vivo. *Am J Physiol.* 226:213–217.

137. Stainsby, W. N., and J. K. Barclay. 1970. Exercise metabolism, O_2 deficit, steady level O_2 uptake and O_2 uptake for recovery. *Med Sci Sports.* 2:177–181.

138. Stamford, B. A., A. Weltman, R. Moffat, and S. Sady. 1981. Exercise recovery above and below anaerobic threshold following maximal work. *J Appl Physiol.* 51:840–844.

139. Stringer, W., R. Casaburi, and K. Wasserman. 1992. Acid-base regulation during exercise and recovery in humans. *J Appl Physiol.* 72(3):954–961.

140. Sullivan, M. J., B. Saltin, R. Negro-Vilar, B. D. Duscha, and H. C. Charles. 1994. Skeletal muscle pH assessed by biochemical and 31P-MRS methods during exercise and recovery in men. *J Appl Physiol.* 77(5):2194–2200.

141. Tesch, P. A., and J. E. Wright. 1983. Recovery from short term intense exercise: its relation to capillary supply and blood lactate concentration. *Eur J Appl Physiol.* 52(1):98–103.

142. Thomas, T. R., B. R. Londeree, and D. A. Lawson, 1994. Prolonged recovery from eccentric versus concentric exercise. *Can J Appl Physiol.* 19(4):441–450.

143. Wasserman, D. H., D. B. Lacy, D. R. Green, P. E. Williams, and A. D. Cherrington. 1987. Dynamics of hepatic lactate and glucose balances during prolonged exercise and recovery in the dog. *J Appl Physiol.* 63(6):2411–2417.

144. Wasserman, D. H., P. E. Williams, D. B. Lacy, D. R. Green, and A. D. Cherrington. 1988. Importance of intrahepatic mechanisms to gluconeogenesis from alanine during exercise and recovery. *Am J Physiol.* 254:E518–525.

145. Wasserman, K., W. L. Beaver, J. A. Davis, J. Z. Pu, D. Heber, and B. J. Whipp. 1985. Lactate, pyruvate, and lactate-to-pyruvate ratio during exercise and recovery. *J Appl Physiol.* 59(3):935–940.

146. Welch, H. G., J. A. Faulkner, J. K. Barclay, and G. A. Brooks. 1970. Ventilatory response during recovery from muscular work and its relation with O_2 debt. *Med Sci Sports.* 2:15–19.

147. Weltman, A., B. A. Stamford, and C. Fulco. 1979. Recovery from maximal effort exercise: lactate disappearance and subsequent performance. *J Appl Physiol.* 47(4):677–682.

148. Williams, R. E., and S. M. Horvath. 1995. Recovery from dynamic exercise. *Am J Physiol.* 268:H2311–2320.

149. Wong, R., G. Lopaschuk, K. Teo, D. Walker, D. Catellier, G. Zhu, D. Burton, R. Collins-Nakai, and T. Montague. 1992. In vivo skeletal muscle metabolism during dynamic exercise and recovery: assessment by nuclear magnetic resonance spectroscopy. *Can J Cardiol.* 8(8):819–824.

150. Yates, J. W., J. T. Kearney, M. P. Noland, and M. W. Felts. 1987. Recovery of dynamic muscular endurance. *Eur J Appl Physiol.* 56(6):662–667.

151. Yudkin, J., and R. D. Cohen. 1974. The contribution of the kidney to the removal of a lactic acid load under normal and acidotic conditions in the conscious cat. *Clin Sci Mol Med.* 46:8P.

Selected Readings

Brooks. G. A. 1991. Symposium: Current concepts in lactate exchange. *Med Sci Sports Exerc.* 23(8):895–943.

Bowers, R. W., and E. L. Fox. 1992. *Sports Physiology.* Dubuque, IA: Wm. C. Brown.

Katz, A., and K. Sahlin. 1990. Role of oxygen in regulation of glycolysis and lactate production in human skeletal muscle. In Pandolph, K. B. (ed.), *Exercise and Sports Sciences Reviews*, vol. 18 (American College of Sports Medicine). Baltimore: Williams and Wilkins.

Maclaren, D. P. M., H. Gibson, M. Parry-Billings, and R. H. T. Edwards. 1989. A review of metabolic and physiological factors in fatigue. In Pandolph, K. B. (ed.), *Exercise and Sports Sciences Reviews,* vol. 17 (American College of Sports Medicine). Baltimore: Williams and Wilkins.

Stainsby, W. N., and G. A. Brooks. 1990. Control of lactic acid metabolism in contracting muscle and during exercise. In Pandolph, K. B. (ed.), *Exercise and Sports Sciences Reviews,* vol. 18 (American College of Sports Medicine). Baltimore: Williams and Wilkins.

4

Measurement of Energy, Work, and Power

One of the most valid means of determining a person's ability to perform physical exercise is to measure the maximal amount of energy he or she can expend. This can be done indirectly by determining one's ability to consume oxygen during maximal exercise. The exercise is usually performed using a cycle ergometer or treadmill, which permits a change in work rate from light to moderate to exhaustive (maximal) activity. The amount of oxygen consumed (often expressed in liters*) by the individual during maximal work can be converted into energy units such as **kilocalories (kcal)** or **kilojoules (kJ)**, work units such as **kilogram-meters (kg-m)**, and power units such as **kg-m per minute (kg-m · min^{-1})†** or **watts (W)**.

These are the conversions used most often in clinical practice, in studies of human performance, and in scientific journals. The American College of Sports Medicine favors the use of kilojoules (kJ = 1000 J) for both energy and work expressions and watts for power expression.

Understanding energy expenditure, how it is measured, and how it relates to activity, work, and power

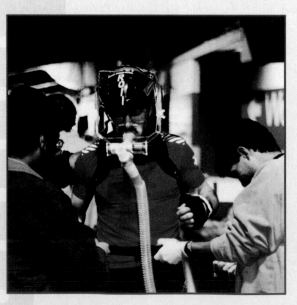

will make you much more knowledgeable about your chosen profession—whether it be physical education, athletics, physical therapy, cardiac rehabilitation, or some other allied health profession. As we have learned in the last two chapters, it is *energy* and the way in which it is expended and restored that allows for continued human movement. At this point, if you clearly see how energy, work, and power interrelate, and how they can be converted from one to another, you are well on your way to understanding energy measurements and their relationship to exercise.

---

*A liter equals 1.057 quarts.
†The negative 1 means the same as "per min" or divided by minutes. The raised dot means multiply. Another illustration: 3.5 mL/kg/min = 3.5 mL/kg · min^{-1} = 3.5 mL · kg^{-1} · min^{-1}. They all mean the same thing!

The major concepts to be learned from this chapter are as follows:

- Energy, work, and power are functionally related, because energy is the capacity to perform work, and power is work per unit of time.
- The direct measurement of energy involves the measurement of heat production, whereas the indirect measurement of energy in the human involves the measurement of oxygen consumption.
- The heat (caloric) equivalent of oxygen consumed depends on the energy nutrient oxidized by the aerobic system.
- An estimation of the energy (oxygen) cost of anaerobic exercise requires measurement of resting, exercise and recovery oxygen consumption, whereas for aerobic exercise, only oxygen consumption at rest and during exercise are required.
- A variety of tests and testing protocols are available to assess anaerobic and aerobic power. Aerobic power can be determined directly by measuring oxygen consumption or can be indirectly estimated using field tests, prediction equations, or metabolic equations.
- The efficiency of the human body while performing various activities is represented by the ratio of work output (kcal) to work input (kcal), which is expressed as a percent.
- Various methods (accelerometers, heart rate by radio telemetry) can be used to measure (estimate) the energy cost of various activities.

Ergometry

To study the energetics of physical activity, suitable measurement devices that are reliable and valid are required. Such devices are named **ergometers** (ergo = work, meter = measure). Reliability of these devices is very important and refers to our ability to consistently reproduce the exact same work condition with a high degree of confidence. For example, following a ten-week jogging program, we observe that a subject's heart rate while exercising at 75 watts is lower during the second test than the first. Such an observation is realistic, representing the effect of the training program on the cardiovascular system rather than a difference in test conditions. A few of the more common ergometers that are available to the exercise physiologist are described below.

Treadmill

Motor-driven treadmills consist of a walking/running surface, similar to a conveyor belt, and a means of controlling both the speed and elevation for uphill walking or running. Some models are adaptable to provide a simulated downhill run. Other adaptations include underwater treadmills (wherein the walking/running surface is submerged in a water tank) and treadmills with extremely wide surfaces that allow for activities such as in-line skating.

Stationary Cycle

The cycle ergometer, or stationary cycle, imposes resistance against a pedaled flywheel through either the mechanical loading of weights onto a platform or through increasing tension on a belt to increase friction. Alternately, resistance can be electronically imposed by increasing magnetic resistance against the flywheel. Incidentally, Åstrand and Rodahl point out that rather than referring to the ergometer as a stationary "bicycle," it should properly be called a cycle ergometer, because there is only one wheel.[3]

Swimming Ergometer

Tethered swimming devices have been designed to provide a means of resistance so that the swimmer can remain in one location in the pool. One such apparatus involves attaching a belt or harness to a swimmer. The belt is attached to a cable that runs through a series of pulleys to a loading platform. To maintain his or her position in the water the swimmer must kick and/or stroke to maintain the load platform at a given point.[15] The device can be constructed in such a manner so that the swimmer can achieve fine gradations in work load. Alternately, in some highly specialized exercise physiology laboratories, such as the Olympic Training Center in Colorado Springs, Colorado, one may find a swimming flume (figure 4.1). This device is comprised of a large tank of water and machinery which generates and controls a current of water to swim against.

Other Devices

The above-named devices are the most commonly available. Other types include upper-body ergometers, ski ergometers ("skimills," see figure 4.1), rowing ergometers, and staircase ergometers. One important feature of any ergometer that is intended for either research or physiologic testing is that it must be able to quantify work rate. To accomplish this, care must be taken to ensure that the device remains calibrated.[63] This requirement may exclude many of the mechanical and seemingly more sophisticated ergometers and exercise machines found in many public and private health clubs.

Energy, Work, and Power

To fully appreciate our topic, energy cost of performance, we need to know the meaning of and relationships among energy, work, and power.

Energy and Work

As discussed in chapter 2, **energy** is the *capacity to perform work*. During exercise we convert chemical energy to mechanical energy and heat; whether it is something as simple as putting a smile on our face or completing the coordinated movement of clearing the cross-bar in the pole vault. The energy needed for us to perform movement is derived from the chemical energy in the food we eat, which is ultimately converted by the body to ATP.

The physicist defines **work** *as the application of a force through a distance*. For example, if you raised a book weighing 1 kilogram vertically 1 meter, the work performed would have been 1 kilogram-meter (kg-m) or 9.8 joules.* One kg-m is defined as the work done when a constant force of 1 kg is exerted on a body that moves a distance of 1 meter in the same direction as the force. Work may be expressed in the following formula:

$$W = F \times D$$

Where:

W = work
F = force (remember, the force must be constant)
D = the distance through which the force is applied (distance is the length of the path through which the body moves while the force is acting on it)

---

*Joule is the SI (le Système Internationale) unit for work. See table 4.1.

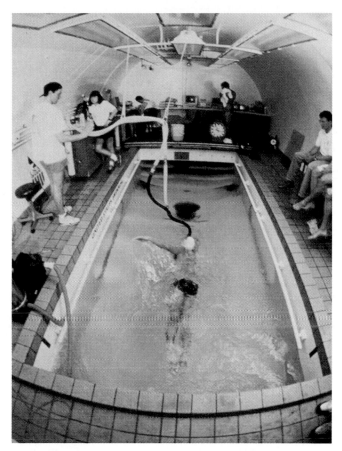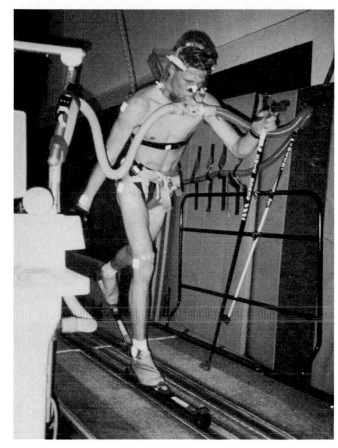

Figure 4.1

Two sport-specific testing ergometers: swimming flume (left) and skimill (right).

Photographs courtesy of Dr. Randall Wilber, U.S. Olympic Training Center, Colorado Springs, Colorado, and Dr. Phil Watts, Northern Michigan University, Marquette, Michigan.

Another example of work would be to perform a pull-up. If the person weighed 70 kg and if the bar were 0.75 meter above the chin, then the amount of work performed during the pull-up would be as follows:

$$W = F \times D$$
$$W = 70 \text{ kg} \times 0.75 \text{ meters}$$
$$W = 52.5 \text{ kg-m}$$

Work may be expressed in different terms or units. Table 4.1 contains a number of work and energy units that enable us to convert one to another depending on how we wish to express our final measurement. Please note that work can be also expressed in terms of kilocalories (kcal). When we discuss oxygen consumption later in this chapter, you will learn that it too can be converted to kcal. The knowledge of this relationship will enable us to make determinations about the energy (caloric) cost of various activities.

Using table 4.1, determine how many joules of work the person performed completing the pull-up. Also, how many kilocalories did the person expend in doing one pull-up?*

table 4.1

Energy and work units

1 kg-m*	= 9.8 joules†
1 kilocalorie (kcal)	= 426.85 kg-m
	= 4.186 kilojoules (kJ)
1 joule (J)	= 1 Newton-meter (Nm)
1 kilojoule (kJ)	= 1000 joules (J) = 0.23889 kcal

*A kilogram-meter (kg-m) represents the work performed when 1 kilogram is moved 1 meter.

†A joule (J) is the SI unit for work and represents the application of a force of 1 Newton (N) through a distance of 1 meter (m).

*Answer: 1 kg-m = 9.8 joules (table 4.1); therefore, work = 514.5 joules (or 0.5145 kJ). The energy expenditure was about 0.12 kcal!

4.2

Relationships among various power units

	Horsepower	kg-m · min^{-1}	ft-lb · min^{-1}	Watts	kcal · min^{-1}	kJ · min^{-1}
1 horsepower	1.0	4,564.0	33,000	745.7	10.694	44.743
kg-m · min^{-1}	0.000219	1.0	7.233	0.16345	0.00234	9,800
ft-lb · min^{-1}	0.00003	0.1383	1.0	0.0226	0.000324	0.0013563
1 watt	0.001341	6.118	44.236	1.0	0.014334	0.060
kcal · min^{-1}	0.0936	426.85	3086	69.767	1.0	4.1860
kJ · min^{-1}	0.02235	0.000102	737.30	16.667	0.2389	1.0

Power

Power is used to express work done in a unit of time or as the *rate* of performing work. It may be written as:

$$P = \frac{W}{t} \text{ or } \frac{(F \times D)}{t}$$

Where:

$$P = \text{Power}$$
$$t = \text{Time}$$

In the aforementioned example, if the book weighing 1 kg were raised 1 meter in 1 second, power would be expressed as 1 kg-m per second. By the same token, if the pull-up were performed in 0.5 second, the power produced would be:

$$P = \frac{W}{t}$$
$$P = \frac{52.5 \text{ kg-m}}{0.5 \text{ second(s)}}$$
$$P = 105 \text{ kg-m} \cdot \text{s}^{-1}$$

Table 4.2 contains a number of ways in which power may be expressed.

From the above discussion it is necessary that the student understand (a) the meaning of energy, work, and power and (b) that the six forms of energy (see chapter 2) can be converted from one form to another. Knowledge of these concepts is important so that we can discuss:

1. How work by a person can be measured by directly assessing the amount of heat the body gives off while performing various tasks.
2. How measurement of heat is employed in determining the energy values of food—in other words, how much energy (in kilocalories) is in a soft drink, an average-sized potato, or a slice of pizza. This information is vital to the understanding of proper weight-control programs.
3. How the exercise physiologist uses an indirect method of measuring energy by determining the amount of oxygen consumed or used.

Direct Measurement of Energy: Heat Production

When energy is expended by the human body while resting or during work or exercise, heat is liberated. Food is the sole source of this heat energy. Hence, the metabolism of the so-called **energy nutrients** (carbohydrates, fats, proteins),* and their corresponding caloric values, should be equivalent to the amount of heat the body liberates. This demonstrates the first law of thermodynamics: *When mechanical energy is transformed into heat energy or heat energy into mechanical energy, the ratio of the two energies is a constant quantity (the principle of the conservation of energy).* It is an observable fact, then, that the expenditure of a fixed amount of energy will always result in the production of the same amount of heat. To demonstrate the first law of thermodynamics, a scientist by the name of Max Rubner, in the latter part of the 1800s, built a chamber containing circulating water on the outside (figure 4.2). A dog was placed inside the chamber in order to measure both heat production and metabolism of the animal. Heat production by the dog in the chamber (called a *bomb calorimeter*) was measured by noting the change (increase) in temperature of the circulating water. Each increase in water temperature of 1° C per kilogram of water is equivalent to 1 kcal of energy. The term *bomb* comes from the shape of the chamber (bomb) and *calorimeter* means the measurement of heat (expressed in calories). Concurrently, metabolism was indirectly determined by measuring the oxygen consumed by the dog in breaking down the energy nutrients.

---

*Alcohol and vitamins both contain carbon atoms and, therefore, when ignited in a bomb calorimeter, release energy. However, the energy in vitamins cannot be released by the body in a usable manner. The energy in alcohol, although able to be released by the body, is *not* essential for life.

4.3

Energy equivalents of the energy nutrients and alcohol

Food	O_2 kcal · L^{-1}	CO_2 kcal · L^{-1}	Energy (bomb calorimeter) kcal · gm^{-1}	Net energy (physiological values)* kcal · gm^{-1}
Carbohydrate	5.05	5.05	4.10	4.02
Protein	4.46	5.57	5.65	4.20
Fat	4.74	6.67	9.45	8.98
Alcohol	4.86	7.25	7.1	7.00
Mixed diet	4.83	5.89	—	—

*In the body there is a loss of kcal to digestion as follows: carbohydrate, 2%; fat, 5%; and protein, 8%, plus a 17% loss in urine. For alcohol there is a small loss in urine and exhaled air.

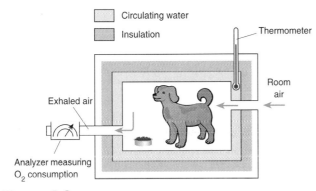

Figure 4.2

Calorimeter for measuring heat energy. The calorimeter allows simultaneous measurement of heat production and metabolism. Oxygen consumption (indirect measurement of metabolism) equals heat production (direct measurement) by the animal as reflected in an increase of temperature of the circulating water.

The results of these early experiments demonstrated unequivocally that energy produced through the metabolism of the energy nutrients is equal to the heat produced by the body. We can conclude, then, that energy expended by an individual doing any kind of work is exactly equal to the heat energy set free through body metabolism. For example, if we were to convert the measured oxygen consumption (VO_2*) of an individual riding a stationary cycle inside a bomb calorimeter large enough to accommodate a human into kilocalories (table 4.3), we would find that the amount

of energy as determined through the measurement of VO_2 would *equal* the amount of heat given off by the body during the exercise.

By the same token, if we wanted to determine the amount of energy contained in an average-sized potato, a soft drink, or a medium-sized pizza, we would simply ignite and burn the food item in the calorimeter. The increase in temperature of the circulating water would be equivalent to the energy or caloric value of the food. In fact, this is how caloric values for various foods are determined.

The use of the bomb calorimeter is referred to as the *direct method* in the measurement of energy. This is true because heat production, a specific form of energy, is being directly determined. On the other hand, when we measure the VO_2 required in metabolizing food, we use an *indirect method* in determining energy. These are two different methods to go about finding the same energy value.

Indirect Measurement of Energy: Oxygen Consumption

Many scientists have now demonstrated that the amount of O_2 consumed at rest or while performing work, when expressed in heat equivalents (kcal), will be equal to the heat produced by the body as determined directly in a calorimeter. Therefore, the measurement of VO_2 is an indirect measure of energy. To express VO_2 in units that are equivalent to those used for heat (i.e., kcal), we must know which energy nutrient is being metabolized. This is because the precise energy equivalent is related to the chemical composition of the energy nutrient (table 4.3). Simplifying this for our purposes, when either carbohydrate, fat, or protein is

*VO_2 = volume of oxygen (O_2) expressed as a unit of work. If a dot is placed above the V (e.g., $\dot{V}O_2$), then this indicates the rate of O_2 consumed per minute—a measure of power.

ignited in the bomb calorimeter, the energy yield is ~ 5 *kcal per every liter* of O_2 used ($kcal \cdot L^{-1}$).

From table 4.3 we can also see that, in terms of *kcal per gram* of energy nutrient metabolized, there is a slight difference in the energy yield between when food is metabolized (physiologically) in the body and when it is burned in the bomb calorimeter. Experiments conducted by Atwater demonstrated this and showed that the lower (net) energy values associated with the body's metabolism are due, in part, to loss of energy due to digestion. For carbohydrate, fat, and protein, the loss of kcal due to digestion is 2%, 5%, and 8%, respectively. For protein, there is an additional loss of kcal in the urine because, in addition to carbon, hydrogen, and oxygen, all protein also contains nitrogen. The body eliminates the nitrogen not as a free gas, like carbon dioxide, but instead as urea. As a result, a portion of the energy in the protein molecule is lost.

In the above discussion, we first focused on the energy released in terms of kilocalories per liter of O_2 because during exercise the athlete is more concerned with getting sufficient O_2 and less concerned with the quantity of food. Please note, however, that on a *per-gram basis*, fats yield more than twice as many kcal than either proteins or carbohydrates (table 4.3). For daily use, it is appropriate to round the Atwater values for fat, protein, and carbohydrates to 9 $kcal \cdot gm^{-1}$, 4 $kcal \cdot gm^{-1}$, and 4 $kcal \cdot gm^{-1}$, respectively. One practical application of these values might be weight loss; specifically, reducing the total grams of fat in one's diet is an excellent first step in reducing calorie intake.

For example, one medium-sized baked potato with one-quarter cup of low fat (1% fat) cottage cheese for topping contains a total of 180 calories and approximately 1 gram of fat. If, however, we took that same potato and made it into french fries, it would now contain 340 calories and *18 grams* of fat. The major difference in calories (160) between the two methods of serving the potato is the difference in grams of fat (17 grams) from frying. For someone who eats just one potato per week, this can equate to 8,000 extra calories per year!

Why more heat or energy is liberated from fats as compared with carbohydrates on a per-gram basis is easy to explain. Remember from chapter 2 that energy is released when water is formed (combining hydrogen and oxygen). There are more hydrogen atoms per oxygen atom in fat than in carbohydrates. For example, a typical carbohydrate, glucose, has the formula $C_6H_{12}O_6$ and a typical fat, palmitic acid, is $C_6H_{32}O_2$. As a consequence, there are more hydrogen atoms in fat to combine with oxygen in forming water (H_2O). Therefore, when the body uses a given amount of fat, more energy is released than when it metabolizes the same amount of carbohydrates.

The question that logically should confront us at this time is: If we have measured the VO_2 used in performing a given exercise task, how do we know which food was metabolized so that we can assign the proper caloric value? In the first place, it would be rare indeed if a person were

using only fat, protein, or carbohydrate exclusively. Rather, *a person exercises on a mixed diet* (predominantly carbohydrates and fats), and it is through measuring not only VO_2 but also the volume of carbon dioxide produced (VCO_2) that permits us to know the mixture of foods being metabolized. This issue is addressed in detail on page 82, but first we must describe the methods and uses of assessing aspired gases.

Measurement of the Energy Cost of Exercise

Let us imagine we were given the problem of measuring the energy expenditure for a given exercise. What procedures do we need to know, and what equipment do we need? In the absence of a bomb calorimeter, we must turn to the indirect measurement of energy expenditure: the assessment of VO_2. Then we need to know whether the exercise being performed is anaerobic or aerobic. If the exercise is anaerobic (i.e., involves both the aerobic and anaerobic energy systems throughout the duration of the exercise), then we need to measure the VO_2: (1) at rest, (2) during exercise, and (3) in recovery. If, however, the exercise can be performed in an aerobic steady-state, then only the VO_2 at rest and during the steady-state exercise period need be measured.

The measurement of resting VO_2 is necessary because this value must be subtracted from the oxygen measured during exercise and, if needed, during recovery to determine the oxygen cost of the exercise alone. This is called the **net oxygen cost of exercise.** For anaerobic activities, the measurement of oxygen in recovery is needed because the amount of oxygen consumed during exercise reflects only the energy supplied through the aerobic system. The recovery oxygen reflects the amount of energy required during exercise through the anaerobic system.* Therefore:

$$Net \; O_2 \; cost \; of \; anaerobic \; exercise \; =$$
$$(Exercise \; VO_2 - Resting \; VO_2) \; +$$
$$(Recovery \; VO_2 - Resting \; VO_2)$$

Holly[37] provides a detailed description of procedures for measuring VO_2 for manual systems. With the manual system, **Douglas bags** or meteorological balloons may be used to collect the exhaled gas for volume measurement and analysis. The originally designed collection bags, rubber-lined and covered with canvas, were named after physiologist C. G. Douglas. Figure 4.3 shows a manual collection system, utilizing a meteorological balloon, used to measure a subject's VO_2. Samples of expired air are collected during rest, exercise, and, if needed, recovery. Several bags may be needed to cover both exercise and recovery periods. Small

---

*Although convention includes recovery oxygen in the calculation of the net oxygen cost of anaerobic exercise, the validity of it reflecting, in a quantitative way, the anaerobic energy released during exercise, is questionable (chapter 3).

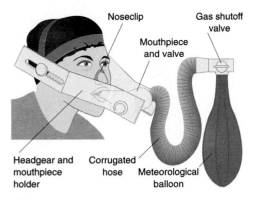

Figure 4.3

Illustration of a gas collection system utilizing a meteorological balloon.

gas samples are taken from each bag and analyzed for CO_2 and O_2 concentrations. Following sample analysis, the entire volume of each bag is determined by directing the gas through a gas meter (the small amount removed for CO_2 and O_2 analysis is added to the metered reading). These measurements are needed to calculate the amounts of oxygen consumed and carbon dioxide produced. At this time you need not go through the actual calculations of VO_2 and VCO_2; you can learn how to do this by reading appendixes C and D.

In summary, the following equipment and supplies are needed to assess the metabolic response to exercise:

1. Two-way non-rebreathing valve, mouthpiece, noseclip, and head gear
2. Tubing
3. Gas collection bags
4. An oxygen analyzer
5. A carbon dioxide analyzer
6. A gas meter or flowmeter for quantifying ventilation or the total volume of collected gas
7. Calibration gases
8. A mercury barometer (mm Hg) and thermometer (°C)

The basic principle of the Douglas bag or meteorological bag method is still in use in contemporary laboratories and "rests on a very secure foundation."[4] However, in the 1970s, semi-automated[65] and automated on-line[66] metabolic measuring systems were developed. In fact, continued advances in electronic, sensor, and computer technology over the past 10 years has led to systems that provide breath-by-breath analysis, fit on a desktop, are lightweight and portable, and can transmit information by telemetry.[10,18,49,50] Figure 4.4 illustrates examples of these various systems. By way of analogy, the metabolic cart is to the clinical exercise physiologist or sport physiologist as a hammer is to the carpenter. Such equipment is the "tool of our trade." A common feature of many of the automated systems is that the measurement of the input variables (barometric pressure, temperature, ventilation, and CO_2 and O_2 concentrations) can be

monitored continuously and in any desired time frame. In addition, the results can be viewed "on line" while the subject is still exercising or recovering.

Computing the Net Oxygen Cost of Anaerobic Exercise

The following describes a test protocol where exercise is performed at an intensity that brings the subject to exhaustion in five minutes. A 5-minute resting collection is made prior to exercise followed by the 5-minute exercise test and a 45-minute recovery period.

In this example let us assume that, on analysis of the gas in the collection balloons, we found that during

- the 5-minute rest period, the subject consumed 1.5 L of O_2 (a rate of 0.3 L · min^{-1});
- the 5-minute period of exhausting exercise, the subject consumed 17.0 L of O_2; and
- the 45-minute recovery period, the subject consumed 25.0 L of O_2

How do we compute the *net* O_2 cost of the exercise?

Begin by subtracting resting VO_2 from that consumed during exercise. Since the duration (in minutes) for both of these conditions was the same (five minutes), no adjustment is needed for differences in time.

17.0 liters − 1.5 liters = 15.5 liters

The 15.5 liters represents net exercise VO_2, or the amount that is over and above that consumed during rest. Also, do you see that the 1.5 liters came from the resting O_2 consumption *rate* of 0.3 L · min^{-1} multiplied by the 5-minute period of exercise time? Remember that the *rate of consumption × time = volume.*

From the recovery oxygen (25 L of O_2), we must also subtract that amount that would have been used if the subject were resting for the 45 minutes. The resting $\dot{V}O_2$ rate is the same (0.3 L · min^{-1}), but in this case it is multiplied by 45 minutes to yield a resting equivalent of 13.5 liters. Subtracting this from the recovery oxygen consumption yields the *net* recovery oxygen:

25 liters − 13.5 liters = 11.5 liters

Therefore, the *net oxygen cost of the anaerobic exercise* would be equal to net exercise plus net recovery oxygen values, or

Net exercise VO_2 = 15.5 liters
Net recovery VO_2 = <u>11.5 liters</u>
Net O_2 cost   = 27.0 liters

For this example, how many kilocalories of energy were expended?*

---

*Answer: remember from page 78 that 1 liter of oxygen consumed equals approximately 5.0 kcal; therefore, 5.0 kcal · L^{-1} × 27.0 L = 135 kcal.

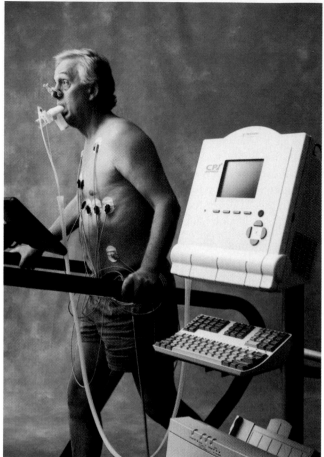

A

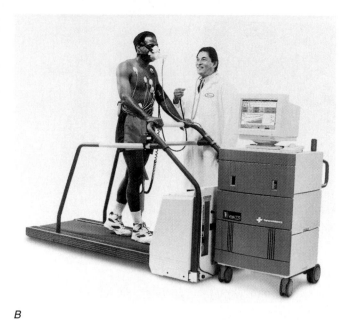

B

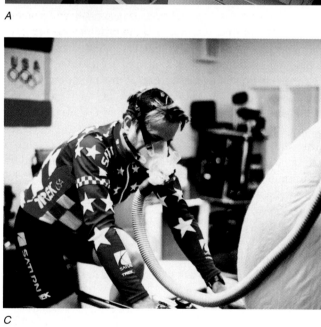

C

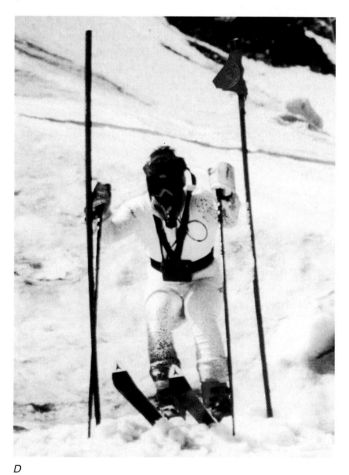

D

Figure 4.4

Examples of various gas collection systems and analyzers used for assessing oxygen consumption.

(Photographs courtesy of: (A) Medical Graphics Corporation; (B) SensorMedics Corporation; (C) Dr. Randall Wilber, U.S. Olympic Training Center; (D) Vacumetrics Inc., Vacu-Med; (E) AeroSport.)

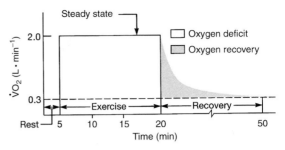

Figure 4.5

Time course of oxygen consumption during rest, submaximal aerobic exercise, and recovery. $\dot{V}O_2$ (volume of oxygen used per unit of time) can be measured any time during steady-state. Subtracting resting $\dot{V}O_2$ from this amount permits us to report the net cost of the exercise in liters per minute.

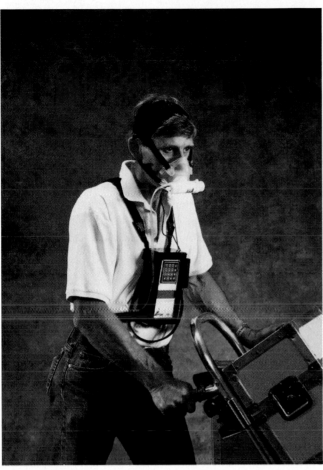

E

Computing the Net Oxygen Cost of Aerobic Exercise

If the exercise is submaximal and can be performed in an aerobic steady-state, the measurement of net oxygen cost is considerably simplified. You will recall that during submaximal exercise, a steady-state of VO_2 occurs, as noted in figure 4.5. The assumption is made that, during steady-state exercise, all the energy required for the exercise is being supplied aerobically. Therefore, the net oxygen cost of the steady-state exercise can be determined simply by (1) measuring the resting $\dot{V}O_2$, and (2) measuring the oxygen consumed during the steady-state period for any one minute.

Recognizing these basic physiological considerations, let us proceed with the actual determination of the net O_2 cost for our subject who is jogging in steady-state for 10 minutes on a treadmill at 9.7 km · hr^{-1} (6 miles per hour). We assume that the subject is capable of jogging at this speed in a steady-state condition—an easy task for endurance-trained athletes.

To accomplish this, the resting $\dot{V}O_2$ is determined as before. When the subject begins to jog, no $\dot{V}O_2$ measurements are made because the steady-state period has not as yet been reached. Once steady-state is reached (usually in 3 to 4 minutes—see figure 4.5), VO_2 is measured over a 1 minute period (sometimes over 2 minutes). Again, either the Douglas bag method or an automated metabolic measurement system may be used to determine the gas volume and O_2 and CO_2 concentrations. The resting $\dot{V}O_2$ value is then subtracted from the steady-state $\dot{V}O_2$ value to determine the net oxygen cost of the exercise on a per-minute basis. (Note: In the scientific literature and in most clinical exercise physiology laboratories, it has become "common practice" to exclude this important step when reporting $\dot{V}O_2$.)[*] Finally, for the total net oxygen cost, the net cost per minute is multiplied by the total exercise time, in minutes.

Returning to our example, suppose that the steady-state $\dot{V}O_2$ determined while jogging at 9.7 km · hr^{-1} on the treadmill was 2.8 liters per minute, and the resting $\dot{V}O_2$ was 0.3 liters per minute. Current practice would report the gross oxygen cost per minute as 2.8 liters. Because the exercise duration was 10 minutes, the *gross* oxygen cost of the entire steady-state exercise bout would be:

$$2.8 \text{ L} \cdot \text{min}^{-1} \times 10 \text{ minutes} = 28 \text{ liters}$$

However, the *net* oxygen cost would be 25 liters [(2.8 L · min^{-1} − 0.3 L · min^{-1}) × 10 min]. Do you see the important difference?

Two other points need to be mentioned at this time. First, the net oxygen cost when expressed *per minute* is a *power* measure ($\dot{V}O_2$). By the same token, when the net oxygen cost is expressed for the total exercise period, it is a *work* measure (VO_2). The two are differentiated from one another by the presence or absence of a dot above the V. In the previous example we gave for anaerobic exercise (p. 79), the total net oxygen cost was 27 liters. Because the

---

[*]When aerobic capacity for an athlete or patient is reported, it generally *includes* the resting metabolism. For example, a $\dot{V}O_2$ max of 60 mL · kg^{-1} · min^{-1} (4.2 L · min^{-1} for a 70 kg person) usually includes the resting level of about 0.3 L · min^{-1}.

exercise lasted 5 minutes, the average net power input* was $27/5 = 5.4$ L of O_2 *per minute*. Using both what you learned previously about the caloric equivalent of 1 L of O_2 (~ 5 kcal $\cdot$ L^{-1}) and the information in table 4.2, we can convert to a more conventional power unit (e.g., watts); in this case 1,884 W.

Conversely, for the example concerning aerobic exercise, the net oxygen cost was 25 liters, about the same as that for the anaerobic exercise. However, the total aerobic exercise time was 10 minutes, and thus the average net power input was $25/10 = 2.5$ L of O_2 per minute. Again using ~ 5 kcal $\cdot$ L^{-1}, and converting to watts, this equals 872 W or less than half the power input of the anaerobic exercise. In other words, although approximately the same *total work* was performed (27 L of O_2 vs. 25 L of O_2), the power or rate of work performed was much different between the two exercises (1,884 W vs. 872 W). This points out the importance of understanding the difference between power and work.

Second, $\dot{V}O_2$ and $\dot{V}O_2$ max, the volume of O_2 consumed per minute during a maximal exercise effort, are usually expressed in absolute (L $\cdot$ min^{-1}) or relative (mL $\cdot$ kg^{-1} $\cdot$ min^{-1}) terms. The proper phrase for this is *aerobic power*. The assessment of aerobic power both via the measurement of $\dot{V}O_2$ and by estimating it is discussed later in this chapter and in appendix F.

The Caloric Equivalent of Oxygen: The Respiratory Exchange Ratio (R)

Now that we've discussed the procedures and equipment needed to measure VO_2, we can return to our discussion about identifying which energy nutrient is being metabolized. Remember, the precise caloric value of 1 L of O_2 consumed depends on which type of food is being metabolized. To begin, we must first define a new term called the **respiratory exchange ratio (R)**,[†] which is the ratio of the volume of carbon dioxide expired per unit of time ($\dot{V}CO_2$) to the volume of oxygen consumed during the same time interval.

$$R = \frac{\dot{V}CO_2 \text{ produced}}{\dot{V}O_2 \text{ consumed}}$$

Relative to identifying which energy nutrient is being used, the R should only be determined under steady-state conditions or at rest.

Carbohydrate

A carbohydrate is an energy nutrient that contains carbon, hydrogen, and oxygen ($C_6H_{12}O_6$). Every molecule of carbohydrate contains the proper proportions of hydrogen and oxygen to form water (twice as much hydrogen as oxygen). Therefore, all of the oxygen that is consumed at rest or during steady-state exercise is used in the oxidation of carbon.

$$C_6H_{12}O_6 + 6O_2 \rightarrow 6CO_2 + 6H_2O$$

According to the law of Avogadro (see also appendix C), equal volumes of gases at the same temperature and pressure contain an equal number of molecules. As a result, if an individual were on a diet of pure carbohydrates and, therefore, metabolized only carbohydrates, then:

$$1 \text{ mole } C_6H_{12}O_6 + 6 \text{ moles } O_2 = \\ 6 \text{ moles } CO_2 + 6 \text{ moles } H_2O$$

or

$$R = \frac{VCO_2}{VO_2} = \frac{6VCO_2}{6VO_2} = 1$$

In this instance 6 moles of CO_2 are produced as a consequence of 6 moles of O_2 being used in the oxidation of a carbohydrate.

Earlier in this chapter you learned that 1 L of oxygen consumed liberates ~ 5 kcal of energy. Remember, however, that this value represents an approximation; the actual caloric equivalent varies according to the measured R (table 4.4).

Fat

When fat is oxidized, O_2 must combine with not only carbon to form CO_2 but also with much hydrogen to form water. This is because the amount of hydrogen compared to oxygen in fat far exceeds a 2:1 relationship. As a result, more O_2 is consumed than CO_2 is produced and, as we would expect, R is less than 1. For example, if only a fat, such as Palmitic acid ($C_{16}H_{32}O_2$) were completely oxidized, then:

$$C_{16}H_{32}O_2 + 23O_2 \rightarrow 16CO_2 + 16H_2O$$

or

$$R = \frac{16CO_2}{23O_2} = 0.70$$

Although fat contains more than twice the chemical energy of carbohydrate (9 kcal $\cdot$ $gram^{-1}$ vs. 4 kcal $\cdot$ $gram^{-1}$), it requires more O_2 to release it. In this example, 16 moles of CO_2 are produced when 23 moles of O_2 are used to oxidize 1 mole of palmitic acid. The ratio is $16CO_2/23O_2 = 0.70$. Checking table 4.4, we see that *one liter (L) of oxygen consumed will liberate 4.686 kcal of energy* when fat is metabolized in the body or burned in a bomb calorimeter.

---

*Note our use of the term *input* here to denote energy that was expended or put "into" the performance. The term work *output* will show up later during calculations of efficiency.

†A single cell respires, whereas the whole animal breathes. At the cellular level $\dot{V}CO_2/\dot{V}O_2$ is usually referred to as the respiratory quotient (RQ). At the level of the lungs, $\dot{V}CO_2/\dot{V}O_2$ is termed the respiratory exchange ratio (R).

table 4.4

Caloric equivalent (kcal · L^{-1} of oxygen) and percentage of total calories provided by carbohydrate and fat at each nonprotein R*

Nonprotein respiratory exchange ratio (R)	kcal of energy per liter of oxygen consumed	Percentage of calories derived from	
		Carbohydrates	Fats
0.70	4.686	0.00	100.00
0.71	4.690	1.10	98.90
0.72	4.702	4.76	95.2
0.73	4.714	8.40	91.60
0.74	4.727	12.00	88.00
0.75	4.739	15.60	84.40
0.76	4.751	19.20	80.80
0.77	4.764	22.30	77.20
0.78	4.776	26.30	73.70
0.79	4.788	29.90	70.10
0.80	4.801	33.40	66.60
0.81	4.813	36.90	63.10
0.82	4.825	40.30	59.70
0.83	4.838	43.80	56.20
0.84	4.850	47.20	52.80
0.85	4.862	50.70	49.30
0.86	4.875	54.10	45.90
0.87	4.887	57.50	42.50
0.88	4.899	60.80	39.20
0.89	4.911	64.20	35.80
0.90	4.924	67.50	32.50
0.91	4.936	70.80	29.20
0.92	4.948	74.10	25.90
0.93	4.961	77.40	22.60
0.94	4.973	80.70	19.30
0.95	4.985	84.00	16.00
0.96	4.998	87.20	12.80
0.97	5.010	90.40	9.58
0.98	5.022	93.60	6.37
0.99	5.035	96.80	3.18
1.00	5.047	100.00	0.00

*Based on data from Zuntz and Schumberg in Lusk.[44]

Protein

Proteins are completely burned in the bomb calorimeter, yielding 5.65 kcal · g^{-1} (table 4.3). As previously mentioned, however, the same is not true when protein is metabolized in the body because nitrogen and a small amount of sulfur residue are excreted in the urine and feces. Consequently, less energy is available when protein is metabolized in the body than when it is burned in the calorimeter. Therefore, energy production in the body from protein is about 4.20 kcal · gram^{-1}, whereas in the calorimeter it averages 5.65 kcal · g^{-1}. Because of this difference, special

consideration must be taken when using R to determine the type of energy nutrient being metabolized. This is of added significance when using R to assign the caloric value to each liter of oxygen that the body is using.

Mixed Diet

If the body metabolized only fats and carbohydrates (and no protein), then R would represent the relative or proportional use of these two energy nutrients because there is only a negligible loss of energy from digestion. For example, an R of 1.00 would indicate to us that only carbohydrates are being metabolized, and an R of 0.70 would mean only fats. And any ratio between these two values would give us the relative combinations of the two foods being metabolized. This is important because during exercise the relative use of carbohydrate and fat varies with intensity of effort, with higher intensity activities resulting in an R value closer to 1.0. During prolonged submaximal exercise, the percentage of fat utilized tends to increase gradually over time, and R may decrease accordingly.

Because proteins are part of our diet, they, too, are metabolized in the body. Fortunately, scientists long before us have measured the excretion of nitrogen and have determined the amount of protein that was oxidized.[44] Subtracting the oxygen required and the carbon dioxide produced when protein is oxidized *from* the total VO_2 yields an R value commonly referred to as the *nonprotein R*. In this manner, we can assign the proper caloric value to each liter of oxygen being consumed by the individual. Table 4.4 contains these nonprotein R values and using this we need only measure the oxygen consumed and the carbon dioxide produced to arrive at the proper caloric value for each liter of oxygen consumed. If this were not the case, nitrogen excretion values would have to be obtained and more cumbersome calculations made. On the other hand, because protein utilization is so low during exercise, R and nonprotein R are usually quite similar.

To determine the amount of energy expended when performing a task or during exercise, we need to know the value of R to determine the caloric value for the amount of O_2 consumed. As an illustration, let us assume that 2 L of O_2 were consumed per minute during 15 minutes of road cycling (a total of 30 L of O_2). From table 4.4, assuming that the only source of food fuel was carbohydrate (R = 1.0), the caloric value for the 30 L of O_2 consumed would represent $30 \times 5.05 = 151.5$ kcal of energy expended. When R is not measured, we can assume it to be 0.83 (4.83 kcal $\cdot L^{-1}$ of O_2 consumed) at rest. Otherwise, during exercise exceeding 70% of aerobic capacity, we can assume that 1 L of O_2 equals 5 kcal. In fact, if approximate values can be used, it is appropriate to use the 5.0 kcal $\cdot L^{-1}$ value for all your computations (rest and exercise) because of the small (7% to 8%) difference that exists between an R = 0.70 and an R = 1.0 (4.686 kcal $\cdot L^{-1}$ vs. 5.047 kcal $\cdot L^{-1}$, respectively).

Other Factors Affecting R

There are times when R can be affected by factors other than the oxidation of food. These factors must be considered when interpreting R:

1. **Hyperventilation** (increased air entering the lungs from rapid and deep breathing), which may be voluntary or may sometimes occur under psychological stress, results in higher-than-normal quantities of CO_2 being eliminated through the lungs. In such an instance, because the volume of CO_2 represents the numerator in the equation for R, the R value would exceed 1.0.

2. During the first minute or so of submaximal aerobic exercise, several changes occur as the body responds to exercise, which results in a brief period of hyperventilation. This, too, causes a person to blow off more CO_2 relative to the amount of O_2 consumed, causing R to briefly approach or exceed 1.0. After a steady-state period is achieved, in about 3 minutes, the VCO_2 produced more closely represents what is occurring in the cells as a consequence of the metabolism of fats and carbohydrates. Thus, to accurately measure the R of a given activity, steady-state conditions should be achieved before making any observations.

3. During short-term, exhaustive exercise (or immediately after stopping exercise), R may exceed 1.0 and go as high as 1.3 because of the buffering of lactic acid, which causes large quantities of CO_2 to be released. Relative to primary energy nutrient and energy use, it is appropriate in this case to consider R = 1.0. In other words, carbohydrate is the primary food source, and each liter of O_2 would be equivalent to 5.05 kcal.

4. During the middle and latter recovery periods from exercise, CO_2 production is dramatically decreased, whereas O_2 consumption remains elevated. Thus R may decrease to levels below resting for several minutes to several hours, depending on how long and how hard the exercise bout was performed.[56]

Protocols for Assessing Fitness

An individual's ability to run, jump, sprint, or cross-country ski depends, in part, on skill level and motivation. Success also depends on stamina or muscular strength. Some activities (e.g., jumping, sprinting, blocking, and others like them) represent short-duration, sudden, "all-out" tasks and require that the individual be able to generate considerable mechanical power. The development of such power is related to muscular strength and to the amount and rate of ATP produced via the anaerobic metabolic pathways (i.e., ATP-PC system and anaerobic glycolysis). An individual's ability to generate power during these activities is referred to as **anaerobic power** or fitness. On the other hand, a person's ability to endure activities such as running and cross-country skiing (at intensities between 40% and up to 80% to 85% of peak) over a long period of time is related to **aerobic power** ($\dot{V}O_2$ or cardiorespiratory fitness). In this case, the ATP needed to perform the work is predominantly derived through the aerobic metabolic pathways.

table 4.5

Maximal anaerobic performance obtained in males using the Wingate anaerobic test

Activity	Class	Peak power (watts)	Peak power (watts · kg^{-1})	Mean power (watts)	Mean power (watts · kg^{-1})
Speed skating	National	—	17.0	—	15.0
Sprint cycling	Olympic	1126	14.5	836	10.7
Volleyball	National	1192	13.3	—	—
Power lifting	National	—	12.6	—	9.4
Gymnastics	National	—	12.3	—	9.1
Ice hockey	Professional	—	12.0	—	9.5
Wrestling	National	—	12.0	—	9.4
Trained (24 year old)	Physical education student	803	12.0	—	9.2
Ice hockey	Olympic	—	11.7	—	9.6
Running (10,000 m)	—	—	11.4	—	9.3
Football (defensive backs, receivers)	Professional	1098	11.4	904	9.3
Running (ultramarathon)	—		11.3		8.9
Alpine skiing	International	845	11.1	718	9.4
Football (lineman)	Professional	1331	10.8	1047	8.5
Running (800 m)	—	—	10.0	—	8.3
Running (2 miler)	—	—	9.3	—	8.0
Active (23 year old)	Normal	700	9.2	563	7.3
Untrained (53 year old)	Normal	644	8.2	538	6.7
Patients with heart disease	—	609	6.7	519	6.0

Compiled from various sources by Clinton A. Brawner and Steven J. Keteyian. Reprinted by permission.

Measuring anaerobic and aerobic power are important techniques used in the study of exercise physiology, human performance, and certain diseases. Whereas anaerobic power is a measure of an individual's ability to produce power in a local muscle site, independent of blood and O_2 supply, aerobic power characterizes the ability of the entire body to respond to exercise. A successful 500-m elite world-class ice speed skater will complete their event in less than 42 seconds and will require a high level of anaerobic fitness in their legs but not their arms. On the other hand, the $\dot{V}O_2$ of a distance runner reflects the ability of the lungs, blood, heart, muscles, and other organs and organ systems to *transport and utilize O_2*. Measuring anaerobic and aerobic fitness helps not only to characterize an individual's ability to perform a certain task but it can also be used to quantify the effect of a change in training regimen on performance.

Assessing Anaerobic Power

Tests that reflect or quantify one's ability to produce ATP through the ATP-PC system and anaerobic glycolysis have changed greatly over the past 25 years. Described below is the Wingate test[7], one method now commonly used to assess anaerobic power. Appendix F describes other, less used methods of assessing anaerobic performance, some of which have been available for more than 75 years.

The Wingate anaerobic test was developed at the Wingate Institute in Israel in the 1970s. Over the years the testing protocol and equipment (usually a cycle ergometer) have been greatly refined. Following practice and a proper period of warm up, subjects exercise at maximal speed, usually for 30 seconds. They do so against a fixed supramaximal braking force equivalent to 2 to 4 times maximum. Braking force is based on the level and type of previous training, age, and to a lesser extent, gender. Subjects receive vocal encouragement to ensure a supramaximal effort. Variables such as peak power, average (mean) power, and total work are assessed. Peak power is usually obtained within the first 5 seconds of the test and reported in watts. Mean power represents the average power achieved over the full test and is computed by dividing the total work completed during the test (reported in J, watts, or kg-m) by the duration of the test. Table 4.5 shows peak power and mean power for a variety of male athletes, expressed both in watts and in watts · kg^{-1} of body weight. Generally, elite female athletes are 5% to 15% lower than their sport-specific male counterpart.

To better understand the Wingate test and its units of measure, we present the following example. A 25-year-old professional football player (offensive lineman; body weight = 130 kg) undergoes a 30-second Wingate test and achieves a peak power of 1500 watts (11.5 watts · kg^{-1}) and a total work of 21,000 J. To determine mean power (in watts), we must first convert 21,000 J per 30 sec to kg-m (1 kg-m = 9.8066 J; table 4.1), then multiply by 2 to get power in kg-m *per minute*. When done, divide by 6.118 (table 4.2) to determine watts.

$$\text{Mean power} = 21,000/9.8066 \times 2$$
$$= 4,282.8 \text{ kg-m} \cdot \text{min}^{-1}$$
$$= 4,282.8/6.118 = 700 \text{ watts}$$

Higher peak power and mean power values during Wingate testing are associated with the ability to achieve a higher rate of ATP production through the ATP-PC system and anaerobic glycolysis and therefore a higher concentration of muscle lactate at peak exercise. And, as you might guess, there is a good relationship between mean power and peak power and both the percentage of fast-twitch (Type II) fibers present in skeletal muscle and their metabolic capabilities.[8,41] If the test duration is extended beyond 30 seconds (e.g., to 40 to 60 seconds), then total work would be increased and perhaps becomes more reflective of anaerobic capabilities, while still minimizing the contribution of aerobic metabolism.[30]

Within the past 15 years, various modifications and/or additions to the concept of sudden, strenuous exercise have been instituted. For example, instead of fixing braking force, McCartney and coworkers[46,47] used a constant-velocity cycle ergometer (e.g., set at 60 rpm) during 30 to 45 seconds of all-out exercise. Controlling pedal rate as they did may help control for the possible confounding effects of a varying pedal rate, allowing persons to achieve a higher maximal power output.

Additionally, to more completely describe the anaerobic qualities of an activity, the assessment of *accumulated O$_2$ deficit*[48] was recently added to 30 seconds of all-out testing.[30] Defined as the difference between calculated O$_2$ demand for a supramaximal activity and measured VO$_2$, Medbo and associates determined that the accumulated O$_2$ deficit is reflective of ATP production via the ATP-PC system and glycolysis.[48]

Two final notes about anaerobic testing. First, unlike cardiorespiratory fitness, which remains essentially unchanged from childhood through young adulthood, anaerobic performance improves from childhood through 30 years of age.[39] Second, although the Wingate test (and other anaerobic tests) can help distinguish persons with well-developed anaerobic capabilities from those with lesser abilities (sprinters vs. distance runners), it is not always a good predictor of success in athletic competition. For example, mean power output obtained during the Wingate test in highly trained ice-speed skaters is correlated with a skater's "on ice" personal best performance. However, mean power output does not always predict success in competition.[26] This is because, at such a high level of competition and among similarly trained athletes, other factors such as technique, strategy, intrinsic motivation, and prior racing experience often differentiate success.

Assessing Aerobic Power

Over the years the utilization and attention given to assessing aerobic power has far exceeded that given to anaerobic power. One reason for this is the many applications associated with assessing aerobic power. Like anaerobic testing, aerobic testing can help describe the characteristics of the elite athlete and evaluate the effects of training and detraining. In addition, aerobic testing can assess the effects of exposure to altitude and pollution and the effect of ergogenic aids.[38] However, unlike anaerobic power, determining one's level of cardiorespiratory fitness also has both general health and clinical applications.

Determining an individual's level of cardiorespiratory fitness (aerobic power) can best be accomplished through the direct measurement of $\dot{V}O_2$, as described elsewhere in this chapter and in appendixes D and F. In the majority of cases, it is measured using one of the ergometers mentioned at the beginning of this chapter. Remember that such testing devices provide the tester with both the opportunity to impose quantifiable work rates and the ability to reproduce the exact same test conditions, if needed, at some time in the future. Among elite athletes, selecting the correct ergometer is important because results can be influenced by the device selected. For example, a world-class cyclist will have a lower max $\dot{V}O_2$ if a treadmill is used for testing versus a cycle ergometer. For this reason, some human performance laboratories, such as those at the U.S. Olympic Training Centers, use sport-specific testing ergometers. *However, in the nonathletic population, max $\dot{V}O_2$ determined on a treadmill is usually 5% to 15% higher than that achieved during cycle ergometry.* Generally, in the United States most exercise physiology laboratories and clinical exercise testing facilities use a treadmill rather than a cycle ergometer. This may differ from Europe where the use of the cycle ergometer is also popular.

Regardless of the ergometer selected, all aerobic fitness test protocols (*graded exercise tests*) have three common features. *First*, optimal test duration should be between 6 and 12 minutes. This is accomplished by selecting a protocol that best fits the fitness level of the person being tested (table 4.6). The method of selecting the correct protocol can be based on both formal (see appendix F) and less formal methods. With respect to the latter, once a test administrator has gained experience with testing a variety of populations, he or she can often ask key questions (exercise habits, type of occupation, health history) that will help them select the correct protocol.

Table 4.7 provides an example of a continuous running test for a recreational runner who can complete a 10-kilometer race in about 42 to 45 minutes. The speed could be set at 8 miles per hour, approximating the average

4.6

Two commonly used exercise test protocols showing treadmill speed, grade, and minutes of exercise*

Bruce Protocol

Stage	Speed (miles · hr^{-1})	Grade (%)	Cumulative time (min)
I	1.7	10	1–3
II	2.5	12	4–6
III	3.4	14	7–9
IV	4.2	16	10–12
V	5.0	18	13–15

Naughton Protocol

Stage	Speed (miles · hr^{-1})	Grade (%)	Cumulative time (min)
I	3.0	2.5	1–2
II	3.0	5.0	3–4
III	3.0	7.5	5–6
IV	3.0	10.0	7 8
V	3.0	12.5	9–10
VI	3.0	15.0	11–12
VII	3.0	17.5	13–14
VIII	3.0	20.0	15–16

*Can be used both for apparently healthy persons and for patients with known heart disease.

4.7

Example of a treadmill protocol to measure the aerobic capacity of a runner capable of running 10K in 42 to 45 minutes

Stage	Time min	Speed mph (kph)	Grade %
Warm-up	Variable (3 to 5 min)	6 (9.7)	0
1	0 to 3	8 (12.9)	0
2	3 to 6	8 (12.9)	4
3	6 to 9	8 (12.9)	6
4	9 to 12	8 (12.9)	8
5	?	8 (12.9)	10

10-km running pace for this individual. Note, however, that if this same protocol were used for a sedentary office worker, it would result in a test that is stopped before their electrocardiogram (ECG) or blood pressure are adequately assessed. For this person, a walking protocol that starts slower and progresses with smaller increases in grade may be more favorable and allow for a sufficient amount of time to evaluate ECG, blood pressure, and max $\dot{V}O_2$.

Second, an exercise test can be either *continuous* or *discontinuous*. Just like the name implies, during continuous tests, the subject begins to exercise and continues to do so until the test is stopped because of (1) fatigue, (2) a pre-

determined end-point is reached, or (3) a sign or symptom is observed or reported. In a discontinuous test the subject exercises for a specified period of time (e.g., 3 minutes), then a period of rest is given (2 to 5 minutes) before the test is restarted at a higher work rate. In both tests, $\dot{V}O_2$, heart rate, blood pressure, and/or an ECG are usually measured at rest, before exercise, during exercise, at peak exercise, and in recovery.

Third, in most laboratories today, the continuous test is more frequently used than the discontinuous test. However, continuous tests can be conducted using either a *steady-state or a ramp* protocol. As the name suggests, a steady-state protocol consists of several exercise stages (usually 2 to 4 minutes), which allow the person to achieve a submaximal steady-state response before work rate is increased. Obviously, as the person being tested nears maximum, a steady-state response is less likely, and with further increases in work rate, fatigue eventually results. Tests of this type are especially useful if data obtained during submaximal exercise from one test will be compared to another test.

For example, a physician may use a continuous steady-state test to assess the therapeutic effect of a recently prescribed blood pressure medication in a person identified as having high blood pressure. To accomplish this, blood pressure is measured at the end of each 3-minute stage of the second test and compared to values taken at the same work rate during the first test, which was completed before the patient was started on his medication.

If, however, submaximal response is not of interest and, instead, only maximal values are, (e.g., peak $\dot{V}O_2$, peak heart rate, peak work rate), then a ramp protocol serves quite well. In the ramp protocol, work rate is literally "ramped up" throughout the test, such as 15 to 25 watts added every minute of the test. In this protocol a submaximal steady-state response is not achieved.

Measured Maximal Oxygen Consumption

The measurement of **oxygen consumption** during exercise is the most valid means of determining a person's maximal aerobic power (max $\dot{V}O_2$). It is generally accepted as the best measure of the functional ability of the cardiorespiratory system—thus, of cardiorespiratory fitness. Max $\dot{V}O_2$ reflects the body's ability to transport and utilize O_2. The physiological basis for this concept is discussed in greater detail in chapters 9 and 12. Briefly, changes in ventilation, perfusion (blood gas exchange of O_2 at the capillary/alveoli interface), central transport (heart rate and stroke volume), and/or peripheral utilization (tissue extraction) can all influence $\dot{V}O_2$ max.

Max $\dot{V}O_2$ is dependent on age, gender, and body size/body composition. Both females and males reach their maximal aerobic power around 15 to 20 years of age (figure 4.6). For the majority of the population, there is a gradual decline of max $\dot{V}O_2$ with age (about 10% per decade), which begins around age 30. This decline, however, more reflects increased inactivity with age, since many studies show that the rate of decline can be markedly reduced if one maintains a regular exercise regimen.

The max $\dot{V}O_2$ of females is ~ 15% to 25% below that of males (figure 4.6). Reasons for this are likely twofold.[40] First, females have more essential body fat than males (14% to 15% vs. 5% to 7%, respectively). However, because the metabolism of the active muscles dictates, in part, one's max $\dot{V}O_2$, much of the gender difference in max $\dot{V}O_2$ is abolished when it is expressed per unit of leg volume (figure 4.7). Second, the hemoglobin concentration of females

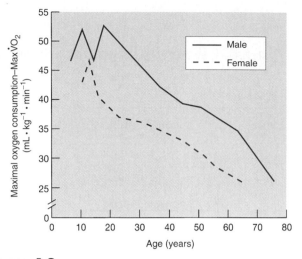

Figure 4.6

The maximal aerobic power (max $\dot{V}O_2$) of males and females from 6 to 75 years of age.

(Based on data from Drinkwater et al.,[24] Robinson,[57] and Robinson.[58])

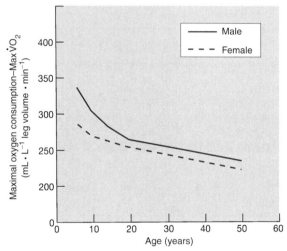

Figure 4.7

The maximal aerobic power (max $\dot{V}O_2$) of males and females from 5 to 50 years of age. In this case, max $\dot{V}O_2$ was measured on a bicycle ergometer and the active muscle mass estimated by leg volume measurements. (Leg volume is a measure of the volume of leg bone plus volume of the leg muscle. Because leg bone volume does not account for much of the total, leg volume primarily reflects leg muscle volume or mass.) Notice how little difference there is between sexes when max $\dot{V}O_2$ is expressed in mL of oxygen per liter of leg volume.

(Based on data from Davies et al.[20])

is ~ 5% to 20% (5% to 10% in trained athletes, 10% to 20% in untrained) lower than in males. Hemoglobin is the compound found in red blood cells and it transports O_2 from the lungs to the skeletal muscles. It stands to reason, therefore, that a reduced hemoglobin concentration would

4.8
table

Maximal aerobic power ($\dot{V}O_2$) in various trained and untrained adults

Activity	Class	Male (L · min^{-1})	Male (mL · kg^{-1} · min^{-1})	Female (L · min^{-1})	Female (mL · kg^{-1} · min^{-1})
Cross-country skiing	National	5.54	77.7	3.81	63.0
Running (distance)	Olympic	4.76	74.7	—	—
Running (marathon)	Team Nike	4.86	74.4	3.62	68.1
Triathlon	Elite/national	—	—	3.70	65.6
Running (mile or 1500 m)	Team Nike	5.0	72.5	3.27	63.1
Cycling	Olympic	5.2	71.1	3.7	62.6
Biathlon	National	5.23	68.9	3.62	61.1
Figure skating	Elite	4.18	66.7	2.81	56.8
Speed skating (short track)	National	4.22	64.3	—	—
Triathlon	Competitive	4.8	63.7	3.1	51.4
Running (400 m)	National	4.64	63.0	—	—
Field hockey	International	4.64	61.8	—	—
Soccer	Professional	4.60	60.9	—	—
Rowing	Olympic	5.54	59.6	—	—
Altitude mountaineering	—	4.30	57.9	3.44	55.2
Volleyball	National	5.08	56.7	—	—
In-line skating	Competitive	3.91	53.6	—	—
Alpine skiing	International	4.07	53.2	2.93	46.4
Football (defensive backs, receivers)	Professional	4.26	50.1	—	—
Race walking	International	—	—	2.51	49.9
Running (master's)	Competitive	—	—	2.53	45.8
Football (lineman)	Professional	5.06	43.0	—	—
Wheelchair racing	National	2.49	38.1	—	—
Untrained (51 year old)	Normal	2.28	28.4	1.42	22.3
Patients with heart disease	—	1.75	20.4	1.03	15.0
Cardiac transplant patients	—	1.33	17.5	—	—

Compiled from various sources by Clinton A. Brawner and Steven J. Keteyian. Reprinted by permission.

also contribute to the lower max $\dot{V}O_2$ observed when comparing trained or untrained age-matched males and females. In the real world of athletic performance, however, the only meaningful relationship is between max $\dot{V}O_2$ and body weight because in most exercises and sports, movement of total body weight greatly impacts power output. Therefore, there is little question that females are at a distinct disadvantage (figure 4.6).

Absolute and relative comparative values for both trained and untrained men and women are shown in table 4.8.

Our discussion about the measurement of $\dot{V}O_2$ would be incomplete if we did not mention the criteria used to determine whether or not a true max $\dot{V}O_2$ was achieved. As stated previously, a general guideline during graded exercise testing is to have the performer reach voluntary (volitional) fatigue within 6 to 12 minutes. A maximum value is felt to be achieved when one or more of the following criteria are achieved.[37,38,62]

1. A further increase in work rate results in no further increase (a plateau) in $\dot{V}O_2$. This might equate to a change in $\dot{V}O_2$ of less than 150 mL · min^{-1} (or 2.1 mL · kg^{-1} · min^{-1}) or less (as shown in figure 4.8).*
2. The R exceeds 1.10 to 1.15.
3. If measured, post-exercise blood lactate exceeds 8 to 10 mM.

It is important to point out that factors such as age and type of testing protocol create variability for each of the criteria. As a result, they cannot be universally applied in the field of exercise physiology.[38] Additionally, by itself the near attainment or attainment of age-predicted maximal

---

*In the original work, Taylor, Buskirk, and Henschel[62] specified the criterion under conditions involving a series of 3-minute, 7-mph tests with increments in grade of 2.5% conducted over a period of several days. Thus, day 1 would be at 3.5% grade, day 2 at 6% grade, and so on. The increment in oxygen consumption, under these conditions, was normally about 300 mL · min^{-1}.

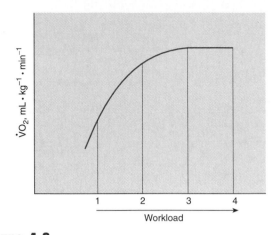

Figure 4.8
Determining the point at which maximal aerobic capacity has been reached. A primary criterion for such a determination depends on the individual's inability to consume additional oxygen when the work load is increased.

4.9

Equations to predict max $\dot{V}O_2$ using two common field tests

1. **Rockport one-mile fitness walking test***
   - $\dot{V}O_{2max}$ (in mL $\cdot$ kg^{-1} $\cdot$ min^{-1}) = 132.853
     $-$ (0.0769 $\times$ body weight) $-$ (0.3877 $\times$ age)
     $+$ (6.315 $\times$ gender) $-$ (3.2649 $\times$ time)
     $-$ (0.1565 $\times$ HR)
2. **Cooper 12-minute test**
   - $\dot{V}O_{2max}$ (in mL $\cdot$ kg^{-1} $\cdot$ min^{-1}) = 3.126
     $\times$ (meters walked and/or run in 12 min.) $-$ 11.3

*body weight = in lbs; gender = 0 for female and 1 for male; time = in min.; and heart rate (HR) is taken at the end of the walk
Adapted from American College of Sports Medicine[2]

heart rate is not a suitable criterion. As a result, it is not uncommon to see the term *peak $\dot{V}O_2$* used when at least one of the above three criteria are not met. However, use of *peak $\dot{V}O_2$* in this manner may be different from what was originally intended, which was *the highest value achieved under a specific set of circumstances or conditions.*[59] Reasons for not achieving a true maximum might include age, certain disease states, lack of motivation, symptoms such as chest pain or lightheadedness, ECG changes, or early fatigue.

The American College of Sports Medicine has defined protocols, procedures, and precautions for exercise testing apparently healthy individuals, persons classified at high risk, and patients with known diseases.[2]

Estimating Aerobic Power

When it is neither feasible nor prudent to measure oxygen consumption, there are various methods available to estimate or predict it. Several of these techniques are mentioned below; however, a drawback inherent to them all is the possible variability that exists (at best 3 to 4 mL $\cdot$ kg^{-1} $\cdot$ min^{-1}) between predicted $\dot{V}O_2$ and measured max $\dot{V}O_2$. If the intent is to simply classify an individual's aerobic power for general purposes or obtain a broad estimate of energy expenditure, then these tests serve well. If, on the other hand, we are trying to monitor the impact of a new training regimen among competitive athletes or to determine the effect of a yet unproven drug therapy, then direct measurement of $\dot{V}O_2$ is preferred.

The least expensive method available to predict max $\dot{V}O_2$ without directly measuring it involves *field tests*, such as the Cooper 12-minute test and the Rockport one-mile fitness walking test. Equations have been developed (table 4.9) for these tests, which provide a somewhat accurate es-

timate of an individual's fitness level. Other advantages of these tests include ease of administration and the ability to assess a large number of persons at one time. There are, however, shortcomings, which include reliance on subject motivation, the confounding effects of a submaximal (versus maximal) pacing effort, and as mentioned above, the difference that exists between estimated and measured max $\dot{V}O_2$. Also, in the absence of ECG and blood pressure monitoring, safety of testing certain people may also be a concern.

The Cooper test requires that the person walk and/or jog as far as possible in 12 minutes. The measured distance is used to determine max $\dot{V}O_2$. The Rockport test is slightly more complex and involves having the individual walk one mile as fast as possible. Immediately after the walk, a 15-second pulse rate is measured, and based on this value and the individual's age, body weight, one-mile time, and gender, a max $\dot{V}O_2$ is predicted.

In the hospital or clinical setting, the equipment needed to directly measure $\dot{V}O_2$ is often unavailable. In this instance, max $\dot{V}O_2$ can be predicted using equations specific to the exercise protocol used. Prediction equations can be either *generalized* or *population specific* and usually involve variables such as total exercise time, age, health status, and activity level. Examples of three equations developed to predict $\dot{V}O_2$ using the Bruce protocol are shown in table 4.10. The accuracy of any equation is improved the closer the population used to develop the equation "fits" the person being tested (gender, age, and fitness level).

The estimation of max $\dot{V}O_2$ can also be accomplished by extrapolating information obtained during submaximal exercise to predicted maximum. Two different methods to accomplish this are the YMCA protocol[31] and the Åstrand-Ryhming test.[4] Both procedures use a cycle ergometer, rely

4.10
table

Estimated or predicted max $\dot{V}O_2$ based on total exercise time during a graded exercise test using the Bruce protocol

Men:[52]*
$$\dot{V}O_2max \ (mL \cdot kg^{-1} \cdot min^{-1}) = 4.326 \times (\text{exercise time in minutes}) - 4.66$$

Women:[53]†
$$\dot{V}O_2max \ (mL \cdot kg^{-1} \cdot min^{-1}) = 0.073 \times (\text{exercise time in seconds}) - 3.9$$

Generalized:[25]‡
$$\dot{V}O_2max \ (mL \cdot kg^{-1} \cdot min^{-1}) = 14.8 - 1.38 \times (\text{exercise time in minutes}) + 0.45 \times (\text{time}^2) - 0.012 \times (\text{time}^3)$$

*Based on 51 healthy men between the ages of 35 and 55.
†Based on 49 healthy women between the ages of 20 and 42.
‡Based on 200 men.

4.11
table

Approximate energy requirements in METs for stationary cycling

Body Weight		Exercise Rate (kg-m · min⁻¹ and watts)						
kg	**lb**	**300** **50**	**450** **75**	**600** **100**	**750** **125**	**900** **150**	**1050** **175**	**1200 (kg-m · min⁻¹)** **200 (watts)**
50	110	5.1	6.9	8.6	10.3	12.0	13.7	15.4
60	132	4.3	5.7	7.1	8.6	10.0	11.4	12.9
70	154	3.7	4.9	6.1	7.3	8.6	9.8	11.0
80	176	3.2	4.3	5.4	6.4	7.5	8.6	9.6
90	198	2.9	3.8	4.8	5.7	6.7	7.6	8.6
100	220	2.6	3.4	4.3	5.1	6.0	6.9	7.7

on the linear relationship between heart rate and $\dot{V}O_2$, and represent tests that can be used in both men and women of various ages. The YMCA protocol involves several stages of submaximal exercise and advances work rate based on heart rate response. The Åstrand-Ryhming method represents a single stage test of 6 minutes. Both tests are described in appendix F, and students are encouraged to undergo one or both of these tests to estimate their own peak power output, caloric expenditure, and max $\dot{V}O_2$.

In each of the above examples, the primary objective was to determine maximal $\dot{V}O_2$. There are, however, many situations when determination of an individual's $\dot{V}O_2$ during *submaximal* exercise at a specified work rate is of interest. For example, estimating energy expenditure (kcal) during steady-state cycling, walking, or jogging can contribute greatly to one's overall weight management plan. To make

such a determination, we rely on various equations that have been developed from laboratory data obtained during exercise.[2] To appreciate their use, tables 4.11 and 4.12 present the already computed approximate energy requirement for stationary cycling and horizontal and/or grade walking in *METs*. When using these equations, the tester must keep in mind that they are appropriate for steady-state submaximal aerobic exercise only.

The Concept of the MET

Another way to express the energy cost of activity is to report the work effort in terms of a MET.[2] The term **MET** is an acronym that stands for "Metabolic Equivalent." One MET is defined as the energy expenditure ($\dot{V}O_2$) expressed as a mL · kg⁻¹ · min⁻¹ (or L · min⁻¹) while *sitting quietly*.[1]

4.12

Approximate energy requirements in METs for horizontal and grade walking

% Grade	mi · h^{-1}	1.7	2.0	2.5	3.0	3.4	3.75
	m · min^{-1}	45.6	53.7	67.0	80.5	91.2	100.5
0		2.3	2.5	2.9	3.3	3.6	3.9
2.5		2.9	3.2	3.8	4.3	4.8	5.2
5.0		3.5	3.9	4.6	5.4	5.9	6.5
7.5		4.1	4.6	5.5	6.4	7.1	7.8
10.0		4.6	5.3	6.3	7.4	8.3	9.1
12.5		5.2	6.0	7.2	8.5	9.5	10.4
15.0		5.8	6.6	8.1	9.5	10.6	11.7

4.13

METs values associated with common occupational and leisure physical activities[1]

	METs value		METs value
Assembly line worker	3.5	Mowing lawn (power mower)	4.5
Bowling	3.0	Painter	4.5
Bus driver	3.0	Security guard	2.5
Carpenter	6.0	Skiing	
Desk worker	1.5	(downhill, light)	5.0
Farmer	5.0	(nordic)	7.0
Fire fighter	12.0	Snow removal	
Gardening	5.0	(hand shovel)	6.0
Golf		(blower)	4.5
(carrying clubs)	5.5	Steel worker	8.0
(with cart)	3.5	Swimming (laps, slow)	8.0
Hunting	6.0	Tennis (general)	7.0
Machine tool operator	4.0	Walking (3.0 mph)	3.3

In short, a MET is resting $\dot{V}O_2$. For the average adult, 1 MET is *approximately* 3.5 mL of O_2 consumed per kilogram of body weight per minute (1 MET = 3.5 mL · kg^{-1} · min^{-1}). It is also approximately 1 kcal · kg^{-1} body weight · hr^{-1}. This constant can also be used to estimate a subject's resting $\dot{V}O_2$. For example, a subject weighing 80 kg would likely have a resting $\dot{V}O_2$ of about 280 mL · min^{-1} (3.5 mL · kg^{-1} · min^{-1} × 80 kg) or 0.280 L · min^{-1}. Obviously, if greater accuracy is required, $\dot{V}O_2$ should be measured.

MET*s* (plural) means multiples of one's resting metabolism. An exercise requiring 10 METs simply means that the oxygen cost of an activity is 10 times resting $\dot{V}O_2$, or 3.5 mL · kg^{-1} · min^{-1} × 10, which equals 35 mL · kg^{-1} · min^{-1}. For a person who weighs 70 kg, this would represent an absolute $\dot{V}O_2$ of 2.45 L · min^{-1} (70 kg × 35 mL · kg^{-1} · min^{-1} = 2450 mL · min^{-1}, or 2.45 L · min^{-1}).

Working the math in the other direction, when presented with a measured $\dot{V}O_2$ you can still define any exercise in terms of METs. For example, how many METs were required during the treadmill run mentioned on page 81 (assume that the subject weighed 70 kg)? You will recall that the overall $\dot{V}O_2$ for the exercise was 2.8 L · min^{-1}; therefore, $\dot{V}O_2$ on a per kilogram of body weight basis would be 2800 mL ÷ 70 kg = 40 mL · kg^{-1} · min^{-1}. Because

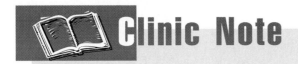

After completing an exercise stress test, patients often ask "How did I do?" or "Did I pass?" Interpreting test results involves a variety of issues, including the effect of a prescribed medication on controlling chest pain, determining the presence or absence of myocardial ischemia* (usually caused by blockages in the arteries that supply the heart itself with much needed oxygen and nutrients), and/or quantifying one's aerobic power or cardiorespiratory fitness level.

Reviewing with the patient whether a certain medication was effective or whether or not myocardial ischemia exists is important, but it is outside the scope of this chapter. Interpreting their fitness level, however, is directly related to the topic at hand.

Whether aerobic power (max $\dot{V}O_2$) is directly measured or estimated, the value must be interpreted for the patient in an understandable and meaningful manner. Doing so can be somewhat difficult for both the patient and the clinician if the patient is unfamiliar with terms like mL of O_2 consumed per kg of body weight per minute or multiples of resting energy expenditure (METs).

A simple approach used in the Henry Ford Hospital Cardiac Rehabilitation Unit, one that is both quantifiable yet easily understandable, involves a unitless scale of

2 to 24. For example, a score of 22 and above would represent the fitness level of an elite aerobically trained athlete, while a score of 5 to 6 is common for the recovering heart patient. This scale is actually based on METs, but the patient need not know this. A peak MET level of 24 approximates a $\dot{V}O_2$ of 84 mL $\cdot$ kg^{-1} $\cdot$ min^{-1} (24 $\times$ 3.5 mL $\cdot$ kg^{-1} $\cdot$ min^{-1}), and a value of 2 represents a $\dot{V}O_2$ of 14 mL $\cdot$ kg^{-1} $\cdot$ min^{-1}. You simply inform the patient, for example, that on a scale of 2 to 24 (with above 15 being representative of very highly fit people and below 6 or 7 reflecting poorer fit people), he or she has a fitness level of X. Students are encouraged to divide the values (per kg body weight) shown in table 4.8 by 3.5 to see how nicely they fall between 2 and 24. A fitness level above which good health is ensured has not yet been definitively identified; however, it is reasonable to expect that persons who exercise moderately (30 minutes per day, 4 to 5 days per week) will attain a fitness level of 8 *or more* on our scale of 2 to 24. (Remember, this means 8 or more METs; we just don't confuse the patient with our elaborate definitions). This concept of a unitless scale of 2 to 24 can be used in various age groups, with men or women, and among trained and untrained persons. Its accuracy is as good as the method used to determine aerobic fitness (direct measurement or prediction equation) and can be applied to whatever set of population-specific or generalized norms the clinician chooses.

*Myocardial = heart, and ischemia = lack of oxygen; therefore, myocardial ischemia literally means temporary lack of oxygen to the heart muscle itself.

---

1 MET is approximately 3.5 mL $\cdot$ kg^{-1} $\cdot$ min^{-1}, the O_2 cost in this example equals 11.4 METs (40 mL $\cdot$ kg^{-1} $\cdot$ min^{-1} $\div$ 3.5 mL $\cdot$ kg^{-1} $\cdot$ min^{-1}). Table 4.13 provides the MET values previously determined for a variety of occupational and leisure activities.[1]

The Utility of MET Estimates

In some situations where one person is helping guide the exercise or work habits of another person, such as in an adult fitness program or an out-patient cardiology clinic, the use of MET estimates can be advantageous. For example, 10 weeks after suffering an uncomplicated heart attack, a 45-year-old patient asks his doctor if he can return to his full-time job of being a house painter. To make this determination the physician needs to answer two questions. First, what is the approximate MET (energy) level of painting?

Second, at what peak MET (energy or fitness) level can the patient safely exert himself? In other words, does he now have the physical capacity or fitness to do his job—or is more exercise conditioning needed before he returns to work?

To answer the first question we turn to table 4.13 and learn that while actively painting the patient will experience a work intensity of approximately 4.5 METs. To answer the second question we need to determine the patient's peak MET level by either measuring $\dot{V}O_2$ using a metabolic cart or by estimating it with an exercise test protocol prediction equation (e.g., table 4.10). As a general rule of thumb, and given no medical problems to the contrary, clinicians generally allow patients to return to a moderate level occupation (such as painting) when the most strenuous part of their job represents less than 75% of their peak MET ability. In this example, the patient's peak MET level would need to

table

4.14

Efficiency while performing various exercise activities

Exercise activity	Efficiency (percent)		References
	Male	Female	
Horizontal walking	19.6–35.2	—	Donovan and Brooks[23]
Inclined walking	20.6–43.0	—	Donovan and Brooks[23]
Swimming (freestyle)	2.9–7.4	2.7–9.4	Pendergast et al.[51]
Rowing	13.0	17.0	Hagerman et al.[33,34]
Rowing	10–20	—	DiPrampero et al.[21]
Ice skating	11.0	—	DiPrampero et al.[22]
Cycling (level)	24.4–34.4	—	Gaesser and Brooks[29]
Cycling (uphill)	19	—	Swain and Wilcox[61]
Arm ergometry	16	—	Quinn et al.[55]
Combined arm and leg ergometry	18	—	Quinn et al.[55]
Stepping machine (stair climber)	23	24	Butts et al.[12]

be 6.0 METs or more for the 4.5 MET level associated with painting to be less than 75% of peak.

Before proceeding, let's consider the limitations associated with using one standard or estimated MET value for all. In this case the MET equivalent of 3.5 mL $\cdot$ kg^{-1} $\cdot$ min^{-1} is a constant that is applied to both men and women, girls and boys, young and old, the obese and thin, and persons with low and high fitness levels. Intuitively, this observation raises the questions, how well can a standard value apply to such diverse groups? Clearly, when using METs there is a loss of precision. If, in fact, a precise value is needed, then it should be measured.

Computation of Efficiency

Our ability to perform certain tasks and activities is related, in part, to the amount of energy we waste in trying to complete the task. When more of the energy we expend goes into work output versus being lost as heat, then performance is optimized. Scientists refer to this concept as **efficiency** (expressed as a percentage), and it is defined as the ratio of work output over work input (energy expenditure) times 100, or:

$$\% \text{ Efficiency} = \frac{\text{Useful work output}}{\text{Energy expended}} \times 100$$

All machines must be less than 100% efficient because of friction. That is to say, the *useful* work output will always be less than the work input. The doctrine of the conservation of energy implies that although it is possible to convert one form of energy to another, *one can neither create nor destroy energy*. Remember, machines do *not* create or destroy energy; they merely convert it from one form to another. During the conversion, some energy is *always* lost (wasted). If this were not the case, we could develop a perpetual motion machine. A steam plant, for example, may operate at 5%, or even less, efficiency because heat is lost through radiation, conduction, and exhaust steam. Turbines and automobile engines operate at about 20% to 25% efficiency, whereas a diesel engine may produce an output to input ratio of 30 to 35%.

In the metabolic sense, we are also interested in work output (kcal produced) and energy expended (kcal). Thus:

$$\% \text{ Efficiency} = \frac{\text{Useful work output (\textbf{kcal})}}{\text{Energy expended (\textbf{kcal})}} \times 100$$

Fortunately, as you have learned, we can convert various work units into energy units. Thus, work output expressed in kg-m can be converted to kilocalories (kcal) or kilojoules (kJ), as can energy expenditure or cost (originally expressed as VO_2).

Keep in mind that we are dealing with work units in these efficiency equations. If work output (numerator) and work input (denominator) are both expressed per unit of time (minutes), they become expressions of power. Efficiency would be the same whether work units, power units, or energy units are used, as long as the same unit is used in both the numerator and denominator of the equation. For example, do not mix kJ with kcal or kg-m with watts in the same equation.

In certain instances, such as road cycle racing or ice-speed skating, it is not possible to quantify actual work

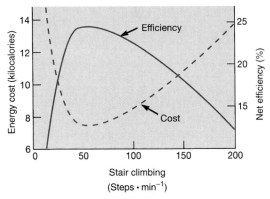

Figure 4.9

Influence of speed in climbing stairs on energy cost and efficiency. The cost is lowest and efficiency highest when 50 steps per minute were climbed.

(Data from Lupton.[43])

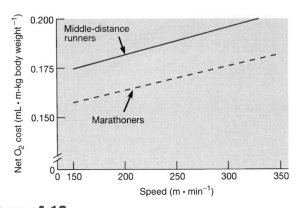

Figure 4.10

Differences in running efficiencies between middle-distance runners and marathon runners. Marathon runners are about 5 to 10 percent more efficient than middle-distance runners.

(Based on data from various sources as compiled by Fox and Costill.[28])

accomplished or power. It is appropriate, in these situations, to use the phrase *economy of movement*, which describes the $\dot{V}O_2$ needed to maintain a given velocity of movement.[16]

Returning to efficiency, what then is the efficiency of the human "machine"? Usually the performance of large muscle activities, such as walking, running, and cycling, results in an efficiency of 20% to 25% (table 4.14). There are, of course, individual differences that are due to body size, gender, fitness level, and skill in performing a given task. In addition, in activities where there is considerable *resistance to movement*, such as cycling, in-line skating, cross-country skiing, ice skating, rowing, and swimming, efficiencies are generally lower than 20%.[21,22,33,34,51] Resistance to movement is the drag encountered by the athlete and his or her equipment while moving through the environment.[16] The extent of drag or resistance to movement is related to the amount of exposed surface area and velocity (e.g., more drag is encountered while in-line skating at 27.4 km · hr^{-1} vs. 22.5 km · hr^{-1}). Also, drag is dependent on the environmental medium (air vs. water), such that the efficiency of swimming is generally less than 10% (table 4.14).[51] This is why techniques meant to improve aerodynamics/hydrodynamics have become so popular and important over the past 10 years—techniques such as changes in body position, drafting, and streamlining equipment.

As discussed, gender can influence efficiency, and just this issue was addressed in a study conducted by Daniels and Daniels,[19] where 20 female and 45 male U.S. Olympic hopeful middle- and long-distance runners underwent comparisons for $\dot{V}O_2$ during exercise. Average max $\dot{V}O_2$ was 14% higher in males (75.4 mL · kg^{-1} · min^{-1}) than in females (66.2 mL · kg^{-1} · min^{-1}), and at matched running velocities of 268, 290 and 310 m · min^{-1}, male runners were ∼ 6% to 7% more economical (consumed less O_2)

than their female counterparts. The better aerobic profile ($\dot{V}O_2$, economy of movement) among the elite male versus female athletes led to their faster race or running velocities.

A classic study by Lupton[43] (figure 4.9) clearly demonstrates the influence of speed on efficiency (in this case economy, since velocity is being used in place of energy output) while climbing stairs. Note that 50 steps per minute produces the highest efficiency (lowest energy cost). The same concept is also true for cyclists (level ground or uphill), where efficiency is highest at pedal rates between 60 to 85 rpm.[9,11,14,61] As summarized by Berry and coworkers,[9] reasons for the improved efficiency at lower (60 to 85 rpm) versus higher (100 to 120 rpm) pedal speeds may include a lower muscular friction at the lower pedal speeds, the recruitment of additional muscles to stabilize the trunk during higher pedal speeds, and/or the increased recruitment of less efficient fast-twitch fibers at higher pedal speeds.

Efficiency is also different among athletes who participate in the same type of activity but subspecialize in different events. Figure 4.10 nicely demonstrates this using runners: middle-distance versus marathon.[28] Efficiency is represented by the net oxygen cost of running at various velocities (m · min^{-1}) and is expressed as mL of oxygen per horizontal meter (m) run and per kg of bodyweight (mL · m-kg body weight^{-1}). Remember, the higher the net oxygen cost at a given velocity between two individuals, the lower the efficiency. Marathon runners are about 5% to 10% more efficient, on average, than middle-distance runners. This advantage, though small for runs of short duration, would be an important consideration during the $2\frac{1}{2}$ hours required to run a good marathon race. For example, a 10% greater efficiency equates to a "savings" of about 60 L of oxygen consumed, or 300 kcal of heat produced per marathon race!

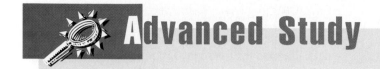

The formula provided in the body of the text refers to gross efficiency. If, in the denominator, we were to subtract resting energy expenditure from energy expended during exercise (work input), we then get net efficiency.

% Net efficiency =
$$\frac{\text{Useful work output (kcal)}}{\text{Energy expended (kcal) } \textit{less} \text{ that expended at rest}} \times 100$$

Additionally, if we compare the relationship between change in work rate to change in $\dot{V}O_2$, we then get delta efficiency. Delta efficiency is measured during exercise and computed as follows:

% Delta efficiency =
$$\frac{\begin{array}{c}\text{The work currently being performed } \textit{less} \text{ that} \\ \text{performed at the previous work rate (kcal)}\end{array}}{\begin{array}{c}\text{Energy expended } \textit{less} \text{ that expended} \\ \text{at the previous work rate (kcal)}\end{array}} \times 100$$

For example, let's say the $\dot{V}O_2$ while cycling increased from 1.2 L · min^{-1} at the first work rate of 75 watts to 1.8 L · min^{-1} at the second work rate of 125 watts; then the ratio for delta efficiency equals 50 watts/0.6 L · min^{-1}

of oxygen. We must then convert 50 watts to kcal · min^{-1} (1 watt = 0.014 kcal · min^{-1}, see table 4.2) and 0.6 L · min^{-1} to kcal (1 L of oxygen consumed = ~ 5.0 kcal) to get a delta efficiency of:

$$\frac{50 \text{ watts}}{0.6 \text{ L} \cdot \text{min}^{-1}} = \frac{0.7 \text{ kcal} \cdot \text{min}^{-1}}{3 \text{ kcal} \cdot \text{min}^{-1}}$$
$$= 0.233 \times 100 = 23\%$$

Delta efficiency is unaffected by body mass (obesity or weight loss) and reflects a more contemporary measure or definition of muscle efficiency.[9,54,55] It is, however, related to the percentage of Type I (red- or slow-twitch) skeletal muscle fibers. Coyle and associates[17] explored this idea and found that delta efficiency increased as the percentage of Type I fibers present in the cyclist's leg muscles increased (figure 4.11). This suggests that persons with a high percentage of Type I fibers are more efficient than persons with a low percentage of the same fibers. Extrapolating their data to the extremes, to 0% Type I fibers and 100% Type I fibers, the authors predicted that the efficiency of Type I fibers is twice that of Type II (white- or fast-twitch) fibers, at 27% versus 13%, respectively.

Other Factors Affecting Efficiency

In addition to those we have discussed, there are other factors that affect the efficiency and economy of human movement. Many of these have been grouped as *structural factors* and *optimal phenomena* by Cavanagh and Kram.[13] Structural factors include total body mass, distribution of body mass, variations in the distance of insertions of key muscles from joint centers, and variations in muscle fiber orientation and length.

Additionally, observations were made of several types of human movement in which biomechanical variables had been manipulated. Such manipulations produce energy cost curves that have a point of least energy cost. Cavanagh and Kram characterized these points as optimal phenomena, some of which include the following.

1. $\dot{V}O_2$ and power output during cycling are affected by seat height.
2. As mentioned previously, pedal frequency affects energy cost during cycling.
3. Changes in stride length while running at a given speed affects energy cost.

4. Energy cost ($\dot{V}O_2$) during downhill running or walking is lowest at a -5% grade.
5. For each person a speed of walking exists at which efficiency is optimized ($\dot{V}O_2$ is lowest). For most people this optimal speed is between 3.3 and 3.7 mph.

Common and Modified Methods for Assessing Energy Cost in the Field

In the appropriately equipped laboratory the measurement of efficiency (work output/work input) during exercise is really quite straightforward. The methods associated with measuring efficiency using a cycle ergometer or a treadmill are detailed in appendix G. However, throughout sports and our daily lives, situations arise that limit the ability of the scientist to easily quantify work, power, or energy. In these instances somewhat different approaches must be employed, several of which are described on the next page.

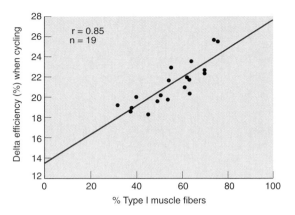

Figure 4.11

The relationship between percent Type I skeletal muscle fibers and delta efficiency while cycling at 80 rpm.

(From Coyle et al.[17])

Measurement of Energy Cost for Sprinting and Other High-Intensity Activities

Imagine the difficulty associated with having a technician run along the track holding a Douglas bag, just to gather a sprinter's exhaled air. An alternate approach might be one where resting VO_2 is determined using a Douglas bag and then, during the sprint, subjects *hold their breath* until they are finished. Immediately upon stopping they hold their nose and direct all exhaled air into a series of Douglas bags.

More than 30 years ago this method was used to measure the energy cost and performance time associated with the open and closed swimming turns.[27] In that study six male swimmers completed both open and closed turns without taking a breath. Immediately upon stopping, they exhaled into a Douglas bag for 15 minutes. The data showed no significant difference between the two turns relative to net energy cost (recovery oxygen − resting oxygen), but the closed turn was performed significantly faster.

What do we do when the event is the 400 m race? Few scientists are physically able to run alongside an elite athlete with Douglas bag in hand to collect exhaled air! Alternately, no athlete can hold their breath for the entire time needed to run 400 m! In this instance, the net recovery oxygen may be used as a *relative* indicator of exercise intensity.

Just such a method was used to compare the 400-yard freestyle using the open versus closed turns.[32] Subjects were required to swim 400 yards in ∼ 4 minutes and 50 seconds. Oxygen consumption was measured at rest and for 30 minutes following the swim. Average net recovery oxygen for the open and closed turn was 4.7 L and 5.1 L, respectively. Although the open turn swim resulted in a smaller recovery oxygen, the difference was not statistically significant.

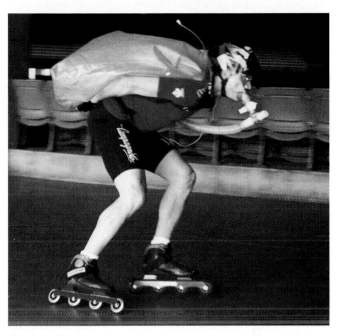

Figure 4.12

The measurement of energy cost during a given activity can pose certain methodologic problems. One method to overcome such difficulties is attaching a Douglas bag to the subject so expired air can be collected during the activity. Contents of the bag are then analyzed soon after collection.

(Photograph courtesy of Fedel Performance, Inc., and Henry Ford Health System)

One other method to consider is the attachment of a Douglas bag to the back of the subject being tested, along with a mouthpiece and a controlling valve (figure 4.12). When the subject turns the valve to direct air into the bag, a miniaturized timer is activated. When the valve is closed, the timer is deactivated. With the exact collection time known, the contents of the bag are then analyzed using the manual or automated method. A possible shortcoming associated with this approach: to what extent does wearing the apparatus impact test results (both aerodynamically and psychologically)?

Measurement of Energy Cost Using a Motion Sensor

Although motion sensors date back some 500 years to the time of Leonardo da Vinci, continued interest to measure caloric expenditure in the field led to the development and application of a new technology. These devices contain motion sensors, or accelerometers, that measure acceleration in a vertical plane or three-dimensionally.[5,6] Usually attached to the subject at the waist, they contain a very small computer programmed to convert acceleration to activity counts or energy expenditure (kcal). Several studies have been conducted to determine the validity of such instruments as compared to the direct measurement of $\dot{V}O_2$, and most of the research has been conducted on walking and running. Regarding these devices, they appear acceptable in well-motivated subjects and are capable of accurately assessing changes in velocity during walking.[6,35,60] However, such devices have difficulty discriminating between running speeds of 8 to 12.8 km · h^{-1} and tend to overestimate energy expenditure during walking (3.2 to 8 km · h^{-1}) and running.[6,36] This difference between estimated energy expenditure and actual (measured) energy expenditure is usually greater in men than in women,[36] most likely because of differences in body weight.

Measurement of Energy Cost Using Telemetry

The scientists at the National Aeronautics and Space Administration (NASA), prior to initiating programs designed to probe an organism's physiological reactions to space, devised instrumentation that could radio back to the space center such information as respiration, heart rate, and blood pressure. Today, the field of physiological radio transmission called **telemetry** is so well advanced that many college and human performance laboratories are equipped for transmitting numerous variables such as heart rate, body temperature, blood pressure, and $\dot{V}O_2$. Of these, the most common for estimating energy expenditure is the ability to transmit heart rate. This is of interest because during moderate submaximal exercise, heart rate is linearly related to $\dot{V}O_2$ and, therefore, to kcal. Figure 4.13 graphically illustrates this relationship.

Many heart rate monitors involve the placement of two chest electrodes that are attached by wires to a transmitter (worn around a subject's waist), which transmits an FM signal to a receiver. The receiver is connected to an oscilloscope/ECG recorder, which is then monitored by someone in the area. In fact, many cardiac rehabilitation programs today use this technology to monitor and supervise the response of recovering heart patients during exercise therapy. Further advances in technology have led to modifications of heart rate monitors. For many of these devices, a strap placed around an individual's chest is capable of "picking up" heart rate and transmitting it to a receiver worn on the subject's wrist (figure 4.14). The data is displayed and/or stored in the wrist receiver, which can then be "downloaded" at a later time to a larger computer for analysis. In fact, storing data on the person using the ample memory capabilities within the receiver has provided exercise scientists with increased flexibility to study activities "from a distance," in different environments (e.g., under water), and in various test conditions. Heart rate monitors have been shown to have acceptable accuracy when compared to direct wire measures of heart rate.[42]

The use of heart rate-based telemetry allows us to estimate the $\dot{V}O_2$ of numerous physical and sports activities that otherwise would be difficult to determine. In general,

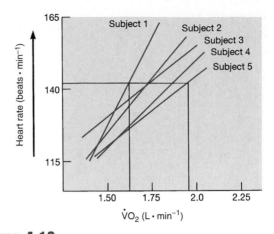

Figure 4.13

Relationships among work load, $\dot{V}O_2$, and heart rate. As the work load or $\dot{V}O_2$ increases, so does heart rate in a linear (straight line) manner. Notice the variability among subjects; however, for any given subject a defined relationship exists.

the higher the exercise heart rate, the greater the intensity of the exercise and, therefore, the greater the $\dot{V}O_2$. However, heart rate is also influenced by other factors, such as temperature, apprehension, and excitement. For example, data obtained from telemetry of heart rate in coaches while they were coaching revealed that heart rate increased considerably (greater than 150 beats · min^{-1}) during critical game situations, even though physical activity was minimal.[45] Also, astronauts aboard the space shuttle at the time of re-entry demonstrate elevations of heart rates (up to 150 beats · min^{-1}), even though physical effort is of little consequence at the time.

To determine energy cost from heart rate while playing racquetball, field hockey, soccer, or some other activity, we would proceed as follows:

1. Have each subject exercise on an ergometer (e.g., cycle or treadmill) at gradually increasing work loads to maximum.
2. At each work load, measure heart rate and oxygen consumption.
3. Using a statistical technique called regression, plot this relationship on a graph, as shown in figure 4.13.

To estimate $\dot{V}O_2$ during the activity we utilize the heart rate-$\dot{V}O_2$ regression line developed for the subject. For example, using figure 4.13, if the heart rate from telemetry for subject 1 were 142 beats · min^{-1} while playing soccer, then $\dot{V}O_2$ at that particular time would equal about 1.6 L · min^{-1} (or 8 kcal · min^{-1}). Please note that a separate regression line must be established for each individual. For example, at the same heart rate (142 beats · min^{-1}), the $\dot{V}O_2$ for subject 5 would be 1.96 L · min^{-1}. At best, the heart rate method provides only a crude assessment of energy expenditure.[35]

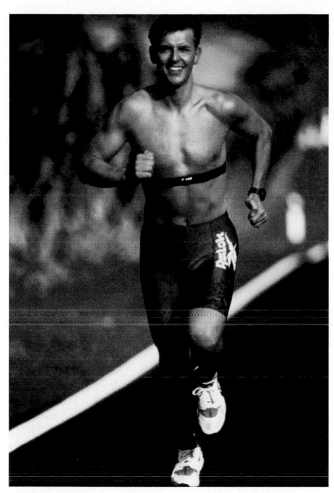

Figure 4.14

Subject fitted with a transmitter for heart rate telemetry (monitoring). The receiver, on the subject's wrist, displays heart rate information and stores data for "downloading" to a computer at a later time. This type of equipment allows the subject to perform the activity unencumbered.

(Photograph courtesy of Polar Electro Inc.)

Ancillary Considerations in Measuring Energy Expenditure

Certain ancillary considerations should be kept in mind when measuring and interpreting the energy cost of activities. Factors such as body size, environmental condition or climate, fitness level, anxiety, hormones, and disease state can all have an effect. Discussing each in detail is beyond the scope of this text but it is fair to say that any one may influence results and thus should be accounted for. For example, for every 1° C increase in body temperature caused by a fever, there is an approximate 11% increase in $\dot{V}O_2$.

Of the previously mentioned factors, body mass is worthy of further discussion. A larger person will simply expend more energy in moving his or her body a given distance than will a smaller person. As a result, expressing energy expenditure in terms of body mass is sometimes more appropriate, particularly when making comparisons. For example:

Work: kilogram-meters per kilogram of body weight ($kg\text{-}m \cdot kg^{-1}$)

Energy: kilocalories per kilogram of body weight ($kcal \cdot kg^{-1}$)

Power: kilogram-meters per kilogram of body weight per minute ($kg\text{-}m \cdot kg^{-1} \cdot min^{-1}$)

Energy: $\dot{V}O_2$ in milliliters per kilogram of body weight per minute ($mL \cdot kg^{-1} \cdot min^{-1}$) or kilocalories per kilogram of body weight per minute ($kcal \cdot kg^{-1} \cdot min^{-1}$)

Body weight is usually expressed in kilograms (kg), a metric unit not as familiar to us as pounds. A table converting body weight from pounds to kilograms is given in appendix E. One pound equals 0.454 kg and 1 kg equals 2.205 pounds. For practice, convert your own body weight in pounds into kilograms.

On occasion, body surface area rather than body weight is used for expressing energy per unit of body size. This is generally the case when expressing energy expenditure (in kcal) during heat balance experiments. The reason for this is that the amount of heat gained and/or lost by the body is more a function of total body surface area than just body weight. The body surface area is estimated from both body weight and height. For example, a person who weighs 70 kg (154 pounds) and who is 180 cm in height (5 feet, 11 inches) has a body surface area of 1.87 square meters. The body surface area can be calculated from a nomograph, which is also contained in appendix E. Once again, for practice, determine your own body surface area.

Average Energy and Work Values

To be comfortable and fluent in the field of exercise physiology you should commit to memory certain common energy values for various levels of exercise. For example, in sitting and reading this book, $\dot{V}O_2$ is between 250 and 300 $mL \cdot min^{-1}$, or between 3.5 and 4.5 $mL \cdot kg^{-1} \cdot min^{-1}$; and heat production is between 1.2 and 1.5 $kcal \cdot min^{-1}$. At the same time, about 6 to 8 L of air are being ventilated per minute. Your resting heart rate is likely between 60 and 80 $beats \cdot min^{-1}$.

Knowing such values forms a baseline for understanding intensity of work. For example, exercise requiring an $\dot{V}O_2$ of 4.5 $L \cdot min^{-1}$ would mean little if one did not realize that 0.3 L (300 mL) is required at rest. Exercise requiring such a high $\dot{V}O_2$ is 15 times more intensive than is resting. So, too, a person ventilating 140 L of air per minute during exercise is moving about 20 times more air through

4.15

Classification of physical work for six males, 22 to 47 years of age

Classification of work	Heart rate (beats · min^{-1})	Metabolic rate				
		$\dot{V}O_2$ (L · min^{-1})	$\dot{V}O_2$ (mL · kg^{-1} · min^{-1})	METs	Heat (kcal · min^{-1})	
1. Rest	< 80	< 0.40	< 4.0	1	< 2.0	
2. Light						
a. Mild	< 100	< 0.75	< 10.5	< 3	< 4.0	
b. Moderate	< 120	< 1.50	< 21.0	< 6	< 7.5	
3. Heavy						
a. Optimal	< 140	< 2.0	< 28.0	< 8	< 10.0	
b. Strenuous	< 160	< 2.5	< 35.0	< 10	< 12.5	
4. Severe						
a. Maximal	< 180	< 3.0	< 42.0	< 12	< 15.0	
b. Exhausting	> 180	> 3.0	> 42.0	> 12	> 15.0	

Data adapted from Wells et al.[64]

From J. G. Wells, B. Balke, and D. D. Van Fossen, "Lactic Acid Accumulation During Work: A Suggested Standardization of Work Classification." in Journal of Applied Physiology, *1957, 10:51–55. Copyright© 1957 American Physiological Society, Bethesda, MD. Reprinted by permission.*

his or her lungs than is required for resting metabolism. At the same time their heart rate may have been elevated only three times above the resting levels.

Table 4.15 contains average energy and related values that allow us to better understand the physiological requirements of performance. Memorizing a few of these values will be well worthwhile.

Summary

Energy, work, and power are functionally related. Energy is defined as the capacity to perform work, whereas work (W) is the application of a force (F) through a distance (D), or

$$W = F \times D$$

Power (P) is work performed per unit of time (t), or

$$P = W/t = (F \times D)/t.$$

The direct quantification of energy in humans involves the measurement of heat production, whereas the indirect method involves the measurement of oxygen

consumption (VO_2). Energy produced through the metabolism of foodstuffs is equal to the heat produced by the body.

Determination of the energy oxygen cost of anaerobic exercise involves measurement of VO_2 at rest, during exercise, and in recovery. The total oxygen consumed during exercise and recovery, less the resting VO_2, is called the net oxygen cost of exercise. During steady-state aerobic exercise, only resting and exercise VO_2 need be measured. In this case, the net oxygen cost is equal to the oxygen consumed during exercise minus resting VO_2. Another unit used to express the energy or oxygen cost of exercise is called the MET. One MET is defined as the amount of oxygen required per minute under quiet resting conditions and is equal to 3.5 ml of oxygen consumed per kilogram of body weight per minute (mL · kg^{-1} · min^{-1}).

The $\dot{V}O_2$ can be expressed in energy units (kilocalories = kcal) by knowing the respiratory exchange ratio (R). R is the ratio of the amount of carbon dioxide produced per minute ($\dot{V}CO_2$) over the $\dot{V}O_2$ per minute, $R = \dot{V}CO_2/\dot{V}O_2$, and indicates which foodstuffs are being metabolized. If carbohydrate is being metabolized, then

4.15

table

Classification of physical work for six males, 22 to 47 years of age (*continued*)

| Ventilation | | | | |
Volume (L · min^{-1})	Rate (breaths · min^{-1})	R	Lactic acid in multiples of resting value	Length of time work can be sustained
< 8	< 12	0.78	16–18 mg · 100 mL^{-1} blood	
< 20	< 14	0.85	Normal	Indefinite
< 35	< 15	0.85	Within normal limits	8 hours daily on the job
< 50	< 16	0.9	1.5×	8 hours daily for few weeks (seasonal work, military maneuvers, etc.)
< 60	< 20	0.95	2.0×	4 hours two or three times a week for a few weeks (special physical training)
< 80	< 25	< 1.0	5–6×	1 to 2 hours occasionally (usually in competitive sports)
> 120	> 30	> 1.0	6× or more	Few minutes; rarely

R = 1.0, and 1 L of oxygen consumed equals 5.05 kcal of heat produced. If R = 0.71, then fat is being metabolized, and 1 L oxygen consumed equals 4.68 kcal of heat produced. Other factors that affect R besides the type of foodstuffs metabolized are: (1) hyperventilation (overventilation of the lungs), which leads to excessive carbon dioxide loss; (2) buffering of lactic acid during exhaustive exercise, which also leads to release of large quantities of CO_2; and (3) the continued elevation of $\dot{V}O_2$ during recovery from exercise.

Percent efficiency is defined as the ratio of work output over work input (energy expenditure). Efficiency is simply the percentage of chemical energy converted to mechanical energy, with the remainder lost as heat. The efficiency of large muscle activities, such as walking, running, and cycling is usually 20 to 25%. Because of the water resistance, swimming has a very low efficiency of approximately 10%. Efficiency is most easily measured on either a bicycle ergometer or an inclined treadmill.

Modified methods of reflecting energy cost include measuring only the recovery $\dot{V}O_2$, motion sensors, and estimating $\dot{V}O_2$ from heart rate measurements. The latter method relies on the linear or direct relationship between heart rate and $\dot{V}O_2$ during submaximal exercise. $\dot{V}O_2$ can be estimated during the actual performance of activities because heart rate can be transmitted by FM radio waves (telemetry) to a receiver monitored by a person(s) some 10 to 100 feet away.

Energy expenditure of weight-bearing activities (e.g., walking or running) should be expressed relative to body size (body weight), whereas in heat-balance studies, energy expenditure should be expressed in kilocalories per unit of body surface area.

Questions

1. Define the terms *energy*, *work*, and *power* using words rather than formulas. Express *work* and *power* with formulas.
2. Explain the difference between direct and indirect calorimetry.
3. What measurements are needed when indirectly measuring the energy expenditure of a given exercise via oxygen consumption?

4. What oxygen consumption measures are needed to compute the net oxygen cost of anaerobic and aerobic exercise?

5. What is the respiratory exchange ratio and how is it used in the indirect measurement of energy?

6. Explain the Wingate test (procedure and measurement units) used for assessing anaerobic power.

7. Discuss the positive and negative attributes of assessing aerobic power using field tests, the direct measurement of oxygen consumption, METs, and prediction equations.

8. Explain efficiency and indicate how the efficiency of a human is measured.

9. Compare and contrast efficiency versus economy of movement.

10. How might you proceed in measuring the energy cost of running the 100-yard dash?

11. What are the physiological considerations that allow you to estimate energy cost through heart-rate telemetry?

12. How are body size and the performance of work related?

References

1. Ainsworth, B. E., W. L. Haskell, A. S. Leon, D. R. Jacobs, Jr., H. J. Montoye, J. F. Sallis, and R. S. Paffenbarger, Jr. 1993. Compendium of physical activities: classification of energy costs of human physical activities. *Med Sci Sports Exerc.* 25(1):71–80.

2. American College of Sports Medicine. 1995. *Guidelines for Exercise Testing and Prescription*, 5th ed. Philadelphia: Lea and Febiger.

3. Åstrand, P.-O., and K. Rodahl. 1986. *Textbook of Work Physiology: Physiological Basis of Exercise.* New York: McGraw-Hill Book Company.

4. Åstrand, P.-O., and I. Ryhming. 1954. A nomogram for calculation of aerobic capacity (physical fitness) from pulse rate during submaximal work. *J Appl Physiol.* 7:218–221.

5. Ayen, T. G., and H. J. Montoye. 1988. Estimation of energy expenditure with a simulated three-dimensional accelerometer. *J Ambulatory Monitoring.* 1:293–301.

6. Balogun, J. D., A. Martin, and M. A. Clendenin. 1989. Calorimetric validation of the Caltrac accelerometer during level walking. *Phys Therapy.* 69:501–509.

7. Bar-Or, O. 1987. The Wingate anaerobic test, an update of methodology, reliability and validity. *Sports Medicine* 4:381–394.

8. Bar-Or, O., R. Dotan, O. Inbar, A. Rothstein, J. Karlsson, and P. Tesch. 1980. Anaerobic capacity and muscle fiber type distribution in man. *Int J Sports Medicine.* 1(2):82–85.

9. Berry, M. J., J. A. Storsteen, and C. M. Woodard. 1993. Effects of body mass on exercise efficiency and VO_2 during steady-state cycling. *Med Sci Sports Exerc.* 25(9):1031–1037.

10. Bigard, A.-X., and C.-Y. Guezennec. 1995. Evaluation of the Cosmed K_2 telemetry system during exercise at moderate altitude. *Med Sci Sports Exerc.* 27(9):1333–1338.

11. Boning, D., Y. Gonen, and N. Maassen. 1984. Relationship between work load, pedal frequency, and physical fitness. *Int J Sports Med.* 5:92–97.

12. Butts, N. K., C. Dodge, and M. McAlpine. 1993. Effect of stepping rate on energy costs during StairMaster exercise. *Med Sci Sports Exerc.* 25(3):378–382.

13. Cavanagh, P. R., and R. Kram. 1985. Mechanical and muscular factors affecting the efficiency of human movement. *Med Sci Sports Exerc.* 17:326–331.

14. Coast, J. R., R. H. Cox, and H. G. Welch. 1986. Optimal pedaling rate in prolonged bouts of cycle ergometry. *Med Sci Sports Exerc.* 18(2):225–230.

15. Costill, D. L. 1967. Use of a swimming ergometer in physiological research. *Res Q.* 37:564–567.

16. Coyle, E. F. 1995. Integration of physiologic factors determining endurance performance ability. *Exercise and Sport Sciences Reviews.* Baltimore: Williams and Wilkins. p. 25–63.

17. Coyle, E. F., L. S. Sidossis, J. F. Horowitz, and J. D. Beltz. 1992. Cycling efficiency is related to the percentage of type 1 muscle fibers. *Med Sci Sports Exerc.* 24(7):782–788.

18. Crandall, C. G., S. L. Taylor, and P. B. Raven. 1994. Evaluation of the cosmed K_2 portable telemetric oxygen uptake analyzer. *Med Sci Sports Exerc.* 26(1):108–111.

19. Daniels, J., and N. Daniels. 1992. Running economy of elite male and elite female runners. *Med Sci Sports Exerc.* 24(4):483–489.

20. Davies, C., C. Barnes, and S. Godfrey. 1972. Body composition and maximal exercise performance in children. *Human Biol.* 44:195–215.

21. diPrampero, P. E., G. Cortili, F. Celentano, and P. Cerretelli. 1971. Physiological aspects of rowing. *J Appl Physiol.* 31(6):853–857.

22. diPrampero, P. E., G. Cortili, P. Mognoni, and F. Saibene. 1976. Energy cost of speed skating and efficiency of work against air resistance. *J Appl Physiol.* 40(4):584–591.

23. Donovan, C. M., and G. A. Brooks. 1977. Muscular efficiency during steady-state exercise: II. Effects of walking speed and work rate. *J Appl Physiol.* 43(3):431–439.

24. Drinkwater, B., S. Horvath, and C. Wells. 1973. Aerobic power of females, ages 10 to 68. *J Gerentology.* 30(4):385–394.

25. Foster, C., A. S. Jackson, M. L. Pollock, M. M. Taylor, J. Hare, S. M. Sennett, J. L. Rod, M. Sarwar, and D. H. Schmidt. 1984. Generalized equations for predicting functional capacity from treadmill performance. *Am Hrt J.* 107(6):1229–1234.

26. Foster, C., and N. N. Thompson. 1990. The physiology of speed skating. In *Winter Sports Medicine.* Philadelphia: F. A. Davis. p. 221–240.

27. Fox, E. L., R. L. Bartels, and R. W. Bowers. 1963. Comparison of speed and energy expenditure for two swimming turns. *Res Q.* 34:322–326.

28. Fox, E. L., and D. L. Costill. 1972. Estimated cardiorespiratory responses during marathon running. *Arch Environ Health.* 24:315–324.

29. Gaesser, G. A., and G. A. Brooks. 1975. Muscular efficiency during steady-rate exercise: effects of speed and work rate. *J Appl Physiol.* 38(6):1132–1139.

30. Gastin, P. B., D. L. Costill, D. L. Lawson, K. Krzeminski, and G. K. McConell. 1995. Accumulated oxygen deficit during supramaximal all-out and constant intensity exercise. *Med Sci Sports Exerc.* 27(2):255–263.

31. Golding, L. A., C. R. Myers, and W. E. Sinning. 1989. *Y's Way to Physical Fitness*, 3rd ed. Champaign: Human Kinetics, p. 89–124.

32. Hagerman, F. C. 1962. A comparison of oxygen debts in swimming the 400-yard freestyle while using the open and closed turns. Masters's thesis, The Ohio State University, Columbus, OH.

33. Hagerman, F. C., M. Connors, J. A. Gault, G. R. Hagerman, and W. J. Polinski. 1978. Energy expenditure during simulated rowing. *J Appl Physiol.* 45(1):87–93.

34. Hagerman, F. C., E. L. Fox, M. Connors, and J. Pompei. 1974. Metabolic responses of women rowers during ergometric rowing. *Med Sci Sports.* 6(1):87.

35. Haskell, W. L., A. S. Leon, C. J. Casperson, V. F. Froelicher, J. M. Hagberg, W. Harlan, J. O. Holloszky, J. G. Regensteiner, P. D. Thompson, R. A. Wahburn, and P. W. F. Wilson. 1992.

Cardiovascular benefits and assessment of physical activity and physical fitness in adults. *Med Sci Sports Exerc.* 24 (6 suppl.):S201–S220.

36. Haymes, E. M., and W. C. Byrnes. 1993. Walking and running energy expenditure estimated by Caltrac and indirect calorimetry. *Med Sci Sports Exerc.* 25(12):1365–1369.

37. Holly, R. G. 1993. Fundamentals of cardiorespiratory exercise testing. In American College of Sports Medicine, *Resource Manual for Guidelines for Exercise Testing and Prescription*, 2nd ed. Philadelphia: Lea and Febiger, p. 247–257.

38. Howley, E. T., D. R. Bassett, Jr., and H. G. Welch. 1995. Criteria for maximal oxygen uptake: review and commentary. *Med Sci Sports Exerc.* 27(9):1292–1301.

39. Inbar, O., and O. Bar-Or. 1986. Anaerobic characteristics in male children and adolescents. *Med Sci Sports Exerc.* 18(3):264–269.

40. Joyner, M. J. 1993. Physiological limiting factors and distance running: influence of gender and age on record performances. In Holloszy, J. O. (ed.), *Exercise and Sport Sciences Reviews.* Baltimore: Williams and Wilkens, pp. 103–133.

41. Kaczowski, W., D. L. Montgomery, A. W. Taylor, and V. Klissouras. 1982. The relationship between muscle fiber composition and maximal anaerobic power and capacity. *J Sports Med.* 22:407–413.

42. Kalkwarf, H. J., J. D. Haas, A. Z. Belko, et al. 1989. Accuracy of heart-rate monitoring and activity diaries for estimating energy expenditure. *Am J Clin Nutr.* 49:37–43.

43. Lupton, H. 1923. Analysis of effects of speed on mechanical efficiency of human movement. *J Physiol.* 57:337.

44. Lusk, G. 1928. *Science of Nutrition*, 4th ed. Philadelphia: W. B. Saunders, p. 65.

45. McCafferty, W. B., J. A. Gliner, and S. M. Horvath. 1978. The stress of coaching. *Phys Sportsmed.* 6(2):66–71.

46. McCartney, N., G. J. F. Heigenhauser, and N. L. Jones. 1983. Power output and fatigue of human muscle in maximal cycling exercise. *J Appl Physiol.* 55(1):218–224.

47. McCartney, N., G. J. F. Heigenhauser, A. J. Sargeant, and N. L. Jones. 1983. A constant-velocity cycle ergometer for the study of dynamic muscle function. *J Appl Physiol.* 55(1):212–217.

48. Medbo, J. I., A.-C. Mohn, I. Tabata, R. Bahr, O. Vaage, and O. M. Sejersted. 1988. Anaerobic capacity determined by maximal accumulated O₂ deficit. *J Appl Physiol.* 64(1):50–60.

49. Melanson, E. L., P. S. Freedson, D. Hendelman, and E. Debold. 1996. Reliability and validity of a portable metabolic measuring system. *Can J Appl Physiol.* 21:109–119.

50. Novitsky, S., K. R. Segal, B. Chatr-Aryamontri, D. Guvakov, and V. L. Katch. 1995. Validity of a new portable indirect calorimeter: the Aerosport TEEM 100. *Eur J Appl Physiol.* 70:462–467.

51. Pendergast, D. R., P. E. diPrampero, A. B. Craig, D. R. Wilson, and D. W. Rennie. 1977. Quantitative analysis of the front crawl in men and women. *J Appl Physiol.* 43(3):475–479.

52. Pollock, M. L. 1976. A comparative analysis of four protocols for maximal treadmill stress testing. *Am Heart J.* 92(1)39–46.

53. Pollock, M. L., C. Foster, D. Schmidt, C. Hellman, A. C. Linnerud, and A. Ward. 1982. Comparative analysis of physiologic responses to three different maximal graded exercise test protocols in healthy women. *Am Heart J.* 103(3):363–373.

54. Poole, D. C., G. A. Gaesser, M. C. Hogan, D. R. Knight, and P. D. Wagner. 1992. Pulmonary and leg VO₂ during submaximal exercise: applications for muscular efficiency. *J Appl Physiol.* 72(2):805–810.

55. Quinn, T. J., R. Kertzer, and W. B. Olney. 1992. Physiologic responses of patients with cardiac disease to arm, leg, and combined arm and leg work on an air-braked ergometer. *J Cardiopulmonary Rehabil.* 12:244–253.

56. Quinn, T. J., N. B. Vroman, and R. Kertzer. 1994. Post exercise oxygen consumption in trained females: effect of exercise duration. *Med Sci Sports Exerc.* 26(7):908–913.

57. Robinson, P. 1974. *The Physiological Effects of Chronic Heavy Physical Training on Female Age-Group Swimmers.* Doctoral Dissertation. Columbus: Ohio State University.

58. Robinson, S. 1938. Experimental studies of physical fitness in relation to age. *Arbeitsphysiol.* 19:251–323.

59. Rowell, L. B. 1974. Human cardiovascular adjustment to exercise and thermal stress. *Physiol Rev.* 54:75–103.

60. Sallis, J. F., M. J. Buono, J. J. Roby, D. Carlson, and J. A. Nelson. 1990. The Caltrac accelerometer as a physical activity monitor for school-age children. *Med Sci Sports Exerc.* 22:698–703.

61. Swain, D. P., and J. P. Wilcox. 1992. Effect of cadence on the economy of uphill cycling. *Med Sci Sports Exerc.* 24(10)1123–1127.

62. Taylor, H. L., E. Buskirk, and A. Henschel. 1955. Maximal oxygen intake as an objective measure of cardiorespiratory performance. *J Appl Physiol.* 8:73–80.

63. von Dobeln, W. 1954. A simple bicycle ergometer. *J Appl Physiol.* 7:222.

64. Wells, J. G., B. Balke, and D. D. Van Fossan. 1957. Lactic acid accumulation during work. A suggested standardization of work classification. *J Appl Physiol.* 10:51–55.

65. Wilmore, J. H., and D. L. Costill. 1974. Semiautomated systems approach to the assessment of oxygen uptake during exercise. *J Appl Physiol.* 36:618.

66. Wilmore, J. H., J. A. Davis, and A. C. Norton. 1976. An automated system for assessing metabolic and respiratory function during exercise. *J Appl Physiol.* 40:619.

Selected Readings

Consolazio, C. F., R. E. Johnson, and L. J. Pecora. 1963. *Physiological Measurements of Metabolic Functions in Man.* New York: McGraw-Hill.

Ellestad, M. H. 1996. *Stress Testing: Principles and Practice*, 4th ed. Philadelphia: F. A. Davis. pp. 11–42, 169–198.

Foster, C., N. N. Thompson, and A. C. Snyder. 1993. Ergometric studies with speed skaters: evolution of laboratory methods. *J Strength and Cond Res.* 7(4):193–200.

Inbar, O., O. Bar-Or, and J. S. Skinner. 1996. *The Wingate Anaerobic Test.* Champaign: Human Kinetics.

Knuttgen, H. G. 1978. Force, work, power, and exercise. *Med Sci Sports.* 10(3):227–228.

McConnel, T. R. 1995. Value of gas exchange analysis in heart disease. *J Cardiopulmonary Rehabil.* 15:257–261.

Williams, K. R. 1985. The relationship between mechanical and physiological energy estimates. *Med Sci Sports Exerc.* 17:317–325.

section 2

Neuromuscular Concepts

Neuromuscular refers to both the nervous and the muscular systems. Therefore, in this section we will direct our attention to the structure and function of nerves, the nervous system, and the muscles as they apply to physical activity and sport. Our primary purpose in studying neuromuscular physiology is to learn how muscles respond to stimuli and, in particular, to gain some understanding about the way in which we learn motor skills. Such information should help us to become better health professionals, teachers, coaches, and trainers, to say nothing of allowing us to better appreciate the complex internal communication system that is part of each of us.

In chapter 5, we will study the structure and function of nerves and the nervous system. There are two kinds of nerves: *sensory* and *motor*. Sensory nerves—also referred to as afferent nerves—convey information from the periphery (e.g., skin, limbs) to the central nervous system (brain and spinal cord). Motor nerves—also called efferent nerves—convey signals from the central nervous system to effector organs (e.g., skeletal muscle).

In chapter 6, we will study the structure and function of skeletal muscle. The more than 600 skeletal muscles of the human body constitute about 40% of the necessary total body weight. The muscles are useful, of course, because they are able to produce motion, the most fundamental function of the muscular and skeletal systems (musculoskeletal system). The action of muscles on the bony levers permits us to stand erect, carry out our activities of daily living, and perform an almost unending variety of sports activities. This miraculous motion of the musculoskeletal system is governed to a large extent by the strength and endurance of the muscles.

The following chapters are contained within this section:

5

Nervous Control of Muscular Movement

For purpose of study we may first divide the nervous system into the sensory, central, and motor portions. Sensory nerves receive stimuli from such areas as the surface of the skin (pain, cold, heat, and pressure), the eyes, nose, ears, and tongue.

The spinal cord, which extends from the base of the skull to the second lumbar vertebra, and the brain compose the **central nervous system (CNS).** The primary functions here are to integrate incoming stimuli, to modify these stimuli (if necessary), to control motor movements, to store information (memory), and to generate thoughts or ideas.

The **autonomic nervous system** (meaning self-controlled, or functioning independently) is generally considered by itself and is that portion of the nervous system that helps to control activities such as those involving the internal organs, urinary output, body temperature, heart rate, adrenal gland secretion, and blood pressure. Although involuntary, many of these functions are influenced by emotions.

Overall, the nervous system performs three basic functions: (1) *excitability,* which results in a signal from a receptor—for example, the retina of the eye becomes excited from a light source; (2) *conduction,*

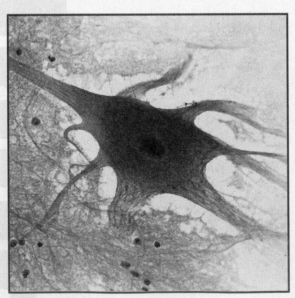

which takes place as the stimulus or signal is transmitted over nerve fibers, either to the CNS (sensory) or from the CNS (motor) to effector organs; and (3) *integration and regulation,* which take place within the CNS, allowing for controlled, coordinated motor responses.

Our purpose in this chapter is to describe how excitation takes place, the method whereby stimuli or signals are conducted, and how the CNS integrates all messages into coordinated performance. This information will give us a better understanding of how a motor skill is learned, how it is stored, and how it is recalled when the appropriate stimulus is applied.

Basic Structure of the Nerve
Basic Function of the Nerve

The Nervous System and Motor Skills

Summary

The major concepts to be learned from this chapter are as follows:

- The central nervous system is comprised of the brain and spinal cord and allows for reflex and voluntary control of movements.
- The autonomic nervous system is comprised of sympathetic and parasympathetic parts that allow involuntary reflex adjustments of bodily functions.
- The basic functional and anatomical unit of a nerve is the neuron, which consists of a cell body, or soma; several short fibers, called dendrites; and a longer fiber, called an axon.
- A nervous impulse or action potential is an electrical disturbance at the point of stimulation of a nerve that is self-propagated along the entire length of the axon.
- A simple reflex arc involves a sensory signal traveling by way of an afferent, or sensory, nerve to the spinal cord and stimulating an efferent, or motor, nerve, causing a muscular response.
- The connection of one nerve to another is called a synapse, whereas the connection of a nerve to a muscle is a special synapse called a neuromuscular junction or myoneurojunction.
- Nervous impulses are relayed from nerve to nerve and from nerve to muscle by chemical transmitter substances released at the ends of the nerve.
- Motoneurons can be excited and inhibited depending on the algebraic summation of impinging stimuli arriving from a variety of central and peripheral sources.
- Proprioceptors are sense organs found in muscles, tendons, and joints that transmit information about muscle contraction, contractile unit tension, and limb position to the central nervous system.
- Muscle spindles play an especially important role in stretch reflexes, muscle tone, and overall quality of movement.
- Three areas of the brain most involved with the selection and execution of voluntary movements are (1) cerebral cortex motor areas, (2) basal ganglia/thalamus, and (3) cerebellum.
- The cerebellum serves as a most important "comparator" to indicate whether intended movements are satisfactorily completed.
- Acquiring motor skills, called motor learning, is specific and likely involves the formation of an engram, a permanent trace left in neural tissue protoplasm by a repeated practice stimulus.
- Memorized motor skill programs (engrams) are stored in the sensory area of the cerebral cortex, which works in cooperation with the cerebellum; engrams have been viewed as "memory drums" that can be replayed on demand.

Basic Structure of the Nerve

The basic functional and anatomical unit of a nerve is the **neuron,** or **nerve cell.** Its structure is shown in figure 5.1. The neuron consists of (1) a **cell body,** or **soma;** (2) several short nerve fibers, called **dendrites;** and (3) a longer nerve fiber, called an **axon.** Although technically both dendrites and axons are nerve fibers, the term *nerve fiber* is generally used in reference to an axon. The dendrites transmit nerve impulses toward the cell body, whereas the axon transmits them away from the cell body.

In large nerve fibers, such as those innervating most skeletal muscles, the axon is surrounded by a **myelin sheath** (figure 5.1). The sheath is composed mainly of lipid (fat) and protein. Nerve fibers containing a myelin sheath are referred to as **myelinated nerve fibers,** whereas those devoid of the sheath are called **nonmyelinated nerve fibers.** The myelin sheath is not continuous along the entire length of the fiber but rather is laid down in segments with small spaces between segments. These spaces are called the **nodes of Ranvier.** We will later see that the myelin sheath and the nodes of Ranvier play important roles in how quickly the nerve impulse is transmitted along the axon.

Basic Function of the Nerve

The information sent from the periphery to the CNS by the afferent nerves is concerned with various kinds of sensations: heat, light, touch, smell, pressure, and so on. The connections of the sensory nerves with the CNS serve to supply us with the perception of these various sensations and to trigger, under certain circumstances, appropriate motor responses.[10] An example of the latter would be the rapid reflex withdrawal of your finger from a lighted candle or a sharp tack.

To complete such a reflex response, motor nerves from **motoneurons (motor neurons)** are also required. These nerves originate in the CNS and terminate in effector organs, such as skeletal muscles. When stimulated, the motor nerves cause the muscles they innervate or act upon to contract. Thus, in brief, when you accidentally place your finger on a hot object, the heat-sensitive receptors located in the skin send information via the sensory nerves to the CNS. Once in the CNS (in this case, in the spinal cord), the sensory nerves relay the information to the appropriate motor nerves which in turn send impulses to the muscles in the arm; the muscles contract, and the finger is automatically and rapidly withdrawn from the hot object. A similar reflex involving pressure-responsive pain receptors prevents injury to the finger when pricked by a sharp tack, as shown in figure 5.2.

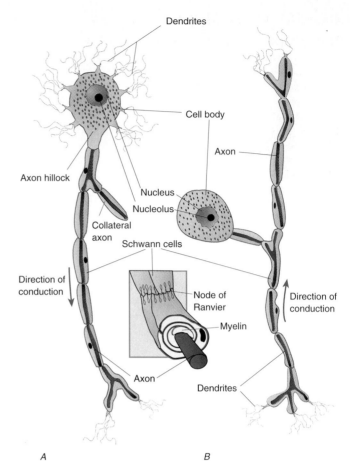

A   *B*

Figure 5.1

The structure of two kinds of neurons (*A*) A motor neuron and (*B*) a sensory neuron. For the motor neuron, note the cell body, or soma, containing the nucleus, the long axon fiber that conducts impulses *away from* the cell body, and the numerous short dendrites that receive impulses from other neurons. For the sensory neuron, note that impulses are conducted *toward* the cell body.

The Nerve Impulse

The information transmitted and relayed by the sensory and motor nerves is in a form of electrical energy referred to as the **nerve impulse.** A nerve impulse can be thought of mainly as an electrical disturbance at the point of stimulation of a nerve that is self-propagated along the entire length of the axon. The actual means by which a nerve impulse is generated and propagated in response to a **stimulus**—a change in the environment that modifies the activity of cells—may be summarized as follows: when a nerve fiber is at rest, sodium ions (Na^+) are most heavily concentrated on the outside of the nerve membrane, causing the inside of the nerve to be electrically negative relative to the outside of the nerve (figure 5.3*A*). Thus, an electrical gradient or difference exists between the inside and outside of the nerve fiber. This is referred to as the **resting membrane poten-**

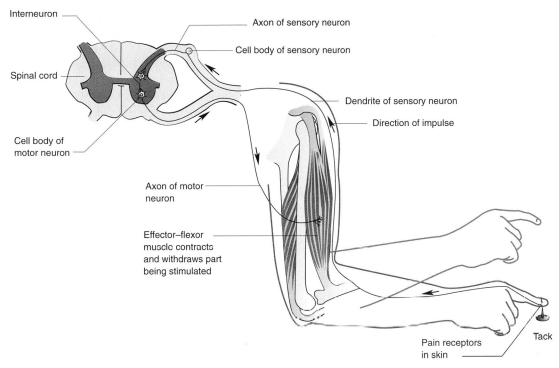

Interneuron

Axon of sensory neuron

Cell body of sensory neuron

Spinal cord

Dendrite of sensory neuron

Direction of impulse

Cell body of motor neuron

Axon of motor neuron

Effector–flexor muscle contracts and withdraws part being stimulated

Pain receptors in skin

Tack

Figure 5.2

The reflex arc. When your finger touches a sharp tack, the pain receptors in the finger receive the stimulus, which is then transmitted by means of the afferent (sensory) nerve fiber to the spinal cord. The stimulus is passed along via an interneuron to the cell body of a motor neuron, which then transmits impulses to the appropriate muscles, and the hand is quickly withdrawn.

tial. When a sufficient stimulus is applied to the nerve, the nerve cell membrane depolarizes and becomes highly permeable to sodium ions as they leak into the inside of the nerve. As a result, the outside of the nerve now becomes negative and the inside positive (figure 5.3*B*). In other words, an adequate stimulus causes a reversal of polarity of the nerve. Such a reversal in polarity is referred to as an **action potential.**

In addition to the action potential, a local flow of current is created in the membrane at the site where the stimulus was applied. This current is self-regenerating in that it flows to adjacent areas of the nerve causing each area to also undergo a reversal of polarity, which in turn evokes a new action potential and a local flow of current (figure 5.3*C*). This process is repeated over and over again until the action potential has been propagated the entire length of the nerve fiber. All this happens very quickly in nerves, but it does matter whether they are myelinated or nonmyelinated.

On some nerve fibers the myelin sheath, if present, insulates that part of the nerve it surrounds from electrical disturbances. Therefore, a nerve impulse can be neither generated nor propagated over that part of the fiber covered by the myelin. Instead, the nerve impulse is propagated only at the nodes of Ranvier—that is, from node to node over the entire length of the fiber. This jumping from node to node, referred to as **saltatory conduction,** serves to greatly in-

crease the conduction velocity of the nerve impulse. For example, the **nerve conduction velocity** of large myelinated fibers typical of those innervating skeletal muscles is 60 to 100 meters per second (135 to 225 miles per hour). In nonmyelinated fibers of the same diameter, conduction velocity is only 6 to 10 meters per second (13.5 to 22.5 miles per hour). Myelinated fibers conduct ten times faster!

Nerve-to-Nerve Synapses

The preceding discussion was concerned with how an action potential is transmitted along a single nerve fiber (axon), such as a motoneuron that innervates a skeletal muscle. Because there are literally billions of nerve cells within the nervous system, the next question to answer is how nervous information, such as an action potential, is passed on from one nerve cell to another.

The connection of an axon of one nerve cell to the cell body or dendrites of another is called a **synapse.** Before reading on, go back to figure 5.1 for a moment and notice the multiple, fine branches located on the end of the axon of the neuron. These represent what are called **synaptic knobs.** These knobs are important in relaying nervous information from one neuron to another. For example, in figure 5.4 a close-up view of a nerve-to-nerve synapse is shown.

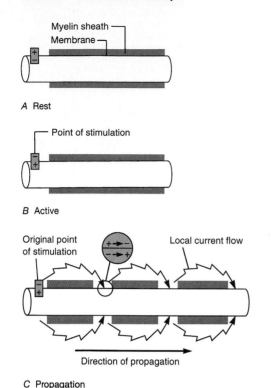

A Rest

B Active

C Propagation

Direction of propagation

Figure 5.3

Generation and propagation of the nerve impulse. *A.* At rest, the outside of the nerve is positive. *B.* A stimulus causes a reversal of polarity or action potential and a local flow of current. *C.* The local flow of current evokes a new action potential and flow of current in adjacent areas of the axon.

(From Fox.[8])

The axon of a presynaptic neuron approaches the soma of a postsynaptic neuron (called an axon-somatic synapse). The nervous information is relayed across the **synaptic cleft** or gap by means of a **chemical transmitter substance.** The chemical transmitter is stored in vesicles within the synaptic knobs. Mitochondria are also found within the knobs, as ATP generated by the aerobic system is required to synthesize new transmitter substance. Continuous synthesis of transmitter substance is necessary, because only a relatively small amount can be stored in the vesicles at any one time.

As an impulse reaches the synaptic cleft, the chemical transmitter is discharged, and depending on the type of transmitter released, either the postsynaptic membrane (neuron) is excited and an electrical potential is created, or the postsynaptic membrane is inhibited and is said to become hyperpolarized. In the first case, an increase in electrical potential (in millivolts [mV]) in the postsynaptic neuron from its resting membrane potential is called the **excitatory postsynaptic potential (EPSP).** If the voltage increase is adequate (increase of about 11 mV above the resting potential of −70 mV), the neuron will fire, sending the impulse, or stimulus, on its way. If the EPSP is less than

11 mV, the neuron will not discharge; consequently, the stimulus will be lost. The minimal electrical level at which a neuron will depolarize (transmit an impulse) is called the *threshold for excitation* (figure 5.5).

In the second case, where the chemical transmitter causes hyperpolarization, the postsynaptic neuron is actually inhibited from eliciting an action potential. In other words, an **inhibitory postsynaptic potential (IPSP)** is said to be created within the neuron. Hyperpolarization refers to the strengthening of the resting membrane potential (e.g., from −70 mV to −75 mV), thus making it more difficult to achieve threshold or initiate action potential.

Excitatory and Inhibitory Transmitter Substances

One of the excitatory transmitters is **acetylcholine (ACh).** As we will see next, ACh is also the excitatory chemical transmitter at the neuromuscular junction. Other excitatory transmitter substances include: (1) **norepinephrine,** (2) **dopamine,** and (3) **serotonin.** At least two chemical substances are thought to be inhibitory transmitters: (1) **gamma-aminobutyric acid (GABA),** which is suspected to be the main inhibitory transmitter in the brain; and (2) **glycine,** a simple amino acid,* which is thought to be the main inhibitory transmitter in the spinal cord. Both excitatory and inhibitory transmitters work in the same general manner, causing a change in permeability in the membrane of the postsynaptic neuron. The excitatory transmitters increase the membrane's permeability to sodium ions (Na^+), whereas the inhibitory transmitters increase the permeability to potassium (K^+) and chloride (Cl^-) ions. Recall that an influx of Na^+, if great enough, elicits an action potential. On the other hand, an increased permeability to only K^+ and Cl^- leads to a strengthening of the resting membrane potential (hyperpolarization).

Figure 5.5 shows some of these concepts of action potential spike development in nerve (and muscle) cells in generalized graphical form. The resting membrane potential is −70 mV, and the events are occurring in fractions of a second (msec). The prefix *milli-* means one-thousandths of a volt or second, so these are very small electrical events that happen very quickly. Two inadequate attempts (shown as I and I′) were made to depolarize the cell membrane, but they were too weak and the excitation threshold for the cell was not reached. The third attempt led to depolarization because the events, although of the same strength, were more closely spaced and could build on one another. Consequently, a **depolarization** spike occurred because of the inrushing of Na^+ across the membrane. Note that the inside of the cell reached +30 mV; however, this event was short-lived because of the continued activity of an ATP-driven sodium-potassium pump that pumped K^+ out of the cell. This latter process is referred to as cell **repolarization.**

---

*Amino acids are the building blocks of protein (see chapter 15).

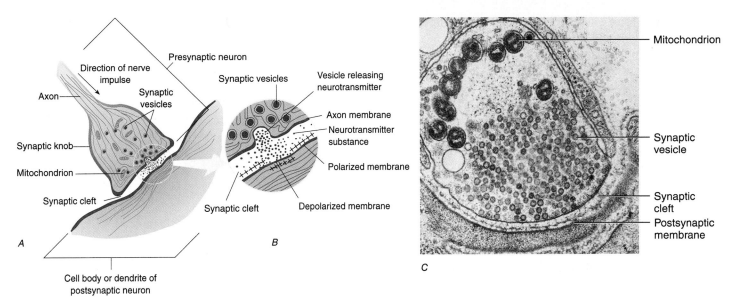

Figure 5.4

A, When a nerve impulse reaches the synaptic knob at the end of an axon, *B*, synaptic vesicles release a neurotransmitter substance that diffuses across the synaptic cleft. *C*, A transmission electron micrograph of a synaptic knob filled with synaptic vesicles.

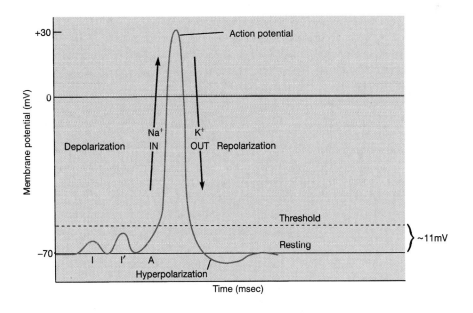

Figure 5.5

General example of an action spike in a nerve cell. Two inadequate (I and I') changes in the resting membrane potential are followed by an adequate (*A*) alteration so the excitation threshold is reached. The depolarization spike (action potential) is caused by alteration in membrane semipermeability and an in-rushing of Na⁺. Repolarization results from K⁺ being pumped back out of the cell by the ATP driven Na⁺/K⁺ pump. Note hyperpolarization from overshoot of this mechanism.

It frequently leads to a brief overshoot in which the cell membrane potential goes below the resting baseline starting level, called **hyperpolarization.**

The above is a generic picture of an action potential generation by all neural cells. The fact that they depolarize in this manner is known as "all-or-nothing firing," i.e., the single or combined stimulus is either adequate and the nerve "fires" or it is inadequate and it does not fire. Nothing in between, all-or-nothing. This all-or-nothing action potential firing concept will show up again in chapter 6 as it also relates to motoneurons and motor units. At this time consider the questions of whether muscle or nerve cells would fire more easily (excitable state) or with more difficulty (inhibited state) if the resting membrane potential started out closer or further away from the excitation threshold. Because it requires about 11 mV to reach threshold, it only makes sense that closer would be easier and further away would be more difficult—right? Might you think of examples where stimulating or suppressing drugs and medications might influence the excitability of nerve and muscle cells? How about caffeine as a stimulant and ethyl alcohol as a depressant?

Spatial and Temporal Summation

Each stimulus received at the synaptic cleft may not by itself be strong enough to affect the postsynaptic neuron. However, provided a minimal number of stimuli are received from various presynaptic terminals (axons) simultaneously, or within a short time of one another, they will summate, causing excitation or inhibition of the postsynaptic neuron. The additive effect of these various stimuli is called **spatial summation.** If successive discharges from the same presynaptic terminal occur within about 15 milliseconds of one another, they too will summate and, if strong enough, will cause a neuronal effect. This is called **temporal summation.**

Excitation versus Inhibition

Most neurons are constantly bombarded with excitatory and inhibitory stimuli (figure 5.6). The net effect of these stimuli on the neuron is determined by their algebraic sum because the two types of stimuli oppose each other. For example, if excitatory stimuli outnumber inhibitory stimuli to the extent that the threshold for excitation of the postsynaptic neuron is reached, then an action potential is elicited, and the impulse continues on its way. However, if this difference between the two stimuli is not great enough to reach the threshold, the neuron will not fire, and the stimulus is not passed on. You will learn in chapter 6 that the smaller motoneurons that service Type I muscle fibers have a lower excitation threshold and fire off before the larger motoneurons of Type II fibers. This is known as the size principle of motor unit recruitment.

Examples of excitation are numerous and are quite familiar to most of us: the contraction of a muscle results from excitation of its motoneuron. The reflex arc mentioned previously, for instance, involved sensory stimuli exciting a motor neuron so that the finger was rapidly withdrawn from the tack point. In addition, as pointed out in chapter 6, the central nervous system component of muscular fatigue is thought to function as a result of the facilitatory (excitatory) influence of the CNS on the motor system.

The function of inhibitory neurons is not only to allow us to overcome excitatory impulses that we consciously wish to oppose, but also—more importantly—to exclude unimportant nonconscious stimuli, especially those elicited through the sensory receptors. Just imagine the number of impulses that would have to be processed by the CNS if inhibition were absent. To mention a few:

1. Continual sensations of pressure from sitting, standing, and lying.

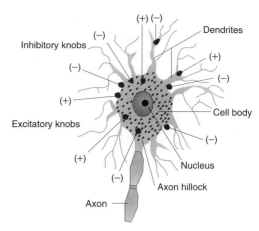

Figure 5.6

Most neurons are constantly bombarded with excitatory (+) and inhibitory (−) stimuli. The net effect of these stimuli on the neuron is determined by their algebraic sum because the two types of stimuli oppose each other ($-6 + 4 = -2$).

2. Sensations of touch from our clothing.
3. Innumerable sounds we do not care to be bothered with.
4. Light alone sends tremendous numbers of impulses to the retina that are of no concern (we see only what we wish to see).
5. Stimulation from minor variations in heat and cold are ignored by the CNS through the inhibitory neuronal mechanism.
6. Odors are about us constantly and perhaps only those coming from the kitchen before dinner are worthy of processing; many others are inhibited and should be.

Stop for a moment and look about you; listen and then ponder the countless number of stimuli coming to the CNS from the environment and from your peripheral nerve endings that are (and should be) inhibited. Inhibition of extraneous impulses allows you to concentrate on the contents of this book, thus enabling you to become a better exercise physiologist, coach, trainer, physical educator, or fitness specialist—we hope! Without the inhibitory mechanism the poor brain probably would be stimulated right out of its cranium!

Later in this chapter (p. 119), we discuss another example of the inhibitory mechanism, the Golgi tendon organs, which when stimulated cause inhibition of muscular contraction. Also, in chapter 6 we will look at the idea that, under most circumstances, muscular strength is inhibited by the CNS.

Nerve-to-Muscle Synapse— The Neuromuscular Junction

Figure 5.7 illustrates the anatomical features of a motor nerve embedded into a muscle fiber. This union is called the **neuromuscular junction** or **myoneural junction** or **motor**

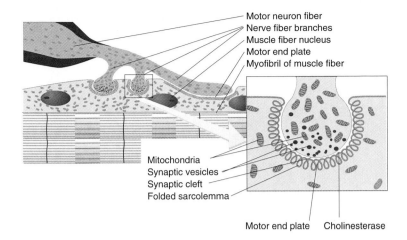

Motor neuron fiber
Nerve fiber branches
Muscle fiber nucleus
Motor end plate
Myofibril of muscle fiber

Mitochondria
Synaptic vesicles
Synaptic cleft
Folded sarcolemma

Motor end plate   Cholinesterase

Figure 5.7

The neuromuscular junction. The point at which the motor nerve fiber invaginates the muscle fiber is called the endplate (enlargement). Transmission of the neuronal impulse across the synaptic cleft is made possible through the secretion of a acetylcholine. The cholinesterase breaks down acetylcholine, thus preventing further excitation of the muscle following stimulation for that immediate time period.

endplate. Transmission of the neuronal impulse across the synaptic cleft is made possible through the release of the chemical transmitter acetylcholine (ACh), from the presynaptic membrane. ACh diffuses through the cleft and then reaches the postsynaptic surface where a receptor is located. Acetylcholinesterase, which is homogenously distributed in the cleft, deactivates the acetylcholine by chemically breaking it down. This prevents further excitation of the muscle fiber following stimulation for that immediate time period. The synaptic endplate current at the neuromuscular junction has been mathematically modeled to provide a better understanding of the described events.[9]

The manner in which a stimulus is transmitted from the nerve to the muscle fiber is very similar, as you will see, to the way in which an impulse is transmitted from nerve to nerve through the neuronal synapse. Apparently, the major difference is that there is no inhibition mechanism at the neuromuscular junction.

As mentioned in chapter 6, a muscle fiber receives only one nerve fiber (figure 5.8). However, the large alpha fiber of an efferent (motor) neuron divides into numerous smaller fibers and innervates as many as 200 muscle fibers. An individual nerve fiber plus all the muscle fibers it innervates is called a *motor unit* (figure 5.9). This is the final output pathway of the motor system.[21] As an impulse arrives at the neuromuscular junction, acetylcholine is released; the impulse is then able to cross the synapses, creating electrical potentials in the muscle fibers. Such a potential, as we just learned in our discussion of the neuronal synapse, is called an *excitatory postsynaptic potential* (EPSP), as it relates to individual fibers and motor unit potentials (MUPs).[7] In the spinal cord, the motor neuron innervating various muscle fibers may receive impulses from several nerve fibers (figure 5.10). If the EPSP is too small the motor neuron will not depolarize and the muscle fiber will not contract; but when the EPSP rises to a certain level, depolarization occurs and the associated muscle fibers contract. All or nothing!

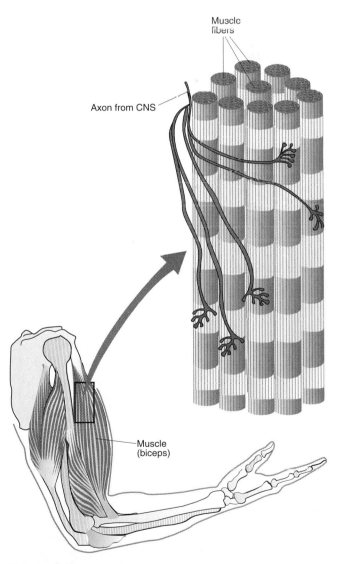

Muscle fibers

Axon from CNS

Muscle (biceps)

Figure 5.8

Structure of skeletal muscle. Each muscle fiber is innervated by the axonal branch of a single axon.

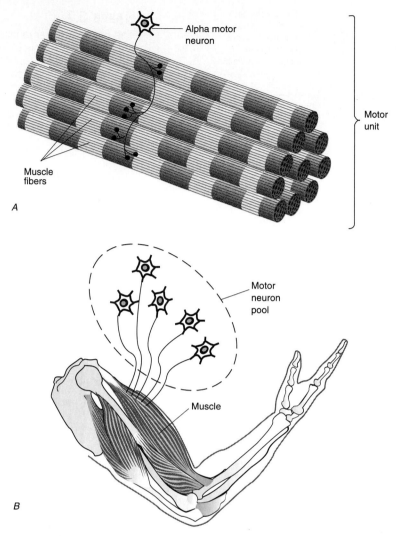

Alpha motor
neuron

Motor
unit

Muscle
fibers

A

Motor
neuron
pool

Muscle

B

Figure 5.9

A motor unit and motor neuron pool. (*A*) A motor unit is an alpha motor neuron and all the muscle fibers it innervates. (*B*) A motor neuron pool is all the alpha motor neurons that innervate one muscle.

As previously illustrated in the description of the neuronal synapse, this progressive increase in size of the EPSP as a result of a number of impulses is called *spatial summation*. In addition, successive discharges from the same presynaptic terminal will summate, eliciting an increased EPSP, provided that the discharges occur in rapid succession (within 15 milliseconds of each other). As before, this mechanism is called *temporal summation*. "Temporal" alludes to timing, and timing is of the essence here.

To illustrate, suppose impulse A is initiated in the brain, and impulse B comes from a pain receptor in the skin. You decide to get a tan from a sun lamp, and in a few minutes impulses from A + B inform you (spatial summation) that the heat is too great; you turn off the lamp or perhaps move farther from it. Conversely, you might fall asleep while under the lamp, in which case impulse A, which originated in the brain, could not be activated. Impulse B is not sufficiently strong by itself to arouse muscular activity (i.e., to create an adequate EPSP to fire the neuron). As a result, you remain asleep while the sun lamp continues to slowly bake your tissue. When you do awaken, in all probability you will have received serious burns. Similarly, by inhibiting activation of brain cells, sleep, anesthetics, and too much alcohol prevent adequate stimulation of recipient neurons.

Figure 5.11 shows how the motor neurons that service different muscles are distributed in the ventral horn (gray matter) of the spinal cord. Note that there are specific locations for muscles according to their contractile function (flexion vs. extension) and anatomical location (axial vs. distal). Before leaving this discussion, let us consider the impulse firing rates of single motor units within various muscles of the human body. These rates are highly variable with an average of 30 impulses per second (Hz units, pronounced *Hertz*) for the biceps brachii and an

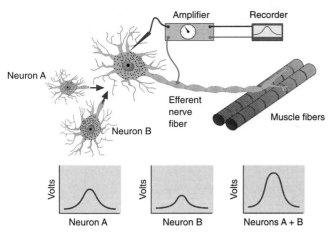

Figure 5.10

Diagram demonstrating measurement of a nerve impulse. One electrode is placed in the soma, the other on the efferent nerve fiber. Upon stimulation from either neuron A and/or neuron B, the impulse is amplified and printed on the recorder. For example, the impulse from neuron A is recorded and appears in the insert as does the impulse from neuron B; the combined effect results in the summation of both impulses (A + B).

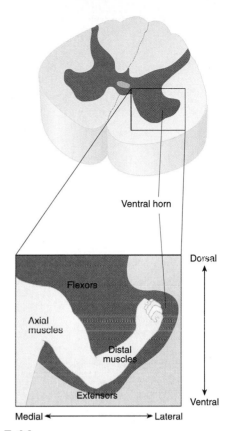

Figure 5.11

Distribution of lower motor neurons in the ventral horn. Motor neurons controlling flexors lie dorsal to those controlling extensors. Motor neurons controlling axial muscles lie medial to those controlling distal muscles.

average of 10 Hz for the soleus muscle.[2] The biceps muscle of the arm contains ~50% or more of Type II fibers, while the soleus is primarily comprised of Type I fibers. These impulse frequencies match up well with the general type of muscle being stimulated (i.e., a high firing rate for the fast-contracting [Type II] muscle and a low rate for the slow-contracting [Type I] muscle). The discharge frequencies for individual motor units of the tibialis anterior muscle of the lower leg are approximately 10 Hz[17] for low-level sustained contractions. Other studies of the thumb adductor pollicis muscle indicate that maximal electrical stimulation through the ulnar nerve at rates as high as 50 to 80 Hz produced rapid fatigue, whereas a stimulation rate of 20 Hz produced fatigue curves similar to those for maximal voluntary contractions.[3] The maximum discharge frequency of this latter muscle also has been shown to relate closely to the percentage of **maximum voluntary contraction (MVC)** that is being performed. The average discharge frequency ranges from 35 to 55 Hz.[23]

Measures of the amplitude and duration of MUPs have been made using needle electrodes that are superficially positioned and inserted deeper into muscles. The MUPs of brachial biceps muscle in healthy human subjects show higher amplitudes and longer durations distally than in the middle of the muscle.[7] This is believed to be caused by a greater temporal (time-related) dispersion of muscle fiber action potentials at a greater distance from the endplate zone. Other studies indicate that there are differences in how quickly the EPSPs spread from the endplates.[25] Na^+ currents are used as an index of membrane excitability and the speed of spreading electrical potentials. Type II fibers

have larger Na^+ currents on the endplate border and at a distance of 200 microns from the endplate. These larger Na^+ currents also subside more quickly in Type II fibers. This fits with other things you will be learning about differences between Type II and Type I fibers. In this case, the rapid spread of EPSPs and their quicker turn off would enable Type II fibers to operate at higher firing frequencies for brief periods of time.

In summary, motor units receive impulse volleys at a rate that relates to the makeup of their constituent fiber types with an overall range between approximately 10 and 60 Hz. Not surprisingly, these reports indicate a higher rate of firing when more force is being applied. This is one important way to gradate the strength of muscle contractions. Likewise, we might expect that the spread of EPSPs from the endplate is faster in Type II fibers as opposed to Type I fibers, consistent with their functional differences. Now we are aware of membrane structural differences that relate to their having distinctive Na^+ channel properties—a clear line for future research.

A very important aspect of coordinated muscle contractions is shown in figure 5.12—namely, **reciprocal inhibition.** If you think about it, it is essential that the an-

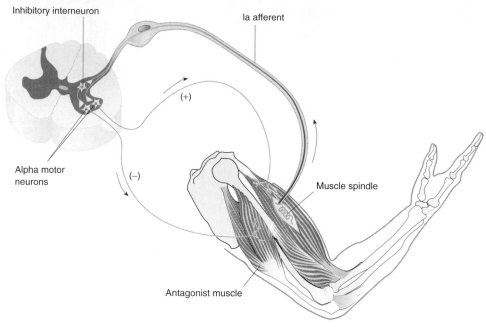

Inhibitory interneuron

Ia afferent

(+)

(−)

Alpha motor
neurons

Muscle spindle

Antagonist muscle

Figure 5.12

Reciprocal inhibition of flexors (+) and extensors (−) of the same joint for a simple stretch reflex.

tagonist muscles relax when the agonists contract. This allows for smooth, unrestricted movement. This is shown here as a simple reflex, but reciprocal inhibition occurs as well during voluntary movement reflex, such as walking or running. In fact, failure of antagonists to relax at the correct time can result in their being partially torn when the agonists undergo forceful contraction. Ouch!

Muscle Sense Organs

There are several types of sense organs in muscle. The pain resulting from exercising too vigorously after long disuse (muscle soreness, p. 35) or from torn muscle fibers are good examples of muscle sense organs at work. These pain receptors, which are few in number, are found not only in the muscle fibers themselves but also in the wall of arteries that supply the muscle cells and in the connective tissues that surround the fibers.

Proprioceptors

Other kinds of sense organs found within the muscles and joints are called **proprioceptors.** The function of proprioceptors is to conduct sensory reports to the CNS from (1) muscles, (2) tendons, (3) ligaments, and (4) joints. These sense organs are concerned with **kinesthesis**—or kinesthetic sense—that, in general, unconsciously tells us where our body parts are in relation to our environment. Their

contributions enable us to execute a smooth and coordinated movement, no matter whether we are putting a golf ball, hitting a home run, or simply climbing an unfamiliar flight of stairs without stumbling. They also help us to maintain a normal body posture and muscle tonus. The tendency for the lower jaw to drop, the head to droop forward, and the knees to buckle because of the effects of gravity are all counterbalanced by the so-called antigravity muscles, which relay information regarding position in space. How do these sense organs or proprioceptors function? We can begin to answer this question by first describing how each type of sense organ sends specific sensory information to the CNS. There are three important muscle sense organs concerned with kinesthesis: muscle spindles, Golgi tendon organs, and joint receptors.

The Muscle Spindle

Muscle spindles are perhaps the most abundant type of proprioceptor found in muscle. Briefly, **muscle spindles** (also called *stretch receptors*) send information to the CNS concerning the degree of stretch of the muscle in which they are embedded. This provides the muscles with information, for example, as to the exact number of motor units needed to contract to overcome a given resistance; the greater the stretch, the greater the load and the greater the number of motor units required. The spindles are important in the control of posture and, with the help of the gamma system, in voluntary movements.[19]

Structure of the Spindle

The structure of the muscle spindle is given in figure 5.13. It is nothing more than several modified muscle fibers contained in a capsule, with a sensory nerve spiraled around its center. These modified muscle cells are called **intrafusal fibers** to distinguish them from the regular or **extrafusal fibers.** The center portion of the spindle is not capable of contracting, but the two ends contain contractile fibers. The thin motor nerves innervating the ends are of the gamma type and are thus called **gamma motor nerves** or **fusimotor nerves.** When they are stimulated, the ends of the spindle contract and pull against the center region. The larger motor nerves innervating the regular or extrafusal fibers are called **alpha motor nerves.** When they are stimulated, muscle fibers contract in the usual manner.

Function of the Spindle

As mentioned previously, the spindle is sensitive to length or stretch. Therefore, because the spindle fibers are found throughout the muscle and lie parallel to the regular fibers, when the whole muscle is stretched, the center portion of the spindle is also stretched. This stretching activates the sensory nerve (**annulospiral nerve**) located there, which then sends impulses to the central nervous system. In turn, these impulses activate the alpha motor neurons that innervate the regular muscle fibers, and the muscle contracts. If the muscle shortens when it contracts, the spindle also shortens, thus stopping its flow of sensory impulses; the muscle then relaxes. The spindle is sensitive to both the rate of change in length and to the final length attained by the muscle fibers. The functional significance of these two types of sensitivity can be illustrated by a muscle engaged in a steady contraction, as when the elbow is flexed steadily against a load (for example, when holding a book). The type of stretch placed on the muscle because of the load is called *tonic stretch* and is concerned with the final length of the muscle fibers. If the load is light, the fibers will be stretched only moderately, and the frequency of discharge of the sensory impulses from the spindle will be low. Thus, only a few motor units are called on in keeping the load steady.

If there is an unexpected increase in the load being held, such as by adding another book, the muscle will again be stretched. This is evidenced by the fact that the forearm will be lowered because of the added load. The ensuing reflex contraction initiated by the spindle will reposition the forearm to its original level. However, there will be some overcompensation—that is, at first the contraction will be greater than needed. The greater and more abrupt the increase in load, the greater the frequency of discharge of the spindle, the greater the contraction, and the greater the overcompensation. In other words, with this type of stretch, called *phasic stretch,* the spindle is responding to the rate or velocity of the change in length and not to the length per se. Another example of phasic stretch is given in the following discussion (stretch reflex).

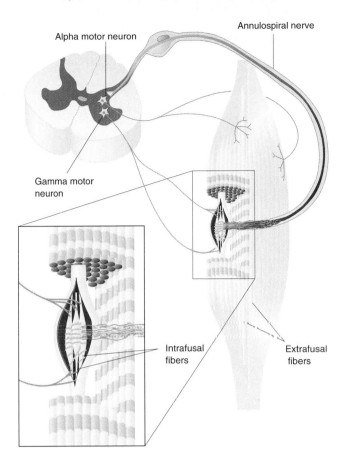

Figure 5.13

Muscle spindle showing its relationship to regular extrafusal muscle fibers that are innervated by the alpha motor neuron fibers. The gamma motor neuron fibers go to the intrafusal muscle fibers located at the ends of the centrally located "sensitive" portion of the stretch receptor. When stretched, afferent sensory impulses are sent back to the CNS via the annulospiral nerve.

The Gamma System

There is one other way in which the spindle can be stretched. You will recall (figure 5.13) that the ends of the spindle fibers are innervated by gamma motor neurons. These gamma neurons can be stimulated directly by the motor centers located in the cerebral cortex of the brain via their pyramidal tract nerve connections to the spinal cord. (Look ahead to figure 5.14.) When stimulated in this manner, the ends of the spindle contract, thus stretching the center portion and stimulating the sensory nerve. In other words, the muscle spindle can be activated by itself, apart from the rest of the muscle. This special neural arrangement is called the **gamma system** or **gamma loop.** This kind of setup provides a very sensitive system for the execution of smooth, voluntary movements. Furthermore, studies have suggested that the gamma neurons have a recruitment order much the same as alpha motor neurons.[5] Although all the functional interrelationships in producing precise voluntary movements

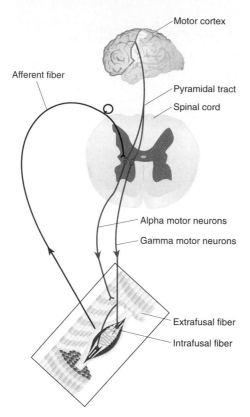

Figure 5.14

Connections to the central nervous system of the muscle spindle. The spindle is sensitive to stretch. It can be stretched when the entire muscle is stretched or when the gamma motor neurons are stimulated by the motor cortex (gamma loop). In either case, sensory impulses from the spindle are sent to the spinal cord, stimulating the alpha motor neurons, and the muscle contracts. Also, direct stimulation of the alpha motor neurons from the motor cortex is possible.

are not completely understood, this combined recruitment is called **alpha-gamma coactivation.** When thinking about voluntary movements and alpha-gamma coactivation, consider that gamma firing occurs just a bit prior to alpha activation. This puts an initial stretch bias on the sensory system resulting in some firing from the annulospiral nerve. One way to stop this backflow of sensory impulses is to contract (shorten) the whole muscle to precisely the proper amount, making a perfect matchup of "gamma-alpha" activation (note reversal of terms to emphasize order of firing) and a turnoff of backflow. If the matchup is imperfect, the initial bias would not be completely removed. In this event, the continued backflow of afferent impulses would signal the alpha motoneurons to send additional impulse volleys. The muscle would undergo further contraction with a concomitant decrease in sensory backflow. This process would be continued until all the initial bias is removed.[26] Remember that these processes occur very rapidly but, at the same time, do require some time for completion.

For an example of how the gamma system (sometimes called the gamma loop) works, let us go back to the person voluntarily holding a book in a fixed position, elbow flexed to 90 degrees. We stated that the tonic stretch on the entire muscle created by the load provides information that keeps the load (book) in a relatively fixed position. However, in addition, the gamma neurons are stimulated by impulses sent down directly from the motor cortex. The ends of the spindle contract, the sensory nerve sends impulses back to the central nervous system, and additional information is provided concerning the number of motor units that are required to maintain the original voluntarily initiated position. This additional information provides the refinement that is needed for a smooth, rather than a jerky, movement.

In summary, there are three ways that the muscle spindle can activate the alpha motor neurons that cause the muscle to contract: (1) by tonic stretch, (2) by phasic stretch, and (3) by the gamma system or gamma loop. All of these controls work together to provide for effective, coordinated, and smooth movement.

Muscle Spindles, Muscle Tone, and Stretch Reflex

Place your forearm on the desk in a completely relaxed and slightly flexed position. In feeling the muscles, even though relaxed, you will notice a resiliency rather than a flabbiness. Maintaining this relaxation, have a partner gently extend your forearm (a little powder on the desk will minimize resistance). Your partner will observe a small amount of muscular resistance not related to conscious effort, assuming of course that you are maintaining complete relaxation. This characteristic of resiliency and resistance to stretch in the relaxed resting muscle is called **muscular tonus,** or **tone.**

Now, if you were to sever the efferent or motor nerves (ventral roots) that service these muscles, they would lose tonus and become flaccid. Furthermore, if the dorsal roots containing sensory fibers from these muscles were cut, tonus would also be obliterated. Such experiments have clearly illustrated that muscular tonus is maintained through reflex activity of the nervous system and is not an intrinsic characteristic of the muscle itself. However, some scientists[1] have evidence to suggest that there are at least two components of muscle tone: (1) *active*—as just mentioned, due to partial contraction of the muscles through activity of the nervous system; and (2) *passive*—due to the natural elasticity or turgor of muscular and connective tissues, which is independent of nervous innervation. Incidentally, muscles with more than normal tone are referred to as *spastic.*

The basic neural mechanism for maintenance of active muscle tonus is the **stretch reflex,** or the **muscle spindle reflex.** As we have just learned, when a muscle is stretched, impulses are discharged from the muscle spindles. As shown in figure 5.15, afferent fibers from these spindles enter the spinal cord and form a synapse with the

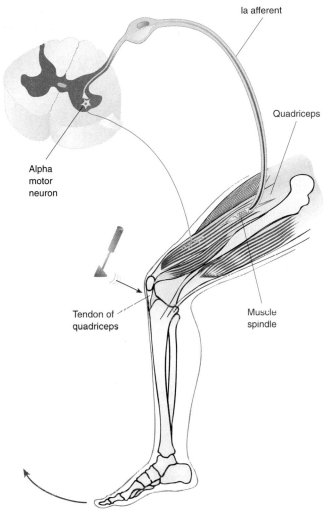

la afferent

Quadriceps

Alpha
motor
neuron

Tendon of
quadriceps

Muscle
spindle

Figure 5.16

The knee-jerk reflex. Tapping the patella tendon stretches the quadriceps muscles and the muscle spindles therein. Sensory impulses are sent to the spinal cord via the Ia afferents, which cause the alpha motor neurons innervating the quadriceps muscles to fire; the muscles contract, and the lower leg extends.

motor nerve cells located there. Axons from these motor neurons conduct impulses to the motor endplates in the same muscle fibers, and this activation produces increased tension, or tonus, in the muscle fibers.

Golgi Tendon Organs

Golgi tendon organs are proprioceptors encapsulated in tendon fibers and are located near the junction of the muscle and tendon fibers (musculotendinous junction). Their structure is shown in figure 5.16. Like the spindles, the Golgi tendon organs are sensitive to stretch. However, they are much less sensitive than the spindles and therefore require a strong stretch before they are activated. Actually,

because of their location with respect to the muscle fibers, the Golgi tendon organs are activated mainly by the stretch placed on them by the contraction of the muscles in whose tendons they lie. Given such a stretch, sensory information is sent to the central nervous system, causing the contracted muscle to relax. In other words, in contrast to the spindles, which are facilitatory (i.e., they cause contraction), stimulation of the tendon organs results in inhibition of the muscles in which they are located. This can be interpreted as a protective function in that during attempts to lift extremely heavy loads that could cause injury, the tendon organs cause a relaxation of the muscles.

A good example of the tendon organs in action is given by arm wrestling. Studies have suggested that the loss of the contest sometimes occurs when the tendon organ inhibition overcomes the voluntary effort to maintain contraction.[22] In addition, the "breaking point" in muscle strength testing might be related to inhibition caused by the tendon organs. If this is the case, maximal strength would be dependent on the ability to voluntarily "override" the inhibition function of the tendon organs.[22]

The spindles and Golgi tendon organs work together, the former causing just the right degree of muscular tension to effect a smooth movement and the latter causing muscular relaxation when the load is potentially injurious to the muscles and related structures.

Joint Receptors

The joint receptors are found in tendons, ligaments, periosteum (bone), muscle, and joint capsules. They supply information to the central nervous system concerning the joint angle, the acceleration of the joint, and the degree of deformation brought about by pressure. The names of some of the joint receptors are the *end bulbs of Krause,* the *Pacinian corpuscles,* and *Ruffini end organs.* All this information plus that from other receptors (e.g., sight, touch, and sound) is used to give us a sense of awareness of body and limb position, as well as to provide us with automatic reflexes concerned with posture.

The Nervous System and Motor Skills

Now we will direct our attention to the motor responses that are fundamental to the execution of motor skills. Figure 5.17 is a cross-sectional diagram of the essential anatomical parts of the spinal cord. The afferent nerve enters the spinal column through the *dorsal* (rear) *root* and forms synaptic junctions with several neurons (called *internuncial neurons*). The efferent nerve leaves the spinal cord by way of the *ventral* (front) *root* to the effector muscle. Injury to the ventral root (efferent) fibers affects the muscle or

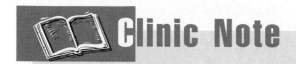

You can test your neuromuscular stretch reflexes by exerting a quick forceful tap with a rubber reflex hammer to the tendon. Three such examples are given as follows.

Biceps Reflex

Flex your forearm 90 degrees and have a partner support it; have the partner place his or her thumb over the tendon of insertion of the biceps (tubercle of radius). Now strike the thumb with the hammer; the force is transferred to your biceps tendon. The biceps muscle will contract, flexing the forearm. (Note: spinal cord segment servicing the muscle biceps brachii is C5–C6 [i.e., fifth and sixth cervical vertebrae].)

Triceps Reflex

Support your arm in a similar fashion as in the biceps reflex. When the triceps tendon of insertion (olecranon process of ulna) is struck directly with the hammer, the triceps will contract, extending the forearm. (Note: spinal cord segment servicing the muscle triceps brachii is C6–C7 [i.e., sixth and seventh cervical vertebrae].)

Patellar Reflex

Sit comfortably on the edge of a table, with your legs dangling and relaxed. Strike the patellar tendon with a sharp blow. The quadriceps femoris muscles will contract, causing extension of the leg (see figure 5.15). (Note: spinal cord segment servicing the four quadricep muscles is L2, L3, L4 [i.e., second, third, and fourth lumbar vertebrae].)

In each reflex, stimulation of the muscle spindles by rapping the tendon with a sharp, firm blow conveys information to the CNS, where motor stimuli are relayed to the appropriate muscle and contraction of the muscle is initiated. A positive response (i.e., lack of contraction for the specified muscle) is indicative of a malfunction or lesion at the level of the spinal cord servicing that particular muscle (e.g., biceps brachii—fifth or sixth cervical vertebrae). Likewise, the absence of limb reflexes might indicate a disruption of a normal function in the sensory afferent or motor efferent nerve systems due to injury or disease. Team physicians and trainers frequently conduct basic reflex tests to determine whether an injured athlete has experienced nerve damage. Similar reflex testing can be used to check for CNS hyperexcitability or depression caused by the possible presence of drugs and medications in the body.

---

muscles supplied with these motor fibers. Severing the nerve results in total paralysis.

The majority of afferent fibers entering the spinal cord do not form a synapse with an efferent fiber and leave at the same level, as depicted in the common reflex arc; rather, they split into ascending and descending branches that travel up and down the cord (figure 5.18). These long reflex paths connect receptors of the feet with those of the hand, and by the same token, the splitting of the ascending and descending fibers allows impulses to be received and discharged as required by the complexity of the movement. Such a vast array of interneurons and connections from the toe to the brain permit the CNS to function as a coordinating unit regardless of movement complexity.

Simple movements, such as removing a finger from a heated surface, are handled by the spinal cord reflex pattern, whereas the more complicated movements involve higher levels of the cord and the brain. Generally speaking, the motoneurons in the spinal cord effect the contraction patterns of the muscles, and the higher centers program the sequence of contraction.

Voluntary Control of Motor Functions

The cerebral cortex and the cerebellum are the centers employed in learning new skills.[8] These areas of the brain initiate voluntary control of movement patterns. Figure 5.19 illustrates the motor area of the brain, which also is designated as area 4. This area contains the pyramidal, or Betz cells. Upon electrical stimulation to this area, motor movements are elicited—hence the term **primary motor cortex.** Area 4 is now often referred to as **M1.** It is here that each region of the body is controlled by clusters of nerve cells for that specific region (foot, trunk, fingers, tongue, and so on). Evidence also suggests that a given cell in this area participates in movements of various directions and that a movement in a particular direction will involve the activation of a whole population of M1 cells.[12]

The **pyramidal tract** or **corticospinal tract** is made up of the long axons of the pyramidal cells and is the route used to send impulses from the motor cortex down to the motoneurons of the spinal cord, referred to as the anterior, or lower, motoneurons. From here, they form spinal nerves

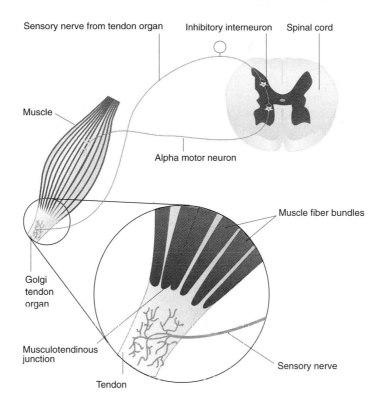

Figure 5.16

The Golgi tendon organ. When a contracted muscle is forcefully stretched, the sensory nerve of the tendon organ is stimulated. Impulses are sent to the spinal cord, where a synapse is made with an inhibitory interneuron that inhibits the alpha motor neuron, and the muscle relaxes.

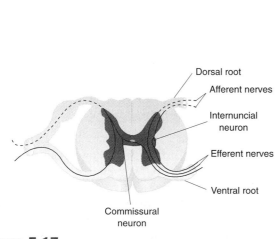

Figure 5.17

Essential anatomical parts of the spinal cord. The afferent (sensory) nerve enters the cord through the dorsal root and synapses with internuncial neurons. The efferent (motor) nerve leaves the cord by way of the ventral root to the effector muscle.

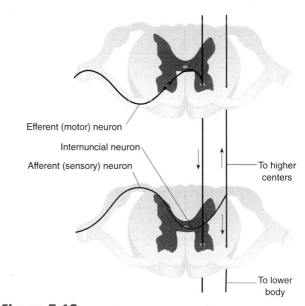

Figure 5.18

The majority of afferent fibers entering the cord do not form synapses with efferent fibers and leave at the same level of the cord; rather, they split into ascending and descending branches, which travel up and down the cord.

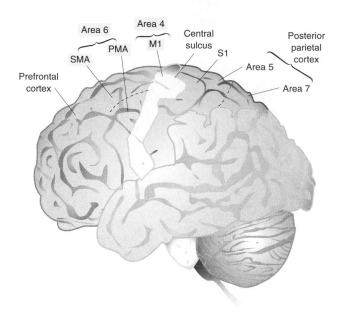

Figure 5.19

Areas of the neocortex intimately involved in the planning and instruction of voluntary movement. Areas 4 and 6 constitute the motor cortex. Area 4 is also called M1 or *primary motor cortex*. Area 6 is made up of the *premotor area* (PMA) and the *supplemental motor area* (SMA).

(comprised of the long axons of alpha and gamma motoneurons) and are distributed to their respective skeletal muscles (figure 5.20). Most of the pyramidal tract fibers cross over before entering the spinal cord so that the right motor cortex controls the muscles of the left side of the body and vice versa. The presence of this anatomical relationship is very apparent in stroke victims. Damage to the right brain is seen as muscular dysfunction on the left side of the body.

Figure 5.21 illustrates the area of the body affected when particular portions of the motor cortex are stimulated. The size of the area represented is related to the discreteness of movement. For example, the tongue, thumb, fingers, lips, and vocal cords are represented by large areas where only minimal stimuli are required to contract a single muscle or perhaps even a single fasciculus. In the abdominal area, however, groups of muscles rather than single muscles are contracted upon stimulation of the pyramidal area.

The current view is that during voluntary movements, pyramidal cell firing in the brain will drive a group of muscles so that a limb will move toward a desired position or "goal." This is accomplished by a burst of firing that occurs just before and during the movement. The bursts encode two important aspects of any movement—namely, force and direction. In the following discussion, we will see that there are other important neuronal circuits that can modify and refine these gross directives for voluntary movements. That is to say, a neural means for deciding on the "best" move to

make and to receive some comparative feedback regarding the movement execution and outcome. All this has much to do with sports skill acquisition.

Premotor Area for Learning Specialized Motor Skills

The area just forward to the motor area, cortical area 6, is probably the "sports skills area" of the brain. The **premotor area (PMA)** is in the lateral portion of this region, and the **supplemental motor area (SMA)** is in the medial portion. We believe that these areas are especially concerned with the acquisition of specialized motor skills. These two areas appear to perform similar functions but on different groups of muscles. While the PMA connects with reticulospinal neurons that innervate proximal motor units, the SMA sends axons that innervate distal motor units directly. If even small bits of these areas are surgically removed or electrically ablated, coordinated skill movements are difficult to develop. This appears to be especially true for tasks that require remembering sequences that follow a specific timing of movements.[14]

Area 6 plays another very important role in the performance of sports skills. Namely, area 6 lies at the junction where signals encoding what actions are desired are converted into signals that specify how the actions are to be carried out. The signals that converge on area 6 are coming from the prefrontal and parietal cortex (see figure 5.19). These signals allow for input related to decision making, abstract thought, and the anticipation of the consequences of action. Anyone who has played sports can relate to all of these types of "thoughts" occuring just prior to or during the performance of a favorite move that will "fool" their opponent or end with a score. Much of the decision process relates to what the performer knows has worked well in the past. Selecting the right move or making one up at the time is a clear mark of a highly skilled performer. This all relates to the matter of motor "memory" and the ability to choose a learned skill from a repertoire of tricks.

Basal Ganglia and Thalamus

The extrapyramidal tract is the route used to send impulses from the premotor area down to the lower motoneurons of the spinal cord (figure 5.20). The premotor area also has several subcortical connections, such as the corpus striatum which is made up of the caudate nucleus and putumen portions of the **basal ganglia.**[4,13] Two other major connections are through the globus pallidus of the basal ganglia and through the ventral lateral nucleus of the **thalamus.** These connections provide a loop where information passes from the cortex through the basal ganglia and thalamus and then back to the premotor cortex, particularly to the SMA. An important function of this loop is the selection and initiation of chosen movements. The premotor area also receives input

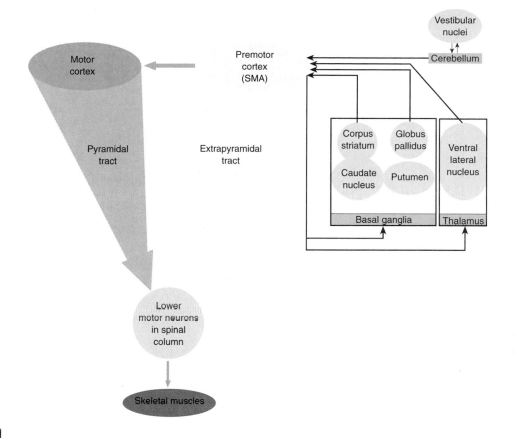

Figure 5.20

The neural pathways of the pyramidal and extrapyramidal tracts to motor neurons in the spinal column. Note the subcortical loop connections from the premotor cortex to the basal ganglia and thalamus and then back to the SMA. Also note the cerebellar input to the premotor cortex.

from the **cerebellum.** This latter part of the brain, as we will see next, is responsible for the coordination of movement patterns involving large groups of muscles.

The Cerebellum

The **cerebellum** receives information when a motor stimulus has occurred regardless of the stimulus source. This is accomplished by axons from various regions of the motor and sensory cortex being connected to clusters of cells in the pons, called the pontine nuclei, which in turn feed the cerebellum. Information from the lateral cerebellum is then looped back to the motor cortex via relay pathways in the ventral lateral nucleus of the thalamus. Two important functions of this loop between the motor cortex and cerebellum are (1) proper execution of voluntary, planned, multijoint movements; and (2) instruction of the primary motor cortex with respect to movement force, timing, and direction. A third important cerebellar function that relates to motor learning is that of "comparator"—i.e., a function of comparing what has happened to what was intended. When this comparison is less than perfect, some adjustments can be made via the cerebellar circuits.

For example, a voluntary movement such as punting a football is initiated. Impulses are transmitted downward through the pyramidal tract to excite the appropriate muscles. Impulses are also simultaneously transmitted to the cerebellum (figure 5.22). As the signals arrive at the muscles, proprioceptors (muscle spindles, Golgi tendon organs, and joint receptors) send the "punting" signal back to the cerebellum. The cerebellum then compares this proprioceptive information to what was intended, and elicits an impulse (correction factor) via the motor cortex. The corrective movement (fine adjustment) is then executed.

Here we have an example of one of the many fascinating but extremely complicated feedback circuits that begin in the motor cortex and return to it via proprioceptors and the cerebellum. This servomechanism type of feedback has been compared to control systems such as those used in industry, guided missiles, automatic pilot mechanisms, and anti-aircraft guns. For example, the guided missile continuously transmits radar signals that are received and fed to a computer. The computer, which is analogous to the cerebellum, monitors the signals and compares them to a prewritten program. In this manner, it can detect any errors in the

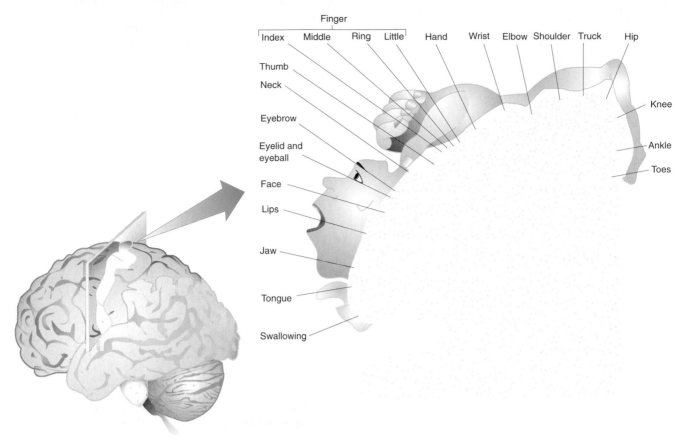

Figure 5.21

When particular portions of the motor cortex are stimulated, certain areas of the body are affected. The size of the area represented is related to the discreteness of movement. For example, the tongue, thumb, big toe, and lips are represented by large areas where only minimal stimuli are required to contract a single muscle.

missile's path and radio a correction signal. In somewhat the same fashion, the cerebellum compares the information from the motor cortex to the execution of the football punt. The "error" is calculated by the cerebellum, and a correction is immediately relayed to the motor cortex.

The cerebellum can be programmed during the course of learning a new sports skill. You will recall from your own experiences that at first, the movements are unsure, jerky, and highly variable with evidence of poor timing and lack of coordination. Performers spend much of their practice time thinking through movements and trying to develop both an improved level of execution and a proper "feel." With repeated practice, however, the movements tend to smooth out and can be repeated again and again, and all without much conscious thought. This is indirect evidence that a new motor program has been learned. Appropriate movement sequences can be generated on demand without having to think them through. You just do them. The cerebellum, then, functions as the unconscious overseer[6] to be certain that newly learned movement skills are properly executed and makes adjustments if they are not. More on this follows in the discussion on motor engrams.

Dampening Effect

It is in the preceding manner that the cerebellum exerts a dampening effect on such pendular movements as the golf swing and throwing and kicking a ball. As the arm or leg moves, momentum is developed with a resulting tendency for the limb to overshoot its mark. The dampening or "correcting" effect is administered by the cerebellum so that the limb stops at the intended position.

Similarly, the cerebellum predicts eventual limb position. The incoming information from the proprioceptors is used by the cerebellum to guide all body parts during the performance of a skill. Through the motor cortex the cerebellum exerts control over both the antagonist and agonist muscles.

Perception of Speed

The cerebellum also allows us to perceive the speed with which we approach objects and with which objects approach us. Without such perception, we would bang into walls and chairs and would miss the shuttlecock or tennis lob. For example, the football player, performing an agility run through

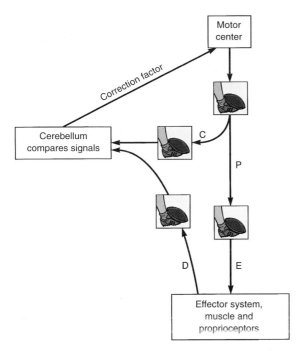

Figure 5.22

When a voluntary movement, such as punting a football, is initiated, impulses are transmitted downward through the pyramidal tract (P) and eventually to the muscles (E). Impulses are also transmitted to the cerebellum (C). As the signals arrive at the muscles, proprioceptors send the "punting" signal back to the cerebellum (D). The cerebellum then compares the two sets of information and elicits an impulse (correction factor) via the motor cortex, where the original stimulus was initiated; the movement is then considered to be completely executed.

a maze of blocking dummies, is guided by the cerebellum so that he does not run into a dummy but rather cuts sharply to either the right or the left at the appropriate time.

Two other variables that the brain takes into account are the speed of limb movements and the effect of gravity on limb positioning.[24] Consideration of these variables is important to programming the proper sequence of muscular contractions and relaxations needed to produce a desired limb movement in sports.

In addition, the cerebellum aids in establishing equilibrium through interpreting changes as revealed by the semicircular canals in the ears. Just as the cerebellum aids in predicting the speed with which we approach an object, it also predicts body positions as a consequence of rotational movements of the head.[6] For example, **tonic neck reflexes** are useful to young children under the age of 4 to 6 months to help them correct losses of balance. These reflexes also are present in persons with certain neurological dysfunctions or those who are well below average in motor skills and coordination. They apparently are not present in normal adults even during the performance of selected activities that would be expected to elicit them.[11]

Sensory Input and Motor Skills

A currently prevalent theory suggests that in the sensory area of the brain, a skill that has been practiced a sufficient number of times becomes memorized and that when the individual wishes to perform the given skill, he or she calls on this particular motor pattern, which is immediately "replayed." Psychologists have referred to these memorized motor patterns as **engrams.** An engram is a permanent trace left by a stimulus in the tissue protoplasm. By practicing the tennis forehand stroke hundreds to thousands of times, for example, this stimulus, over a period of practice sessions, changes the protoplasmic configuration of certain cells in the sensory portion of the brain. The resulting "realignment" is an engram, or a motor memory pattern, for that special skill. The engram now becomes a part of the person's sensory portion of the brain and on the appropriate stimulus can be recalled for immediate use.

The sensory engram involves a proprioceptor feedback servomechanism. Neuronal pathways from proprioceptors pass through the cerebellum to the sensory areas of the cerebral cortex and then to the motor cortex. Each center can modify the response to the muscles that perform the motor act. Once learned, the engram is stored and becomes available for use whenever the act is to be performed. In drinking from a glass, the proprioceptors from fingers, hand, and arm convey messages to the CNS. Here the previously stored engram is used as the model. When and if deviations from the stored engram occur, a correction is made through the release of additional motor signals from the motor cortex as "told" to it by the cerebellum.

Engrams for extremely rapid movements are stored in the motor area of the brain and are referred to as **motor engrams.** Engrams stored in the sensory portion of the brain, which are for slower motor acts, operate through the feedback servomechanism previously described in our discussion of the cerebellum; engrams in the motor area (frontal lobe) can be effected without sensory feedback. Typing or rapid movements at the keyboard do not allow sufficient time for a servomechanistic feedback.

Henry's Memory Drum

Research has cast doubt on the widely accepted theory that motor ability is completely general. This theory states that if one excels in a certain sport, the ability shown there will carry over into other activities. The range of skills displayed by the high-school athlete who excels in a number of sports has been cited, although perhaps erroneously, as proof of this theory. Relying on the "obvious," we have permitted ourselves to conclude that motor ability is truly general or nonspecific, whereas the contrary is probably true. Athletes who excel in several sports may owe more to their motivation and to their numerous activity experiences than to any carry-over of acquired skills from one sport to another.

Also, they may be endowed with many specific sports aptitudes rather than any great amount of general motor ability.

Research by Franklin Henry and his colleagues at the University of California has shown that the simple ability to perform a given neuromotor skill is no indication that the performer will be equally capable of performing other such skills; in other words, motor ability is specific to a task rather than general.[15,16] His reasoning led to the theory that neuromotor coordination patterns are stored in the mind on what we might call a memory drum. Whenever a specific movement pattern is needed, the stimulus causes the storage center or memory drum to "play back" the particular learned skill. Hence, the movement is performed automatically. Such learned skills as playing the piano, running, walking, throwing, and eating are all performed without conscious thought; the memory drum simply plays them back on demand.

The entire process might be likened to the functioning of a computer. According to this theory, the program (or recorded movement pattern) has been learned previously and stored on a file (memory drum or motor memory), ready to be selected and released when needed. Such a program consists of a set of nonconscious instructions that direct the necessary nerve impulses to the appropriate muscles in a coordinated sequence, thus causing the desired movement. The "read-out time," or performance times, varies somewhat, depending on the length and complexity of the movement. A program in process of being "read out" cannot be changed before it has been completed, in conformity with the all-or-none law of physiology. Some of the findings that lend support to this theory are as follows:

1. Individual differences in ability to make a fast arm movement are about 70% specific to the particular movement being made. For example, a person who can perform a certain arm movement rapidly is not necessarily able to perform other movements of the same arm with equal speed.
2. Reaction time lengthens with increased movement complexity.
3. Little or no relationship exists between static strength and speed of movement. This seems to indicate that speed of movement depends more on the quality of the impression of the memory drum than on the muscular strength of the limb.
4. A fast limb movement, once underway, cannot be changed in its direction, nor can it be stopped partway through unless it was originally programmed to be stopped rather than completed.
5. Motor-oriented programming results in slower movement and greater reaction latency than sensory-oriented programming. For instance, concentration on the movement to be made (motor orientation) rather than on the starting signal (sensory orientation) tends to result in slower reaction time, as conscious control of motor movement interferes with the reading out of the programmed impulses.

6. The component parts of a skill are first learned discretely and are gradually combined into a continuous pattern on the memory drum. When a skill deteriorates, as is the case in aging[18] or long disuse, one notices that the combined pattern breaks up and reverts to the separate movements.
7. Research over a period of many years has shown that the relationship between different motor skills is usually quite low.

We suggest you read the work of McCullagh et al. for a more detailed review of this topic.[20]

Summary

The central nervous system (CNS) comprises the brain and spinal cord, the latter extending from the base of the skull to the second lumbar vertebrae. This electrical conduction system allows for both reflex contractions (cord level) and voluntary controlled movements (entire system).

The basic functional and anatomical unit of the nervous system is the neuron, which consists of a cell body, or soma, several short nerve fibers called dendrites, and a longer nerve fiber called an axon.

The information transmitted and relayed by nerves is in a form of electrical energy that is referred to as the nerve impulse or action potential. A nerve impulse is an electrical disturbance at the point of stimulation of a nerve that self-propagates along the entire length of the axon.

A finger being quickly withdrawn from a hot flame or a sharp tack as a consequence of a painful sensation exemplifies a simple reflex arc. The sensory signal travels by way of an afferent, or sensory, nerve fiber to the spinal cord and makes contact with a motor nerve fiber; the appropriate muscles are stimulated, and the hand is withdrawn.

The connection of an axon of one nerve to the cell body or dendrites of another is called a synapse. When an impulse arrives at the synapse, a chemical transmitter substance is released from the synaptic knobs at the end of the axon. If it is an excitatory transmitter, such as acetylcholine (ACh), the adjoining nerve fiber is brought closer to the firing threshold; if it is an inhibitory transmitter, such as gamma-aminobutyric acid (GABA), the adjoining fiber is hyperpolarized or moved further away from the firing threshold. Such an inhibitory mechanism permits the CNS to select or reject stimuli.

At the neuromuscular junction, where the motor nerve invaginates the muscle fiber, a similar synaptic arrangement exists. However, all stimuli are transmitted across the neuromuscular junction by the transmitter ACh, as inhibition does not occur here.

The selection and performance of voluntary movements involves an interplay between the premotor cortex, basal ganglia, thalamus, and motor cortex along with the cerebellum, which acts as a "comparator" to ensure that intended movements are carried out.

In muscles (muscle spindles), tendons (Golgi tendon organs), ligaments, and joints (joint receptors) are located proprioceptors that transmit information about the completeness of desired muscle contractions, tension on the contractile unit, and changes in joint angles to the CNS. These are also called kinesthetic receptors because they provide information about the location of the limbs and the body in an environment and thereby aid in performing movements.

The learning of a motor skill is a complex and not completely understood process. It mainly takes place in the cerebral cortex and the cerebellum. Signals dealing with the particular skill originate in the motor cortex and are transmitted to the muscles. A "copy" of this information to the muscles is also fed to the cerebellum. As movement of the muscles is initiated, proprioceptors relay the program status back to the cerebellum, which sends a corrected signal to the motor cortex if necessary; the skill is then completed.

Motor learning is a term used to describe the acquisition and retention of new motor skills. The newly acquired skill is called an *engram,* which is viewed as a permanent trace left in neural tissue protoplasm by repeated stimulation during practice sessions.

Henry's memory drum theory of neuromotor reaction provides some hypotheses about how skills are memorized. Most important evidence supports the concept of specificity, which states that the learning of motor skills is specific rather than general. There is little if any carryover from one sport to another unless skills are nearly identical.

Questions

1. What are considered to be the three basic functions of the nervous system?
2. Diagram and label the parts of a nerve cell.
3. Describe how a nerve transmits a nervous impulse along its axon.
4. What is a reflex arc?
5. How are signals transmitted from one nerve fiber to another?
6. How does inhibition at the neuronal synapse occur? Of what value is the inhibitory mechanism?
7. Diagram the myoneural junction and the related anatomical parts.
8. Explain how a signal is transmitted across the myoneural junction.
9. What are proprioceptors, where are they located, and how do they function?
10. Explain muscle tonus.
11. What is the stretch reflex, and how might we test for it?
12. Where is the "sports skill area" of the brain located?
13. Outline the manner in which a voluntary skill is performed.
14. Which three areas of the brain are most involved in voluntary movements?
15. Describe the special role that the cerebellum plays as a "comparator."
16. What is meant by the "dampening effect" exerted through the cerebellum?
17. Define a motor engram.
18. Outline Henry's memory drum theory of motor learning.

References

1. Basmajian, J. V. 1974. *Muscles Alive,* 3d ed. Baltimore: Williams and Wilkins.
2. Bellemare, F., J. J. Woods, R. Johansson, and B. Bigland-Ritchie. 1983. Motor-unit discharge rates in maximal voluntary contractions of three human muscles. *J Neurophysiol.* 50(6):1380–1392.
3. Bigland-Ritchie, B., D. A. Jones, and J. J. Woods. 1979. Excitation frequency and muscle fatigue: electrical responses during human voluntary and stimulated contractions. *Exper Neurology.* 64:414–427.
4. Brooks, D. J. 1995. The role of the basal ganglia in motor control: contributions from PET. *J Neurol Sci.* 128 (1):1–13.
5. Burke, D., K. E. Hagbarth, and N. F. Skuse. 1978. Recruitment order of human spindle endings in isometric voluntary contractions. *J Physiol* (London). 285:101–112.
6. Denise, P., and C. Darlot. 1993. The cerebellum as a predictor of neural messages—II. Role in motor control and motion sickness. *Neuroscience.* 56(3):647–655.
7. Falck, B., E. Stalberg, and C. Bischoff. 1995. Influence of recording site within the muscle on motor unit potentials. *Muscle Nerve.* 18(12):1385–1389.
8. Fox, E. L. 1984. *Sports Physiology,* 2d ed. Philadelphia: W. B. Saunders, p. 72.
9. Friboulet, A., and D. Thomas. 1993. Reaction-diffusion coupling in a structured system: application to the quantitative simulation of endplate currents. *J Theor Biol.* 160(4):441–455.
10. Gatz, A. 1979. *Manter's Essentials of Clinical Neuroanatomy and Neurophysiology,* 3d ed. Philadelphia: F. A. Davis, p. 121.
11. Geddes, D., and W. O'Grady. 1979. Manifestation of tonic neck reflexes in normal adults during physical activity. *Am Corr Ther J.* 33:184–187.
12. Georgopoulos, A. P. 1994. Behavioral neurophysiology of the motor cortex. *J Lab Clin Med.* 124:766–774.
13. Graybiel, A. M., T. Aosaki, A. W. Flaherty, and M. Kimura. 1994. The basal ganglia and adaptive motor control. *Science* 265(5180):1826–1831.
14. Halsband, U., N. Ito, J. Tanji, and H. J. Freund. 1993. The role of premotor cortex and the supplementary motor area in the temporal control of movement in man. *Brain* 116:243–266.
15. Henry, F. M. 1960. Influence of motor and sensory sets on reaction latency and speed of discrete movements. *Res Q.* 31:459.
16. Henry, F. M., and D. E. Rogers. 1960. Increased response latency for complicated movements and a "memory drum" theory of neuromotor reaction. *Res Q.* 31:448.
17. Kato, M., K. Murakami, K. Takahashi, and H. Hirayama. 1981. Motor unit activities during maintained voluntary muscle contraction at constant levels in man. *Neurosci Letters* 25:149–154.
18. Keen, D. A., G. H. Yue, and R. M. Enoka. 1994. Training-related enhancement in the control of motor output in elderly humans. *J Appl Physiol.* 77(6):2648–2658.

19. Loeb, G. E. 1984. The control and responses of mammalian muscle spindles during normally executed motor tasks. *Exercise Sport Sci Rev.* 12:157–204.

20. McCullagh, P., M. R. Weiss, and D. Ross. 1989. Modeling considerations in motor skill acquisition and performance: An integrated approach. *Exercise and Sports Sciences Reviews* 17:475–513.

21. Miles, T. S. 1994. The control of human motor units. *Clin Exp Pharmacol Physiol.* 21(7):511–520.

22. O'Connell, A., and E. Gardner. 1972. *Understanding the Scientific Bases of Human Movement.* Baltimore: Williams and Wilkins, p. 209.

23. Petrofsky, J. S., and C. A. Phillips. 1985. Discharge characteristics of motor units and the surface EMG during fatiguing isometric contractions at submaximal tensions. *Aviat Space Environ Med.* 56:581–586.

24. Ross, E. D., and M. Muhlbauer. 1983. Speed of movement, gravity, and the neural coordination of muscular actions. *Electromyogr Clin Neurophysiol.* 23:385–392.

25. Ruff, R. L., and D. Whittlesey. 1993. Na$^+$ currents near and away from endplates on human fast and slow twitch muscle fibers. *Muscle Nerve.* 16(9):922–929.

26. Suzuki, S., and R. S. Hutton. 1976. Postcontractile motoneuronal discharge produced by muscle afferent activation. *Med Sci Sports.* 8(4):258–264.

27. Svendenhag, J., B. G. Wallin, and G. Sundlöf. 1984. Skeletal muscle sympathetic activity at rest in trained and untrained subjects. *Acta Physiol Scand.* 120:499–504.

Readings

Armstrong, D. M., and D. E. Marple-Horvat. 1996. Role of the cerebellum and motor cortex in the regulation of visually controlled locomotion. *Can J Physiol Pharmacol.* 74:443–455.

Donoghue, J. P., and J. N. Sanes. 1994. Motor areas of the cerebral cortex. *J Clin Neurophysiol.* 11:328–396.

Georgopoulos, A. P. 1996. On the translation of directional motor cortical commands to activation of muscles via spinal interneuronal systems. *Brain Res Cogn Brain Res.* 3:151–155.

Lang, W., P. Hollinger, A. Eghker, and G. Lindinger. 1994. Functional localization of motor processes in the primary and supplementary motor areas. *J Clin Neurophysiol.* 11:397–419.

Tanji, J., and H. Mushiake. 1996. Comparison of neuronal activity in the supplementary motor area and primary motor cortex. *Brain Res Cogn Brain Res.* 3:143–150.

6

Skeletal Muscle: Structure and Function

For clinicians, physical educators, and coaches to adequately plan and conduct programs designed to increase muscular strength, endurance, and flexibility, they need a knowledge of the muscular system. They should know structure, both gross and microscopic, to understand function; and although much more research is needed, they should know the most recent views on how a muscle contracts and what causes a muscle to fatigue. The purpose of this chapter, then, will be to discuss both the structure and function of skeletal muscle. We will give considerable coverage to muscle fiber types because of the veritable explosion of research on this topic over the past three decades.[44] We also will explore the concept of **muscle plasticity,** which is defined as adaptive changes in muscle fibers brought on by disuse, injury, aging, or specific types of overload training.[47] That is to say, muscle is malleable and can be shaped to best meet the time and circumstantial needs of the individual.

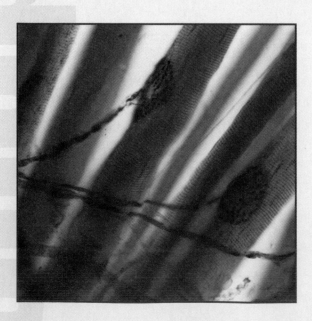

Structure—The Basis for Contraction

Function of Skeletal Muscle

Summary

The major concepts to be learned from this chapter are as follows:

- The structure of skeletal muscle forms the basis for understanding how it contracts.
- The basis for skeletal muscle function is the motor unit, defined as a single motor nerve (motorneuron) and the muscle fibers (cells) it innervates.
- Muscular strength gradations are possible by varying the number of motor units contracting at any given time and by varying the frequency of contraction of individual motor units.
- There are two kinds of motor units: one containing Type I (slow-twitch) muscle fibers and the other containing Type II (fast-twitch) muscle fibers.
- Type I fibers have a high aerobic capacity and are used preferentially for endurance activities whereas Type II fibers have a high anaerobic capacity and are used preferentially for sprintlike activities.
- Histochemical staining allows further subdivision of Type II fibers into IIA (oxidative-glycolytic), IIB (glycolytic), and IIC (unclassified) categories, referred to as phenotypes.
- Differences in muscle fiber phenotypes are due to their differences in myofibrillar protein isoforms, chiefly the amount of heavy versus light myosin chains that are present.
- The isoforms control the Ca^{++} activated rate of shortening and maximal velocity of shortening, with Type I fibers being less responsive and Type II fibers being more responsive.
- Numerous factors control protein expression and synthesis of isoforms, which ultimately determine the functional properties of muscle fiber phenotypes.
- Some of these controlling factors have neurotrophic, myogenic, temperature, fatigue, hormonal, and metabolic regulatory signal origins.
- Motor units are preferentially recruited during exercise following a motorneuron "size principle"; small ones first, large ones last.
- Type I motor units are recruited for low-intensity exercise, Type IIA for more prolonged, higher-intensity exercise, and Type IIB for all-out, maximal efforts.
- With endurance training, the most common adaptation is an increase in the aerobic capacity of both Type I and II fibers and shifts to higher ratios of IIA:IIB fibers.
- The peak force generated by a muscle decreases, and the peak power increases with increasing velocities of movement.
- For any given velocity of movement, the peak force and peak power produced are greater the higher the percentage distribution of Type II fibers in the muscle.
- The most probable sites of local muscular fatigue are the neuromuscular junction, the muscle itself (contractile mechanism), and the central nervous system (brain and spinal cord).

Structure—The Basis for Contraction

A great deal of the knowledge of muscle contraction has been gathered in the past 30 years. For the most part, information about the structural changes that occur when a resting muscle cell is actively contracted has been obtained by use of the electron microscope. It is imperative that we first understand muscle structure so that the theory as to how a muscle contracts will be easier to comprehend.

Connective Tissues

Skeletal muscle is composed of many thousands of individual contractile fibers bound together by a sheath of connective tissues. That portion of connective tissue that covers each muscle fiber or cell is called the **endomysium.** Just inside and attached to the endomysium is the muscle cell membrane or **sarcolemma.** The sarcolemma is not a connective tissue, so we will talk more about it later. The inside of the muscle cell is composed of a specialized protoplasm called **sarcoplasm** (*sarco* means "flesh") or **cytoplasm** (cell fluid). Numerous muscle cells (fibers) are grouped together to form muscle bundles or **fasciculi.** These bundles, containing various numbers of muscle fibers, are in turn held together by a connective tissue referred to as the **perimysium.** Encasing the entire muscle (or all the muscle bundles) is yet another connective tissue component, called the **epimysium.** The structural units of muscle and their associated connective tissues are given in table 6.1 and illustrated in figure 6.1.

Tendons

The intramuscular network of connective tissues coalesces and becomes continuous with the dense connective tissue of the tendons at each end of a muscle. These tendons are rigidly cemented to the outermost covering of bone, the **periosteum,** and thereby serve to connect the skeletal muscles to the bony skeleton. The muscle fibers themselves do not come into direct contact with the skeleton; thus the tremendous tension developed by muscles is borne entirely by their tendinous attachments. There are several advantages to this arrangement. If muscle fibers were attached directly to bone, they would be subject to considerable damage each time the muscle contracted. Tendons not only are much tougher than muscles but are also composed of "nonliving" fibers, which are metabolically inactive compared to muscle tissue. Furthermore, because tendons are stronger than muscles, a relatively small tendon can withstand the tension developed by a relatively large muscle. Consider their relative sizes when muscle undergoes unbelievable enlargement, as in the case of competitive body builders, but the connecting tendons remain quite small.

table 6.1

Structural units of skeletal muscle and their corresponding connective tissues

Structural unit	Connective tissue
Muscle fiber or cell	Endomysium
Muscle bundle (fasciculus)	Perimysium
Entire muscle	Epimysium

Blood Supply

Muscles are richly supplied with blood vessels. Arteries and veins enter and exit the muscle along with the connective tissues and are oriented parallel to the individual muscle fibers. They branch repeatedly into numerous arterioles, capillaries, and venules, forming vast networks in and around the endomysium (figure 6.2). In this manner each fiber is assured of an adequate supply of freshly oxygenated blood from the arterial system and of the removal of waste products such as carbon dioxide via the venous system. In sedentary men and women, an average of three to four capillaries surround each muscle fiber, whereas in male and female athletes, five to seven capillaries surround each fiber.[56,93] This is a most important adaptation for aerobic endurance performance.

The amount of blood required by skeletal muscle depends, of course, on its state of activity. During maximal exercise the muscles may require as much as 100 times more blood than when resting. Besides the large number of capillaries that supply each muscle fiber, there are other ways in which this blood-flow requirement can be met. For example, the alternating contraction and relaxation of active muscle causes periodic squeezing of the blood vessels. This pumping or milking action, called *muscle pump,* speeds up the return of blood to the heart, ultimately increasing the amount of fresh blood that can be oxygenated and then returned to the muscles. During exercise, constriction of the arteries supplying blood to the inactive areas of the body (such as the gut, kidney, and skin)—and dilation of those to the active skeletal muscles—also aid in regulating muscle blood flow. We will discuss these important muscle pump and shunting mechanisms again in chapter 9.

Nerve Supply

The nerves supplying a muscle contain both **motor** (efferent) and **sensory** (afferent) **fibers,** and usually enter and leave the muscle along with the blood vessels (see figure 6.2). The efferent fibers branch out repeatedly throughout

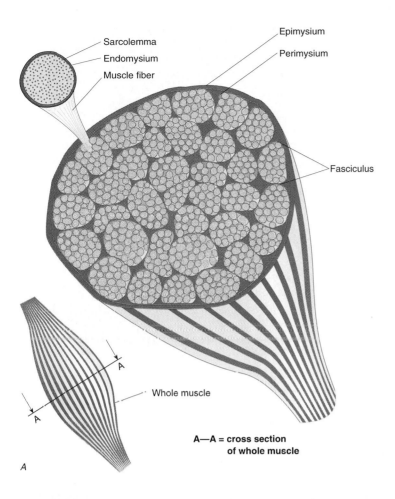

Sarcolemma
Endomysium
Muscle fiber

Epimysium
Perimysium

Fasciculus

Whole muscle

A—A = cross section
of whole muscle

A

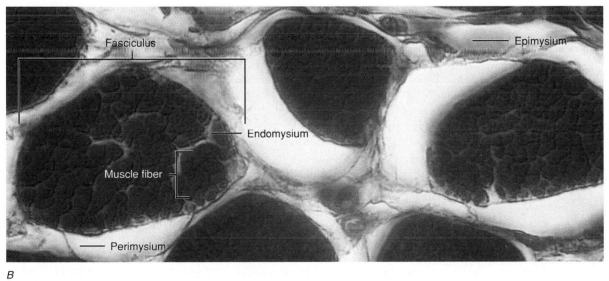

Fasciculus

Epimysium

Endomysium

Muscle fiber

Perimysium

B

Figure 6.1

A. Relationship between connective tissues and the cell membrane (sarcolemma) of skeletal muscle. *B.* Scanning electron micrograph of a fascicle (fasciculus) surrounded by its connective tissue sheath, the perimysium. Muscle fibers within the fascicle are surrounded by endomysium (320x).

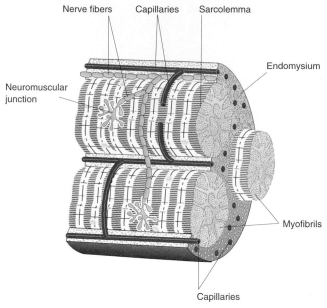

Figure 6.2

The nerves supplying a muscle usually enter the muscle along with the blood vessels. They branch out repeatedly through the connective tissue framework of the muscle, thus reaching all the muscle fibers.

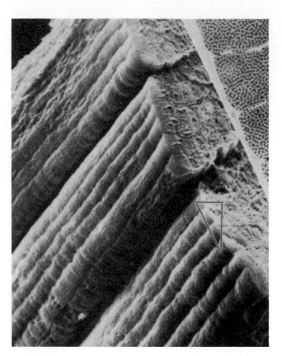

Figure 6.3

Scanning electron micrograph of insect flight muscle showing three very large muscle fibers or cells. The individual myofibrils making up the fibers are also clearly outlined. The inset in the upper right-hand corner is a light micrograph of the same tissue in transverse (cross) section.

(From Smith, D. S.: Muscle. New York, Academic Press, 1972, p. 10.)

the connective tissue framework of the muscle, thus reaching all the muscle fibers. The motor nerves, which when stimulated cause muscle fibers to contract, originate in the central nervous system (spinal cord and brain). The point of termination of a motor nerve (axon) on a muscle fiber is known as the **neuromuscular (myoneural) junction** or the **motor endplate** (p. 112). By definition, a motor nerve and all of the individual muscle fibers it innervates is called a motor unit. Motor nerves constitute about 60% of the nerves associated with a muscle. The sensory nerves, which make up the remaining 40%, convey information concerning pain, tension, and muscle contraction from the muscle and tendon sensory receptors to the central nervous system. The muscle and tendon sense organs as well as other aspects of the nerve supply to muscle were discussed in detail in the preceding chapter.

Structure of the Muscle Cell

The scanning electron microscope provides us with detailed insights about the make-up and arrangement of muscle fibers. Fiber sections viewed at magnifications 10,000 times their original size are used to provide photographs called **electron micrographs.** These can be further enlarged during printing to give even further magnifications—e.g., 225,000 times.[98] Figure 6.3 is for insect flight muscle, but there is great similarity across various animal species including human beings.

To further appreciate the microscopic structure of a muscle cell, we can tease out a fiber from the sartorius muscle of a frog. After placing this single fiber (cell) under a light microscope, we can observe regularly alternating light and dark striations (figure 6.4). Because of these striations, skeletal muscle is sometimes referred to as striated or striped muscle. Inside the sarcolemma is the sarcoplasm, which we mentioned earlier. Subcellular components, such as nuclei and mitochondria, are suspended in this reddish, viscous fluid. The sarcoplasm also contains myoglobin, fat, glycogen, phosphocreatine, ATP, and hundreds of threadlike protein strands called **myofibrils.** Within these myofibrils, the contractile units, called **sarcomeres** (German word for *small boxes*), are housed. The contractile unit contains **myofilaments** named **myosin** (thick ones) and **actin** (thin ones). These contractile proteins are found in a special arrangement to one another (i.e., each myosin is surrounded [think three-dimensional] by six or more actins).

The Myofibrils

As mentioned, the myofibrils (figure 6.4) are characterized by alternating light and dark areas. In fact, it is the geometrical arrangement of all these light and dark areas of the myofibrils that gives the fiber its overall striated appearance. The

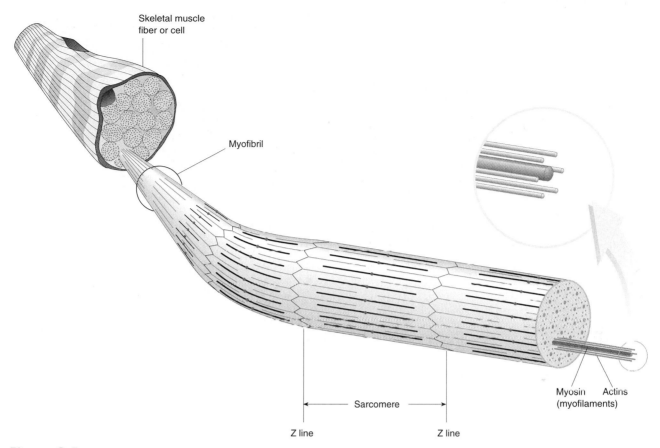

Skeletal muscle
fiber or cell

Myofibril

Myosin   Actins
(myofilaments)

Sarcomere

Z line   Z line

Figure 6.4

Skeletal muscle showing microscopic delineation of fiber, myofibril, and myofilaments. Note the striations in both the fiber and the myofibril; these alternating light and dark bands are caused by the geometric arrangement of the protein filaments—myosin and actin.

light areas are called **I bands,** the dark areas, **A bands** (figure 6.5). In the middle of each I band is a dark line, the **Z line** (from the German *zwischen* meaning "between"). The bands, which are composed of protein filaments, are so named because of what happens to the velocity of a light wave as it passes through them. For example, when a light wave passes through the A band, its velocity is not equal in all directions (i.e., it is *anisotropic*). When a light wave is passed through the I band, the velocity of the emerging light is the same in all directions and thus is *isotropic*.

The Sarcoplasmic Reticulum and T-Tubules

As shown in figure 6.5, surrounding the myofibrils is a net-like system of tubules and vesicles, collectively referred to as the **sarcoplasmic reticulum (SR).** The **longitudinal tubules** of the SR are so named because they run parallel (longitudinally) to the myofibrils. The longitudinal tubules terminate at either end into vesicles sometimes referred to as the **outer vesicles** or **cisterns** (see figure 6.5). The outer vesicles are where calcium ions (Ca^{++}) are stored, one of

the substances required for contraction within the myofibrils. This reticular pattern is repeated regularly along the entire length of the myofibrils. The outer vesicles of one reticular pattern are separated from those of another by a group of tubules called the transverse tubules (because they run transversely to the myofibril), the T system, or simply the T-tubules. The T-tubules, although functionally associated with the sarcoplasmic reticulum are known to be anatomically separate from it. They are extensions or invaginations of the muscle cell membrane, the sarcolemma. The two outer vesicles and the T-tubule separating them are known as a *triad.*

The entire function of the sarcoplasmic reticulum and T-tubules is not known.[99] However, it is known that the triad is of particular importance in muscular contraction. For example, the T-tubules are responsible for spreading the nervous impulse from the sarcolemma inward to the deep portions of the fiber. The outer vesicles of the reticulum contain large amounts of calcium (Ca^{++}). As the impulse travels over the T-tubules and "communicates" with the outer vesicles, Ca^{++} is released into the cytoplasm. The fractional volume of the reticulum system and tubules has been

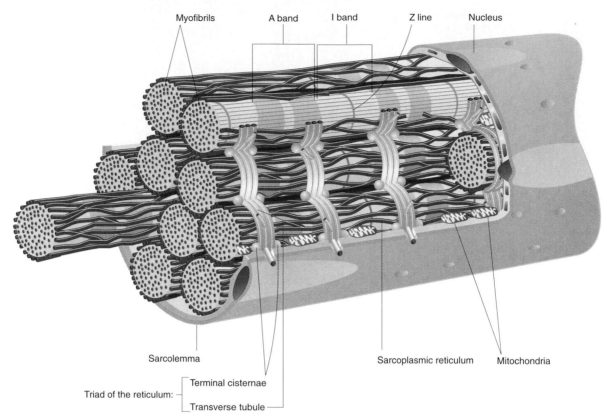

Figure 6.5

The sarcoplasmic reticulum and transverse tubules form a netlike system of tubules and vesicles surrounding the myofibrils. The outer vesicles store large quantities of calcium ions (Ca^{++}), one of the ingredients required for the contractile process. The transverse tubules are concerned with conduction of the nervous impulses deep into the myofibrils. The two outer vesicles (terminal cisternae) and the transverse tubule separating them are known as a triad.

determined to be about 5% of the total volume of a muscle fiber. With chronic exercise training, this volume increases by about 12% on the average,[14] providing for a more effective spread of depolarization and Ca^{++} release. We will discuss shortly the importance of both the spreading of the nervous impulse and the release of Ca^{++} in the actual contractile process. Right now, let us go on with the microscopic structure of muscle.

The Protein Filaments

The I and A bands are made up of two different protein filaments, a thinner filament called actin and a thicker one called myosin. Their arrangement within the myofibrils is shown in figures 6.4 and 6.6. As can be seen, the I band is composed entirely of the thinner actin filaments. They are not continuous within one sarcomere (i.e., between two Z lines); rather, they are anchored to the Z lines at each end of the sarcomere and partly extend into the A band region. The latter band, although composed mainly of the thicker myosin filaments, also contains a small amount of actin. The so-called **H zone** is caused by the slight variation in shading resulting from the absence of actin filaments in the

middle of the A band. The Z lines adhere to the sarcolemma, lending stability to the entire structure, and presumably keep the actin filaments in alignment. The Z lines may also play a role in the transmission of nervous impulses from the sarcolemma to the myofibrils.

A closer look at the actin or thin filament is presented in figure 6.7. The protein actin consists of globular (spheroidal) molecules linked together to form a double helix. Such a pattern is very similar in appearance to a twisted strand of beads. Actins do not merely participate as passive "cables" to be pulled on during muscular contraction but are chemically and mechanically involved in the contraction process.[60] And although the thin filament is called the actin filament, it actually contains two other important proteins, **tropomyosin** and **troponin.** The tropomyosin is a long, thin molecule that lies on the surface of the actin strand. The ends of the tropomyosin molecules are embedded in globular molecules of troponin (figure 6.7).

The myosin filaments have tiny protein projections on each end that extend toward the actin filaments (figure 6.7). These are called **cross-bridges,** and together with the actin filaments they play a very important role in the contraction process. As shown, there are actually two cross-bridge heads

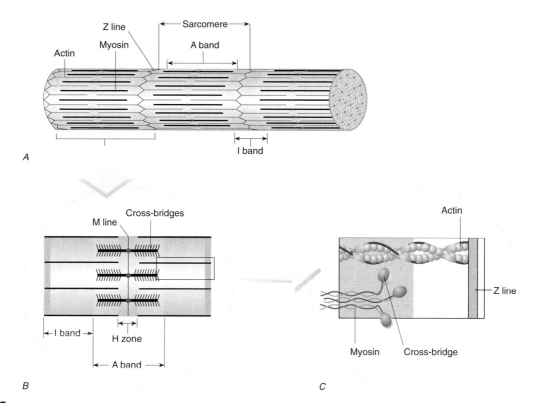

Figure 6.6

The Myofibril—the contractile unit of skeletal muscle. *A.* Note that the A band is composed of two protein filaments (actin and myosin). The I band contains actin filaments only. *B.* A closer look at the myosin filament, which projects in cross-bridging fashion toward the actin filament. The H zone (in the middle of the A band) is a result of the absence of actin filaments. *C.* A magnified view of a single myosin cross-bridge as it projects toward a single actin filament.

(From Fox[33])

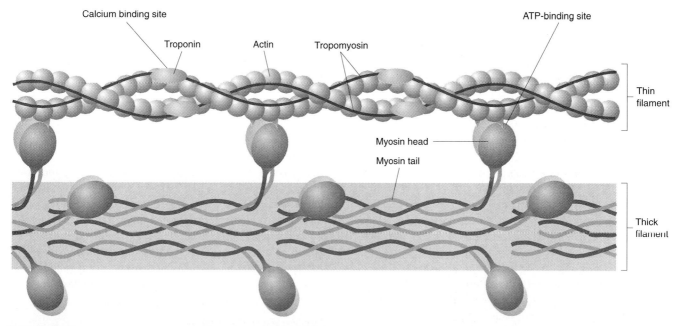

Figure 6.7

Close-up of actin (thin) and myosin (thick) filaments. The actin filament actually contains two other proteins important in the contractile process: troponin and tropomyosin. The head of the myosin filament is called the cross-bridge.

attached to one long tail in each myosin molecule. The tails aggregate to form the backbone of the thick filament. The heads are globular in appearance and contain the sites for actin binding and ATP splitting (hydrolysis). These cross-bridge heads or simply cross-bridges are the energy transducing (chemical to mechanical) components of the contractile machinery. As we will soon see, the cyclic interaction of the cross-bridges is responsible for the sliding of the actin filaments past the myosin filaments during muscle force generation.[21]

The Sliding Filament Theory of Muscular Contraction

The structural arrangement of skeletal muscle presented above has led to a **sliding filament theory** of muscular contraction proposed by H. E. Huxley.[54] As the name of the theory implies, one set of filaments is thought to slide over the other, thus shortening the muscle. This is illustrated in figure 6.8. Note that the lengths of the actin and myosin filaments do not change during contraction, but rather the former merely slide over the latter toward the center of the sarcomere. This leads to a shortening of the I band but not of the A band and to disappearance of the H zone. The sliding filament theory is somewhat analogous to the way in which a telescope shortens: the overall length of the telescope (muscle) decreases as one section (actin) slides over the other (myosin), with neither section itself shortening.

The exact manner in which this sliding process is effected has yet to be completely elucidated. However, it is thought that the myosin cross-bridges form a type of chemical bond with selected sites on the actin filaments. This forms a protein complex called **actomyosin.** When actomyosin is extracted from muscle and ATP is added, it will contract as it does in living muscle.

The mechanical and physiological events underlying the sliding filament theory of muscular contraction can be conveniently divided into five phases: (1) rest, (2) excitation-coupling, (3) contraction (shortening and tension development), (4) recharging, and (5) relaxation. Keep in mind that this is a theoretical model, and researchers continue to verify and refute various aspects of the model. For example, there is an ongoing search for the actual mechanism by which depolarization of the sarcolemma is communicated across the small gap between the T-tubules and the cisterns of the SR system so Ca^{++} is released to the cytoplasm.[99] Other researchers are interested in which specific part of the cross-bridge is involved in the contractile process,[112] and how to account for the elastic nature of cross-bridges.[102] Still others are researching the possibility that the major role of the troponin-tropomyosin complex is to prevent the weakly binding ATP cross-bridges found in relaxed fibers from going on to more strongly binding states in the presence of Ca^{++}.[97] And so the search continues, but let us take a closer look at this theoretical model under the

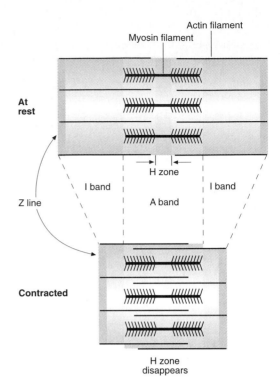

Figure 6.8

The sliding filament theory. When the sarcomeres of a muscle contract as compared to rest: (1) the H zone disappears because the actin filaments slide over the myosin filaments toward the center of the sarcomere; (2) the I band shortens because the actin filaments attached to the Z lines on either side of the sarcomere are pulled toward the center; (3) the A band does not change in length; and (4) neither the myosin nor the actin filaments change in length because of the sliding or interdigitation mechanics.

(From Fox[33])

different phases mentioned here. These phases are described in figure 6.9, parts *A* through *E*.

Rest

Under resting conditions, the cross-bridges of the myosin filaments extend toward but do not interact with the actin filaments. An ATP molecule is bound to the end of the cross-bridge. At rest this complex is referred to as an *"uncharged" ATP cross-bridge complex.* As mentioned previously, calcium as Ca^{++} is stored in large quantities in the vesicles of the sarcoplasmic reticulum. In the absence of free Ca^{++}, the troponin and tropomyosin of the actin filament work together to inhibit the myosin cross-bridge from binding with actin (i.e., actin and myosin are said to be uncoupled).

Excitation-Coupling

When an impulse from a motor nerve reaches the motor endplate, acetylcholine is released, stimulating the generation of an impulse (action potential) in the sarcolemma of

Figure 6.9

Proposed mechanism of the sliding filament theory. *A.* At rest, uncharged ATP cross-bridges are extended, actin and myosin are uncoupled, and Ca^{++} is stored in the reticulum. *B.* During excitation-coupling, stimulation releases Ca^{++}, which then binds to troponin, "turning on" actin active sites; actomyosin is formed. *C.* During contraction, ATP is broken down, releasing energy that swivels the cross-bridges; actin slides over the myosin, tension is developed, and the muscle shortens. *D.* During recharging, ATP is resynthesized, and actin and myosin uncouple and are recycled. *E.* When stimulation ceases, Ca^{++} is restored to the reticulum by a calcium pump, and the muscle relaxes.

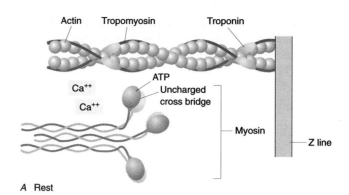

A   Rest

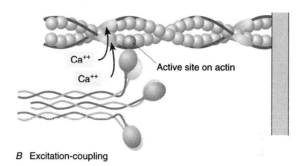

B   Excitation-coupling

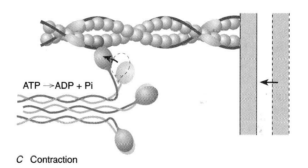

C   Contraction

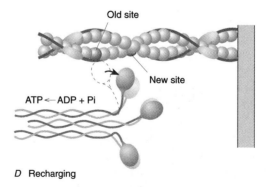

D   Recharging

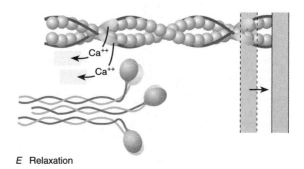

E   Relaxation

the muscle fiber (p. 113). This impulse quickly spreads throughout the fiber by way of the T-tubules. En route, they trigger the release of Ca^{++} from the vesicles of the reticulum. The Ca^{++} is immediately bound (taken up) by the troponin molecules on the actin filaments. This results in what is referred to as the "turning on" of active sites on the actin filament. The turning on is a result of the Ca^{++} ions triggering changes in the conformation (structure) of both troponin and tropomyosin.[18] Simultaneously, but in an unknown manner, the "uncharged" ATP cross-bridge complex is changed into a "charged" ATP cross-bridge complex. The turning on by Ca^{++} of the active sites on the actin filament and the "charging" of the ATP cross-bridge complex mean that the two proteins are mutually attracted to each other. This results in a physical-chemical coupling of actin and myosin (i.e., in the formation of the actomyosin complex). Such a complex, as we will see, is force-generating.

Contraction

The formation of actomyosin activates an enzyme component of the myosin filament called *myosin ATPase.* Myosin ATPase, as you might guess, causes ATP to be broken down into ADP and Pi (inorganic phosphate) with the release of large amounts of energy. This released energy allows the cross-bridge to swivel to a new angle[54] or to collapse[22] in such a way that the actin filament to which it is attached slides over the myosin filament toward the center of the sarcomere. Thus the muscle develops tension and shortens.

Recharging

A single myosin cross-bridge may "make and break" with active sites on the actin filaments hundreds of times in the course of a one-second contraction. To do this, the myosin cross-bridge must be recharged. The first step in recharging is the breaking of the old bond between the actin and the myosin cross-bridge. This is accomplished by reloading the myosin cross-bridge with a new ATP molecule. (The resynthesis of ATP was discussed in chapter 2.) Once a new ATP is reloaded, the bond between the myosin cross-bridge and the active site on the actin filament is broken; the ATP cross-bridge is freed from the actin.* The cross-bridge as well as the active site are thus made available for recycling.

Relaxation

When the flow of nervous impulses over the motor nerve innervating the muscle ceases, Ca^{++} is unbound from troponin and is actively pumped (calcium pump) back into storage in the outer vesicles of the sarcoplasmic reticulum. Removal of Ca^{++} alters the troponin-tropomyosin interaction, "turning off" the actin filament such that ATP cross-bridge complexes are no longer able to form. The ATPase activity of myosin is also turned off, and no more ATP is broken down. The muscle filaments return to their original positions, and the muscle relaxes.

The contraction process described in figure 6.9*C* is for shortening contractions where the Z lines are pulled toward the middle of the sarcomere, called **concentric contraction.** This would be the type of contraction performed by the biceps muscles of the upper arms during the lifting or **positive work** (against gravity) portion of a chin-up. By contrast, during the lowering or **negative work** (assisted by gravity) portion, the actin filaments are viewed as sliding outward from the middle of the sarcomere. That is to say, controlled elongation of muscles back toward their original resting length also is possible. This muscle action is called **eccentric contraction.** In both cases the ATP cross-bridge complexes are made and broken as the actin filaments are either "pulled in" or "let out" depending on need. In **isometric action** or **static contractions,** where there is no visible muscle shortening, the actins remain in their same relative position while ATP cross-bridges are recycled to provide **tension.**

Other questions about the relative positioning of actins and myosins and the formation of cross-bridges should be addressed. Because we know that muscle tone is present in relaxed muscle, does this mean that some cross-bridges have formed and are recycling without producing movements? The likely answer is yes, with perhaps as many as 30% of cross-bridges being attached when muscle is in a state of relaxation.[122] When muscle sarcomeres are stretched out or compressed, does this hinder the number of cross-bridges that can be attached? This also seems true, as only 50% of the cross-bridges are functional when the sarcomere is stretched too far, so as to eliminate overlap of the actins and myosins, or when they are progressively hindered under conditions of osmotic compression.[5] Finally, do the cross-bridges recycle (make and break) at a faster rate and use proportionally more ATP when they are exerting more isometric tension? Once again the answer appears to be yes. When the Huxley model is considered and it is

assumed that one molecule of ATP is hydrolyzed per cycle of the cross-bridge, the rate constant for dissociating (breaking) the cross-bridges is proportional to the ratio of actomyosin ATPase to isometric tension.[67] This means that, when exerting higher levels of static tension, the cross-bridges recycle more quickly.

By way of summary, the contractile events of a muscle can be compared to the firing of a gun.[81] The gun must first be loaded by placing an appropriate cartridge (ATP) in a specific chamber (myosin cross-bridge). This combination (uncharged ATP cross-bridge) is converted to a readied form by cocking the gun (charged ATP cross-bridge). When the trigger is squeezed (calcium turning on actin sites), the ATP is rapidly broken down, releasing large amounts of energy. Work is done on the bullet (myosin cross-bridge). The process is completed by ejection of the spent cartridge (ADP + Pi) and reloading with another cartridge (ATP).

Table 6.2 contains a summary of the sequence of events thought to occur during muscular contraction according to the sliding filament theory.

Function of Skeletal Muscle

The main function of skeletal muscle is contraction, the result of which is movement. In physical education, athletics, and clinical rehabilitation, it is generally the quality of the movement that is important. Therefore, it is appropriate at this time to discuss some of the basic functions of muscle as they relate to movement. For example, how is the strength graded within a given muscle? Do all muscle fibers have the same functional capacities? What is the relationship between the force produced by a muscle and the speed of movement? What factors are involved in muscular fatigue?

The Motor Unit

If we were to count the number of motor nerves entering a muscle and to calculate the number of muscle fibers within the muscle, we would find that a great difference exists between the two. There are about a quarter of a billion separate muscle fibers that make up the skeletal musculature in humans, but there are only about 420,000 motor nerves. Inasmuch as the number of muscle fibers greatly exceeds the number of nerve fibers and keeping in mind the fact that every muscle fiber is innervated, we see that the nerve fibers must branch repeatedly. In other words, a single motor nerve fiber innervates anywhere from 1 to 5 to 150 to 500 or more muscle fibers. All the muscle fibers served by the same motor nerve contract and relax at the same time, working as a unit. For this reason, the single motor nerve (motorneuron) and the muscle fibers it innervates are called the **motor unit** (figure 6.10). Therefore, the motor unit *is* the basic functional unit of skeletal muscle.

The ratio of muscle fibers innervated by a single motor nerve is not determined by the size of the muscle, but

---

*If ATP is not available, as in the case after death, the cross-bridges remain attached to the actin, and the muscle is said to be in *rigor.* This is thought to be the maximal force-producing state.

6.2

Summary of events occurring during muscular contraction according to the sliding filament theory

1. Rest	(a) Uncharged ATP cross-bridges extended
	(b) Actin and myosin uncoupled
	(c) Ca^{++} stored in sarcoplasmic reticulum
2. Excitation-coupling	(a) Nerve impulse generated
	(b) Ca^{++} released from vesicles
	(c) Ca^{++} saturates troponin, turning on actin
	(d) ATP cross-bridge "charged"
	(e) Actin and myosin coupled $\rightarrow$ actomyosin
3. Contraction	(a) ATP $\xrightarrow{ATPase}$ ADP + Pi + energy
	(b) Energy swivels cross-bridges
	(c) Muscle shortens $\rightarrow$ actin slides over myosin
	(d) Force developed
4. Recharging	(a) ATP resynthesized
	(b) Actomyosin dissociates $\rightarrow$ actin + myosin
	(c) Actin and myosin recycled
5. Relaxation	(a) Nerve impulse ceases
	(b) Ca^{++} removed by calcium pump
	(c) Muscle returns to resting state

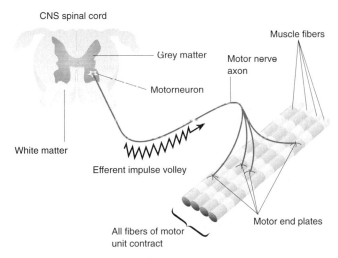

Figure 6.10

Motor unit of skeletal muscle. A single motor nerve from the central nervous system is shown innervating several muscle fibers through the motor endplates (neuromuscular junctions). The F:N ratio is only 4 in this example. All fibers of a motor unit undergo contraction on arrival of an impulse volley (i.e., if the motorneuron fires, all the fibers it innervates contract).

rather by the precision, accuracy, and coordination of its movement. Muscles that are called on to perform fine and delicate work, such as the eye muscles, may have as few as one muscle fiber in a motor unit; muscles used for rather heavy work, such as the quadriceps, may have hundreds or even thousands of muscle fibers per motor unit. By way of summary, a high **fiber:nerve ratio (F:N ratio)** is associated with gross movements requiring considerable force, whereas a low F:N ratio exists where very precise, low force, or fine tension outputs are required of muscles.

A muscle fiber contracts either completely or not at all. In other words, a minimal stimulus that is sufficient to depolarize the motorneuron causes the individual muscle fiber it innervates to contract to the same extent that a stronger stimulus does. This phenomenon is known as the **all-or-none law.** Because a single neuron supplies many muscle fibers in the formation of the motor unit, it naturally follows that the entire motor unit will also function according to the all-or-none law. Although this law of physiology holds true for the individual muscle fibers and motor units, it does not apply to the muscle as a whole. It is possible, therefore, for the muscle to exert forces of graded strengths, ranging from a barely perceptible contraction to the most vigorous type of contraction. This voluntary capability is called muscle strength **gradation.**

The Motor Unit and Strength Gradations

The capability of strength gradation is important to everyday activities as well as to sport performance. Essentially, without the capability to vary the strength of muscular contractions, smooth, coordinated movement patterns would be virtually impossible. Can you imagine, for example, the outcome of brushing your teeth with the same muscular force used to lift a 50-kilogram weight?

How is the strength of a muscle graded? There are basically two ways this is accomplished: (1) by varying the number of motor units contracting at any given time, referred to as **multiple motor unit summation** or recruitment; and (2) by varying the frequency of contraction of individual motor units, referred to as **wave summation.** It is conceptually important here to envision that both of these processes can be evoked at the same time, allowing for gradations in force production that range from very weak efforts to maximal, all-out efforts.

Multiple Motor Unit Summation

As mentioned previously, a motor unit adheres to the all-or-none law (i.e., given an adequate stimulus, it contracts maximally). It follows that the strength of a muscle can be graded depending on whether one motor unit is contracting or several units are contracting simultaneously.

Actually, in determining the final tension or strength developed by a muscle, both the number of motor units contracting at any one time and the size or number of muscle fibers within each unit (i.e., the F:N ratio) are important. In most muscles, the number of fibers within a motor unit varies. For example, a muscle may have a total of 25 motor units, with one motor unit having as few as 25 or as many as 500 fibers, and the average having 200 fibers. Assuming that each fiber can produce a tension of 5 grams, the smallest tension that can be produced by a *single motor unit* is 1 motor unit $\times$ 25 fibers $\times$ 5 g = 125 g ($\frac{1}{8}$ of a kg). By the same token, the largest tension that can be produced by the contraction of a single motor unit is 1 motor unit $\times$ 500 fibers $\times$ 5 g = 2500 g (2.5 kg). Therefore, depending only on the size of the motor unit and not the number, the strength of the muscle can be graded anywhere between .125 ($\frac{1}{8}$) and 2.5 kg. The maximal tension of the entire muscle is developed when *all* its motor units contract, which in this case would result in a tension of 25 motor units $\times$ 200 fibers $\times$ 5 g = 25,000 g (25 kg). Thus, the full range of strength gradations of the muscle would be between $\frac{1}{8}$ and 25 kg.

The relationship between the tension or strength of a muscle and the number of motor units contracting is shown in figure 6.11.

Wave Summation

A motor unit responds to a single stimulus (nerve impulse) by giving a **twitch,** a brief period of contraction followed by relaxation. A recording of such a twitch is shown in figure 6.12. When a second stimulus is applied to the motor unit before it completely relaxes from the previous twitch, the two twitches are said to *summate* so that the tension developed by the motor unit is now greater than that produced by a single twitch alone. If the stimuli are repeated regularly at a high enough frequency, summation continues until the individual twitches are completely fused. Under these con-

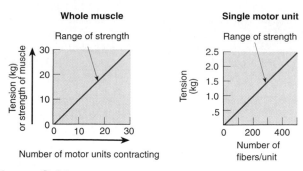

Figure 6.11

Multiple motor unit summation. The tension or strength of a muscle can be graded depending on both the size and the number of motor units contracting at any one time.

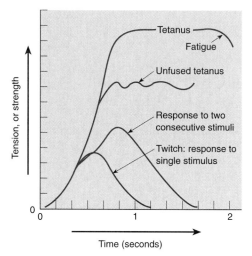

Figure 6.12

Wave summation. A motor unit responds to a single stimulus (nerve impulse) by giving a twitch (i.e., a brief period of contraction followed by relaxation). When a second stimulus is applied to the motor unit before it completely relaxes from the previous twitch, the two twitches summate so that the tension developed is greater than that produced by a single twitch alone. If the stimuli are repeated, summation continues until the individual twitches are completely fused (tetanus). Eventually fatigue occurs and tension is reduced.

ditions, the motor unit is said to be in **tetanus,** with tension maintained at a high level as long as the stimuli continue or until fatigue sets in (figure 6.12). The tension developed during tetanus as a result of wave summation can be three to four times greater than that for a single twitch.

Asynchronous Summation of Motor Units—Smooth Contractions

During a maximal contraction, all the motor units, and thus all the fibers within a muscle, contract and summate more or less synchronously. However, during submaximal contractions, motor units contract and summate asynchronously—in other words, some are contracting (twitching) while others are relaxing. As each motor unit comes into play, it fuses with the twitches of the other already contracting units, thus producing a continued contraction of any given strength that is smooth and nonjerky.

The degree of synchronization of motor units during various levels of muscular efforts is now being studied in humans in relation to weight-resistance training.[77] Although this type of training appears to increase the synchronization of motor units, the significance of this change with respect to performance is not yet clearly understood. There also are indications that motor unit firing rate, recruitment, and degree of synchronization decrease during sustained submaximal isometric contraction to fatigue.[73] Interestingly, this decrease in discharge rate of motor units during fatigue occurs even though the excitatory drive to the motorneuron pool is increased.[37] This phenomenon is not fully understood and has been referred to by Marsden as "muscle wisdom," a possible protective mechanism that occurs during fatigue.

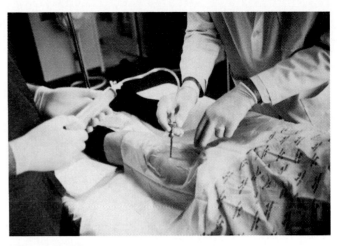

Figure 6.13

Muscle tissue needle biopsy procedure performed under local anesthesia.

(Photo courtesy of Henry Ford Health System.)

Different Kinds of Motor Units—Type I (Slow-Twitch) and Type II (Fast-Twitch) Fibers

All skeletal muscle motor units function in the same general manner as described previously. However, not all motor units contain muscle fibers that have the same metabolic or functional capabilities. For example, whereas all motor units, and thus all muscle fibers, can perform under both aerobic and anaerobic conditions, some are better equipped biochemically and structurally to work aerobically, while others are better equipped to work anaerobically. In humans the aerobic-type fibers have at different times been called Type I, red, tonic, slow-twitch (ST), or slow-oxidative (SO); the anaerobic-type fibers have been called Type II, white, phasic, fast-twitch (FT), or fast-glycolytic (FG).[24,25,41,79] A further subdivision of the Type II fibers into IIA (FT$_A$, fast-oxidative-glycolytic, FOG), IIB (FT$_B$, fast-glycolytic, FG), and IIC (FT$_C$, undifferentiated, unclassified, intermediate, interconversion) can also be made.[12,61,100]

For now, we will use the fiber-type designations that are being used in the research literature for the four main fiber types—namely, **Types I, IIA, IIB, and IIC.** But let's keep in mind the usefulness of the corresponding designation system that indicates the relative speed of contraction and the predominant sources of energy production associated with each phenotype. That is to say, SO (slow-oxidative) for Type I, FOG (fast-oxidative-glycolytic) for Type IIA, FG (fast-glycolytic) for Type IIB, and unClassified for the IIC phenotype. There is considerable recent research interest in the functional significance of this subdivision that allows for a metabolic continuum to exist within muscles. This continuum ranges from fibers that are mainly oxidative, through combined oxidative-glycolytic ones, and on to those that are principally glycolytic. It also acknowledges the existence of some fibers that cannot be classified and

about which we need to know more in terms of their functional role in exercise responses and training adaptations.

A major recent advance in the field of muscle fiber types has been the discovery of **myogenic factors** that regulate the properties specific to the fiber—i.e., **phenotypic properties.**[52] The fibers have different forms of myofibrillar and other proteins called **isoforms,** and consequently they have different speeds and power production during contraction. Chief among these are their differences in **myosin heavy chains,** which modify the two main regulatory steps in the cross-bridge formation cycle. The first step controls the rate of force development, while the second controls the maximal velocity of shortening. As expected, calcium (Ca^{++}) is involved in all of this since it initiates force development in muscle by increasing the rate of attachment of cross-bridges. Type I have a lower threshold for Ca^{++}-activated force (cross-bridges form more easily) but a lesser force response to Ca^{++}. On the other hand, Type II fibers have a higher threshold for Ca^{++} (cross-bridges not so readily formed) and a steeper force to Ca^{++} response. These differences are largely attributable to Type II fibers having troponin with a higher Ca^{++} binding capacity and a faster process of cross-bridge attachment. Since all of these intracellular structures are proteins, it has been concluded that muscle fiber types reflect a complex interaction of multiple sources of control of **protein expression,** and the net effect of this control ultimately defines the fiber's functional properties.[104]

Method of Classifying Fiber Types

The classification of fiber types is done by histochemical analysis of a sample of muscle tissue obtained by a needle biopsy procedure. This procedure, which is relatively painless, involves the insertion of a pencil-size needle through a 1.0 cm incision in the skin and fascia (see figure 6.13). The

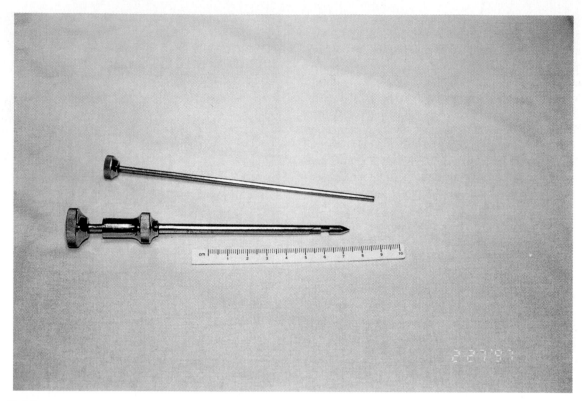

Figure 6.14

Bioptome instrument used to obtain muscle tissue biopsy samples for analysis.

incision is made under topical anesthesia. The needle (or bioptome, figure 6.14) is pushed into the muscle and a small window-like opening is filled with tissue. An internal cutting blade snips off the tissue, which usually weighs only 20 to 40 mg. The biopsy sample is then either mounted in an embedding medium and frozen using solutions of isopentane and liquid nitrogen or simply quickly frozen using liquid nitrogen. The analysis involves chemically staining the tissue for the presence of various oxidative and glycolytic enzymes as well as an enzymatic indicator of muscle fiber contraction speed. This latter enzyme is myofibrillar adenosine triphosphatase or **myosin ATPase (m-ATPase).** These tissue preparations and analyses are performed in well-equipped clinical and research laboratories.

When the stained muscle sample is viewed in cross section with a light microscope, it looks like the one shown in figure 6.15. All muscle fibers within any given motor unit are of the same type. For example, Type I motor units contain only Type I fibers, and Type II units only Type II fibers. Also, as indicated in figure 6.15, the fibers of Type I and Type II motor units are mixed together in the muscle, giving it a checkerboard appearance.

Carefully examine the slide shown in figure 6.15, which was prepared from the vastus lateralis muscle (outer thigh region) of a human subject. The vastus lateralis and the gastrocnemius (calf muscle) are commonly used in stud-

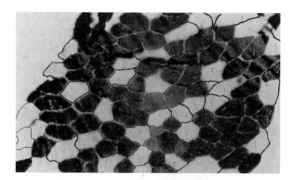

Figure 6.15

When a stained muscle sample is viewed in cross section, it has a checkerboard appearance, because the fibers of Type I and Type II motor units are mixed together in the muscle. In this human muscle sample from the vastus lateralis, the darkly stained fibers are Type I and those lightly stained are Type II. (Note: fine lines showing boundaries were added.)

ies of human muscle fiber typing. The slide has been touched up by an artist to allow you to more easily distinguish the individual cell boundaries. What would you estimate the ratio of dark stained Type I to lightly stained Type II fiber areas to be? Perhaps 2:1 or about 66% Type I and 33% Type II? Check this by assuming for the moment that all the

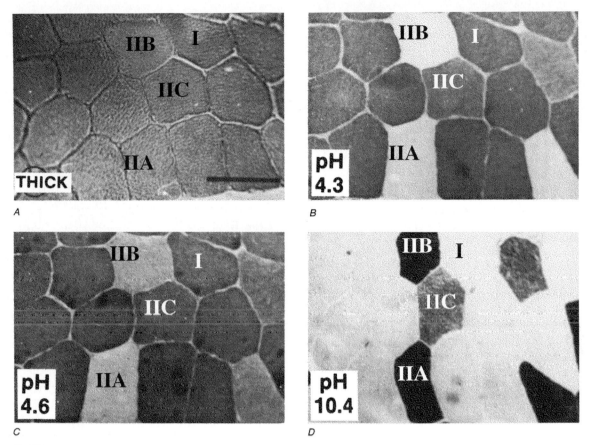

Figure 6.16

Serial cross sections of human vastus lateralis muscle fibers. Part *A* shows thick sections (40–50 μm) where all fibers appear to be the same. Other photos show the same muscle fibers stained for m-ATPase activity after different preincubation pH treatments; *B.* high acid of pH 4.3; *C.* intermediate acid of pH 4.6; and *D.* basic solution of pH 10.4. Type I, IIA, IIB, and IIC fibers are identified. Bar in *A* = 100 μm.

(Modified from Staron, et al.[100])

fibers are the same general shape and have the same diameters. Count the approximate number of each fiber type. Do you get about 90 Type I and 45 Type II, a 2:1 ratio? Although an exercise scientist would project the slides to enlarge the fibers and then take great pains to measure their actual circumferences and calculate the areas occupied by the two major fiber types, you have done much the same thing. You have just "fiber typed" this muscle sample. It is primarily comprised of Type I fibers; probably from the leg of an endurance athlete or a person who might have a good chance of success in endurance events. Why might we conclude this?

As mentioned previously, Type II fibers can be further subdivided.[11] To do this, slides of serial cross sections from the same muscle biopsy are preincubated in solutions that differ in their alkalinity (high pH, such as 10.4) or acidity (medium pH, such as 4.6; or lower pH, such as 4.3). You should recall here the inverse relationship between pH and hydrogen ion concentrations in that a lower pH indicates a more acid solution and vice versa (i.e., a pH of 4.3 is more

acid than a pH of 4.6). The serial slides, which can be thought of as slices of a loaf of bread, are then stained for myosin ATPase, an enzyme that identifies their contractile speed. In this case dark staining indicates stability of the m-ATPase within the muscle fiber. Likewise, intermediate staining indicates the presence of some stable enzyme, whereas light staining indicates nearly complete breakdown or lability of the enzyme as a result of the specific preincubation treatment.

Figure 6.16 shows such a series of slides for human vastus lateralis muscle. Slide *A* indicates four selected muscle fibers marked Type I, IIA, IIB, and IIC. These fibers all look similar when cut in thick sections (40–50 μm), prepared with fixatives, and viewed under a light microscope. The bar indicates a length of 100 μm (100 micrometers or $\frac{1}{10}$ of a millimeter). To gain a better "feel" for the actual diameters of the fibers, mark off one millimeter on a piece of paper and attempt to draw ten distinct and separate pencil lines (simulating individual muscle fiber widths) within the boundaries. Use a very sharp pencil. Small, aren't they?

The second, *B,* third, *C,* and fourth, *D,* slides in figure 6.16 were cut much thinner (only 10 μm) and were assayed for m-ATPase activity after three different preincubation pH treatments (4.3, 4.6, and 10.4, respectively) as shown. The Type I fiber stained dark after both high and intermediate acid treatments (pH 4.3 and 4.6) but stained light after the basic treatment (pH 10.4). The m-ATPase of the Type I fiber was acid stabile but basic labile. Conversely, the Type IIA fiber stained light after the acid treatments (pH 4.3 and 4.6) but dark after basic treatment (pH 10.4). The m-ATPase of the Type IIA fiber was basic stabile and acid labile.

Next, the Type IIB fiber stained light after the high acid treatment (pH 4.3), intermediate after the intermediate acid treatment (pH 4.6), and dark after basic treatment (pH 10.4). The Type IIB fiber is acid labile and basic stabile, just like the Type IIA fiber, but displays a major difference in that its m-ATPase also shows some stability after exposure to intermediate acid (pH 4.6). Perhaps it is easiest to recall that the IIB fiber shows intermediate stain intensity after intermediate acid treatment. These relationships are summarized in figure 6.17.

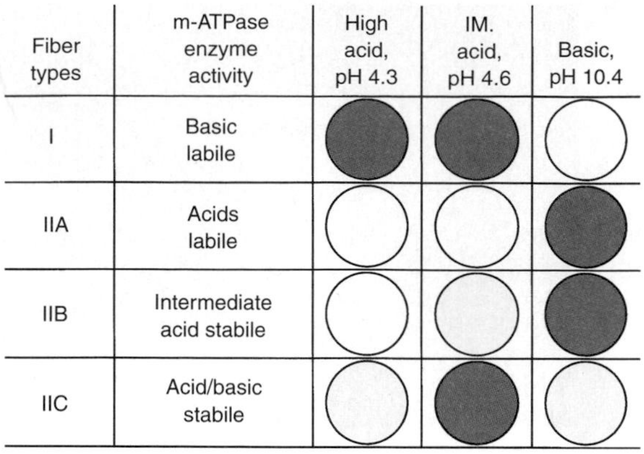

Finally, note the uniqueness of the IIC fiber in that it stained quite dark over the entire range of pH treatments. It appears that the m-ATPase of the IIC fibers possess some of the stability characteristics common to the m-ATPase found in all the other fiber types. This is what has led scientists to regard the IIC fiber as an undifferentiated, less specialized fiber. Before becoming too concerned about these fibers we should keep in mind that IIC fibers usually make up only 0 to 2% and no more than 5% of the total fiber population in human muscle.[100] For that reason, they are more of academic than practical interest to us here.

Distribution of Type I and Type II Fibers

Studies of fiber distribution in postmortem samples of muscles from infants and young children through age 8 have been reported and summarized.[114] The predominant fiber type in limb and trunk muscles of the early fetus is the primitive, undifferentiated, IIC fiber. Fiber differentiation then occurs so that the histochemically identifiable I, IIA, and IIB fibers are eventually all present. The maturation rates for the various fiber types, however, are different. For example, Type I fibers first appear after the nineteenth week of gestation, but the great majority of fibers during the twentieth through the twenty-sixth weeks are Type IIA and IIB. That is to say, the Type I fibers lag behind in their development before birth. By 36 weeks there are numerous IIA and IIB fibers and only a few of the original undifferentiated IIC fibers. You might say that all of the maturational differentiation that occurs in the womb occurs at the expense of the IIC fibers.

After birth, there is wide variation in the number of Type I and II fibers, a pattern that persists through the first

Fiber types	m-ATPase enzyme activity	High acid, pH 4.3	IM. acid, pH 4.6	Basic, pH 10.4
I	Basic labile	●	●	○
IIA	Acids labile	○	○	●
IIB	Intermediate acid stabile	○	◐	●
IIC	Acid/basic stabile	○	●	○

Figure 6.17

m-ATPase staining patterns reflecting labile/stabile characteristics for different fiber types after preincubation in high acid (pH 4.3), intermediate acid (pH 4.6), and basic (pH 10.4) solutions. Note "reverse staining" pattern for Type I vs. Type IIA fibers, intermediate staining for Type IIB fibers in intermediate acid, and a wide range of pH stability for Type IIC fibers.

year of life. Generally speaking, after the first year of life, more than 50% of the fibers are of Type I. Thereafter the greatest changes are not in the distribution of fibers but in their size. Unlike adults, who display wide variation in fiber size for a given muscle, fiber diameters do not vary much in children. The quadriceps muscle of the anterior thigh is an exception with these fibers being consistently larger than those of other muscles after the age of 2 years. This difference is presumably due to the heavy loads placed on these muscles for locomotion and getting up and down from the floor. In normal children, Type I fibers tend to be of similar size or larger than Type II fibers, and there is concern for muscle disease if they are smaller. As expected, fiber size correlates well with age; older children having larger muscle fiber diameters. There is no difference in muscle fiber size between boys and girls through age 8, and any gender differences may not become apparent until puberty. Adult fiber size is usually attained by the age of 12 to 15 years.

In summary, differentiation of IIC fibers into Type I, IIA, and IIB fibers is a process that begins in the womb as neurological and muscular systems mature and as limb, diaphragm, and trunk muscles begin to function. After birth, there is a great increase in Type I fibers so important to maintaining spinal posture, locomotion, and improved endurance. Once the fiber types are established in approximately equal percentages within muscles—about 50% Type I and 50% Type II—the major changes will be in fiber diameter, with adult fiber size attained in the early teen years. These developmental, maturation, and age-related concepts must be remembered when fiber typing is considered as a "screening" tool to identify potentially outstanding young athletes as discussed later.

The proportions of the different types of fibers in adult human muscles vary to a great extent. However, generally the majority of our muscles contain an approximately equal mixture of Type I and II fibers, although there are specific muscles that are considered to be predominantly either Type I or II. For example, the soleus contains 25% to 40% more Type I fibers than the other leg muscles, and the triceps contain 10% to 30% more Type II fibers than the other arm muscles.[63] The arrangement of muscle fibers within the fascicle bundles is very consistent with a high proportion of Type IIB fibers on the border near the perimysium.[85] Mostly Type I fibers make up the layer just below, with Type IIA fibers rather uniformly distributed throughout all layers of the fasciculus.

A study of the various fibers in muscle samples from four young men who had died suddenly indicates similar variability in distribution averages.[26] The soleus (24% Type I) and vastus lateralis (57% Type II) muscles of the leg were quite different in their compositions, whereas the biceps brachii (55% Type II) and the lateral and long heads of the triceps brachii (60% Type II) of the arm were quite similar. A difference in fiber type distribution within the same arm muscle was evident because the medial head of the triceps brachii contained only 40% Type II fibers.

In another study, comparisons of shoulder deltoideus to leg vastus lateralis and gastrocnemius muscles of elite orienteers showed that they contained approximately the same percentage of Type I fibers, about 68%.[61] This is of interest because the legs receive a much greater training stimulus than the shoulder muscles in this gruelling sport, which involves running over a wide variety of outdoor terrain. Marked differences existed, however, for Type IIA and IIB distributions in leg versus shoulder muscles. Leg muscles contained unequal distributions of about 26% Type IIA and 3% Type IIB fibers, whereas shoulder muscles contained more equal distributions of 14% Type IIA and 17% Type IIB. Type IIC percentages were small in all muscles, ranging from 0% to 4%.

Taken collectively, these findings indicate that the composition of fiber types varies within different regions of the same muscle, between different muscles within the same person, and certainly within the same muscles of different people. Considerable variability also exists among Type II fiber subgroups (A, B, and C) for muscles in different regions of the body. It is important to have an awareness of these variations in fiber distributions as we consider such distributions in athletes and their potential impact on performance.

The distribution of Type I and II fibers in muscles of different groups of male and female athletes is shown in figure 6.18. Although there is some degree of individual variation, on the average, endurance athletes tend to have greater percentages of Type I fibers, whereas nonendurance athletes have greater percentages of Type II fibers than their nonathletic counterparts. Although not shown in this figure, there also is evidence that the "trained" muscles of endurance athletes have higher percentages of Type I fibers than muscles that they use less.[105]

In addition, the relationship between the maximal aerobic power (max $\dot{V}O_2$) of male athletes and male nonathletes and their percentage of distribution of Type I fibers is given in figure 6.19. Notice that the max $\dot{V}O_2$ is higher with higher percentages of Type I fibers in both groups. This makes sense, because Type I fibers have a greater potential for aerobic metabolism than do Type II fibers. Notice also that for a given percentage of Type I fibers above 40%, the max $\dot{V}O_2$ is higher in athletes. We will discuss this further later.

Two major questions have been raised concerning the distribution of fiber types among athletes and the relationship between the percentage of Type I fibers and the max $\dot{V}O_2$: (1) does training cause a change in the percentage of distribution of Type I and II fibers, and (2) is the increase in max $\dot{V}O_2$ that can be induced by training genetically limited by the percentage of Type I fibers one is born with? The answer to the first question is no.[43] The majority of evidence still suggests that the only way to effectively change a Type I fiber to a Type II fiber, or vice versa, is to **cross-innervate** the two fibers.[80] Cross-innervation means that the nerve originally innervating one fiber is transplanted to innervate the other, and vice versa. The result is that each fiber then takes on the original characteristics of the other. In other words, the motor nerve to a muscle has been shown to have an influential effect (called a *trophic effect*) on the eventual functional capabilities of that muscle fiber.

More recent studies indicate that the motorneuron can exert only a limited control over fiber properties at the motor unit level.[47,104] Other factors such as muscle architecture, mechanical loading, and intrinsic factors preset during development also influence the muscle plasticity adaptations that take place. Still other suggested influences over plasticity changes include the "acute" effects of exercise induced fatigue, changes in muscle temperature,[94] and cytoplasmic signals from metabolic systems working to regulate energy balance.[71] As we will discuss later, training causes an increase in the size and functional capacities of the respective fiber types but apparently does not cause conversion from one type to another. It is clear from the above review that the search continues for the factor or factors that drive these known adaptations.

In answering the second question, both the distribution of fiber types and the magnitude of the max $\dot{V}O_2$ are genetically determined to a very large extent. However, as shown in figure 6.19, the max $\dot{V}O_2$ is higher for athletes than for nonathletes at any given percentage of Type I fibers above 40%. This could be interpreted to mean that training also has a significant influence on the magnitude of the max $\dot{V}O_2$ over and above that pre-set by the percentage of Type I fibers. Therefore, a direct answer to the second question is no, the genetic limit set on the percentage of distribution of Type I fibers does not entirely limit the magnitude of the max $\dot{V}O_2$ resulting from training.

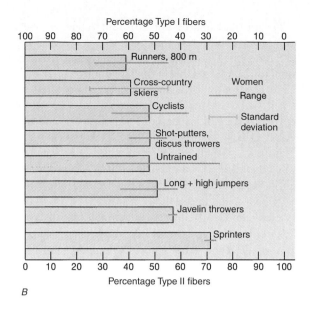

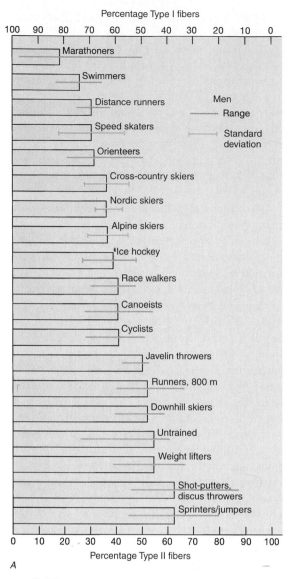

Figure 6.18

The distribution of Type II and Type I fibers in muscles of different groups of *A.* male and *B.* female athletes. Although there is some degree of variation, on the average, endurance athletes tend to have greater percentages of Type I fibers, whereas nonendurance athletes have greater percentages of Type II fibers than their nonathletic counterparts.

(Based on data from Burke et al.,[12] Costill et al.,[19] Gollnick et al.,[41] Komi et al.,[68] and Thorstensson et al.[111])

Functional Differences between Type I and Type II Fibers

As indicated earlier, Type I fibers have a relatively large aerobic capacity and a relatively small anaerobic capacity compared with Type II fibers. This is true even when the higher oxidative capabilities of the IIA fibers are considered; in other words, an oxidative hierarchy exists with Type I > Type IIA > Type IIB.[100] In fact, in humans, none of the Type II subgroups has as high an oxidative capacity as the Type I fibers.[27] Muscles comprised mainly of Type I fibers also display different metabolic responses to graded rhythmic exercise than those comprised of a mixture of Type I and Type II or primarily Type II fibers.[78] The main differences are that muscles having mostly Type I fibers display a faster Pi and a faster PC recovery. These differences and other structural, biochemical, and functional relationships are summarized in table 6.3.

A remarkable aspect of the research underlying this summary is how well the structural and functional findings have consistently supported one another. This gives credence to the adage "anatomical structure supports function." Note first the sharp contrasts between characteristics for the Type I versus combined Type IIA and IIB fibers. For the most part, they are opposites. A few exceptions are mitochondrial density, capillary density, myoglobin content, and

6.3

Structural and functional characteristics of Type I and Type II (IIA and IIB) muscle fibers

Characteristics	Fiber Type		
	I	IIA	IIB
Neural Aspects			
Motorneuron size	Small	Large	Large
Motorneuron recruitment threshold	Low	High	High
Motor nerve conduction velocity	Slow	Fast	Fast
Structural Aspects			
Muscle fiber diameter	Small	Large	Large
Sarcoplasmic reticulum development	Less	More	More
Mitochondrial density	High	High	Low
Capillary density	High	Medium	Low
Myoglobin content	High	Medium	Low
Energy Substrates			
Phosphocreatine stores	Low	High	High
Glycogen stores	Low	High	High
Triglyceride stores	High	Medium	Low
Enzymatic Aspects			
Myosin-ATPase activity	Low	High	High
Glycolytic enzyme activity	Low	High	High
Oxidative enzyme activity	High	High	Low
Functional Aspects			
Twitch (contraction time)	Slow	Fast	Fast
Relaxation time	Slow	Fast	Fast
Force production	Low	High	High
Energy efficiency, "economy"	High	Low	Low
Fatigue resistance	High	Low	Low
Elasticity	Low	High	High

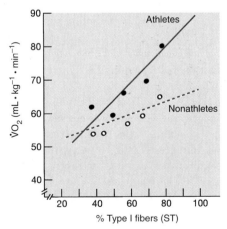

Figure 6.19

Relationship between maximal aerobic power (max $\dot{V}O_2$) of male athletes and male nonathletes and their percentage of distribution of slow-twitch (Type I) muscle fibers. The max $\dot{V}O_2$ is higher with higher percentages of Type I fibers in both groups; for a given percentage of Type I fibers above 40%, the max $\dot{V}O_2$ is higher in athletes.

(Based on data from Bergh et al.[9])

triglyceride stores, where IIA fibers are more similar to Type I fibers. Next, let us review the various characteristics of the fibers, keeping in mind the important known general relationship between structure and function.

The smaller motorneurons have a lower excitation threshold, which means the motor units comprised of Type I fibers will be recruited first. According to Henneman, this concept is referred to as the **size principle** of motor unit recruitment.[117] Type I motor units are used during low-intensity exercise and the Type IIA motor units are recruited for higher intensity or more prolonged exercise. The Type IIB fibers are recruited for all-out force production or as other fibers display fatigue.[116] Motor nerve conduction velocity refers to the speed with which impulses travel down the axons of motor nerves. The slower velocities of Type I fibers are consistent with their use for maintaining posture and slower, less intense movements where speed is not critical. On the other hand, the fast velocities of Type IIA and IIB fibers are consistent with quicker, more forceful muscle contractions where speed and power are critical to performance. For example, the slow positional adjustments made by a basketball rebounder before a free throw will have less influence than an explosive powerful vertical jump in determining whether she or he gets the ball after a missed shot. But both movements are important to a successful outcome so Type I motor units and then Type II motor units are preferentially recruited depending on need. Can you think of other examples?

The muscle fiber diameter characteristics in table 6.3 best describe general differences in fiber size for limb and postural muscles. For example, postural muscles of the back contain many small, Type I fibers, whereas the Type I fibers of limb muscles are larger. In fact, in children and women, Type I fibers in limb muscles may be as large or larger than Type II fibers.[114] In men, the limb Type II fibers are more hypertrophied and usually the same size or larger than the Type I fibers. The generally larger size of the Type II fibers allows them to contain more protein contractile filaments, which can produce higher forces. This larger size is accompanied by the development of a more extensive sarcoplasmic reticulum, the structural network so important to the rapid release of Ca^{++} throughout the length and breadth of the fiber.

Other structural differences such as a higher mitochondrial density (i.e., more mitochondria per unit of cell volume) and higher myoglobin content in Type I versus Type IIB fibers reflects their differences in support of aerobic metabolism. Type I fibers have a distinct advantage over Type IIB fibers when it comes to production of ATP through oxidative processes because the mitochondria, capillaries, and myoglobin are all present in larger quantities. Additionally, the vascular beds of Type I muscles have a higher blood flow at rest. However, they show less of an increase in blood flow during exercise in that they lack the functional vasodilative response more common to Type II muscles. Type IIA fibers also have a high density of mitochondria and a substantial presence of capillaries and myoglobin to support the oxidative aspects of their metabolic function. As muscle fibers increase in size with training, there is a linear increase in the average number of capillaries that surround them.[55] This holds for all three fiber types and represents a most important adaptation.

Perhaps it is not surprising that the energy substrates and enzyme differences (table 6.3) between Type I and Type II fibers closely follow the descriptive scenario that is unfolding. The phosphocreatine stores are high in Type II fibers where the demand for quick, high force outputs are common and are low in Type I fibers where the reverse is true. Likewise, glycogen stores in Type II fibers are higher than in Type I fibers, although limb Type I fibers may still contain considerable amounts of intramuscular glycogen.[30] Generally speaking, the Type II fibers are ready to deliver high force outputs and have the backup reserves to provide additional energy from stored PC or are capable and ready to provide ATP through glycolysis. The concentrations of glycogen, ATP, and PC have been studied in single human muscle fibers from the quadriceps femoris muscles of sub-

jects who received 64 seconds of intermittent electrical stimulation. This treatment produces a short-term maximal muscle contraction. Although both Type I and II fibers were recruited, the breakdown of glycogen (glycogenolysis) occurred in only the Type II fibers.[48]

Conversely, the Type I and IIA fibers have higher quantities of stored triglycerides that they can use to produce ATP under more relaxed oxidative conditions. Not unexpectedly, the presence of oxidative and glycolytic enzymes and their specific activities reflect these differences in substrate availability. Note the reverse patterns for Type I versus combined Type IIA and IIB fibers under the heading of enzymatic aspects (table 6.3). At this point, having high levels of substrate without the needed enzymes to speed reactions along would not make much sense, because they cannot be utilized effectively.

Finally, let us consider the functional aspects of different fiber types in table 6.3. Note that the fast-twitch contraction times match up with high m-ATPase activity levels in Type II fibers and slow times with low levels in Type I fibers. These are the functional and related enzymatic bases upon which Type I (slow) and Type II (fast) fibers were originally named. Type II contraction times to peak tension are about twice as fast as Type I times (0.05 seconds versus 0.10 seconds), and the relaxation times (return to one-half of peak tension) also are proportionally faster. The force output under repetitive electrical stimulation, which would be similar to an impulse volley during voluntary movement, is much greater for Type II fibers because they wave summate and tetanize more quickly.[117]

Type I fibers, however, are more energy efficient, because they produce more force during dynamic contraction for the quantity of energy used. Type I fibers also are more "economical," which means they produce more static or isometric force per unit of energy used.[88] Because of this and the many structural and metabolic support systems described above, the Type I fibers are comparatively resistant to fatigue. Even the known differences in elasticity of the different fiber types fit the picture. Type I fibers have more collagen, which is the building block of connective tissue.[70] This means that Type I fibers are less elastic and "stiffer" than Type II fibers. This does not really hinder the function of the Type I fibers because they are contracting more slowly. Greater elasticity helps the Type II fibers, however, because they can initiate rapid, forceful contractions without undue hindrance. This is referred to as a "higher compliance" of Type II muscle. Once again, an impressive matchup between muscle structure and function exists.

The functional significance of the different biochemical and physiological characteristics of Type I and II fibers during exercise is indicated by the fact that Type II fibers are preferentially recruited for performing short, high-intensity work bouts, such as sprinting. By the same token, Type I fibers are preferentially recruited during long-term endurance types of activity.[42,43] This is shown in figure

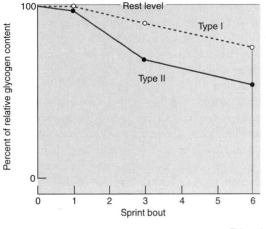

A

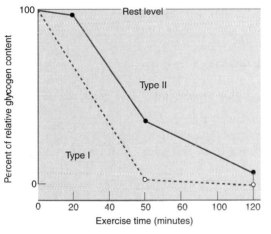

B

Figure 6.20

Glycogen content of Type I and Type II muscle fibers during *A.* sprint exercises and *B.* endurance exercises. The glycogen content decreased sooner and to a greater extent in the Type II fiber during sprint bouts but sooner and to a greater extent in the Type I fiber during endurance exercise. This suggests that the Type II fibers are preferentially recruited for performing short, high-intensity work bouts, whereas the Type I fibers are preferentially recruited during long-term, endurance types of activities.

(Based on data from Bollnick et al.[42,43])

6.20, in which the glycogen content of both fiber types of human muscle was qualitatively estimated during sprint and endurance exercises. The glycogen content decreased sooner and to a greater extent in the Type II fiber during sprint bouts but sooner and to a greater extent in the Type I fiber during endurance exercise, thus suggesting preferential recruitment.

One other factor is noticeable in figure 6.20. The initial glycogen level does not limit sprint-like performance because at exhaustion the glycogen content in both fiber types is still substantial. On the contrary, the glycogen, particularly in the Type I fibers, is completely used up after two hours of exhaustive endurance exercise. In this case, the initial glycogen level limits performance. More will be said about this later.

There has been further research on muscle glycogen depletion as evidence for preferential recruitment of Type I, IIA, and IIB fibers.[116] Subjects worked at 75% of their maximum oxygen uptake ($\dot{V}O_2$ max) on a treadmill or bicycle ergometer until they reached exhaustion. Muscle biopsies were taken from the lateral portion of the quadriceps. Not unexpectedly, the glycogen content of the combined Type IIA and IIB fibers at rest was 16% greater than the Type I fibers. What was surprising was that the Type I and IIA fibers showed the same glycogen depletion rates from the start of exercise, indicating that both fiber types were being recruited. The glycogen content of combined Type IIA and IIB, and IIB alone, was unchanged at first. A later decrease in combined Type IIA and IIB and finally in IIB indicated a difference in "threshold force" for recruiting these fibers.

In summary, the intensity of the exercise was adequate to cause initial recruitment of both Type I and IIA fibers. Although the exercise intensity remained unchanged at 75% of max $\dot{V}O_2$, the effects of the fatigue required the recruitment of Type IIB fibers so that work could be continued. These findings do not invalidate earlier observations that, generally speaking, Type I fibers are recruited during low-intensity exercise and Type II fibers during high-intensity exercise. More importantly, they indicate that Type I fibers are always recruited first and depending on the intensity, duration, or fatigue that occurs, Type IIA and IIB fibers are called into play. For moderate-intensity exercise, Type I and IIA, then IIB are used if activity is continued. For high-intensity exercise, Type I, IIA and IIB are used in more rapid recruitment order. For all-out power performances, all fibers are recruited as quickly and completely as possible. Now let us consider some applications of these and other recent research findings related to muscle fiber types and typing.

Applications of Research

There has been much research interest in recent years in muscle fiber typing, training adaptations within different fiber types, the impact of different types of training programs on fibers, and how fiber typing might be used as a screening tool. Before beginning this review of selected findings, the reader is reminded that the composition of fibers in adult muscles is determined by a process of differentiation and maturation that begins before birth and is not completed until the teenage years.[114] Furthermore, the distribution of fiber types can vary greatly within the same muscle, between different muscles within the same body, and among the same muscles from different people.[26,61]

Also recall that during the process of preferential recruitment the Type I fibers are always recruited regardless of exercise intensity, whereas the Type II fibers are recruited only during prolonged activity leading to fatigue, or for higher intensity exercise and all-out power efforts.[45,116]

Sprinters versus Distance Runners

There has been a long-standing interest in characterizing the fiber-type profiles of athletes who excel in the performance of sprint versus endurance-type events.[34] There has been little inconsistency in these reports, which indicates higher percentages of Type II fibers in sprinters and higher percentages of Type I fibers in endurance athletes. It follows that the muscle enzyme profiles of these athletes is consistently in the direction of greater anaerobic enzymes in the sprinters and greater aerobic enzymes in the endurance performers. For example, individual human muscle fibers from the vastus lateralis muscles of age-matched endurance-trained and strength-trained athletes have been studied. The Type I fibers from the endurance-trained groups showed significant differences in their isoenzyme profiles in that they contained more of the type of lactate dehydrogenase (LDH) found in the heart muscle (H-LDH) of most vertebrates. This is indicative, on an individual fiber basis, of a higher oxidative capacity, suggesting that endurance training causes a favorable metabolic adaptation that allows muscle to cope with increased energy demands during prolonged exercise.[2]

Interest subsequently has been directed toward track-and-field athletes who compete in the middle-distance running events and jumping or throwing events that require explosive power. These latter athletes do not display clear distinctions in their muscle fiber makeup and in fact are represented by a wide range of fiber compositions.[19] These findings suggest that although training dictates the ultimate capacity for endurance, success in either sprint or distance running is in part determined by muscle fiber composition. Because middle-distance runners, jumpers, and throwers have relatively low muscle enzyme activities and highly variable fiber compositions, it is less likely that any clear predictions of performance success can be made on the basis of muscle fiber typing alone. We must therefore look beyond genetic endowment.

Male versus Female Athletes

What about differences in comparative muscle fiber compositions and size of fibers between male and female athletes? Female athletes have larger fibers than control subjects but smaller fibers than male athletes who perform similar events.[19,86] This holds for Type I, IIA, and IIB fibers. By contrast, there are no apparent differences in fiber type distribution or histochemical properties between the sexes.[19,86] Generally speaking, the same high percentages of Type I fibers and associated enzymes and high Type II fibers and associated enzymes are present in endurance run-

ners and sprinters, respectively, regardless of whether they are male or female. Studies of elite female track-and-field athletes confirm these earlier findings regarding fiber composition relative to specific events—comparative smaller size of fibers and difficulty in clearly characterizing middle-distance runners.[49]

An additional finding is that in women, the size of Type I relative to Type II fibers tends to be greater than in men. The fiber size trends, however, with respect to event specialization are identical in women and men: events requiring greater power and less endurance are associated with a greater relative size of Type II fibers. This relationship in relative size exists because the Type II fibers are smaller in athletes specializing in endurance events and the Type I fiber size is similar for the different types of athletes.[49]

In summary, muscle fiber distribution and enzymatic characteristics are quite similar for men and women. Athletes of both sexes have larger fibers than control subjects, male athletes have larger fibers than female athletes, and female athletes tend to have larger Type I to Type II fiber size ratios.

Training and Fiber Number

Questions about what happens to the number of each fiber type with training have been of interest to coaches and trainers of recreational and competitive athletes alike. It now seems clear that any increase in muscle size is due to increases in the size of fibers (**hypertrophy**) rather than to any increase in fiber number due to splitting (**hyperplasia**).[46] That is to say, muscle fiber number is fixed early in life and any increases or decreases in muscle weight occur via hypertrophy or atrophy of existing fibers. Furthermore, it appears that the percentages of each fiber type are determined during the process of pre- and postnatal differentiation and maturation as discussed earlier.

Shifts in Fiber Types

There is limited evidence that some shifts in fiber types can be induced by specific training programs during the growing phase in juvenile research animals.[117] In this study, a static overload was placed on muscles by cutting the tendons of synergists while dynamic exercise was simulated by having animals jump to reach a food reward. The static overload enhanced conversion of Type IIA to IIC fibers whereas the dynamic exercise slowed this conversion process. A study of adult human subjects who cross-country skied 18.5 miles per day with a 25-kg backpack, 6 days per week for 8 weeks produced some similar results.[95] There was a 6% decrease in combined Type IIA and IIB fibers and a 4% increase in IIC fibers in their triceps muscles. Such studies have kept alive the notion that Type IIC fibers may be transitional fibers in the process of conversion of Type II to Type I fibers.[62] Although we must await further insight on this matter, the majority of evidence would indicate that Type I fibers remain as Type I fibers and Type II fibers as Type II fibers regardless of the type of training that is imposed.

One exception is the experimental procedure of muscle-nerve cross-innervation mentioned earlier. A formerly fast-twitch muscle can be made to take on the structural, enzymatic, and metabolic characteristics of a slow-twitch muscle, and vice versa, by cutting their respective nerves and cross attaching them. This procedure has helped us to understand the importance of nerve impulse patterns in determining the structure and function of muscles, the neurotrophic effect. At the same time, it has little potential for application and we are left with the impression that the distribution of Type I and II fibers cannot be altered to any significant degree by training.

Substrate Shifts with Training

Because the distribution of Type I and Type II fibers cannot be significantly altered, researchers have begun to look more closely at substrate differences and metabolic shifts that might occur within fiber types with specific training.[108] These differences and shifts reasonably could provide some advantages to athletes in their various sports. For example, individual fibers teased out of freeze-dried samples of human muscles contain similar amounts of glycogen regardless of fiber type whereas the Type I fibers contain more neutral fat in the form of triglycerides.[27] Other studies of muscle biopsies taken four to six seconds after static and dynamic exercise indicate that lactic acid accounts for most of the intracellular acids that are formed.[50] In these studies, phosphocreatine levels showed a nonlinear negative relationship to the level of lactic acid produced during exercise, and lactate content was generally higher in Type II fibers after contraction. This means that as PC levels were being depleted during prolonged exercise, more Type II fibers were being recruited. ATP was being synthesized through anaerobic metabolic pathways so that activity could be continued, but at the expense of producing increased amounts of intracellular lactic acid.

The importance of this likely rests with the observation that both the lactate threshold (chapter 7) and work load that produce the onset of blood lactate accumulation, called W_{OBLA}, are higher in subjects who have large Type I fiber percentages.[57,58] The advantage of this is that subjects with more Type I fibers can use them to perform low-intensity exercise or the early phases of moderate- to high-intensity exercise before having to recruit Type II fibers as exercise is prolonged, the intensity is increased, or fatigue begins to occur. It is easy to see that having a larger percentage of Type I fibers would provide an advantage for many sports. At the same time one might argue that having more Type II fibers would provide an advantage for throwing, jumping, or other power sports. But we have already discussed that little, if anything, can be done to alter their numbers. This causes us to consider what might be done

through training to alter the size and internal make up of existing fibers to better meet the specific needs of different sports. This is the direction that has the greatest potential for application, so let's consider two specific aspects: metabolic shifts that can occur within muscle fibers as a result of training and the influence that progressive exercise training has on muscle fibers.

Metabolic Shifts with Training

One of the most apparent metabolic shifts that occurs with training is a shift toward a greater oxidative potential and capacity. This shift toward an enhanced oxidative capacity holds true for all fiber types and is accompanied by increases in mitochondrial volume density near the sarcolemma.[53] That such shifts occur in Type I fibers regardless of the type of training relates, once again, to their being recruited on the initiation of all activities independent of intensity. Significant shifts toward oxidative metabolism also occur in Type IIA and IIB fibers. For example, female field hockey athletes have a higher percentage of oxidative (Type I plus IIA) fibers than untrained student controls, 83% versus 46%.[86] Also, the oxidative potential was increased in both Type I and II fibers in older male subjects who had not trained for two years prior to their being studied.[40] They pedaled a cycle ergometer at a work load that required 75% of maximum aerobic capacity for 1 hour per day, 4 days per week, over a 5-month period. A similar study indicates that part of the observed shifts might be due to a gradual conversion of Type IIB to Type IIA fibers, which are more oxidative.[1] These findings, that Type II fibers have the ability to adapt metabolically to high oxidative demands, hold for elite orienteers who have been shown to have higher ratios of Type IIA to IIB fibers.[61] It is of interest and perhaps not unexpected that with the described endurance training, the glycolytic capacity increased in only the Type II fibers.[40] It is apparent from this that a real advantage to training is the shift in oxidative metabolic capacity that occurs within all fibers and some specific improvement in the glycolytic capacity of the Type II fibers.

Impact of Strength Training

The impact of strength training programs on fiber types[119] might help explain some of the highly variable responses that coaches, trainers, and rehabilitation specialists see when they put different people on the "same" program. Compared to distance runners, weight lifters have a significantly lower percentage of Type I fibers, 40% versus 70%, and a higher percentage of Type IIA, 40% versus 23%, and Type IIB fibers, 22% versus 4%.[100] Compared to control subjects, and irrespective of fiber type, weight lifters have more muscle fiber mitochondria but a lower intrafiber lipid content. This, plus the fact that control subjects have nearly twice as many IIB fibers as weight lifters, may indicate the power of inactivity as a fiber type determinant.[100] Inactive people have many glycolytic IIB fibers that can change toward more oxidative IIA fibers if they start a weight training program. Sounds like changes that take place with endurance-training programs, doesn't it?

The above contrasts weight lifters to inactive control subjects but does not answer the question of what happens to inactive subjects when they are put on a weight-training program. It appears that systematic strength training increases the Type I to Type II fiber area ratio, an indication of the specific effect of heavy training loads on Type II muscle fibers.[109] Studies on young women subjects indicate a decrease in Type IIB and an increase in Type IIA fibers following 18 weeks of intensive resistance training.[118] Keep in mind that the area represented by the different fiber types is being considered here and there are inconsistencies in findings. For example, no changes in Type I or Type II fiber areas have been found for either accommodating resistance or weight resistance training programs. This occurred although both training methods effectively increased the strength and muscle mass of the subjects.[84] Perhaps the explanation rests in that training can cause the intracellular components of all fiber types to increase proportionally with an increase in their fiber size.[118] For example, increases in the absolute volume of myofibrils, intermyofibrillar space and mitochondrion could account for large improvements in performance, even though the relative areas occupied by the enlarged fibers remained the same.

As mentioned earlier, inactive control subjects have greater numbers of Type IIB fibers, but they are small in size. This leaves relatively more potential for hypertrophy with strength training (i.e., increase size and area within the Type II fiber pool). This is an important concept in the face of findings that five to six months of heavy resistance training produced a 98% increase in maximum elbow extension strength accompanied by increases in the fiber areas of both Type II (39%) and Type I (31%) fibers.[74]

Once again, it is more difficult for the Type I fibers to compete in the hypertrophy contest if they are larger in the beginning. No correlation has been found between the magnitude of changes in fiber size and increases in maximal strength following heavy weight training.[74] This is consistent with earlier findings that showed only low to moderate correlations between maximum strength measurements and limb girth or estimated cross-sectional area. Dynamic strength increases relative to muscle cross section, however, have been positively correlated to the relative content of Type II fibers.[23] This latter finding supports the concept of specificity of training and indicates further that a high content of Type II fibers in muscles may be a prerequisite for a successful strength-training program. The best outcome likely will be achieved when subjects start with a high percentage of atrophied Type II fibers and are trained with loads greater than 20 repetitions at 50% of their maximum strength (e.g., 6 repetitions at 80% of maximum). The fact that subjects vary so greatly from these ideal starting conditions provides a most plausible explanation for the wide variability in strength gains and hypertrophic change with standard weight-training programs.

Limited data on bodybuilders indicates that they may differ from weight trainers in terms of functional strength.[96] Bodybuilders also display a greater overall fiber size than elite Olympic weight lifters or power lifters. But the ratio of Type II to Type I area has been shown to be greater in the competitive weight lifters. The differences appear to be the result of different types of resistance training that is practiced over a long period of time.[107]

As expected, body builders have larger muscles than male and female physical education students. Yet their maximal strength expressed per unit of cross-sectional area is no greater. These findings are based on measures of maximal isokinetic torque of knee extensor and elbow flexor and extensor muscles made at angular velocities of 30, 90, and 180 degrees per second. Some of the body builders had been using anabolic steroids, and they willingly submitted to needle biopsy measures of their thigh muscles, but not to biopsy measures of their arm triceps muscles. It is apparent that more research is needed to sort out true differences in the structure and function of muscles of body builders and weight trainers.

Fiber Types and Injuries

There is some evidence that muscles composed of Type I fibers are more susceptible to exercise injuries than are muscles composed of Type II fibers.[91] These data are from rats and mice that were exposed to a single bout of exercise by running them on a motor-driven treadmill for several hours. The differences in injury levels between the major muscle types is likely due to the process of selective recruitment discussed earlier. Increasing the duration of running increased the level of exercise injuries, whereas endurance training prior to the administration of the strenuous exertion reduced the exercise injuries. In summary, it appears that Type I fibers are injured more easily during the performance of low-intensity, long-duration exercise. Less is known about the fiber types that might be injured during high-intensity or all-out efforts.

The Aging Process

Type II fibers display the greatest fiber atrophy during the aging process with concomitant losses in oxidative capacity.[87] This may be the result of a selective degeneration of the largest and fastest conducting motorneurons, which innervate the high-threshold Type II fibers as described by Rexed in 1944. These changes may ultimately be a reflection of progressive disuse as people purposely and unknowingly participate in less vigorous activities as they age.[72] There has been some study of the effects of strength-training programs in reversing the progressive atrophy of the Type II fibers. Eighteen sedentary males ranging in age from 22 to 65 years participated in a 60- to 80-minute, low-resistance, high-repetition, circuit training program, twice a week for 15 weeks. Older subjects showed increases in fiber size for both Type I and Type II fibers but no significant improvements in isokinetic strength measures of their knee extensor muscles. This supports the contention that muscle fiber atrophy is not the primary explanation for strength declines with age.[72]

Screening Athletes by Fiber Typing

A final research application that has been discussed much more than it has ever been practiced in the United States is the use of fiber typing as a screening and guidance measurement for young athletes. The idea would be to take muscle biopsy samples from children who show potential for elite sports performance and then, based on their having predominantly Type I or Type II fibers, guide them into sports where they have the best chance of excelling. Let us examine some reasons why this idea has intuitive merit but, at the same time, has never caught on in the United States.

We should first recall that the number of Type I and Type II fibers are not fixed until some period during the teen years. This presents a problem because of individual variations in maturation rates so that there would be no assurance that the ratios of Type I and Type II fibers would truly reflect the numbers finally attained. This will remain a problem until adequate normative data are available to allow accurate prediction of final distributions from measurements made earlier in the young athlete's life. Second, the technical and logistical aspects of any meaningful broad screening approach must be considered. Although muscle biopsy procedures are considered to be relatively safe in the hands of well-trained clinicians, there is some associated risk of soreness, swelling, hematoma, and infection. Consequently, the procedures would need to clear human subjects research review committees and signed consent would have to be obtained from the parents of minors. A combination of these factors would inhibit the implementation of any widespread screening and guidance program.

Even if screening and guidance programs could be conducted, there are many problems of interpretation that would need to be addressed. A major concern here would be the damaging effect that a misinterpretation caused by measurement error could have in stifling the interest or motivation of an otherwise promising young athlete when they are told that they lack the "right stuff." Advocates of such programs would need to keep in mind the variability in fiber composition that exists in different regions of muscles and between different muscles of the same body. Although some studies indicate that genetics may be operating in the process of selection and attraction of elite endurance athletes,[61] we should be mindful of a limited ability to predict running performance times on the basis of fiber composition.[32] In the former study, adult male elite orienteers had the same percentage of Type I fibers in their lesser trained upper body muscles as they did in their more highly trained leg muscles. This suggests that training had not caused the high per-

centage of Type I fibers (about 68%), but that individuals were "selected" with the best prerequisites for high oxidative capacity. The latter study reports only modest correlation coefficients of $r = -0.52$, -0.54, and -0.55 between Type I percentages and performance times for running 1, 2, and 6 miles, respectively. Much stronger relationships existed between max $\dot{V}O_2$ measures and run times: $r = -0.84$, -0.87, and -0.88, and it was concluded that max $\dot{V}O_2$, not fiber composition, is the primary determinant of cross-sectional differences in running performance. Keep in mind that these studies are for adult athletes. In younger athletes, the added variability due to differences in levels of growth, development, and maturation would make future performance prediction even more complex and difficult.

The finding that distance running performance relates better to max $\dot{V}O_2$ than to muscle fiber composition points to a final major argument against the use of fiber typing for success prediction and guidance in competitive athletics. The point being that the magnitude of a max $\dot{V}O_2$ measurement reflects a number of physiological functional adaptations rather than a single morphological measurement. In fact, the magnitude even represents the level of motivation of the subjects and their ability to endure exertional stress and pain related to fatigue. These individual characteristics, which are difficult, if not impossible, to quantitate, are the factors that often separate gold medal winners from other competitors who are of the same caliber. This, coupled with the fact that a considerable range of fiber composition percentages exist for any athletic group (see figure 6.18) makes us wary of preselection and guidance solely on fiber typing. There are too many other factors operating that can influence performance.

Does this mean that efforts to screen and guide young athletes into activities where they have the best chance for success should be discontinued? The answer is no, and it is clear that youth sports coaches do this each time they line up aspiring young athletes to determine who can best run sprints or longer distances. Likewise, as they note the developing somatotypes, heights, and weights of their young charges and make "eyeball measurements" of the children's parents, they are formulating screening and guidance strategies. In this regard, coaches might do well to explore more fully the existing genetic basis for performance by interviewing both the parents and grandparents about sports activities in which they innately excelled.

The advantage of field tests such as time trials for running, distance trials for jumping and throwing, and trials for regional body strength are obvious. First, they circumvent many of the administrative and logistical problems described above for clinical and laboratory tests. More importantly, they have a high level of face validity; they test aspects of performance that clearly can be related to the sports event itself. This is easily understood by the athletes and parents. Furthermore, test results reflect performance of the young athletes as a functioning organism at a particular point in time. This includes their levels of motivation, maturation, growth and development, and numerous other compensating factors that are integrated into a final performance score. Field tests are relatively easy to administer so that frequent retests can be conducted. All of this reduces the false-negative risk of screening future champions out of a sport on the basis of their lacking a single genetic predictor of success such as a favorable muscle fiber composition.

Future applications of such clinical and laboratory tests may not reside with the screening and guidance of youthful athletes but with the better understanding of differences in the performance levels of elite athletes. They already will have survived screening and self-selection trials but the objective remains of how to best assist them in achieving their full performance potential.

Muscle Force-Velocity and Power-Velocity Relationships

In physical education activities, athletics, and rehabilitation, muscular force and power are most often applied through a range of motion (e.g., during limb movement). Thus, it is important to understand some of the basic concepts underlying the relationship between muscular force and speed (velocity) of movement and muscular power and speed of movement.

The Force-Velocity Curve: Influence of Fiber-Type Distribution

The relationship between muscular force and speed of movement is shown in figure 6.21. Muscular force when applied over a range of motion is measured as torque.* In the figure, the peak torque an individual produced at the relatively slow speed of 57 degrees $\cdot$ s^{-1} was used as a reference. All subsequent torque measurements were expressed as its fraction and denoted as % torque (vertical axis). The movement performed was leg extension. Two important features of the force-velocity relationship should be noted.

1. The peak torque generated by a muscle decreases with increasing velocities of movement. In other words, the greatest torque is produced at the slowest speeds of movement. This is true regardless of the fiber-type distribution (figure 6.21A).
2. At any given velocity of movement, the torque produced is greater the higher the percentage of distribution of Type II fibers in the muscle (figure 6.21A and B). By the same token, at any given torque produced, the velocity of movement is greater the higher the percentage of distribution of Type II fibers.

The preceding relationships point out that Type II fibers are capable of producing greater peak muscular ten-

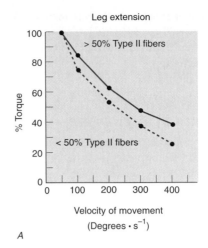

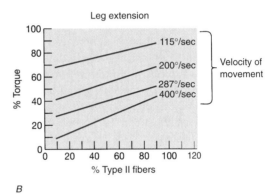

Figure 6.21

Muscle force-velocity relationships. *A.* The peak torque (force) generated by a muscle decreases with increasing velocities of movement (i.e., the greatest torque is produced at the slowest speeds of movement). *B.* At any given velocity of movement, the torque produced is greater the higher the percentage of distribution of Type II fibers in the muscle. The data were obtained during leg extension movements.

(Based on data from Coyle et al.[20])

sion and a faster rate of tension development than are Type I fibers. The biochemical and physiological properties related to these contractile dynamics are the fiber's myosin ATPase activities (p. 139) and their rates of calcium release and uptake from the sarcoplasmic reticulum.[17] Both of these properties are higher within the Type II fiber than in the Type I fiber.[117] Note that Type II fiber percentages are used as the basis for plotting changes in percent torque in figure 6.21B. Other studies have shown no correlation between similar expressions of torque and the percentage of Type I fibers.[96] Likewise, there is no significant correlation between Type I fiber percentages and decreases in torque with faster movement speeds as shown in figure 6.21A.[96]

The preceding information has some practical importance to physical education and athletics. For example, a high percentage of Type II muscle fibers would seem

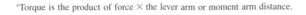

*Torque is the product of force $\times$ the lever arm or moment arm distance.

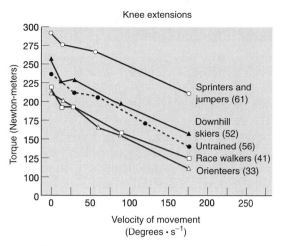

Figure 6.22

Muscle force-velocity curves for various groups of athletes. The curve for the power athletes (sprinters and high jumpers), who have the greatest percentage of Type II fibers (in parentheses), is significantly above those of the other groups, whereas the curves for the endurance athletes, who have the lowest percentage of Type II fibers, are significantly below the others. The data were obtained during knee extension movements.

(Based on data from Thorstensson et al.[111])

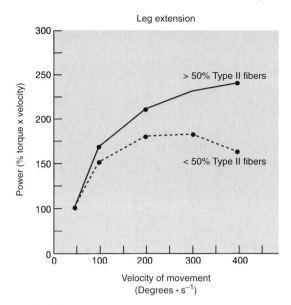

Figure 6.23

Muscle power-velocity relationships. The peak power generated by a muscle increases exponentially with increasing velocities of movement, and at any given velocity of movement, the peak power generated is greater the higher the percentage of distribution of Type II fibers in the muscle. The data were obtained during leg extension movements.

(Based on data from Coyle et al.[70])

advantageous for athletes who participate in power-type events. That this is actually the case can be seen from figure 6.22, in which force-velocity curves for various groups of athletes are shown. The curve for the power athletes (sprinters and high jumpers) is significantly above those of the other groups, whereas the curves for the endurance athletes (race walkers and orienteers) are significantly below the others. In fact, these latter curves are even below the curve for the untrained group.

The sprinters and jumpers have the highest percentage of Type II fibers (61%), whereas the race walkers (41%) and orienteers (33%) have the lowest. Although this was expected, the percentage of Type II fibers in the untrained group (56%) is very close to that of the sprinters and jumpers (61%), yet the magnitudes of the force-velocity curves are quite different. This suggests that training, per se, can significantly influence the force-velocity curve. (For more on training, see pp. 353–361.)

The Power-Velocity Curve: Influence of Fiber-Type Distribution

Studies of elite female athletes indicate similar Type I:Type II fiber ratios.[49] Sprinters had 39:61, pentathletes 54:46, middle-distance runners 63:37, and distance runners 73:27 percentage ratios. Decreases in leg extensor torque-velocity plots were also related to whether the athletes had < 50% or > 50% Type II fibers as was shown for other subjects in figure 6.21A. Unlike earlier reports, there was no decline in

torque when movement velocity was increased from 0 to 96 degrees $\cdot$ s^{-1}. This is additional evidence that training can alter force-velocity curves toward an enhanced performance.

The relationship between muscular power and speed of movement is shown in figure 6.23. The measurements were obtained during leg extension movements and are from the same group of subjects for which torque measurements are shown in figure 6.21. Recall that power is defined as the amount of work performed per unit of time. In the figure, it is the product of the percentage of torque produced and the velocity of the movement. As with the torque measurements, there are two points to notice.

1. The peak power generated by a muscle increases exponentially with increasing velocities of movement. This is to say, the increase in power is more rapid at lower speeds of movement and less rapid at higher speeds. In fact, as shown by the lower curve, the power generated may level off or actually start to decrease at very high velocities of movement.

2. At any given velocity of movement, the peak power generated is greater the higher the percentage of distribution of Type II fibers in the muscle. As mentioned before, this relationship is attributable to the biochemical and physiological differences between Type I and Type II fibers.

With respect to application, in figure 6.24, power-velocity curves for various groups of athletes are presented. These are the same groups of athletes for whom

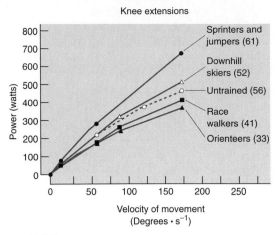

Figure 6.24

Muscle power-velocity curves for various groups of athletes. Peak muscular power is greater at any given velocity of movement in athletes who participate in the so-called power events and who have relatively greater distributions of Type II fibers (percentage in parentheses). The data were obtained during knee extension movements.

(Based on data from Thorstensson et al.[111])

force-velocity curves are given in figure 6.22. Again, it is clearly evident that peak muscular power is greater at any given velocity of movement for athletes who participate in the so-called power events and who have relatively greater distributions of Type II fibers. For example, the peak power generated at a velocity of movement of 180 degrees · s^{-1} was found to be 81% greater in sprinters and jumpers than in orienteers.

Local Muscular Fatigue

Muscle fatigue has been defined as a decline in maximal force generating capacity and as a common response to muscular activity.[115] Although much research has been devoted to muscular fatigue, neither the exact sites or causes of fatigue are very well understood. Interestingly, fatigue can be viewed as an important, if not essential, contributor to the overall stimulus for muscles to improve their strength[89] or to make other structural or metabolic adaptations. Miller et al.[76] point out that both metabolic factors and impairment of neural activation appear to play a role in human muscle fatigue. By measuring EMG, metabolites, and force during fatiguing exercise and recovery, they estimated the contribution of different factors which produce fatigue. The inter-individual variability in metabolic and EMG changes in these studies is high even under the most favorable of standardized isometric exercise conditions.[8] With this as background, we will start our discussion with the influences of fiber-type distribution on fatigue and then proceed to the possible sites and causes of local muscular fatigue.

Influence of Fiber-Type Distribution on Muscular Fatigue

Earlier, in table 6.3 (p. 149), we mentioned that Type II fibers are more easily fatigued than are Type I fibers. Another advantage of having more Type I fibers is that glycogen resynthesis is faster during recovery from exhaustive exercise.[13] In humans, one of the ways in which muscle fatigue is quantified is by recording the decrease in peak tension (torque) of a muscle group during a given number of repetitions of very rapid contractions performed through a range of motion. The decline in peak tension of the muscle is taken as a measure of fatigue. As an example, figure 6.25 shows the results of such an experiment following 50 repetitions of knee extensions. Each repetition was performed at a fast speed of movement (180 degrees · s^{-1}), and the muscle group studied was the vastus lateralis. These results show that muscular fatigue (as indicated by the magnitude of decline in peak tension) was greater (1) the greater the percentage of distribution of Type II fibers in the muscle (figure 6.25A) and (2) the greater the Type II fiber area of the muscle (figure 6.25B). Because of the biochemical and physiological differences between Type I and Type II fibers, the preceding information—as we will see next—is particularly important in helping to understand some of the causes of muscular fatigue.

Possible Sites and Causes of Muscular Fatigue

In the body, a muscle or muscle group may fatigue because of failure of any one or all of the different neuromuscular mechanisms involved in muscular contraction. For example, the inability of a muscle to contract voluntarily could be due to failure of the following:

1. The *motor nerve* innervating the muscle fibers to transmit nervous impulses.
2. The *neuromuscular junction* to relay the nervous impulses from the motor nerve to the muscle fibers.
3. The *contractile mechanism* itself to generate a force.
4. The *central nervous system* (i.e., the brain and spinal cord) to initiate and relay nervous impulses to the muscle.

Most research concerning local muscular fatigue has previously focused on the neuromuscular junction, the contractile mechanism, and the central nervous system. The possibility of the motor nerve as the site and cause of fatigue is not very great. Fitts[28] now believes that the primary sites (note use of the plural here) of fatigue appear to be within the muscle cell itself and for the most part do not involve the central nervous system or the neuromuscular junction. In his view, the major hypotheses of fatigue center on disturbances in the surface membrane, excitation-contraction coupling, or metabolic events. Since uncertainty clearly exists here, we have elected to review this

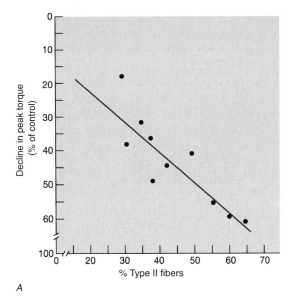

A

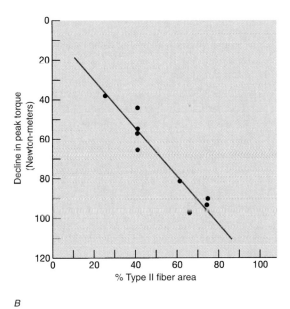

B

Figure 6.25

A. Muscular fatigue, as measured by decline in peak torque, is greater the greater the percentage of distribution of Type II fibers in the muscle; and *B.* the greater the percentage of distribution of the Type II fiber area of the muscle. The data were obtained during knee extension movements.

(Data in A from Thorstensson and Karlsson,[110] data in B from Tesch et al.[106])

matter in a more comprehensive way rather than restricting it as suggested by Fitts.

1. *Fatigue at the Neuromuscular Junction.* There is some evidence both for [15,69,101] and against [2,29,30,69,75,83] the idea that local muscular fatigue is caused by failure at the neuromuscular junction. This type of fatigue appears to be more common in Type II motor units[69,101] and may account, in part, for the greater fatigability of these fibers when compared with Type I fibers. Failure of the neuromuscular junction to relay nervous impulses to the muscle fibers is most likely due to a decreased release of the chemical transmitter, acetylcholine, from the nerve ending. (More on acetylcholine and chemical transmitters is given on p. 110.)

2. *Fatigue within the Contractile Mechanism.* Several factors have been implicated in fatigue of the contractile mechanism itself. Some of them are as follows:

   a. *Accumulation of Lactic Acid.* Fatigue due to lactic acid accumulation had been suspected for many years.[31,51,64,65,66] However, it was not until the late 1970s that a relationship between intramuscular lactic acid accumulation and decline in peak tension (a measure of fatigue) was established.[28,105] This relationship is shown in figure 6.26*A* for isolated frog sartorius muscle[30] and in figure 6.26*B* for intact human vastus lateralis muscle.[106] Whereas establishment of these relationships does not in itself prove conclusively that lactic acid causes fatigue, it does lend considerable support to the idea. Surprisingly, in the classic experiments conducted by A. V. Hill and colleagues over 60 years ago[51] from which the hypothesis that lactic acid causes muscular fatigue originated, lactic acid accumulation in the muscle was never even measured!

   The lactic acid accumulation in the human vastus lateralis is represented as the ratio of lactic acid concentrations in Type II to Type I fibers (horizontal axis of figure 6.26*B*). This means that as the ratio increases, more lactic acid is being produced in Type II fibers in comparison with Type I fibers. This greater ability to form lactic acid might be one contributing factor to the higher anaerobic performance capacity of the Type II fibers.[106] Notice also that as the lactic acid Type II:Type I ratio increases, the peak tension of the muscle decreases. This may be interpreted to mean that the greater fatigability of Type II fibers is related to their greater ability to form lactic acid.

   The idea that lactic acid accumulation is involved in the fatigue process is further strengthened by the fact that there are at least two physiological mechanisms whereby lactic acid could hinder muscle function. Both mechanisms depend on the effects lactic acid has on intracellular pH or hydrogen ion (H^+) concentration. With increases in lactic acid, H^+ concentration increases and pH decreases. On one hand, an increase in H^+ concentration hinders the

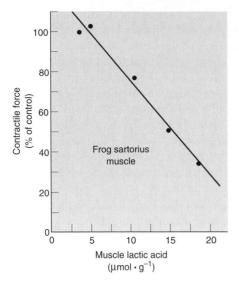

A

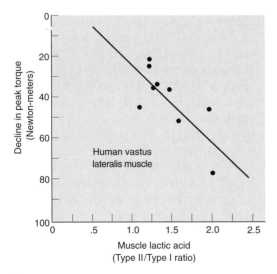

B

Figure 6.26

A. Relationship between intramuscular accumulation of lactic acid and decline in peak tension (a measure of muscular fatigue) for isolated frog sartorius muscle and *B.* for intact human vastus lateralis muscle.

(Data in A from Fitts and Holloszy,[30] data in B from Tesch et al.[106])

excitation-coupling process (figure 6.9*B*) by decreasing the amount of Ca^{++} released from the sarcoplasmic reticulum[35] and interfering with the Ca^{++}-troponin binding capacity.[82] On the other hand, an increased H^+ concentration also inhibits the activity of phosphofructokinase, a key enzyme involved in anaerobic glycolysis.[113] Such an inhibition slows glycolysis, thus reducing the availability of ATP for energy.

b. *Depletion of ATP and PC Stores.* Because ATP is the direct source of energy for muscular contraction, and PC is used for its immediate resynthesis, intramuscular depletion of these phosphagens results in fatigue. However, studies with humans[65,66] have been conclusive that exhaustion cannot be attributed to critically low phosphagen concentrations in muscle. A similar conclusion was reached from a study conducted on isolated frog sartorius muscle.[30] Some of the results of this study are shown in figure 6.27. As can be seen, the largest decrease in the concentration of ATP and PC occurred in the first two minutes of contraction, before there was a decline in peak tension of the muscle. When the muscle was fully fatigued (after 15 minutes of contraction), there was still 76% of the resting concentration of ATP available to the muscle. In addition, the concentrations of both ATP and PC increased very rapidly within the first several minutes of recovery, but muscular force changed very little. This further indicates that phosphagen availability and muscular fatigue are not highly correlated.

Despite the preceding information, the possibility that ATP and PC might still be involved in the fatigue process cannot be completely dismissed. For example, studies have suggested that during contractile activity, the concentration of ATP in the region of the myofibrils might decrease more markedly than in the muscle as a whole.[30] Therefore, ATP could be limited within the contractile mechanism even though there is only a moderate decrease in total muscle ATP content. Another possibility is that the energy yield in the breakdown of ATP rather than the amount of ATP available is limiting for muscular contraction. For example, the amount of energy liberated when 1 mole of ATP is broken down to ADP + Pi has been calculated to decrease almost 15%, from 12.9 kilocalories (kcal) at rest to as low as 11.0 kcal after exhaustive exercise.[90] The reason for this decrease might be related in part to large increases in intracellular H^+ concentration, primarily due to lactic acid accumulation. Also noteworthy is that subjects can maintain their power outputs better during a short duration (10 seconds), high-intensity cycle ergometer test if they have ingested 20 g of creatine per day over a 6-day period.[6] In this study the total muscle creatine (C plus PC) at rest was significantly increased, which would argue for the involvement of [PC] in muscle fatigue.

c. *Depletion of Muscle Glycogen Stores.* Earlier, it was mentioned that during prolonged exercise

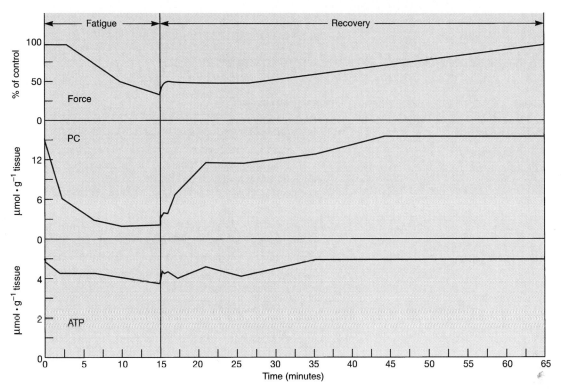

Figure 6.27

Relationship between muscular fatigue (decline in peak force) and intramuscular concentrations of ATP and PC in isolated frog muscle. The largest decrease in the concentration of ATP and PC occurred in the first two minutes of contraction before there was a decline in peak tension of the muscle. When the muscle was fully fatigued (about 15 minutes of contraction), there was still 76% of the resting concentration of ATP available to the muscle.

(Based on data from Fitts and Holloszy.[30])

(e.g., 30 minutes to 4 hours) the muscle glycogen stores within some of the fibers (mainly Type I fibers) are nearly completely depleted (figure 6.20). It is thought that such severe glycogen depletion is a cause of contractile fatigue.[92] This is thought to be true even though plenty of free fatty acids and glucose (from the liver) are still available as fuels to the muscle fibers. Apparently, these other fuels cannot fully cover the energy demand of the glycogen-depleted muscle fibers.[92] As with lactic acid and fatigue, a definite cause-and-effect relationship between muscle glycogen depletion and muscular fatigue has not been determined.

d. *Other Factors.* Some additional but less well-understood factors that may contribute to muscular fatigue are lack of oxygen[39,121] and inadequate blood flow[7] to the muscle fibers. Also, the reasons that greater and longer lasting fatigue occurs after eccentric exercise[16] and that fatigue affects isometric force production less than isokinetic force production[59] remain to be explained. The fact that women have significantly longer endurance times than men when

performing sustained submaximal isometric handgrip exercise still awaits an adequate explanation.[120]

3. *The Central Nervous System and Local Muscular Fatigue.* **Central neural fatigue** during exercise is defined as a decrease in muscle force attributable to a decline in motorneuronal output.[36] This central fatigue develops during many forms of exercise and may have a number of mechanisms that contribute to its development. For example, motorneurons may be inhibited by group III and IV afferents from fatiguing muscles, along with a decrease in muscle spindle facilitation. The output from these afferents may be greater when the work rate does not match up well with the preferred rate of the performer (e.g., pedalling speed is too slow).[103] Also, motor cortical output may be less than optimal. In any case, in conscious humans, fatiguing muscular contractions are accompanied by a decrease in discharge rate of alpha motorneurons.[38] This close association between alpha motorneuron discharge rate and the generation of force by skeletal muscle has been called "muscle wisdom." It is believed to ensure that during fatigue, the central neural drive to skeletal muscle matches

6.4

table

Summary of possible sites and physiological mechanisms involved in local muscular fatigue

Site of fatigue	Proposed mechanism
1. Neuromuscular junction	(a) Decreased release of acetylcholine at nerve ending
2. Contractile mechanism	(a) Decreased Ca^{++} released from sarcoplasmic reticulum and reduced Ca^{++}-troponin binding capacity due to increased H^+ concentration caused by lactic acid accumulation
	(b) Depletion of ATP + PC stores and/or decreased energy yield per mole of ATP broken down
	(c) Depletion of muscle glycogen stores
	(d) Lack of oxygen and inadequate blood flow
3. Central nervous system	(a) Local disturbances caused by contractile fatigue signals the brain to send inhibitory signals to the motor system—resulting in a further decline in muscular work output

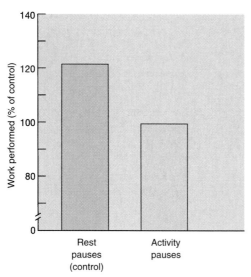

Figure 6.28

Repeated bouts of exhaustive work consisting of rhythmical lifting of weights were performed with either the elbow flexor muscles or the flexors of the middle finger. Pauses lasting two minutes spent either at complete rest (control) or while physically active were alternated between the work bouts. The amount of work performed when active pause periods were used was 22% greater than when complete rest periods were used.

(Based on data from Asmussen and Mazin.[4])

that needed to generate the required force. Also, it may serve as an important mechanism to decrease or to postpone full-blown central neural fatigue.

Research has been conducted by Asmussen and associates[3,4] into the role of a central nervous system component in local muscular fatigue. He and his staff performed a very clever series of experiments in which repeated bouts of exhaustive work consisting of rhythmical lifting of weights were performed with either the elbow flexor muscles or the flexors of the middle finger. Pauses lasting two minutes spent either at complete rest (control) or while physically active were alternated between the work bouts. The active pause periods consisted of performing what was referred to as "diverting activities" (i.e., physical activity performed with nonfatigued muscles). The results of one of these experiments[4] are shown in figure 6.28. The amount of work performed when diverting activities were used during the pause periods was 22% greater than when complete rest was used. Further experiments in the same series of studies[3] showed that similar results were obtained when (1) the diverting activities were performed simultaneously with the exhaustive bouts of work, (2) the circulation to the muscles involved in both the exhaustive and diverting exercises was occluded, (3) mental work was used as the diverting activity, and (4) exhausting work was performed with open compared with closed eyes (more work was performed with the eyes open). These results led to the conclusion that recovery from local muscular fatigue is influenced by a central nervous system factor that is independent of the local blood flow.

Physiologically, how might such a mechanism work? Although the exact mechanism is not known, it is proposed that as a muscle fatigues, the local disturbances that occur within its internal environment are signaled back to the central nervous system (brain) via sensory nerves. In turn, the brain sends out inhibitory signals to the nerve cells in the motor system, resulting in a declining muscular work output.

During a rest pause, the local disturbances tend to be restored in the muscles, and the fatigue gradually diminishes or disappears. If a diverting activity is performed during a pause period, other signals from the periphery or from the brain itself will impinge on the facilitatory areas of the brain. Consequently, facilitatory impulses will be sent to the motor system leading to better muscular performance or to a faster recovery from fatigue.[3] The local disturbances in the contractile mechanism of the muscle that initiates this series of events are most likely those discussed earlier (i.e., lactic acid accumulation and depletion of ATP + PC and muscle glycogen).

As has been indicated from the preceding discussion, local muscular fatigue is complex, having several etiologies, and is not as yet well understood. The most likely causes of muscular fatigue are summarized in table 6.4.

Summary

The connective tissues of skeletal muscle are the endomysium, surrounding the fibers or cells, the perimysium, surrounding the fascicle bundles, and the epimysium, encasing the entire muscle. The cell membrane of the muscle fiber is called the sarcolemma. These connective tissues become continuous with the connective tissue of the tendons, which connect the skeletal muscles to the bony skeleton.

Muscles are richly supplied with blood vessels. On the average, three to four capillaries surround each fiber in sedentary men and women, whereas five to seven surround each fiber in male and female athletes.

Muscles contain both motor and sensory nerves. Motor nerves originate in the central nervous system (brain and spinal cord) and when stimulated, cause the muscles to contract. The termination of a motor nerve on a muscle fiber is known as the neuromuscular junction. Sensory nerves convey information concerning pain and orientation of body parts from the muscle to the central nervous system.

Each muscle fiber or cell contains hundreds of threadlike protein strands called myofibrils, within which the contractile unit is housed. The light and dark striations of the myofibrils are called the I and A bands, respectively. The bands contain two protein filaments, actin and myosin. Actin filaments also contain the proteins troponin and tropomyosin. Myosin filaments have tiny protein projections called cross-bridges, which extend toward the actin filaments.

The sarcoplasmic reticulum is a network of tubules surrounding each myofibril. It aids in spreading the nervous impulse throughout the muscle and in storing and releasing calcium (Ca^{++}), both of which are important in the contractile and recovery processes.

Muscular contraction, according to the sliding filament theory, results when the actin filaments are pulled over the myosin filaments, thus producing tension and shortening the muscle. Both shortening and tension development depend on (1) the breakdown of ATP for energy; (2) Ca^{++}-troponin binding for activation of the actin filaments; and (3) the coupling of myosin to actin (formation of actomyosin).

The single motor nerve and the muscle fibers it supplies are called the motor unit, which is the basic functional unit of skeletal muscle. The motor unit functions according to the all-or-none law, meaning that it contracts maximally or not at all. Strength gradations are possible by (1) varying the number of motor units contracting at any given time, called recruitment or multiple motor unit summation; and (2) by varying the frequency of contraction of individual motor units, called wave summation.

The muscle fibers within a given motor unit may be either slow-twitch (Type I) or fast-twitch (Type II) fibers, but not both. Generally speaking, motor units comprised of Type II fibers can be further subdivided into Type IIA, IIB and IIC categories, which represent an aerobic to anaerobic metabolic continuum.

Type I fibers have the highest aerobic capacity whereas Type IIA fibers are both oxidative and glycolytic. Type IIB fibers have only a high capacity for anaerobic, glycolytic metabolism. Type IIC fibers are an unclassified, nondifferentiated type which are very few in number.

A combination of neurotrophic, myogenic, fatigue, temperature, metabolic control signal, and hormonal factors have been implicated in determining the properties specific to the different fiber types; these are called *phenotypic properties.*

A key phenotypic property that regulates the rate of force development and velocity of shortening is the presence of different forms of myofibrillar protein called *isoforms.*

Two isoforms found in Type II fibers that contribute to their higher and faster force output are more myosin heavy chains and troponin, which has a higher Ca^{++}-binding capacity and a faster process of cross-bridge attachment.

During exercise there is preferential recruitment of fiber types based on the "size principle" of their motorneurons: small ones first, large ones last. Type I fibers are recruited first for low-intensity, endurance exercise. Type IIA fibers and then Type IIB fibers are recruited as exercise duration is extended, intensity is increased, or fatigue occurs.

All available fibers are recruited for all-out power efforts. Sprint athletes tend to have a predominance of Type II fibers and endurance athletes a predominance of Type I fibers. Middle-distance runners, throwers, and jumpers display a wider range of fiber type compositions.

Major adaptations with endurance training include increases in the aerobic capacity of Type I and Type IIA fibers and a shift toward a higher ratio of Type IIA:Type IIB fibers. Weight training produces some similar effects but also stimulates Type II fibers to enlarge. In neither case do fibers switch from one fiber type to the other, nor do they increase in number. The muscle fiber distributions and enzymatic characteristics of male and female athletes are quite similar.

Heredity strongly influences final adult muscle fiber composition in a process that begins before birth, shows considerable change during the first year of life, and is completed during the teenage years. This and other logistic, safety, and cost factors along with concern over the validity and reliability of the measurement results, inhibit the widespread use of fiber typing as a useful tool to screen and guide young athletes into sports that are "best" for them.

The peak force generated by a muscle decreases and the peak power increases with increasing velocities of movement. For any given velocity of movement, the peak force and peak power produced are greater the higher the percentage of distribution of Type II fibers in the muscle.

The most probable sites of local muscular fatigue are the neuromuscular junction, the muscle itself (contractile mechanism), and the central nervous system. Fatigue at the neuromuscular junction, which might be more common in Type II fibers, is probably due to a decreased release of chemical transmitter, acetylcholine, from the nerve ending.

Fatigue within the contractile mechanism may be caused by one or more of the following: (1) accumulation of lactic acid, (2) depletion of ATP and PC stores, (3) depletion of muscle glycogen stores, and (4) lack of oxygen and inadequate blood flow. Recovery from local muscular fatigue is quickened by a central nervous system factor that involves irradiation of facilitatory impulses of the motor system.

Questions

1. What are the structural units and associated connective tissues of skeletal muscle?
2. Describe the nerve and blood supplies to muscle.
3. Draw and label a diagram of a sarcomere. Include the I band, A band, H zone, and Z lines.
4. Describe the structure and function of the sarcoplasmic reticulum and T-tubule system.
5. What proteins make up the thick and thin filaments? What is their functional significance?
6. Define the sliding filament theory of muscular contraction.
7. Describe in detail how the myosin cross-bridges are thought to form a bond with selected sites on the actin filaments during an isotonic contraction.
8. Describe the structure and function of the motor unit.
9. How is the strength of a muscle graded?
10. Explain how our movements are made smooth and non-jerky.
11. What are the major functional differences between Type I and Type II muscle fibers or motor units?
12. Discuss the distribution of muscle fiber types in various groups of athletes.
13. What is the functional significance of Type I and Type II fibers with respect to sprint and endurance exercises?
14. What is the "size principle" of motor unit recruitment?
15. What relationships exist between exercise intensity and the "types" of motor units recruited?
16. Describe the force-velocity and power-velocity curves. How does fiber-type distribution affect these curves?
17. Discuss some of the causes of local muscular fatigue.

References

1. Andersen, P., and J. Henriksson. 1977. Training induced changes in the subgroups of human type II skeletal muscle fibres. *Acta Physiol Scand.* 99:123–125.
2. Apple, F. S., and P. Tesch. 1989. CK and LD isoenzymes in human single muscle fibers in trained athletes. *J Appl Physiol.* 66:2717–2720.
3. Asmussen, E., and B. Mazin. 1978. A central nervous component in local muscular fatigue. *Eur J Appl Physiol.* 38:9–15.
4. ———. 1978. Recuperation after muscular fatigue by "diverting activities." *Eur J Appl Physiol.* 38:1–7.
5. Bachouchi, N., and J. E. Morel. 1989. Behaviour of the crossbridges in stretched or compressed muscle fibres. *J Theor Biol.* 141:143–157.
6. Balsom, P. D., K. Sonderlund, B. Sjodin, and B. Ekblom. 1995. Skeletal muscle metabolism during short duration high-intensity exercise: influence of creatine supplementation. *Acta Physiol Scand.* 154:303–310.
7. Barclay, J. K., and W. N. Stainsby. 1975. The role of blood flow in limiting maximal metabolic rate in muscle. *Med Sci Sports.* 7(2):116–119.
8. Bendahan, D., Y. Jammes, A. M. Salvan, M. Badier, S. Confort-Gouny, C. Guillot, and P. J. Cozzone. 1996. Combined electromyography—31P-magnetic resonance spectroscopy study of human muscle fatigue during static contraction. *Muscle Nerve.* 19:715–721.
9. Bergh, U., A. Thorstensson, B. Sjödin, B. Hulten, K. Piehl, and J. Karlsson. 1978. Maximal oxygen uptake and muscle fiber types in trained and untrained humans. *Med Sci Sports.* 10(3):151–154.
10. Brooke, M. H., and K. K. Kaiser. 1970. Muscle fibre types: how many and what kind? *Arch Neurol.* 23:369–379.
11. ———. 1970. Three "myosin adenosine triphosphatase" systems: the nature of their pH lability and sulfhydryl dependence. *J Histochem Cytochem.* 18:670–672.
12. Burke, F., F. Cerny, D. Costill, and W. Fink. 1977. Characteristics of skeletal muscle in competitive cyclists. *Med Sci Sports.* 9:109–112.
13. Casey, A., A. H. Short, E. Hultman, and P. L. Greenhaff. 1995. Glycogen resynthesis in human muscle fibre types following exercise-induced glycogen depletion. *J Physiol.* 483:265–271.
14. Cirrito, J. F. 1979. *Fractional Volumetric Changes in the Ultra Structure of Sarcoplasmic Reticulum in Rat Skeletal Muscle due to Chronic Exercise.* Doctoral dissertation, The Ohio State University, Columbus, OH.
15. Clamann, H. P., and K. T. Broecker. 1979. Relationship between

force and fatigability of red and pale skeletal muscles in man. *Am J Phys Med.* 58(2):70–85.

16. Clarkson, P. M., and D. J. Newham. 1995. Associations between muscle soreness, damage and fatigue. *Adv Exp Med Biol.* 384:457–469.

17. Close, R. I. 1972. Dynamic properties of mammalian skeletal muscles. *Physiol Rev.* 52(1):129–197.

18. Cohen, C. 1975. The protein switch of muscle contraction. *Sci Am.* 233(5):36–45.

19. Costill, D., J. Daniels, W. Evans, W. Fink, G. Krahenbuhl, and B. Saltin. 1976. Skeletal muscle enzymes and fiber composition in male and female track athletes. *J Appl Physiol.* 40:149–154.

20. Coyle, E. F., D. L. Costill, and G. R. Lesmes. 1979. Leg extension power and muscle fiber composition. *Med Sci Sports.* 11(1):12–15.

21. Craig, R. 1985. First sight of crossbridge crystals. *Nature.* 316:16–17.

22. Davies, R. 1963. A molecular theory of muscle contraction: calcium dependent contractions with hydrogen bond formation plus ATP-dependent extensions of part of the myosin-actin crossbridges. *Nature.* 199:1068–1074.

23. Dons, B., K. Bollerup, F. Bonde-Petersen, and S. Hancke. 1979. The effect of weight lifting exercise related to muscle fiber composition and muscle cross-sectional area in humans. *Eur J Appl Physiol.* 49:95–106.

24. Dubowitz, V., and A. Pearse. 1960. A comparative histochemical study of oxidative enzymes and phosphorylase activity in skeletal muscle. *Histochemistry.* 2:105–117.

25. Edström, L., and B. Nyström. 1969. Histochemical types and sizes of fibers of normal human muscles. *Acta Neurol Scand.* 45:257–269.

26. Elder, G. C. B., K. Bradbury, and R. Roberts. 1982. Variability of fiber type distributions within human muscles. *J Appl Physiol: Respirat Environ Exerc Physiol.* 53(6):1473–1480.

27. Essen, B., E. Jansson, J. Henriksson, A. W. Taylor, and B. Saltin. 1975. Metabolic characteristics of fibre types in human skeletal muscle. *Acta Physiol Scand.* 95:153–165.

28. Fitts, R. H. 1994. Cellular mechanisms of muscle fatigue. *Physiol Rev.* 74:49–94.

29. Fitts, R.H., and J. O. Holloszy. 1977. Contractile properties of rat soleus muscle: effects of training and fatigue. *Am J Physiol.* 233(3):C86–C91.

30. ———. 1976. Lactate and contractile force in frog muscle during development of fatigue and recovery. *Am J Physiol.* 231(2):430–433.

31. Fletcher, W. W., and F. G. Hopkins. 1907. Lactic acid in mammalian muscle. *J Physiol* (London). 35:247–303.

32. Foster, C., D. L. Costill, J. T. Daniels, and W. J. Fink. 1978. Skeletal muscle enzyme activity, fiber composition and VO$_2$ max in relation to distance running performance. *Eur J Appl Physiol.* 39:73–80.

33. Fox, E. L. 1979. *Sports Physiology.* Philadelphia: W. B. Saunders, pp. 89, 90, 106–107.

34. Fridén, J., M. Sjöström, and B. Ekblom. 1984. Muscle fibre type characteristics in endurance trained and untrained individuals. *Eur J Appl Physiol.* 52:266–271.

35. Fuchs, F., V. Reddy, and F. N. Briggs. 1970. The interaction of cations with the calcium-binding site of troponin. *Biochem Biophys Acta.* 221:407–409.

36. Gandevia, S. C., G. M. Allen, and D. K. McKenzie. 1995. Central fatigue. Critical issues, quantitation and practical implications. *Adv Exp Med Biol.* 384:281–294

37. Garland, S. J., R. M. Enoka, L. P. Serrano, and G. A. Robinson. 1994. Behavior of motor units in human biceps brachii during a submaximal fatiguing contraction. *J Appl Physiol.* 76:2411–2419.

38. Garland, S. J., and M. P. Kaufman. 1995. Role of muscle afferents in the inhibition of motoneurons during fatigue. *Adv Exp Med Biol.* 384:271–278.

39. Gladden, L. B., B. R. MacIntosh, and W. N. Stainsby. 1978. O$_2$ uptake and developed tension during and after fatigue, curare block, and ischemia. *J Appl Physiol.* 45(5):751–755.

40. Gollnick, P. D., R. B. Armstrong, B. Saltin, C. W. Saubert, IV, W. L. Sembrowich, and R. E. Shepherd. 1973. Effect of training on enzyme activity and fiber composition of human skeletal muscle. *J Appl Physiol.* 34(1):107–111.

41. Gollnick, P., R. Armstrong, C. Saubert, K. Piehl, and B. Saltin. 1972. Enzyme activity and fiber composition in skeletal muscle of untrained and trained men. *J Appl Physiol.* 33(3):312–319.

42. Gollnick, P., R. Armstrong, C. Saubert, W. Sembrowich, R. Shepherd, and B. Saltin. 1973. Glycogen depletion patterns in human skeletal muscle fibers during prolonged work. *Pflugers Arch.* 344:1–12.

43. Gollnick, P., R. Armstrong, W. Sembrowich, R. Shepherd, and B. Saltin. 1973. Glycogen depletion pattern in human skeletal muscle fiber after heavy exercise. *J Appl Physiol.* 34(5):615–618.

44. Gollnick, P. D., and D. R. Hodgson. 1986. The identification of fiber types in skeletal muscle: a continual dilemma. *Exerc Sport Sci Rev.* 14:81–104.

45. Gollnick, P. D., K. Pichl, and B. Saltin. 1974. Selective glycogen depletion pattern in human muscle fibers after exercise of varying intensity and at varying pedal rates. *J Physiol.* 241:45–47.

46. Gollnick, P. D., B. F. Timson, R. L. Moore, and M. Riedy. 1981. Muscular enlargement and number of fibers in skeletal muscles of rats. *J Appl Physiol.* 50(5):936–943.

47. Gordon, T., and M. C. Pattullo. 1993. Plasticity of muscle fiber and motor unit types. *Exerc Sport Sci Rev.* 21:331–362.

48. Greenhaff, P. L., J. M. Ren, K. Soderlund, and E. Hultman. 1991. Energy metabolism in single human muscle fibers during contraction without and with epinephrine infusion. *Am J Physiol.* 260:E713–718.

49. Gregor, R. J., V. R. Edgerton, J. J. Perrine, D. S. Campion, and C. DeBus. 1979. Torque-velocity relationships and muscle fiber composition in elite female athletes. *J Appl Physiol.* 47(2):388–392.

50. Harris, R. C., K. Sahlin, and E. Hultman. 1977. Phosphagen and lactate contents of m. quadriceps femoris of man after exercise. *J Appl Physiol.* 43(5):852–857.

51. Hill, A. V., and P. Kupalov. 1929. Anaerobic and aerobic activity in isolated muscle. *Proc Roy Soc* (London), Series B, 105:313–322.

52. Hoh, J. F. 1992. Muscle fiber types and function. *Curr Opin Rheumatol.* 4:801–808.

53. Howard, H., H. Hoppeler, H. Claassen, O. Mathieu, and R. Straub. 1985. Influence of endurance training on the ultrastructural composition of the different muscle fiber types in humans. *Pflugers Arch.* 403:369–376.

54. Huxley, H. 1969. The mechanism of muscular contraction. *Science.* 164(3886):1356–1366.

55. Ingjer, F. 1979. Capillary supply and mitochondrial content of different skeletal muscle fiber types in untrained and endurance-trained men. A histochemical and ultrastructural study. *Eur J Appl Physiol.* 40:197–209.

56. ———. 1978. Maximal aerobic power related to the capillary supply of the quadriceps femoris muscle in man. *Acta Physiol Scand.* 104:238–240.

57. Ivy, J. L., R. T. Withers, P. J. Van Handel, D. H. Elger, and D. L. Costill. 1980. Muscle respiratory capacity and fiber type as determinants of the lactate threshold. *J Appl Physiol.* 48(3):523–527.

58. Jacobs, I., and P. Kaiser. 1982. Lactate in blood, mixed skeletal muscle, and FT or ST fibres during cycle exercise in man. *Acta Physiol Scand.* 114:461–466.

59. James, C., P. Sacco, and D. A. Jones. 1995. Loss of power during fatigue of human leg muscles. *J Physiol.* 484:237–246.

60. Janmey, P. A., S. Hvidt, G. F. Oster, J. Lamb, T. P. Stossel, and J. H. Hartwig. 1990. Effect of ATP on actin filament stiffness. *Nature.* 347:95–99.

61. Jansson, E., and L. Kaijser. 1977. Muscle adaptation to extreme endurance training in man. *Acta Physiol Scand.* 100:315–324.

62. Jansson, E., B. Sjödin, and P. Tesch. 1978. Changes in muscle fibre type distribution in man after physical training: a sign of fibre type transformation? *Acta Physiol Scand.* 104:235–237.

63. Johnson, M. A., J. Polgar, D. Weightman, and D. Appleton. 1973. Data on distribution of fibre types in thirty-six human muscles. An autopsy study. *J Neurol Sci.* 18:111–129.

64. Karlsson, J., F. Bonde-Petersen, J. Henriksson, and H. G. Knuttgen. 1975. Effects of previous exercise with arms or legs on metabolism and performance in exhaustive exercise. *J Appl Physiol.* 38:763–767.

65. Karlsson, J., and B. Saltin. 1970. Lactate, ATP, and CP in working muscles during exhaustive exercise in man. *J Appl Physiol.* 29(5):598–602.

66. ———. 1971. Oxygen deficit and muscle metabolites in intermittent exercise. *Acta Physiol Scand.* 82:115–122.

67. Kerrick, W. G., J. D. Potter, and P. E. Hoar. 1991. The apparent rate constant for the dissociation of force generating myosin crossbridges from actin decreases during Ca^{2+} activation of skinned muscle fibers. *J Muscle Res Cell Motil.* 12:53–60.

68. Komi, P., H. Rusko, J. Vos, and V. Vihko. 1977. Anaerobic performance capacity in athletes. *Acta Physiol Scand.* 100:107–114.

69. Komi, P. V., and P. Tesch. 1979. EMG frequency spectrum, muscle structure, and fatigue during dynamic contractions in man. *Eur J Appl Physiol.* 42:41–50.

70. Kovanen, V., H. Suominen, and E. Heikkinen. 1984. Collagen of slow twitch and fast twitch muscle fibres in different types of rat skeletal muscle. *Eur J Appl Physiol.* 52:235–242.

71. Kushmerick, M. J. 1995. Bioenergetics and muscle cell types. *Adv Exp Med Biol.* 384:175–184.

72. Larsson, L. 1982. Physical training effects on muscle morphology in sedentary males at different ages. *Med Sci Sports Exerc.* 14(3):203–206.

73. Loscher, W. N., A. G. Cresswell, and A. Thorstensson. 1994. Electromyographic responses of the human triceps surae and force tremor during sustained isometric plantar flexion. *Acta Physiol Scand.* 152:73–82.

74. MacDougall, J. D., G. C. B. Elder, D. G. Sale, J. R. Moroz, and J. R. Sutton. 1980. Effects of strength training and immobilization on human muscle fibres. *Eur J Appl Physiol.* 43:25–34.

75. Merton, P. A. 1954. Voluntary strength and fatigue. *J Physiol* (London). 123:553–564.

76. Miller, R. G., J. A. Kent-Braun, K. R. Sharma, and M. W. Weiner. 1995. Mechanisms of human muscle fatigue. Quantitating the contribution of metabolic factors and activation impairment. *Adv Exp Med Biol.* 384:195–210.

77. Milner-Brown, H. S., R. B. Stein, and R. G. Lee. 1975. Synchronization of human motor units: Possible roles of exercise and supraspinal reflexes. *Electroenceph Clin Neurophysiol.* 38:245–254.

78. Mizuno, M., N. H. Secher, and B. Quistorff. 1994. 31P-NMR spectroscopy, rmsEMG, and histochemical fiber types of human wrist flexor muscles. *J Appl Physiol.* 76:531–538.

79. Morris, C. 1968. Human muscle fiber type grouping and collateral re-innervation. *J Neurol Neurosurg Psychiatr.* 32:440–444.

80. Munsat, T. L., D. McNeal, and R. Waters. 1976. Effects of nerve stimulation on human muscle. *Arch Neurol.* 33:608–617.

81. Murray, J., and A. Weber. 1974. The cooperative action of muscle proteins. *Sci Am.* 230(2):58–71.

82. Nakamura, Y., and S. Schwartz. 1972. The influence of hydrogen ion concentration on calcium binding and release by skeletal muscle sarcoplasmic reticulum. *J Gen Physiol.* 59:22–32.

83. Nilsson, J., P. Tesch, and A. Thorstensson. 1977. Fatigue and EMG of repeated fast voluntary contractions in man. *Acta Physiol Scand.* 101:194–198.

84. O'Hagan, F. T., D. G. Sale, J. D. MacDougall, and S. H. Garner.

1995. Comparative effectiveness of accommodating and weight resistance training modes. *Med Sci Sports Exerc.* 27:1210–1219.

85. Pernus, F., and I. Erzen. 1991. Arrangement of fiber types within fascicles of human vastus lateralis muscle. *Muscle Nerve.* 14:304–309.

86. Prince, F. P., R. S. Hikida, and F. C. Hagerman. 1977. Muscle fiber types in women athletes and non-athletes. *Pflugers Arch.* 371:161–165.

87. Proctor, D. N., W. E. Sinning, J. M. Walro, G. C. Sieck, and P. W. Lemon. 1995. Oxidation capacity of human muscle fiber types: effects of age and training status. *J Appl Physiol.* 78:2033–2038.

88. Rall, J. A. 1985. Energetic aspects of skeletal muscle contraction: implications of fiber types. *Exercise Sport Sci Rev.* 13:33–74.

89. Rooney, K. J., R. D. Herbert, and R. J. Balnave. 1994. Fatigue contributes to the strength training stimulus. *Med Sci Sports Exerc.* 26:1160–1164.

90. Sahlin, K., G. Palmskog, and E. Hultman. 1978. Adenine nucleotide and IMP contents of the quadriceps muscle in man after exercise. *Pflugers Arch.* 374:193–198.

91. Salminen, A. 1985. Lysosomal changes in skeletal muscles during the repair of exercise injuries in muscle fibers. *Acta Physiol Scand.* 124 (Suppl 539):5–31.

92. Saltin, B. 1975. Adaptive changes in carbohydrate metabolism with exercise. In Howald, H., and J. Poortmans (eds.), *Metabolic Adaptation to Prolonged Physical Exercise.* Basel, Switzerland: Birkhäuser Verlag, pp. 94–100.

93. Saltin, B., J. Henriksson, E. Nygaard, and P. Andersen. 1977. Fiber types and metabolic potentials of skeletal muscles in sedentary man and endurance runners. *Ann NY Acad Sci.* 301:3–29.

94. Sargeant, A. J. 1994. Human power output and muscle fatigue. *Int J Sports Med.* 15:116–121.

95. Schantz, P., R. Billeter, J. Henriksson, and E. Jansson. 1982. Training-induced increase in myofibrillar ATPase intermediate fibers in human skeletal muscle. *Muscle Nerve.* 5:628–636.

96. Schantz, P., E. Randall-Fox, W. Hutchison, A. Tydén, and P. O. Åstrand. 1983. Muscle fibre type distribution, muscle cross-sectional area and maximal voluntary strength in humans. *Acta Physiol Scand.* 117:219–226.

97. Schoenberg, M. 1988. The kinetics of weakly- and strongly-binding crossbridges: implications for contraction and relaxation. *Adv Exp Med Biol.* 226:189–202.

98. Sjöström, M., S. Kidman, K. H. Larsén, and K. A. Ångquist. 1982. Z- and M-band appearance in different histochemically defined types of human skeletal muscle fibers. *J Histochem Cytochem.* 30(1):1–11.

99. Somlyo, A. P. 1985. Excitation-contraction coupling: The messenger across the gap. *Nature.* 316:298–299.

100. Staron, R. S., R. S. Hikida, F. C. Hagerman, G. A. Dudley, and T. F. Murray. 1984. Human skeletal muscle fiber type adaptability to various workloads. *J Histochem Cytochem.* 32(2):146–152.

101. Stephens, J., and A. Taylor. 1972. Fatigue of maintained voluntary muscle contraction in man. *J Physiol* (London). 220:1–18.

102. Stewart, M., A. D. McLachlan, and C. R. Calladine. 1987. A model to account for the elastic element in muscle crossbridges in terms of a bending myosin rod. *Proc Roy Soc.* (London) 229:381–413.

103. Takaishi, T., Y. Yasuda, and T. Moritani. 1994. Neuromuscular fatigue during prolonged pedalling exercise at different pedalling rates. *Eur J Appl Physiol.* 69:154–158.

104. Talmadge, R. J., R. R. Roy, and V. R. Edgerton. 1993. Muscle fiber types and function. *Curr Opin Rheumatol.* 5:695–705.

105. Tesch, P. A., and J. Karlsson. 1985. Muscle fiber types and size in trained and untrained muscles of elite athletes. *J Appl Physiol.* 59:1716–1720.

106. Tesch, P., B. Sjödon, A.Thorstensson, and J. Karlsson. 1978. Muscle fatigue and its relation to lactate accumulation and LDH activity in man. *Acta Physiol Scand.* 103:413–420.

107. Tesch, P. A., A. Thorstensson, and B. Essen-Gustavsson. 1989.

Enzyme activities of FT and ST muscle fibers in heavy-resistance trained athletes. *J Appl Physiol.* 67:83–87.

108. Thomson, J. A., H. J. Green, and M. E. Houston. 1979. Muscle glycogen depletion patterns in fast twitch fibre subgroups of man during submaximal and supramaximal exercise. *Pflugers Arch.* 379:105–108.

109. Thorstensson, A. 1976. Muscle strength, fibre types and enzyme activities in man. *Acta Physiol Scand.* (Suppl 443):7–45.

110. Thorstensson, A., and J. Karlsson. 1976. Fatiguability and fibre composition of human skeletal muscle. *Acta Physiol Scand.* 98:318–322.

111. Thorstensson, A., L. Larsson, P. Tesch, and J. Karlsson. 1977. Muscle strength and fiber composition in athletes and sedentary men. *Med Sci Sports.* 9:26–30.

112. Tregear, R. T. 1986. Muscle contraction: crossbridges, force and motion. *Nature.* 321:563.

113. Trivedi, B., and W. H. Danforth. 1966. Effect of pH on the kinetics of frog muscle phosphofructokinase. *J Biol Chem.* 241:4110–4112.

114. Vogler, C., and K. E. Bove. 1985. Morphology of skeletal muscle in children. *Arch Pathol Lab Med.* 109:238–242.

115. Vollestad, N. K. 1995. Metabolic correlates of fatigue from different types of exercise in man. *Adv Exp Med Biol.* 384:185–194.

116. Vollestad, N. K., O. Vaage, and L. Hermansen. 1984. Muscle glycogen depletion in type I and subgroups of type II fibers during prolonged severe exercise in man. *Acta Physiol Scand.* 122:433–441.

117. Vrbova, G. 1979. Influence of activity on some characteristic properties of slow and fast mammalian muscles. *Exercise Sport Sci Rev.* 7:181–213.

118. Wang, N., R. S. Hikida, R. S. Staron, and J. A. Simoneau. 1993. Muscle fiber types of women after resistance training—quantitative ultrastructure and enzyme activity. *Pflugers Arch.* 424:494–502.

119. Watt, P. W., G. Goldspink, and P. S. Ward. 1984. Changes in fiber type composition in growing muscle as a result of dynamic exercise and static overload. *Muscle Nerve.* 7:50–53.

120. West, W., A. Hicks, L. Clements, and J. Dowling. 1995. The relationship between voluntary electromyogram, endurance time and intensity of effort in isometric handgrip exercise. *Eur J Appl Physiol.* 71:301–305.

121. Wilson, B. A., and W. N. Stainsby. 1978. Relation between oxygen uptake and developed tension in dog skeletal muscle. *J Appl Physiol.* 45(2):234–237.

122. Yu, L. C., and B. Brenner. 1989. Structures of actomyosin crossbridges in relaxed and rigor muscle fibers. *Biophys J.* 55:441–453.

Selected Readings

Buchthal, F., and H. Schmalbruch. 1980. Motor unit of mammalian muscle. *Physiol Rev.* 60(1):90–142.

Klug, G. A., and G. F. Tibbits. 1988. The effect of activity on calcium-mediated events in striated muscle. *Exercise and Sports Sciences Reviews.* 16:1–59.

Otten, E. 1988. Concepts and models of functional architecture in skeletal muscle. *Exercise and Sports Sciences Reviews.* 16:89–137.

section 3

Cardiorespiratory Considerations

In chapter 2 we discussed the importance of oxygen with respect to the production of ATP. For this to occur, oxygen must be transported from the environment, through our lungs, and to the muscles. It is in the mitochondria of our skeletal muscles that oxygen is consumed to yield the ATP needed for work and play. The transport of oxygen (and the removal of carbon dioxide) involves the respiratory and circulatory systems (cardiorespiratory system). In the respiratory system, the movement of air in and out of the lungs takes place, along with the exchange of oxygen and carbon dioxide between the lungs and the blood. In the circulatory system, the transport of oxygen and carbon dioxide by the blood occurs, as does gas exchange between blood and muscle.

In section 3 we shall study the functional components of the respiratory and the circulatory systems (chapters 7, 8, and 9). We will also discuss the processes by which gas transport and blood flow are regulated (chapter 10).

To facilitate your studies we draw heavily upon six key or basic equations that are often used in cardiac and respiratory physiology. These equations are explained in this section and summarized nicely in a student study guide provided as *Appendix H*. The six equations you need to become well familiar with are:

$$\dot{V}_E \ (L \cdot min^{-1}) = V_T \times f$$

$$\dot{Q} \ (L \cdot min^{-1}) = heart\ rate \times stroke\ volume$$

$$P_{mean} \ (mm\ Hg) = diastolic\ blood\ pressure + \tfrac{1}{3}\ pulse\ pressure$$

$$T_S P_R \ (mm\ Hg \cdot L^{-1} \cdot min^{-1}) = P_{mean} \div \dot{Q}$$

$$a - \overline{v}O_2\ diff\ (mL \cdot L^{-1}) = arterial\text{-}mixed\ venous\ O_2\ difference$$

$$\dot{V}O_2 \ (L \cdot min^{-1}) = \dot{Q} \times a - \overline{v}O_2\ diff$$

Finally, much of the information found in this section serves as a foundation for additional material discussed elsewhere in this book. This section also prepares students for advanced training in exercise science and future studies in the clinical disciplines. All in all, this section should make a valuable contribution to your professional preparation.

The following chapters are contained within this section:

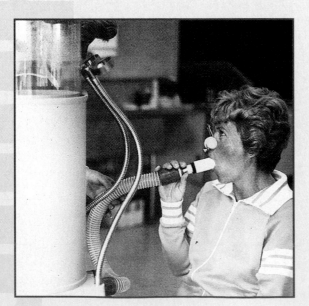

chapter seven

7

Pulmonary Ventilation and Mechanics

The movement of air into and out of the lungs is accomplished by a well developed system capable of accommodating both the resting individual and the competing Olympic athlete. While sitting and reading this text, you require that $\sim$ 5 L to 10 L of air be exchanged per minute. On the other hand, the competing Olympic athlete may demand well over 150 L of air each minute. The lungs, therefore, are "intended for exercise,"[17] capable of exchanging O_2 (and CO_2) at levels that are 15 to 30 times those observed at rest. In fact, the complex task of "acquiring" the O_2 necessary to sustain life, let alone to sustain exercise, begins within the pulmonary system. That is why many pulmonary physiologists believe their field of study is one of the most important areas of human function. Without debating the issue, it is safe to say that, indeed, the study of pulmonary ventilation and mechanics represents an important topic—one that should prove to be both challenging and intellectually satisfying.

Our study of pulmonary or respiratory exercise physiology includes the mechanical properties of the lung, alveolar ventilation, the respiratory regulation of pH, and several special topics. While studying this material you may find it helpful to refer to appendix A, which includes a standardized list of cardiorespiratory symbols as well as examples of typical pulmonary function values often measured in adult fitness, clinical, and research laboratories.

The Lung—Structure and Function

Ventilatory Mechanics

Standard Lung Volumes, Capacities, and Measures

Minute Ventilation

Lactate Threshold and Its Detection Using Gas Exchange

Unique Issues Related to the Respiratory System and Pulmonary Gas Exchange

Respiratory Regulation of pH

Summary

The major concepts to be learned from this chapter are as follows:

- A primary responsibility of the lungs and the entire respiratory system is to facilitate the exchange of O_2 and CO_2 between the ambient external environment and the internal environment of our body.
- The exchange of O_2 and CO_2 occurs in the alveoli and is regulated by the partial pressure of these gases in both alveoli air and pulmonary capillary blood.
- Ventilation is brought about through activity of the respiratory muscles, which are skeletal muscles located within the thoracic (rib) cage but not in the lungs themselves.
- During exercise, ventilation may be 15 to 30 times greater than at rest.
- In a healthy individual, exercise capacity is not normally limited by ventilation.
- Alveolar ventilation, ventilation of the tiny air sacs (alveoli) in the lungs, ensures adequate oxygenation of the blood as well as removal of CO_2.
- During exercise, lactate threshold can indirectly be identified by gas exchange using the V-slope method.
- The respiratory system aids in the regulation of the H^+ concentration in the blood and cerebrospinal fluid by changing the rate and depth of breathing.
- The two greatest sources contributing to the decrease in pH during exercise are carbonic acid, secondary to the metabolic production of CO_2, and lactate from anaerobic glycolysis.
- Alkali reserve refers to the amount of HCO_3^- available to buffer dissolved CO_2

The Lung—Structure and Function

A primary purpose of the lungs and of the entire respiratory system is to facilitate the exchange of O_2 and CO_2 between the external environment we live in and the internal environment of our body. This is accomplished by (a) the movement of air in and out of the lungs (ventilation) and (b) the movement (**diffusion**)* of O_2 and CO_2.

The actual processes of moving O_2 into the blood and CO_2 into the soon-to-be exhaled air occurs at the level of the **alveoli** (singular, **alveolus**). The alveoli are tiny (microscopic) structures—sometimes called air sacs—that are in very close contact with the pulmonary capillaries. There are literally millions of alveoli, providing a vast surface area for gas exchange to take place. Figure 7.1A shows the various organs that comprise the respiratory system as well as where the alveoli are located within it.

The diffusion of O_2 and CO_2 across the alveoli-pulmonary capillary interface is regulated by the partial pressure† of these gases within both alveolar air and pulmonary capillary blood. Each gas "moves" or is driven from an area of higher partial pressure to an area of lower partial pressure, until equilibrium is achieved. The pressure gradients associated with air and blood during inspiration and exhalation are shown in figure 7.1B. A more in-depth discussion of gas exchange (diffusion, partial pressure, and pressure gradients) is presented in chapter 8 on pages 196–199.

Ventilatory Mechanics

The entire process of getting O_2 to the exercising muscles must first begin with moving air into the lungs. And, ultimately, changes in intrapulmonary pressure lead to this movement of air. Specifically, variations in the size or volume of the thoracic cage due to contraction and relaxation of the respiratory muscles results in changes in intrapulmonary pressure (i.e., the pressure inside the lungs). The mechanisms responsible for this are described next.

Movement of the Thoracic Cage—The Respiratory (Ventilatory) Muscles

Figure 7.2 shows the thoracic cavity and the main respiratory muscles. These muscles include the diaphragm and the intercostal muscles. The lungs themselves are passive contributors to the respiratory movements of breathing because they contain no respiratory muscles.

---

*Diffusion is the random movement of molecules, in this case gas molecules.
†Partial pressure expresses the pressure of a gas in a gas mixture (air) or a liquid (blood).

Muscles of Inspiration

During quiet (resting) inspiration or inhalation, the size of the thoracic cage is increased longitudinally (neck to abdomen) by contraction of the diaphragm muscle; it is increased transversely (left to right) and anteriorially-posteriorly (front to back) by contraction of the external intercostal muscles. The diaphragm, the principal muscle of inspiration[19] is a large, dome-shaped muscle innervated by the left and right phrenic nerves. Stimulation of the phrenic nerve during inspiration causes the diaphragm to contract or flatten (i.e., its domed portion is lowered), thus increasing the longitudinal diameter of the thoracic cavity. Contraction of the diaphragm contributes up to three-fourths of the total air we inhale with each breath or *tidal volume* (V_T).[19,22,53]

The intercostal muscles (see insert in figure 7.2) lie between successive ribs (*intercostal* means "between ribs") and consist of two layers. The fibers of the external layer (the external intercostal muscles) are so arranged that when they contract, the ribs are lifted and rotated outward, thus increasing the transverse and anterior-posterior diameters of the thoracic cavity.

The larger V_T that occurs during exercise (i.e., from 0.5 L at rest to more than 2.0 L during exercise) is also caused by contraction of accessory inspiratory muscles, all of which further increase the size of the rib cage.[15] For example, contraction of the scalene muscles elevates the first two ribs, and contraction of the sternocleidomastoid muscles elevates the sternum (front of thorax). During maximal exercise, contraction of the trapezius muscle and the extensor muscles of the back and neck may also facilitate inspiration.

Muscles of Expiration

Simple relaxation of the diaphragm and external intercostal muscles during quiet expiration or exhalation permits the thoracic cage to return to its original size. In other words, expiration under resting conditions is passive and independent of the expiratory muscles. This happens because during inspiration the elastic tissues of the lungs and the walls of the thorax (connective tissue, cartilage, and muscle) are stretched, thus storing potential energy. Therefore, reduction in the size of the thoracic cage during normal expiration results from the elastic recoil of these tissues brought about by the release of stored energy.

During exercise, expiration is usually active, facilitated by contractions of the expiratory muscles—especially the *abdominal* group (rectus and transverse abdominus muscles and abdominal obliques).[22] Contraction of these muscles increases pressure inside the abdomen by decreasing the anterior-posterior size of the abdomen and depressing the lower ribs. These movements force the diaphragm upward and into the thoracic cavity. The *internal intercostal muscles* are also muscles of expiration. Their fibers (see insert in figure 7.2) and movements are diametrically opposed

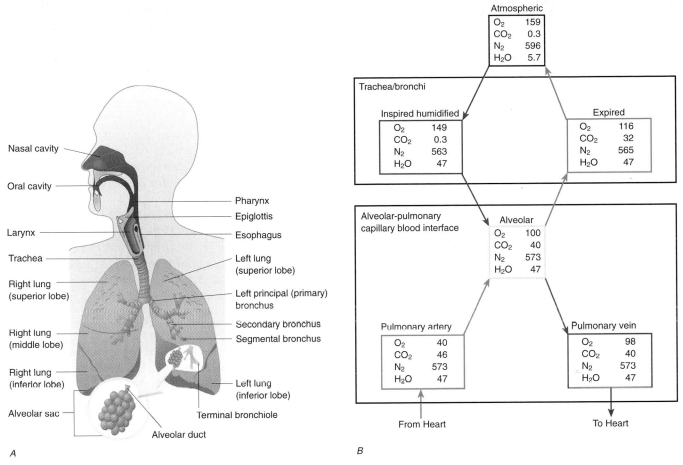

A

B

Figure 7.1

A. The gross and microscopic anatomy of the respiratory or pulmonary system. The inset is a section of lung tissue showing many smaller alveoli and a larger alveolar duct. The pulmonary capillaries run in the walls of the alveoli and are not visible.
B. The distribution of partial pressures (mm Hg) in air and pulmonary capillary blood during resting inspiration and expiration.

to those of the external intercostals, and when active, they lower the ribs and move them closer together. All these actions aid in reducing the size of the thorax and thus facilitate the act of expiration.

The Respiratory Muscles and Training

Because the respiratory muscles are skeletal muscles, it appears that their strength and endurance can be increased with training programs.[10,26] This is particularly true if the training programs are limited to the ventilatory muscles.[5,29,30] Such changes in strength and endurance may be partly responsible for the lower ventilatory response to exercise observed in some athletes.[30] Increases in the strength and endurance of the respiratory muscles as a result of training might also explain the slightly greater lung volumes ($\sim$ 4% to 15%) sometimes observed in athletes, especially swimmers.[13]

A summary of the major respiratory muscles and their actions during rest and exercise is contained in table 7.1.

Pressure Changes

At the beginning of this chapter, we explained that changes in thoracic cavity size or volume result in changes in intrapulmonary pressure. These changes ultimately lead to the movement of air into and out of the lungs.

The Pleural Cavity

The lungs are not directly attached to the inner walls of the thorax. Rather, they are "connected" by a thin film of fluid, called *serous fluid,* which covers and is secreted by the inner surfaces of two thin serous membranes, collectively known as the **pleurae** (singular, **pleura**). The outer surface of one pleura has two components: the part that lines the thoracic wall, which is called the *parietal pleura* (*parietal* means "wall"), and the part that covers the diaphragm, which is called the *diaphragmatic pleura.* The outer surface of the other pleura covers the lungs; this is the *visceral* pleura (*visceral* pertains to internal organs). The "potential

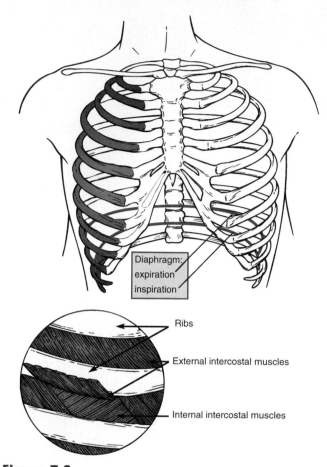

Figure 7.2

The ventilatory muscles. The diaphragm and the intercostal muscles (insert) are the principal muscles of respiration.

space" between these two pleurae is called the *pleural cavity*. The thin film of serous fluid is located within this cavity. Through this fluid connection, any movements and resulting pressure changes that occur in the thorax are reflected directly in the lungs. These relationships are shown in figure 7.3.

Intrapulmonary and Intrapleural Pressures

As the previous discussion indicates, expansion of the thorax leads to expansion of the lungs. And whenever a given volume of gas is suddenly expanded, the space between gas molecules becomes greater, in effect reducing their pressure. Thus, during inspiration, *intrapleural pressure* (pressure within the pleural space) is reduced such that intrapulmonary pressure is also reduced to below atmospheric pressure, causing air to flow into the lungs. As air fills the lungs, intrapulmonary pressure rises, and when it is equal

again to atmospheric pressure (at end-inspiration), airflow ceases. The opposite is true during expiration. Passive or active compression (or both) of the thorax raises intrapleural pressure such that intrapulmonary pressure eventually exceeds atmospheric pressure, and air flows out of the lungs. At end-expiration, intrapulmonary pressure is again equal to atmospheric pressure, and there is no movement of air.

Hopefully you've noticed that changes in intrapleural (or intrathoracic) pressure occur in a direction that is similar to the changes that occur inside the lung (intrapulmonary). However, intrapleural pressure is always lower (~ 5 mm Hg) than intrapulmonary and atmospheric pressures. The reason for this is related to the elastic tissues of the lungs and thoracic walls, which create a partial vacuum or subatmospheric pressure in the pleural cavity. The changes that occur in intrapulmonary pressure, in intrapleural pressure, and in lung volume during inspiration and expiration are summarized in figure 7.4.

Standard Lung Volumes, Capacities, and Measures

There are several standard lung volumes and lung capacities with which you should become familiar. *Lung volumes* cannot be further subdivided and include **tidal volume (V_T)**, **residual volume (RV)**, **expiratory reserve volume (ERV)**, and **inspiratory reserve volume (IRV)**.

The *lung capacities,* which result from adding two or more lung volumes, include: **functional residual capacity** (FRC = ERV + RV), **inspiratory capacity** (IC = IRV + V_T), **total lung capacity** (TLC = IC + FRC), and **vital capacity** (VC = IRV + V_T + ERV). Most of these volumes and capacities are used as measures of pulmonary function; therefore, knowledge of them will enable you to better understand respiratory physiology. Most are easily measured with an instrument called a **spirometer.***

Spirometers have changed greatly over the years. Figure 7.5A shows a cutaway drawing of an older, bell-type spirometer, one used to make the spirographs shown in figures 7.5B (untrained) and 7.5C (trained). This particular instrument consists of two metal containers, one inverted over the other. The inverted container is made airtight by sealing it in a column of water. As the person exhales through a hose and into the spirometer, the inverted container, called the bell, moves up, whereas on inhalation, the bell moves down. The up-and-down movements of the bell, which correspond to the volume of air breathed, are

---

*Residual volume (and thus functional residual capacity and total lung capacity) cannot be measured directly with a spirometer. Its measurement is more complex and involves gas dilution or washout methods.

7.1

table

The major respiratory muscles during rest and exercise

Respiratory phase	Muscles acting during rest	Action	Muscles acting during exercise
Inspiration	Diaphragm External intercostals	Flattens Raises ribs Elevates first and second ribs Elevates sternum	Diaphragm External intercostals Scalenes Sternocleidomastoids
Expiration	None	Lowers ribs Depresses lower ribs and forces diaphragm into thorax	Internal intercostals Abdominals

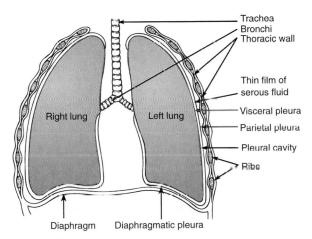

Figure 7.3

The pleural cavity.

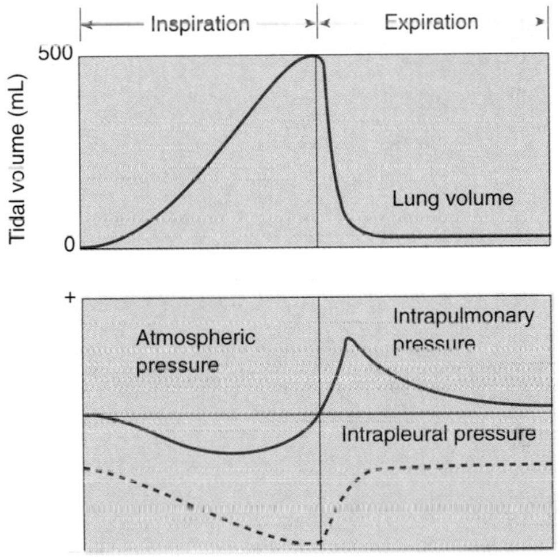

Figure 7.4

Changes in intrapulmonary ("within the lungs") and intrapleural ("between the lung wall and thoracic wall") pressures and lung volume during inspiration and expiration at rest.

recorded on a rotating chart by a marker. Using this older-type instrument, the test supervisor then computes the volumes and capacities by hand. Such a device, although no longer used in clinical pulmonary laboratories, does help students develop a practical understanding of how one lung volume differs from another (e.g., ERV vs. IRV) and of how a lung capacity is a combination of two or more lung volumes.

Today more contemporary, fully automated, desktop spirometers are available. Such devices are simpler to set up, maintain, and use; they also eliminate the need for calculations by hand. Table 7.2 contains a list of the lung volumes and capacities, their definitions, and the approximate

changes they undergo during exercise. Students are encouraged to familiarize themselves with this material.

Although some evidence exists to the contrary,[2] current thinking is that endurance training generally has little, if any, effect on altering lung structure, volumes, or capacities. This holds true for males and females, although the absolute values for females are ~ 20% below those observed for males. With endurance training, TLC and VC may be unchanged or increased slightly (figures 7.5B vs. 7.5C). VT is generally unchanged. However, as a rule swimmers often develop a larger VC than their matched counterparts, possibly resulting from a form of "resistance training" that they undergo while exhaling into the water.[13]

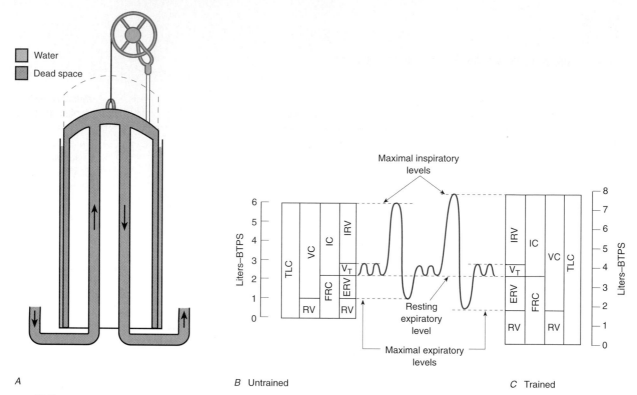

Figure 7.5

A cutaway drawing (*A*) of a spirometer from which spirographic tracings are made. As a person exhales into the spirometer, the inverted container, called a bell, rises; upon inhalation, the bell moves down. Up-and-down movements of the bell are recorded on a kymograph and are referred to as a spirogram. As shown in these spirograms, various lung volumes at rest (except V_T) can be smaller in untrained (*B*) than in trained (*C*) individuals. For definitions and key abbreviations, see table 7.2.

(*Data from untrained subjects from Comroe et al.[12]; data for trained subjects from Holmgren.[24]*)

table 7.2

Definition of lung volumes and capacities, typical values at rest, and their changes during exercise as compared with rest

Lung volume or capacity	Definition	Typical values at rest	Change during exercise
Tidal volume (V_T)	Volume inspired or expired per breath	400–600 mL	Increase
Inspiratory reserve volume (IRV)	Maximal volume inspired from end-inspiration	3100 mL	Decrease
Expiratory reserve volume (ERV)	Maximal volume expired from end-expiration	1200 mL	Decrease
Residual volume (RV)	Volume remaining at end of maximal expiration	1200 mL	Slight decrease
Total lung capacity (TLC)	Volume in lung at end of maximal inspiration	6000 mL	Slight decrease
Vital capacity (VC)	Maximal volume forcefully expired after maximal inspiration	4800 mL	Slight decrease
Inspiratory capacity (IC)	Maximal volume inspired from resting expiratory level	3600 mL	Increase

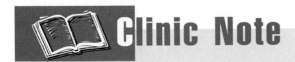

Clinic Note

Pulmonary Disease and Rehabilitation

Two major lung disorders resulting in abnormal spirometry measures are *restrictive* and *obstructive* disorders. Restrictive lung diseases, as the name implies, are related to the inability (restriction) of the lungs to inflate properly. Causes of restrictive lung disease can result from both problems within the lungs proper (e.g., pulmonary fibrosis) or in the chest (e.g., obesity or neuromuscular disorders). Hallmark to patients with restrictive lung disease are reduced lung volumes (total lung capacity, vital capacity, residual volume). Patients with obstructive lung disorders, diseases "obstructing" the ability of the lungs to exhale, may demonstrate a normal or greater than normal total lung capacity and residual volume; however, expiratory flow measures are characteristically reduced—sometimes to less than 50% of normal.

A common expiratory measure used during routine spirometry is forced vital capacity (FVC), which is the amount of air that can be forcefully exhaled from the lungs after maximal inhalation. Of that air, the amount that can be exhaled in the first second is called *forced expiratory volume$_1$* (FEV$_1$). Among healthy males and females FEV$_1$ should generally exceed 3.0 L and 2.0 L, respectively. Clinically, a very useful measure of expiratory flow is the ratio between FEV$_1$ and FVC. In normal persons, this ratio (FEV$_1$/FVC) exceeds 75%. In other words, more than 75% of one's FVC should be exhaled in the first second.

Two diseases that are grouped under the broad classification of chronic obstructive pulmonary disease (COPD) are emphysema and chronic obstructive bronchitis.[4] Patients with *emphysema* have overdistension and destruction of the bronchioles, alveolar ducts, and/or alveoli. The destruction of this and other tissue within the lungs can result in the loss of pulmonary elastic recoil, airflow limitation, and a reduction of the alveolar-capillary surface for gas exchange. Without question, cigarette smoking contributes greatly to causing and worsening emphysema. In fact, approximately one of every two people who smoke cigarettes—that's 50%—go on to develop emphysema.

Chronic obstructive bronchitis is defined as the chronic production of mucus to cause cough with expectoration for at least three months of the year for more than two consecutive years. The airflow obstruction is mainly caused by thickened bronchial walls resulting from excess secretions from both the large and small airways.

These two disorders are not mutually exclusive. For example, a patient with emphysema may meet the clinical criteria for chronic obstructive bronchitis as well. Whatever the underlying problem, the symptom of which most all COPD patients complain—the one that limits their ability to exert themselves for any period of time—is called dyspnea (labored breathing). Ultimately, a vicious cycle takes hold, where decreasing one's level of physical activity to avoid dyspnea leads to further deconditioning—which then leads to even more dyspnea on exertion. Additionally, isolationism, loss of self-confidence, frustration, and depression are commonly associated with COPD.

Until almost the 1970s, the standard therapy for patients with COPD was rest, stopping smoking, and the avoidance of stress (including limiting physical activity). However, many studies over the past two decades have shown that patients with COPD can benefit from a structured, multidimensional program involving education, breathing retraining, and exercise rehabilitation.[40,51] In fact, pulmonary rehabilitation programs are now quite common not only in the U.S. but in many other countries as well.

COPD patients enrolled in pulmonary rehabilitation programs regularly attend classes about energy conservation techniques, proper nutrition, medications, and breathing mechanics. In addition, two or three times per week they participate in a supervised exercise class led by a registered nurse, respiratory therapist, physical therapist, or exercise specialist. During exercise, many of these patients receive supplemental O$_2$ to avoid exercise-induced hypoxemia. As a result of their participation in a pulmonary rehabilitation program, patients generally feel better and go on to experience fewer disease-related hospitalizations. They are also physically able to be more active before experiencing limiting dyspnea. The patients often perceive the above changes as being an improvement in the quality of their lives. However, the gains these patients experience (e.g., increased walking distance or less dyspnea with stairs) do not necessarily translate into improvements in VC, FEV$_1$, or $\dot{V}O_2$ max. Nonetheless, it does not make the functional gains they achieve any less meaningful.

Minute Ventilation

In addition to the lung volumes and capacities discussed previously, another significant measure to introduce is ventilation. Ventilation is composed of two phases: one that brings air into the lungs, called *inspiration,* and one that lets air out into the environment, called *expiration.* **Minute ventilation** refers to the amount (liters) of air we either inspire or expire (but not both) in one minute. Most often it refers to expired ($\dot{V}_E$)* rather than inspired ($\dot{V}_I$) air. This amount can be determined by knowing both (a) the V_T (i.e., how much air we expire in one breath) and (b) the respiratory frequency (f) (i.e., how many breaths we take in one minute). In other words:

$$
\begin{array}{ccccc}
\dot{V}_E & = & V_T & \times & f \\
\text{Minute} & = & \text{Tidal volume} & \times & \text{Respiratory} \\
\text{ventilation} & & & & \text{frequency} \\
(\text{L} \cdot \text{min}^{-1}) & & (\text{L}) & & (\text{breaths per min})
\end{array}
$$

Under normal resting conditions, $\dot{V}_E$ varies considerably from person to person. Usually, we ventilate between 6 and 15 $\text{L} \cdot \text{min}^{-1}$ (BTPS)† at rest. This varies with body size and is a smaller amount in women. V_T and respiratory frequency vary even more than $\dot{V}_E$. This is easy to understand because there are many combinations of V_T and frequency that yield the same minute ventilation. At rest, typical values for V_T and frequency are 400 mL to 600 mL and 10 to 25 breaths per minute, respectively.

Ventilation and Exercise

$\dot{V}_E$ increases during exercise and the increase is directly proportional to increases in $\dot{V}O_2$ and $\dot{V}CO_2$ by the working muscles. This is shown in figure 7.6 for trained and untrained young men. Only at the extremes of exercise intensity do we see that $\dot{V}_E$ is disproportional to $\dot{V}O_2$ (figure 7.6A); however, this is not the case with $\dot{V}CO_2$ (figure 7.6B), which indicates that $\dot{V}_E$ is related more to CO_2 removal than to $\dot{V}O_2$, at least under maximal exercise.[50] The fact that ventilation increases much more than $\dot{V}O_2$ (indicated by the curved portion of the two lines in figure 7.6A) also tells us that $\dot{V}_E$ does not normally limit aerobic capacity (max $\dot{V}O_2$). Specifically, during maximal exercise when further increases in $\dot{V}O_2$ are no longer observed, most healthy persons can still achieve further increases in $\dot{V}_E$.

We must point out, however, that research over the past 15 years has shown that among some elite athletes, the pulmonary system may indeed limit $\dot{V}O_2$ max. This results

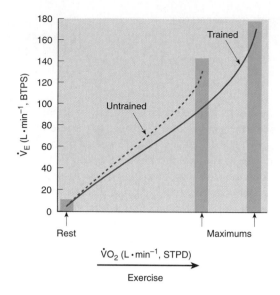

A

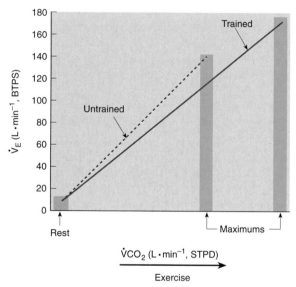

B

Figure 7.6

Effects of exercise on minute ventilation ($\dot{V}_{EBTPS}$) in trained and untrained subjects. The close relationship of $\dot{V}_E$ to $\dot{V}O_2$ is shown in *A* and to $\dot{V}CO_2$ in *B*. Note that $\dot{V}_E$ is disproportional to $\dot{V}O_2$ but not to $\dot{V}CO_2$ at maximal and near maximal values.

partly from a reduced transit time of the red blood cell through the pulmonary capillary beds, which occurs in some athletes during high intensity exercise.[17] This reduction in transit time means an insufficient amount of time exists for equilibrium to occur between gases in alveolar air and capillary blood. As a result, the partial pressure of O_2 in arterial blood (PO_2) falls slightly during exercise.

One other point to note in figure 7.6 is that trained subjects tend to have a lower $\dot{V}_E$ at any given exercise work load ($\dot{V}O_2$) or $\dot{V}CO_2$. This lower ventilatory response to exercise (or higher ventilatory efficiency), although often observed among athletes,[8,35] is most pronounced in endurance

---

*The measurement of $\dot{V}_E$, via either the Douglas bag method or a fully automated metabolic cart, is described in chapter 4.
†Body Temperature and Pressure Saturated. The procedures for calculating BTPS and STPD are given in appendix C.

athletes.[32] The physiological reason for this is not entirely known; however, it may be related to diminished peripheral receptor stimulation[8,33] or genetic/familial influences.[11,43] (Peripheral receptors are covered in more detail in chapter 10). Regardless of its cause, the lower ventilatory response during submaximal exercise may contribute to outstanding endurance athletic performance.[32]

Ventilation varies not only with work load but also before, during, and after exercise. These changes are shown in figures 7.7*A* and *B*.

Changes before Exercise

During quiet rest, ventilation (V_T and frequency) is regulated by intrinsic ("built-in") respiratory neurons located in the medulla oblongata. However, immediately before exercise begins, there is a relatively small increase in $\dot{V}_E$. Obviously, the increase is not caused by exercise itself; instead, it is caused by "voluntary" stimulation from the higher brain (i.e., cerebral cortex) acting on the respiratory control area in the medulla. This "central command" takes place as one anticipates or "gets ready for" an upcoming exercise bout.

Changes during Exercise

During exercise, there are two major changes in ventilation:

1. A very rapid increase occurs within the first few seconds after the start of exercise (figures 7.7*A* and *B*). This is primarily caused by central command from the higher brain (cortex), although nervous stimuli arising from joint/muscle receptors that are activated when the skeletal muscles begin to move may also be involved.

2. The rapid rise in ventilation soon ceases and is replaced by a slower rise, which in submaximal exercise (figure 7.7*A*) tends to level off (i.e., reach a steady-state value). This slower rise in ventilation is thought to be caused by both central command and chemical stimuli. The latter represents a "fine-tuning" effect, which acts in response to changes in the partial pressure of CO_2 (PCO_2) and H^+ concentration in cerebral spinal fluid or arterial blood. These changes in cerebral spinal fluid and blood chemistry stimulate chemoreceptors located in the medulla or in the aorta and/or carotid arteries—the latter two of which, in turn, provide regulatory feedback to the medulla.

During exercise progressed to maximum (figure 7.7*B*), the above described steady-state does not occur; rather, $\dot{V}_E$ continues to increase until exercise is terminated. Maximal exercise ventilation (max $\dot{V}_E$) can reach values exceeding 200 and 145 $L \cdot min^{-1}$ (BTPS) in male and female athletes,

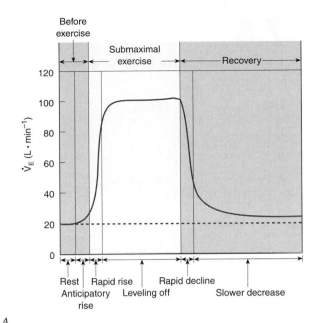

A

B

Figure 7.7

Minute ventilation ($\dot{V}_E$) increases even before exercise begins. Immediately after exercise starts, ventilation increases rapidly, then either levels off (submaximal exercise as shown in *A*) or continues to increase (maximal exercise as shown in *B*). During recovery, ventilation decreases more rapidly at first, then gradually toward resting values.

respectively. This represents about a 15- to 30-fold increase over resting values. In untrained athletes, where max $\dot{V}O_2$ and $\dot{V}CO_2$ are lower, max $\dot{V}_E$ is also lower. Along with this lower max $\dot{V}_E$ is a lower ventilatory efficiency; in other words, untrained males or females have a greater $\dot{V}_E$ at a given $\dot{V}O_2$ than do trained males or females (figure 7.6*A*).

table 7.3

Ventilatory changes before, during, and after exercise

Phase	Change	Controlling mechanism
1. Rest	—	Central and peripheral chemoreceptors influencing intrinsic pattern established by the medulla
2. Before exercise	Moderate increase	↑ Central command (cerebral cortex)
3. During exercise a. Immediate	Rapid increase	↑ Central command and possibly ↑ neural stimuli to medulla caused by activation of muscle/joint receptors
b. Mid	Steady-state or slower rise	Central or peripheral chemoreceptors reacting to ↑ PCO_2 and ↓ pH in blood or cerebral spinal fluid
c. End	Continued or rapid (hyperventilation) increase	Same as above, with possible additional input from ↑ blood potassium, ↑ blood catecholamines, ↑ body temperature, and ↑ central command
4. Recovery a. Immediate	Rapid decrease	↓ Central command
b. Later	Slower decrease toward rest	↓ Input from central and peripheral chemoreceptors as PCO_2 and pH normalize

These increases in $\dot{V}_E$ are made possible by increases in both the depth (V_T) and frequency of breathing. However, V_T tends to level off or plateau at ∼ 65% of one's VC, meaning that further increases in $\dot{V}_E$ during heavy work are predominantly caused by further increases in breathing frequency alone.[17] During all-out maximal exercise, V_T among some elite athletes may be five to six times greater than at rest, exceeding 3.0 L per breath! At the same time respiratory frequency may exceed 60 per min. The increase in V_T results from the equal utilization of both IRV and the ERV.[27]

Changes during Recovery

During recovery from exercise, there are again two major changes (figure 7.7 *A* or *B*):

1. As soon as exercise is stopped, there is a sudden decrease in ventilation. This results from a decrease in central (voluntary) command from the higher brain.
2. After the sudden decrease in ventilation, there is a gradual or slower decrease toward resting values. The more severe the work, the longer it takes for ventilation to return to resting levels. This decrease is proportional to the decrease in receptor stimulation that occurs as PCO_2 and pH levels in the cerebral spinal fluid and/or blood return to pre-exercise values.

A summary of these ventilatory changes is given in table 7.3. We will discuss their control in more detail in chapter 10.

Alveolar Ventilation and Dead Space

Not all the fresh air we inspire each minute takes part in the gas exchange that occurs within the capillaries that perfuse the lungs. Only the portion of fresh air that reaches the alveoli, called **alveolar ventilation** ($\dot{V}_A$), assists with the oxygenation of pulmonary capillary blood (and removal of CO_2). The volume of fresh air that does not participate in gas exchange is referred to as dead space ventilation (V_D). The space (nose, mouth, pharynx, larynx, trachea, bronchi, and bronchioles) it occupies in the pulmonary system is called **anatomical dead space.** Thus:

$$\dot{V}_E = \dot{V}_A + \dot{V}_D$$

V_D is difficult to measure in humans, particularly during exercise. In fact, V_D may double during exercise because of dilation of the respiratory passages. However, because V_T also increases, an adequate $\dot{V}_A$ is maintained.

It should now be clear that $\dot{V}_E$ alone does not indicate whether $\dot{V}_A$ is adequate. Instead, $\dot{V}_A$ is dependent on three factors: (1) depth of breathing (V_T), (2) rate of breathing (frequency), and (3) V_D. For example, in figure 7.8A and B, resting $\dot{V}_E$ is 6.0 L · min^{-1}. However, in figure 7.8A, V_T is 0.5 L and respiratory frequency is 12 breaths · min^{-1}. This differs from figure 7.8B, where V_T is reduced to 0.25 L and frequency is increased to 24 breaths · min^{-1}. If V_D in each case is 0.15 L, then 0.35 L of fresh air will enter the alveoli per breath in figure 7.8A, but only 0.10 L will enter the alveoli in figure 7.8B. This means that $\dot{V}_A$ in figure 7.8A

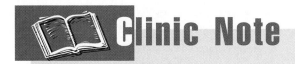

Clinic Note

Asthma is a very common disorder, affecting 4% to 5% of the U.S. population. The common denominator underlying an asthmatic attack is hyperirritability of the tracheobronchial tree, which leads to bronchoconstriction and a dramatic decrease in air flow. Although the precise mechanism responsible for increased airway reactivity is unknown, several precipitating stimuli have been identified. These include allergens such as pollens; pharmacologic stimuli (e.g., aspirin); infections; air pollutants (e.g., ozone); occupational exposure to metals such as platinum, chrome, and nickel; emotional stress; and exercise.

In fact, of the above-mentioned precipitating factors, exercise is one of the more common culprits. However, exercise as a stimulus for asthma differs from other naturally occurring factors like antigens and viral infections because it does not produce long-term ramifications—nor does it alter future airway reactivity. For many patients with asthma, exercise provides the first clue that they have the disorder. When followed over a period of time, patients with true exercise-induced asthma begin to manifest asthmatic events at times other than exercise. Additionally, exercise-induced asthma (sometimes called exercise-induced bronchoconstriction) more often than not occurs after

exercise has stopped, reaching a peak response as soon as 5 minutes after exercise. Such a response may require up to 30 minutes before full recovery is achieved.

Exercise-induced asthma seems to be influenced by a variety of factors, including minute ventilation, air temperature, and the water content of inspired air. For example, for the same inspired air conditions, vigorous running may precipitate a more severe attack than walking. Alternately, walking or skating in cold, dry air may be more provocative of an attack than walking or swimming in an environment with warm, moist air. Finally, it appears that the underlying mechanism leading to airway obstruction may not be contraction of the bronchial smooth muscle alone. It may also result from hyperemia or engorgement of the small blood vessels supplying the bronchial tree.

Effective treatment strategies include medications meant to open the airways (bronchodilators) as well as those aimed at stabilizing the cells (mast cells) that produce the chemicals that initiate bronchoconstriction. Additionally, prevention is very important, which means avoiding or controlling those factors (i.e., air temperature and humidity) that can precipitate or trigger an asthmatic attack.

---

will be $4.2 \text{ L} \cdot \text{min}^{-1}$, adequate to ensure the sufficient exchange of gases at the alveolar-capillary interface. On the other hand, $\dot{V}_A$ in figure 7.8B will be reduced to only $2.4 \text{ L} \cdot \text{min}^{-1}$, a value that is low and associated with inadequate gas exchange, even at rest.

These relationships also point out why doubling V_D during exercise does not necessarily lead to decreased $\dot{V}_A$, provided that V_T and frequency increase proportionally. For example, if during moderate exercise:

$$\dot{V}_E = 40 \text{ L} \cdot \text{min}^{-1}$$
$$V_T = 1.6 \text{ L} \cdot \text{breath}^{-1}$$
$$V_D = 0.3 \text{ L} \cdot \text{breath}^{-1}$$
$$\text{frequency} - 25 \text{ breaths} \cdot \text{min}^{-1}$$

Then:

$$\dot{V}_A = (V_T - V_D) \times f$$
$$= (1.6 - 0.3) \times 25 = 32.5 \text{ L} \cdot \text{min}^{-1}$$

This volume of inspired air actually reaches the alveoli, which, along with an approximate threefold increase in pulmonary capillary blood volume, helps ensure that alveolar and capillary O_2 levels reach equilibrium during exercise.

Lactate Threshold and Its Detection Using Gas Exchange

During incremental exercise to exhaustion, $\dot{V}O_2$ increases in a linear fashion. However, the simultaneous measurement of blood lactate during the same exercise bout shows no change in this blood chemistry until $\dot{V}O_2$ exceeds $\sim 50\%$ or more of maximum.[16] The point where the nonlinear increase in blood lactate occurs during exercise is called the **lactate threshold,** or onset of blood lactate accumulation.

Assessing changes in blood lactate concentration during exercise requires that a very small sample of blood ($\sim 25 \ \mu\text{L}$) be obtained at rest and periodically during incremental exercise. At rest, blood lactate is approximately $0.5 \text{ mmol} \cdot \text{L}^{-1}$ to $1.0 \text{ mmol} \cdot \text{L}^{-1}$,* and during or

---

*$1 \text{ mmol} \cdot \text{L}^{-1}$ of lactic acid = 9 milligrams (mg) per 100 mL of blood. Therefore, a resting lactate level of $0.6 \text{ mmol} \cdot \text{L}^{-1} = 5.4 \text{ mg} \cdot 100 \text{ mL}^{-1}$ of blood. An exercise value of $4 \text{ mmol} \cdot \text{L}^{-1} = 36 \text{ mg} \cdot 100 \text{ mL}^{-1}$ of blood.

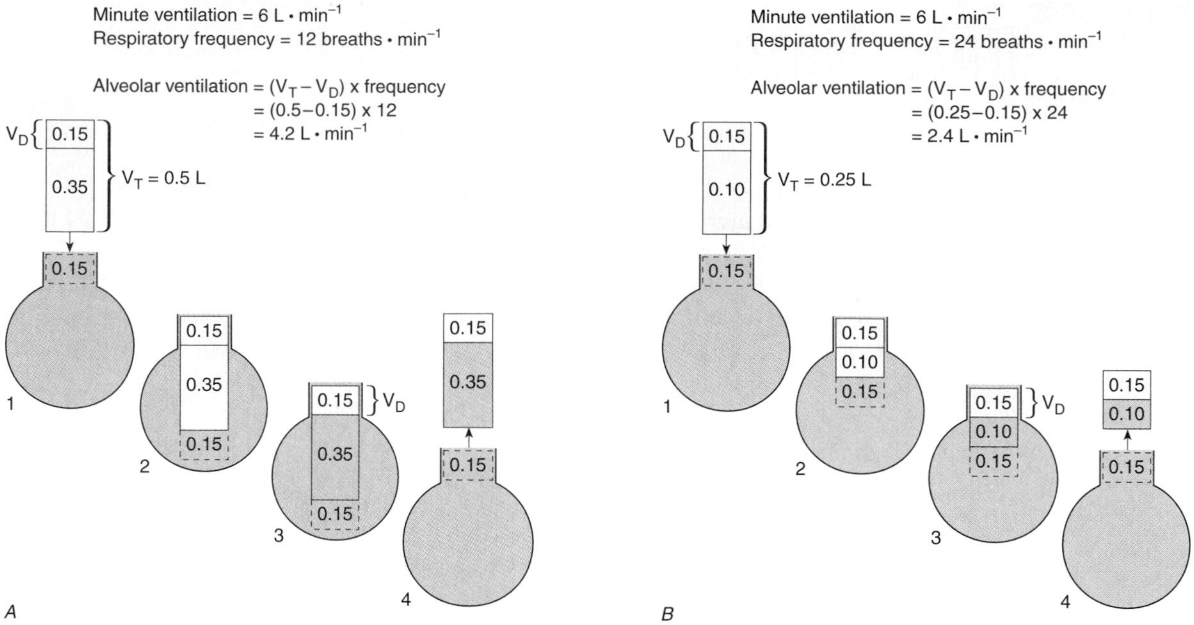

Minute ventilation = 6 L · min⁻¹
Respiratory frequency = 12 breaths · min⁻¹

Alveolar ventilation = $(V_T - V_D)$ × frequency
= (0.5 − 0.15) × 12
= 4.2 L · min⁻¹

V_D { 0.15
0.35 } V_T = 0.5 L

Minute ventilation = 6 L · min⁻¹
Respiratory frequency = 24 breaths · min⁻¹

Alveolar ventilation = $(V_T - V_D)$ × frequency
= (0.25 − 0.15) × 24
= 2.4 L · min⁻¹

V_D { 0.15
0.10 } V_T = 0.25 L

A

B

Figure 7.8

Effects of tidal volume (V_T) and frequency of breathing on alveolar ventilation. The large circles represent alveoli; the necks of the circles represent the respiratory passages or dead space volume (V_D); the yellow blocks, fresh air (high in O_2, low in CO_2); pink areas, alveolar gas (low in O_2 and high in CO_2). Numbers inside blocks represent gas volumes, in liters. In *A* and *B*, both minute ventilation and dead space are equal. However, in *A* more fresh air reaches the alveoli than in *B* because the breaths are deeper but not as frequent. The numbers under the alveoli designate respiratory phases: (1) pre-inspiration, (2) inspiration, (3) end-inspiration, and (4) end-expiration.

(Modified and redrawn from Comroe et al.[12])

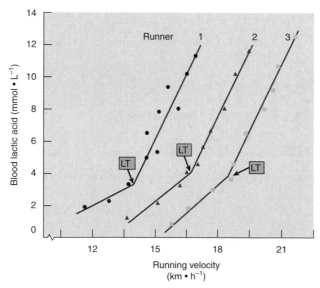

Figure 7.9

The detection of the lactate threshold involves measurement of blood lactic acid levels at different exercise intensities, such as while running on a treadmill at various speeds, as shown here. The running speed at which the lactate threshold (LT) is found (∼ 4 mmol · L⁻¹) varies from one athlete to another. Runner 1 is an example of a beginner who is totally untrained; runner 2, an experienced but only average competitor; and runner 3, a highly experienced international competitor.

following exercise it may exceed 10 to 12 mmol · L⁻¹. In fact, among elite, motivated athletes, lactate may even approach 14 to 16 mmol · L⁻¹ during exhaustive exercise. Figure 7.9 shows the detection of the lactate threshold among runners with three different levels of fitness. Note that in each runner lactate threshold occurred at a blood lactate value between 3 and 5 mmol · L⁻¹, which, for most athletes, coincides with a $\dot{V}O_2$ between 50% and 90% of maximum. However, the exercise pace (or absolute $\dot{V}O_2$) at which it occurs is generally higher in highly trained individuals than in untrained and lesser trained individuals (figure 7.9).

Some investigators equate or feel that lactate threshold is related to an event called **anaerobic threshold.**[54,55,56] Anaerobic threshold is defined as the exercise $\dot{V}O_2$ above which anaerobic energy production via glycolysis accelerates to supplement (not replace) aerobic energy production. This increase in skeletal muscle glycolysis is caused by a muscle oxygen content (end-capillary PO_2) that is insufficient or unable to keep pace with O_2 demand, resulting in the inability of the mitochondrial membrane shuttle to accept H^+ at a pace that is commensurate with production of NADH via glycolysis. In the end, pyruvate in the cytoplasm reacts with NADH + H^+ to form lactic acid, which accumulates first in the muscle and then in the blood.

We must point out, however, that other scientists feel the existence of an anaerobic threshold to be physiologi-

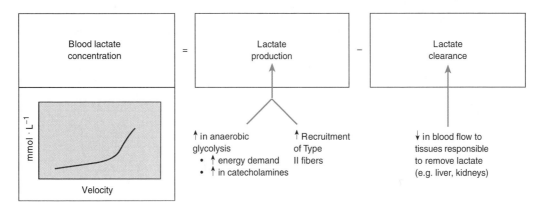

Figure 7.10

Lactate turnover at rest and during exercise is a function of those factors that affect *both* lactate production and lactate clearance.

cally incorrect.[6,7,48] They believe that a critical-capillary PO_2 is not an issue and that an increase in anaerobic glycolysis is not the only factor that can lead to the observed lactate threshold phenomenon. Figure 7.10 depicts other factors that might contribute to the disproportionate increase in blood lactate concentration during exercise.

For example, while the metabolically more active skeletal muscles are producing lactate during exercise, other organs are involved with clearing it from the blood. Two sites where this occurs include the liver and the kidneys. Therefore, factors that restrict the ability of these two organs to clear lactate would lead to its build-up in the blood. One such factor is blood flow, which is normally decreased in the liver and the kidneys during exercise. As exercise intensity increases from light to moderate to heavy, blood flow is progressively diverted away from the metabolically less active organs (i.e., kidney, liver, and gastrointestinal tract) in favor of the metabolically more active skeletal muscles.

Another factor influencing blood lactate concentration during exercise is the type of skeletal muscle recruited during activity.[46] Specifically, Type II fibers, or those better equipped for intensive, short-duration exercise, demonstrate a greater activity of a certain muscle-specific form of the enzyme lactate dehydrogenase (LDH) that facilitates the conversion of pyruvate to lactate. This differs from Type I fibers, the fibers better equipped for endurance-type activities, which have a type of LDH (heart-specific) that more readily converts lactate to pyruvate. Again, during incremental exercise progressed from mild to moderate to heavy work, Type I fibers are generally recruited first, followed by the recruitment of Type II fibers. The recruitment of Type II fibers, however, can occur when O_2 availability to the mitochondria is still sufficient (person is still aerobic). As a result, their increased involvement contributes to an increase in first muscle and then blood lactate—despite the skeletal muscles still functioning in a predominant aerobic exercise state. The "take home" message here is an appreciation that

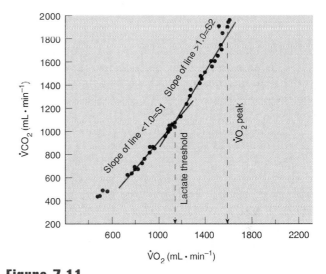

Figure 7.11

Determination of lactate threshold using the V-slope method. Patient is a 63-year-old male who suffered a heart attack in July 1996, with subsequent coronary artery angioplasty in September 1996. Exercise test was performed in November 1996, just prior to entering cardiac rehabilitation. Peak $\dot{V}O_2$ was 1590 mL · min^{-1} and estimated lactate threshold occurred at a $\dot{V}O_2$ of 1150 mL · min^{-1}, or approximately 72% of peak.

blood lactate concentration during exercise is simply not the result of anaerobic glycolysis alone.

Despite the debate as to whether or not anaerobic threshold reflects lactate threshold, the fact remains that a lactate threshold does exist. And, from a practical point-of-view, this threshold can often be non-invasively identified using the V-slope method.[3,18,34,49]

As figure 7.11 shows, the V-slope method involves plotting $\dot{V}CO_2$ as a function of $\dot{V}O_2$, data easily collected during an exercise test performed with the simultaneous measurement of gas exchange. Notice how during the early and mid portions of exercise, $\dot{V}O_2$ increases at a rate that is greater than the increase in $\dot{V}CO_2$ [therefore, the slope of

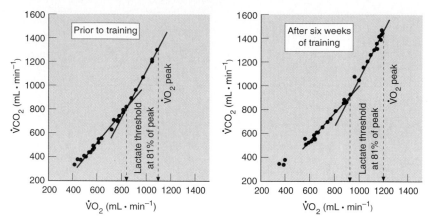

Figure 7.12

Use of the V-slope method to estimate lactate threshold before and after a six-week endurance exercise training program.

the line (S1) is less than 1.0]. As exercise continues and intensity is increased, $\dot{V}CO_2$ then increases at a rate that is greater than the increase in $\dot{V}O_2$. In this case the slope of the line (S2) is now greater than 1.0. The intersection of these two lines (S1 and S2) can easily be identified[18] and often coincides with, or is just slightly higher than, the measured blood lactate threshold.

Lactate threshold (via direct measurement of blood samples or V-slope method) can be, and has been for years, used by coaches to guide exercise intensity and improve human performance.[20,31] Additionally, clinicians use the lactate threshold (mostly via the V-slope method) as a means to evaluate severity of illness and treatment efficacy in patients with certain heart or lung diseases. For example, figure 7.12 shows the effect of a 6-week exercise training program on lactate threshold using the V-slope method in a 46-year-old female patient with stable heart failure. Notice that in both curves estimated lactate threshold occurred at a similar relative $\dot{V}O_2$, ~ 80% of peak. However, after six weeks of training, it occurred at a higher absolute value (shifted from 880 mL · min^{-1} to 970 mL · min^{-1}). In this patient, exercise therapy resulted in a 10.1% increase in peak $\dot{V}O_2$ (1090 mL · min^{-1} to 1200 mL · min^{-1}) and a 10.2% increase in $\dot{V}O_2$ at estimated lactate threshold, with no change in relative lactate threshold expressed as a percent ($\dot{V}O_2$ at threshold/peak $\dot{V}O_2 \times 100$).

The sport related applications of using lactate threshold are described in chapters 11 and 12. In elite athletes exposed to years of intense training, gains in peak $\dot{V}O_2$ become harder and harder to achieve as one nears their "ceiling" for aerobic potential. These athletes instead strive to increase "that point" during exercise where lactate threshold occurs. In fact, among elite athletes, relative lactate threshold may occur at a $\dot{V}O_2$ approximating 85% to 90% of maximum. Also, endurance athletes, such as marathon runners, often run their entire event at a pace that is within 5% of lactate threshold. Thus, improving one's lactate threshold through training can improve performance without necessarily experiencing equal gains in peak $\dot{V}O_2$.[37]

Unique Issues Related to the Respiratory System and Pulmonary Gas Exchange

Much of what we have covered so far is concerned with the basics of exercise physiology and the respiratory system. Having learned this, we must now move on and discuss several other important issues—issues that are relevant regardless of whether or not one finds himself working in a human performance laboratory or a clinical exercise testing center.

Common Terminology

Several terms are used in cardiopulmonary laboratories and pulmonary medicine that students should become familiar with. These terms, and their application to sport and clinical exercise physiology, are described in the following discussions.

Hyperventilation

The increase in $\dot{V}_E$ that occurs during progressive exercise is called *hyperpnea* (i.e., increased ventilation). Such an increase is normal and proportional to both the increased energy demands associated with exertion and the need to maintain arterial PCO_2. However, there is a point during the latter (near end) stages of exercise where $\dot{V}_E$ may become disproportionally greater than the increase in work load or energy demand. That response is referred to as **hyperventilation.**

In addition to exercise, hyperventilation can also be induced voluntarily while resting or it may occur involuntarily during periods of anxiety. Hyperventilation results from increases in either or both the frequency of breathing or the depth of breathing (V_T). When performed at rest, hyperventilation can decrease arterial PCO_2 from 40 mm Hg to less than 20 mm Hg (called *hypocapnia,* or low CO_2 levels in arterial blood). This "blowing-off" of CO_2 via hyperventilation at rest can drive the respiratory exchange ratio or R ($\dot{V}CO_2/\dot{V}O_2$, see chapter 4, pp. 82) above 1.0, thus invalidating the use of this measure as a means to estimate fuel source (fats or carbohydrates).

Relative to the hyperventilation that occurs during exercise, refer back to figure 7.6A. Notice that both trained and untrained persons exhibit a disproportional increase in $\dot{V}_E$ during heavy (toward the end of) exercise. Resulting from the "blowing-off" of CO_2, R can approach if not exceed 1.3 during or immediately following very strenuous exercise.

The precise reason for the hyperventilation that occurs with heavy exercise is unknown. Such a response is likely caused, at least in part, by the decrease in arterial pH (increase in H^+) that occurs secondary to increasing lactic acid production in the skeletal muscle. An increase in arterial H^+ concentration stimulates chemoreceptors and results in hyperventilation, thus the term *respiratory compensation.* The end result is a lowering of arterial PCO_2. However, a hyperventilation response during exercise has also been shown to occur in humans who cannot produce appreciable amounts of lactic acid (McCardle's syndrome).[23] And, as reviewed by Forster and Pan,[21] other factors have been linked to the hyperventilation response, including central (cerebral) command, hyperkalemia (increased blood potassium levels), increased body temperature, and increased plasma catecholamine (epinephrine and norepinephrine) levels. It is possible that several of these and other factors may act in concert to result in the hyperventilation that occurs during heavy exercise.

Before leaving the topic of hyperventilation there are two controversial sport (swimming) applications that deserve mention. Both include the use of voluntary hyperventilation at rest to decrease arterial PCO_2 and, therefore, temporarily incapacitate one's physiologic drive for breathing. The end result is that one's ability to hold her or his breath is improved. The first application involves both hyperventilation and a common theory that increasing the number of swimming strokes taken per breath improves stroke mechanics, thus providing an "edge" during competition (especially among the sprint events). However, since less O_2 is being inhaled because of fewer breaths, arterial PO_2 levels can fall (*arterial hypoxia*)[47]—which represents a potential danger.

The second group of swimmers are those involved with underwater swimming, such as persons attempting to set new distance records. In this instance not only is the drive to breathe lowered by pre-exercise hyperventilation, but it is willfully suppressed so they can stay under water longer. These actions, in combination with the fall in arterial PO_2 mentioned earlier, can cause a person to pass out from hypoxia. Craig documented 25 cases of drowning and 35 cases of near-drowning in which individuals were trying to either set new distance records for underwater swimming or were diving while holding their breath.[14] All

7.4

Rating scale to evaluate severity of dyspnea*

+1 Mild; some labored or difficulty with breathing noticeable to patient but not observer

+2 Mild; difficulty with breathing that is noticeable to observer

+3 Moderate difficulty with breathing that is nonlimiting

+4 Severe difficulty with breathing to the extent that activity must be diminished or discontinued

*Adapted from the American College of Sports Medicine.[1]

individuals in the report were known to be good swimmers, and each person who survived confirmed that they had learned just prior to the accident of the "possible value" of hyperventilation. It is unfortunate that the victims had not also "learned" of the possible consequences of such a practice.

Dyspnea

Dyspnea refers to the sensation of difficulty or labored breathing. Dyspnea can be brought on with exercise, be present at rest, or can come on suddenly while sleeping. Broadly speaking, dyspnea occurs when the demand for ventilation is out of proportion to a person's ability to respond to that demand. Because it is a subjective phenomenon, it is difficult to measure and, therefore, the factors responsible for it are poorly understood. For patients with heart failure, chronic bronchitis, and emphysema, dyspnea can be the symptom limiting their ability to exercise. This differs from normal healthy persons who ordinarily discontinue exercise because of leg or generalized fatigue.

Table 7.4 details a standardized scale used in clinical practice, one designed to help pulmonary patients quantify the extent of their dyspnea during an activity. Using this scale, changes in a dyspnea score can be used to assess changes in disease state or the effects of a rehabilitative or medical intervention.

Second Wind

All of us who have exercised have probably experienced getting our **second wind** at one time or another. It is generally characterized by a sudden transition from a rather ill-defined feeling of respiratory distress or fatigue during the early portion of exercise to a more comfortable, less stressful feeling during later exercise. Such an "adjustment" occurs without us having to change exercise intensity or pace.

The apparent distress experienced just prior to getting one's second wind is manifested in a variety of ways, such as dyspnea; rapid, shallow breathing (*tachypnea*); chest pain; throbbing headache; or pain in various muscles.[28]

Physiologically, no one knows exactly what the causative mechanism for second wind really is. One study designed to investigate this phenomenon[28] found that second wind was experienced at different times during exercise by different subjects (between 2 and 18 minutes during a 20-minute treadmill run). Also, in 90% of the subjects second wind was associated with more comfortable breathing, in 70% with relief or partial relief of muscular fatigue or pain in the legs, and in 35% with simultaneous relief from both leg and chest pain.

A review of this phenomenon revealed several possible causes; these include:[45] (1) relief from breathlessness caused by slowed ventilatory adjustments early in the exercise; (2) removal (oxidation) of lactic acid that accumulated early in the exercise because of a delayed increase in blood flow to the working muscles; (3) relief from local muscle fatigue, particularly of the respiratory muscles; and (4) psychological factors. Other possibilities include a sudden redistribution of blood flow to the diaphragm, catecholamine release leading to increased contractility, and an improved efficiency of diaphragm contractility resulting in a decreased energy demand for the same force output.[42]

Stitch in the Side

Another phenomenon familiar to many athletes, and to anyone else who starts an exercise program following a long period of inactivity, is a "stitch in the side." The symptom most associated with this phenomenon is a sharp pain in the side or "under" the rib cage. Like second wind, it occurs early during exercise and can subside as exercise continues. However, unlike second wind, the pain can be so severe that exercise intensity must be reduced or stopped altogether. Although the exact cause of such pain is unknown, it has been suggested that lack of oxygen (hypoxia or anoxia) in the respiratory muscles (particularly in the diaphragm and intercostal muscles) is involved.

Oxygen Cost of Ventilation and Cigarette Smoking

The work required of the ventilatory muscles to overcome both the elastic recoil of the lungs and the resistance to airflow offered by the respiratory passages is minimal at rest. This is because V_T and respiratory frequency are also minimal, and expiration is passive. Under these conditions, the amount of O_2 consumed by the ventilatory muscles constitutes no more than 1% to 2% of total body $\dot{V}O_2$. During exercise, however, increases in V_T and frequency and

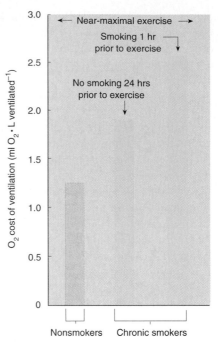

Figure 7.13

The oxygen cost of ventilation in chronic cigarette smokers is greatly increased during near-maximal exercise, particularly if a few cigarettes are smoked within an hour prior to exercise. Abstinence from smoking 24 hours before exercise decreases the cost of ventilation but does not decrease it to the nonsmokers levels.

(Based on data from Rode and Shephard[41] and Shephard.[44])

involvement of more respiratory muscles means that the O_2 cost of ventilation also increases. In fact, the $\dot{V}O_2$ of the respiratory muscles during heavy exercise may constitute 8% to 10% of total body $\dot{V}O_2$.[36,44] As mentioned earlier, trained persons, especially athletes, have a higher ventilatory efficiency (require less O_2 when ventilating the same amount of air) than do untrained persons (figure 7.6A).

Another factor impacting ventilatory efficiency during exercise is that of cigarette smoking. To overcome the nicotine-induced increase in airway resistance caused by bronchoconstriction, the respiratory muscles must work harder (consume more O_2) to ventilate a given amount of air. As shown in figure 7.13, when only a few cigarettes were smoked within one hour prior to heavy exercise, the O_2 cost of ventilation in chronic smokers was found to be over twice that of nonsmokers.[41] (In one subject who smoked 1 to 1½ packs per day for 27 years, the difference was nearly four times that of the nonsmokers!) If no cigarettes were smoked for 24 hours prior to exercise, the oxygen cost of ventilation among smokers was ~ 25% lower, but still about 55% higher than in nonsmokers.[41,44]

This information has two practical implications. First, the added cost of ventilation caused by chronic cigarette smoking can rob the working muscles of a large percentage

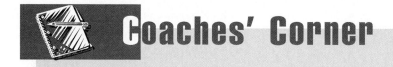

Coaches' Corner

Nasal Breathing

By their very nature, many competitive athletes are willing to try any technique that claims to, or does, aid performance. One such device is the now quite popular Breathe Right® nasal strip.

When attached across the bridge of the nose, this device lifts the soft-tissue area above the flare of each nostril, producing somewhat of a spring-action as it attempts to "straighten itself out." The end result is a very mild pulling action that opens the nasal passages and reduces nasal airway resistance by 30%.[9] Initially developed for persons with obstructive sleep apnea,* many professional athletes now use it to hold their nasal passages open and make breathing easier. Such use is observed most often among those athletes who participate in anaerobic-type events (e.g., football and basketball).

Although no direct claims have been made by the manufacturer stating that the device actually improves athletic performance, they do state that the "benefits from the Breathe Right nasal strip appear to be more readily detected during recovery (from exercise)."[9] One belief among endurance athletes (and among some coaches) is that the increased nasal airflow will improve O_2 delivery and, therefore, lead to (1) less reliance on anaerobic glycolysis, and (2) a greater peak $\dot{V}O_2$. On the contrary, at present there is no definitive scientific evidence that the Breathe Right device provides an

"ergogenic effect" that aids either endurance (aerobic) or anaerobic performance. Specifically, no significant improvements in $\dot{V}O_2$, ventilation, tidal volume, frequency of breathing, power output or respiratory exchange ratio have been observed during submaximal exercise, peak exercise, or in recovery from exercise.[25,38,52]

Testing 16 college-age varsity athletes, Trocchio et al.[52] had subjects perform two maximal cycle ergometer tests while measuring expired gases. One test was conducted using the Breathe Right device and the other without. Although all 16 subjects stated that they felt the device in some way "opened up" their nasal passages, peak $\dot{V}O_2$ was 44.0 mL · kg^{-1} · min^{-1} without the device and 43.8 mL · kg^{-1} · min^{-1} while wearing the device. Virtually no difference. One likely reason for the absence of a beneficial effect during endurance exercise is that the oxygen-carrying hemoglobin in our blood is normally fully saturated with O_2 (chapter 8) even without the Breathe Right device. Research investigating the Breathe Right device during recovery from anaerobic events is now underway; research is also being conducted to identify what causes some athletes to be "responders" and others to be "nonresponders" to the device.

Although no physiologic evidence presently exists supporting the use of the Breathe Right device, perhaps there is a psychologic advantage associated with being able to breathe easier. This feeling, in and of itself, may be the reason some athletes choose the device, especially among those who suffer from nasal congestion (e.g., those with nasal allergies).

Persons with obstructive sleep apnea experience 30 or more episodes during a seven-hour sleep in which oral-nasal airflow ceases for 10 or more seconds.

---

of their potential O_2 supply. During maximal exercise, this could lead to a corresponding reduction in performance. During submaximal exercise this could lead to the earlier (and possibly greater) reliance on anaerobic glycolysis and thus premature fatigue.

Second, a large part of the increase in the O_2 cost of ventilation among chronic smokers can be substantially reduced with a relatively short period of abstinence from cigarettes. Therefore, smokers who plan to exert themselves (e.g., swim, shovel snow, play weekend softball) can lessen the physiologic cost of breathing by not smoking for part, if not all, of the day preceding exercise. The same logic is applied in many hospital-based stress testing laboratories and cardiac rehabilitation programs, where patients who smoke are asked to abstain from cigarette smoking for a minimum of five hours prior to their appointment.

In addition to the obvious short-term disadvantages cited here, the health consequences associated with chronic cigarette use (e.g., various cancers, emphysema, and heart disease) provide even greater reasons for not smoking.

Marijuana Smoking and Exercise Performance

Ethical, legal, and any medicinal issues aside, present estimates are that ~ one-fourth of the U.S. residents between 20 and 25 years old use marijuana at least once annually. The pharmacologic effects that occur at rest as a result of marijuana smoking include a rapid heart rate, bronchodilation, and an increase in limb blood flow. Because of these changes at rest, some have postulated that marijuana

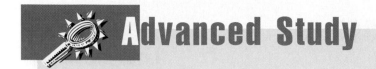

One of the many environmental air pollutants we are exposed to when breathing smog is ozone (O_3). O_3 is a potent oxidizing agent known to cause a reduction in FEV_1, tracheal irritation, and cough. However, it was not until 1984, following the Olympic games in Los Angeles, that we began to see an increase in exercise-related research on this topic. One reason for the sharp increase in such research is that exercise has been shown to accentuate or worsen the negative effects of O_3. These effects include impairment of pulmonary function, along with symptoms of respiratory discomfort (e.g., cough and shortness of breath). The current National Ambient Air Quality Standard for O_3 is less than 0.12 parts per million (ppm); however, it is not uncommon for certain urban cities like Los Angeles to often exceed 0.20 ppm during the summer months.

The degree to which exercise accentuates the negative effects associated with O_3 is dependent on the O_3 concentration in the ambient air, the intensity of exercise, and the duration of the exercise bout (exposure time). With respect to intensity of exercise, moderate to heavy exercise leads to a greater $\dot{V}_E$ (60 L · min^{-1} to 100 L · min^{-1}) than does light or moderate exercise (30 L · min^{-1} to 60 L · min^{-1}), which means more O_3 is brought into the respiratory system and in contact with respiratory tissue. Therefore, well-trained athletes who are able to sustain a high $\dot{V}_E$ for a prolonged period of time may actually be more susceptible to the negative effects of O_3 exposure. However, the response to O_3 exposure from exercise can vary greatly from one individual to another. Exercising in hotter versus moderate environments appears to worsen O_3-induced respiratory discomfort.

The performance consequences of O_3 exposure during exercise include a reduction in exercise duration and decreases in maximal work rate, $\dot{V}O_2$ (5% to 15%), heart rate, and $\dot{V}_E$. The reasons responsible for these reductions are not well understood. Subject discomfort (difficulty breathing, cough, airway irritation, and chest soreness) seems to be of prime importance, yet physiologic factors such as abnormalities in O_2 diffusion at the alveolar-capillary interface and an increased energy requirement for respiratory muscular effort cannot be ruled out. Clearly, the interaction between exercise and O_3 environments and the effect of O_3 on exercise performance are two areas worthy of continued research. Additional knowledge could impact both the competitive athlete as well as the leisure jogger who is simply trying to maintain good health.

---

smoking might enhance exercise performance. As you can imagine, however, not a lot of scientific information is available about the acute effects of marijuana smoking on exercise performance.

In a study of 12 healthy young adults (9 males and 3 females), Renaud and Cormier[39] asked their subjects to undergo two maximal exercise cycle tests. One test was started 10 minutes after subjects finished smoking a marijuana cigarette containing 7 mg of marijuana · kg of body weight.$^{-1}$ The other test was conducted on a separate day and without the prior use of marijuana. Smoking was associated with a marked increase in resting heart rate from 94 beats · min^{-1} to 120 beats · min^{-1}! And this marijuana-induced elevation in higher heart rate persisted through 80% of peak exercise. Also, marijuana smoking reduced exercise time by 6.2% and had no positive or negative effect on maximal heart rate, $\dot{V}O_2$ or $\dot{V}_E$. During the latter stages of exercise, at workloads between 60% and 80% of maximum, both $\dot{V}_E$ and breathing frequency were increased with marijuana use. The authors concluded that acute marijuana use reduced maximal exercise performance, resulting in the pre-mature achievement of max $\dot{V}O_2$. Their study, however, did not address how intensity of exercise or level of fatigue were perceived with and without marijuana use, two variables that might be altered given the known psychotropic effects of the drug.

Respiratory Regulation of pH

Molecules that contribute H^+ to a solution and raise its H^+ concentration are called acids. Alternately, a base contributes a hydroxyl ion (OH^-) capable of combining with H^+, such that the H^+ concentration of a solution is lowered. If the amount of H^+ exceeds the amount of OH^-, the solution is acidic. If the amount of OH^- exceeds the amount of H^+, the solution is basic (or alkaline). To express the acidity or alkalinity of a solution, one first determines the amount of H^+ present, with the resulting number expressed as the pH of a particular solution. A pH of 7.0 is considered neutral, this means the concentration of H^+ equals the concentration

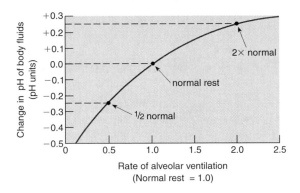

Figure 7.14

Hyperventilation at a rate twice normal (rest) will cause the blood and body fluid pH to increase as much as 0.25 pH units. On the other hand, when alveolar ventilation is reduced to one-half normal, the pH decreases by about 0.25 pH units.

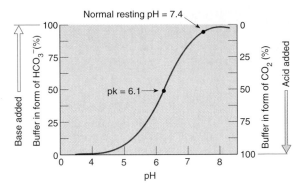

Figure 7.15

A buffer system. An increase in the concentration of HCO_3^- (bicarbonate or base added) causes a rise in pH of the solution, and an increase in dissolved CO_2 (acid added) decreases the pH.

of OH^-. At rest, blood pH is slightly alkalinic at ~ 7.4. However, during brief bouts of exhaustive exercise it can become quite acidic, falling as low as 6.8. Left unchecked, a decrease in muscle (and subsequently blood) pH can impair exercise performance by, for example, interfering with muscle force production and/or the enzymes involved with both aerobic and anaerobic metabolism.

The sources that can decrease pH during exercise are many, with the two greatest contributors being (1) the carbonic acid (H_2CO_3) derived from the CO_2 produced during aerobic metabolism, and (2) the lactic acid (LA^+) from anaerobic glycolysis. These two sources are detailed in the following reactions.

Aerobic: $CO_2 + H_2O \longleftrightarrow H_2CO_3 \longleftrightarrow H^+ + HCO_3^-$
Anaerobic Glycolysis: $LA^+ + HCO_3^- \longrightarrow$
$$H_2O + CO_2 + \text{Lactate}$$

Note that in both cases CO_2 is involved, which, being a gas, provides an opportunity for respiration to help influence blood pH. Earlier in this chapter we mentioned that chemoreceptors in the medulla oblongata of the brain and in peripheral arteries (aorta/carotid bodies) are sensitive to changes in cerebral spinal fluid and/or blood H^+ and PCO_2 concentrations. Other mechanisms beside the respiratory system that also help buffer or regulate blood pH during exercise include blood (protein, hemoglobin, and HCO_3^-) and intracellular (proteins and phosphate groups) buffers.

The increase in muscle CO_2 from aerobic metabolism drives the first of the above two equations to the right. Specifically, CO_2 is converted to H_2CO_3, which then dissociates to H^+ and bicarbonate (HCO_3^-). This ultimately leads to a decrease in pH. Second, the lactic acid produced via anaerobic glycolysis also lowers pH (and increases arterial PCO_2). Increases in arterial and cerebral spinal fluid H^+ concentration stimulate the chemoreceptors to increase pulmonary ventilation, which then facilitates the removal (blowing off) of CO_2. The elimination of CO_2 in this

manner causes H^+ concentration to decrease and pH to rise (driving the first reaction to the left). All-in-all, the intact respiratory system represents a responsive entity, one capable of controlling arterial PCO_2 and pH.

For example, alterations in the rate and depth of respiration (i.e., in alveolar ventilation) can immediately affect changes in body fluid pH. As shown in figure 7.14, hyperventilation at rest that is twice the rate of normal will cause the blood and body fluid pH to increase as much as 0.25 pH units. On the other hand, when alveolar ventilation is reduced to one-half normal, such as is the case when blood pH is above 7.4, the pH decreases by about 0.25 pH units.

Alkali Reserve

The degree to which the pH of the body fluids is affected by the buildup of CO_2 and the subsequent formation of carbonic acid (H_2CO_3) depends on the amount of HCO_3^- available for the buffering operation. Actually, the pH of the body fluids is related to the ratio of the concentration of HCO_3^- to the amount of dissolved CO_2. By formula:

$$pH = pK + \log \left[\frac{HCO_3^-}{CO_2} \right]$$

The abbreviation "pK" refers to a constant of a buffer, which for the bicarbonate buffer system is equal to 6.1. This means that when the concentration of HCO_3^- is equal to the amount of dissolved CO_2 (for a ratio of 1:1), the pH of the solution (in this case, the body fluids) will be 6.1.* Normally, however, at rest the ratio of HCO_3^- to CO_2 is 20:1, for a pH of 7.4 (pH = 6.1 + $\log_{10}$ 20 = 6.1 + 1.3 = 7.4). As shown in figure 7.15, an increase in the concentration of HCO_3^- (base

---

*When the concentration of HCO_3^- ions and dissolved CO_2 are equal, the ratio of HCO_3^-:CO_2 = 1; the log of 1 = 0; therefore, pH = pK = 6.1.

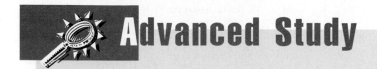

Generally, the kidneys do not help regulate blood pH during exercise. However, at other times they do play a very important role with respect to blood pH. The principal way that the kidney accomplishes this is by increasing or decreasing the bicarbonate ion (HCO_3^-) concentration in blood. The important steps in this process are as follows:

1. CO_2 from the extracellular fluids and from the epithelial cells of the kidney tubules combines with water (in the presence of the enzyme, carbonic anhydrase) to form carbonic acid ($CO_2 + H_2O \rightarrow H_2CO_3$) within the tubule cells.

2. H_2CO_3 dissociates into a HCO_3^- and a H^+. The H^+ is actively transported or secreted into the lumen of the kidney tubules and is eventually excreted in the urine as water. Additionally, the newly formed HCO_3^- diffuses into the extracellular fluid, soon to be available to serve in the blood's buffering action of H^+.

As mentioned earlier, the kidneys do not play an important role in regulating blood pH during exercise. This is because the renal mechanisms described here take 3 to 4 hours or more to effectively respond to a change in blood chemistry.

---

added) causes a rise in pH, whereas an increase in dissolved CO_2 (acid added) decreases the pH. In the body the amount of bicarbonate ions available for buffering is called the **alkali reserve.**

Some sport scientists have investigated the concept of taking doses of bicarbonate to increase alkali reserve and delay fatigue during prolonged, heavy exertion. Using ingested or intravenous bicarbonate as an ergogenic aid is discussed in chapter 18.

Summary

The lungs and the entire respiratory system are responsible for the exchange of O_2 and CO_2 between the ambient external environment and the internal environment of our body. The exchange of O_2 and CO_2 occurs at the alveoli-pulmonary capillary interface.

The principal muscles of inspiration are the diaphragm and the external intercostal muscles at rest, with added help from the scalene and sternocleidomastoid muscles during exercise. Expiration is passive at rest and is facilitated by the abdominal and internal intercostal muscles during exercise. The strength and endurance of the respiratory muscles can be increased through exercise training programs.

Air rushes into the lungs when the intrapulmonary and intrapleural pressures decrease because of contraction of the inspiratory muscles. During expiration, these pressures are reversed, and air is forced out of the lungs and back into the environment.

There are several lung volumes and measures that students should familiarize themselves with, including vital capacity, tidal volume, and respiratory rate. These

measures and others are assessed using a spirometer, and in general, they are influenced little, if at all, by regular exercise training.

The movement of air into and out of the lungs is called pulmonary ventilation. Ventilation is composed of two phases: inspiration and expiration. Minute ventilation is the amount of air we either exhale or inhale in one minute. At rest, this amounts to between 6 and 15 liters. During maximal exercise, this can increase to over 200 liters in males and 145 liters in females. Ventilation changes before, during, and after exercise. In most persons, minute ventilation does not limit exercise performance.

Alveolar ventilation ensures adequate oxygenation of the pulmonary capillary blood and carbon dioxide removal. The volume of air that remains in the respiratory passages and does not participate in gas exchange is called anatomical dead space. Alveolar ventilation is dependent on the depth and frequency of breathing and on the size of the dead space.

The lactate threshold is that exercise intensity (work or oxygen consumption) during which a nonlinear increase in blood lactate concentration is observed. Lactate threshold is influenced by factors that affect both lactate production and clearance. Using the V-slope method, it can be indirectly detected via gas exchange assessed during progressive exercise.

Hyperventilation can be voluntarily induced at rest or can occur during exercise. Relative to exercise, it is that point where the increase in minute ventilation is disproportionately greater than the increase in energy demand. Second wind is thought to be related to adjustments in ventilation and metabolism that occur some time early on in exercise. Its exact cause, however, is not known. Stitch in the side is a sharp pain along the lower rib cage that also occurs soon after exercise is initiated. It may be caused by ischemia of the respiratory muscles, for which there is no simple remedy. Both cigarette smoking and marijuana smoking can influence physiologic responses and performance during exercise. Chronic cigarette smoking increases the oxygen cost of ventilation.

The respiratory system aids in the regulation of hydrogen ion concentration of body fluids by changing the rate and depth of ventilation. When body fluid pH increases, ventilation decreases, retaining CO_2; when body fluid pH decreases, ventilation increases to blow off CO_2. The degree to which the pH of the body fluids is affected by the build up of CO_2 depends on the amount of HCO_3^- available for the buffering operation. In the body, the amount of HCO_3^- available for buffering is called the alkali reserve.

Questions

1. Name the respiratory muscles of inspiration and expiration at rest and during exercise. Are they affected by exercise training programs?
2. Describe intrapulmonary and intrapleural pressure changes as they relate to the movement of air into and out of the lungs at rest.
3. Define tidal volume, breathing frequency, vital capacity, residual volume, and total lung capacity. How are tidal volume and breathing frequency changed during an exercise bout? Quantify your answer whenever possible.
4. What contribution does expiratory reserve volume and inspiratory reserve volume make relative to the changes in tidal volume that you described in question 3?
5. What are the phases of ventilation, and what two factors comprise the minute ventilation?
6. Describe the nature of the ventilatory changes: (a) immediately before exercise, (b) during exercise, and (c) during recovery from exercise.
7. How much air do we expire per minute at rest and during maximal exercise?
8. Define alveolar ventilation and dead space, and explain their roles in providing adequate ventilation.
9. Alveolar ventilation depends on what three factors?
10. A person's minute ventilation during exercise is $100 \text{ L} \cdot \text{min}^{-1}$, anatomical dead space is $0.4 \text{ L} \cdot \text{breath}^{-1}$, and tidal volume is $2.0 \text{ L} \cdot \text{breath}^{-1}$. What is their breathing frequency and alveolar ventilation?
11. Describe factors that might influence lactate production or clearance during exercise and, therefore, blood lactate concentration.
12. How might lactate threshold, assessed either directly using blood samples or indirectly via the V-slope method, be a better indicator of improved performance among elite athletes than peak $\dot{V}O_2$?
13. Discuss the possible causes of second wind and stitch in the side.
14. Discuss the effects of chronic cigarette smoking and abstinence from smoking on the O_2 cost of ventilation.
15. As one moves from light to moderate to heavy exercise, explain how the respiratory system aids in the regulation of acid-base balance.

References

1. *ACSM Guidelines for Exercise Testing and Prescription, 4th ed.* Philadelphia: Lea and Febiger.
2. Bachman, J., and S. Horvath. 1968. Pulmonary function changes which accompany athletic conditioning programs. *Res Q.* 39:235–239.
3. Beaver, W. L., K. Wasserman, and B. J. Whipp. 1986. A new method for detecting anaerobic threshold by gas exchange. *J Appl Physiol.* 60(6):2020–2027.
4. Berman, L. B., and J. R. Sutton. 1986. Exercise for the pulmonary patient. *J Cardiopulmonary Rehabil.* 6:52–61.
5. Bradley, M. E., and D. E. Leith. 1978. Ventilatory muscle training and the oxygen cost of sustained hyperpnea. *J Appl Physiol.* 45(6):885–892.
6. Brooks, G. A. 1985. Anaerobic threshold: review of the concept and directions for future research. *Med Sci Sports Exerc.* 17(1):22–31.
7. Brooks, G. A., T. D. Fahey, and T. P. White. 1996. *Exercise Physiology,* 2d ed. Mountain View, CA: Mayfield. pp.189–193.
8. Byrne-Quinn, E., J. V. Weil, I. E. Sodal, G. F. Filley, and R. F. Grover. 1971. Ventilatory control in the athlete. *J Appl Physiol.* 30(1):91–98.
9. CNS, Inc. February 6, 1996. Exercise studies with Breathe Right nasal strips. Minneapolis, MN.
10. Coast, J. R., P. S. Clifford, T. W. Henrich, J. Stray-Gundersen, and R. L. Johnson, Jr. 1990. Maximal inspiratory pressure following maximal exercise in trained and untrained subjects. *Med Sci Sports Exerc.* 22(6):811–815.
11. Collins, D. D., C. H. Scoggin, C. W. Zwillich, and J. V. Weil. 1978. Hereditary aspects of decreased hypoxic response. *J Clin Invest.* 21:105–110.
12. Comroe, J., R. Forster, A. DuBois, W. Briscoe, and E. Carlsen. 1962. *The Lung,* 2d ed. Chicago: Year Book Medical.
13. Cordain, L., and J. Stager. 1988. Pulmonary structure and function in swimmers. *Sports Medicine.* 6:271–278.
14. Craig, A. B. 1974. Summary of 58 cases of loss of consciousness during underwater swimming and diving. *Med Sci Sports.* 8(3):171–175.
15. Cumming, G. 1969. Correlation of athletic performance with pulmonary function in 13- to 17-year-old boys and girls. *Med Sci Sports.* 1(3):140–143.
16. Davis, J. A. 1985. Response to Brooks' manuscript. *Med Sci Sports Exerc.* 17(1):32–34.
17. Dempsey, J. A. 1986. Is the lung built for exercise? *Med Sci Sports Exerc.* 18(2):143–155.
18. Dickstein, K., S. Barvik, T. Aarland, S. Snapinn, and J. Millerhagen. 1990. Validation of a computerized technique for detection of the gas exchange anaerobic threshold in cardiac disease. *Am J Cardiol.* 66:1363–1367.
19. Farkas, G. A., F. J. Cerny, and D. F. Rochester. 1996. Contractility of the ventilatory pump muscles. *Med Sci Sports Exerc.* 28(9):1106–1114.
20. Farrell, P. S., J. H. Wilmore, E. F. Coyle, J. E. Billings, and D. L. Costill. 1979. Plasma lactate accumulation and distance running performance. *Med Sci Sports.* 11(4):338–344.

21. Forster, H. V. and L. G. Pan. 1991. Exercise Hypernea. In Crystal, R. G. and J. B. West (eds). *The Lung, Scientific Foundations,* vol. 2. New York, NY: Raven Press. pp. 1553–1564.

22. Grimby, G., J. Bunn, and J. Mead. 1968. Relative contribution of rib cage and abdomen to ventilation during exercise. *J Appl Physiol.* 24(2):159–166.

23. Hagberg, J. M., E. F. Coyle, J. E. Carroll, J. M. Miller, W. H. Martin, and M. H. Brooks. 1982. Exercise hyperventilation in patients with McArdle's disease. *J Appl Physiol.* 52:991–994.

24. Holmgren, A. 1967. Cardiorespiratory determinants of cardiovascular fitness. *Can Med Assoc J.* 96:697–702.

25. Huffman, M. S., M. T. Huffman, D. D. Brown, J. C. Quindry, and D. Q. Thomas. 1996. Exercise responses using the Breathe Right external nasal dilator. *Med Sci Sports Exerc.* 28(5-Suppl):S70.

26. Johnson, B. D., E. A. Aaron, M. A. Babcock, and J. A. Dempsey. 1996. Respiratory muscle fatigue during exercise: implications for performance. *Med Sci Sports Exerc.* 28(9):1129–1137.

27. Johnson, B. D., and J. A. Dempsey. 1991. Demand vs. capacity in the aging pulmonary system. In J. O. Holloszy (ed). *Exercise and Sports Sciences Reviews.* 19:171–210. Baltimore: Williams and Wilkins.

28. Lefcoe, N., and M. Yuhasz. 1971. The "second wind" phenomenon in constant load exercise. *J Sports Med Phys Fit.* 11:135–138.

29. Leith, D. E., and M. E. Bradley. 1976. Ventilatory muscle strength and endurance training. *J Appl Physiol.* 41(4):508–516.

30. Leith, D. E., B. Philip, R. Gabel, H. Feldman, and V. Fencl. 1979. Ventilatory muscle training and ventilatory control. *Am Rev Respir Dis.* 119(2):99–100.

31. MacDougall, J. D. 1977. The anaerobic threshold: its significance for the endurance athlete. *Can J Appl Sport Sci.* 2:137–140.

32. Martin, B. J., K. E. Sparks, C. W. Zwillich, and J. V. Weil. 1979. Low exercise ventilation in endurance athletes. *Med Sci Sports.* 11(2):181–185.

33. Martin, B. J., J. V. Weil, K. E. Sparks, R. E. McCullough, and R. F. Grover. 1978. Exercise ventilation correlates positively with ventilatory chemoresponsiveness. *J Appl Physiol.* 45(4):557–564.

34. Mickelson, T. C., and F. C. Hagerman. 1982. Anaerobic threshold measurements of elite oarsmen. *Med Sci Sports Exerc.* 14(6):440–444.

35. Miyamura, M., T. Yamashina, and Y. Honda. 1976. Ventilatory responses to CO_2 rebreathing at rest and during exercise in untrained subjects and athletes. *Jap J Physiol.* 26:245–254.

36. Otis, A. The work of breathing. 1964. In Fenn, W., and H. Rahn (eds.), *Handbook of Physiology.* Sec. 3, Respiration, vol. 1. Washington, D.C.: American Physiological Society, p. 463.

37. Peronnet, G., E. Thibault, C. Rhodes, and D. C. McKenzie. 1987. Mechanisms and patterns of blood lactate increase during exercise in man. *Med Sci Sports Exerc.* 19(6):610–615.

38. Quindry, J. C., D. D. Brown, M. S. Huffman, M. T. Huffman, and D. Q. Thomas. 1996. Exercise recovery responses using the Breathe Right nasal dilator. *Med Sci Sports Exerc.* 28(5-Suppl):S70.

39. Renaud, A. M., and Y. Cormier. 1986. Acute effects of marihuana smoking on maximal exercise performance. *Med Sci Sports Exerc.* 18(6):685–689.

40. Ries, A. L. 1993. Position paper of the American Association of Cardiovascular and Pulmonary Rehabilitation: scientific basis of pulmonary rehabilitation. In G. Connors and L. Hilling (eds.). *Guidelines for Pulmonary Rehabilitation Programs.* Champaign, IL: Human Kinetics. pp. 73–101.

41. Rode, A., and R. Shephard. 1971. The influence of cigarette smoking upon the oxygen cost of breathing in near-maximal exercise. *Med Sci Sports.* 3(2):51–55.

42. Scharf, S. M., H. Bark, D. Heimer, A. Cohen, and P. T. Macklem. 1984. "Second wind" during inspiratory loading. *Med Sci Sports Exerc.* 16(1):87–91.

43. Scoggin, C. H., R. D. Doekel, M. H. Kryger, C. W. Zwillich, and J. V. Weil. 1978. Familial aspects of decreased hypoxic drive in endurance athletes. *J Appl Physiol.* 44(3):464–468.

44. Shephard, R. 1966. The oxygen cost of breathing during vigorous exercise. *Q J Exp Physiol.* 51:336–350.

45. Shephard, R. 1974. What causes second wind? *Physician Sports Med.* 2(11):37–42.

46. Skinner, J., and T. McLellan. 1980. The transition from aerobic to anaerobic exercise. *Research Quarterly.* 51:234–248.

47. Stager, J. M., L. Cordian, J. Malley, and J. Wigglesworth. 1989. Arterial desaturation during arm exercise with controlled frequency breathing. *J Swimming Research.* 5(1):5–10.

48. Stainsby, W. N. 1986. Biochemical and physiological bases for lactate production. *Med Sci Sports Exerc.* 18(3)341–343.

49. Sue, D. Y., K. Wasserman, R. B. Moricca, and R. Casaburi. 1988. Metabolic acidosis during exercise in patients with chronic obstructive pulmonary disease. *Chest.* 94(5):931–938.

50. Sutton, J. R., and N. L. Jones. 1979. Control of pulmonary ventilation during exercise and mediators in the blood: CO_2 and hydrogen ion. *Med Sci Sports.* 11(2):198–203.

51. Swerts, P. M. J., L. M. J. Kertzers, E. Terpstra-Lindeman, and E. F. M. Wouters. 1992. Exercise training as a mediator of increased exercise performance in patients with chronic obstructive disease. *J Cardiopulmonary Rehabil.* 12:188–193.

52. Trocchio, M., J. W. Wimer, A. W. Parkman, and J Fischer. 1995. Oxygenation and exercise performance-enhancing effects attributed to the Breathe-Right nasal dilator. *Journal of Athletic Training.* 30(3):211–214.

53. Wade, O. 1954. Movements of the thoracic cage and diaphragm in respiration. *J Physiol.* (London) 124:193–212.

54. Wasserman, K., J. E. Hansen, D. Y. Sue, B. J. Whipp, and R. Casaburi. 1994. *Principles of Exercise Testing and Interpretation,* 2d ed. Philadelphia: Lea and Febiger.

55. Wasserman, K., and M. B. McIlroy. 1964. Detecting the threshold of anaerobic metabolism. *Am J Cardiol.* 14:844–852.

56. Wasserman, K., B. J. Whipp, S. N. Koyal, and W. L. Beaver. 1973. Anaerobic threshold and respiratory gas exchange during exercise. *J Appl Physiol.* 35(2):236–243.

57. West, J. B. 1974. *Respiratory Physiology—The Essentials.* Baltimore: Williams and Wilkins, p. 4.

Selected Readings

Adams, W. C. 1987. Effects of ozone exposure at ambient air pollution episode levels on exercise performance. *Sports Medicine.* 4:395–424.

Dressendorfer, R. H., C. E. Wade, and E. M. Bernauer. 1977. Combined effects of breathing resistance and hyperoxia on aerobic work tolerance. *J Appl Physiol.* 42(3):444–448.

Grimby, G. 1969. Respiration in exercise. *Med Sci Sports.* 1(1):9–14.

Kaufman, M. P. and H. V. Forster. 1996. Reflexes controlling circulatory, ventilatory and airway responses to exercise. In Rowell, L. B. and J. T. Shepard (eds.) *Handbook of Physiology.* New York: Oxford University Press, chapter 10.

Milic-Emili, J., J. Petit, and R. Deroanne. 1962. Mechanical work of breathing during exercise in trained and untrained subjects. *J Appl Physiol.* 17:43–46.

Roussos, C., M. Fixley, D. Gross, and P. T. Macklem. 1979. Fatigue of inspiratory muscles and their synergic behavior. *J Appl Physiol.* 46(5):897–904.

Waldrop, T. G., F. L. Eldridge, G. A. Iwamoto, and J. H. Mitchell. 1996. Central neural control of respiration and circulation during exercise. In Rowell, L. B., and J. T. Shepard (eds.) *Handbook of Physiology.* New York: Oxford University Press, chapter 19.

8

Gas Exchange and Transport

We saw in the last chapter that pulmonary ventilation (more accurately, alveolar ventilation) supplies the alveoli with fresh air, which is high in O_2 and low in CO_2. Venous blood, on the other hand, is low in O_2 and high in CO_2. Thus, gas exchange between the alveolar air and venous blood (which occurs at the alveolar-pulmonary capillary membrane or interface) loads and unloads the blood with O_2 and CO_2, respectively. After being transported via the circulation, O_2 and CO_2 are again exchanged, this time between the arterial blood and the tissues (e.g., muscle) at the **tissue-capillary membrane.** Here, O_2 in the blood is given up to the tissues, and CO_2 in the tissues is given up to the blood. This chapter discusses how these gases are exchanged and how they are carried in the blood.

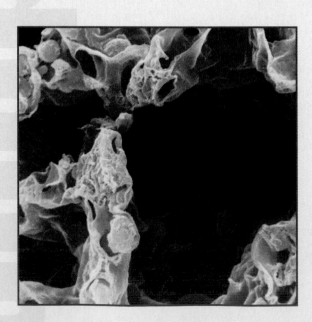

Gas Exchange—Diffusion

Gas Transport

Summary

Key Terms

The major concepts to be learned from this chapter are as follows:

- Gas exchange between the lungs and blood (alveolar-capillary membrane) and between the blood and tissues (tissue-capillary membrane) takes place through diffusion, a physical process involving the random movement of molecules.
- The single most important factor affecting gas diffusion is the partial pressure gradient of the gases involved. Partial pressure refers to the pressure exerted by a single gas in a gas mixture or in a liquid.
- The partial pressure of oxygen is highest in the lungs and lowest in the tissues, whereas the partial pressure of carbon dioxide is highest in the tissues and lowest in the lungs.
- Diffusion of a gas always takes place from an area of higher to an area of lower partial pressure.
- Other factors influencing gas exchange are the length of the diffusion path, the number of red blood cells or the hemoglobin concentration, and the surface area available for diffusion.
- During exercise, the diffusion of oxygen and carbon dioxide across the alveolar-capillary and tissue-capillary membranes increases.
- Oxygen and carbon dioxide are transported by the blood, mainly in chemical combination with hemoglobin. However, a small amount is carried in plasma (dissolved in solution).
- Factors affecting the saturation of hemoglobin with oxygen (at rest and during exercise) are the partial pressure of oxygen, the temperature of the blood, blood pH, and the amount of carbon dioxide in the blood.

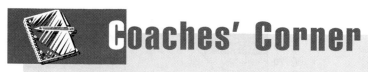

Coaches' Corner

Supplemental O_2 and Performance

It's Monday Night Football on ABC! It's late in the third quarter, and the Chargers have the ball on the Chiefs' 10 yard line—threatening to score on third down. After the snap the quarterback drops back to pass, he looks left then throws a soft screen pass to the right . . . toward a halfback who is wide open coming out of the backfield. But wait—out of nowhere comes the Chiefs' strong-side defensive safety who intercepts the pass and runs 90 yards in the other direction for a touchdown.

Seconds later, as the television camera moves in to show the home-viewing audience the still jubilant Chiefs' sideline, we see the defensive safety who intercepted the pass now with an O_2 mask clamped over his face . . . breathing deeply in hopes of speeding along his recovery from that vigorous 90-yard run. The questions here are: does the use of supplemental O_2 in this fashion greatly improve O_2 transport? does it aid recovery? does it improve subsequent performance? The answer to all three questions is no.

Although inhaling O_2-rich gas increases the partial pressure of O_2 in inspired air and therefore increases the pressure gradient between alveolar PO_2 and

pulmonary capillary PO_2, where is the increased O_2 supposed to go? At rest, during exercise, and in recovery, arterial Hgb is almost fully saturated with O_2; therefore, little more can be carried to the skeletal muscles via this route. That leaves driving more O_2 into the plasma (dissolved in solution), which does occur, but its effect in healthy individuals is useless both at rest and during recovery when O_2 demand is low. On the other hand, studies conducted in the 1950s through 1970s showed that breathing O_2-enriched gases during exercise slightly improved endurance and lowered minute ventilation and blood lactate accumulation. But think about it. To reap these benefits, the athlete would have to wear a face mask and carry a separate O_2 source (tank) during his or her endurance event. In the end, whatever gains might be derived from breathing O_2-enriched gas during exercise are offset by the impracticality of the technique. And since no benefits are gained through its use before or after exercise, this approach is really quite limited. But, then again, it sure looks great on television!

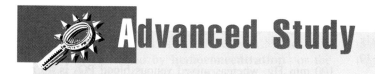

Advanced Study

O_2 at Altitude

As one moves from sea level ($P_B = 760$ mm Hg) to higher elevations, P_B is reduced (i.e., the weight of the surrounding air is reduced because there is less air). At the top of Pikes Peak in Colorado (modest altitude, 4300 m or 14,100 feet) P_B is ~ 460 mm Hg, which results in a lower atmospheric PO_2 (~ 90 mm Hg) and, therefore, in a lower alveolar PO_2 (~ 53 mm Hg). Hiking in and around the summit impacts the blood's O_2-carrying ability because less O_2 is available to combine with Hgb. In this example both Hgb concentration and its affinity for O_2 are intact.

Ignoring any hemoconcentration effect for the moment, the $\%SO_2$ may be computed as follows.

$$\%SO_2 = 86\% = \frac{15.0 \text{ g} \cdot \text{dL}^{-1} \times 1.15}{15.0 \text{ g} \cdot \text{dL}^{-1} \times 1.34} = \frac{17.2 \text{ vol}\%}{20.1 \text{ vol}\%} \times 100$$

Notice in the numerator that Hgb is not fully saturated with O_2, carrying only 1.15 mL of $O_2 \cdot$ g of Hgb^{-1} versus the usual value of 1.34 mL $\cdot$ g of Hgb^{-1}. Again, this reduction results from the lower alveolar PO_2 (~ 53 mm Hg), which means less O_2 is available to combine with the Hgb that passes through the lungs in pulmonary capillary blood. The end result from this hypoxia is that the hiker experiences increased ventilation and early fatigue with exertion.

$20.1 \times 0.75 = 15$ vol%. The difference between the two, called the **arterial mixed venous oxygen difference (a − $\overline{v}O_2$ diff)**,* represents how much O_2 is extracted or consumed by the tissues from each 100 mL of blood perfusing them. Using the values given above from figure 8.11A the a − $\overline{v}O_2$ diff (shaded in red) is:

$$19.5 - 15.0 = 4.5 \text{ mL of } O_2 \cdot 100 \text{ mL}^{-1} \text{ of blood flow}$$

Most of the O_2 transported by Hgb during rest is thus kept in reserve, which will come in handy during exercise, as we shall soon see.

The second thing we should notice is the shape of the curve. The upper part of the curve is almost flat. This means that a large change in PO_2 in this portion of the curve is associated with only a small change in the amount of O_2 held by Hgb. For example, if arterial blood PO_2 were increased from the normal 100 mm Hg (such as by breathing pure O_2 at sea level), only 0.5 vol% of O_2 is added to Hgb. This small amount, plus the additional O_2 dissolved in plasma, represents only an 11% increase in the amount of O_2 transported to the tissues. Therefore, normally, arterial PO_2 is maintained at close to optimal levels, and the use of pure O_2 at sea level during exercise will not greatly increase O_2 transport. Conversely, if arterial PO_2 were decreased from 100 to 70 mm Hg (as by ascent to a moderate altitude of $\sim$ 10,000 feet or 3000 m), %SO_2 would decrease from 97.5% to 93%. Quite a difference, yet one that is still associated with only a small change (decrease) in the amount of O_2 carried to the tissues, $\sim$ 1 vol%. In this case, the flat upper part of the curve helps protect against inadequate oxygenation of blood, despite somewhat substantial decreases in PO_2. Such a small loss should not affect resting conditions but would likely impact one's maximal exercise performance.

The steep middle and lower portions of the curve likewise reflect protective functions, but of a different kind. In this portion of the curve (below a PO_2 of about 50 mm Hg), a small change in PO_2 is associated with a large change in Hgb saturation. Therefore, a small decrease in tissue PO_2 enables the tissues to extract a relatively large amount of O_2. For example, if tissue PO_2 decreased from 40 to 10 mm Hg, %SO_2 decreases from 75% to 13%, a difference of 13.5 vol% that can be extracted by the tissues. The steep middle

and lower portions of the curve, then, protect the tissues by favoring dissociation of O_2 from Hgb despite small decreases in PO_2. During exercise, the PO_2 of active skeletal muscles may approach 5 mm Hg.

The HgbO₂ Curve during Exercise

Our discussion of the $HgbO_2$ dissociation curve would not be complete unless we included the effects of pH (H^+), temperature, and CO_2 on O_2 transport. Increases in the blood's H^+ concentration (which decreases pH), temperature, and CO_2 cause a shift of the $HgbO_2$ dissociation curve to the right.[17,18] This is shown in figure 8.11B (solid line). The curve represented by the dashed line is the same as that in figure 8.11A and is included as a reference line. During exercise, increased CO_2 and lactic acid production lower blood pH, and increased heat production raises blood temperature. Therefore, the curve, shifted to the right in figure 8.11B, is applicable under exercise conditions. More importantly, instead of visualizing the $HgbO_2$ curve as a static entity, picture it as a constantly shifting curve whose position on the graph is dependent on (1) whether the blood in question is in pulmonary capillaries or tissue capillaries and (2) what changes have occurred in blood pH, CO_2, and temperature.

Significance of the Shift in the Dissociation Curve

What does this shift mean? A close look at the curve reveals that the greatest amount of shift occurs in the steep middle and lower portions (e.g., between $PO_2 = 20$ and 50 mm Hg). On the other hand, at a PO_2 between 90 and 100 mm Hg, very little shift occurs. During exercise, these differences are extremely important for two reasons. First, in the lungs, the loading of pulmonary capillary blood with O_2 is not greatly affected by the rightward shift. Second, at the muscle site more O_2 is made available (dissociates from Hgb) at a given PO_2. For example, suppose that during exercise arterial blood PO_2 equaled 100 mm Hg, and mixed venous blood PO_2 equaled 30 mm Hg. If there were no shift in the $HgbO_2$ dissociation curve, the a − $\overline{v}O_2$ diff (i.e., the amount of O_2 given up to the tissues, shaded in red and yellow in figure 8.11B) would be:

$$19.5 \text{ vol\%} - 11.6 \text{ vol\%} = \textbf{7.9 mL of } O_2 \cdot \textbf{100 mL of blood flow}^{-1}$$

With the shift of the curve to the right the a − $\overline{v}O_2$ diff (shaded in red, yellow, and green) is now:

$$19.0 \text{ vol\%} - 8.8 \text{ vol\%} = \textbf{10.2 mL of } O_2 \cdot \textbf{100 mL of blood flow}^{-1}$$

This represents an $\sim$ 30% [(10.2 − 7.9) ÷ 7.9] increase in the amount of O_2 available to the tissues. During maximal

---

*Notice the bar above the v in a − $\overline{v}O_2$ diff. This bar refers to average or "mixed" venous blood. The best location to obtain such a sample would be the right ventricle or pulmonary artery, where blood is sufficiently mixed and representative of an average venous sample for the entire body. This approach requires the use of special catheters. A little less complex, yet still not without discomfort, is obtaining a sample of arterial blood. Such a sample can be obtained from *any* artery in the body (e.g., brachial artery), since each has not yet reached its target tissue where it will unload O_2. As you can see, the direct measurement of a − $\overline{v}O_2$ diff is quite an invasive procedure. (Given $\dot{V}O_2$ and cardiac output, the noninvasive calculation of a − $\overline{v}O_2$ diff is possible using the Fick equation; see chapter 9.)

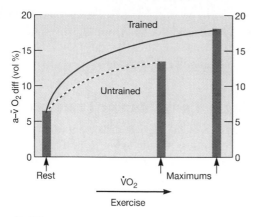

Figure 8.12

Effects of exercise on arteriovenous oxygen difference (a − $\bar{v}O_2$ diff) for trained and untrained subjects. During exercise, the muscles extract a greater amount of O_2 from a given quantity of arterial blood. Training improves this capacity.

exercise, this shift, plus the greatly lowered PO_2 of the active muscles, may increase the a − $\bar{v}O_2$ diff 3 to 3.5 times that at rest (figure 8.12).

Transport of Carbon Dioxide by Blood

Like oxygen, carbon dioxide is carried by the blood (figure 8.13) in physical solution (dissolved) and in chemical combination. Also, as in O_2 transport, the amount of dissolved CO_2 constitutes only a small percentage (about 5%) of the total transported; the majority (95%) is carried in chemical combination. However, the chemical reactions that CO_2 undergoes (principally in the red blood cells) are quite different from those of O_2. In blood, CO_2 reacts chemically both with water, to form a weak acid called *carbonic acid,* and with blood proteins (principally, the globin of Hgb), to form **carbamino compounds.**

Dissolved Carbon Dioxide

What we discussed earlier about dissolved O_2 is also applicable to dissolved CO_2. Briefly:

1. The amount of CO_2 dissolved in blood (arterial and venous) and in tissues is dependent on its solubility and partial pressure.
2. Dissolved CO_2 is relatively unimportant as a transporting mechanism.
3. Dissolved CO_2 determines blood and tissue PCO_2 and therefore is important in cardiorespiratory regulating mechanisms.

Transport of CO_2 in Chemical Combination

Carbonic Acid and the Bicarbonate Ion

As CO_2 diffuses into tissue-capillary blood, it immediately reacts with water in plasma and red blood cells to form carbonic acid (H_2CO_3), according to the following reaction:

$$CO_2 + H_2O \rightleftharpoons H_2CO_3$$

For this reaction to occur with any great speed, an enzyme called **carbonic anhydrase** is required. In plasma, this enzyme is absent, but in red blood cells, it is highly concentrated. Therefore, the formation of H_2CO_3 takes place principally within the blood cells.

As quickly as H_2CO_3 is formed, it ionizes; in other words, it dissociates into a hydrogen ion (H^+) and a **bicarbonate ion (HCO_3^-)** as follows:

$$H_2CO_3 \rightleftharpoons H^+ + HCO_3^-$$

The complete reaction, then, is more accurately written as:

$$CO_2 + H_2O \rightleftharpoons H_2CO_3 \rightleftharpoons H^+ + HCO_3^-$$

Thus, as shown by this reaction, CO_2 is carried in the blood in the form of HCO_3^-. The double arrows in the equation mean that the reactions are reversible. It proceeds to the right as CO_2 is added (by diffusion) to tissue-capillary blood, and it proceeds to the left when CO_2 diffuses from the blood into the alveoli. Although the formation of HCO_3^- occurs mostly within the red blood cell, it is transported primarily by plasma. This is because as the concentration of HCO_3^- increases in the red blood cell (but not in plasma) it diffuses into the plasma.*

The small amount of H^+ formed when H_2CO_3 dissociates will increase the acidity of venous blood (↓ pH) if they are not buffered. (This is one of the reasons why an increase in CO_2 production is associated with an increase in acidity.) In plasma, H^+ is buffered (i.e., taken out of circulation) by plasma proteins. Inside the red blood cell, where most of the H^+ is formed, Hgb serves as the buffer. It is interesting to note that Hgb is a better buffer than is oxyhemoglobin. This means that as O_2 dissociates from Hgb and diffuses into the tissues, the buffering of H^+ is facilitated. In turn, more HCO_3^- can be formed and more CO_2 carried without a substantial change in blood acidity. Furthermore, remember that an increase in blood acidity shifts the $HgbO_2$ dissociation curve to the right. This favors not only the release of O_2 at the tissue, but also the "freeing-up" of Hgb, which is the better buffer.

---

*As HCO_3^- diffuses from the red blood cell into plasma, chloride ion (Cl^-) diffuses from plasma into the red blood cell. This is called the *chloride shift* and serves to maintain the ionic balance between red blood cells and plasma.

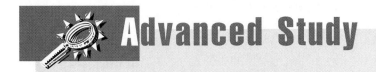

Advanced Study

2,3-DPG and O₂ Transport

The red blood cell has no nucleus and no mitochondria. As a result, its metabolic needs are fewer than most other cells. What little energy is needed is used to maintain cell shape and preserve the concentrations of various ions inside the cell. The energy required to accomplish these tasks is derived from anaerobic glycolysis, with one by-product being 2,3-Diphosphoglycerate (2,3-DPG). Increases in 2,3-DPG occur in response to two conditions: exposure to altitude and anemia; in other words, tissue hypoxia. Its presence facilitates the dissociation of O_2 from Hgb at the tissue level (shifts curve to the right).

Historically, the role of 2,3-DPG during an acute exercise is not without controversy. One study involving a group of trained runners and a group of sedentary control subjects showed no significant difference between groups in the levels of 2,3-DPG at rest; however, levels were higher in the runners after a 50 minute run.[12] In 1986 Mairbauri et al.[14] reported that neither moderate or heavy exercise increased 2,3-DPG levels, confirming that the rightward shift in the $HgbO_2$ dissociation curve during exercise results from changes in other blood factors (pH, temperature). More importantly, significant changes in the concentration of 2,3-DPG generally take several hours to occur, making it an unlikely candidate to influence O_2 transport during an acute bout of exercise.

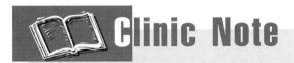

Clinic Note

Carboxyhemoglobin

In the last chapter we discussed the harmful effects of cigarette smoking on airway resistance. As you might guess, cigarette smoking also impacts O_2 transport by interfering with the amount of O_2 that can be carried by Hgb. One of the by-products inhaled in the smoke from burning tobacco is carbon monoxide (CO). Carbon monoxide has an affinity for Hgb that is 200 to 250 times higher than that of O_2. This means that the partial pressure of CO need be only 1/250 of that of O_2 to combine equally with Hgb. Therefore, when both CO and O_2 are present in alveolar air, CO acts much more quickly to combine with Hgb, forming a compound called carboxyhemoglobin (HgbCO). Once CO has combined with Hgb, it is impossible for $HgbO_2$ to be formed because CO combines with the same chemical unit of Hgb (heme) that ordinarily would combine with O_2. As a result, the O_2-carrying capacity of blood is reduced.

For example, the normal blood level of HgbCO in nonsmokers is 1% to 2%; however, among heavy, chronic smokers it may reach 12%. Such values can be associated with complaints of mild headaches and shortness of breath on moderate exertion. For a smoker with a HgbCO of 12%, the amount of O_2 bound to one gram of Hgb is reduced—from its normal level of $1.34 \, mL \cdot g^{-1}$ to $\sim 1.18 \, mL \cdot g^{-1}$. Therefore, $\%SO_2$ is reduced as follows:

$$\%SO_2 - 88\% - \frac{15.0 \, g \cdot dL^{-1} \times 1.18}{15.0 \, g \cdot dL^{-1} \times 1.34} = \frac{17.7 \, vol\%}{20.1 \, vol\%} \times 100$$

A patient with CO poisoning, such as an unfortunate victim caught in a house fire, is treated by giving pure O_2 or 95% O_2 with 5% CO_2. Victims can also be given O_2 in a hyperbaric chamber because it is able to raise inspired PO_2 to 2000 mm Hg and, therefore, force into solution (dissolve in plasma) all the O_2 required by the body while at rest (up to 6 vol%).

Besides cigarette smoking and house fires, CO can also enter the lungs as an air pollutant. Concentrations as high as 115 ppm have been reported for ambient air in areas of high-density automobile traffic. People who exercise in these areas may develop HgbCO levels exceeding 5%, which can increase ventilation during exercise training and reduce $\dot{V}O_2$ max.

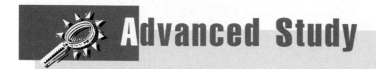

Advanced Study

Blood Doping

In chapters 4 and 9 we define aerobic power as the ability of the body to transport and utilize O_2. In the person with a normal blood Hgb level, the word "transport" in this definition mostly refers to cardiac output (chapter 9). However, as discussed in this chapter, we also know that the transport of O_2 is partly influenced by the amount of Hgb in blood.

In the arena of competitive, world-class athletics, the issue of improving performance by increasing the ability of the blood to transport more O_2 has, at times, received wide-spread attention. For example, in the 1968 Olympic games in Mexico City, the winners of many of the endurance footraces tended to hail from countries or regions that are considered highlands (those athletes were familiar with performing at altitude). This led to a resurgence of research aimed at increasing the O_2-carrying capacity of blood through a variety of techniques called **blood doping.**

In the 1970s and 1980s, blood doping involved removing blood from the athlete (two separate units of blood several weeks apart), then separating the red blood cells from the whole blood and freezing them for re-infusion at some time in the future (a time just prior to athletic competition). This meant that ~ 400 mL of their own red blood cells were used in the process. One study of this technique involving 6 male runners showed an increase in hematocrit from 41.5% to more than 47%.[4] This means that Hgb increased from ~ 13.8 g $\cdot$ dL^{-1} to ~ 15.7 g $\cdot$ dL^{-1}, increasing the actual O_2 content of Hgb as follows.

Pre-infusion of red blood cells:

$$13.8 \text{ g} \cdot \text{dL}^{-1} \times 1.34 \text{ mL } O_2 \cdot \text{g Hgb}^{-1} = 18.4 \text{ vol\%}$$

Post-infusion of red blood cells:

$$15.7 \text{ g} \cdot \text{dL}^{-1} \times 1.34 \text{ mL } O_2 \cdot \text{g Hgb}^{-1} = 21.0 \text{ vol\%}$$

The 14% increase in actual Hgb content from 18.4 vol% to 21.0 vol% was associated with a significantly faster 10 km run time and an approximate 10 beat per minute decrease in submaximal exercise heart rate—clearly a beneficial or ergogenic effect.

In the late 1980s, another blood doping technique came on the scene, this one involving the injection of a hormone approved by the Food and Drug Administration for use in patients receiving dialysis secondary to kidney failure. This hormone (erythropoietin), naturally produced by the kidneys for the purpose of stimulating the bone marrow to manufacture more red blood cells, can also be manufactured in the laboratory (rEPO). Ekblom and Berglund[7] gave rEPO to 15 healthy men three times per week for six weeks and showed that hematocrit increased from 45% to 50%. This increase was associated with an 8% increase in peak $\dot{V}O_2$.

Although we have shown that both of these blood doping methods lead to polycythemia (an increase in red blood cells), we are quick to point out that both are also banned by the United States Olympic Committee as a means of enhancing athletic performance. More importantly, both practices place the athlete at an increased risk for a variety of health-related complications, not the least of which is a stroke resulting from thrombi (blood clot). This concern is especially true for rEPO, where the dose-response relationship (the more drug given, the greater the response) can drive hematocrit beyond 55%, increasing the viscosity of blood (resistance to flow) to dangerously elevated levels. Unfortunately, accurate information about the side effects and complication rates associated with blood doping among athletes is difficult to find because these methods are usually practiced secretly and in an unmonitored fashion.

Carbamino Compounds

Plasma proteins and Hgb, besides serving as buffers, also play another important role in the direct transport of CO_2. This role involves their chemical reaction with CO_2, forming what are referred to as carbamino compounds. In these reactions, H^+ are also formed and must be buffered (as described on page 208). Formation of carbamino compounds takes place mainly in the red blood cells, by the reaction of CO_2 with Hgb—yielding carbaminohemoglobin. CO_2 reacts with the protein fraction (globin) of the Hgb molecule and not with the heme (iron) group, as is the case with O_2. This means that Hgb alone is capable of chemically combining with, and thus transporting, O_2 and CO_2 simultaneously. However, Hgb alone is capable of combining with more CO_2 than $HgbO_2$. Therefore, as in the bicarbonate ion mechanism, the unloading of O_2 at the tissue-capillary membrane facilitates the loading of CO_2, and vice versa.

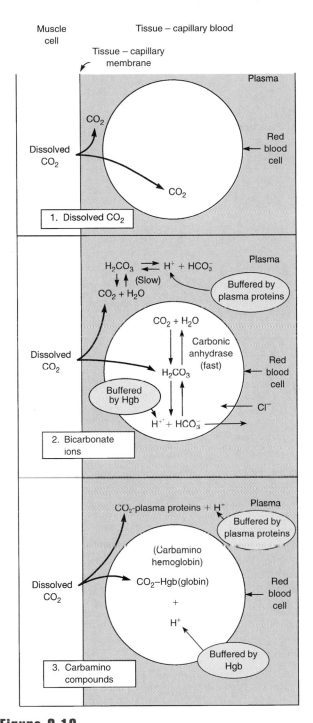

Figure 8.13

Carbon dioxide transport. Carbon dioxide is transported in physical solution as (1) dissolved CO_2 or in chemical combination as (2) bicarbonate ions and (3) carbamino compounds.

Again, the transport mechanisms for CO_2 as it diffuses from the tissues into tissue-capillary blood are summarized in figure 8.13. As CO_2 diffuses from the pulmonary-capillary blood to the alveoli, all reactions are reversed,

8.1

Oxygen and carbon dioxide content of blood at rest and during exercise

Transport mechanism	O_2 or CO_2 content (Milliliters per 100 mL whole blood)		
	Arterial blood	Mixed venous blood	$a - \bar{v}O_2$ difference
Rest ($\dot{V}O_2 = 0.246\ L \cdot min^{-1}$, $\dot{V}CO_2 = 0.202\ L \cdot min^{-1}$)			
Total O_2	19.8	15.18	4.62
In solution	0.3	0.18	0.12
As $HgbO_2$	19.5	15.0	4.5
Total CO_2	48.0	51.8	3.8
In solution	2.3	2.7	0.4
As HCO_3^-	43.5	45.9	2.4
As carbamino compounds	2.2	3.2	1.0
Heavy exercise ($\dot{V}O_2 = 3.2\ L \cdot min^{-1}$, $\dot{V}CO_2 = 3.03\ L \cdot min^{-1}$)			
Total O_2	21.2	5.34	15.86
In solution	0.3	0.06	0.24
As $HgbO_2$	20.9	5.28	15.62
Total CO_2	45.0	60.0	15.0
In solution	2.1	3.1	1.0
As HCO_3^-	40.8	53.2	12.4
As carbamino compounds	2.1	3.7	1.6

$a - \bar{v}O_2$ diff) is only 3.4 times that at rest (15.86 vol% ÷ 4.62 vol%). This is enough to increase $\dot{V}O_2$ from 0.246 to 0.84 $L \cdot min^{-1}$ (0.246 × 3.4), a favorable change but one that is inadequate to fully meet the O_2 demands of exercise. To accomplish this, blood flow must also be increased, as we shall see in chapter 9.

Summary

Gas exchange at the alveolar-capillary and tissue-capillary membranes occurs through the process of diffusion (random motion of molecules) and is primarily dependent on the partial pressure gradients of the gases involved. Gases always diffuse from an area of higher to an area of lower partial pressure. The partial pressure of a gas (as expressed in Dalton's law) is the pressure of a single gas either in a gas mixture or in a liquid and depends on the amount of gas present and the total barometric pressure.

Besides being affected by partial pressure gradients, gas exchange can be affected by: (1) the length of the diffusion path, (2) the number of red cells or the hemoglobin concentration, or both, and (3) the surface area available for diffusion.

During exercise, the diffusion capacity increases because of the opening of more alveoli and capillaries, thus increasing the surface area. Generally, athletes have larger diffusion capacities at rest and during maximal exercise than do nonathletes. During an acute bout of exercise, plasma volume decreases, which produces a hemoconcentration effect. As the result of chronic exercise training, both blood volume and plasma volume are expanded or increased.

Oxygen is carried in small amounts in plasma and in large amounts by the red blood cells. In the plasma, it is carried in solution and is responsible for the partial pressure of oxygen in the blood. In the red blood cell, it is chemically united with hemoglobin. Five factors affect the saturation of Hgb with O_2: (1) the partial pressure of O_2 in the blood, (2) the temperature of the blood, (3) the pH of the blood, (4) the amount of CO_2 in the blood, and (5) the concentration of 2,3-diphosphoglycerate in the red blood cell. During exercise, the first four factors change in a fashion that favors the release of O_2 to the working muscles. The relationships among these factors may be shown by what is called the oxyhemoglobin dissociation curve.

Like oxygen, carbon dioxide is carried both in physical solution and in chemical combination. By far the greater amount of CO_2 is transported in chemical combination, just like oxygen. Carbon dioxide combines with water in the blood to form carbonic acid and with blood proteins (including Hgb) to form carbamino compounds.

Questions

1. What is meant by the partial pressure of a gas?
2. Describe the relationship between partial pressure and concentration of gases in a gas mixture.
3. Discuss the partial pressure of a gas in a liquid.
4. What is the physiological significance of dissolved oxygen and carbon dioxide?
5. Discuss all factors affecting gas exchange.
6. How does diffusion capacity change during an acute bout of exercise or with exercise training?
7. What is meant by: (a) the oxygen-carrying capacity of Hgb, and (b) the percent saturation of Hgb?
8. Relative to both rest and exercise, explain the significance of the shape of the oxyhemoglobin dissociation curve with respect to gas exchange and transport.
9. During exercise, there are increases in blood acidity, temperature, and CO_2. How do these factors affect the dissociation curve?
10. Describe the ways in which CO_2 is transported from muscle tissue to the lungs.
11. Relate CO_2 transport to acid-base balance.

References

1. Åstrand, P. O. 1952. *Experimental Studies of Physical Working Capacity in Relation to Sex and Age.* Copenhagen: Ejnar Munksgaard.
2. Åstrand, P., T. Cuddy, B. Saltin, and J. Stenberg. 1964. Cardiac output during submaximal and maximal work. *J Appl Physiol.* 19:268–274.
3. Åstrand, P. O., B. Eriksson, I. Nylander, L. Engstrom, P. Karlbert, B. Saltin, and C. Thoren. 1963. Girl swimmers. Acta Paediat. (Suppl):147.
4. Brien, A. J., and T. L. Simon. 1987. The effects of red blood cell infusion on 10-km race time. *JAMA* 257:2761–2765.
5. Carroll, J. F., V. A. Convertino, C. E. Wood, J. E. Graves, D. T. Lowenthal, and M. L. Pollock. 1995. Effect of training on blood volume and plasma hormone concentrations in elderly. *Med Sci Sports Exerc.* 27:79–84.
6. Eichner, E. R. 1992. Sports anemia, iron supplements, and blood doping. *Med Sci Sports Exerc.* 24:S315–S318.
7. Ekblom, B., and B. Berglund. 1991. Effect of erythropoietin

administration on maximal aerobic power. *Scand J Med Sci Sports.* 1:88–93.
8. Green, H. J., L. L. Jones and D. C. Painter. 1990. Effects of short-term training on cardiac function during prolonged exercise. *Med Sci Sports Exerc.* 22:488–493.
9. Guyton, A. C., and J. E. Hall. 1996. *Textbook of Medical Physiology,* 9th ed. Philadelphia: W. B. Saunders. pp. 298–300.
10. Holmgren, A., and P. Åstrand. 1966. DL and the dimensions and functional capacities of the O_2 transport system in humans. *J Appl Physiol.* 21(5):1463–1470.
11. Kaufmann, D., E. Swenson, J. Fencl, and A. Lucas. 1974. Pulmonary function of marathon runners. *Med Sci Sports.* 6(2):114–117.
12. Lijnen, P., P. Hespel, S. Van Oppens, R. Fiocchi, W. Goossens, E. Vanden Eynde, and A. Amery. 1986. Erythrocyte 2,3-diphosphoglycerate and serum enzyme concentrations in trained and sedentary men. *Med Sci Sports Exerc.* 18(2):174–179.
13. Magel, J., and K. Andersen. 1969. Pulmonary diffusing capacity and cardiac output in young trained Norwegian swimmers and untrained subjects. *Med Sci Sports.* 1(3):131–139.
14. Mairburi, H., et al. 1986. Regulation of red cell 2,3-DPG and $HB-O_2$ affinity during acute exercise. *Eur. J Appl Phyiol.* 55:174–180.
15. Newman, F., B. Smalley, and M. Thompson. 1961. A comparison between body size and lung function of swimmers and normal school children. *J Physiol.* (London). 156:9P.
16. Reuschlein, P., W. Reddan, J. Burpee, J. Gee, and J. Rankin. 1968. Effect of physical training on the pulmonary diffusing capacity during submaximal work. *J Appl Physiol.* 24(2):152–158.
17. Shappell, S., J. Murray, A. Bellingham, R. Woodson, J. Detter, and C. Linfant. 1971. Adaptation to exercise: role of hemoglobin affinity for oxygen and 2,3-diphosphoglycerate. *J Appl Physiol.* 30(6):827–832.
18. Thompson, J., J. Dempsey, L. Chosy, N. Shahidi, and W. Reddan. 1974. Oxygen transport and oxyhemoglobin dissociation during prolonged muscular work. *J Appl Physiol.* 37(5):658–664.

Selected Readings

Comroe, J. 1974. *Physiology of Respiration,* 2d ed. Chicago: Year Book Medical.

Comroe, J., R. Forster, A. DuBois, W. Briscoe, and E. Carlsen. 1962. *The Lung,* 2d ed. Chicago: Year Book Medical, pp. 111–161.

Forster, R. 1957. Exchange of gases between alveolar air and pulmonary capillary blood: Pulmonary diffusing capacity. *Physiol Rev.* 37:391–452.

Guyton, A. C., and J. E. Hall. 1996. *Textbook of Medical Physiology,* 9th ed. Philadelphia: W. B. Saunders.

Levitzky, M. G. 1991. *Pulmonary Physiology,* 3d ed. New York: McGraw-Hill, Inc.

Weibel, E. 1973. Morphological basis of alveolar capillary gas exchange. *Physiol Rev.* 53(2):419–495.

Wasserman, K., J. E. Hansen, D. Y. Sue, B. J. Whipp, and R. Casaburi. 1994. *Principles of Exercise Testing and Interpretation,* 2d ed. Philadelphia: Lea & Febiger.

9
Cardiovascular System: Function and Exercise Responses

Each day, virtually all people participate in some type of physical activity. For some, this may mean making their bed or preparing meals. For others, this might entail high-intensity exertion, such as running a 1500 m race. Common to all activities is the involvement of the cardiovascular system. The cardiovascular responses that take place can be brief and "relatively" minor, such as an increase in heart rate as one stands up from a chair and walks from one room to another. Alternately, cardiovascular responses can be quite complex, to the extent that blood flow during intense mountain biking is increased and preferentially directed toward the more metabolically active skeletal muscles. And while much is already known about how the cardiovascular system adapts or responds to an acute bout of exercise, many key questions still remain unanswered. A thorough knowledge of cardiovascular physiology, its many terms, and acute exercise responses will help serve persons entering careers in medicine, rehabilitation, sport physiology, coaching, and athletic training. As you can see, the implications are quite widespread.

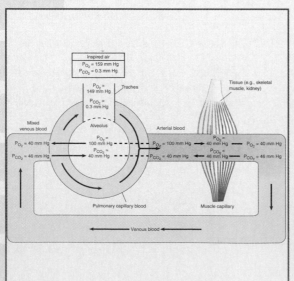

Before proceeding, recall from the previous chapter that to fully meet gas transport (O_2 and CO_2) demands during exercise, an increase in blood flow or the amount of blood delivered to the active muscles must occur. The two major changes responsible for the increase in blood flow are (1) an increase in **cardiac output** (i.e., the amount of blood pumped per minute by the heart) and (2) a redistribution of blood flow from less active organs to the more active skeletal muscles. The above changes allow us to accomplish the tasks we desire, whether they are simple or pushing the limits of human performance.

chapter overview

key terms

The major concepts to be learned from this chapter are as follows:

- The heart is two muscular pumps in one: the left heart, which pumps blood to the body tissues (systemic system), and the right heart, which pumps blood to the lungs (pulmonary system).
- The individual cardiac muscle fibers are interconnected so that they function (contract) together as one large unit.
- Cardiac tissue has the property of autorhythmicity, which is the ability to self-generate electrical impulses in a rhythmical fashion.
- Like any other muscle or organ, the heart also requires a blood supply, called the coronary circulation. This circuit involves two primary arteries: the left main coronary artery and the right coronary artery.
- Changes in electrical activity (voltage) across the myocardium can be graphically displayed as a function of time via an electrocardiogram. Such a recording can be made while at rest and during exercise.
- The two major components of cardiac performance are stroke volume (the amount of blood pumped per beat) and the heart rate. Both increase during exercise and, therefore, increase cardiac output. During exercise, several mechanisms operate to maintain and increase stroke volume during exercise, which include an increase in venous return and an increase in myocardial contractility.
- The redistribution of blood flow during exercise involves more vasoconstriction of the arterioles supplying the inactive areas of the body and less vasoconstriction of the arterioles in the active muscles. The latter is caused, primarily, by increases in local temperature, CO_2, and lactic acid levels, and by a decrease in O_2.
- The ability of the body to transport and utilize oxygen represents the best overall measure of cardiorespiratory function. It involves stroke volume, heart rate, and the oxygen content difference between arterial and mixed venous blood.
- The study of physical laws, as they relate to blood flow, is called hemodynamics.

Blood Flow Changes

As previously mentioned, the transport of gases (O_2 and CO_2) to and from the working muscles involves an increase in cardiac output and a redistribution of blood away from the inactive muscles and organs toward the active muscles. Before detailing these changes we will start with a review of the heart and the cardiac cycle.

The Heart and Cardiac Cycle

The heart is made up of a number of components: cardiac muscle, valves, great vessels, pacemaker and electrical conducting system, coronary vessels, autonomic nervous system innervation, and a fibroserous sac surrounding the heart called the *pericardium*. Its major function is to pump blood through the circulatory system so that the tissues can be adequately perfused. Before discussing the exercise aspects of the circulatory system, we must first address three major areas: (1) the anatomy (structure) and physiology (function) of the heart, (2) the cardiac cycle—the electrical and mechanical aspects of the heart muscle, and (3) cardiac performance.

Anatomy and Physiology of the Heart

Figure 9.1*A* shows an illustration of a human heart. As you can see, it is really two pumps, separated by a common septum. The right side of the heart consists of the right atrium and ventricle, and the left side of the heart consists of the left atrium and ventricle. The right side receives blood from the body and then pumps it to the lungs via the *pulmonary* circulation or circuit. The left side receives blood from the lungs and then pumps it throughout the rest of the body via the *systemic* circulation or circuit. The septum prevents blood on the left side from mixing with blood on the right side and vice versa. It is the left sided pump that is responsible to pump blood to the skeletal muscles during physical activity or exercise.

In both pumps the thin-walled atria (plural for atrium) stretch to accommodate blood returning to the heart, allowing ~80% of the blood they receive to passively pass through into the thick-walled ventricles that lie below. The atria then simultaneously contract, completing the last 20% of ventricular filling. Soon after this, the ventricles contract and propel blood into the pulmonary and systemic circuits.

Heart Valves and Direction of Blood Flow

Blood from the head and upper extremities and from the trunk and lower extremities returns to the right atrium via the *superior and inferior vena cava,* respectively. At the same time, oxygenated blood is returning to the left atrium from the lungs via the pulmonary veins. Blood entering the

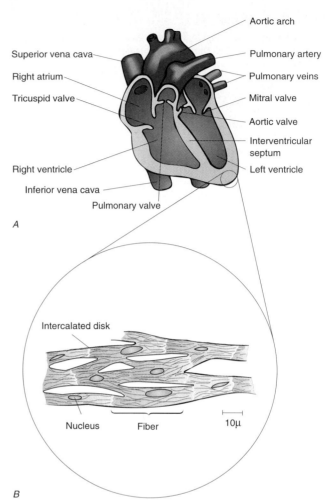

Figure 9.1

The human heart. *A.* The heart consists of four main chambers, the left atrium and left ventricle (left heart) and the right atrium and right ventricle (right heart). The left heart pumps blood to the body tissues and the right heart to the lungs. *B.* Schematic diagram of the heart muscle (myocardium) showing the intercalated discs and syncytial arrangement of fibers.

right ventricle from the right atrium passes through the *tricuspid valve,* while blood entering the left ventricle from the left atrium passes through the *mitral valve.* When the right ventricle contracts, the tricuspid valve closes preventing the retrograde or backward flow of blood into the right atrium. This forces the *pulmonic valve* open, causing blood to be ejected into the pulmonary arteries and toward the lungs. At the same time, the left ventricle contracts and the *mitral (bicuspid) valve* closes to prevent retrograde blood flow into the left atrium, instead directing blood through the *aortic valve* and into the systemic arterial circuit. Incidentally, if a valve is damaged or does not close properly, retrograde blood flow can occur, causing a noise that can be easily heard using a stethoscope. This type of noise is one cause of a *heart murmur.*

Microscopic Structure of Heart Muscle

In some ways cardiac or heart muscle, called the *myocardium,* is similar to skeletal muscle. For example, it is striated containing myofibrils and actin and myosin protein filaments. In fact, the actual contraction of the myocardium is thought to occur according to the sliding filament theory of muscular contraction as outlined in chapter 6.

However, in other ways, cardiac muscle is quite different from skeletal muscle. In cardiac muscle the cells are shorter and contain a higher myoglobin and mitochondria content. Energy in cardiac cells is produced predominately through aerobic pathways, using glucose, lactate and free-fatty acids as the fuel sources. Additionally, all the individual myocardial fibers or cells are anatomically connected, in series or end-to-end, by what are referred to as *intercalated discs* (figure 9.1*B*). These discs are actually nothing more than cell membranes that fuse together and form a "gap junction," the electrical resistance of which is quite low compared to other areas of the fiber's cell membrane. Through these gap junctions, ions are able to readily diffuse, allowing electrical impulses (i.e., action potentials) to travel longitudinally from one fiber to the next. Because all the fibers of heart muscle are interconnected, the heart acts as if it were one large fiber.

The entire heart muscle follows the all-or-none law, whereas with skeletal muscle, only the individual motor units and their associated fibers follow this law. Such an arrangement is referred to as a *functional syncytium* (or myocardial cross bridging), *functional* in the sense that when one cardiac fiber contracts, all fibers contract, and a *syncytium* because all the fibers are interconnected. Actually, there are two functional syncytia, one for the atria and one for the ventricles. This means that first the atria contract together and then the ventricles—an arrangement that results in the synchronous movement of blood through the heart, quite an effective pumping action.

Conduction System of the Heart

The heart has an inherent contractile rhythm of its own. That is to say, if all nerves regulating the heart are severed, the heart continues to generate a depolarizing impulse that causes it to contract in a rhythmical fashion. Normally, this automaticity originates in a specialized area of cardiac muscle fibers referred to as the **sinoatrial node (S-A node).** However, all heart tissue has this property. The S-A node (with an intrinsic depolarization rate of 60 or more per min) is located in the superior wall of the right atrium, immediately anterior to the opening of the superior vena cava (figure 9.2). Despite its location in the right atrium, the S-A node serves both the right and left sides of the heart. The ability of S-A nodal fibers to "self-excite" and generate a depolarization wave that will eventually activate the entire myocardium is caused by the fact that the cell membrane of these fibers is naturally "leaky" to sodium ions. This means that the resting potential of S-A nodal fibers is (1) only −55

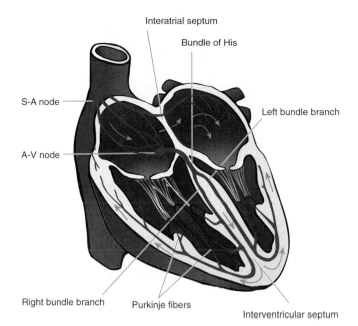

Figure 9.2

The intrinsic electrical conduction system of the heart. The S-A node is considered the primary pacemaker of the heart because the cardiac impulse is normally initiated there at a rate of 60 to 100 impulses per minute.

mV versus −85 mV in other cardiac cells and (2) constantly moving closer to the threshold for discharge of −40 mV. Because the S-A node depolarizes at a rate that is faster than all other areas of the heart, it is referred to as the *pacemaker* of the heart.

From the S-A node, the electrical impulse spreads throughout the atria (both right and left), some of it traveling along three specialized pathways called internodal tracts. These pathways are designed to move the impulse more quickly throughout the atria than if it had to travel across atrial muscle alone. Next, the impulse that originated from the S-A node activates another specialized area of cardiac tissue referred to as the **atrioventricular node (A-V node).** The A-V node, if not first activated by an S-A node generated depolarization wave, has the intrinsic ability to depolarize on its own at a rate of 40 to 60 beats · min^{-1}. It is also located in the right atrium, near the atrioventricular junction (figure 9.2). The A-V node briefly delays the transmission of the cardiac impulse from the atria into the ventricles. This delay of approximately 0.10 sec allows sufficient time for the atria to finish filling the ventricles before ventricular contraction begins.

From the A-V node, the depolarization wave progresses into the proximal end of the interventricular septum via more specialized conducting cells called the *Bundle of His.* The Bundle of His then divides into the *right bundle* and *left bundle branches,* which conduct the electrical impulse to the right and left ventricles, respectively. The right and left bundles give off many subbranches that eventually terminate in the *Purkinje system.* These fibers spread

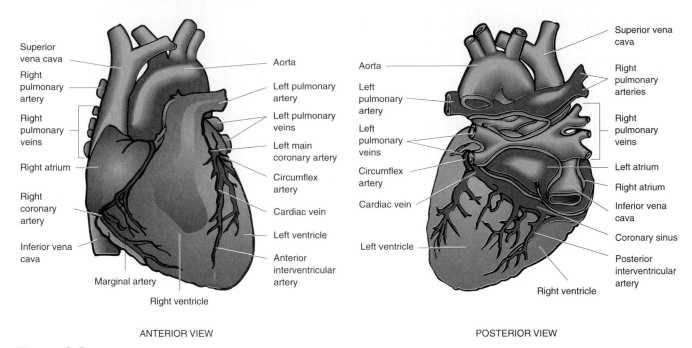

ANTERIOR VIEW   POSTERIOR VIEW

Figure 9.3

The coronary circulation. The heart muscle is supplied by two major arteries, the left main and right coronary arteries. The arteries and veins give off many branches as they encircle the heart.

throughout the entire ventricular myocardium to stimulate a "coordinated" contraction.

Blood Supply to the Heart

Like any living tissue, the cardiac muscle requires a blood supply of its own to provide it with oxygen and remove waste products. The blood supply to the heart is referred to as the *coronary circulation,* which is shown in figure 9.3. The heart muscle is supplied by two arteries, the left main coronary artery and the right coronary artery. Each artery originates from an *ostium* or opening in the wall of the aorta, at a point that is just above the aortic valve. The two major branches of the left main coronary artery are the *circumflex branch* (serving the lateral-posterior wall of the heart) and the *anterior interventricular (or anterior descending) branch.* The *right coronary artery* supplies most of the right ventricle, as well as the posterior side of the heart in 80% to 90% of people. All along the way, branches are given off such that the entire myocardium is supplied with a rich vascular network.

The coronary veins run alongside the arteries (figure 9.3). Most of the venous blood flow (~75%) drain into a very large vein referred to as the *coronary sinus.* From this vessel venous blood flows directly into the right atrium of the heart.

A unique feature about the coronary arteries and coronary blood flow is the large amount of oxygen extracted by the myocardium, even when a person is resting. For example, of the blood perfusing peripheral organs and tissues (e.g., muscle), ~25% to 30% of the available O_2 is extracted under resting conditions. In contrast to this, ~75%

of the O_2 available in the arterial blood perfusing the heart is extracted by myocardial tissue. As a consequence, when cardiac work increases during exercise, the demand for increased O_2 is not satisfied by big increases in O_2 extraction. Instead, there is an increase in coronary blood flow. For example, coronary blood flow increases from ~250 mL $\cdot$ min^{-1} at rest to ~1000 mL $\cdot$ min^{-1} at maximum exercise—a some fourfold increase.

The Cardiac Cycle

The cardiac cycle refers to the *electrical* and *mechanical* changes (pressure and volume changes) that occur in the heart during and following a single heartbeat. These include the contraction and relaxation of the myocardium, as well as pressure and volume changes. The contractile phase of the cardiac cycle is referred to as **systole** and the relaxation phase as **diastole** or **diastasis.** That portion of time within the cardiac cycle associated with systole is referred to as the *systolic time interval* and that portion of time associated with no electrical or mechanical activity (relaxation) is termed the *diastolic time interval.* Generally, at rest, the systolic time interval represents ~⅓ of the total cardiac cycle time. This means if one complete cardiac cycle takes one second, then the systolic time interval would be ~.33 sec. Therefore, at rest, the diastolic time interval is ~⅔ of the cardiac cycle.

Electrical Events in the Heart

The conduction system of the heart and the flow of the electrical impulse throughout the myocardium have already been described. Change in electrical activity (voltage) can

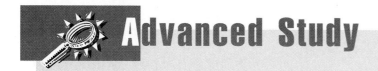

Advanced Study

Angiogenesis

Whether or not cardiac tissue experiences ischemia (temporary lack of oxygen) during exertion is dependent on the balance between myocardial oxygen demand and myocardial oxygen supply. Simply, when O_2 demand exceeds O_2 supply, ischemia results. One factor that can affect O_2 supply is a blockage in one or more of the coronary arteries, such as that caused by atherosclerosis. This can limit blood flow to a certain region of the heart and produce ischemia.

In response to a long-standing blockage in a coronary artery causing ischemia, the body often adapts by developing a new microvasculature around the blockage—called collateral vessels. Such vessels can help restore, in part, myocardial O_2 supply. This growth of new blood vessels, called *angiogenesis,* is not uncommon since ischemia is a stimulus for the release of angiogenic factors (small peptides such as fibroblast growth factor and angiogenin). New vessel growth usually appears in the form of a capillary loop or a small arteriole.

Well, along these same lines, several research studies have investigated the effects of exercise training on coronary artery angiogenesis or new collateral development. Using animal models (dog and pig) with experimentally induced coronary artery blockages, an increase in collaterals have been shown to occur with exercise training. In humans, however, definitive evidence that exercise training develops collaterals in the presence or absence of ischemia is lacking. Among patients with coronary atherosclerosis, it appears that exercise training may enhance or facilitate pharmacologic- (drug-) induced angiogenesis.[34] Most important, it is clinically unadvised to routinely ask patients with known exercise induced myocardial ischemia to willingly exercise in an ischemic state in hopes of improving collateral growth.

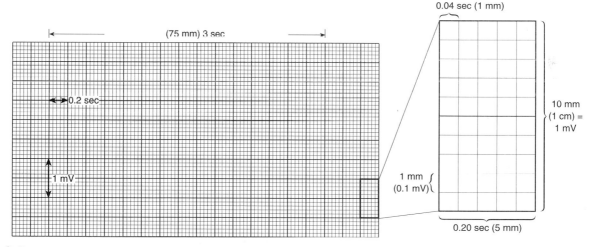

Figure 9.4

Typical ECG paper with its grid pattern and units of measurement specified. Time intervals are for a paper speed set at $25\ mm \cdot s^{-1}$.

be graphically recorded as a function of time using a recording called an **electrocardiogram (ECG).** The ECG is recorded by placing electrodes on the surface of the body that are connected to an amplifier and a recorder called an electrocardiograph.

The electrical activity of the heart is recorded on specially marked paper called ECG paper. Observe figure 9.4 as we describe these special markings to you. ECG recorders are designed to run in the horizontal direction at designated paper speeds; which is usually $25\ mm \cdot s^{-1}$. Looking at the paper you can see a grid pattern consisting of very small square boxes (1 mm × 1 mm) and larger boxes made up of 25 small ones (5 mm × 5 mm). Horizontally, five of the large boxes represents 25 mm and thus a time of 1 second when paper speed is $25\ mm \cdot s^{-1}$. This arrangement allows for the conversion of distance in mm to time in seconds. At a paper speed of $25\ mm \cdot s^{-1}$, each small box (1 mm) = 0.04 seconds and each larger

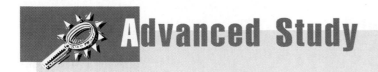

Advanced Study

Coronary Artery Blood Flow

There is a relationship between coronary artery blood flow and heart rate. Generally, at rest, ~20% of total coronary artery blood flow occurs during systole (myocardial contraction), much less than the 80% that occurs during diastole. Why is there such a difference? The most important reason has to do with the action of the ventricle muscle or wall. During systole, the distal coronary arterioles and capillary beds are physically closed down or occluded because of the forces acting upon them by the contracting heart muscle. This markedly limits perfusion of the myocardium during systole. However, during diastole (i.e., when the heart is "relaxed") the mechanical forces and pressure inside the ventricle wall are much lower (e.g., 5 to 10 mm Hg), far below the pressure within the coronary arteries at this time. As a result, the arteries and arterioles remain open and blood flows to nourish the heart muscle itself.

During exercise, as heart rate increases, both the systolic and diastolic time intervals shorten. However, the decrease in the diastolic interval time is much more pronounced than is the decrease in the systolic time interval. And since the coronary arteries predominately fill during diastole, it makes sense then that with increased heart rates—blood flow to certain areas of the cardiac muscle ((i.e., endocardium) will be somewhat diminished. Among healthy persons this does not ordinarily pose a problem because total blood flow is sufficiently increased—almost fourfold. However, among patients with a blockage within one or more of their coronary arteries, it is no wonder that an increase in heart rate (and the associated decrease in blood flow resulting from a shortened diastolic filling time) can result in myocardial ischemia.

---

box (5 mm) = 0.2 seconds. How many seconds is represented by 50 mm? By 75 mm?[*]

In the vertical direction, the small squares are calibrated to represent voltage. When an ECG recorder has been standardized, 1 millivolt (mV) is represented by 10 mm of vertical deflection (1 mV = 1 cm). By convention, an upward deflection is termed positive, and a downward deflection is termed negative. A deflection that is partly positive and partly negative is called *biphasic*. That part of the ECG that is flat means there is no change in voltage current (no positive or negative deflection), and it is said to be *isoelectric* or *baseline*. Taking the combined measurement of time intervals in the horizontal direction and voltage in the vertical direction provides for a moving record of the heart's electrical activity—the ECG.

As mentioned above, electrodes placed on the skin surface are used to detect the heart's electrical activity. Using switches built into the ECG machine itself, these electrodes can be made to act either as a positive pole electrode or as a distant ground electrode. When cardiac muscle is depolarized and a *depolarization wave* moves across the myocardium (atria or ventricles) and toward a positive skin electrode, a positive deflection is recorded on the ECG paper. Conversely, a negative deflection appears on the ECG when the depolarization wave travels away from a positive electrode.

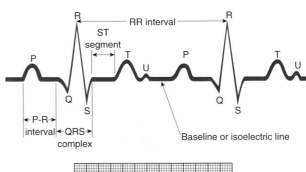

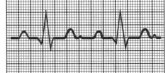

Figure 9.5

Normal, resting ECG for two complete heartbeats or cardiac cycles. The P wave results from atrial depolarization, the QRS complex from ventricular depolarization, and the T and U waves result from ventricular repolarization. The PR interval, ST segment and RR interval are discussed in the text.

STANDARD ECG MEASUREMENTS. Before contraction of cardiac muscle can occur, depolarization must spread through the muscle to initiate the chemical process of contraction. An example of a normal resting ECG for two complete cardiac cycles or heart beats is shown in figure 9.5. The ECG waves and intervals and their relationship to atrial and ventricular contraction are summarized as follows:

---

[*]50 mm × 0.04 s · mm^{-1} = 2 s; 75 mm × 0.04 s · mm^{-1} = 3 s.

9.1
The electrocardiographic leads and electrode placements

Lead	Position of Electrodes
Standard limb leads (bipolar)	
I	Right arm and left arm
II	Right arm and left leg
III	Left arm and left leg
Augmented leads (unipolar)	
aV_R	Right arm
aV_L	Left arm
aV_F	Left leg
Chest leads (unipolar)	
V_1	4th intercostal space, right side of sternum
V_2	4th intercostal space, left side of sternum
V_3	5th intercostal space, left side (between V_2 and V_4)
V_4	5th intercostal space, left side (mid-clavicular line)
V_5	5th intercostal space, left side (anterior axillary line)
V_6	5th intercostal space, left side (mid-axillary line)

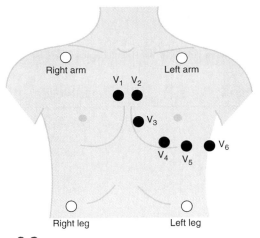

Figure 9.6
Electrocardiographic (ECG) electrode placement used during exercise testing.

- The *P wave* represents atrial depolarization and occurs at the beginning of atrial contraction.
- The *PR interval,* measured from the beginning of the P wave to the beginning of the QRS complex, represents the time that it takes for the depolarization wave to spread from the S-A node, across the atria, through the A-V node, and into the ventricles.
- The *QRS complex* represents ventricular depolarization and occurs at the beginning of ventricular contraction.

    1. The Q wave (when present) is the first negative deflection following the P wave and, depending on the electrode or lead chosen, may reflect initial activation of the ventricular septum.
    2. The R wave is the first positive deflection and represents depolarization of the vast majority of the ventricle.
    3. The S wave is a negative deflection that follows the R wave; it is the last part of the ventricles to get activated.

- The *ST segment,* measured from the end of the QRS complex to the beginning of the T wave, represents the beginning of ventricular repolarization.
- The *T wave* represents the later, more rapid, stages of ventricular repolarization.
- The *U wave,* which is often not observed, follows the T wave and represents the final component of ventricular repolarization.
- The *RR interval* represents the time for one complete cardiac cycle or beat. At a paper speed of $25 \text{ mm} \cdot \text{s}^{-1}$, one need only divide 4500 by the sum (in mm) of three consecutive RR intervals to obtain an accurate determination of heart rate (frequency of contractions per min).

THE TWELVE-LEAD ELECTROCARDIOGRAM. Usually performed while the person is resting in the supine position, the standard ECG consists of three sets of recordings that yield a total of 12 leads. Table 9.1 indicates where the electrodes are placed on the skin for each of the 12 leads. Leads I, II, and III are called *bipolar* leads, which means one lead is electrically designated as a positive monitoring electrode while the other is electrically designated as a negative reference electrode. The augmented voltage (aV) leads and the chest or precordial leads are *unipolar,* which means one electrode is connected to the positive monitoring terminal while two or more of the limb leads are connected via resistors to the negative/neutral terminal all at the same time. Figure 9.6 depicts where the electrodes are placed during exercise testing (see later exercise electrocardiogram discussion).

9.2

Five general pieces of information made available by an electrocardiogram (ECG)

Variable	Definition
Rate	Frequency of contractions (cardiac cycles) per minute. Normally, there is a 1:1 ratio between atrial and ventricular contractions. This means for every atrial contraction there is a corresponding ventricular contraction.
Arrhythmia	Denotes an abnormal cardiac rhythm, which can mean a variable rhythm, a rhythm that is too fast (tachycardia) or too slow (bradycardia), premature beats originating from an area other than the S-A node, or a change in the normal 1:1 ratio between atrial and ventricular contractions (now 2:1 or 3:1).
Axis	The general direction and magnitude of the heart's electrical activity during contraction, expressed as a vector. Separate vectors (axes) can be determined for both atrial (P wave) and ventricular (QRS complex) contractions.
Hypertrophy/ enlargement	Hypertrophy refers to an increase in left or right ventricular muscle mass, usually caused by some type of overload (pressure or volume) stress. Enlargement most often refers to an increase in left or right atrial chamber size.
Infarction	An area of necrotic (dead) tissue due to prolonged ischemia. A myocardial infarction (heart attack) results from complete, prolonged occlusion of a coronary artery—which had previously perfused a certain region of the myocardium with blood.

The twelve-lead system allows the analyst to view a single electrical event from twelve different positions simultaneously. Imagine standing in front of a large Sequoia tree that is many feet across and appears to be without damage. However, all you can see is that portion of the tree that is in your field of vision. To see the left, right, or back sides of the tree you must walk around it. Once on a different side you may discover a huge scar left by a limb that was felled, possibly by lightning or high winds from years past. Well, the twelve-lead ECG system allows you to see all sides of the heart simultaneously. The type of information made available by the ECG is detailed in table 9.2.

Under resting conditions, a normal sinus rhythm represents 60 to 100 cardiac cycles per minute. A heart rate less than 60 b · min^{-1} is called **bradycardia,** and a rate greater than 100 b · min^{-1} and less than 250 b · min^{-1} is called **tachycardia.** Heart rates in excess of 250 b · min^{-1} are called flutter or fibrillation, a life-threatening problem if occurring in the ventricles. Among untrained patients with heart disease a heart rate below 60 b · min^{-1} might be of concern. However, among well trained athletes, especially endurance athletes, it is not uncommon to find a marked normal physiological bradycardia approaching 40 b · min^{-1}. And while some tachycardias are abnormal or even life-threatening, others are not. For example, during exercise we all experience an increase in rate, approaching 200 b · min^{-1} in some young persons. The vast majority of the time this type of tachycardia is a sinus tachycardia, meaning that the impulses to depolarize the myocardium originated from the S-A node. It is by no means abnormal.

THE STRESS OR EXERCISE ELECTROCARDIOGRAM. Although a great deal of information can be obtained from an ECG conducted on an individual while at rest, additional information about the heart's abilities and limitations can also be obtained if an ECG is performed while the person is exercising. To accomplish this a stress ECG is usually conducted in a laboratory, clinic, hospital or physician's office, as part of a symptom-limited* graded exercise stress test. Normal, exercise-related changes[13] that appear on the ECG include a decrease in the RR interval (as rate increases), a shortened PR interval, a slightly taller P wave, a general decrease in the height of the R wave, a slight decrease in the duration of the QRS, and an initial increase in

---

*Symptom-limited, graded exercise test means that the subject or patient continues to undergo increasing levels of exertion until symptoms such as fatigue, chest discomfort, or shortness of breath limit their ability to continue. Obviously, if the person supervising the test observes blood pressure or ECG abnormalities, the test is also stopped.

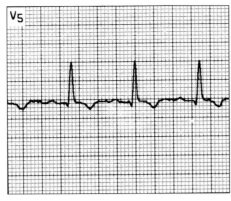

A Rest

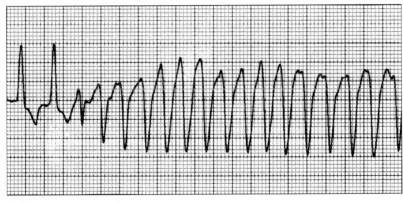

B Recovery from exercise

Figure 9.7

ECG tracings (lead V_5) from a 56-year-old male who sustained a heart attack approximately six months prior to this exercise test. *A*. Tracing is from pre-exercise ECG and shows sinus rhythm (rate = 88 b · min^{-1}). *B*. Tracing was recorded 30 seconds after exercise was stopped. Note that the shape of the QRS complex changes because the depolarization wave now originates in the ventricles. This is a life-threatening arrythmia called ventricular tachycardia. It was quickly and successfully treated with advanced emergency care.

T wave amplitude which then decreases near maximum effort. Some of the various protocols and instrumentation used to conduct a graded exercise test were described in chapter 4.

The shortened PR interval is worth exploring because it represents a unique property of the heart's conduction system called *dromotropicity* (conduction time). For example, recall that the PR interval reflects the time required for the electrical wave of activation to pass from the S-A node, across the atria, be delayed at the A-V node (PR segment), and then "meet-up with" the ventricular myocardium. Normally the PR interval is less than 0.2 sec and, as mentioned above, it is common for it to shorten during exercise—let's say from 0.16 to 0.14 sec. This shortening of the PR interval represents a *positive dromotropic effect,* which means there was a decrease in conduction time. (Similarly, the slightly shortened QRS duration during exercise means conduction time for ventricular depolarization is decreased—another positive dromotropic effect.) One reason that the PR interval decreases during exercise is the pres-

ence of elevated concentrations of catecholamines. These agents reach the myocardium via both the direct release by the sympathetic nerves that innervate the heart (norepinephrine only) and/or what is released elsewhere (epinephrine and norepinephrine) in the body and then transported to the heart by the blood. Therefore, catecholamines are said to have a positive dromotropic effect. Conversely, any agent or medication that lengthens conduction time is said to have a *negative dromotropic effect.*

Two of the many important pieces of information derived from a stress ECG are discussed below.[13]

• First, in most everyone heart rate and rhythm are regular at rest—and rate increases normally, without irregularity, during progressive exercise. There are others, however, who demonstrate a normal heart rate and rhythm at rest, only to have it suddenly speed up or become irregular (called an arrhythmia) during exercise (figure 9.7). A sudden tachycardia or irregular heart rhythm with exercise often originates from an area of the heart other than the S-A node, for example the atria (atrial or supraventricular arrhythmia) or the ventricles (ventricular arrhythmia). A stress ECG might be used to quantify the nature and severity of the arrhythmia and once this is accomplished, a physician may then order additional tests and/or prescribe, if needed, a medication to control it. Depending on the type of arrhythmia, another exercise ECG may then be ordered to assess whether or not the particular treatment chosen by the physician was, in fact, effective.

- Second, you overhear your favorite uncle who, at 48 years old, tells one of your parents that he has been experiencing chest discomfort and pain while rushing through the airport to catch a plane. When he stops and rests for a moment the discomfort goes away. Your uncle goes on to say that at first he simply tried to ignore the problem, attributing it to letting himself get out-of-shape. However, since his job demands that he travel a lot and he continues to experience the discomfort, it simply could no longer be overlooked. As a result, your uncle went to see a physician who performed a resting twelve lead ECG, the results of which were "perfectly normal." Just to be on the safe side, however, the physician asked your uncle to undergo a graded exercise stress test.

What precisely is it that the doctor suspects is causing the problem in the above example? And what could possibly show up on the stress ECG that was not present on the resting ECG?

To answer the first question, the doctor is concerned that there might be a blockage in one of the coronary arteries (see page 218) that supply blood, oxygen, and nutrients to the myocardium. Such a blockage does not present a problem when your uncle is resting, because the metabolic demands placed on the heart are low at that time. However, the blockage can be limiting when, during an activity such as rushing through the airport, the oxygen demanded by the now more metabolically active heart exceeds the amount of blood (and oxygen) that can get past the blockage in the coronary artery. This temporary lack of oxygen to heart tissue creates a condition called **myocardial ischemia.** For many people who experience the problem the typical symptom they experience is chest pain or discomfort known as *angina pectoris.* As discussed in chapter 14, the cause of the blockage is usually a deposition of cholesterol, which occurs over time and effects the innermost lining of the coronary artery (coronary artery disease caused by atherosclerosis). Ultimately, atherosclerosis decreases the size of the opening or lumen of the coronary artery and restricts blood flow.

Well, if myocardial ischemia is what the physician suspects is the problem, what is it about the stress ECG that will help him or her make the diagnosis? The answer lies in the ST segment portion of the ECG. Recall from our previ-

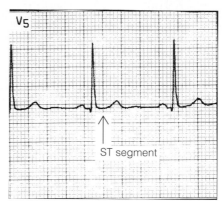

A Rest

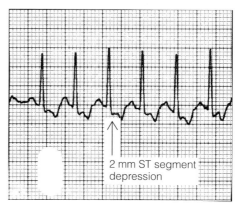

B Peak exercise

Figure 9.8

ECG tracings (lead V_5) from a 65-year-old male who underwent coronary artery bypass surgery in 1993. Tracing *A* is from a pre-exercise ECG and shows a normal sinus rhythm (rate = 69 b · min^{-1}). ST segments are at baseline. Tracing *B* was taken from a peak exercise ECG and shows 2 mm of ST segment depression that is strongly suggestive of exercise induced myocardial ischemia.

ous discussion that the ST segment starts at the end of the QRS complex and finishes at the beginning of the T wave. Note in figure 9.8*A* that the ST segment in lead V_5 at rest is normal, right up to baseline. However, at peak exercise (figure 9.8*B*) the ST segment in lead V_5 is depressed, approximately 2 mm below baseline. Such a change in lead V_5 is quite compatible with exercise-induced myocardial ischemia. And, although other disorders can cause chest pain or discomfort (e.g., reflux esophagitis), if one considers both factors (ST depression with exercise and chest pain that is brought on by exertion and relieved by rest) the probability that your uncle is experiencing myocardial ischemia due to atherosclerosis exceeds 90%.

Mechanical Events—Pressure and Volume Changes

As previously mentioned, the heart alternately contracts and relaxes in a rhythmical fashion resulting from the changes in electrical activity. During this cycle of systole and

9.3
Summary of events during the cardiac cycle

Line numbers (refer to figure 9.9)	Phase of cardiac cycle	Pressure/volume changes
1	Beginning of ventricular systole	Ventricular pressure greater than atrial pressure
1–2	Isometric ventricular contraction	Ventricular pressure rises rapidly; little change in aortic and atrial pressures
2	—	Ventricular pressure greater than aortic pressure
2–3	Ventricular ejection	Ventricular and aortic pressures reach peaks, then begin to decrease; little change in atrial pressure; rapid decrease in ventricular volume
3	Beginning of diastole	Ventricular pressure less than aortic pressure
3–4	Isometric relaxation	Ventricular pressure decreases rapidly; little change in aortic and atrial pressures
4	—	Ventricular pressure lower than atrial pressure
4–5	Diastole	Little change in ventricular and atrial pressures, aortic pressure decreasing gradually; rapid increase in ventricular volume
5–6	Diastole-atrial contraction	Small increases in ventricular and atrial pressures; little change in aortic pressure; small increase in ventricular volume

diastole, both the pressure and volume of blood within the left ventricle fluctuate as shown in figure 9.9. The upper two curves depict pressure changes within the aorta and left ventricle. The third curve shows changes in left ventricular blood volume. Note that as the ventricle begins to contract (see QRS complex at bottom of figure 9.9), the mitral valve is closed and ventricular pressure rises sharply. This happens before the aortic valve opens and any change in ventricular blood volume occurs. As pressure in the ventricle continues to increase and exceed aortic pressure, the aortic valve is opened allowing blood to be ejected from the ventricle into the aorta—quite rapidly during early ejection and then slower during later ejection.

The important features or events within the cardiac cycle are summarized in table 9.3. Remember, these changes are for the left heart. However, they are essentially the same for the right heart, except that the pressures within the pulmonary arteries and right ventricle are much lower, about one-sixth of that in the aorta and left ventricle.

Cardiac Performance

Two major determinants of cardiac performance are **stroke volume** and heart rate. And although it is tempting to consider each factor relative to its own influence on the heart, this is simply not correct. Instead, it is important to remember that the intact, functioning heart is a dynamic organ, one where both stroke volume and heart rate often "act

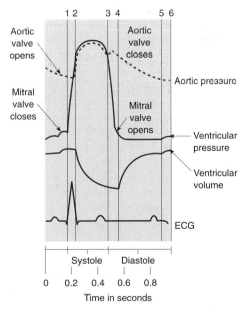

Figure 9.9

Electrical and mechanical changes in the left heart during the cardiac cycle. The upper two curves depict pressure changes in the aorta and left ventricle, respectively. The middle curve shows changes in the volume of blood in the left ventricle. The bottom curve represents the ECG recording. The numbered, vertical lines correspond to different, important events of the cycle, which are detailed in Table 9.3.

Source: Data from Barbara R. Landau, Essential Human Anatomy and Physiology, *1976, Scott, Foresman & Company.*

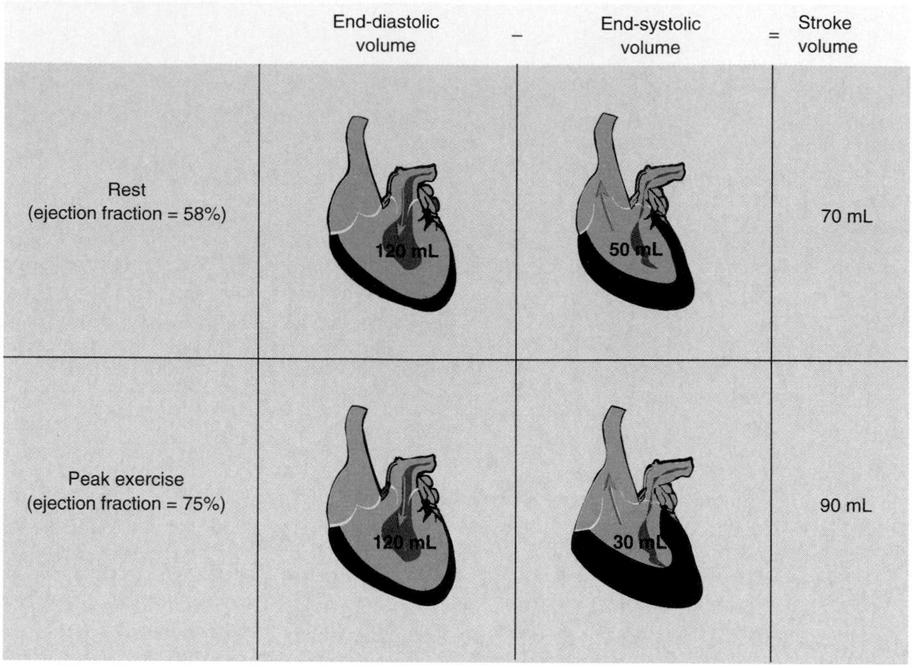

Figure 9.10

Left ventricular end-diastolic volume, end-systolic volume, stroke volume and ejection fraction at rest and during exercise. Note that stroke volume increases in this example due to a better emptying of the left ventricle at the end of systole. This is due to increased myocardial contractility with exercise.

together" to optimize ventricular performance. Before detailing how these factors contribute to cardiac performance during exercise, a brief explanation of each is appropriate. If needed, the reader is encouraged to review several other resources for a more in-depth description of stroke volume and heart rate.[4,19,23,42]

Stroke Volume

Stroke volume is the amount of blood (mL) pumped by the heart per stroke or beat of the heart. The stated value is usually made in reference to the left ventricle and except for any very short-term differences between the left and right sides of the heart, the value for the left ventricle is usually the same as the right ventricle. The resting, sitting* stroke volume of untrained male subjects averages between 70 and 90 mL · beat^{-1}, and with training it may approach 100 to 120 mL · beat^{-1} (figure 9.10). Among untrained females resting stroke volume may be between 50 and 70 mL · beat^{-1}, whereas among trained females it may be between 70 and 90 mL · beat^{-1}.

One common instrument used to measure stroke volume is an echocardiograph machine, which is described in

chapter 11 (page 289) and an example of which is provided in chapter 12 (figure 12.13). In addition to other variables, this instrument can measure both left ventricular end-systolic and end-diastolic volumes. Once these volumes are determined, stroke volume can be computed using the following simple equation:

Stroke volume = End-diastolic volume −

End-systolic volume

Left ventricular end-diastolic volume literally means the amount of blood in the left ventricle at the very end of diastole, just prior to the next contraction. And left ventricular end-systolic volume means the amount of blood that remains in the left ventricle just after the heart has finished contracting, just before it begins to refill. Figure 9.10 depicts these measures using actual values. It also introduces another new term called *ejection fraction,* which is the percentage of end-diastolic volume ejected with each systole. At rest, ejection fraction should be above 55%. Note that ejection fraction is a percentage (not an absolute number) and it is computed as follows:

Ejection fraction =

$$\frac{\text{End-diastolic volume} - \text{End-systolic volume}}{\text{End-diastolic volume}} \times 100 =$$

$$\frac{\text{Stroke volume}}{\text{End-diastolic volume}} \times 100$$

---

*Stroke volume is lower in the upright or sitting position when compared with the lying or supine position. In the upright position, more blood pools in the extremities and less returns to the heart. As a result, stroke volume decreases. Because most exercise is performed in the upright position, this will be the position of reference unless otherwise noted.

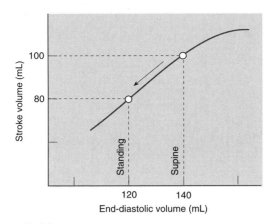

Figure 9.11

The Frank-Starling mechanism showing that a change in left-ventricular end-diastolic volume results in a change in stroke volume, such as occurs when moving from the supine to standing position.

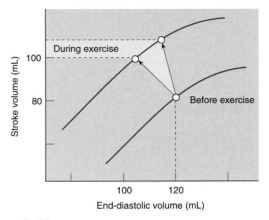

Figure 9.12

Example of the Frank-Starling mechanism and the effects of an agent that has a positive inotropic effect. In this case the agent might be norepinephrine which increases in the blood during exercise. Norepinephrine causes a shift in the Frank-Starling curve upward and/or to the left. This means that for any given end-diastolic volume, there is a greater emptying of the ventricle because of an increase in myocardial contractility. Stroke volume is increased as a result.

Two of the primary factors affecting stroke volume are *preload* and *inotropic state*. Each is briefly discussed below. A third factor called *afterload* (the average tension or force the ventricles must generate during systole to overcome the load opposing the ejection of blood by the ventricles), will not be discussed because its influence upon stroke volume during dynamic exercise is really quite negligible.[23,42]

PRELOAD. In the late 1800s and early 1900s, the separate contributions of two scientists (Otto Frank and Ernest Starling) did much to advance our understanding of the factors that influence stroke volume. The **Frank-Starling mechanism** (Law of the Heart) involves a change in cardiac performance (stroke volume*) as a function of the **preload** or stretch placed on the cardiac muscle just prior to contraction. Figure 9.11 shows that as end-diastolic volume is changed, in this case from 140 to 120 mL because of a "pooling" of blood in the legs that occurs when changing from the supine (laying down) to upright positions, there is a change in stroke volume. In this example there is a decrease in preload and stroke volume as we descend a single ventricular function curve. Conversely, if for some reason there is an increase in blood volume returning to the heart, then we would move up the function curve and stroke volume (and stroke work) would increase.

Obviously, the heart can only pump what blood it takes in; therefore, **venous return** (and its maintenance during exercise) is very important relative to setting preload state. Several factors that effect preload during exercise are discussed later in this chapter (page 229).

INOTROPIC STATE. Another major factor controlling stroke volume is inotropicity or contractility. **Inotropic** is defined as a shift of the Frank-Starling curve either upward to the left (increased contractility or positive inotropic effect) or downward to the right (decreased contractility or negative inotropic effect). A change in inotropic state means a greater or lesser force of contraction at a given end-diastolic volume (preload). The end result is that more blood (positive effect) or less blood (negative effect) is squeezed out, which leads to an increase or decrease in stroke volume, respectively.

Using norepinephrine again as an example (figure 9.12), an increase affects the heart by increasing the force of contraction without any change in end-diastolic volume. This exemplifies why catecholamines are said to have a positive inotropic effect. A change in ejection fraction is sometimes used as a marker or index of a change in inotropic state or contractility.

Heart Rate

Throughout our daily lives we are constantly reminded about the important role that heart rate plays in cardiac performance. The pounding in our chest we feel after slamming on the car brakes to avoid a traffic accident or the rapid beating or flutter we feel while waiting for an important job interview represent only a few of many such examples. As you might guess, in the intact heart changes in rate markedly influence cardiac performance. At rest, heart rate is regulated by the parasympathetic nervous system (i.e.; vagus nerve), which is discussed in detail in chapter 10.

---

*Technically, stroke work is the correct term to be used here, where stroke work = stroke volume × mean ejection pressure, and where mean ejection pressure can be approximated as mean arterial pressure (see page 237). For our purposes, however, we will take a much more simplified approach and just use stroke volume.

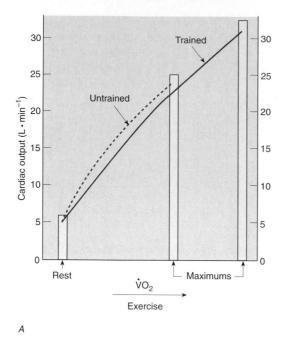

A

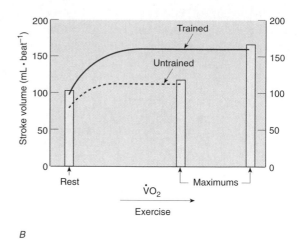

B

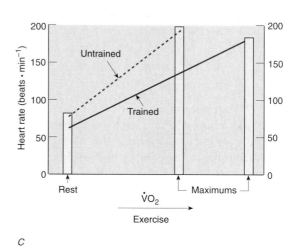

C

Figure 9.13

A, Cardiac output, *B,* stroke volume, and, *C,* heart rate during exercise in trained and untrained subjects. Cardiac output and heart rate are closely related to V̇O₂ over the entire range from rest to maximal exercise; maximal stroke volume is usually reached at a submaximal exercise V̇O₂. Cardiac output is the product of stroke volume times heart rate.

When discussing heart rate it is important that you familiarize yourself with two key terms.

The first term is **chronotropic,** which is defined as an increase or decrease in heart rate. An agent, such as epinephrine (adrenaline), which increases heart rate is said to have a positive chronotropic effect. Conversely, any agent or factor that decreases heart rate is said to have a negative chronotropic effect. For example, associated with a program of regular endurance-type exercise is a decrease in resting heart rate; therefore, exercise training is said to have a negative chronotropic effect.

The second term we need to introduce is *pulse rate,* which refers to the frequency of pulses we are able to palpate (feel) in any artery (e.g., radial in the wrist or carotid in the neck) or on the chest wall (apical pulse). Heart rate and pulse rate are usually the same value. However, among some patients with a very fast heart rate, a very slow heart rate, or an irregular heart rhythm, not all contractions of the heart are forceful enough so that an equal number of pulse

beats are felt in the peripheral artery. A description of how to measure pulse rate is given in chapter 11, page 276.

Cardiac Performance during Exercise

Cardiac output (Q̇) is defined as the amount of blood ejected per minute by the heart, specifically, by the left ventricle. It is computed as the product of heart rate (HR) and stroke volume (SV):

$$\underset{(\text{L} \cdot \text{min}^{-1})}{\dot{Q}} \quad = \quad \underset{(\text{beats} \cdot \text{min}^{-1})}{\text{HR}} \quad \times \quad \underset{(\text{mL} \cdot \text{beat}^{-1})}{\text{SV}}$$

The increase in cardiac output that occurs during exercise to maximum is shown in figure 9.13*A* for trained and untrained male subjects. As shown, this increase is closely related to V̇O₂ (and thus to work load) over the entire range from rest to maximum. At rest, there is little difference in cardiac output between trained and untrained subjects, with average values ranging between 5 and 6 L · min^{-1}. While exercising at similar submaximal work rates, the cardiac outputs of untrained subjects may be slightly higher than[9,10,20,53] or the same as trained subjects.[22,44]

Maximal cardiac outputs in trained male subjects can reach values in excess of 30 L · min^{-1}. This represents a five- to sixfold increase over resting values. In fact, it is not unusual to find highly trained endurance athletes who achieve maximal cardiac outputs near 40 L · min^{-1}.[11] By the same token, untrained male subjects who have lower aerobic capacities have lower maximal cardiac outputs (about 20 to 25 L · min^{-1}). In general, the higher the maximal cardiac output, the higher the maximal aerobic power (max $\dot{V}O_2$), and vice versa.

The changes in cardiac output described above for men are similar to those for women.[2,31] However, in comparison with men, women tend to have a slightly higher cardiac output when exercising at the same $\dot{V}O_2$.[2,16] This difference amounts to between 1.5 and 1.75 L · min^{-1}. The reason for this difference is probably due to the women's lower oxygen-carrying capacity of blood, resulting from lower levels of hemoglobin (page 202). Also, the maximal cardiac output of both trained and untrained women is generally lower than that of their male counterparts.

The large increases in cardiac output observed during exercise are brought about through increases in (1) stroke volume and (2) heart rate. For example, if during heavy exercise stroke volume was 160 mL (0.16 L) · beat^{-1} and heart rate was 185 beats · min^{-1}, cardiac output would be:

$$\dot{Q} = SV \times HR$$
$$= 0.16 \text{ L} \cdot \text{beat}^{-1} \times 185 \text{ beats} \cdot \text{min}^{-1}$$
$$= 29.6 \text{ L} \cdot \text{min}^{-1}$$

Stroke Volume

The relationship of stroke volume to exercise $\dot{V}O_2$ is shown in figure 9.13B. During both arm[30] and leg exercise, stroke volume increases during the progression from rest to moderate work,[3,7,30,52] after which it may stay the same or continue to increase. However, in most cases, it appears that stroke volume plateaus at a $\dot{V}O_2$ ~40% to 60% of maximum.[3,52] This applies to both trained and untrained male and female subjects.

During maximal exercise stroke volume in untrained males may approach 100 to 120 mL · beat^{-1}. For trained males this value is higher, approaching 150 to 170 mL · beat^{-1}. In fact, among elite, highly trained endurance athletes, maximal stroke volume may reach or even exceed 200 mL · beat^{-1}![10] Thus, the primary contributing factor for the much larger cardiac output observed in endurance trained athletes is an increase in maximal stroke volume. Maximum heart rates are generally similar in both trained and untrained individuals, whereas the maximum stroke volume of an athlete may approach twice that of the nonathlete.

For women, the values for stroke volume are generally lower than those for men under all conditions. For example, maximal stroke volumes for untrained and trained females are usually between 80 and 100 mL · beat^{-1} and 100 and 120 mL · beat^{-1}, respectively. At a submaximal work load requiring the same oxygen consumption, stroke volume will be lower in the female than in the male, due, primarily, to the smaller heart volume of the female. The mechanisms responsible for the increase in stroke volume during exercise involve at least two of the factors described earlier—preload (Frank-Starling mechanism) and inotropic state.

Preload

Several studies have shown that left ventricular end-diastolic volume does not increase during exercise,[5,17,50] and so the contributory role of the Frank-Starling mechanism to the increase in stroke volume has been questioned. However, an echocardiographic study conducted in our laboratory comparing young endurance-trained athletes (cyclists and swimmers) to age-matched nonactive controls showed that during submaximal exercise, left-ventricular end-diastolic volume did increase among the trained athletes (figure 9.14A-C[48]). Although this study did not prove that the Frank-Starling mechanism, which we know is important in the intact heart at rest, is evoked during exercise, it did provide strong indirect evidence. Additional evidence comes from Younis et al.,[56] who used a special test called radionuclide ventriculography during upright exercise to show that end-diastolic volume increased during exercise in both patients who had previously received a cardiac transplant and in normal older persons who did not undergo heart surgery. It was through the Frank-Starling mechanism, rather than a decrease in end-systolic volume, that stroke volume increased in these subjects during exercise. Possibly, and likely more true for young persons who are not well trained, the major role of the Frank-Starling mechanism during exercise is to help maintain stroke volume at pre-exercise levels.

VENOUS RETURN. Ultimately, an increase in stroke volume (and cardiac output) is dependent on the amount of blood returned to the right heart via the systemic venous system, thus called *venous return*. An increase in cardiac output to 30 L · min^{-1} or more during maximal exercise means that the venous return must also increase by that same amount. Those events responsible for increasing venous return during exercise are the muscle pump, the respiratory pump, and venoconstriction.

1. *The Skeletal Muscle Pump—the Second Heart.* The *muscle pump* is a true pump that results from the mechanical action produced by rhythmical muscular contractions. It is a major determining factor of venous return. As the muscles contract and compress surrounding veins, the driving pressure for blood flow through the muscle increases, causing the blood within the veins to be propelled toward the heart.[42]

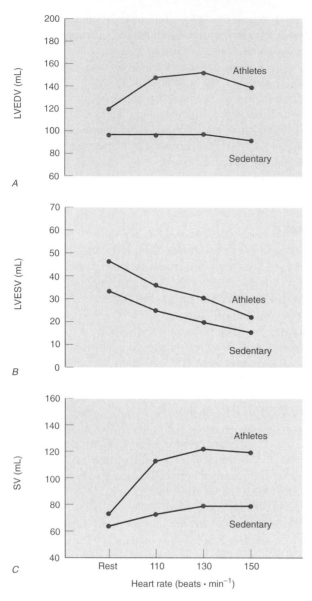

Figure 9.14

Changes in left ventricular (LV) end-diastolic volume (EDV), end-systolic volume (ESV) and stroke volume (SV) among endurance-trained athletes and sedentary adults at rest and while exercising at heart rates of 110, 130 and 150 b · min⁻¹.

Source: Data from Schairer, et al., "Left Ventricular Response to Submaximal Exercise in Endurance-trained Athletes and Sedentary Adults" in American Journal of Cardiology, 1992, 70:430–433.

Blood is prevented from flowing backward in the veins in the limbs because they contain numerous valves that permit flow only in one direction—toward the heart. When the muscles relax, blood fills the veins again and with the next muscular contraction, more blood is forced toward the heart. The muscle pump is important when walking, running, and performing other dynamic activities that involve the alternating contraction and relaxation of the skeletal muscles. It is sometimes viewed as a second pump,

on the venous side of the circuit, having the capacity to generate flow toward the heart, which rivals left ventricular action to pump blood away from the heart. If the two were not similar, cardiac output would not rise sufficiently. During weight lifting or other types of exercises that are static or require sustained muscular contractions that compress and occlude the veins, the muscle pump does not operate effectively and venous return is actually hindered.

2. *The Respiratory and Abdominal Pumps.* Another mechanical action that promotes venous return is provided by the respiratory pump. With this pump, the veins of the thorax and abdomen are emptied toward the heart during inspiration and refilled during expiration. One reason for this is that intrathoracic pressure decreases during inspiration (becomes more subatmospheric; page 174), and this serves to widen the pressure gradient between the right atrium and that point where the inferior vena cava enters the thorax through the diaphragm. The end result is the acceleration of blood flow within the vena cava, which facilitates the return of blood toward the heart. Also, the flattening of the diaphragm during inspiration increases abdominal pressure, which causes the veins contained within the abdomen to be forcefully emptied centrally or toward the heart (abdominal pump). The above pressure effects are reversed during expiration, and the veins fill again with more venous blood. Thus, merely by breathing, venous return is enhanced. This pump is more effective the greater the respiratory rate and the greater the depth of breathing, such as during exercise.

3. *Venoconstriction.* A third way in which venous return is likely enhanced during exercise is through **venoconstriction,** a reflex constriction or narrowing of the small veins and venules draining the muscles. Venoconstriction reduces the volume capacity of the systemic venous system, and, as a result, blood is moved "out" toward the heart. This action is one of the many that is initiated and controlled by the sympathetic nervous system, which is described in detail in chapter 10.

Inotropic State (Contractility)

At rest, only about 55% to 60% of end-diastolic volume is normally ejected during each ventricular systole. (This is ejection fraction, see figure 9.10.) During exercise, a more forceful contraction (positive inotropic effect) develops, as evidenced by an ejection fraction that can approach 75%. This increase in myocardial contractility can as much as double stroke volume, by more completely emptying the ventricles[37,51], resulting in a lower end-systolic volume. Changes in inotropic state are mediated through autonomic nervous system and hormonal influences (chapters 10 and 17).

Both the maintenance of end-diastolic volume (and/or its increase) and the increase in contractility during exercise are sufficient to offset a small increase in afterload that occurs during exercise. The net effect is an increase in stroke volume during exercise.

Heart Rate

In both highly trained female and male endurance athletes resting heart rate may approach 40 b · min^{-1} or less. During exercise, heart rate increases linearly with increasing work rate or $\dot{V}O_2$—and maximal heart rate is slightly lower, if any, in trained versus untrained persons (figure 9.13C). Among eighteen to thirty year old persons, maximal heart rate may approach or exceed 200 b · min^{-1}, and thereafter, it generally decreases with age. Once maximal stroke volume is achieved, which generally occurs between 40% and 60% of maximum work rate, further increases in cardiac output are caused by increases in heart rate alone.

During submaximal exercise, females tend to have a higher heart rate at any given work rate than their male counterparts. As mentioned previously, this is because females tend to have a greater cardiac output and smaller stroke volume for the same $\dot{V}O_2$. (Remember, $\dot{Q} = SV \times HR$.) Following exercise, heart rate follows a two-phase recovery pattern. Initially (i.e., within seconds up to two minutes), heart rate decreases rapidly after exercise is stopped (Phase I response), which is followed by a slower decline to near pre-exercise values over the next 2 to 10 minutes (Phase II response). The autonomic nervous system and hormonal factors that regulate heart rate response during exercise and in recovery are discussed in chapter 10.

A relatively slow heart rate coupled with a relatively large stroke volume indicates an efficient circulatory system. This is true because for a given cardiac output, the heart does not beat as often. For example, consider an endurance trained athlete whose cardiac output during exercise is 20 L · min^{-1} and stroke volume is 150 mL · beat^{-1} (0.15 L · beat^{-1}). In this example heart rate is computed as follows:

$$HR = \frac{\dot{Q}}{SV} = \frac{20 \text{ L} \cdot \text{min}^{-1}}{0.15 \text{ L} \cdot \text{beat}^{-1}} = 133 \text{ b} \cdot \text{min}^{-1}$$

Compare the above heart rate of 133 b · min^{-1} to the one computed below for an untrained subject exercising at the same cardiac output. In this second example, stroke volume is lower at 120 mL · beat^{-1}.

$$HR = \frac{\dot{Q}}{SV} = \frac{20 \text{ L} \cdot \text{min}^{-1}}{0.12 \text{ L} \cdot \text{beat}^{-1}} = 167 \text{ b} \cdot \text{min}^{-1}$$

Thus, for a given cardiac output, a slower beating heart (133 vs. 167 b · min^{-1}) with a larger stroke volume (150 vs. 120 mL · beat^{-1}) means the heart requires less oxygen—which indicates improved efficiency.

Measurement of heart rate or pulse rate in the laboratory or in the field is relatively simple. And, given the relationship between heart rate and $\dot{V}O_2$ (or work rate), one can see why it represents the single most used index of circulatory function during exercise. As a trainer, researcher, or clinician, one can use heart rate response to (1) guide intensity or severity of exercise and (2) assess the effects of an exercise training regimen. However, these uses should be applied on an individual basis only, because heart rate responses to both acute exercise and exercise training can (and do) vary considerably from one person to another.

Cardiac Output during Prolonged Exercise

Changes in cardiac output, stroke volume, and heart rate for *short-term (5 to 10 minutes) submaximal* exercise are shown in figure 9.15. Like $\dot{V}O_2$ and pulmonary ventilation, in each case there is a sharp rise at the onset of exercise followed by a more gradual rise and then a leveling off or steady-state plateau.

During prolonged submaximal work (over 30 to 60 minutes) in a warm environment, cardiac output is maintained over the course of the exercise, but stroke volume and heart rate are not.[12,45] As shown in figure 9.16, stroke volume gradually decreases and heart rate gradually increases as exercise progresses. This is sometimes referred to as **cardiovascular drift**.[21,25,39,47] Because the changes are opposite in direction and equal in magnitude, cardiac output remains fairly constant. Thus, in prolonged efforts, it is not surprising to find near maximal heart rates by the end of the performance. As an example, it has been estimated that during a $2\frac{1}{2}$ hour marathon race, in which the energy requirements are about 75 to 85% of maximum, heart rate was maximal for as long as 1 hour or so.[14]

The reasons behind the increase in heart rate and decrease in stroke volume during prolonged exercise have to do with both body temperature and plasma volume. During moderate intensity exercise in a warm environment, blood is distributed to both the skin and the active skeletal muscles. The increase in cutaneous blood flow helps lessen, through conduction, convection, and evaporation (chapter 19) the increase in body core temperature. However, because of this, less blood is returned to the heart. Additionally, recall from chapter 8 that during exercise fluid (water) moves from the blood into the surrounding cells and tissue. This is due, in part, to an increase in mean arterial pressure and the compression of venules due to muscle action. This shift in blood fluid decreases plasma volume, which reduces further the amount of blood returned to the heart. This decrease in plasma volume can be made worse if inadequate fluid intake is present. The net effect from the above mentioned increase in cutaneous blood flow and decrease in plasma volume is a decrease in venous return, a smaller left ventricular end-diastolic volume, a decrease in stroke volume and, if left uncompensated, a decrease in cardiac

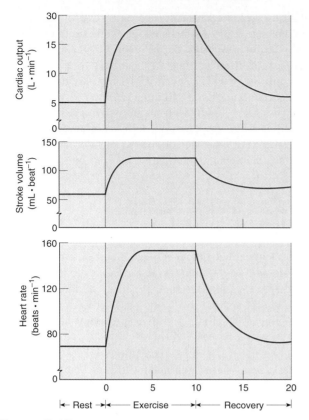

Figure 9.15

Pattern of change in cardiac output (top), stroke volume (middle), and heart rate (bottom) during short-term (5 to 10 minutes) submaximal exercise. There is a sharp rise at the onset of exercise, followed by a steady state response, then a sharp decline as exercise stops.

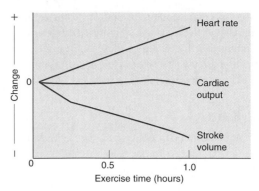

Figure 9.16

During prolonged exercise, heart rate increases steadily while stroke volume decreases. This is referred to as "cardiovascular drift." Because these changes are equal in magnitude and opposite in direction, cardiac output remains stable.

rebreathing) has been extensively studied across a variety of patient populations and, at present, represents the most often used noninvasive method.[35]

Distribution of Blood Flow

Figure 19.17 shows the approximate percentages of the total cardiac output distributed to the skeletal muscles, in comparison with other organs, at rest and during exercise. At rest, ~20% of the total systemic flow is distributed to the muscles, with the majority going to the visceral organs (gastrointestinal tract, liver, spleen, and kidneys), the heart, and the brain. However, during exercise there is a redistribution of blood flow so that the metabolically more active skeletal muscles receive the greatest proportion of the cardiac output.[18,39,40,41] In fact, during maximal exercise the working muscles may receive as much as 85 to 90% of the total blood flow. This means that, with a cardiac output of $25 \text{ L} \cdot \text{min}^{-1}$, more than $22 \text{ L} \cdot \text{min}^{-1}$ of blood would go to the muscles.

This redistribution of blood flow during exercise results from both *vasoconstriction* of the larger arterioles supplying the metabolically less active tissues (e.g., the visceral organs and the uninvolved skeletal muscles) and *vasodilation* (i.e., less vasoconstriction) of the arterioles (especially the terminal arterioles or metarterioles) supplying the metabolically more active skeletal muscles. Figure 9.18 presents a schematic of the vasculature discussed above.

The vasoconstriction in nonactive tissues begins to play an important role usually at heart rates greater than $100 \text{ b} \cdot \text{min}^{-1}$, and is mostly due to an increase in both neural (sympathetic adrenergic) input to the arteriolar smooth muscles and increased plasma norepinephrine. Norepinephrine enters the blood following its release from

output. However, to compensate for any drop in stroke volume and to maintain cardiac output during exercise, a compensatory increase in heart rate occurs. This phenomena explains why higher heart rates are observed during prolonged exercise at the same intensity, especially in a hot versus a cool climate.

One final point about cardiac output during exercise, prolonged or otherwise. Specifically, its measurement during steady-state exercise can be problematic. Although direct, invasive methods are preferred during exercise, the application of such methods requires special and costly equipment, a sterile setting, and properly trained personnel. As a consequence, invasive measurement is not used in the typical exercise physiology laboratory. Alternate methods for assessing cardiac output during exercise have been explored and, when used in the manner for which they were intended, reasonably valid estimates of cardiac output can be made—at less cost and with less subject discomfort. Three alternate methods used for assessing cardiac output and stroke volume during exercise are echocardiography, Doppler flowmetry, and CO_2 rebreathing. The latter (CO_2

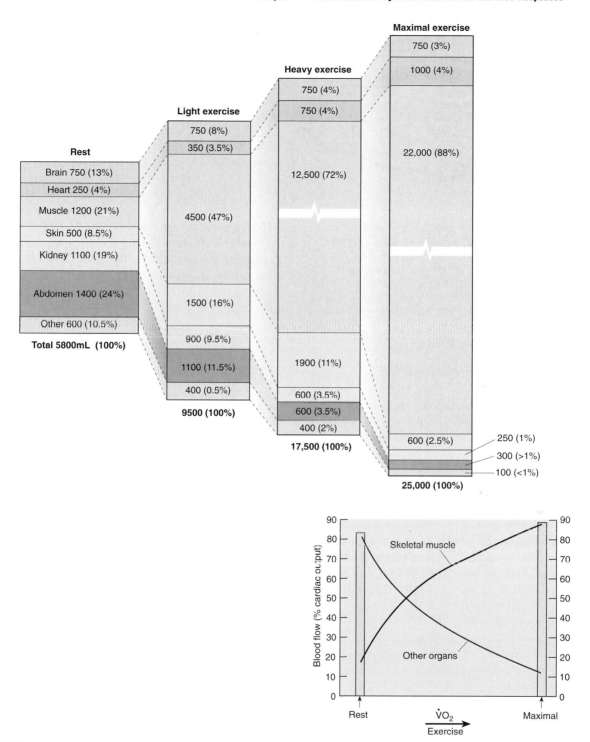

Figure 9.17

Distribution pattern of cardiac output through the various organs of the body during rest and exercise. Cardiac output to each area is expressed in milliliters and as a percentage of the total blood flow. The insert illustrates the percentage of blood flow to the muscles versus the combination of all other organs.

(Modified from Chapman and Mitchell.[8])

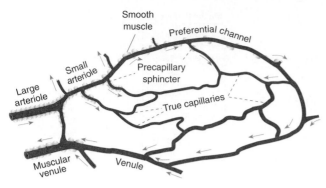

Figure 9.18

A schematic presentation of a capillary bed. Blood from a larger arteriole passes into a series of smaller arterioles (terminal or metarterioles), which lie between the larger arteriole and the capillary. After leaving the capillaries, blood enters the venules before returning to the general circulation. Note the change in the density of the smooth muscle surrounding a vessel as one moves from the larger arterioles to the capillaries.

the adrenal medulla and the sympathetic post-ganglionic nerve endings.

The vasodilation of arterioles and metarterioles and increase in blood flow (*exercise hyperemia*) that occur in active skeletal muscles is due, in part, to the following.

1. A local effect caused by an increase in temperature, CO_2, potassium ions, hydrogen ions, and adenosine and lactic acid levels and a decrease in O_2, particularly as the exercise continues. It may not be that any one of these factors predominates but instead, several of these chemical changes act in concert to result in vasodilation.[19,33] For example, the loss of potassium ions from inside the muscle cell may contribute to vasodilation soon after exercise has begun, only to become less important later on as other factors "take over."[26]

2. The release of vasodilatory substances called *endothelial-derived relaxing factors* (the most studied of which is nitrous oxide) from the innermost layer of an arterial blood vessel, the intima. The intima is comprised of a single layer of endothelium cells that also serves as a smooth surface over which blood elements can pass. Nitrous oxide is released in response to a change in both local chemistry (increase in norepinephrine or decrease in O_2 levels) and physical stimuli (increase in blood flow or sheer stress),[26,32,33] both of which are altered during an exercise bout. Nitrous oxide seems to act on both the larger conducting arteries, as well as the smaller arterioles. The precise degree to which it influences local blood flow within the intact, active muscle is, at present, being intensely studied.[32,33] Discrepancies between studies relative to the role of nitrous oxide may be due to study design issues such as the nature

of the isolated muscle preparation being studied and differences in fiber type composition and fiber recruitment.[33]

3. An initial sympathetic cholinergic reflex response in the arterioles of active muscles, which occurs before and at the very beginning of exercise.

As might be suspected, the above changes are coordinated with the nervous system and hormonal factors that mediate the increased stroke volume, heart rate, and venous return.

In addition to the above, absolute blood flow to the heart (because it too is an active muscle) likewise increases during exercise as a result of vasodilation,[36] whereas blood flow to the brain is maintained at resting levels.[57] Relative to cutaneous blood flow, after core temperature reaches a certain level the hypothalamus acts to increase blood flow to the skin, which will then decrease if exercise is pushed to maximum.

Cardiorespiratory Function— The Whole Picture

As mentioned in chapter 4, the ability of the body to transport and utilize O_2 (i.e., aerobic power, max $\dot{V}O_2$) represents the best overall measure of cardiorespiratory function. To illustrate this point functionally, we need to examine the classic Fick equation (Adolph Fick, 1870):

$$\dot{Q} = \frac{\dot{V}O_2}{\text{a-}\overline{v}O_2 \text{ diff}}$$

where:

$\dot{Q}$ = cardiac output (L $\cdot$ min^{-1})
$\dot{V}O_2$ = oxygen consumption (L $\cdot$ min^{-1})
a-$\overline{v}O_2$ diff = arterio − mixed venous O_2 diff (mL $\cdot$ L^{-1})

Rearranging and simplifying the Fick equation, we get the following:

cardiorespiratory fitness = oxygen transport ×
                                    oxygen utilization

or

$$\dot{V}O_2 = (\text{HR} \times \text{SV}) \times \text{a-}\overline{v}O_2 \text{ diff}$$

Broadly, in this equation cardiac output (HR × SV) represents O_2 transport and a-$\overline{v}O_2$ diff represents O_2 utilization. Obviously, other factors such as pulmonary ventilation and hemoglobin concentration can also influence $\dot{V}O_2$, but given normal pulmonary function and a normal hemoglobin level, these factors are rarely limiting.

Some examples of O_2 transport and utilization at rest and during maximal exercise for untrained and endurance trained male subjects are given in table 9.4. Notice how each variable contributes toward increasing the amount of O_2 consumed. Using the untrained subjects as an example, the O_2 consumed during maximal exercise (3100 mL $\cdot$

9.4

Components of the oxygen transport system at rest and during maximal exercise for untrained subjects and endurance athletes

Condition	$\dot{V}O_2$ (mL · min^{-1})	=	Stroke volume (L · beat^{-1})	×	Heart rate (beats · min^{-1})	×	a-$\bar{v}O_2$ diff (mL · L^{-1})
Untrained							
Rest	300	=	0.075*	×	82	×	48.8
Maximal exercise	3100	=	0.112	×	200	×	138.0
Endurance athletes							
Maximal exercise	5570	=	0.189	×	190	×	155.0

*Usually expressed in mL · beat^{-1}, e.g., 0.075 L · beat^{-1} = 75 mL · beat^{-1}. (Data for untrained subjects from Ekblom et al.,[10] and data for endurance athletes from Ekblom and Hermansen.[11]

min^{-1}) is ten times greater than that found during rest (300 mL · min^{-1}). This increase is accomplished by a 3.6-fold increase in cardiac output, brought about by a 1.5-fold increase in stroke volume and a 2.4-fold increase in heart rate. Additionally, there is a 2.8-fold increase in the a-$\bar{v}O_2$ diff.

Be sure to also notice the differences between the untrained and highly trained endurance athletes at maximal exercise. The endurance athletes were international competitors in long-distance and cross-country running and cycling. They were members of the Swedish National teams and had been training for several years. In this comparison, maximal heart rate was quite similar between the two groups (190 b · min^{-1} vs. 200 b · min^{-1}) and there is only a modest increase (12%) in maximal a-$\bar{v}O_2$ diff for the endurance trained athletes. However, the biggest difference is in the magnitude of the stroke volume. The stroke volume in the endurance athletes is 70% higher than that of the untrained subjects! Such a large difference clearly points out that the most important component of the oxygen transport system is stroke volume.

Circulatory Mechanics— Hemodynamics

So far we have discussed only some of the physiological mechanisms that modify blood flow during exercise. Full comprehension of how these mechanisms occur is incomplete without a basic understanding of the physical laws that govern fluid (blood) flow. The study of these physical laws, as they relate to blood flow, is called **hemodynamics.**

The two major hemodynamic factors that we need to consider are (1) **blood pressure** or the driving force that tends to move blood through the circulatory system and (2) resistance to flow or the opposition offered by the circulatory system to this driving force. The relationship of these factors to blood flow or cardiac output is shown in the following hemodynamic equation:

$$\text{cardiac output} = \frac{\text{blood pressure}}{\text{resistance}}$$

To better apply the above equation to our study of hemodynamics in the systemic circuit we need to rearrange it algebraically as follows:

$$P_{mean} = \dot{Q} \times T_S P_R$$

where:

P_{mean}* = is the mean blood pressure during a complete cardiac cycle

$T_S P_R$ = total systemic peripheral resistance

In the above equation, P_{mean} increases with increases in cardiac output or resistance and decreases with decreases in cardiac output or resistance. Right now let us discuss blood pressure and resistance in more detail.

Blood Pressure

As we have mentioned, blood pressure is the pressure exerted by the blood against the inside of the arterial walls. It is also the force that moves the blood through the circulatory

*A pressure gradient or differential determines the rate of blood flow. The pressure differential for the entire systemic circulatory system is P_{mean} minus the pressure in the right atrium. Because the latter is generally zero, P_{mean} alone can be used.

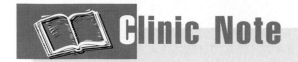

Clinic Note

Cardiac Rehabilitation

Up until the late 1960s and early 1970s, the average hospital stay experienced by a patient recovering from an uncomplicated myocardial infarction (heart attack) was 21 days. And, at that time, their hospital stay consisted mainly of strict bed rest. The prevailing idea back then was to allow sufficient time for the damaged area of the heart to heal by "scarring over."

However, following a patient's discharge from the hospital to their home many complained of marked exercise intolerance and weakness. Questions were then raised as to whether or not the activity restrictions imposed on the patients while in the hospital (and continued when at home) actually contributed to their deconditioning and symptoms of exercise intolerance. Fortunately, we have learned much over the past 30 years—to the point that many patients who experience an uncomplicated myocardial infarction are now discharged from the hospital after only four to six days! And, following initial stabilization in the hospital, the activities they are allowed to engage in are progressively increased, so that many patients walk freely on their ward and some even try a flight of stairs before going home.

Once patients have returned home, regular exercise training is prescribed for many, often through the use of a formal cardiac rehabilitation program. In addition to serving patients recovering from a heart attack, these programs also care for patients with stable angina pectoris, patients with stable heart failure, and those who have undergone either coronary artery bypass surgery or coronary angioplasty. In many cases, the rehabilitation program is begun days to just a few weeks after the patient is discharged from the hospital. Such programs are often called Phase II cardiac rehabilitation.* These programs are usually supervised by registered nurses, exercise specialists, or physical therapists and involve, at least initially, having the patient undergo continuous or intermittent ECG monitoring to ensure they are training at a level that is safe for their given medical condition.

After having "graduated" from Phase II, patients are then expected to adhere to regular exercise habits on their own. Some patients who so enjoyed the group support offered by the exercise class environment choose to enroll into another program, one with less clinical supervision and ECG monitoring—often called Phase III cardiac rehabilitation.

The effectiveness of cardiac rehabilitation programs to improve fitness, decrease subsequent heart attacks, and improve a patient's feeling of well-being and symptoms has been well established.[55] In fact, among these patients a regular exercise program has been shown to improve exercise capacity by 15% to 25%, as well as reduce subsequent fatal myocardial infarctions by 25% over the next three years.

However, changes within the profession now dictate that cardiac rehabilitation programs should no longer represent an "exercise only" service. Instead, these programs also incorporate intensive bio-behavioral components meant to favorably modify the "other" risk factors that place a person at higher risk for another event. Factors such as elevated cholesterol, continued cigarette smoking, unsuccessful weight management, poor nutritional habits, and their failure to effectively manage stress. Just like advances in cardiology that have brought us shortened hospital stays and new medications and techniques meant to prevent a second heart attack, cardiac rehabilitation represents an effective component of a patient's overall care.

---

*Phase I cardiac rehabilitation usually encompasses the education and exercise therapy that patients receive while hospitalized. This service has become increasingly difficult to deliver because of the shortened length of hospital stays.

---

system. More important, however, is the concept that blood, as does any other fluid, flows along pressure gradients—from an area of higher pressure to one of lower pressure. For example, as shown in figure 9.19, blood flows from the left ventricle of the heart into the aorta (the main artery of the systemic circuit), because as the ventricle contracts it exerts a pressure that is higher than exists in the aorta (figure 9.9 and table 9.3). Blood flows from the aorta through the remaining systemic blood vessels (arteries, arterioles, capillaries, venules, and veins) and finally arrives in the right side of the heart because of the pressure gradient that exists along the systemic vascular tree. This is true for pulmonary blood flow as well, except that here the pressures are lower in magnitude.*

---

*Although the pressure differential in the pulmonary circuit is lower than in the systemic circuit, blood flow is the same because pulmonary resistance is also lower.

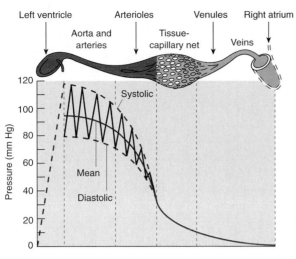

Figure 9.19

Blood pressure differential along the systematic vascular tree. Blood always flows from an area of high pressure to one of low pressure. Note also that the pressure (and thus the flow of blood) fluctuates in the arteries and arterioles, but that it is steady in the capillaries. Systolic pressure is the highest pressure obtained, diastolic the lowest; and mean pressure is computed as one-third pulse pressure + diastolic pressure.

Systolic and Diastolic Pressures

Figure 9.19 also shows that the pressure fluctuates in the cardiovascular system, with the highest values noted in the left ventricle during systole. During any cardiac cycle the highest arterial pressure obtained during the contraction phase is called the **systolic pressure.** As blood drains from the arteries during ventricular diastole, the intra-arterial pressure decreases to a minimum **(diastolic pressure).** These pressure fluctuations are minimized and, in fact, are absent in the capillaries, because the arteries are elastic rather than rigid. Thus, their walls stretch during systole and recoil during diastole. The elasticity of the arteries plus an added arterial resistance to flow insures a steady flow of blood in the capillaries. This has real meaning, because it is in the capillaries that diffusion of gases and other nutrients takes place.

Mean Arterial Pressure

You probably noticed in the hemodynamic equation on page 235 that P_{mean} or mean arterial pressure was used instead of systolic or diastolic blood pressure. P_{mean} is the most important circulatory pressure because it, more than any other, determines the rate of blood flow through the systemic circuit and it best reflects the pressure perfusing the tissue at any given moment.

The precise determination of P_{mean} is not simple. It is not merely the average or mean value of systolic and diastolic pressures. This is because diastole usually lasts longer than systole. P_{mean} can be easily estimated using the following equation:

$$P_{mean} = \text{diastolic pressure} + \tfrac{1}{3} \text{ pulse pressure}$$

where:

$$\text{pulse pressure} = \text{systolic pressure} - \text{diastolic pressure}$$

For example, if the systolic pressure were 125 millimeters of mercury (mm Hg) and the diastolic pressure 80 mm Hg, then P_{mean} would be estimated as follows:

$$\begin{aligned}
P_{mean} &= 80 \text{ mm Hg} + \tfrac{1}{3}(125 \text{ mm Hg} - 80 \text{ mm Hg}) \\
&= 80 \text{ mm Hg} + \tfrac{1}{3}(45 \text{ mm Hg}) \\
&= 80 \text{ mm Hg} + 15 \text{ mm Hg} \\
&= 95 \text{ mm Hg}
\end{aligned}$$

Following a single bout of exercise, systolic, mean, and diastolic pressures often return to pre-exercise levels within minutes. And, in some instances these pressures may actually fall below pre-exercise levels resulting in what is called *post-exercise hypotension.* This hypotension has been well described and can reach 10 to 12 mm Hg below resting systolic values and 5 to 7 mm Hg below resting diastolic values. These changes can remain in effect for up to four hours.[54]

Resistance to Flow

Resistance to blood flow is caused by friction between the blood and the walls of the blood vessels. The greater this friction, the greater the resistance to flow. Vascular friction depends on (1) the *viscosity* (or thickness) of the blood, (2) the *length* of the blood vessel, and (3) the *diameter* of the blood vessel. For example, an increase in the number of red blood cells, such as what occurs with the illegal use of blood doping agents, increases blood viscosity, which in turn causes greater vascular friction and resistance to flow. By the same token, the longer the vessel, the greater the vascular surface that is in contact with the blood and the greater the resistance.

Additionally, when the luminal diameter of the vessel changes, resistance to flow also changes. For instance, the smaller the diameter of a vessel the greater the portion of blood that is in contact with the walls of the vessel, and as a result, the greater will be the friction. The opposite is true for vasodilation. To clarify, resistance to flow varies inversely to the fourth power of the vessel radius. In other words, if the radius (which is one-half the diameter) of the vessel doubles, resistance decreases 16 times; if the radius is halved, resistance increases 16 times! For this reason changes in vessel diameter (increase = vasodilation; decrease = vasoconstriction) that occur primarily in the arterioles, control, to a very large degree, blood flow through the systemic circuit. (Present estimates are that $\sim\tfrac{2}{3}$ of T_SP_R is attributable to arteriolar tone.) At rest, the sympathetic nervous system is the predominant factor that influences vessel diameter and, therefore, T_SP_R.

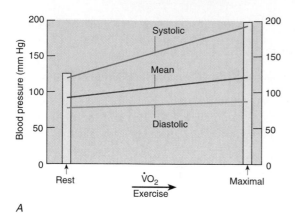
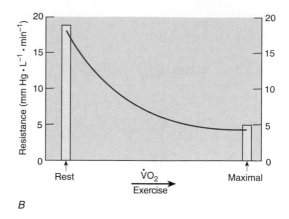

A

B

Figure 9.20

A, Changes in blood pressure and, *B,* resistance to flow during exercise. Blood pressure increases linearly during exercise as a result of an increase in cardiac output (heart rate and stroke volume), whereas resistance decreases because of less vasoconstriction in the active muscles.

Changes in Pressure and Resistance during Exercise

Shown in figure 9.20*A* are systemic blood pressures at rest and during exercise. Common systolic and diastolic pressures at rest might be 120 and 80 mm Hg, respectively, with a mean pressure of about 93 mm Hg.

During exercise, systolic pressure increases and may exceed 200 mm Hg. Such an increase results from (1) the increase in cardiac output (i.e., increases in stroke volume and heart rate) and (2) an increase in vascular resistance among the less metabolically active tissues. As shown in figure 9.20*A,* although the increase in systolic pressure can be quite dramatic, there is only a modest increase in P_{mean} and little change, if any, in diastolic pressure. The lesser changes in P_{mean} and diastolic pressure during exercise are caused by the decrease in peripheral resistance that develops because of the vasodilation of arterioles supplying blood to the active skeletal muscles. This means that more blood will drain from the arteries through the arterioles and into the muscle capillaries, thus minimizing changes in diastolic pressure. In fact, among well-trained endurance athletes exercised to maximum, it is not uncommon for diastolic blood pressure to drop below 60 or even 50 mm Hg.

Although resistance to blood flow cannot be directly measured in humans, it can be indirectly calculated using the formula:

$$T_S P_R = \frac{P_{mean}}{\dot{Q}}$$

If cardiac output at rest is 5 L · min^{-1} and P_{mean} at rest is 93 mm Hg, then total systemic resistance to blood flow must be 93 mm Hg / 5 L · min^{-1} = 19 mm Hg / L^{-1} · min^{-1} (figure 9.20*B*). At maximal exercise, if P_{mean} is 126 mm Hg and cardiac output is 30 L · min^{-1}, then total systemic resistance would be 126 / 30 = 4.2 mm Hg / L^{-1} · min^{-1}.

This represents a 4.5-fold decrease from what was observed at rest.

Here's a tough question—one of logic and of function: Why, if cardiac output increases during exercise and total systemic resistance decreases, does P_{mean} increase? Wouldn't the changes, being in opposite directions, offset one another and result in no change in P_{mean}? Clearly, we know that P_{mean} does increase, at a rate approximating one-third the increase in systolic pressure (figure 9.20*A*). The answer to our question relates to the fact that the increase in cardiac output is greater than the decrease in total systemic peripheral resistance.

$$\uparrow P_{mean} = \uparrow \uparrow \uparrow \dot{Q} \times \downarrow \downarrow T_S P_R$$

This means that even during extreme exercise, when resistance is low and you would think the large arterioles are as wide open as they can be, they are instead still somewhat constricted. In fact, if the large arterioles were to dilate fully during heavy exercise, it would take a cardiac output approaching 60 L · min^{-1} to prevent a decrease in P_{mean} during exercise.[43] Such a value has not been reported, not even among champion athletes. This is why some physiologists prefer to use the phrase *less vasoconstriction* in place of vasodilation. Such a phrase better reflects what is actually occurring, in that during maximal exercise, the arterioles within the exercising muscles take on a state of less vasoconstriction rather than undergoing vasodilation.

Other Issues Related to the Cardiovascular System

Before summarizing this chapter, it is important that several other topics, all of which are related to cardiac function, be introduced.

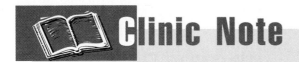

Clinic Note

Blood Pressure during Exercise

During a graded exercise stress test, blood pressure is generally measured every two or three minutes. Why do we do this? What is it about blood pressure responses that we are so interested in? Well, one important reason is safety. According to the American College of Sports Medicine, a systolic pressure exceeding 260 mm Hg or a diastolic pressure greater than 115 mm Hg are two reasons for stopping the test.[1]

There is another very important reason for measuring blood pressure during exercise, which is to screen for severe ischemia or triple vessel coronary artery disease (significant disease in all three arteries of the heart) among patients with suspected or known heart disease. To illustrate, let's pretend we are observing a graded exercise test being performed on Mr. W.D., a 52-year-old male who was discharged from the hospital approximately two weeks ago after recovering from a heart attack. Since returning home Mr. W.D. has been mildly walking 10 minutes twice a day and he is now planning to enroll in a cardiac rehabilitation program. While at home he has experienced one or two bouts of chest discomfort during activity, but nothing like the chest pain and squeezing he felt when he had his heart attack.

Prior to the exercise test, Mr. W.D.'s resting (sitting) blood pressure was 126/80 mm Hg. At minutes three and six of exercise, the blood pressure appropriately increased to 130/82 mm Hg and 138/82 mm Hg, respectively. At minute nine of the test the blood pressure is 128/86 mm Hg, leading the test supervisor to ask that the pressure again be measured. This time, systolic pressure is even lower—similar to pre-exercise values, at 126/86 mm Hg. Mr. W.D. now begins to complain of the vague chest discomfort he occasionally experienced at home. At the same time, his ECG demonstrates 1.5 mm of ST segment depression indicative of myocardial ischemia (page 224). Having confirmed that systolic pressure has, in fact, decreased, the exercise test is stopped. The obvious question here is, What could be so ominous about the decrease in systolic pressure that it warranted the discontinuation of exercise? To answer the question we must again review the following equation:

$$P_{mean} = HR \times SV \times T_SP_R$$

Next, let's make three assumptions. First, as expected, T_SP_R did decrease. Second, during the exercise test systolic pressure was the indicator of P_{mean}. This is generally a safe assumption since, given the absence of any real change in diastolic pressure (80 to 86 mm Hg), the increase in P_{mean} then occurs at a rate that is $\sim\frac{1}{3}$ the increase in systolic pressure (see also figure 9.20A). Third, heart rate was measured throughout the test via ECG and we observed that it increased as exercise workload increased.

Recall from the adjoining text that P_{mean} increases because the increase in cardiac output is greater than, and offsets, the decrease in T_SP_R. If cardiac output did not increase sufficiently there would be a fall in systolic pressure (and P_{mean}), just as was noted during this test. Therefore, the failure of cardiac output to increase can only be due to either a decrease in heart rate or stroke volume. Well, we have ECG evidence that heart rate did increase during the stress test. By the process of elimination, we now know that stroke volume must have *decreased* during exercise.

How can this be? Well, in patients like Mr. W.D., the first thing one would suspect would be exercise induced myocardial ischemia. In this case, the ischemia he experienced was so severe that it actually hindered left ventricular function to the point that contractility was impaired. In other words, the left ventricle could not effectively pump blood. In fact, among patients with severe coronary artery disease who demonstrate a drop in systolic pressure with exercise along with ST segment depression, additional tests (e.g., cardiac catherization) are often ordered on the assumption that coronary artery bypass surgery may be needed. Such surgery has been shown to prolong life in patients with severe (triple vessel) disease. This means that mortality in these patients is quite high over the next year unless bypass graft surgery is used as an intervention.

Generally, in most exercise testing laboratories, a systolic blood pressure that first increases with exercise but then falls more than 10 to 15 mm Hg and/or below resting values is used as a criterion for stopping a graded exercise test.

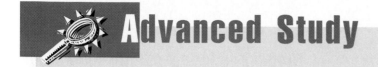

Advanced Study

Measuring Blood Pressure

Knowledge of a patient's blood pressure at rest and during exercise provides valuable information about cardiovascular hemodynamics, future risk, disease status, and the effectiveness of therapy. Therefore, its accurate measurement is essential. Unfortunately, a variety of errors are commonly introduced into blood pressure measurement, some of which include the use of the wrong sized (too big or too small) pressure cuff, equipment that is no longer calibrated, improper patient preparation, and improper tester skills.

Proper methods for the indirect measurement of blood pressure in the brachial artery at rest include the following:[1,38]

1. Seat (back against the chair, feet flat on the floor) the patient or subject in a quiet, calm environment for a minimum of five minutes.

2. Wrap an appropriately sized and known to be calibrated cuff firmly around the upper arm at heart level. The cuff should be aligned so that the center of the bladder inside the pressure cuff is directly over the brachial artery.

3. Place the earpieces of a stethoscope into the ear canals, angled forward to fit snugly. Palpate the brachial artery and place the head of the stethoscope over the brachial artery pulse, which should be felt just above and medial to the bend in the elbow. Press on the head of the stethoscope firmly, but not too tightly, so that its entire circumference is in direct contact with the skin.

4. While looking at the manometer, quickly inflate the cuff to 200 mm Hg or approximately 20 mm Hg greater than estimated systolic pressure. Slowly loosen (open) the inflator bulb valve and deflate the bladder at 2 mm Hg per sec until you hear the first Korotkoff sound. The value on the manometer corresponding to the first appearance of a Korotkoff sound represents systolic blood pressure.

5. Continue to deflate the cuff, now at a rate of 2 mm Hg per pulse beat. Listen carefully for a change in the audible sounds. Make a mental note of the manometer values that correspond to when you heard both the muffling of the a Korotkoff sounds (fourth Korotkoff sound) and then the complete disappearance of sound (fifth Korotkoff sound). At rest the fourth and fifth sounds may occur at the same time, representing diastolic pressure. If both

sounds are heard separately, which commonly occurs after exercise because of the high velocity flow, then it is usually the fourth Korotkoff sound that is used for diastolic pressure. Round off all values to the nearest 2 mm Hg.

It is good practice to obtain more than one measure during each sitting. However, at least one minute should be allowed between each measurement. It may also be helpful to obtain readings from both arms or while the patient is lying down or standing. Such information can provide additional information about hemodynamics and disease state. Also, the measurement of blood pressure during exercise can provide even more information. However, obtaining accurate values during exercise is difficult for a variety of reasons, such as extraneous noise from the exercise equipment and movement of the arm.

One question that may come to mind after reading the above is—what exactly produces the Korotkoff sounds that are heard when measuring blood pressure? Part of the answer lies in how blood flows through our blood vessels. Normally, blood flows in parallel laminar layers, with each layer equivalent to the approximate thickness of a red blood cell. Interestingly, these layers flow at different velocities, with those layers located nearer to middle of the vessel (in the axial stream) flowing much faster than the outer layers located closer to the inner artery wall. However, laminar flow can be disrupted so that multidirectional, nonlayered, or turbulent flow occurs. Turbulent flow is associated with audible sounds that can be heard by a stethoscope. Turbulent flow can occur at a bifurcation where one artery branches into two, as the result of very high velocity blood flow, or where there is a disruption/narrowing of the vessel secondary to a blockage or an aneurysm.

Putting it all together, when the blood pressure cuff is inflated, the bladder inside the cuff applies pressure to the upper arm muscles. In turn, these muscles compress the brachial artery and occlude the vessel so that no blood flows into the lower arm. As the pressure in the cuff bladder is slowly released, it reaches a point where the highest pressure generated during systole is eventually able to overcome the resistance imposed by the now deflating cuff. When blood first starts to push through the semi-occluded artery, it encounters the stationary blood distal to the pressure cuff. This creates

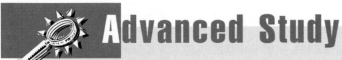

turbulence and the first Korotkoff sound heard by the stethoscope. As the pressure in the cuff continues to decrease, the pulsating sound will still be audible because of the turbulent flow caused by the cuff's continued but decreasing occlusion of the brachial artery. Finally, when the cuff no longer occludes the artery, laminar flow in the artery is re-established, resulting in the muffling of the Korotkoff sounds or its disappearance. The latter is our measure of diastolic blood pressure.

Be aware that a single recorded blood pressure value greater than 140/90 mm Hg does not mean that an individual has high blood pressure. The confirmation of true clinical hypertension requires several blood pressure readings taken over several different office visits. Clearly, much practice with measuring blood pressure (both at rest and during exercise) is required before an individual should feel qualified and confident to accurately obtain a blood pressure reading in the clinical, research, or public health settings.

Hypertension

When systolic and/or diastolic blood pressure is chronically elevated at rest it is called **hypertension** or high blood pressure. Values taken over several examination visits that exceed 140 mm Hg and 90 mm Hg are generally classified as systolic and diastolic hypertension, respectively.[38] At present, approximately 24% of the entire U.S. population has high blood pressure, the prevalence of which is highest among black males at 32%.[6] It has been estimated that 12% of all persons die as a direct result of hypertension. Clinical problems that are related to high blood pressure include heart failure, renal failure, stroke, and heart attack.

From our basic hemodynamic equation, we know that the $P_{mean} = \dot{Q} \times T_S P_R$; therefore, it is easy to see that hypertension is a result of either an increased cardiac output and/or an increased systemic peripheral resistance. An increased resistance can be caused by a number of factors, some of which include problems associated with kidney function. A common type of high blood pressure is called *essential hypertension*. It has no known cause and, therefore, no known cure. Another type of high blood pressure, one that is associated with fluctuations—such that sometimes the readings are elevated during examination and at other times the readings are normal—is called *labile hypertension*.

Although the treatment of hypertension often involves the use of medications designed to decrease plasma volume (e.g., diuretics) or reduce afterload, regular and moderate exercise training has also been shown to lead to a sustained decrease in both systolic and diastolic blood pressure. Two excellent papers on this topic indicate that an ~10 mm Hg decrease in systolic blood pressure and an ~8 mm Hg decrease in diastolic blood pressure can be expected among persons with moderate hypertension who undergo regular exercise training.[27,54] Thus, more and more, clinicians recommend that a patient with high blood pressure first initiate a regular and moderate activity program before starting drug therapy. Assessed over time, exercise training may lower a patient's blood pressure to the point that less medication, or possibly no medication, might be needed for treatment. Additionally, it is important to point out that improvements in blood pressure are achieved with moderate intensity (40% to 70% of $\dot{V}O_2$ max) exercise. Vigorous (>70% $\dot{V}O_2$ max) exercise intensity is not required or may not be as beneficial.[24]

Rate-Pressure Product— Myocardial Oxygen Consumption

Throughout this text we have used the terms max $\dot{V}O_2$ and peak $\dot{V}O_2$ to define the aerobic capacity of the body as an intact, whole organism. We must remember, however, that these terms represent a summation of activity throughout the entire body. A measurement of max $\dot{V}O_2$ at the mouth using a metabolic cart or Douglas bags (chapter 4) does not isolate or quantify for us the contributing amounts from specific organs—such as the metabolically more active skeletal muscles vs. the metabolically less active kidneys or colon. Well, it is possible to measure O_2 consumption across a specific organ by directly measuring the blood flow and O_2 content in the arteries and veins supplying and draining the tissue. To accomplish this, however, involves invasive procedures requiring catheters and controlled conditions that are not routinely available in most exercise physiology laboratories.

table 9.5

Cardiorespiratory responses of 10 moderately active males (average age = 51 years) following four minutes of submaximal exercise performed at 30 watts

	Heart rate (beats · min^{-1})	Stroke volume (mL · beat^{-1})	Cardiac output (L · min^{-1})	Systolic blood pressure (mm Hg)	Rate-pressure product × 10^3 (mm Hg · beat^{-1} · min^{-1})
Arm	97	107	10.3	169	16.4
Leg	92	115	10.3	148	13.6

Based on data from Keteyian et al.[28]

Invasive studies conducted in the 1950s and 1960s that involved the placement of catheters in the coronary arteries and coronary sinus (vein) of various subjects showed that, even at rest, the heart consumes ~70% of the O_2 brought to it in arterial blood. As a result, to accommodate the increased myocardial demand for O_2 that occurs during exercise, the heart must greatly increase coronary circulation some fourfold, from 250 mL · min^{-1} to 1000 mL · min^{-1}.[13] Factors influencing myocardial O_2 demand or consumption, both at rest and during exercise, include: (1) heart rate (the more frequently the heart contracts the more O_2 it requires), (2) left ventricular size (the greater the stretch on the myocardial muscle fibers the more energy [O_2] required), and (3) myocardial contractility (force of contraction).

Fortunately, prior studies[46] have shown that traditional catheter-type invasive methods could be avoided and that myocardial oxygen consumption could be reliably estimated using a noninvasive method—the simple product of heart rate × systolic blood pressure. The term applied to this method is **rate-pressure product.** What this all means is that myocardial oxygen consumption can be estimated using variables easily obtained during a standard graded exercise test.

During exercise, rate-pressure product increases in direct proportion to increases in heart rate and systolic pressure. When applied to the clinical care of patients with coronary artery disease, we are now able to estimate the myocardial oxygen consumption. For instance, let's review the actual case of a 58-year-old sedentary female who, until one month prior, had been without symptoms (chest pain) since undergoing coronary artery bypass surgery five years ago. To assess the extent of this patient's problem, a graded exercise stress test was completed where it was found that her evidence of ischemia (i.e., chest pain, ST segment de-

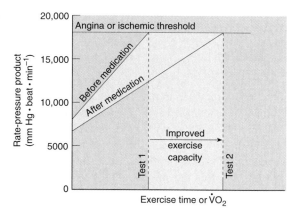

Figure 9.21

Rate-pressure product (heart rate × systolic blood pressure) is a good reproducible marker of myocardial oxygen demand or consumption. Among patients with ischemic heart disease, it is an important measurement in clinical exercise physiology. Note certain medications and therapies can lower blood pressure and heart rate response during exercise, allowing a patient to exercise longer or to a higher $\dot{V}O_2$ before being at their ischemic threshold.

pression) occurred at an exercise rate-pressure product of ~19,300 mm Hg · beat · min^{-1} (heart rate of 140 beats · min^{-1} × systolic pressure of 138 mm Hg). A medication was prescribed to slow heart rate and blunt blood pressure response during exercise (a so-called beta-blocker), which, during follow-up testing, allowed the patient to exercise longer before she achieved the same rate pressure product (figure 9.21). For this patient it meant she could now perform her routine activities of living without experiencing chest pain. It doesn't mean that her disease was cured.

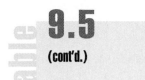

9.5

(cont'd.)

$\dot{V}O_2$ (L · min^{-1})	Ventilation (L · min^{-1})	Respiratory exchange ratio	Blood lactate (mmol · L^{-1})
0.84	28.7	1.01	4.3
0.73	21.0	0.85	2.8

Additionally, this patient entered a cardiac rehabilitation program and her exercise prescription was written such that her training intensity was set sufficiently below her "ischemic threshold". The use of the rate pressure product in treating patients with coronary artery disease represents an important tool in clinical exercise physiology.

Comparative Responses during Arm vs. Leg Exercise

Although several studies were conducted in the 1960s detailing the physiologic responses to arm exercise, it wasn't until the 1980s that this area of exercise physiology received the attention it deserved. Clearly, the response to both submaximal and peak arm exercise differs from what is observed during submaximal and peak leg exercise. Learning about these differences is of practical importance, if one considers activities such as snow shoveling or raking leaves—two tasks that are commonly performed and require vigorous arm involvement.

Upper Extremity Exercise— Submaximal Responses

As shown in table 9.5, arm exercise at a submaximal work rate (30 watts) is performed at a greater cost than is leg exercise performed at the same work rate.[15] Specifically, heart rate, systolic blood pressure, rate-pressure product, $\dot{V}O_2$, minute ventilation, respiratory exchange ratio, and blood lactate concentration are all higher during arm when compared to leg exercise. The increase in stroke volume, however, is less during arm than during leg exercise. Since equal amounts of work (e.g., 30 watt) are conducted with both arm and leg exercise, there is no difference in cardiac output.

The above described differences in cardiorespiratory and hemodynamic responses to arm versus leg exercise have been consistently observed in healthy males and females,[15] patients with coronary artery disease,[49] patients having undergone cardiac transplant,[30] and patients with stable heart failure.[28] The factors responsible for these differences include a lower mechanical efficiency of the arms, a smaller muscle mass employed by the arms, a greater rise in plasma catecholamines during arm exercise, increased corticomedullary (central command) activity, and/or a compensatory response to the smaller increase in stroke volume that occurs with arm exercise.

Upper Extremity Exercise—Responses to Maximal Exercise

Among apparently healthy people and a variety of patient populations, cardiorespiratory responses to maximal leg exercise are greater than the responses observed during maximal arm exercise (table 9.6). The factors responsible for these elevated differences during leg exercise include muscle fiber recruitment patterns, the larger muscle mass engaged in the activity, and fitness level. Given the above information, it is important to point out that a measured value for either the arms or the legs should not be used to predict the metabolic or hemodynamic responses of the other. Simply stated, peak $\dot{V}O_2$ measured during leg exercise cannot be used to predict peak $\dot{V}O_2$ during arm exercise.

Additionally, for each variable shown in table 9.6 the absolute arm or leg response is generally greater among apparently healthy persons than those with heart disease. Such differences may be due to disease state, cardiac innervation, abnormalities of autonomic function, and fitness level. However, when peak arm response is expressed as a percentage of peak leg response, there are only small differences between the different groups presented (table 9.7).

table 9.6

Cardiorespiratory responses of healthy normals, patients with heart failure, and patients with cardiac transplant to peak arm and leg exercise

	Power output (watts)	Heart rate (beats · min^{-1})	Rate-pressure product × 10^3 (mm Hg · beat^{-1} · min^{-1})	$\dot{V}O_2$ (L · min^{-1})	Ventilation (L · min^{-1})	Respiratory exchange ratio
Normals						
Arm	62	140	28.5	1.5	63.6	1.14
Leg	162	154	32.5	2.28	89.8	1.14
Heart failure						
Arm	43	128	20.5	1.08	51.2	1.15
Leg	101	144	24.1	1.48	66.5	1.15
Cardiac transplant						
Arm	51	135	24.8	1.15	57.2	1.17
Leg	109	145	27.8	1.6	74.0	1.17

Based on data from Keteyian et al.[28,29]

table 9.7

Comparison of peak arm response expressed as a percentage of peak leg response among healthy normals, patients with heart failure, and patients with cardiac transplant

	Power output	$\dot{V}O_2$	Ventilation	Heart rate	Rate-pressure product × 10^3
Normals	39	67	71	92	89
Heart failure	43	74	77	89	85
Cardiac transplant	46	72	77	93	92

Based on data from Keteyian et al.[28,29]

Summary

The heart is a muscular pump that circulates the blood (oxygen and nutrients) through the circulatory system. The direction of blood flow is controlled by unidirectional valves located in the heart. The myocardium (heart muscle) is a syncytium of interconnected fibers that allows a depolarization wave to uniformly spread throughout the heart so that all fibers contract in unison.

The heart has an inherent depolarization rate that originates in the sinoatrial node (S-A node) in the right atrium, then spreads across the atrium to the atrioventricular node (A-V node), the Bundle of His, the left and right bundle branches, and from there, throughout both ventricles via the Purkinje fiber system.

The left and right coronary arteries are the major arteries supplying blood to the myocardium. They branch repeatedly throughout the entire heart muscle. The great and lesser veins return the venous blood of the heart to the right atrium via the coronary sinus. At rest the heart extracts ~75% of the O_2 available in arterial blood; therefore, increased myocardial demand for O_2 during exercise is met by dramatic increases in coronary blood flow.

The cardiac cycle refers to the electrical and mechanical changes that occur in the heart during contraction (systole) and relaxation (diastole). The electrical activity of the heart can be detected via surface electrodes on the body and is recorded as an electrocardiogram (ECG). The hemodynamic events of primary interest during systole and diastole involve pressure changes in the aorta, left atrium, and left ventricle.

Two major determinants of cardiac performance are stroke volume and heart rate. Two major factors affecting stroke volume are preload and myocardial contractility.

To fully meet gas transport demands during exercise, two major blood flow changes are necessary; they are: (1) an increase in cardiac output and (2) a redistribution of blood flow from inactive organs to the active skeletal muscles.

The increase in cardiac output ($\dot{Q}$) with exercise is brought about through increases in stroke volume (SV) and heart rate (HR). Their mathematical relationship is $\dot{Q} = SV \times HR$. The increase in stroke volume generally plateaus at $\sim 50\%$ of maximum $\dot{Q}$. Heart rate increases linearly with increasing work load and $\dot{V}O_2$ in both trained and untrained subjects.

A slow heart rate coupled with a relatively large stroke volume, characteristic of the athlete, indicates an efficient circulatory system. For a given cardiac output, a slower beating heart with a larger stroke volume requires less oxygen.

Cardiac output is ultimately dependent on venous return, the heart pumping only what is returned back to it. During exercise, the muscle and respiratory pumps plus venoconstriction help in increasing the venous return.

The redistribution of blood flow that occurs during exercise, so that the active muscles receive the greatest proportion of the cardiac output, results from (1) vasoconstriction of the arterioles supplying the metabolically less active areas of the body (visceral organs and nonworking skeletal muscles) and (2) vasodilation of the arterioles supplying the metabolically more active skeletal muscles. The vasodilation is due to an initial reflex sympathetic nervous system response; a local effect caused by changes in CO_2, potassium ions, hydrogen ions, adenosine, lactate, and O_2 levels; and, possibly, an increase in endothelial-derived relaxing factors (e.g., nitrous oxide).

The ability of the body to transport and utilize O_2 can be mathematically expressed after re-arranging the Fick equation as follows:

$$\dot{V}O_2 = SV \times HR \times a\text{-}\overline{v}O_2 \text{ diff}$$

where

$$SV = \text{stroke volume}$$
$$HR = \text{heart rate, and}$$
$$a\text{-}\overline{v}O_2 = \text{arterial-mixed venous oxygen difference}$$

The main difference in the oxygen transport system between trained and untrained subjects is a larger stroke volume.

The study of the physical laws that govern blood flow is called hemodynamics. The two main hemodynamic factors are blood pressure and resistance to flow. Mean arterial pressure determines the rate of blood flow through the systemic circulation. Resistance to flow is caused by friction between the blood and the walls of the vessels. The most important determinant of resistance is arteriolar tone. During exercise, systolic pressure substantially increases, mean pressure modestly increases, diastolic pressure generally is unchanged, and resistance decreases.

Modest, regular exercise training has been shown to favorably lower both systolic and diastolic pressures in patients with high blood pressure (hypertension).

Questions

1. Describe the flow of blood through the heart, identifying the major structures along the way, and the function associated with each structure.
2. Provide two examples how cardiac muscle differs from skeletal muscle. One example must include how the heart operates as a functional syncytium.
3. Name the important coronary arteries that ensure that the heart receives its own supply of oxygen and nutrients.
4. What is an ECG and how is it recorded? Identify three important measures we are able to obtain from it.
5. Define bradycardia and tachycardia.
6. If an agent or drug is said to have a negative chronotropic effect, what does this mean?
7. What part of the exercise ECG is used as an indicator of myocardial ischemia? Define myocardial ischemia.
8. State the two major determinants of cardiac performance that were discussed in this chapter.
9. Is the Frank-Starling mechanism involved with increasing stroke volume during exercise?
10. To what extent does an increase in inotropicity affect stroke volume during exercise? Please explain.
11. What is the usual response of stroke volume during a progressive bout of exercise to maximum? What is the usual response of heart rate during the same bout of exercise? How are these changes related to an increase in cardiac output?
12. Give some values for cardiac output at rest and during maximal exercise for (a) untrained males and females and (b) trained males and females.
13. Identify and describe three factors used to help maintain venous return during exercise.
14. Define cardiovascular drift.
15. Explain how the blood flow is redistributed during exercise and how changes within the local chemistry of the arterioles influence blood flow.
16. Using the Fick equation, explain how $\dot{V}O_2$ is related to the body's ability to transport and utilize O_2.

17. Define systolic, pulse, mean, and diastolic blood pressures and explain how and why they change during a single bout of exercise.
18. Identify and describe two factors mentioned in the chapter that influence resistance to blood flow.
19. Rate-pressure product is the product of what two variables? And rate-pressure product estimates what component of heart function?

References

1. American College of Sports Medicine. 1995. *Guidelines for Exercise Testing and Prescription,* 5th ed. Philadelphia: Lea and Febiger, pp. 95–97.
2. Åstrand, P., T. Cuddy, B. Saltin, and J. Stenberg. 1964. Cardiac output during submaximal and maximal work. *J Appl Physiol.* 19:268–274.
3. Bevegard, S., U. Freyschuss, and T. Strandell. 1966. Circulatory adaptation to arm and leg exercise in supine and sitting position. *J App Physiol.* 21:37–46.
4. Braunwald, E. (ed.). 1992. *Heart Disease: A Textbook of Cardiovascular Medicine,* 4th ed., vol. 1. Philadelphia: W. B. Saunders.
5. Braunwald, E., A. Godblatt, D. Harrison, and D. Mason. 1963. Studies on cardiac dimensions in intact unanesthetized man. III: Effects of muscular exercise. *Circ Res.* 13:448.
6. Burt, V. L., P. Whelton, E. J. Roccella, C. Brown, J. A. Cutler, M. Higgins, M. J. Horan, D. Labarthe. 1995. Prevalence of hypertension in the U.S. adult population: Results from the third national health and nutrition examination survey, 1988–1991. *Hypertension.* 25:305–313.
7. Chapman, C. B., J. N. Fisher, and B. J. Sproule. 1960. Behavior of stroke volume at rest and during exercise in human beings. *J Clin Invest.* 39:1208–1213.
8. Chapman, C. B., and J. H. Mitchell. 1965. The physiology of exercise. *Sci Am.* 212(5):88–96.
9. Clausen, J. 1969. Effects of physical conditioning. A hypothesis concerning circulatory adjustment to exercise. *Scand J Clin Lab Invest.* 24:305.
10. Ekblom, B., P. Åstrand, B. Saltin, J. Stenberg, and B. Wallstrom. 1968. Effect of training on circulatory response to exercise. *J Appl Physiol.* 24(4):518–528.
11. Ekblom, B., and L. Hermansen. 1968. Cardiac output in athletes. *J Appl Physiol.* 25(5):619–625.
12. Ekelund, L., and A. Holmgren. 1964. Circulatory and respiratory adaptation during long-term, non-steady state exercise, in the sitting position. *Acta Physiol Scand.* 62:240–255.
13. Ellestad, M. H. (ed.). 1996. *Stress Testing: Principles and Practice,* 4th ed. Philadelphia: F. A. Davis Co.
14. Fox, E., and D. Costill. 1972. Estimated cardiorespiratory responses during marathon running. *Arch Environ Health.* 24:315–324.
15. Franklin, B. A. 1985. Exercise testing, training, and arm ergometery. *Sports Med.* 2:100–119.
16. Freedson, P., V. L. Katch, S. Sady, and A. Weltman. 1979. Cardiac output differences in males and females during mild cycle ergometer exercise. *Med Sci Sports.* 11(1):16–19.
17. Gorlin, R., L. Cohen, W. Elliott, M. Klein, and F. Lane. 1965. Effect of supine exercise on left ventricular volumes and oxygen consumption in man. *Circulation.* 32:361.
18. Grimby, G. 1965. Renal clearance during prolonged supine exercise at different loads. *J Appl Physiol.* 20:1294–1298.
19. Guyton, A. C., and J. E. Hall. 1996. *Textbook of Medical Physiology,* 9th ed. Philadelphia: W. B. Saunders.
20. Hanson, J., B. Tabakin, A. Levy, and W. Nedde. 1968. Long-term physical training and cardiovascular dynamics in middle-aged men. *Circulation.* 38:783–799.
21. Hartley, L. H. 1977. Central circulatory function during prolonged exercise. *Ann NY Acad Sci.* 301:189–194.
22. Hartley, L., G. Grimby, A. Kilbom, N. Nilsson, I. Åstrand, B. Ekblom, and B. Saltin. 1969. Physical training in sedentary middle-aged and older men. III: Cardiac output and gas exchange at submaximal and maximal exercise. *Scand J Clin Lab Invest.* 24:335–344.
23. Janicki, J. S., D. D. Sheriff, J. L. Robotham, and R. A. Wise. 1996. Cardiac output during exercise: contributions of the cardiac, circulatory, and respiratory systems. In Rowell, L. B. and J. T. Shephard (eds.), *Handbook of Physiology.* New York: American Physiology Society, chap. 17.
24. Jennings, G. L., G. Deakin, P. Korner, I. Meredith, B. Kingwell, and L. Nelson. 1991. What is the dose-response relationship between exercise training and blood pressure? *Ann Med.* 23:313–318.
25. Johnson, J. M. 1977. Regulation of skin circulation during prolonged exercise. *Ann NY Acad Sci.* 301:195–212.
26. Johnson, P. C., P. D. Wagner, and D. F. Wilson. 1996. Regulation of oxidative metabolism and blood flow in skeletal muscle. *Med Sci Sports Exerc.* 28(3):305–314.
27. Kelley, G. and Z. V. Tran. 1995. Aerobic exercise and normotensive adults: a meta-analysis. *Med Sci Sports Exerc.* 27(10):1371–1377.
28. Keteyian, S. J., C. R. C. Marks, C. A. Brawner, A. B. Levine, T. Kataoka, and T. B. Levine. 1996. Responses to arm exercise in patients with compensated heart failure. *J Cardiopulmonary Rehabil.* 16:366–371.
29. Keteyian, S. J., C. R. C. Marks, A. B. Levine, F. Fedel, J. Ehrman, T. Kataoka, and T. B. Levine. 1994. Cardiovascular responses of cardiac transplants to arm and leg exercise. *Eur J Appl Physiol.* 68:441–444.
30. Keteyian, S. J., C. R. C. Marks, A. B. Levine, T. Kataoka, F. Fedel, and T. B. Levine. 1994. Cardiovascular responses to submaximal arm and leg exercise in cardiac transplants. *Med Sci Sports Exerc.* 26(4):420–424.
31. Kilbom, A., and I. Åstrand. 1971. Physical training with submaximal intensities in women. II: Effect on cardiac output. *Scand J Clin Lab Invest.* 28:163–175.
32. McAllister, R. M. 1995. Endothelial-mediated control of coronary and skeletal muscle blood flow during exercise: introduction. *Med Sci Sports Exerc.* 27(8):1122–1124.
33. McAllister, R. M., T. Hirai, and T. I. Musch. 1995. Contribution of endothelium-derived nitric oxide (EDNO) to the skeletal muscle blood flow response to exercise. *Med Sci Sports Exerc.* 27(8):1145–1151.
34. McKirnan, M. D. and C. M. Bloor. 1994. Clinical significance of coronary vascular adaptations to exercise training. *Med Sci Sports Exerc.* 26(10):1262–1268.
35. Marks, C., V. Katch, A. Rocchini, R. Beekman, and A. Rosenthal. 1985. Validity and reliability of cardiac output by CO_2 rebreathing. *Sports Medicine.* 2:432–446.
36. Messer, J., R. Wagman, H. Levine, W. Neill, N. Krasnow, and R. Gorlin. 1962. Patterns of human myocardial oxygen extraction during rest and exercise. *J Clin Invest.* 41:725–742.
37. Michielli, D. W., R. A. Stein, N. Krasnow, J. R. Diamond, and B. Horwitz. 1979. Effects of exercise training on ventricular dimensions at rest and during exercise. *Med Sci Sports.* 11(1):82.
38. Reeves, R. A. 1995. Does this patient have hypertension? How to measure blood pressure. *JAMA.* 273(15):1211–1218.
39. Rowell, L. 1974. Human cardiovascular adjustments to exercise and thermal stress. *Physiol Rev.* 54(1):75–159.
40. Rowell, L., J. Blackmon, and R. Bruce. 1964. Indocyanine green clearance and estimated hepatic blood flow during mild to maximal exercise in upright man. *J Clin Invest.* 43:1677–1690.

41. Rowell, L., J. Blackmon, R. Martin, J. Mazzarella, and R. Bruce. 1965. Hepatic clearance of indocyanine green in man under thermal and exercise stresses. *J Appl Physiol.* 20:384–394.

42. Rowell, L., D. S. O'Leary, and D. L. Kellog, Jr. 1996. Integration of cardiovascular control systems in dynamic exercise. In Rowell, L. B. and J. T. Shephard (eds.), *Handbook of Physiology.* New York: American Physiology Society, chap. 17.

43. Saltin, B. 1987. Physiologic adaptation to physical conditioning. *Acta Med Scand. Suppl.* 711:11–24.

44. Saltin, B., G. Blomqvist, J. Mitchell, R. Johnson, K. Wildenthal, and C. Chapman. 1968. Response to exercise after bed rest and after training. *Circulation.* 38(Suppl. 7):1–78.

45. Saltin, B., and J. Stenberg. 1964. Circulatory response to prolonged severe exercise. *J Appl Physiol.* 19:833–838.

46. Sarnoff, S. J., et al. 1959. Hemodynamic determinants of oxygen consumption of the heart with special reference to the tension-time index. In Rosenbaum, F. F. (ed.), *Work and the Heart.* Paul B. Hoeber, Harper & Bros., New York.

47. Sawka, M. N., R. G. Knowlton, and J. B. Critz. 1979. Thermal and circulatory responses to repeated bouts of prolonged running. *Med Sci Sports.* 11(2):177–180.

48. Schairer, J. R., P. D. Stein, S. Keteyian, F. Fedel, J. Erhman, M. Alam, J. W. Henry, and T. Shaw. 1992. Left ventricular response to submaximal exercise in endurance-trained athletes and sedentary adults. *Am J Cardiol.* 70:930–933.

49. Schwade, J., C. G. Blomqvist, and W. Shapiro. 1977. A comparison of the response to arm and leg work in patients with ischemic heart disease. *American Heart Journal.* 94(2):203–208.

50. Simon, G., H. H. Dickhuth, J. Starger, C. Essig, W. Kindermann, and J. Keul. 1980. The value of echocardiography during physical exercise. *Int Sport Sci.* 1(11) (Abstr.):900.

51. Slutsky, R., J. Karliner, D. Ricci, G. Schuler, M. Pfisterer, K. Peterson, and W. Ashburn. 1979. Response of left ventricular volume to exercise in man assessed by radionuclide equilibrium angiography. *Circulation.* 60(3):565–571.

52. Stenberg, J., P. O. Åstrand, B. Ekblom, J. Royce, and B. Saltin. 1967. Hemodynamic response to work with different muscle groups, sitting and supine. *J Appl Physiol.* 22:61–70.

53. Tabakin, B., J. Hanson, and A. Levy. 1965. Effects of physical training on the cardiovascular and respiratory response to graded upright exercise in distance runners. *Br Heart J.* 27:205–210.

54. Tipton, C. M. 1991. Exercise, training, and hypertension: An update. *Exercise and Sport Sciences Reviews,* vol. 18. Baltimore: Williams and Wilkins, pp. 447–505.

55. Wenger, N. K., E. S. Froelicher, L. K. Smith, et al. 1995. *Cardiac Rehabilitation.* Clinical Practice Guideline No. 17. Rockville, MD: U.S. Department of Health and Human Services, Public Health Service, Agency for Health Care Policy and Research and the National Heart, Lung, and Blood Institute. AHCPR Publication No. 96–0672.

56. Younis, L. T., J. A. Melin, J. C. Schoevaerdts, M. V. Dyck, J. M. Detry, A. Robert, C. Chalant, and M. Goenen. 1990. Left ventricular systolic function and diastolic filling at rest and during upright exercise after orthotopic heart transplantation: comparison with young and aged normal subjects. *J Heart Transplant.* 9:683–692.

57. Zobl, E., F. Talmers, R. Christensen, and L. Baer. 1965. Effect of exercise on the cerebral circulation and metabolism. *J Appl Physiol.* 20:1289–1293.

Selected Readings

American College of Sports Medicine. 1993. Physical activity, physical fitness, and hypertension. *Med Sci Sports Exerc.* 25:i–x.

Dubin, D. 1997. Rapid Interpretation of EKGs, 5th ed. Cover Publishing Co., Tampa.

Griffin, S. E., R. A. Roberts, and V. H. Heyward. 1997. Blood pressure measurement during exercise: a review. *Med Sci Sports Exerc.* 29:149–159.

Hagberg, J. M. 1990. Exercise, fitness, and hypertension. In C. Bouchard, et al., *Exercise, Fitness and Health: A Consensus of Current Knowledge,* Champaign, IL: Human Kinetics, pp. 455–466.

Keul, J. 1973. The relationship between circulation and metabolism during exercise. *Med Sci Sports.* 5(4):209–219.

Opie, L. H. (ed.). 1991. *The Heart: Physiology and Metabolism,* 2nd ed. New York: Raven Press.

Segal, S. S., and D. T. Kurjiaka. 1995. Coordination of blood flow control in the resistance vasculature of skeletal muscle. *Med Sci Sports Exerc.* 27(8):1158–1164.

Vanfraechem, J. H. P. 1979. Stroke volume and systolic time interval adjustments during bicycle exercise. *J Appl Physiol.* 46(3):588–592.

10 Cardiorespiratory Control

In 1934 Sir Joseph Barcroft realized the benefit of forcing a system to perform at high levels of function to understand better how it works. Relative to understanding control of the cardiovascular and respiratory systems, exercise provides the means that "forces them" to operate at a higher level of function. Previous chapters have described the many respiratory and circulatory adjustments that occur during exercise, all of which are designed to meet the increased metabolic demands of working muscles. To do this efficiently, however, all of these adjustments must be initiated, controlled, and coordinated with one another.

The difficult job of orchestrating cardiorespiratory responses is carried out by the central nervous system through the combined efforts of the respiratory and cardiovascular areas located in the brain. These areas constantly receive information from both the motor cortex or a variety of receptors located throughout the body. Then, using this information as a basis, they elicit, if necessary, regulatory changes in pulmonary ventilation and blood flow.

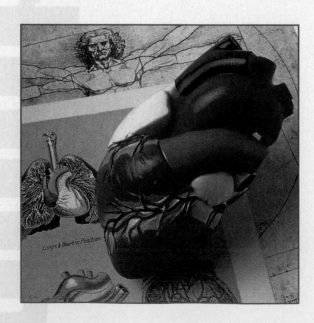

Summary of the Cardiorespiratory System

The Respiratory and Cardiovascular Control Areas

Summary

The major concepts to be learned from this chapter are as follows:

- During rest and exercise, control of the respiratory and circulatory systems is complex.
- Control of respiration and circulation involves the cardiovascular and respiratory areas, which are located in the medulla oblongata of the brain.
- Central, humoral, physical, and peripheral neural stimulation of these areas aids in regulating important cardiorespiratory variables, such as arterial blood pressure and arterial blood PO_2, PCO_2, and H^+ concentration.
- This regulation is accomplished through increases or decreases in heart rate, myocardial contractility, breathing rate and depth, and an increase or decrease in the extent of constriction within blood vessels.
- The response of the cardiorespiratory system during exercise is initially matched to the intensity and type of muscle contractions (static versus dynamic), to the amount of active muscle mass, and later to the fatigue that might be occurring.
- During exercise, primary neural drives to the cardiorespiratory areas include descending impulses from the motor cortex, which are then refined by mechanical-sensitive and chemical-sensitive receptors located in the skeletal muscles, tendons, joints, or major arteries (carotid, aorta).
- Cardiovascular adjustments primarily are made by an increase in sympathetic neural activity and/or a decrease in parasympathetic neural activity. This may include activation of the central portion of the adrenal gland, the medulla, which results in the release of norepinephrine and epinephrine.
- Ventilatory adjustments are made by activation of the phrenic and intercostal nerves to the diaphragm and intercostal muscles.
- These cardiovascular and ventilatory responses may respectively be called the *exercise pressor reflex* and *exercise-induced hyperpnea*.
- Precise regulation is attempted through feedback error impulses sent from peripheral (and possibly central) receptors to signal a need for additional systematic adjustments. The regulation is never perfect.

Summary of the Cardiorespiratory System

Let us begin our discussion of cardiorespiratory control by summarizing the functions of this system. We see from figure 10.1 that the respiratory system first provides a means whereby air is moved into and out of the lungs. This rhythmic to-and-fro movement of air is called *pulmonary ventilation*. Next, the oxygen brought in from the outside environment via pulmonary ventilation is made available to the blood through a vast network of capillaries surrounding the ~ 600 million tiny air sacs or *alveoli* found in the lungs. The blood initially contained within the capillaries is relatively low in oxygen and high in carbon dioxide content. At the *alveolar-capillary membrane,* oxygen diffuses from the air in the alveoli into capillary blood. At the same time carbon dioxide diffuses in the opposite direction (from the capillary blood to alveoli air). The alveolar-capillary membranes, then, represent a functional interface between the respiratory and circulatory systems.

The next important job is the transport of oxygen-rich (*arterialized*) blood to the body's tissues. This task is carried out by the left side of the heart and its associated blood vessels. In figure 10.1 note that one of the tissues that receives blood from the left side of the heart is skeletal muscle. Recall from chapter 6 that skeletal muscle is richly supplied with capillary beds, all of which come in close contact with the individual muscle fibers. At the *tissue-capillary membrane,* a second exchange of gases occurs. This time, oxygen diffuses from the capillaries and into the cells of the tissues. And just like in the lungs, carbon dioxide diffuses in the opposite direction. The exchange of gases at this tissue-capillary interface converts arterial blood to venous blood. The venous blood is then returned to the right heart and then the lungs where the entire process of gas exchange and transport is repeated over and over again.

The Respiratory and Cardiovascular Control Areas

As mentioned in the introduction to this chapter, the difficult task of receiving information relative to pulmonary ventilation and blood flow, integrating it, and then initiating a response to match mechanical and metabolic demand occurs within the respiratory and cardiovascular control areas of the brain. Specifically, the central processing action takes place in networks of nerve cells and their connections, located mostly in the **medulla oblongata** of the brain stem. Anatomically, it is rather difficult to distinguish the cardiovascular control area from the respiratory control area; however, physiologically they are separate. For example, studies have shown that electrical stimulation of certain areas

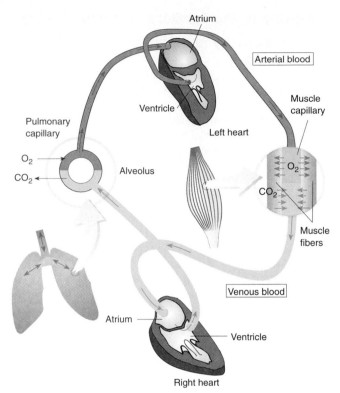

Figure 10.1

The cardiorespiratory system. The respiratory and circulatory systems work intimately together in meeting, under all conditions, the gaseous exchange and transport requirements of the cells.

primarily affects respiration, whereas stimulation of nearby but different areas primarily affects circulation.

The effect on respiration is mainly a change in pulmonary (alveolar) ventilation (i.e., in the rate and particularly in the depth of breathing). Circulatory effects include changes in heart rate, stroke volume (force of contraction or myocardial contractility), the distribution of blood to various organs (vasoconstriction and vasodilation), and venous return (venoconstriction). Although stimulation of the respiratory or cardiovascular areas may affect one system more than the other, they are neurally interconnected, so that each is somewhat informed of the other's activity. Therefore, stimulation of one area will, via its connection with the other, generally affect both ventilation and blood flow. This, of course, makes sense since changes in both systems are usually necessary if the body is to respond in an effective and coordinated manner.

Stimulation of the Cardiorespiratory Control Areas

The cardiorespiratory areas in the brain stem are stimulated by input received from a variety of locations within the body, as shown on the left side of figure 10.2. For our purposes, stimulation refers to an increase in the activity of the

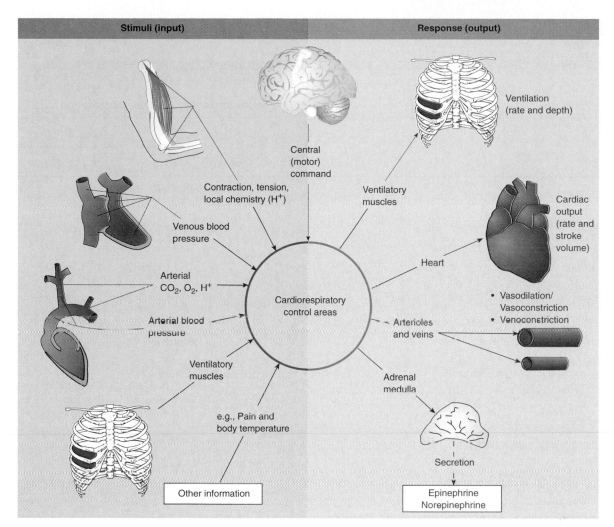

Stimuli (input)

Response (output)

Central (motor) command

Contraction, tension, local chemistry (H⁺)

Venous blood pressure

Arterial CO_2, O_2, H^+

Arterial blood pressure

Ventilatory muscles

e.g., Pain and body temperature

Other information

Ventilatory muscles

Cardiorespiratory control areas

Heart

Arterioles and veins

Adrenal medulla

Ventilation (rate and depth)

Cardiac output (rate and stroke volume)

• Vasodilation/ Vasoconstriction
• Venoconstriction

Secretion

Epinephrine Norepinephrine

Figure 10.2

Nervous control of the cardiorespiratory system. Various kinds of information (stimuli) from all parts of the body are sent to the respiratory and circulatory areas located in the brain stem. Then, using this information, the areas elicit, if necessary, regulatory changes in pulmonary ventilation and blood flow.

nerve cells and connections within these areas. As we will see later, this increased activity leads to regulatory changes in ventilation and blood flow.

Classification of Stimuli

We will group the many incoming stimuli shown in figure 10.2 into four functional classifications: *central command, humoral, physical,* and *peripheral neural.* Be aware that each of these stimuli may not elicit equal, if any, changes in cardiovascular and pulmonary function. Provided below is a brief description of each of the four classifications of stimuli.

Central motor command or, simply, **central command** input to the cardiorespiratory center occurs mostly via neurons that originate in the motor cortex and "irradiate" or "spill over" as they pass through the cardiorespiratory center on their way to initiate a skeletal muscle action.[16] This spill-over action in the medulla can lead to changes in both

ventilation and cardiovascular function. Specifically, central command involves a parallel, simultaneous excitation of neuronal circuits controlling both the locomotor and cardiorespiratory systems.[16] Actions initiated by the cardiorespiratory centers influence neural activity to the heart and blood vessels as well as neural outflow to the motor neurons innervating respiratory muscles. Additionally, central command can be initiated by mental conditions (emotions) integrated by the hypothalamic region of the limbic system.

Humoral stimuli originate from changes in the chemical properties of blood or cerebral spinal fluid, which ultimately influence receptors located elsewhere in the body. Once activated, these receptors provide afferent* neural

---

*Generally, efferent nerve fibers are those that originate from the central nervous system (brain or spinal cord) with the purpose of *effecting* (thus the word *efferent*) an action elsewhere within the body. Afferent fibers are sensory fibers that originate in tissues other than the central nervous system and, once activated by various stimuli (e.g., pain), inform the central nervous system of local conditions.

table 10.1

Action of various stimuli on the cardiorespiratory areas of the brain stem and their effects on respiration and circulation

			Action on Cardiorespiratory Areas	
			Receptor	
Stimuli	**Feedforward**	**Feedback**	**Type**	**Location**
Central command	✓		*	*
Humoral (blood or CSF)				
Increased PCO_2, H^+, K^+	✓?	✓	Chemo	Brainstem, carotid
Decreased PO_2		✓	Chemo	arteries, or aortic
Increased epinephrine and norepinephrine		✓	Chemo	arch
Physical				
Increased pressure		✓	Baro	Aortic arch, carotid arteries
Increased volume		✓	Pressure or stretch	Right atrium/ pulmonary artery
Peripheral neural				
Respiratory muscles		✓	Stretch or mechano	Muscle, joints, tendons
Other skeletal muscle				
Mechanical		✓	Mechano	Muscle
Metabolic		✓	Metabo	

*No receptors involved with feedforward mechanism; CSF = cerebral spinal fluid; ↑ = more vasoconstriction; ↓ = less vasoconstriction.
†Less vasoconstriction generally dominates in *active* skeletal muscle because of vasoactive metabolites.

input to the cardiorespiratory area, which then evokes an appropriate response. The receptors we are referring to are primarily chemoreceptors that are sensitive to changes in fluid chemistry, such as PO_2, PCO_2, K^+ concentration, and/or pH. These chemoreceptors are located in the medulla (called central chemoreceptors) or elsewhere in the body, such as in the aortic bodies of the aorta or in the carotid bodies found at the bifurcation of the carotid arteries. The central chemoreceptors are sensitive to changes in cerebral spinal fluid (and blood) chemistry (mainly PCO_2 and pH), while the aortic and carotid artery chemoreceptors (called peripheral chemoreceptors) are sensitive to changes in blood chemistry (PCO_2, PO_2, and H^+ or K^+ concentrations).

Changes in the physical characteristics of blood (e.g., pressure, volume, temperature) are classified as *physical stimuli*. Among this class of stimuli, there are pressure-sensitive mechanoreceptors (the baroreceptors) located in the aortic arch and carotid arteries. Low pressure baroreceptors—located in the atria, ventricles, pulmonary artery, and pulmonary vein—are also involved. For example, a fall in blood pressure at the level of the aorta alters the

baroreceptors such that it signals the cardiovascular center to initiate corrective actions meant to increase heart rate, contractility, and total systemic peripheral resistance—all of which help to increase blood pressure.

Peripheral neural stimuli are independent of changes in the chemical or physical properties of blood; rather, they originate from changes that take place in the lungs, muscles, joints, tendons, and skin, and result in an afferent neural response being generated toward the cardiorespiratory areas. The feedback information they provide is concerned with (1) changes in the local chemistry (and possibly temperature) in and around the skeletal muscle; (2) muscle contraction and limb movement or tension development; and (3) intense pain, general discomfort and/or the presence of respiratory irritants (hence, the cough and sneeze reflexes). Although all of these neural stimuli are important, we are most interested in those arising from the muscles.

For example, two neural reflex mechanisms originate from skeletal muscles and comprise the **exercise pressor reflex.**[9] Feedback information from the exercise pressor reflex to the cardiorespiratory areas of the medulla occurs

table 10.1 (cont'd.)

	Effects	
	Circulation	
Respiration	Heart rate	Arteriolar tone†
↑↑↑	↑↑↑	↑↑↑
↑↑	↑	↑
↑	↑	↑
↑	↑	↑
↓	↓	↓
↓	↓	↓
↑	↑ ?	?
↑ ? ↑ ?	↑ ↑↑	↑ ↑↑

mainly via Group III and Group IV afferent fibers. Group III fiber nerve endings are primarily activated by deformation (shape) changes in the contracting muscle and are termed **mechanoreceptors.** Group IV fiber nerve endings are primarily activated by metabolic* changes in and around skeletal muscles and are called **metaboreceptors.** Notice our use of the word *primarily* in the previous two sentences. Clearly, the separation between the two receptors is not clean, as a portion of the mechanoreceptors are sensitive to metabolic stimuli and, conversely, a portion of the metaboreceptors are sensitive to mechanical stimuli. We will discuss the exercise pressor reflex further later in this chapter.

One other possible receptor that may contribute to cardiorespiratory regulation—one that is less understood

---

*An insufficient supply of O_2 (poor blood flow) to active muscles during strenuous exercise changes local metabolism such that anaerobic pathways are increasingly relied upon for energy production. This leads to the production of lactate, which increases muscle interstitial H^+ concentration and activates the chemical sensitive metaboreceptors.

than either of the two previously mentioned receptors—is the muscle thermoreceptor.[13] Muscle temperature is normally below 35° C at rest and can exceed 40° C during dynamic exercise—well within the normal firing range of 24° to 44° C for these receptors. One reason for our lack of knowledge about muscle thermoreceptors is the difficulty of experimentally manipulating local muscle temperature while at the same time controlling for the effects that blood that is warmed as it passes through the muscle may have on body core temperature.

Action on the Cardiorespiratory Areas

As indicated in table 10.1, stimuli may act on the cardiorespiratory areas via *feedforward* and/or *feedback* mechanisms. *Feedforward* stimuli act on the cardiorespiratory areas directly via central command (nervous impulses from higher brain centers). *Feedback* stimulation of the cardiorespiratory areas is part of a reflex response that occurs via afferent sensory nerves originating in specialized receptors located throughout the body. In this case the number and frequency of incoming sensory impulses are based on changes in arterial pressure; blood/muscle temperature; blood/muscle PO_2, PCO_2, and H^+ concentrations; muscle contraction; and limb movement. The names and locations of the receptors are summarized in table 10.1 and are schematically shown in figure 10.2.

Innervation of the Cardiorespiratory Apparatus

The innervation of the cardiorespiratory system is shown schematically on the right side of figure 10.2. The motor nerves connected to the ventilatory muscles (p. 172) are called *somatic motor nerves* (*somatic* means "body"). We know that when they are stimulated they affect both the rate and the depth of respiration. In addition, they belong to the voluntary nervous system, like those innervating the other skeletal muscles. This explains why we have some voluntary control over ventilation—in other words, why we can alter our ventilatory behavior such as deep breathing or breath holding at will.

The nerves innervating the heart and blood vessels, on the other hand, are quite different. This is evidenced by the fact that we do not usually have voluntary control over the circulatory system. These particular nerves belong to the involuntary or **autonomic nervous system,** which has two components: the **sympathetic** division and the **parasympathetic** division. The *sympathetic system* stimulates those bodily actions that are needed during an emergency or stressful (exercise usually being a positive form of stress) situation—the so-called "fight, fright, and flight responses." The sympathetic nervous system is sometimes referred to as either the thoracolumbar system or the adrenergic system. The first name is based on the fact that its initial (preganglionic) nerve fibers emerge from all the thoracic and the upper two lumbar levels of the spine. The phrase *adren*ergic nervous system is based on the neurotransmitter released by its terminal (postganglionic) fibers (i.e., **norepinephrine** or *noradrenaline*).

In contrast, the *parasympathetic system* is associated with the conservation and restoration of body resources. Other names given to this division of the autonomic nervous system include the craniosacral system or the cholinergic system. The former refers to the fact that its initial or preganglionic fibers emerge either with various cranial nerves or at the much lower sacral spinal levels. The term *cholin*ergic system comes from the neurotransmitter (i.e., *acetylcholine*) that is secreted from its terminal or postganglionic fibers.

When stimulated, the sympathetic nerves that innervate the heart—pretty much the entire heart (with a proportionately greater amount to the ventricles)—cause increased rate and force of contraction (increased stroke volume). That is why they are referred to as *cardioaccelerator nerves.* Conversely, when stimulated, the parasympathetic nerves (i.e., the vagus nerves) evoke a decrease in heart rate (and to a much lesser extent a decrease in contractility). The cardiac vagus nerves predominantly innervate the sinoatrial and atrioventricular nodes, with some fibers distributed to the two atria and far fewer fibers distributed to the ventricular muscle. The balance or interaction between the cardiac sympathetic and parasympathetic nerves provide for a precise controlling mechanism.

For example, increases in heart rate can result from either a decreased rate of stimulation of the vagus nerves or an increased rate of stimulation of the sympathetic cardioaccelerator nerves, or both. During exercise* there is both parasympathetic withdrawal, which is primarily responsible for the initial increase in heart rate (up to ~ 100 b $\cdot$ min^{-1}), and an increase in sympathetic tone, which becomes more dominant at rates above ~ 100 b $\cdot$ min^{-1}. Conversely, very soon after stopping exercise, immediate stimulation of the vagus nerves obscure the sustained increase in sympathetic activity that is "left over" from exercise and produces a rapid decrease in heart rate.[10]

The nerves innervating the smooth muscles of the arterioles and veins also belong to the autonomic nervous system. For the most part they include sympathetic nerves that, when stimulated, cause arteriolar constriction and venoconstriction—thus the term *sympathetic vasoconstrictor nerves.* We must point out that there are some sympathetic nerves that act on the arterioles of skeletal muscles only, and when stimulated, cause vasodilation (*sympathetic vasodilator nerves*). These nerves are relatively less important than vasoconstrictor nerves and are felt to be most active in the alarm/defense reaction or before and at the very beginning of exercise.

Once activated further during exercise, the "intention" of the sympathetic vasoconstrictor nerves is to produce arteriolar vasoconstriction. Despite this, vasodilation predominates in the metabolically more active skeletal muscles because of the accumulation of locally produced vasodilator agents such as adenosine, lactic acid, hydrogen ions, potassium ions, CO_2, and possibly, nitrous oxide. Thus, both the sympathetic vasoconstrictor nerves that reduce arteriolar size (thus blood flow) to metabolically less active tissues (the visceral organs and nonactive skeletal muscles) and the above-mentioned vasodilation in more active muscles act together to redistribute blood away from inactive tissues and toward active muscles.

Before leaving our discussion about activation of the cardiorespiratory system, we must mention a group of specialized gland cells found within the medulla (central portion) region of the adrenal glands. These cells are similar to sympathetic nerves in that they, too, release norepinephrine. In addition, they release a similar chemical called **epinephrine** *(adrenaline).* These two chemicals are referred to as **catecholamines** and act as hormones because they are released into the blood. They are most often secreted by the adrenal medulla when the sympathetic nerve fibers acting on this area are stimulated. This occurs during alarm or fright, and during exercise.

Generally, the release of epinephrine by the adrenal medulla is greater than the release of norepinephrine (about 80% of what is released is epinephrine); however, during exercise the blood concentration of norepinephrine is higher than epinephrine. The higher level of norepinephrine than epinephrine during exercise results from the fact that $\sim 20\%$ of the norepinephrine released by sympathetic fibers throughout the body "spills over" from neural synaptic clefts and into the blood—instead of being taken back up by the nerve endings. The two organs making the largest spillover contributions to the increase in plasma norepinephrine during exercise are the skeletal muscles and the kidneys. The effects of circulating epinephrine and norepinephrine on both the heart and the smooth muscles of blood vessels and bronchioles are almost identical to the effects produced when sympathetic nerves innervating these tissues are directly stimulated. In addition, these hormones cause numerous other actions throughout the body, such as an increase in metabolic rate, inhibition of the gastrointestinal tract, dilation of the pupils of the eyes, release of glucose into the blood, and the mobilization of fatty acids (see also chapter 17).[5]

Cardiorespiratory Control at Rest and during Exercise

One of the most important functions of any physiological control system is to maintain certain variables at optimal levels. Relative to the cardiorespiratory control system, it strives to maintain ventilation, blood pressure, and blood

---

*At rest the heart is primarily under the influence of the left and right vagus nerves. In fact, the slower heart rates observed among well-trained athletes is due, in great part, to an increase in vagal tone.

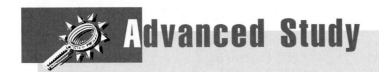

Advanced Study

Adrenergic Receptors

The actions of norepinephrine and epinephrine are not solely due to their presence at the cell membrane. The nature and extent of the actions caused by these two catecholamines also depends on the type and number of *receptors* located in the cell membrane proper. Let us explain.

Picture, if you will, that each receptor acts like a keyhole, while the catecholamines act like a key. The catecholamine (key) must correctly fit into the appropriately configured keyhole (receptor) before it can exert its action on the cell. There are three main types of keyholes that respond to norepinephrine or epinephrine; they are called *alpha receptors, beta$_1$ receptors,* and *beta$_2$ receptors.* And although these receptors influence a myriad of other actions throughout the body, for our purposes it is important to know that stimulation of alpha receptors leads to vasoconstriction of the arterioles nourishing skeletal muscles and the viscera (e.g., gastrointestinal tract) as well as the breakdown of glycogen in the liver (glycogenolysis). Stimulation of beta$_1$ receptors causes increases in heart rate and contractility and the breakdown of fat stores (lipolysis). Stimulation of beta$_2$ receptors cause vasodilation of coronary arterioles and relaxation of the bronchioles (bronchodilation).

Norepinephrine, the chemical that can be either released into circulation by the adrenal medulla or released as a neurotransmitter by postganglionic sympathetic nerve endings, stimulates only alpha receptors and beta$_1$ receptors. *Epinephrine,* on the other hand, which is released into circulation by the adrenal medulla, stimulates all three receptors—alpha, beta$_1$, and beta$_2$.

During moderate exercise norepinephrine is released by sympathetic nerves directly onto the heart, which then interact with (fit into) the beta$_1$ receptors located on cardiac cells. With the help of the beta$_1$ receptors, norepinephrine is then able to exert its full action on the heart—causing an increase in rate and force of contraction. At the same time, norepinephrine is also being released by sympathetic vasoconstrictor nerves onto arteriolar smooth muscle cells in both nonactive skeletal muscle and the viscera. With the help of alpha receptors, we see vasoconstriction and the redirection of blood flow from metabolically less active tissues to the metabolically more active skeletal muscles.

In the 1970s a class of drugs became available called beta-adrenergic blocking agents—beta-blockers for short. These drugs (e.g., inderal, metoprolol, and atenolol) act as agents that block the actions of beta$_1$, beta$_2$, or both receptors simultaneously. Their use in medicine as a means to block the actions of the sympathetic nervous system is now widespread, especially in the treatment of high blood pressure (hypertension) and certain cardiac disorders. For example, for persons who have suffered a heart attack, the daily use of a beta-blocker lowers subsequent heart attack rates by ~ 25%. Let's take a moment and investigate just how these agents work.

Recall from the previous discussion that the beta receptors found on cell membranes act as keyholes and, when filled by the correct key (norepinephrine or epinephrine), initiate a certain action within the cell. If, as the name implies, beta-blockers enter or block cardiac beta$_1$ receptors, they would prevent the catecholamines from "getting in" and exerting their full effect. In this case there is less of an increase in heart rate and less of an increase in contractility. Simply put, the action that the catecholamines were hoping to accomplish is blunted.

Patients who have atherosclerotic blockages within the coronary arteries that supply blood to their heart (ischemic heart disease) have a reduced ability to adequately deliver oxygen to the heart muscle itself. These patients are often treated with beta-blockers. Why? Because during times of stress (and exercise), when the heart is literally being "bombarded" with increased levels of epinephrine and norepinephrine, the use of beta-blockers helps minimize the "oxygen consuming" increases in heart rate and contractility. The end result is that myocardial oxygen demand is lowered (even during exercise) and thus is kept in line with what can be supplied by narrowed coronary arteries.

---

flow at optimal levels while at rest, during exercise, and when exposed to temperature and gravitational extremes. As you might guess, accomplishing this is no simple task— one that is further complicated as metabolic needs change from minute to minute (e.g., going from resting in an air-conditioned gymnasium to running outdoors on a hot day).

Providing a detailed explanation of all the mechanisms involved with maintaining optimal cardiorespiratory function at rest and during exercise is beyond the scope of this chapter. Additionally, the precise roles of the various stimuli influencing cardiorespiratory function have not been fully elucidated. Therefore, in the material that follows we present what we feel are the important factors and actions that predominate. Numerous excellent review articles and original investigations have been published on this topic, many of which have been extensively used to present the material that follows.[6,9,10,11,12,13,14,15,16]

Control at Rest

The most important factors in the maintenance of adequate ventilation and blood flow at rest are changes in arterial blood pressure, PO_2, PCO_2, and H^+ concentrations. As mentioned earlier in this chapter, changes in blood pressure represent a form of *physical stimuli,* while the other three represent *humoral* (chemical) *stimuli.*

For example, when an individual moves from the supine to the standing position, causing blood to "pool" in the lower extremities, there is an initial drop in blood flow to the head and upper body that is associated with a decrease in blood pressure (P_{mean} falls). Loss of consciousness would eventually result if it were not for the fact that this decrease in pressure is quickly sensed by **baroreceptors,** found mostly in the walls of the internal carotid arteries and in the aortic arch (figure 10.3). These pressure-sensitive receptors respond greatest to changes in transluminal (across the walls) stretch. As a result, the firing rate of afferent neural signals generated by the baroreceptors— those that travel to the medulla via the vagus nerves, Hering's nerves, and other nerves—is altered. The end result being: (1) inhibition of parasympathetic input to the myocardium causing an increase in heart rate and possibly contractility (Treppe effect), and (2) an increase in efferent sympathetic vasoconstrictor nerve action (causing an increase in total systemic peripheral resistance).* Specifically, after two to three minutes of standing, you would observe that systolic blood pressure is now only slightly lower than when laying supine, and heart rate may be slightly elevated. Conversely, an increase in mean arterial pressure (e.g., above the 95 to 100 mm Hg value normally maintained at rest) causes an increase in parasympathetic tone (decrease in heart rate) and inhibition of sympathetic vasoconstrictor nerves (less vasoconstriction). This type of control is referred to as a feedback control mechanism.

In addition to the aortic and carotid baroreceptors mentioned here, other stimuli can also affect blood pressure

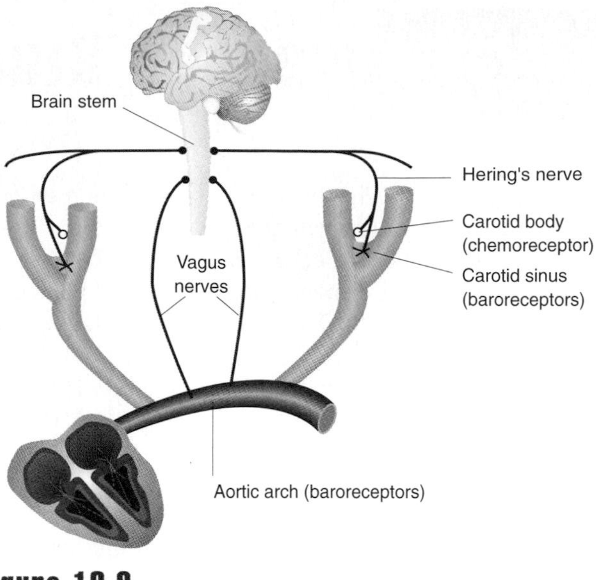

Figure 10.3

The arterial baroreceptor (pressure) and chemoreceptor (PO_2, PCO_2, H^+) feedback systems.

and blood flow. These other mechanisms include (1) the low pressure baroreceptors found in the heart and pulmonary vasculature and (2) chemoreceptors found in the carotid bodies at the bifurcation of the common carotid artery and the aortic bodies that lie just adjacent to the aorta (figure 10.3). The low pressure baroreceptors do not detect changes in pressure, per se, as much as they detect sudden changes in blood volume. However, their importance during exercise remains unclear and, as a result, will not be discussed further.

The chemoreceptors are sensitive to a reduction in PO_2, PCO_2 excess, or H^+ excess. If flow (and pressure) to these receptors falls, there is a drop in O_2 content and a build up of CO_2 and H^+ in and around the receptors. Once stimulated, they, too, send afferent signals to the medulla via Hering's nerves or the vagus nerves. However, relative to blood flow and blood pressure management, the chemoreceptors play a minor role when compared to the baroreceptors. By far, their most important function is to assist with fine-tuning ventilation.

For example, should PO_2 fall precipitously low in the blood (< 55 mm Hg)—like what might occur in the unfortunate victim who is trapped in a house fire and subjected to carbon monoxide inhalation—ventilation increases in response. In addition, changes in PCO_2 and H^+ concentration in arterial blood influence the carotid and aortic chemoreceptors (and the central chemoreceptors found in the medulla) such that corresponding or corrective changes in ventilation (rate and depth) occur. Unlike the way the carotid and aortic chemoreceptors wait until there is a dramatic decrease in PO_2 before they discharge afferent signals, these same receptors are sensitive to small changes in PCO_2 and H^+ concentration.

---

*Recall from chapter 9: $P_{mean} = \dot{Q} \times T_S P_R$

where: $\dot{Q}$ = stroke volume $\times$ heart rate

Therefore, increases in heart rate and stroke volume increase pressure. Also, increases in peripheral resistance in the arms, legs, and viscera redirects some of the blood meant to flow into these areas toward the chest and head. The net effect from the above helps prevent people from losing consciousness when they stand.

Control during Exercise

While changes in arterial pressure, PO_2, PCO_2, and H^+ concentration represent the predominant regulatory stimuli at rest, this may or may not be true during exercise. Specifically, during exercise the threshold for activating some of these stimuli changes.

First, we know from experience that heart rate and ventilation increase even before exercise begins, long before changes in arterial pressure PO_2, PCO_2, and H^+ concentration can occur. For example, in a person who is about to undergo an exercise stress test, heart rate can often be observed to increase at about the same time the treadmill is turned on—literally while he or she is sitting and waiting to move over to the machine. Just the anticipation of exercise and seeing or hearing the treadmill belt move readies the individual for exertion via inhibition of the cardiac vagus nerves.

Second, we know from a physiological standpoint that an increase in heart rate (and in stroke volume) increases arterial blood pressure. If this increased pressure (which is normal during exercise) were to evoke the baroreceptor reflex during exercise in the same manner that it does at rest, heart rate and stroke volume should eventually decrease rather than increase. Fortunately, the baroreceptors are temporarily "turned off"—or more specifically, they are quickly "reset" to a higher threshold when exercise is started. This allows heart rate and blood pressure to increase with little opposition.

Third, changes in arterial PO_2, PCO_2, and H^+ concentration would have to be quite pronounced to account fully for the large increase in pulmonary ventilation that occurs during exercise. In fact, these variables change very little during mild to moderate exercise, even though minute ventilation increases some 3- to 5-fold. During very heavy or maximal exercise, PO_2 may decrease slightly, and H^+ increases—the latter primarily due to lactic acid accumulation. In this case, these changes—particularly in H^+ concentration—likely contribute to the increase in ventilation.

Which stimuli, then, predominate during exercise? Unfortunately, all the stimuli have not as of yet been identified or fully explained. However, there are several that are known to be of primary importance relative to influencing cardiorespiratory function. These include: (1) increased activity of the motor cortex (central command), (2) changes in muscle chemistry, contraction and static tension development, (3) changes in blood H^+ concentration and PCO_2, (4) changes in blood pressure, and (5) increased secretion of norepinephrine and epinephrine from the adrenal medulla. Their effects on ventilation and blood flow are reviewed in table 10.1. Most of these stimuli (particularly the first four) supply information concerning the intensity of exercise rather than the level or magnitude of any particular cardiorespiratory variable. This enables the resulting adjustments in ventilation and blood flow to keep pace with the increased gas exchange and blood transport requirements of the working muscles.

Cardiovascular Control

The response of the cardiovascular system during exercise is matched to the *type* and *intensity* of the activity being performed. For example, during *static-type exercise,* such as holding or pushing a heavy object, the increase in arterial blood pressure is directly related to how much muscle mass is involved (arms versus legs) and to the percentage of effort it represents relative to one's maximal voluntary contraction. The above example differs from *dynamic exercise,* such as swimming, where the increase in blood flow (cardiac output) matches intensity of effort, which is directly related to the amount of oxygen being consumed by the more metabolically active skeletal muscles. In both cases, these (and other) cardiovascular responses are mediated by changes in parasympathetic and sympathetic nervous system activity. Additionally, relative to sympathetic vasoconstrictor nerve activity to both the viscera and the inactive skeletal muscles, we know that such activity is also related to the onset and progression of fatigue in exercising muscles. Now let's take a closer look at just how cardiovascular adjustments are mediated during exercise. To better understand the material that follows, refer to figure 10.4 as needed.[8]

Isometric Exercise

In isometric (static exercise), central command primarily raises heart rate and cardiac output by vagal withdrawal of the parasympathetic nervous system. This results in a reduced release of acetylcholine at the sinoatrial node, allowing heart rate to increase. Additionally, the deformation-sensitive (or stretch-sensitive) mechanoreceptors, which are part of the skeletal muscle exercise pressor reflex (see page 252), may also be involved. These receptors are activated more during the onset of exercise, then they travel, mostly via Group III afferent fibers, to the cardiovascular areas of the medulla. Here they initiate sympathetic activity (which has been clearly demonstrated in animals) to bring about increases in heart rate and arterial pressure. As mentioned, activation of these mechanoreceptors is likely most prominent during the initiation and the early phases of static exercise because their firing rates have been shown to decrease rather quickly as exercise continues.

If vigorous isometric activity is maintained for any length of time (> 1 to 2 min), this leads to lack of oxygen to the contracting muscles and the accumulation of metabolites, such as potassium, adenosine, bradykinin, and (especially) H^+. These agents activate the chemical-sensitive muscle metaboreceptors, which in turn initiate peripheral afferent neural impulses toward the medulla via the slower conducting Group IV (sensory) fibers. These fibers travel through the dorsal root of the spinal cord and then follow ascending pathways to the brain stem. One reason for the delayed activation of the muscle metaboreflex is that the metabolites must first accumulate to sufficient

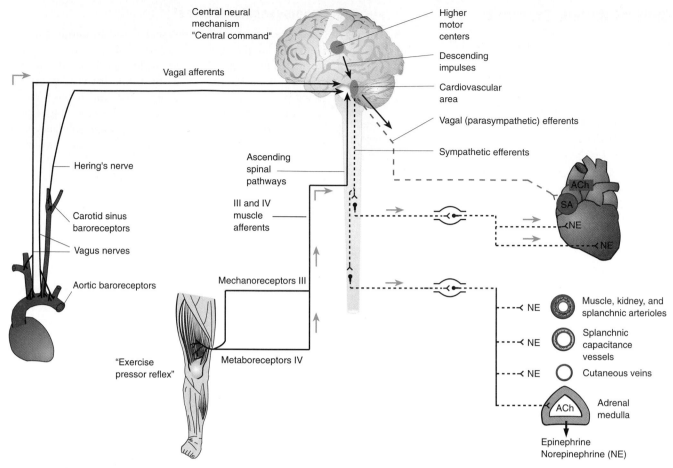

Figure 10.4

Control over the cardiovascular system during exercise. Both descending impulses from the motor region of the cerebrum (central command) and afferent input from the arterial baroreceptors and skeletal muscle receptors impinge on the cardiovascular area of the medulla. This results in reduced parasympathetic activity to the heart and an increase in sympathetic activity to the heart, blood vessels, and adrenal medulla. The end result is an increase in cardiac output and an increase in blood pressure.

concentrations in and around the muscle cell before the receptors are fired. The end result, however, is stimulation of the sympathetic cardioaccelator nerves acting on the sinoatrial node (and other areas) of the heart. Recall that this causes an increase in rate and contractility. The muscle metaboreceptors also lead to stimulation of the sympathetic vasoconstrictor nerves within both the viscera and nonactive skeletal muscle, which in turn causes an increase in blood pressure that may or may not be buffered (refined) by the arterial baroreceptors.

Dynamic Exercise

During the onset of dynamic exercise, the increase in heart rate and cardiac output is first caused by a feedforward, central-command-mediated vagal withdrawal. More importantly, central command also resets (within seconds) the baroreceptors to a higher blood pressure setting or operating point. As long as the increase in heart rate and cardiac

output caused by parasympathetic withdrawal can quickly increase blood pressure to its new operating point, there is no mismatch error between actual arterial pressure and the newly set operating point (no pressure error). Therefore, sympathetic activity does not increase appreciably. However, if the parasympathetically mediated increases in rate and cardiac output are insufficient to raise blood pressure to its new operating level (pressure error), sympathetic activity is initiated, which influences both cardioaccelatory nerves and vasoconstrictor nerves. This demonstrates that the baroreceptor reflex is essential during mild (and possibly during moderate) exercise. If exercise intensity continues to increase, a second mismatch error can develop, this time between blood flow (oxygen) delivery and muscle metabolism needs. This type of error leads to a greater reliance of the skeletal muscles on anaerobic glycolysis for energy production, which in turn activates (due to lactic acid production) the chemical-sensitive metaboreceptors to fire afferent signals. In the end, even more sympathetically mediated

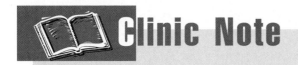

Clinic Note

Exercise and Cardiac Transplant

Among normal healthy persons (figure 10.5A), the increase in heart rate that occurs during progressive, dynamic exercise is due to changes in both blood catecholamines and autonomic nervous system activity. At rest, heart rate is governed by parasympathetic (vagal) activity, and just before and right after exercise is begun, such input is withdrawn, allowing heart rate to increase. As exercise intensity increases and heart rate begins to exceed ~ 100 b · min^{-1}, direct cardiac sympathetic nerve activity is brought "on line" to increase rate even further. At maximal or peak exercise, parasympathetic activity is almost completely absent, and sympathetic activity predominates. In addition, there is an exercise-intensity-related increase in plasma catecholamines (e.g., norepinephrine), which acts to increase rate.

This description of factors regulating heart rate during exercise among healthy persons is more clearly understood when compared to exercise heart rate response in patients who have undergone a cardiac transplant. These patients received a heart from a "consenting donor"—specifically, from a person who was placed on life support after being involved in an unfortunate fatal, trauma-type accident. During this operation, autonomic (parasympathetic and sympathetic) nerves leading to the recipient's original heart are cut and cannot be reattached to the donor heart.

Compare the description of what controls heart rate during exercise in healthy normals (figure 10.5A) to what is shown in figure 10.5B for cardiac transplant recipients. Note that in the absence of vagal control, heart rate at rest in transplant patients now approximates the intrinsic rate of the sinoatrial node (~ 100 b · min^{-1}). As a result, there is little increase in heart rate during early exercise because of vagal withdrawal. Additionally, since there are no direct cardiac sympathetic nerves, eventual increases in rate are caused by increases in blood catecholamines alone. In fact, it is not uncommon for transplant patients to demonstrate higher norepinephrine levels than normals at rest, throughout exercise, and at

peak. It is one way that their bodies compensate for the absence of autonomic innervation. Despite this marked increase in plasma norepinephrine, peak heart rate in cardiac transplant patients is generally lower than that achieved by healthy persons. This is caused by the absence of the sympathetic nerves, which act on the heart directly.

Our comparison between healthy persons and cardiac transplant recipients does not end with the cessation of exercise. Notice in figure 10.5A that among normals, heart rate follows a two-phase recovery pattern after exercise is stopped. Initially, heart rate decreases rapidly—within seconds to 2 minutes (Phase I response)—which is followed by a slower decline over the next 2 to 20 minutes (Phase II response). This rapid decrease in heart rate mainly results from a marked increase in vagal tone to the sinoatrial node, as central command is "turned off" (motor function ceases). Be aware that after exercise, sympathetic activity to the heart remains high because of activation of the muscle metaboreceptors by metabolites and H$^+$ in and around the skeletal muscle cell. The sympathetic activity, however, is overridden by the more dominant parasympathetic input, which causes heart rate to decrease soon after exercise is stopped. The slower (Phase II) decrease in heart rate during later recovery is partly caused by realignment of skeletal muscle O$_2$ demand with O$_2$ supply (muscle metaboreflex is "turned off").

In figure 10.5B (transplant patients) notice that in the absence of parasympathetic input, heart rate remains elevated in recovery. Here the absence of a Phase I response is not due to a sustained increase in cardiac sympathetic input (remember, there is none); instead, it is likely due to (1) the decreasing but still elevated plasma norepinephrine levels and (2) to the inability of the transplanted heart to clear norepinephrine from its tissue. Heart rate does decrease in recovery in these patients but at a much slower pace than is normal.

increases in heart rate, myocardial contractility, and vaso-constriction occur.

The role of the muscle mechanoreceptors during dynamic exercise remains uncertain in humans. One reason is that we (humans) represent a "difficult model" for scientists

to experimentally isolate the function of mechanoreceptors alone. These receptors appear to be only slightly active, if at all, during the transition from rest to mild dynamic exercise, but they may contribute to the increase in sympathetic tone that occurs during strenuous exercise.

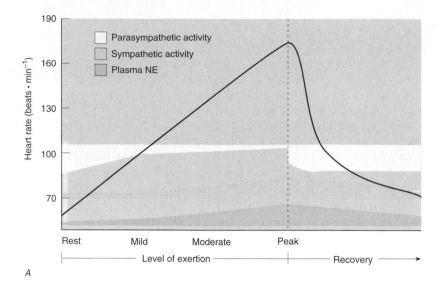

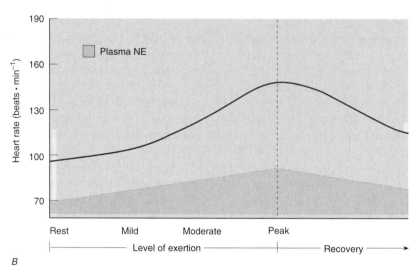

Figure 10.5

Factors contributing to increase in heart rate response during dynamic exercise and recovery among normal healthy persons (*A*) and cardiac transplant patients (*B*). Note the absence of parasympathetic and sympathetic activity in cardiac transplant patients. (NE = norepinephrine.)

Given the previous discussion, it appears that both *central command* and the *exercise pressor reflex (muscle metabo-* and *mechanoreceptors)* play important roles in regulating cardiovascular response to static and dynamic exercise in humans. Specifically, neither mechanism should be singled out as being the most important. In fact, it may be more appropriate that we think of these two neural control mechanisms as being *redundant*. The term *redundant* here means that either mechanism (central command or exercise pressor reflex) can result in a similar cardiovascular response (↑ heart rate, ↑ blood pressure), because both independently impinge on the same regulatory nerves in the medulla. When both mechanisms are functioning normally, there is overlap such that the action evoked by the cardiorespiratory area is commensurate with whichever input

stimuli is greater—central command or peripheral neural input. These regulatory mechanisms are, therefore, felt to be somewhat redundant rather than additive. However, this redundancy is not necessarily bad, given the importance of ensuring adequate blood flow to metabolically active skeletal muscles during exercise.

Pulmonary or Ventilatory Control

An ultimate goal of ventilation is to maintain proper concentrations of O_2, CO_2, and H^+ in the tissues. And, fortunately, the ability of the human body to accomplish this during exercise is really quite exceptional. According to Wasserman et al.,[17] "Despite a manyfold increase in CO_2 production and O_2 consumption during exercise, the ventilatory regulatory mechanisms we possess normally keep

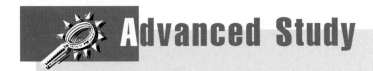

Cardiovascular Control

Of all the discussions in section 3, and quite possibly in the entire book, understanding cardiovascular regulation during dynamic exercise can literally be a nightmare for many students. To ease one's discomfort with this material, we summarize our presentation of cardiovascular control during dynamic exercise by adapting a model put forth by O'Leary.[11]

1. At the onset of exercise there is an increase in heart rate (and contractility) as central command initiates, working through the medulla, a decrease in parasympathetic tone. This allows cardiac output (and blood pressure) to rise. Additionally, there is likely some—not a lot of—sympathetic vasoconstrictor activity to the viscera (e.g., gastrointestinal tract) so that blood can begin to be diverted to the metabolically more active skeletal muscles.

2. At the same time, the operating point for the carotid and aortic artery baroreceptors are quickly reset to a higher level, which likely contributes to an even further decrease in parasympathetic tone. At this point neither the muscle metaboreceptors nor the muscle mechanoreceptors appear to be highly involved.

3. As the intensity of work effort increases beyond a mild level of intensity (heart rates > 100 b · min^{-1}),

cardiac output (heart rate and stroke volume) is increased further because of additional withdrawal of parasympathetic activity and important increases in sympathetic cardiac and vasoconstrictor tone. The increase in sympathetic tone is caused by activation of the muscle metaboreceptor, likely by further involvement of the baroreceptors, and possibly by activation of the muscle mechanoreceptors.

4. At near maximal effort, parasympathetic activity is almost nonexistent, and sympathetic activity exists at greatly increased levels. As a result, heart rate, stroke volume, and cardiac output are all operating maximally. Therefore, any further increase in blood pressure that is needed can only occur via peripheral vasoconstriction—some of which must occur in active skeletal muscle, since it is now receiving the vast majority (> 80%) of total blood flow.

5. Following maximal exercise, heart rate decreases sharply as parasympathetic activity quickly rises after withdrawal of central command. The increase in vagal tone obscures the sustained increase in sympathetic activity, which remains for a period of time because of continued activation of the muscle metaboreceptors.

PCO$_2$ and H$^+$ concentration remarkably constant over a wide range of metabolic rates."

Control mechanisms for the pulmonary or ventilatory system during exercise are shown in figure 10.6. Note first that there are similarities between this control model[3] and that shown for cardiovascular regulation in figure 10.4. For example, the respiratory and the cardiovascular areas of the medulla both receive impulses from (1) the descending higher motor regions of the cerebrum and (2) ascending afferent impulses from the periphery.[18] Although we will go on to explain the specifics of each signal in more detail, in general, we can explain that the rapid rise in ventilation that occurs at the onset of exercise is due to central (motor) command "spill over" from neurons that pass through the medulla on their way to initiate muscular contraction. This central-command-mediated (*feedforward control*) increase in ventilation is then, depending on the type of activity, fine-tuned by peripheral sensors (*feedback control*). Now we will further explore ventilatory regulation during isometric and dynamic exercise.

Isometric Exercise

As mentioned previously, at the onset of exercise there is an increase in ventilation (*exercise hyperpnea*) that is predominantly caused by central command. During progressive isometric exercise (from mild to fatiguing), ventilation increases further as certain motor units are asked to fire more often or as additional motor units are recruited for tension development. During this type of exercise (static), the increase in ventilation is caused more by an increase in tidal volume than by an increase in breathing frequency. Additionally, this increase in ventilation does not appear to be greatly influenced by peripheral chemoreceptors. When isometric contraction is stopped, there is a large, rapid fall in ventilation.

Dynamic Exercise

During dynamic exercise, central (motor) command is, again, the major mediator for the dramatic increase in ventilation (tidal volume and frequency) that occurs at the

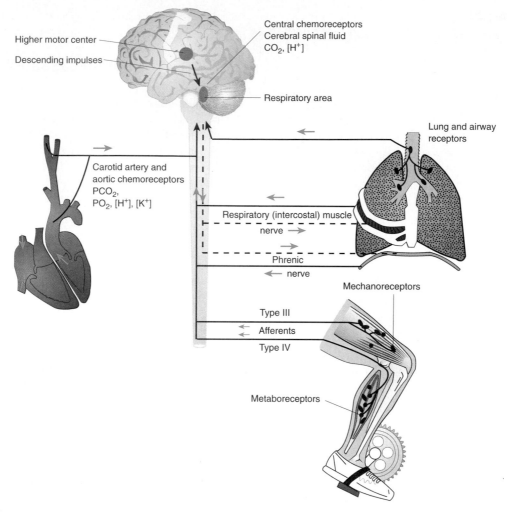

Figure 10.6

Control over the ventilatory system during exercise. The respiratory area is impinged on by descending impulses from the motor region of the brain (central command), from central chemoreceptors, and from a variety of ascending impulses from specialized receptors meant to "fine-tune" exercise hyperpnea. These receptors include the carotid artery body and aortic body chemoreceptors and intercostal muscle and diaphragm afferents. During exercise, ventilation may also be refined by lung and airway receptors and/or skeletal muscle metabo- and mechanoreceptors. The above results in increased neural activity to the diaphragm and intercostal muscles via the phrenic and intercostal nerves, which then increase rate and depth of breathing to regulate arterial PO_2, PCO_2, and pH.

onset of exercise. Increases in rate and depth of breathing are made possible via increased neural activity to the motor neurons that innervate both the intercostal muscles and the diaphragm (phrenic nerve). The extent of the exercise hyperpnea is somewhat commensurate with the magnitude of muscle force production and metabolic rate. Central command likely also contributes throughout exercise to help CO_2 remain constant. In addition, several other mechanisms impinge on the medullary respiratory center and act to "fine tune" ventilatory response (figure 10.6).

The first of these "other" mechanisms involves both central (brain stem) and peripheral chemoreceptors, the latter of which are found in the carotid and aortic arteries. The central chemoreceptors are sensitive to an increase in cerebral spinal fluid PCO_2 or H^+ concentrations. The carotid

artery and aortic chemoreceptors are also sensitive to changes in PCO_2 and H^+ concentrations; however, they are influenced by an increase in potassium and by a dramatic decrease in PO_2 as well. Once central command has provided the major drive to increase ventilation, these chemoreceptors (most important of which are the carotid artery receptors) refine ventilation to minimize changes in PCO_2. Such that, a 1 mm Hg rise in PCO_2 results in an approximate $2 \text{ L} \cdot \text{min}^{-1}$ increase in ventilation.[2]

For the most part, changes (a decrease) in PO_2 during exercise do not greatly contribute to the exercise hyperpnea. However, picture the individual who drives from sea level to an elevation of 3,070 m (10,000 feet). With such a trip, the partial pressure of inspired O_2 is reduced from 150 mm Hg to 100 mm Hg—resulting in a reduction of arterial PO_2

to ~ 66 mm Hg. This big drop in PO_2 stimulates the chemoreceptors found in the carotid bodies of the carotid arteries to fire afferent signals to the respiratory center of the medulla, causing an increase in ventilation.

The diaphragm, the intercostal muscles, and the abdominal expiratory muscles represent the primary muscles of breathing, and each have muscle spindle, Golgi tendon, and Group III and Group IV afferent fibers like other skeletal muscles. Although activation of the respiratory muscle afferents does not provide the primary drive for the exercise hyperpnea, these nerves likely influence ventilation during exercise in several possible ways. For our purposes we will mention only one: breathing efficiency. Although the specifics behind this mechanism are not fully elucidated, afferent fibers from respiratory muscle mechanoreceptors (and possibly from the lungs) provide information to the medulla aimed at regulating efficiency (O_2 cost) of breathing. Specifically, muscle spindle and Golgi tendon organ afferents inform the brain about conditions in the respiratory muscles, which then acts to change neuron firing pattern and rate and depth of breathing among the inspiratory and expiratory muscles and the airway muscles. The desired outcome is a minimization of the work of breathing.

Still other feedback mechanisms provide input to the medulla and as a result may also help refine ventilatory response during exercise. These include (1) the proprioceptors, mechanoreceptors, and metaboreceptors found in the exercising muscles, and (2) mechanoreceptors found within the right ventricles. Clearly, muscle spindle, Golgi tendon, and other joint receptors in and around the active skeletal muscle do provide afferent stimuli to the respiratory center. Additionally, the Group III and Group IV afferent fibers activated by mechanical deformation and changes in local chemistry surrounding skeletal muscles, respectively, are also known to be involved with ventilation. What remains uncertain, however, is the precise role of the above afferent signals relative to regulating ventilation during exercise. It is well accepted that their influence, if any, is certainly less than the carotid artery chemoreceptors. Perhaps these receptors provide redundant control mechanisms when compared to central command. One of the reasons contributing to our lack of precise knowledge about these receptors is the difficulty confronting scientists relative to designing experiments that adequately isolate the specific receptor being studied.

Additionally, some have postulated that an as of yet unidentified receptor in the lung—one designed to detect changes in CO_2 flow (defined as the product of cardiac output $\times$ the concentration of CO_2 in mixed venous blood)—also mediates the exercise hyperpnea. In this case, an increase in CO_2 flow, such as what occurs during exercise when there is an increase in pulmonary blood flow and/or an increase in venous CO_2 content, would initiate afferent feedback to the medulla and result in an increase ventilation. Current thinking, however—despite studies providing evidence both for and against the existence of CO_2 flow-

related receptors—is that a CO_2 flow mechanism (and other lung and airway receptors) do not act to mediate ventilation during exercise.[6] This conclusion is based, in part, on studies completed on patients who have undergone a double lung transplant, a procedure where all afferent fibers to the medulla are cut. Exercising these patients shows a strikingly similar exercise hyperpnea (increase in minute ventilation or alveolar ventilation) when compared to persons with normal intact lungs. This suggests that pulmonary afferents simply do not play an important role during exercise.

During heavy or intense dynamic exercise, the body experiences a hyperventilation, in that the increase in ventilation is disproportionately greater than the increase in work rate. It appears that the accumulation of H^+ in the blood is not the sole factor responsible for triggering this carotid artery chemoreceptor-induced increase in ventilation. Other factors, such as an increase in plasma catecholamines, an increase in blood potassium, and central drive (as more muscles are voluntarily recruited to match work effort) are likely involved as well.

Like cardiovascular regulation during exercise, our discussion about respiratory control during exercise would not be complete without mentioning the concept of redundancy. By themselves, many of the above mechanisms in some manner influence ventilation at rest and/or during exercise. When acting together in the intact human, some of these mechanisms "mask" the affect of another while others act in a redundant fashion. This is especially true if one compares central versus peripheral mechanisms. Like the cardiovascular system, the issue of redundancy is not necessarily a bad problem, given the vital nature of exercise hyperpnea to survival.

Physical Training and Cardiorespiratory Control

Physical training has been shown to affect some of the cardiovascular and ventilatory control mechanisms we have just reviewed. For example, the well-known bradycardia of training is mediated through different mechanisms at rest and during exercise.[4,13] (See also chapter 12, page 312 and 319.) The resting bradycardia is due to enhanced parasympathetic control, whereas the lower heart rate at a given $\dot{V}O_2$ (exertional bradycardia) is mostly the result of a decreased sympathetic drive. In addition, the greater blood flow to working muscles at peak exercise after physical training is likely caused by inhibition of the sympathetic vasoconstrictor nerves innervating arterioles in the exercising muscles. The net effect here is an increase in peak blood flow to active muscles.

Differences between trained and control subjects also exist in the area of ventilatory control, as trained subjects have lower increases in ventilation per unit of $\dot{V}O_2$ or $\dot{V}CO_2$.[7] This means a lower ventilatory response to a given chemical stimuli. Furthermore, hypoxic and hypercapnic ventilatory drives have been shown to be inversely related to $\dot{V}O_2$ max.[1] As is often the case, these training adaptations support the observation of an improved ability to endure exercise.

Summary

Nervous control of the cardiorespiratory system is paramount to the overall functional efficiency of this system; for this reason, we have studied it in some detail. The essential constituents for such control are found in the respiratory and circulatory areas located in the brain stem. Central command, humoral, physical, and peripheral neural stimulation of these areas aids in regulating such important variables as arterial blood pressure, ventilation, and arterial blood PO_2, PCO_2, and H^+ concentration.

Regulation of these variables occurs as a result of adjustments in heart rate, myocardial contractility, breathing rate and depth, and redirection of blood flow via changes in arteriolar tone (more or less vasoconstriction).

Innervation of the cardiorespiratory apparatus involves both the voluntary nervous system (supplying the respiratory muscles) and the involuntary or autonomic nervous system (supplying the heart and blood vessels).

During exercise, the predominant stimuli regulating ventilation, blood pressure, PO_2, PCO_2, and H^+ concentration are (1) increased activity of the motor cortex or central command; (2) changes in muscle chemistry, contraction, or static tension development; (3) increased arterial H^+ concentration and PCO_2; (4) increased blood pressure; and (5) secretion of norepinephrine and epinephrine from the adrenal medulla.

During both static and dynamic exercise, cardiorespiratory responses (heart rate, contractility, ventilation) are initially driven by feedforward central command impulses that spill over and influence the medulla oblongata on their way to initiate muscular contraction. This initial response is then fine tuned using input from a variety of receptors found in the skeletal muscles, respiratory muscles, or the carotid or aortic arteries.

Questions

1. Where in the brain are the centers that regulate respiratory and circulatory function located? Are the responses generated by these two regulatory areas separate or integrated? Explain.
2. Provide descriptive examples of the central, physical, peripheral neural, and humoral stimuli involved with cardiorespiratory control.
3. Discuss the innervation of the cardiorespiratory apparatus. Include in your answer both "arms" of the autonomic nervous system.
4. Outline how blood pressure and blood flow are regulated during exercise. Be sure to include regulatory responses that occur early during exercise as well as those that occur during later exercise.
5. Outline how ventilation is regulated during exercise. Be sure to include regulatory responses that occur early during exercise as well as those that occur during latter exercise.
6. Discuss similarities and differences between the regulation of respiration and circulation during exercise using your answers from questions 4 and 5 above.

References

1. Bryne-Quinn, E., J. V. Weil, I. E. Sodal, G. F. Filley, and R. F. Grover. 1971. Ventilatory control in the athlete. *J Appl Physiol.* 30(1):91–98.
2. Dempsey, J., S. Powers, and N. Gledhill. 1990. Discussion: cardiovascular and pulmonary adaptation to physical activity. In C. Bouchard et al., *Exercise, Fitness and Health: A Consensus of Current Knowledge.* Champaign, IL: Human Kinetics, pp. 206–216.
3. Dempsey, J. A., E. H. Virduk, and G. S. Mitchell. 1985. Pulmonary control systems in exercise: update. *Fed Proc.* 44(7):2260–2270.
4. Frick, M., R. Elovainio, and T. Somer. 1967. The mechanism of bradycardia evoked by physical training. *Cardiologia.* 51:46–54.
5. Guyton, A. C., and J. E. Hall. 1996. *Textbook of Medical Physiology,* 9th ed. Philadelphia: W. B. Saunders, p. 776.
6. Kaufman, M. P., and H. V. Forster. 1996. Reflexes controlling circulatory, ventilatory and airway responses to exercise. In Rowell, L. B. and J. T. Shepard (eds.), *Handbook of Physiology.* New York: Oxford University Press, pp. 381–447.
7. Martin, B. J., K. E. Sparks, C. W. Zwillich, and J. V. Weil. 1979. Low exercise ventilation in endurance athletes. *Med Sci Sports.* 11(2):181–185.
8. Mitchell, J. H. 1985. Cardiovascular control during exercise: central and reflex neural mechanisms. *Am J Cardiol.* 55:34D–41D.
9. Mitchell, J. H. Neural control of the circulation during exercise. 1990. *Med Sci Sports Exerc.* 22:142–154.
10. O'Leary, D. S. 1993. Autonomic mechanisms of muscle metaboreflex control of heart. *J Appl Physiol* 74:1748–1754.
11. O'Leary, D. S. 1996. Heart rate control during exercise by baroreceptors and skeletal muscle afferents. *Med Sci Sports Exerc* 28:210–217.
12. Rowell, L. B., and D. S. O'Leary. 1990. Reflex control of the circulation during exercise: Chemoreflexes and mechanoreflexes. *J App Physiol* 69:407–418.
13. Rowell, L. B., D. S. O'Leary, and D. L. Kellogg. 1996. Integration of cardiovascular control systems in dynamic exercise. In Rowell, L. B., and J. T. Shepard (eds.), *Handbook of Physiology.* New York: Oxford University Press, pp. 770–838.
14. Seals, D. R., and R. G. Victor. 1991. Regulation of muscle sympathetic nerve activity during exercise in humans. *Exercise and Sport Sciences Reviews.* 19:313–349.
15. Victor, R. G., D. R. Seals, and A. L. Mark. 1987. Differential control of heart rate and sympathetic nerve activity during dynamic exercise. *J Clin Invest* 79:508–516.
16. Waldrop, T. G., F. L. Eldridge, G. A. Iwamoto, and J. H. Mitchell. 1996. Central neural control of respiration and circulation during exercise. In Rowell, L. B., and J. T. Shepard (eds.), *Handbook of Physiology.* New York: Oxford University Press, pp. 333–380.
17. Wasserman, K., J. E. Hansen, D. Y. Sue, B. J. Whipp, and R. Casaburi. 1994. *Principles of Exercise Testing and Interpretation,* 2d ed. Philadelphia: Lea and Febiger, p. 42.

18. Weissman, M. L., K. Wasserman, D. J. Huntsman, and B. J. Whipp. 1979. Ventilation and gas exchange during phasic hindlimb exercise in dog. *J Appl Physiol.* 46(5):878–884.

Selected Readings

Asmussen, E., and M. Nielsen. 1955. Cardiac output during muscular work and its regulation. *Physiol Rev.* 35:778–800.

Dempsey, J. A., G. S. Mitchell, and C. A. Smith. 1984. Exercise and chemoreception. *Am Rev Respir Dis.* (129 Suppl)S31–S34.

Hildebrandt, J. R., and J. Hildebrandt. 1979. Cardiorespiratory responses to sudden release of circulatory occlusion during exercise. *Respir Physiol.* 38(1):83–92.

Melcher, A., and D. E. Donald. 1981. Maintained ability of carotid baroreflex to regulate arterial pressure during exercise. *Am J Physiol.* (Heart Circ. Physiol. 10):H838–H849.

Mitchell, J. H., M. P. Kaufman, and G. A. Iwamoto. 1983. The exercise pressor reflex: its cardiovascular effects, afferent mechanisms, and central pathways. *Ann Rev Physiol.* 45:299–342.

Stone, H. L., and I. Y. S. Liang. 1984. Cardiovascular response and control during exercise. *Am Rev Respir Dis.* 129:Suppl S13–S16.

Walgenbach, S. C., and D. E. Donald. 1983. Inhibition by carotid baroreflex of exercise-induced increases in arterial pressure. *Circ Res.* 52:253–262.

Whipp, B. J., S. A. Ward, and K. Wasserman. 1984. Ventilatory responses to exercise and their control in man. *Am Rev Respir Dis.* 129:Suppl S17–S20.

section 4

Physical Training

Over the past century, there have been massive assaults on athletic performance records. For example, the world's best running performances in the marathon and in the 100-meter, 400-meter, and 1500-meter races have all fallen sharply from the 1900s to the present, with an average improvement of about 25%. Similar record-breaking trends have also occurred in competitive swimming, ice speed skating, and most other sport activities. Are the athletes of today that much better trained than their predecessors of just two or three generations past? Or are other factors such as genetics, running surface, nutritional habits, and mental preparation the keys that have unlocked the gateways to record-breaking performances? Without question, improved training techniques and methods, resulting partly from our better understanding of the physiology of exercise, have played a pivotal role.

Section 4 will cover the spectrum of human performance—from sedentary office worker to elite, world-class athlete. Chapter 11 presents information and concepts related to anaerobic training methods for sports and competition. Chapter 12 does the same but focuses its attention on aerobic training or endurance-type sports. In both chapters the physiological consequences associated with the training are discussed in detail. Chapter 13 is similarly structured in that it addresses the training techniques and physiologic effects that lead to improved muscle strength, muscle endurance, and flexibility. Chapter 14 brings forth discussion on what continues to be a most rapidly developing area in exercise physiology: the health aspects of physical activity. Chapter 14 differs from chapters 11 through 13 in that the primary emphasis is not on the extremes of human performance but rather on physical activity—specifically as it relates to improving one's overall health.

In each chapter we integrate our discussion in a manner that addresses both males and females. There are, however, opportunities that allow us to compare and contrast characteristics that are unique to each gender. These are addressed accordingly.

The following chapters are contained within this section:

11
Methods for Anaerobic Training and Physiologic Responses

Except for the occasional softball game or daily trip up and down a flight of stairs, most of us have little day-to-day association with anaerobic activities. Instead, we spend the majority of our day engaging in light-to-moderate home/school-related tasks, or enjoying an aerobic workout. The truth is, most of us simply don't run 400 m races or block opposing linemen on a regular basis.

Despite this fact, it remains important that students develop a good understanding of both the principles of anaerobic training and the physiologic changes that occur as a result. One reason for this might be to better fulfill any personal aspirations you may have to someday coach others who participate in anaerobic activities. The ability of your players to successfully compete will depend on the training program you establish for them. Or, if you plan to enter a career in health care, then consider the 40-year-old recovering heart patient who, prior to suffering an uncomplicated heart attack, served as an active firefighter. Is medical disability all that lies ahead, or is it realistic to assume that he, in time, will be able to return to the job he is trained for? And how about yourself in 10 years—your ability to run up and down the court during a pick-up basketball game will be directly related to your anaerobic capabilities. Learning to recognize which energy system is employed during a given activity and how to develop an effective training regimen is an integral part of your overall education.

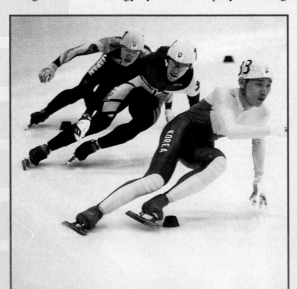

To accomplish this, we will now focus our attention on anaerobic training, which includes having to discuss some concepts that are common to *both* aerobic and anaerobic training. We will limit, however, our discussion about aerobic training, given that it is well covered in chapter 12.

General Considerations

Training Methods for Anaerobic Performance

Application of Training Methods to Various Anaerobic Sports

Physiological Effects of Anaerobic Training

Summary

The major concepts to be learned from this chapter are as follows:

- The basic tenets in any training program are (1) to recognize the major energy system used to perform a specific activity, and (2) through the overload principle, to construct a training program that will develop that particular energy system more than any other will.
- The primary energy system for any activity can be estimated on the basis of its performance time. The overload principle, as applied to anaerobic (sprint) training programs, requires that the training intensity be near maximal.
- Training intensity can be best judged either from the heart rate response to exercise or from the lactate threshold.
- Many athletes now train all year around using off-season, preseason, and in-season training programs.
- Warm-up and cool-down activities and procedures are important in the overall safety and effectiveness of training programs.
- Training programs that develop primarily the ATP-PC system and/or anaerobic glycolysis are available.
- The physiologic responses that result from anaerobic training occur mostly within the skeletal muscles; however, some adaptations occur within the heart. Finally, little information is known about the effects of detraining on anaerobic performance.

General Considerations

There are five general considerations that are important to all training programs:

1. Basic training principles
2. The various training phases
3. Preliminary activities or warm up
4. Cool-down activities
5. Sport-specific training methods

Training Principles

Please note the two key words boldfaced in the following sentence. *To improve one's ability to perform a certain task involves working **specific** muscles or organ systems at an **increased** resistance.* The first key word refers to the principle of **specificity of training,** which means designing and implementing a training program meant to specifically develop the muscles and organs (e.g., heart, lungs) involved in any given sport activity. The second key word refers to the **overload principle**. This means stimulating the involved muscles or organs at an increased level, causing them to adapt and achieve a greater maximal energy potential within each cell. These training principles (table 11.1) apply, to varying degrees, to both anaerobic and aerobic sports and activities. As mentioned in the introduction, our focus here is on the former.

The end result of *overload training* applied to the muscles or organs that are called upon to perform a specific task can be a faster movement, a more forceful movement, or an improved ability to resist fatigue (improved endurance)—specifically, improved performance!

Specificity of Training

Anaerobic power, or anaerobic fitness, represents a local characteristic of a muscle that exists independent of blood and oxygen supply to that muscle. Therefore, all anaerobic training programs must develop the anaerobic energy system or systems within the muscle(s) needed to perform a specific sport. For example, if someone sets out to improve their ability to run 800 meters (predominant systems: anaerobic glycolysis and the ATP-PC system), then, in addition to practicing technique and race strategy, it is important that the muscles of the legs experience the overload during training. Developing the anaerobic energy systems in the arms is of lesser importance, since they have little to do with running. Conversely, for a competitive aerobic activity such as cross-country skiing, both the aerobic energy systems and anaerobic glycolysis become important. In this case, training should include not only the muscles of the legs, but the muscles of the arms and other organs (e.g., heart, lungs) as well. Finally, if only improved general health is desired, then training the aerobic systems may be all that is needed.

table

11.1

Training principles for anaerobic and aerobic sports, activities, and events

Specificity of Training
- Identify the predominant energy system(s)
- Using a sport-specific modality, implement a training regimen meant to develop the predominant energy system(s)

Overload Principle
- Intensity
- Frequency
- Duration

Determining the Predominant Energy System for Anaerobic Sports or Events

How does one know which energy system predominates in various activities and sports? To assist, we present a modification of a broad classification system developed by Mitchell and colleagues (figure 11.1). Please note that activities that possess a moderate to high static component tend to rely on the anaerobic metabolic pathways. Some of these activities, such as throwing, entail very little movement of the body (low dynamic), whereas others, such as boxing, are quite dynamic and repeatedly tax the anaerobic pathways. It stands to reason, then, that training regimens should be designed to develop the anaerobic metabolic pathways. Conversely, training programs for aerobic sports (low static component with moderate-to-high dynamic component) should stress the aerobic energy systems. Obviously, cross-country skiing would stress the aerobic energy systems to a much greater extent than would volleyball and this difference should be reflected in the nature of the training program.

Hopefully, you have also noticed that some activities require significant energy from both the anaerobic and aerobic energy systems. These activities have a moderate static component and a moderate-to-high dynamic component (figure skating, basketball). Obviously, the list of activities given in figure 11.1 is not all-inclusive. You should, however, now be able to generally classify other activities that are not listed, based on their static and dynamic components. Doing so will provide you with a quick reference to the nature of the training program needed to enhance the predominant energy system. Where would you place lacrosse on figure 11.1? How about weight lifting? And here's a tough one—how about orienteering?*

---

*Lacrosse is a sport, much like hockey, that has both static and dynamic components. Therefore, training should include intense development of both the anaerobic and aerobic energy systems. Weight lifting is a highly static event with little dynamic movement. Training for this event is almost entirely anaerobic. Orienteering, a rigorous event more popular in Europe than in the U.S., involves navigating (mostly running) over a wide variety of outdoor terrain and against other competitors. It is highly dynamic, with a very low static component. As such, training should stress the aerobic energy systems.

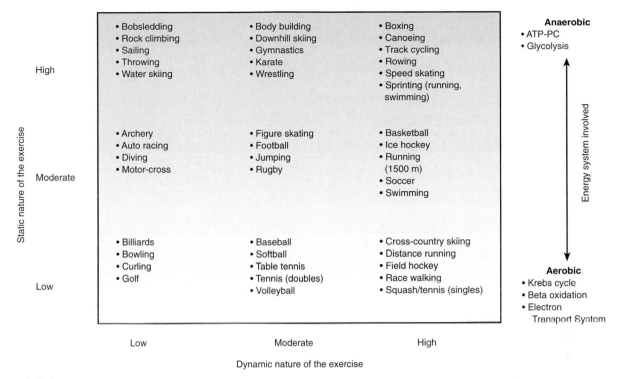

Figure 11.1

Classification of sport activities based on static component, dynamic component, and energy system involved.

Modified from Mitchell et al.[45]

To better quantify the contributions of the different energy systems to energy production across a variety of activities, we present table 11.2. Some activities rely almost exclusively on aerobic energy systems (e.g., marathon), and others are quite anaerobic in nature (e.g., 50 m swim). Additionally, there are still other activities where the predominate energy systems are constantly changing, such as the team sports (e.g., basketball or soccer) or the "kick" at the end of a 1500 m swim.

Using table 11.2 there are three other points we wish to discuss. First, regardless of the type of activity performed, *performance time is related to the energy-yielding systems involved.* For example, a world record time for the men's 5000 m ice speed skating event is approximately 6 minutes and 35 seconds. Similarly, a world record time for the men's 3000 m run is approximately 7 minutes and 10 seconds. Although the type of activity performed for these two sports is quite different (ice skating versus running), the times are similar, and as a result, the energy contribution from the various energy systems are also similar. From a coach's perspective, both ice speed skaters and middle-distance runners should spend approximately 30% to 35% of their time training the ATP-PC and anaerobic glycolysis systems and 65% to 70% of their time training the aerobic systems. *Therefore, the energy sources for a given activity are time- and intensity-dependent.* Whether a person is chopping wood, shoveling snow, performing calisthenics, running, or swimming, the primary source of energy will be dependent on the performance time that can be maintained at a given intensity.

Second, you've probably already noticed that the energy systems in table 11.2 have been grouped as follows: ATP-PC and anaerobic glycolysis, anaerobic glycolysis and aerobic, and aerobic only. This has been done because it is not yet possible to identify the exact percent contribution of any one energy system during any one sport or activity. The one exception to this might be the aerobic system. Since it has been studied more than the others, more information concerning its energy contribution to various sports is available. Given these facts, table 11.2 represents our best estimates to date.

Third, the percentages shown in table 11.2 relate to the proportional contributions from the various energy systems that occur during the performance of a specific activity. For example, in baseball, during the chasing down of a fly ball or running out a triple, the ATP-PC system predominates (80% of total energy derived). Does this mean that a baseball player should spend 80% of his training time developing the ATP-PC system? The answer is obviously no. Baseball is a game in which long periods of low activity are interspersed with bursts of high-intensity sprinting. Sensibly, then, there should be a "good" aerobic base with the ability to use the predominant systems when called upon.

Figure 11.2 presents a summary of the major, intermediate, and minor physiologic factors involved in the specificity of anaerobic training. Notice that all factors contribute to activity improvement but, as indicated by the various colors used, some factors contribute more than others. Also note that aerobic metabolism influences the ATP-PC system. This

table 11.2

Various sports and their predominant energy systems*

Sports or sports activity	% Emphasis by energy system		
	ATP-PC and anaerobic glycolysis	Anaerobic glycolysis and aerobic	Aerobic
1. Aerobic dance	5	15–20	75–80
2. Baseball	80	15	5
3. Basketball	60	20	20
4. Fencing	90	10	negligible
5. Field hockey	50	20	30
6. Football	90	10	negligible
7. Golf	95	5	negligible
8. Gymnastics	80	15	5
9. Ice hockey			
A. Forward, defense	60	20	20
B. Goalie	90	5	5
10. Ice speed skating			
A. 500 m	80	10	10
B. 1000 m	35	55	10
C. 1500 m	20–30	30	40–50
D. 5000 m	10	25	65
E. 10,000 m	5	15	80
11. In-line skating, > 10 km	5	25	70
12. Lacrosse			
A. Goalie, defense, attacker	50	20	30
B. Midfielders, man-down	60	20	20
13. Rowing	20	30	50
14. Skiing			
A. Slalom, jumping	80	15	5
B. Downhill	50	30	20
C. Cross-country	5	10	85
D. Recreational	20	40	40
15. Soccer			
A. Goalie, wings, strikers	60	30	10
B. Halfbacks or sweeper	60	20	20
16. Stepping machine	5	25	70
17. Swimming and diving			
A. Diving	98	2	negligible
B. 50 m	90	5	5
C. 100 m	80	15	5
D. 200 m	30	65	5
E. 400 m	20	40	40
F. 1500 m, 1650 yd	10	20	70

*From E. L. Fox and Donald K. Mathews, *Interval Training Conditioning for Sports and General Fitness.* Copyright © 1974 W. B. Saunders. Reprinted by permission of Donald K. Mathews.

occurs during recovery or between intense exercise bouts, since the aerobic system regenerates ATP-PC stores during these times. This fact represents the science behind why it is important for athletes involved in repetitive anaerobic activities (e.g., a lineman in football) to develop a good aerobic base—a topic we will discuss later in this chapter.

The Overload Principle: Intensity, Frequency, and Duration of Training

Recall from the previous discussion that our second training principle was the overload principle. In weight lifting or weight training this is accomplished by establishing an ath-

table 11.2

Various sports and their predominant energy systems (*continued*)

Sports or sports activity	% Emphasis by energy system		
	ATP-PC and anaerobic glycolysis	Anaerobic glycolysis and aerobic	Aerobic
18. Tennis	70	20	10
19. Track and field			
A. 100, 200 m	95–98	2–5	negligible
B. Field events	95–98	2–5	negligible
C. 400 m	80	15	05
D. 800 m	30	65	05
E. 1500 (mile)	20–30	20–30	40–60
F. 3000 m (2 mile)	10	20	70
G. 5000 m (3 mile)	10	20	70
H. 10,000 m (6 mile)	05	15	80
I. Marathon	negligible	05	95
20. Volleyball	80	05	15
21. Walking	negligible	05	95
22. Wrestling	90	5	5

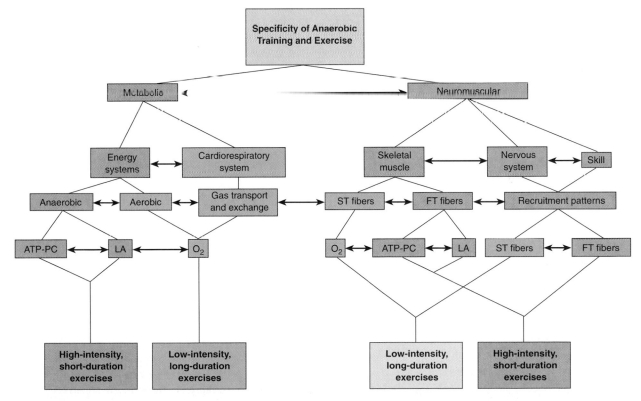

Figure 11.2

A summary of the major (orange), intermediate (dark blue), and minor (green) physiological factors in the specificity of anaerobic training and exercise. The interaction among the various components is indicated by double-headed arrows. LA = anaerobic glycolysis or lactic acid system, ST = slow twitch (Type I) fibers, and FT = fast twitch (Type II) fibers.

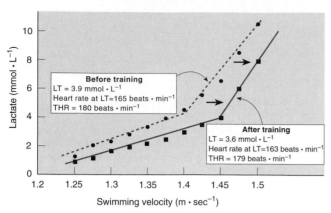

Figure 11.3

Lactate threshold (LT) before and after a 6-week anaerobic swimming program. Note that the lactate curve is shifted to the right with training. In both tests LT, heart rate at LT, and training heart rate were similar. However, as a result of training, the athlete had to swim at a faster pace to achieve her training heart rate.

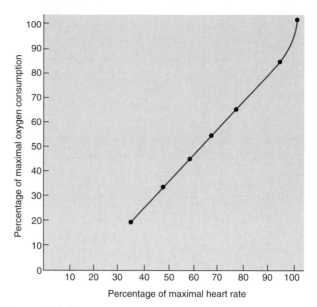

Figure 11.4

The relationship between heart rate and oxygen consumption expressed as a percentage of the maximum for each. Note the generally linear relationship between the two variables.

lete's one repetition maximum (p. 344), then training at a percentage of that level. For aerobic (e.g., running or swimming) and anaerobic training programs (sprinting and wrestling), *intensity, frequency, and duration* of effort are used as the means to stimulate *progressive* overload. Intensity refers to how hard one exercises, frequency refers to how often, and duration can refer either to how long the athlete has been in training (weeks, months) or to the duration of a single exercise bout (minutes, hours). Clearly, the use of these three factors and their subcomponents are more often associated with the development of aerobic training programs (chapter 12). However, they can be applied to anaerobic regimens as well.

Determining Intensity of Anaerobic Training

Of the above three factors, intensity is the most important. Generally, three different methods can be used to help guide intensity of anaerobic training. They are heart rate, blood lactate level, and training pace/velocity. You will soon see, however, that these methods are not distinctly different—instead, they are quite interrelated.

Ultimately, the objective is to "overload" the anaerobic energy pathways during training so as to cause corresponding adaptations that lead to an athlete's improved ability to perform. One marker that is used to indicate whether or not an athlete is, in fact, sufficiently stressing the anaerobic energy systems (i.e., anaerobic glycolysis) is the practice of monitoring blood lactate concentration. However, conducting such testing on a daily or weekly basis is both impractical and costly. Instead, once a specific **lactate threshold** is identified, the corresponding heart rate or training pace associated with the threshold can be used.

For a more complete description of both the science behind lactate threshold and how it is assessed, review

chapter 7, p. 181. Generally, it is that point (threshold) during progressive exercise where there is a marked, disproportionate increase in blood lactate. Among athletes the lactate threshold is approximately 4 millimoles per liter (mmol · L^{-1}).[36,37] It must be emphasized, however, that great individual variation is present. For example, Maglisco states that "in more than 10 years of blood testing, only 50% to 60% of the swimmers" he has trained presented with a lactate threshold approximating 4 mmol · L^{-1}.[38] Therefore, 40% to 50% of his athletes achieved their lactate threshold either above or below the 4 mmol · L^{-1} value. To avoid training athletes too hard (too far above the threshold) or too easy (too far below the threshold), an athlete's own threshold should be identified.

As mentioned previously, pace and/or heart rate at lactate threshold is used to guide an athlete's training intensity. With respect to anaerobic training and the overload principle, this might correspond to a training heart rate that is 5% to 15% above heart rate at lactate threshold. However, as athletes adapt physiologically, they will notice a decrease in heart rate while training at a certain pace. As a result, they must increase their pace (*progressive* overload) to elicit a heart rate that is again ~ 10% above their heart rate at lactate threshold (figure 11.3).

Several times in the preceding discussion we mentioned monitoring heart rate, so it is important to review its response during exercise. Within a wide range of values, heart rate and oxygen consumption (or power output) are related in a linear (straight-line) fashion (figure 11.4). However, at very high work levels, the linear relationship breaks down a bit. Specifically, when maximum

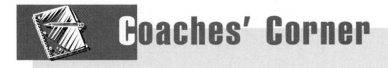

Coaches' Corner

Guiding Anaerobic Intensity

To demonstrate that the three methods of guiding anaerobic exercise training are interrelated, we draw your attention to table 11.3. The data presented in this table were obtained during maximal rowing ergometer tests, completed in December 1995 at the U. S. Olympic Training Center in Colorado Springs, CO. These athletes (12 males between 24 and 31 years of age) compete in the 2000 m sculling event. Depending on the type of event (single, double, quad), race times range from 6 to 7 minutes, which, as you now know, rely heavily on the anaerobic energy systems (i.e., anaerobic glycolysis). Training habits for these athletes include distance training but also much sprint work at a velocity (pace) that elicits a training heart rate 5% to 10% above heart rate at lactate threshold. Average heart rate at lactate threshold for these athletes is 165 beats · min^{-1}, which is approximately 92% of maximum heart rate (180 beats · min^{-1}). This rate corresponds to an average lactate threshold for the group of 3.4 mmol · L^{-1}. In April and May of 1996, as the 1996 Summer Olympics in Atlanta drew closer, these athletes spent an increasing percentage of their practice time training above their lactate threshold.

A few final observations from these data. First, heart rate at lactate threshold varied from one individual to the next, which is not at all uncommon. Second, except for one athlete, lactate threshold was always less than 4.0 mmol · L^{-1}. Third, note how pace and heart rate can be interchanged and used as markers for training an athlete at or just above his or her blood lactate threshold. With training, as the athlete's anaerobic capabilities improved, training velocity or pace was increased to maintain exercise heart rate sufficiently above heart rate at lactate threshold.

table 11.3

Individual and mean data for elite athletes participating in men's sculling

| | Maximal exercise | | | At lactate threshold | | | |
Athlete	Heart rate (beats · min^{-1})	Blood lactate (mmol · L^{-1})	$\dot{V}O_2$ (L · min^{-1})	Heart rate (beats · min^{-1})	Blood lactate (mmol · L^{-1})	$\dot{V}O_2$ (L · min^{-1})	Pace over 500 m (min:sec)
1	193	12.8	5.12	175	4.0	4.77	1:47
2	180	11.9	5.32	156	3.5	4.66	1:46
3	183	11.3	5.84	176	3.0	5.17	1:41
4	171	8.9	5.51	161	3.0	5.11	1:42
5	173	12.4	5.85	159	3.7	5.14	1:43
6	187	14.0	5.17	161	3.3	4.56	1:46
7	177	9.9	5.53	167	3.9	5.03	1:46
8	193	12.9	5.60	173	3.1	4.58	1:45
9	184	11.5	5.93	164	3.5	5.26	1:42
10	182	11.8	5.62	170	3.4	5.06	1:42
11	176	10.5	5.76	165	3.4	5.35	1:42
12	165	12.1	5.24	149	3.5	4.80	1:43
Average	**180**	**11.7**	**5.54**	**165**	**3.4**	**4.96**	**1:44**

Reprinted by permission of Dr. Randy Wilber, U.S. Olympic Committee, Colorado Springs, CO.

Values in shaded area indicate blood lactate threshold for each individual athlete. Data were collected at an elevation of 1800 m (6100 ft).

heart is achieved, further small increases in $\dot{V}O_2$ or power output can still be achieved. For most 20- to 30-year-old athletes, this corresponds to a heart rate at or above 175 to 195 beats $\cdot$ min^{-1}.

To check whether your athletes are attaining the appropriate heart rate during exercise, it is a good idea to teach them to take their pulse rate* occasionally during training sessions. Doing this while exercising is quite difficult; however, the count obtained in a 6-, 10-, or 15-second span immediately following exercise is a reasonable indicator of what the pulse rate was during exercise. To compute pulse rate per minute, a 6-second count is multiplied by 10, a 10-second count by 6, or a 15-second count by 4. Most often, pulse rate is assessed by *palpating* either the radial artery (at the wrist) or carotid artery (in the neck). Both methods are shown in figure 11.5. Only light pressure should be used, particularly at the carotid artery, to avoid triggering rare cardiac abnormalities.[59] When assessing the carotid pulse, be sure to place your fingers on just one side of the neck. It is incorrect to simultaneously palpate both carotid arteries by using two fingers on one side of the neck and your thumb on the other side.

Determining Frequency and Duration of Anaerobic Training

Generally, the more frequent (4 times per week versus 2 times per week) and the longer (16 weeks versus 4 weeks) the training program, the greater the improvement in performance. With respect to a single training session, seldom, if ever, would an athlete spend their entire workout on just anaerobic training. Obviously, some athletes, such as 100-meter sprinters, would spend more of their practice time involved with anaerobic activities than would basketball players. Part of the reason why one's entire practice time cannot be devoted to anaerobic training is that it is simply too strenuous—athletes must allow time for lactate to be cleared from the muscles and to develop the aerobic energy pathways. In fact, a well-developed aerobic system assists with both the clearing of lactate and the regeneration of the ATP-PC stores. Such an adaptation would prove useful during a fast-and-furious ice hockey game, where an athlete goes all-out during his 45- to 60-second shift on the ice, and then must recover quickly while awaiting his next turn. Once again this emphasizes the importance of a solid aerobic foundation or base.

A recommended training frequency for incorporating anaerobic training in the practice schedule of sports that

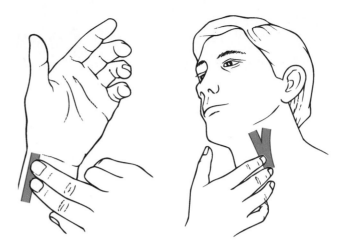

Figure 11.5
The heart rate may be determined by palpating the radial artery (at the wrist) or the carotid artery (in the neck).

have a significant anaerobic component is 3 to 4 days per week. This rule of thumb holds true for most anaerobic-type sports (fencing, wrestling), with the exception of sprint runners, sprint swimmers, and sprint skaters. Here the training frequencies are usually 5 days per week. Generally, only one training session per day is recommended, because two or even three workouts per day do not lead to greater fitness or performance gains.

With respect to duration, athletes who wish to develop the ATP-PC system should focus on repeated sprints that are 25 seconds in duration or less. Development of the anaerobic glycolysis system would involve repeated bouts of 3 to 4 minutes or less. The amount of exercise time within one's daily workout devoted to anaerobic training varies from sport to sport. For example, swimmers involved with 50 m or 100 m events might spend 7% to 10% of their total practice time engaged in anaerobic training, whereas the 1500 m swimmers might spend less than 10%. These values might seem inordinately low, but clearly, the athletes are not able to mentally or physically tolerate much more. A general summary of the guidelines for developing a training regimen for anaerobic activities is shown in table 11.4.

Training Phases

The total training program of athletes is usually separated into three phases: *off-season*, *preseason*, and *in-season*, and the training regimens for each are quite different.

Off-Season Training

Training programs during the off-season vary greatly from one sport to another. Thorough healing of any prior injuries, weight management, and participation in activities and

---

*Heart rate refers to the number of times the heart beats per minute, usually computed from an electrocardiogram. Pulse rate refers to the rate counted by palpating (feeling) a peripheral artery or the chest wall (apical pulse). In most people, heart rate and pulse rate are the same whether measured at rest or during exercise. However, in some patients with either very fast or very slow heart rates or an irregular heart rhythm, not all contractions will be forceful enough so that an equal number of pulse beats are felt in a peripheral artery.

11.4
table

General guidelines for estimating intensity, frequency, and duration of training for an anaerobic (sprint) program

Training factor	Guideline
Intensity	Heart rate that is 5% to 15% above heart rate at lactate threshold
Frequency	3 to 4 days per week
Sessions per day	1 (maybe 2)
Duration	8 to 10 weeks
Duration per session	
ATP-PC system	Repeated work bouts of 25 seconds or less
Anaerobic glycolysis	Repeated work bouts of 3 to 4 minutes or less

recreational games for relaxation and enjoyment are all a must during the off-season. Other areas to be considered:

1. As outlined in chapter 13, a two to three time per week weight-training program—one designed to develop muscular strength, endurance, and power among those muscle groups most directly involved in a specific athletic event.

2. An informal, *low-intensity* cardiorespiratory endurance program performed no more than three to four times per week. Such a program could be administered concurrently with the weight-training program or performed on alternate days. It is meant to develop the "aerobic base" needed to replenish the ATP-PC stores during recovery from anaerobic activity. It may also reduce the likelihood for injury by improving joint, tendon, and ligament integrity. The type of activity chosen for maintaining cardiorespiratory endurance can be sport-specific (runners run and swimmers swim) or cross-training (runners swim and swimmers cycle). A more detailed discussion of cross-training is presented in chapter 12.

3. Skill development in sport-specific activities. For example, in basketball this might include repetitive shooting or ball-handling (dribbling, passing) drills.

Preseason Training

For most sports, formal preseason training begins 8 to 12 weeks prior to competition. During this time the athletes must increase to maximum the capacity of the anaerobic energy system that is predominant for their specific event. The athletes must spend a great deal of time performing their sport (specificity), and doing so using a high-intensity (overload) program. Various training programs are presented later in this chapter. Further advances in individual skill development can still take place, and the off-season weight-training program can be continued. If an athlete's sport requires

a significant aerobic component (e.g., field hockey or soccer), then practice time should be allocated to develop these pathways as well.

Does, in fact, a preseason (or off-season) training program lead to actual improvements in anaerobic performance—such as sprint time? Common sense would answer "yes," but to scientifically address this question Delecluse and co-workers[13] studied the effects of nine weeks of either high-resistance weight-training or high-velocity plyometric training on 100-meter sprint performance. Twenty-four subjects (untrained physical education students, 18 to 22 years of age) were assigned to each of the two training groups. Fifteen additional students served as a nontraining control group.

Subjects in the high-resistance group performed a series of 11 different weight-lifting exercises at maximal speed, two times per week. Subjects in the high-velocity plyometric group performed exercises that are movement- and velocity-specific to sprint running, also two times per week. Examples of these exercises included standing broad jump, vertical jump, hurdle jump, skipping, bounding, hopping, and several others. During training, these exercises were performed with full effort against a specific time, height, or distance criterion. Both training groups also participated in a sprint training workout one time per week. As figure 11.6A indicates, only the plyometric group experienced an improved (faster) 100 m sprint time following training. A major reason for this change was increased acceleration during the first 10 m of the event (figure 11.6B), believed to be due to movement-specific neural adaptations (coordination, specificity of motor recruitment)—an important component that contributes to anaerobic performance. Specifically, maximal acceleration of the whole body during the "take-off" phase of the various plyometric exercises mimicked well the initial acceleration phase of sprinting. Some sprint coaches use high-velocity training as the only overload method for improving sprint performance, while

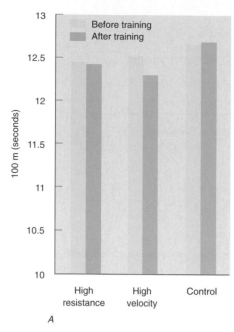

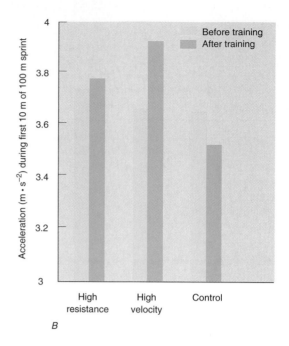

A

B

Figure 11.6

Effects of two types of anaerobic training programs on 100 m sprint time *(A)* and acceleration during first 10 m of 100 m sprint *(B)*. In this study, the resistance weight training group did not improve sprint performance or acceleration. However, the high-velocity training group favorably decreased 100 m sprint time, mostly due to increased acceleration during the first 10 m of the sprint.

(Based on data from Delecluse.[13])

others use it as a "bridge" between high-resistance weight training and sprint training. High-resistance training remains popular among both athletes and coaches, and this study did not exclude the fact that a long-term (> 9 weeks) program would result in faster sprint times.

In-Season Training

Traditionally, in-season training programs for most sports emphasize skill development, team play, and preparation for the next opponent. For the majority of athletes who compete regularly, practice drills, scrimmages, and competition are sufficient to maintain the increases in energy capacities that were obtained through preseason training. However, for those athletes who experience a reduced amount of playing time at practice and/or during events, some additional conditioning is required. This might include (1) one to two days of hard training each week, especially if many days elapse between events; (2) one day of weight training per week; and (3) increased utilization of certain skill activities meant to maintain fitness, such as three-quarter court fast-break (2 on 1, 3 on 2) drills in basketball.

Preliminary Exercise (Warm Up)

Record performances among athletes have occurred without so-called warm up. And some studies have shown that performance without prior warm up is no different than per

formance with prior warm up.[34,42,53] On the other hand, other studies have shown that prior to a heavy workout or competitive performance, warm up should be performed.[3,8,9,29,41,44,47]

There are several physiological reasons for warm-up exercises. These include: (1) increases in body and muscle temperatures, which cause an increase in enzyme activity and thus the metabolic reactions associated with the energy systems;[8,41] (2) increases in blood flow and oxygen availability;[7] and (3) decreases in contraction and reflex time.[58] Some of these changes are shown in figure 11.7. Notice how peak $\dot{V}O_2$ and heart rate during maximal exercise are directly related to muscle temperature. The higher the temperature, the higher the $\dot{V}O_2$ and heart rate. Also note that although work time was not increased at the highest muscle temperature, blood lactic acid was considerably reduced.

The following preliminary exercises are recommended to increase muscle temperature and blood flow:

1. Do not move right into stretching a "cold" muscle or doing calisthenics. First, perform your sport-specific activity at a very, very slow pace (swimmers, swim; sprinters and hurdlers, walk or slowly jog; skaters, skate) for four to five minutes. Doing so will provide the greatest overall effect on total body blood flow and temperature while minimizing muscle tears and injury. Additionally, one's subsequent ability to stretch a muscle will be increased.

2. Follow several of the examples provided in chapter 13 and slowly ("static") stretch the major muscle groups—with a special focus on those that are sport-specific. Remember, one objective of stretching exercises is to increase joint range of motion (to lessen the likelihood of injuring a muscle or connective tissue).

3. Calisthenics differ from stretching exercises because they involve active (i.e., "ballistic") muscular contractions. They contribute to further increases in body and muscle temperatures and, like stretching exercises, should be somewhat sport/muscle-site specific. Two examples include push-ups for upper-body weight lifting and controlled vertical jumps for playing basketball. The use of calisthenics in warm up might not apply to every athlete or every sport. Athletes should be cautioned not to overdo these activities, limiting total time to three to five minutes.

4. The last phase of the warm up should consist of performing component skills that are specific to an athlete's sport. For example, throwing in baseball, wall turns in swimming, free throws in basketball, and coming out of the blocks in sprinting. This kind of practice serves at least two purposes: first, it ensures that physiological factors, such as muscle temperature and blood flow, are optimal; second, it refines both hand-eye and foot-eye coordination and sport-specific neuromuscular patterns.

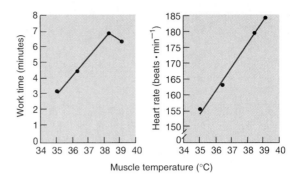

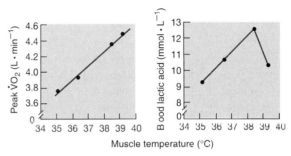

Muscle temperature (°C)

Figure 11.7

Oxygen consumption (peak $\dot{V}O_2$) and heart rate during maximal exercise are directly related to muscle temperature. The higher the temperature, the higher the $\dot{V}O_2$ and heart rate. Although work time is not increased at the highest muscle temperature, blood lactic acid is considerably reduced.

(Based on data from Bergh and Ekblom.[8])

Cool-Down Exercises

Athletes and others who engage in regular physical exercise commonly cool down (i.e., perform light or mild exercise) immediately following competition and training sessions. There are at least two important reasons for such a practice.

1. As pointed out in chapter 3, blood and muscle lactic acid levels decrease more rapidly during active or exercise-recovery than during rest-recovery. Most prior research, however, has made this observation following aerobic exercise. Relative to the effects of active recovery on plasma lactate and subsequent anaerobic performance, Ahmaidi et al.[2] asked 10 males to complete two separate series of exercise; each series was comprised of 5 bouts of intense (6 sec) cycling performed against increasing resistance. In one series of exercise, 5 min of no-activity was given in between each bout of exercise. In the other series, active recovery (~ 32% of $\dot{V}O_2$ max) was used between each bout of exercise. At the highest levels of resistance active recovery was associated with a 20% to 25% lower blood lactate level at the end of recovery, and a 5% to 7% greater power output during the subsequent exercise bout. Thus, the use of an active cool-down period promotes faster recovery

from fatigue, which may be helpful for individuals involved in repetitive events with a strong anaerobic component (3 on 3 basketball or boxing).

2. Mild activity following heavy exercise keeps the muscle pump active and thereby prevents the blood from pooling in the extremities, particularly the legs. Recall (p. 229) that the muscle pump promotes venous return by a milking action caused by the alternate contraction and relaxation of the skeletal muscle. Preventing the pooling of blood not only reduces the possibility of delayed muscular stiffness and soreness, but also reduces the tendency for fainting and/or dizziness.

Our recommendation for types of cool-down activities generally involves the use of warm up activities, but in reverse order. For example, sport-specific skill activities, such as slow running after hard running or free-throw shooting after a basketball scrimmage, might be first. This would be followed by stretching or flexibility exercises that are unique to a specific sport. During this time most athletes will notice that their range of motion in and around a specific joint is generally increased, when compared to similar stretches performed during warm up. This provides further evidence of the effects of an increase in muscle temperature on muscles and connective tissue.

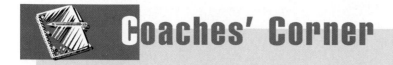

A separate, yet similar athletic training concept involves the principle of **periodization**.[35] This method is defined as "the structured, sequential development of athletic skill or physiologic capacity brought about by organizing training regimens into blocks of time."

Now popular among elite athletes, this practice involves time blocks that can range from a single training session of several hours to countless sessions spread out over several months to even a year of training. These blocks of time are called *macrocycles,* which can be further subdivided into shorter time blocks called *mesocycles.*

For example, the U.S. national weight lifting team may undergo three to four macrocycles over the course of a year, each one preceding a major competition.[35] Each macrocycle begins with an 8 to 10 week mesocycle that emphasizes high-volume, medium-intensity (80% to 90% of maximum) lifting. Such a plan is meant to prepare the athlete's muscles and connective tissue for the even heavier weights in the next mesocycle. During the second mesocycle (4 to 5 weeks), the athlete's goal is to increase strength and power, which is accomplished by having him conduct lifts equivalent to 90% to 100% of maximum capacity. The macrocycle concludes with a third mesocycle, which begins by continuing the extremely high-intensity lifts performed at the end of the second mesocycle. Doing so "carries over" the strength

and power gains achieved by the athlete. The end of the third mesocycle, literally now the week preceding the competition, involves tapering the volume and intensity of lifts to allow the athlete to recover.

Periodization can also involve the sequencing of different training methods, such as establishing a cycle of weight training before shifting to a cycle of sprint training. A study by Sleivert and associates[54] used just this approach to test their hypothesis that an eight-week cycle of weight training completed prior to (and in sequence with) a six-week cycle of sprint training would improve performance parameters to a greater extent than would a 14-week cycle of sprint training alone. The authors theorized that performance would be enhanced if the sport-specific muscles underwent weight training to develop muscle hypertrophy prior to undergoing sprint training, which is designed to recruit the newly acquired muscle mass in a sport-specific manner. Surprisingly, results showed that 14 weeks of sequenced strength-sprint training and 14 weeks of sprint training alone were equally effective in increasing cycle ergometer power output, developing Type I and Type II skeletal muscle hypertrophy, and increasing nerve conduction velocity. One possible explanation for the absence of a clear sequence effect in this study might be that more than just eight weeks of weight training is required before moving into the sprint phase of training.

Training Methods for Anaerobic Performance

Much of the improvement in sports performances over the past century can be attributed to refinement of the training methods used by coaches and athletes. Relative to anaerobic-type sport activities, the principle method for optimizing performance is interval training. Although this method is also useful for improving aerobic performance or $\dot{V}O_2$ max (chapter 12), its application in this chapter will be strictly anaerobic.

Interval Training

Interval training, as the name implies, is a series of repeated bouts of work or exercise alternated with periods of relief. The **work interval** is the portion of interval training that consists of high-intensity exercise, such as a 200 m

swim in a specified time. The **relief interval** is the time in between work intervals (or sets of intervals). The relief interval may include light exercise, such as walking (referred to as **rest-relief**), or it may include mild to moderate exercise (referred to as **work-relief**). Complete rest (no activity) is seldom used during a relief interval. Table 11.5 provides a list of common interval training terms and their definitions; these terms will be used repeatedly throughout this chapter and chapter 12.

Energy Production and Fatigue during Intermittent Work

To understand why interval training has been so successful, we must first recall what we learned in chapters 2 and 4 about energy production. Specifically, a certain amount of energy is required to perform a certain amount of work, regardless of whether the work is performed intermittently or continuously. There is, however, one very important difference.

table 11.5

Terms commonly used with interval training and their associated definitions

Term	Definition
Interval training	A series of repeated bouts of exercise or work alternated with periods of relief.
Work interval	The portion of interval training that consists of high intensity exercise.
Relief interval	The time between work intervals or sets of work-relief intervals.
Rest relief	A relief interval that involves mild or no exercise.
Work relief	A relief interval that involves mild to moderate exercise.
Work-relief ratio	The relationship between work interval and relief interval. For example, a ratio of 1:1½ means that the duration of the relief interval is one-and-one-half times longer than the work interval.
Set	Series of work and relief intervals, such as six 100 m swims.
Repetitions	The number of work intervals in a set.
Training time	The time alloted to complete the work interval (e.g., 200 m run in 36 seconds).
Training distance	The distance to be covered during the work interval.

To illustrate the difference, pay close attention to the following. First, suppose you ran continuously, as far and as hard as you could for one minute. Then compare this to another occasion where you ran just as hard as you did the first time, but this time for only 10 seconds, which is then followed by 30 seconds of relief and repeated six times. Ultimately, you performed the same amount of work (60 seconds at the same intensity) during the two runs; however, the degree of fatigue following intermittent running was likely considerably less.

Let's consider the physiological explanation behind this. The answer lies in the interaction between the ATP-PC system and anaerobic glycolysis during intermittent running as compared to continuous running. During short-duration, intermittent running, the energy supplied via anaerobic glycolysis, is less than what it contributes during continuous running. Conversely, the ATP-PC system contributes more to energy production during intermittent running.[21,39] Ultimately, there will be less lactic acid produced, greater lactic acid cleared, and thus less fatigue associated with the intermittent work. This is true regardless of the intensity of the intermittent work bouts or how long they last.

Replenishing ATP and PC

How is it possible that the ATP-PC system can supply more ATP during the series of intermittent runs as compared with the continuous run? We already indicated that the stores of ATP + PC are exhausted after only a few seconds of all-out running. Remember, however, that between each intermittent run there is a *period of relief*. Therefore, the question that we need to answer is, what is occurring during the relief intervals?

Recall from chapter 3 that during recovery (relief), a major portion of the muscular stores of ATP and PC that

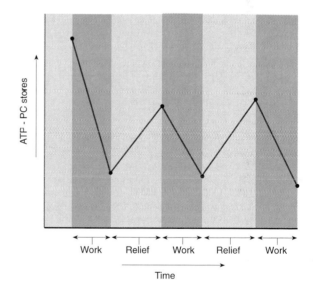

Figure 11.8

During the relief intervals of intermittent work, a portion of the muscular stores of ATP and PC that were depleted during the preceding work intervals will be replenished via the aerobic system.

Source: Data from E. L. Fox and Donald K. Mathews, Interval Training: Conditioning for Sports and General Fitness, *1974, W. B. Saunders, Philadelphia, PA.*

were depleted during the preceding work interval are replenished via the aerobic system.[27,39,49] This is shown in figure 11.8, and it occurs during the fast component of recovery (see chapter 3). In addition, a big portion of the O_2-myoglobin stores are also replenished.[4,5,10] Thus, during each run that follows a relief interval, the replenished ATP, PC, and O_2-myoglobin stores will again be available as an energy source. Consequently, anaerobic glycolysis is

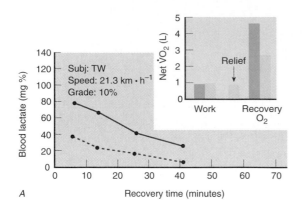

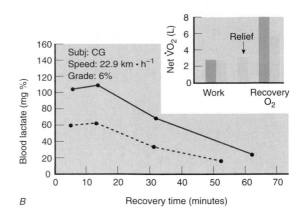

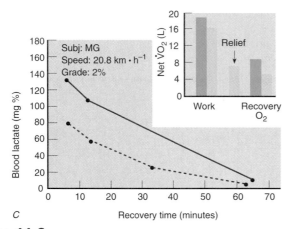

C

Figure 11.9

A. Blood lactate during recovery from a continuous run (solid line) and interval runs (dashed line) involving the same amount of work. In the continuous run, the subject ran for 30 seconds; in the interval run, he ran three intervals of 10 seconds each, with 20 seconds of rest-relief between intervals. Net O_2 consumption ($\dot{V}O_2$) during work, during the rest-relief intervals, and after work (recovery O_2) for the continuous (filled bar) and interval (open bar) runs are also shown. *B.* Similar measurements during and after a continuous run of 60 seconds duration and an interval run of five 12-second runs with 20 seconds of rest-relief between intervals. *C.* A continuous run of 300 seconds duration and an interval run of five 60-second runs with 60 seconds of rest-relief between intervals. Symbols the same as in *A.*

Source: Data from E. L. Fox, et al., "Metabolic Energy Sources During Continuous and Interval Running" in Journal of Applied Physiology, *1969, 27:174–78, American Physiological Society, Bethesda, MD.*

"spared," or called upon less to produce energy, which means that lactic acid will not accumulate as rapidly or to as great an extent (figure 11.9). In contrast, during a continuous 60-second exhaustive run, the phosphocreatine (PC) in the ATP-PC system will be depleted within a matter of seconds.[27,33] Therefore, anaerobic glycolysis will be called upon early in the run to produce ATP, and lactic acid will accumulate to higher levels.

Finally, recent research indicates that recovery from repeated bouts of high-intensity activity is somewhat age-dependent.[26] Eight prepubescent boys (8 to 12 years of age) underwent two 30-second all-out tests on each of three separate days. On each day a different recovery period (1, 2, 10 minutes) was used between tests. Their results were compared to those of eight men (19 to 23 years of age) and showed that power output on the second exercise test was

higher in the boys than in the men, as was $\dot{V}O_2$. Additionally, carbon dioxide production in recovery was lower. The authors concluded that boys recovered faster than the men, likely due to less reliance on anaerobic glycolysis (leading to less acidosis) or faster post-exercise removal of metabolites.

The application of the interval-training method to anaerobic training is where the coach or trainer can best appreciate its true meaning. Specifically, *the savings in fatigue that accompanies intermittent work can be "converted" to an increase in intensity during the next work interval.* This increased intensity (recall the overload principle) is what is used to stimulate improved anaerobic capabilities. The work level during interval training can be as much as two-and-one-half times the intensity of the continuous level before blood lactic acid levels in each of the two methods (intermittent versus continuous) are comparable.[4,10,18,21,39]

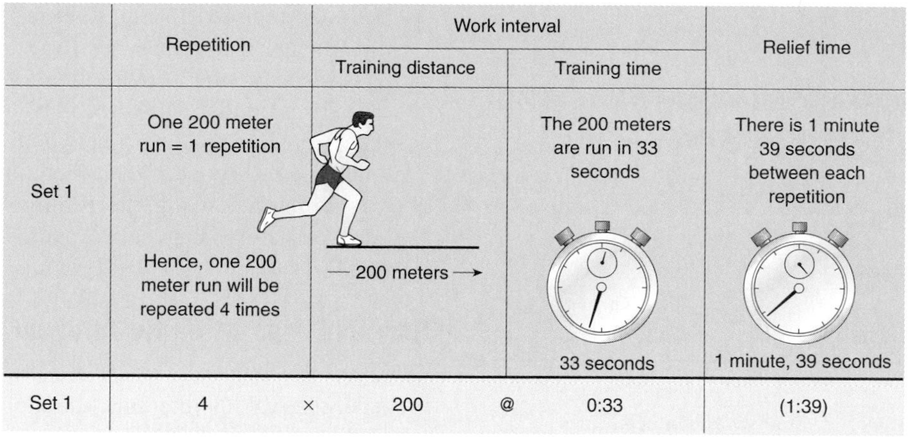

	Repetition	Work interval		Relief time
		Training distance	Training time	
Set 1	One 200 meter run = 1 repetition Hence, one 200 meter run will be repeated 4 times	← 200 meters →	The 200 meters are run in 33 seconds 33 seconds	There is 1 minute 39 seconds between each repetition 1 minute, 39 seconds
Set 1	4	× 200	@ 0:33	(1:39)

Figure 11.10

Interpretation of an interval-training program prescription involving running.

Source: Data from E. L. Fox and Donald K. Mathews, Interval Training: Conditioning for Sports and General Fitness, *1974, W. B. Saunders, Philadelphia, PA.*

Our discussion so far has focused on differences in the duration of the work interval (e.g., six 10-second intervals versus one 60-second bout). The interaction between the ATP-PC system and anaerobic glycolysis during interval training can also be influenced by the type, duration, and intensity of activity imposed during the *relief* interval. Interval work of the same intensity and duration performed using a *rest-relief interval* as compared with *work-relief interval* results in a blood lactic acid level that is higher with the latter.[21] This is because the work performed during the work-relief interval partially blocks the complete replenishment of the ATP-PC stores.[21] Without as much of these stores being renewed, a greater proportion of the energy needed during subsequent work intervals must be supplied via anaerobic glycolysis—resulting in lactate build-up.

An *interval training prescription* outlines the specifics of an athlete's interval-training program. To demonstrate this, let's review the following example taken from one set of a prescription written for a running program (see also table 11.5 and figure 11.10):

One set = 4 × 200 at 0:33 to 1:39

Where:

4 = number of repetitions
200 = training distance in meters
0:33 = training time of work interval in minutes:seconds
1:39 = time of relief interval in minutes:seconds

Selecting the Type of Work for the Work Interval

Interval training prescriptions for athletes must apply an overload during the work interval and do so in a manner that is specific to that athlete's sport. The *overload principle*, as applied to interval training, is accomplished through the manipulation of five variables:

1. Rate and distance of work interval
2. Number of repetitions during each workout
3. Time of relief interval
4. Type of activity during relief interval
5. Frequency of training per week

Rate (Intensity) and Distance of Work Interval

Interval-training prescriptions for anaerobic-type events are made up of medium-duration intervals performed at moderate to hard intensities (ATP-PC system and anaerobic glycolysis) or of short-duration intervals performed at even higher intensities (ATP-PC system).* For most anaerobic activities, the intensity of the work interval can best be written by considering the performance time of the work interval. You will recall that knowing the performance time of an activity allows us to determine the predominant energy system involved (p. 271). (Covering 100 m in 1.5 minutes is an aerobic event; whereas moving the same distance in 14 seconds is an anaerobic endeavor.)

How is a sufficient rate of work determined? There are several methods, some of which were discussed earlier in this chapter.

1. One method is based on the *heart rate* response during the work interval. As mentioned previously, this involves achieving a training heart rate that is 5% to 15% above the heart rate measured at lactate threshold.
2. A second method is based on the number of work intervals (repetitions) that can be performed per set or per the total workout. At a given work rate or pace, if at least five repetitions cannot be performed because of exhaustion, the pace is too intensive. On the other

---

*Interval-training programs made up of long-duration intervals performed at lower intensities are specific for aerobic-type events.

11.6

Guidelines for determining a sufficient work rate for running and swimming interval-training programs

Training distance (meters)		
Run	**Swim**	**Training pace**
50	1½	Seconds slower than best times from moving start
100	25	3
200	50	5
400	100	1 to 4 seconds faster than one-fourth the best times in 1600 m run or 400 m swim
800	200	3 to 4 seconds slower than one-fourth the best times in 1600 m run or 400 m swim

Source: Data from E. L. Fox and Donald K. Mathews, *Interval Training: Conditioning for Sports and General Fitness,* 1974, W. B. Saunders, Philadelphia, PA.

hand, if more than eight repetitions can be performed without difficulty, then the pace is too easy. As an illustration, suppose you are using 400 m as your training distance. The speed of each 400 m run, therefore, should permit between five and eight repetitions per set before undue exhaustion.

3. Wilt[60] has worked out a method for determining a sufficient work rate when structuring the interval-training prescription for sprint running. This method can be applied to other events, such as swimming and ice speed skating, as well. Relative to running, the times for training distances between 50 m and 200 m should be between 1.5 seconds and 5 seconds slower, respectively, than the best time for those distances measured from running starts. For example, if a person can run 50 m from a running start in six seconds, the training time for this distance would be $6 + 1.5 = 7.5$ seconds.

For training distances of 100 and 200 m, add three and five seconds, respectively, to the best times taken from running starts. For training distances of 400 m, the rate of work would be one to four seconds less (i.e., the person must run faster) than one-fourth

the time required to run 1600 m ($\sim$ one mile). As an illustration, if a person ran 1600 m in six minutes (or 360 seconds), the average time for each 400 m would be 90 seconds (360 seconds $\div$ 4 = 90 seconds). Therefore, the training time would be between 86 seconds and 89 seconds.* This method can also be applied to swimming, using the training distances that are approximately one-fourth of those used for running (table 11.6).

Time and Type of Relief Interval

There are two important considerations when dealing with the relief interval: (1) the time (duration) of the relief interval, and (2) the type of activity during the relief interval.

1. *Time of Relief Interval.* Recovery pulse rate following the work interval is a good indication as to whether the individual is physiologically ready for the next interval or next set. For example, for men and women less than 20 years old, both athletic and nonathletic, the pulse rate should drop to at least 140 beats per minute between repetitions and to 120 beats per minute between sets.[19]

Because it is sometimes difficult to use pulse rate to guide the duration of the relief interval, the work-relief ratio method can be used. This will guarantee that heart rates will have recovered to near 120 to 140 beats per minute. With longer work intervals (800 m and over), usually a 1:1 or 1:1½ work-relief ratio is prescribed. For middle-duration intervals (400 m to 600 m), a 1:2 ratio is used. And for shorter work intervals, because of the high intensity, a 1:3 work-relief ratio is prescribed. This means the duration of the relief interval is three times as long as the duration of the work interval.

Knowing these work-relief ratios simplifies administration of the interval-training program, particularly to groups, since it is no longer necessary to measure pulse rate following each work effort. However, pulse checks should periodically be obtained so that work intensity can be increased, decreased, or maintained.

2. *Type of Relief Interval.* As mentioned previously, what you do during the relief intervals is important, for it also relates to the energy system you may wish to develop. The relief interval may be rest-relief (i.e., walking about or flexing arms and legs), work-relief (i.e., light or mild exercise, including rapid walking and maybe jogging), or a combination of rest-relief and work-relief.

Rest-relief intervals should be used with interval-training programs that are designed to modify the ATP-PC

---

*90 seconds − 4 = 86 seconds; 90 seconds − 1 = 89 seconds.

11.7
table

Pertinent information for writing interval-training prescriptions based on training distances

Major energy system	Training distance (meters)		Approximate training time	Sets per workout	Repetitions per set	Work-relief ratio	Type of relief interval
	Run	Swim	(min:sec)				
ATP-PC	50	—	0:10	5	10	1:3, 1:4	Rest-relief (e.g.,
	100	25	< :20	3	8	1:3	walking, flexing)
ATP-PC or anaerobic glycolysis	200	50	0:30–0:45	4	4	1:3	Work-relief (e.g.,
	400	100	1:20–1:30	2	4	1:2	light to mild exercise, jogging)
Anaerobic glycolysis or aerobic	600	125–150	1:45–2:15	1	5	1:2	Work-relief
	800	200	2:30–3:00	2	2	1:1	Rest- or work-relief

Source: Data from E. L. Fox and Donald K. Mathews, *Interval Training: Conditioning for Sports and General Fitness,* 1974, W. B. Saunders, Philadelphia, Pennsylvania.

energy system, which predominates during short-term exhaustive work. Rest-relief intervals help to more quickly restore ATP-PC supplies in the muscles so that intense exercise can again be repeated. When training to improve anaerobic glycolysis, work-relief intervals should be used between work intervals. As you may recall, mild work will inhibit or partially block complete restoration of the ATP-PC energy system. As a consequence, anaerobic glycolysis, rather than the ATP-PC system, will be forced to provide more energy during subsequent work intervals.

Summary of the Interval Training System

There are two clear advantages to using an interval training program. First, it allows the coach or trainer to individualize a precise training program for each athlete, one that is specific to the energy system that predominates for a given sport and to do so at a level of physiologic stress that optimizes gains in performance. Second, interval training programs can be the same day-to-day (allowing the athlete to observe progress) or flexible. The latter is important in that programs can be modified based on travel schedules, training locations and facilities, and training phase (preseason versus in-season).

Before going on to other types of anaerobic training methods, let's summarize the interval-training system.

1. Determine which energy system(s) need(s) to be increased.
2. Select the type of activity to be used during the work interval (cyclists cycle, swimmers swim).

3. Develop a training prescription that provides the correct number of repetitions, sets, work-relief ratio, and type of relief. Table 11.7 provides some typical examples for running and swimming based on training distance (and approximate training time).
4. Provide for an increase in intensity (progressive overload) throughout the training program.

Other Training Methods for Anaerobic Performance

Sprint training, or "speed training" as it is sometimes called, is used by sprinters to develop speed and muscular strength.[60] Part of this is accomplished through improved tolerance to lactate (lactate-tolerance training) via improved pain tolerance to acidosis and/or improved buffering capacity in the blood or muscles.[37] Here, repeated sprints at *all-out, maximal* speed or *supramaximal* effort are performed. For example, during running, about 6 seconds are required to accelerate to maximum speed from a static start. Therefore, the sprinter should run at least 150 to 200 m on each sprint to experience moving at top speed.[60] Also, the duration of each sprint should be long enough to produce severe acidosis. Recovery between repetitions, therefore, must be relatively complete—thus longer recovery intervals are utilized (5 minutes or more). Only 3 to 6 such bouts should be used in any one training session. And this method should be employed sparingly during a season, usually as the athlete heads into their end-of-the-year competition.

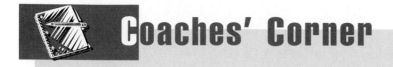

Coaches' Corner

The Most Anaerobic of Athletes

Speed skaters are among the most "anaerobic" of athletes. In Olympic-style ice speed skating, the events range from 500 m to 10,000 m for males and from 500 m to 5,000 m for females and require from 35 sec to 14 min to complete. Blood lactate concentration at the conclusion of the 1000 m and 1500 m events is usually around 25 mmol · L^{-1}, which requires approximately 2 min for completion. Although muscle lactate concentrations have never been measured in speed skaters with blood lactate concentrations as high as the value cited here, it's safe to assume that muscle levels are as high as those ever reported in a variety of other athletes.

Based on the limited amount of data that is available, one can surmise that only modest gains in anaerobic capacity (combined ATP-PC and anaerobic glycolysis systems) are achieved through anaerobic training. Nevertheless, skaters continue to train on the premise that frequent production of high muscle lactate concentrations will lead to adaptations that ultimately permit progressively higher muscle lactate concentrations during competition.

One of their favorite training methods to accomplish this is the "hill tempo." Hill tempos involve running up a very steep hill for predetermined periods of time (usually 30 to 120 sec). However, the goal is to run as hard as possible right from the very start, so that lactate rises as quickly as possible. This means that the majority of the run is completed with already high muscle lactates. A very steep hill is favored because (1) it requires loading of the hip and knee extensors, which are central to the push off in skating, and (2) the high-stride frequency that results from running uphill reduces the period of time during a stride where the athlete is "floating." This phase of the running stride is associated with adequate muscle blood flow, just the opposite of what occurs during skating.

Do hill tempos work? No one knows for sure. However, during hill tempo training elite speed skaters often develop blood lactate levels above 25 mmol · L^{-1}. In fact, Bonnie Blair, certainly one of the best ice speed sprinters of all time, routinely achieved some of the highest post-hill-tempo and post-competition blood lactate levels—when compared to both her male and female colleagues at the time. She was also famous for beating the male skaters on hill tempos—and quite a few of them on the ice too!

Source: Contributed by Carl Foster, Ph. D., Sinai Samaritan Medical Center.

Risks associated with this method include possible overtraining and injury.

As the name implies, **acceleration sprints** involve a gradual increase in speed from slow to moderate and finally to full sprinting.[14,60] For example, a swimmer may swim easily for 50 m, go at a faster pace for 50 m, and then sprint for 50 m. This is followed by 50 m of light recovery activity. The entire scenario is then repeated. Coaches often use it to train athletes how to build intensity throughout a race and how to finish strong.

Application of Anaerobic Training Methods to Various Sports

Whatever method is chosen, it is important to modify its application so that it is sport specific. For example, wide receivers and running backs in football should limit sprint distances to less than 100 yards, offensive and defensive linemen to less than 40 to 50 yards. In both cases, some of the sprint work can include backward as well as lateral running or stop-and-go sprinting. In basketball, stop-and-go sprints (line drills) are common, and an occasional sport-specific application might include performing the drills while dribbling one or two balls. Alternately, have the athletes shoot two free throws immediately afterward—to simulate having to "settle-down" and perform a skill task immediately after an intense exercise period.

These skill-specific variations emphasize movement patterns that are somewhat distinct from the effects of just anaerobic training alone.[15] Interestingly, factors that dictate improvement in performance for high-power output activities (blocking in football) include not only improvement in the anaerobic energy pathways but changes in motor unit recruitment patterns or chemical alterations at the neuromuscular junction as well.[15] Therefore, repeated performance of a specific motor skill or movement pattern can contribute to improved anaerobic performance.

Which training method should be used for which sport? The answer to this lies in how well the various

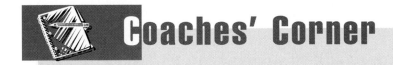

Coaches' Corner

One of the most demanding events in track cycling is the men's 1 km time trial, a race that is conducted using an aerodynamically enhanced bicycle on an outdoor track called a velodrome. This race, sometimes called the "killermeter," is an all-out sprint for 1000 m—and the athletes compete alone against the clock. An Olympic caliber kilo rider will complete the sprint in ~ 63 s to 65 s. As a result, the energy for this grueling event comes almost exclusively from the two anaerobic pathways: the ATP-PC system and anaerobic glycolysis. Without question, anaerobic power and capacity are critical physiological characteristics for success in this event.

The Wingate (p. 85) test is most often used to evaluate Olympic caliber kilo riders at the United States Olympic Training Center in Colorado Springs. Approximate average values achieved by these elite athletes for peak power, average power, and total work are 1375 W, 917 W, and 27.5 kJ, respectively. Compare these values to nonathletic men of similar age and body mass, where peak power, average power, and total work might be 650 W, 465 W, and 15.6 kJ, respectively. For each variable the athletes achieved values nearly twice that of their nonathletic counterparts.

One of the cyclists, a bronze medal winner in the 1992 Barcelona Olympics and a silver medal winner in the 1996 Atlanta Olympics, achieved a peak power of 1394 W, an average power of 957 W, and a total work of 28.7 kJ. In other words, this athlete generated enough power to illuminate 100 lightbulbs (each 60 W) for almost 5 seconds!

Source: Contributed by Randy L. Wilber, Ph.D., U.S. Olympic Committee, Sport Science and Technology.

---

training methods develop the different system(s) employed in a specific sport. Part of the science (and art) of coaching involves selecting the correct training method and then applying it or modifying it so it best develops the ATP-PC or anaerobic glycolysis energy systems.

Physiological Effects of Anaerobic Training

The chronic anatomic, morphologic, physiologic, and psychologic changes that result from repeated exposure to exercise comprise what is called the **training effect.** Without question, more extensive study has been conducted relative to describing the training effect associated with aerobic versus anaerobic exercise. Such an imbalance, however, by no means diminishes the important changes that do occur in response to anaerobic training. We will now discuss the effects of anaerobic training on general anaerobic fitness (peak power, mean power), the skeletal muscle, and the heart.

General Anaerobic Fitness

In chapter 4 we described several tests designed to quantify an individual's ability to produce ATP through the ATP-PC system and anaerobic glycolysis. The most common of these tests, the 30-second Wingate test, has been used in many cross-sectional studies and has demonstrated that athletes involved in anaerobic activities generally possess better anaerobic abilities than either endurance-trained athletes or sedentary patients (see also table 4.5, page 85). At present, however, it remains unclear as to whether or not the Wingate test represents a sensitive enough test that is capable of detecting an individual's "adaptation" to an anaerobic exercise training regimen.

Grodjinowsky and colleagues[25] assessed fifty 11- to 13-year-old boys who were randomly assigned to three groups: sprint training, high-intensity cycling, and a no exercise group. Boys in both of the exercise groups improved peak power output by 5% following just three weeks of training, whereas the control subjects showed no change. In this example, the Wingate test quantified nicely that training was associated with improved anaerobic performance, and no training resulted in no change in anaerobic performance. Conversely, Jacobs et al.[30] showed no change in Wingate test performance following six weeks of supramaximal cycle sprint training in 11 college-age males and females.

A second method for assessing anaerobic fitness uses maximal accumulated oxygen deficit as a measure of overall anaerobic energy release. Medbo and associates[43] showed a 10% improvement following a six-week anaerobic training program. Analyzing the improvement by gender, they found that males improved more than females (17% versus 5%). The authors were unable to explain why the greater increase occurred among the males versus females; however, they did not feel that anaerobic capacity was more trainable in the males.

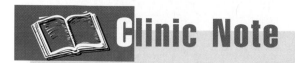

Clinic Note

Anaerobic Performance and Heart Disease

Since the 1970s, the importance of aerobic exercise training as a means to aid patients recovering from a heart attack or from coronary artery bypass surgery has been well recognized. As a result, all conditioning activities to date have focused on assessing and improving a patient's aerobic capacity (peak $\dot{V}O_2$). However, evaluating and training the anaerobic capabilities of patients with coronary artery disease may also be important. For example, some patients may wish to return to jobs (e.g., firefighter, assembly line worker) and activities (e.g., softball, basketball, masters-level hockey) that are anaerobic in nature.

Using a 30-second isokinetic cycle test, a procedure somewhat similar to the Wingate test, Oldridge and colleagues[46] documented that anaerobic performance can also be improved in patients with heart disease. In their study patients were randomly assigned to either aerobic exercise training (n = 12) or to a nonexercise control group (n = 10). Patients assigned to

12 weeks of 5 times per week of endurance/aerobic training demonstrated, as expected, an 18% increase in maximum $\dot{V}O_2$ (from 1.85 L · min^{-1} to 2.19 L · min^{-1}). In addition, a 14% increase in peak anaerobic power output was also shown (from 774 watts to 883 watts). Among the nonexercising controls, both maximum $\dot{V}O_2$ and peak power output were unchanged.

This study represents an initial step in the concept of anaerobic training among eligible patients with stable heart disease. Hopefully, however, you have noticed that anaerobic power (peak power output) was increased using an aerobic regimen. No studies to date have looked at the effects of an anaerobic training program in these patients, leaving to speculation what gains in anaerobic capabilities one might expect if a specific anaerobic regimen were used. Perhaps such a regimen will allow some patients to return to the activities they desire with even greater ability and comfort.

Anaerobic Training and Skeletal Muscle

Relative to training, by now you recognize that success in anaerobic endeavors is associated with the abilities of the skeletal muscles. Changes that occur in these muscles as a result of anaerobic training lead to increased capacities of the ATP-PC system and anaerobic glycolysis to generate ATP. Relative to the ATP-PC system, it is enhanced by two major biochemical changes: either increased stores of ATP and PC in the muscle or increased activity of the key enzymes involved in the ATP-PC system.

Muscular stores of ATP have been shown to increase approximately 25% (from 3.8 to 4.8 mmol · kg^{-1} of wet muscle) following a training program of distance running of 2 to 3 days per week for 7 months.[32] Also, the concentration of PC in the muscles of boys 11 to 13 years of age increased nearly 40% after 4 months of training.[16] Because these phosphagens represent the most rapidly available source of energy for the muscle, their increased storage following training correlates well with the improved execution of activities that require only a few seconds to perform.

As mentioned previously, training also alters several key enzymes of the ATP-PC system.[55,57] Remember that in the ATP-PC system, ATP is continually turned over (i.e.,

broken down and resynthesized). The breakdown of ATP is facilitated by an enzyme called ATPase, whereas its resynthesis is facilitated by the enzymes myokinase (MK) and creatine kinase (CPK). Myokinase catalyzes the reactions involved in replenishing ATP from ADP, and CPK catalyzes the reactions involved in replenishing ATP from PC. In a study on humans,[48] the activities of these enzymes were found to increase following eight weeks of sprint training as follows: ATPase, 30%; MK, 20%; and CPK, 36%. Thus, training not only increases the storage of ATP and PC, but also enhances their rates of turnover. These mutually beneficial changes clearly demonstrate that the rapid release of energy by the muscle cell is alterable through proper (mainly sprint) training programs.

With respect to the effects of training on anaerobic glycolysis, a number of well-designed studies have indicated that several of the key glycolytic enzymes, in addition to glycogen storage are significantly altered by physical training. For example, the activity of one such enzyme, phosphofructokinase (PFK), which is important in the early reactions of glycolysis, doubled following endurance training.[22] In another study, 11 college-age men and women who underwent 6 weeks of sprint training showed a 16% increase in PFK.[30] Other important glycolytic enzymes have also been reported to increase following training.[6,51,56] In addition, it has been shown that the chemical activity of important glycolytic en-

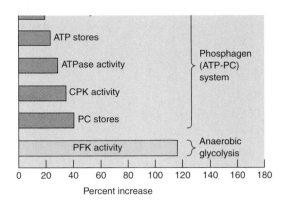

Figure 11.11

The effects of training on the anaerobic potential of skeletal muscle include increases in the activities of the ATP turnover enzymes [ATPase, myokinase (MK), and creatine phospho kinase (CPK)] in muscular stores of ATP and PC, and in glycolytic capacity.

(Based on data from Thorstensson et al.[57]; Karlsson et al.[32]; Eriksson et al.[16]; and Gollnick and King.[24])

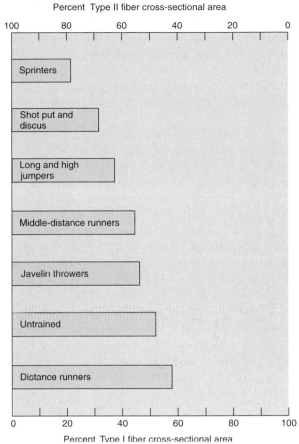

Figure 11.12

Training produces a selective hypertrophy of Type I and II skeletal muscle fibers. The Type I fibers of endurance athletes occupy a greater area of the muscle than do Type II fibers. However, Type II fibers occupy a greater area in sprinters, shot-putters, and discus throwers.

(Based on data from Costill et al.[12])

zymes is much higher in sprint athletes than in endurance athletes.[12] The changes in the ATP-PC system and in the anaerobic glycolysis enzymes as a result of training are shown in figure 11.11. The nature of these changes appears to be similar in both males and females.

Not surprisingly, the adaptations of the skeletal muscle to anaerobic training do not all occur to the same degree in the Type I fiber as compared to the Type II fiber. Some of the differences are as follows:

1. The previously mentioned changes appear to occur more in Type I fibers as compared to Type II fibers.[1] Other researchers, however, feel that the changes in the glycolytic capacity of skeletal muscle appear to be more specific to Type II fibers.[17,23] Obviously, this issue is not yet resolved and requires further investigation.

2. Evidence suggests that there is a selective hypertrophy of Type I and Type II fibers. For example, Type II fibers occupy a greater area in sprinters, shot-putters, and discus throwers (figure 11.12). This information implies a selective hypertrophy that is dependent on the kind of training and/or sport activity performed by the athlete.

3. Most available evidence suggests that there is no interconversion of Type I to Type II fibers as a result of physical training.[16,23,50] However, some evidence indicates that the percentage of Type II fibers increases and the percentage of Type I fibers decreases following anaerobic training.[30,31] Nevertheless, the majority of evidence is still in favor of no true fiber type interconversions caused by sprint training.

Anaerobic Training and the Heart

Although the enlarged heart of the athlete was initially described in the 1800s, it wasn't until the 1970s—following the development of echocardiography*—that the study of the "athlete's heart" began to flourish. Differences in how an athlete's heart structurally adapts or remodels in response to training is related to the type of activity she or he is involved with.[52] For example, compared to nonexercising controls, athletes involved in anaerobic-type activities (sprinters, weight lifters, shot putters) develop a thickening of the septum between the left and right ventricles, a thickening of the posterior wall, and increased left ventricular

---

*A noninvasive (outside the body) method of recording the position and motion of the walls and structures of the heart using ultrasonic waves directed through the chest wall.

mass, with little or no change in left ventricular end-diastolic cavity dimension. These changes are believed to be caused by *pressure overload.* Conversely, endurance-trained athletes (runners, cyclists) develop changes in the heart caused by *volume overload.* These changes include an increase in left ventricular end-diastolic cavity size and only proportional increases in septal and posterior wall thickness.

To demonstrate these differences relative to type of activity, we draw your attention to figure 11.13, an echocardiographic study of 10 runners, 10 wrestlers and 10 nonexercising controls.[11] Compared to controls, the wrestlers showed increases in interventricular septal thickness and left ventricular wall thickness, with no difference in left ventricular end-diastolic dimension. In contrast, the runners showed significant changes in left ventricular end-diastolic dimension only. Similar increases in left ventricular mass were observed among both wrestlers (326 g) and runners (312 g) when compared to controls (216 g).

It should be pointed out that the effect of aerobic and anaerobic training on cardiac dimensions is not clear-cut.[40] Although most studies of athletes show an enlarged heart when compared to nonathletes, several studies have not found differences between aerobically and anaerobically trained athletes.

Detraining

Little research is available relative to the effects of stopping training (**detraining**) on anaerobic performance. Intuitively, and anecdotally, we know that an athlete asked to compete during the off-season does not perform as well as if they had been asked to compete in the middle of their competitive season. In the absence of such information, we can gain some insight into the effects of detraining by looking at the anaerobic capabilities of injured athletes or of individuals with different diseases.[28] These persons represent individuals who, in a sense, are detrained because they do not have sufficient capacity or ability to perform routine activities of daily living.

A simple example would be those individuals who, for whatever reason, must undergo limb immobilization—let's say for a broken arm or an injured knee. Upon removing the cast, it's obvious that the limb is smaller (due to muscle atrophy) and that, until recovered, the limb tires more easily. The latter results from losses of muscle power and endurance. Another example, albeit rare, involves persons with a deficiency in one or more of the enzymes needed for anaerobic glycolysis. The best known of these so-called "metabolic diseases" is McArdle's disease, in which there is an aberration in muscle phosphorylase. Patients with McArdle's disease can engage in mild aerobic activities but are intolerant (pain, cramps) to moderate or high-intensity work.

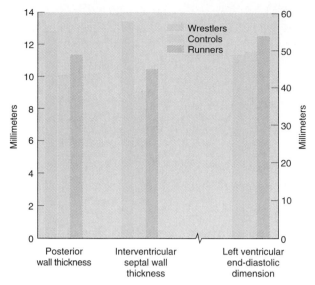

Figure 11.13

Resting echocardiographic measurements of the heart in wrestlers, controls, and runners. The anaerobic athletes (wrestlers) clearly showed changes consistent with "pressure overload," such as a greater posterior wall thickness and interventricular septal wall thickness. The aerobically trained athletes (runners) developed changes caused by volume overload, such as a greater left ventricular end-diastolic volume.

(Based on data from Cohen and Segal.[11])

Summary

The basic tenets in any conditioning or training program are (1) to recognize the major energy source used in performing a given activity, and (2) to construct a program that will develop that particular energy source through the overload principle. The primary energy system for any activity can be estimated on the basis of its performance time.

The overload principle requires that the training intensity be near maximal. For anaerobic-training programs, training intensity can be guided by pace, heart rate, lactate threshold, or combinations of all three methods. For example, the *pace* at which an athlete runs or swims should result in a *heart rate* that is 5% to 15% above the heart rate that he achieved at his *lactate threshold.* Other important overload factors are training frequency and training duration.

Off-season training should consist mainly of weight training and low-intensity aerobic training. Preseason training should contain weight training and high-intensity anaerobic training. In-season training should consist of some aerobic training and weight training as well as skill-related drills, sprint work, scrimmages, and competitive performances.

Warm up prior to any training session promotes increased body and muscle temperatures, which in turn promote increases in muscle metabolism, blood flow, and oxygen availability; and decreases in muscle contraction and reflex times. Warm-up activities should include stretching exercises, calisthenics, and formal activity. Cool down should include similar activities but performed in reverse order. Cool down appears to hasten recovery and reduce soreness.

The interval-training system involves repeated bouts of hard work (work interval) alternated with periods of relief (lighter work or rest). Intermittent work delays fatigue and allows for maximal intensity during the work intervals. Manipulation of the rate and distance of the work interval, the number of repetitions, and the time and type of relief interval provides for a training program that can meet the needs of many athletes and nonathletes. Other training methods to develop the ATP-PC system and anaerobic glycolysis include sprint training, acceleration sprints, and tempo work.

Adaptations of the body to anaerobic training do occur. These include improvement in peak power output and mean power output, increased ATP and PC stores, increased activity of the enzymes involved with both the ATP-PC system and anaerobic glycolysis, and a somewhat selective hypertrophy of the Type II skeletal muscle fiber. Additionally, cardiac mass is generally increased in anaerobically trained athletes when compared to nonexercising controls. This may or may not be associated with an increase in left ventricular wall thickness.

Questions

1. How might you determine which energy system(s) predominate(s) in any sport or activity? Include in your answer why this is important when developing a training program (*hint:* specificity of training).
2. What is meant by the overload principle as applied to anaerobic training programs?
3. Discuss the various methods for guiding exercise intensity during anaerobic training. How can they be used in an interrelated manner during training?
4. What are the different phases of training?
5. A friend of yours plays on the university's basketball team and asks you to set up an off-season conditioning program—please describe your plan.
6. Why are warm-up and cool-down programs important from a physiological standpoint?
7. Define the following terms: *interval training*, *work interval*, and *relief interval*.
8. Physiologically, explain why intermittent work, and thus the interval-training system, can be used to improve anaerobic performance.
9. Explain what type of relief interval (rest-relief, work-relief) you would choose to improve the ATP-PC system and anaerobic glycolysis. Provide the physiologic rationale.
10. Define and discuss two other training programs that can be used to develop the anaerobic system.
11. What physiologic changes occur in (a) the skeletal muscle, (b) the ATP-PC energy system, and (c) anaerobic glycolysis in response to anaerobic training?
12. Why is it important for an "anaerobic" performer to also possess a solid aerobic base?

References

1. *ACSM's Resource Manual for Guidelines for Exercise Testing and Prescription*, 2d ed. 1993. Philadelphia: Lea & Febiger.
2. Ahmaidi, S., P. Granier, Z., Taoutaou, J. Mercier, H. Dubouchaud, and C. Prefaut. 1996. Effects of active recovery on plasma lactate and anaerobic power following repeated intensive exercise. *Med Sci Sports Exerc.* 28(4)450–456.
3. Asmussen, E., and O. Boje. 1945. Body temperature and capacity for work. *Acta Physiol Scand.* 10:1–22.
4. Åstrand, I., P. O. Åstrand, E. Christensen, and R. Hedman. 1960. Intermittent muscular work. *Acta Physiol Scand.* 48:448–453.
5. ———. 1960. Myohemoglobin as an oxygen-store in man. *Acta Physiol Scand.* 48:454–460.
6. Baldwin, K., W. Winder, R. Terjung, and J. Holloszy. 1972. Glycolytic capacity of red, white, and intermediate muscle: adaptive response to running. *Med Sci Sports.* 4:50.
7. Barnard, R., G. Gardner, N. Diaco, R. MacAlpin, and A. Kattus. 1973. Cardiovascular responses to sudden strenuous exercise heart rate, blood pressure, and ECG. *J Appl Physiol.* 34(6):833–837.
8. Bergh, U., and B. Ekblom. 1979. Physical performance and peak aerobic power at different body temperatures. *J Appl Physiol.* 46(5):885–889.
9. Carlile, F. 1956. Effects of preliminary passive warming-up on swimming performance. *Res Q.* 27:143–151.
10. Christensen, E., R. Hedman, and B. Saltin. 1960. Intermittent and continuous running. *Acta Physiol Scand.* 50:269–287.
11. Cohen, J. L., and K. R. Segal. 1985. Left ventricular hypertrophy in athletes: an exercise-echocardiographic study. *Med Sci Sports Exerc.* 17(6):695–700.
12. Costill, D. L., J. Daniels, W. Evans, G. Fink, G. Krahenbuhl, and B. Saltin. 1976. Skeletal muscle enzymes and fiber composition in male and female track athletes. *J Appl Physiol.* 40(2):149–154.
13. Delecluse C., H. V. Coppenolle, E. Willems, M. V. Leemputte, R. Diels, and M. Goris. 1995. Influence of high-resistance and high-velocity training on sprint performance. *Med Sci Sports Exerc.* 27(8):1203–1209.
14. Dintiman, G. 1974. *What Research Tells the Coach about Sprinting.* Washington, D.C.: American Alliance for Health, Physical Education, and Recreation.
15. Edgerton, V. R. 1976. Neuromuscular adaptation to power and endurance work. *Can J Appl Sport Sci.* 1:49–58.
16. Eriksson, B., P. Gollnick, and B. Saltin. 1973. Muscle metabolism and enzyme activities after training in boys 11–13 years old. *Acta Physiol Scand.* 87:485–497.

17. Fink, W., D. L. Costill, J. Daniels, M. Pollock, and B. Saltin. 1975. Muscle fiber composition and enzyme activities in male and female athletes. *Physiologist.* 18(3):213.

18. Fox, E. L. 1975. Differences in metabolic alterations with sprint versus endurance interval training. In Howald, H., and J. Poortmans (eds.), *Metabolic Adaptation to Prolonged Physical Exercise.* Basel, Switzerland: Birkhauser Verlag, pp. 119–126.

19. Fox, E. L., J. Klinzing, and R. L. Bartels. 1977. Interval training: metabolic changes as related to relief-interval heart rates of 120 and 140 beats per minute. *Fed Proc.* 36(3):449.

20. Fox, E. L., and D. K. Mathews. 1974. *Interval Training: Conditioning for Sports and General Fitness.* Philadelphia: W. B. Saunders.

21. Fox, E. L., S. Robinson, and D. Wiegman. 1969. Metabolic energy sources during continuous and interval running. *J Appl Physiol.* 27:174–178.

22. Gillespie, A. C., E. L. Fox, and A. J. Merola. 1982. Enzyme adaptations in rat skeletal muscle after two intensities of treadmill training. *Med Sci Sports Exerc.* 14(6):461–466.

23. Gollnick, P., R. Armstrong, B. Saltin, C. Saubert, W. Sembrowich, and R. Shepherd. 1973. Effect of training on enzyme activity and fiber composition of human skeletal muscle. *J Appl Physiol.* 34(1):107–111.

24. Gollnick, P., and D. King. 1969. Effects of exercise and training on mitochondria of rat skeletal muscle. *Am J Physiol.* 216:1502–1509.

25. Grodjinowski, A., O. Inbar, R. Dotan, and O. Bar-Or. 1980. Training effect on the anaerobic performance of children as measured by the Wingate Anaerobic Test. In K. Berg, and B.O. Eriksson (eds), *Children and Exercise* vol. IX. Baltimore: University Park Press. 139–145.

26. Hebestreit, H., K. Mimura, and O. Bar-Or. 1993. Recovery of muscle power after high-intensity short-term exercise: comparing boys and men. *J Appl Physiol.* 74(6):2875–2880.

27. Hultman, E., J. Bergstrom, and N. McLennan-Anderson. 1967. Breakdown and resynthesis of phosphorylcreatine and adenosine triphosphate in connection with muscular work in man. *Scand J Clin Invest.* 19:56–66.

28. Inbar, O., O. Bar-Or, and J. S. Skinner. 1996. *The Wingate Anaerobic Test.* Champaign: Human Kinetics.

29. Inger, F., and S. B. Stromme. 1979. Effects of active, passive or no warm up on the physiological response to heavy exercise. *Eur J Appl Physiol.* 40:273–282.

30. Jacobs, I., M. Esbjornsson, C. Sylven, I. Holm, and E. Jansson. 1987. Sprint training effects on muscle myoglobin, enzymes, fiber types, and blood lactate. *Med Sci Sports Exerc.* 19(4):368–374.

31. Jansson, E., B. Sjodin, and P. Tesch. 1978. Changes in muscle fibre type distribution in man after physical training. *Acta Physiol Scand.* 104:235–237.

32. Karlsson, J., L.-O. Nordesjo, L. Jorfeldt, and B. Saltin. 1972. Muscle lactate, ATP, and CP levels during exercise after physical training in man. *J Appl Physiol.* 33(2):199–203.

33. Karlsson, J., and B. Saltin. 1970. Lactate, ATP and CP in working muscles during exhaustive exercise in man. *J Appl Physiol.* 29:598–602.

34. Karpovich, P., and C. Hale. 1956. Effect of warming-up upon physical performance. *JAMA* 162:1117–1119.

35. Kearney, J. T. 1996. Training the Olympic athlete. *Scientific American.* June:52–63.

36. Kindermann, W., G. Simon, and J. Keul. 1979. The significance of the aerobic-anaerobic transition for the determination of work load intensities during endurance training. *Eur J Appl Physiol.* 42:25–34.

37. Mader, A., H. Liesen, H. Heck, H. Philippi, R. Rost, P. Schurch, and W. Hollmann. 1976. Zur Beurteilung der Sportartspezifischen Ausdauerleistungsfahigkeit im Labor. *Sportarzt Sportmed.* 27:80–88, 109–112.

38. Maglisco, E. W. 1993. *Swimming Even Faster.* Mountain View: Mayfield Publishing Co.

39. Margaria, R., R. Oliva, P. diPrampero, and P. Cerretelli. 1969. Energy utilization in intermittent exercise of supramaximal intensity. *J Appl Physiol.* 26:752–756.

40. Maron, B. J. 1986. Structural features of the athlete heart as defined by echocardiography. *J Am Coll Cardiol.* 7:190–203.

41. Martin, B. J., S. Robinson, D. L. Wiegman, and L. H. Aulick. 1975. Effect of warm up on metabolic responses to strenuous exercise. *Med Sci Sports.* 7(2):146–149.

42. Mathews, D., and H. Snyder. 1959. Effect of warm up on the 440-yard dash. *Res Q.* 30:446–451.

43. Medbo J. I., and S. Burgers. 1990. Effect of training on the anaerobic capacity. *Med Sci Sports Exerc.* 22(4):501–507.

44. Michael, E., V. Skubic, and R. Rochelle. 1957. Effect of warm up on softball throw for distance. *Res Q.* 28:357–363.

45. Mitchell, J. H., W. L. Haskell, and P. B. Raven. 1994. Classification of sports. *Med Sci Sports Exerc.* 26(10-supplement):S242–S245.

46. Oldridge N. B., N. McCartney, A. Hicks, and N. L. Jones. 1989. Improvement in maximal isokinetic cycle ergometry with cardiac rehabilitation. *Med Sci Sports Exerc.* 21(3):308–312.

47. Pacheco, B. 1957. Improvement in jumping performance due to preliminary exercise. *Res Q.* 28:55–63.

48. Pollock, M. 1973. The quantification of endurance training programs. In Wilmore, J. (ed.), *Exercise and Sport Sciences Reviews*, vol. 1. New York: Academic Press, pp. 155–188.

49. Saltin, B., and B. Essen. 1971. Muscle glycogen, lactate, ATP, and CP in intermittent exercise. In Pernow, B., and B. Saltin (eds.), *Muscle Metabolism during Exercise.* New York: Plenum Press, pp. 419–424.

50. Saltin, B., K. Nazar, D. L. Costill, E. Stein, E. Jansson, B. Essen, and P. D. Gollnick. 1976. The nature of the training response; peripheral and central adaptations to one-legged exercise. *Acta Physiol Scand.* 96:289–305.

51. Saubert, C., R. Armstrong, R. Shepherd, and P. D. Gollnick. 1973. Anaerobic enzyme adaptations to spring training in rats. *Pflugers Arch.* 341:305–312.

52. Shapiro, L. M. 1992. Morphologic consequences of systemic training. In Maron, B. J. (ed), *Cardiology Clinics: The Athletes Heart*, vol. 10. Philadelphia: W. B. Saunders, pp. 219–225.

53. Skubic, V., and J. Hodgkins. 1957. Effect of warm-up activities on speed, strength, and accuracy. *Res Q.* 28:147–152.

54. Sleivert G. G., R. D. Backus, and H. A. Wenger. 1995. The influence of a strength-sprint training sequence on multi-joint power output. *Med Sci Sports Exerc.* 27(12):1655–1665.

55. Smith, D. C., and A. El-Hage. 1978. Effect of exercise training on the chronotropic response of isolated rat atria to atropine. *Experientia.* 34(8):1027–1028.

56. Staudte, H., G. Exner, and D. Pette. 1973. Effects of short-term, high-intensity (sprint) training on some contractile and metabolic characteristics of fast and slow muscle of the rat. *Pflugers Arch.* 344:159–168.

57. Thorstensson, A., B. Sjodin, and J. Karlsson. 1975. Enzyme activities and muscle strength after "sprint training" in man. *Acta Physiol Scand.* 94:313–318.

58. Tipton, C., and P. Karpovich. 1966. Exercise and the patellar reflex. *J Appl Physiol.* 21(1):15–18.

59. White, J. R. 1977. EKG changes using carotid artery for heart rate monitoring. *Med Sci Sports.* 9(2):88–94.

60. Wilt, F. 1968. Training for competitive running. In Falls, H. (ed.), *Exercise Physiology.* New York: Academic Press, pp. 395–414.

Selected Readings

American College of Sports Medicine. 1995. *Guidelines for Exercise Testing and Prescription*, 5th ed. Philadelphia: Lea and Febiger.

Chu, D. A. 1992. *Jumping into Plyometrics*. Champaign, IL: Human Kinetics.

Councilman, J. E., and B. E. Councilman. 1994. *The New Science of Swimming*. Engelwood Cliffs: Prentice-Hall.

Fox, E. L. 1977. Physical training: methods and effects. *Ortho Clin N Am.* 8:533–548.

———. 1978. Methods and effects of physical training. *Pediatric Ann.* 7(10):66–94.

Pelliccia, A., B. J. Maron, F. Culasso, A. Spataro, and G. Caselli. 1996. Athlete's heart in women. *JAMA* 276:211–215.

Shaffer, T. E., and E. L. Fox. 1977. Guidelines to physical conditioning for sports. *Pediatric Basics.* 18:10–14.

Wells, C. L., and R. R. Pate. 1993. Training for performance of prolonged exercise. In Lamb, D. R. and C. Gisolfi (eds.), *Perspectives in Exercise Science and Sports Medicine.* Dubuque: Wm C. Brown Communications.

12

Methods for Aerobic Training and Physiologic Responses

In chapter 11 we discussed the training principles associated with—and the physiologic consequences of—anaerobic sports. In contrast, this chapter focuses on training the aerobic energy pathways—and on the physiologic responses that occur as a result. For those students who have not yet studied chapter 11, we encourage you to review, at minimum, pages 270–274 and pages 276–279 at this time. Doing so will help provide the "foundational theory" behind training principles and phases in general. To a certain extent, this chapter builds upon information previously learned and simply applies it to endurance training.

Like chapter 11, we will again focus our discussion on developing the competitive or elite athlete. We will not discuss training principles and adaptations relative to the development of physical fitness or health improvement among the general population. That information is addressed in chapter 14.

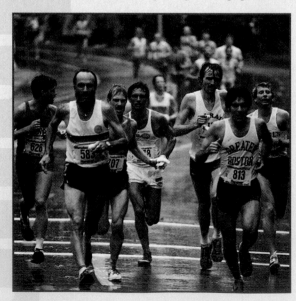

General Considerations

Training Methods for Aerobic Performance

Physiological Effects of Aerobic Training

Other Factors Influencing Training and Training Effects

Summary

The major concepts to be learned from this chapter are as follows:

- Like anaerobic training, aerobic training principles involve specificity of training and overload.
- Training intensity can be guided by heart-rate-based methods or by lactate threshold.
- Training methods for improved endurance performance can include long-duration, moderate-intensity methods; moderate-duration, high-intensity methods; and/or short-duration, very high-intensity methods.
- Endurance training induces physiological changes in almost every system of the body, particularly within the skeletal muscles and the cardiorespiratory system.
- The effects of training are lost after several weeks of detraining.
- Training effects can be maintained with maintenance programs consisting of one or two days of exercise per week.
- For the currently untrained person who was previously trained, the magnitude or rate of regain of the training effects is not greater during a subsequent training program.
- Overtraining and/or staleness are associated with physiologic changes, decrement in performance, fatigue, and disturbances of mood.

General Considerations

In this section we discuss training principles and phases relative to aerobic or endurance-type sport activities.

Training Principles

To improve endurance performance the athlete must work specific muscles or organ systems at an increased resistance. The two key phrases in this statement are *specific* (specificity of training) and *increased resistance* (progressive overload). With respect to endurance performance, recall from chapters 4, 7, and 9 that $\dot{V}O_2$ max and $\dot{V}O_2$ at lactate threshold represent two measures of aerobic fitness. $\dot{V}O_2$ max is the ability of our bodies to transport and utilize oxygen. $\dot{V}O_2$ at lactate threshold reflects the ability of our bodies to generate ATP via predominately aerobic pathways—prior to having to increase reliance on anaerobic metabolism for energy production. Training practices, therefore, should be designed to improve these two measures.

Specificity of Training

All training programs must be designed to develop the specific physiological capacities required to perform a given sport skill or activity. Concerning aerobic or endurance sports, this primarily involves the skeletal muscles, the cardiorespiratory system, and/or neuromuscular function.

At the skeletal muscle level, the athlete, coach, trainer, or therapist must first determine the contribution of the various energy systems to energy production during a given activity. A listing of various activities and the contribution of the different energy pathways is provided in chapter 11 (table 11.2). Generally, most endurance activities rely heavily on the aerobic energy systems of skeletal muscle (Krebs Cycle, electron transport system, and beta-oxidation). However, some activities—such as the 400 m swim, the 1500 run, or playing mid-fielder in soccer—require important contributions from anaerobic glycolysis as well. From a coach's perspective, an appropriate training plan would incorporate aerobic and anaerobic training in a manner that is somewhat proportional to the contribution of the aerobic and anaerobic energy pathways.

The cardiorespiratory or oxygen transport system is responsible for the transport and exchange of oxygen and carbon dioxide between the environment and the working muscles. Because oxygen must be shuttled to the muscles in quantities sufficient to allow energy production to continue via aerobic metabolism, the cardiorespiratory system is more important during low-intensity, long-duration exercises than during very high-intensity, short-duration exercises.

The neuromuscular basis for specificity of training addresses the different motor units or fiber types found in skeletal muscle and their specific recruitment patterns during the performance of various kinds of exercises. While fiber recruitment is controlled mainly by the central nervous system (i.e., the brain and spinal cord), fiber types (Type I [slow-oxidative] and Type IIB [fast-glycolytic]) have metabolic specificity. Recall that Type I fibers have a high aerobic capacity and a low anaerobic capacity whereas Type IIB fibers have a low aerobic capacity and a high anaerobic capacity. Therefore, Type I fibers, and to some extent Type IIA fibers, are predominantly recruited for aerobic-type activities. This level of specificity dictates that the exercises used during a training regimen should simulate as closely as possible the movement patterns required to perform a specific athletic task.

A summary of the major, intermediate, and minor contributing factors involved in the specificity of aerobic training is presented in figure 12.1.

Before leaving our discussion of specificity of training, let's examine two research studies that highlight the importance of this principle. First, the max $\dot{V}O_2$ of three different groups of athletes—rowers, cyclists, and skiers—was first determined while they ran on a treadmill and then while they performed their specific sport (figure 12.2). For each test condition the max $\dot{V}O_2$ was 3% to 5% higher when the athletes were tested while performing their specific sport versus when tested while running. Clearly, training optimized performance of specific muscles and neuromuscular firing patterns, which was not fully transferable to performance during treadmill running.

Second, on two separate days, a group of male college students were tested on a cycle ergometer. One test involved performing *submaximal* exercise with the arms (pedaling with the arms), and the other involved performing *submaximal* exercise with the legs (pedaling with the legs). Testing was repeated after 5 weeks of daily training, where half of the students trained using their arms only and the other half with their legs only.[57,117] The results are shown in figure 12.3. Notice the specificity of responses. For each variable, the magnitude of the posttraining changes were always greater when the submaximal testing was performed with the limbs that underwent training versus the limbs that were untrained. Again, these results emphasize the specific nature of the physiological changes induced by training.

Progressive Overload

The term *progressive overload* can include changes in *intensity, duration,* or *frequency* of activity. Of these three factors, intensity is probably the most important relative to improving both the aerobic energy systems of the skeletal muscle *and* the organs responsible for the transport of oxygen.

Determining Intensity of Aerobic Training

Before proceeding, we must raise two important questions. First, what constitutes an effective training program? For some it may be a change in resting heart rate, weight

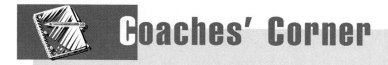

Coaches' Corner

Are Football Players Fit?

We trust that most readers have heard the statement "not all professional athletes are necessarily physically fit." Obviously, one's interpretation depends on their definition of fitness. For example, just prior to his entering training camp in the early 1990s, we measured the peak $\dot{V}O_2$ of a National Football League all-pro running back at 45.2 mL · kg^{-1} · min^{-1}. No matter how you interpret it, for a man in his 20s, this value represents an average level of aerobic fitness. However, by no means did our analysis of his aerobic power infer that he is not a great athlete. In fact, many feel he is one of the greatest running backs of all time. What a peak $\dot{V}O_2$ of 45.2 mL · kg^{-1} · min^{-1} did indicate is specificity of training. As an athlete, he spent the majority of his training time involved with anaerobic-type drills—those that develop world-class neuromuscular coordination, timing, quickness, speed, and explosive power. Therefore, we were not surprised when we did not observe a measured peak $\dot{V}O_2$ indicative of a well-trained, elite endurance athlete.

In fact, the 45.2 mL · kg^{-1} · min^{-1} value we measured was consistent with similar work previously reported by Shields and coworkers.[149] In their study of 167 professional football players, the average max $\dot{V}O_2$ of offensive and defensive lineman was 43.0 mL · kg^{-1} · min^{-1}; for quarterbacks and running backs it was 47.2 mL · kg^{-1} · min^{-1}; and for defensive backs and receivers it was 50.1 mL · kg^{-1} · min^{-1}. Even among their group of professional football players, the concept of specificity of training was evident. Those athletes (lineman) in positions least demanding of aerobic performance exhibited the lowest $\dot{V}O_2$ max; whereas those athletes occupying positions involved with the most running (wide receivers and defensive backs) presented with a slightly higher level of aerobic fitness.

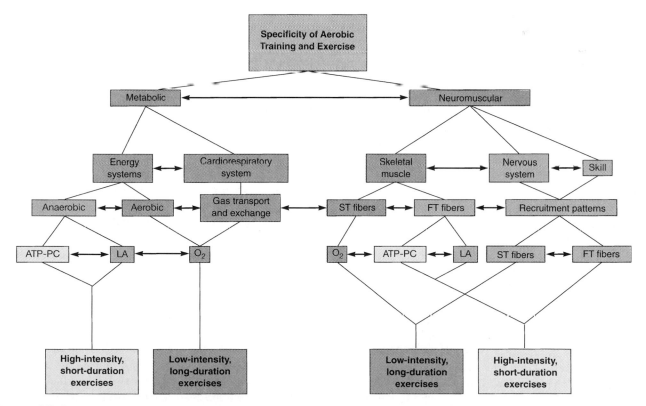

Figure 12.1

A summary of the major (orange), intermediate (blue), and minor (green) physiological factors in the specificity of aerobic training and exercise. The interaction among the various components is indicated by double-headed arrows.

reduction, or an increase in peak $\dot{V}O_2$. For elite athletes it more than likely means improved performance. Therefore, an effective training program is one that safely optimizes an individual's ability to achieve his or her own measure of success or improvement.

Second, we must consider if there is a minimum training intensity or threshold that must be reached before a training effect (physiologic adaptation) is observed. General consensus suggests that such a threshold exists, and among untrained persons it may be as low as 40% to 50% of peak $\dot{V}O_2$. Above this threshold training intensity itself is no longer the sole determining factor. Instead, the total volume of work (intensity, duration, and frequency) becomes the determining factor in fitness development.

During training for endurance-type sports, the general goal is to increase intensity so that $\dot{V}O_2$ falls between 50% to 85% of maximum (figure 12.4). At this level of intensity, repeated bouts of exercise are sufficient to stimulate adaptations within the body. Obviously, well-trained, elite athletes would likely exercise more closely to 85%, maybe even 90%. On the other hand, novices or athletes in the early preseason phase might start in the 70% to 80% range before increasing training intensity over time. That's why it's called *progressive* overload.

Given these facts, and to ensure that $\dot{V}O_2$ during training is at the level we desire, it would seem necessary to measure $\dot{V}O_2$ during each training session—possibly using a metabolic cart or a Douglas bag procedure (page 79). Although doing so would quantify training intensity, it represents both a costly and an impractical approach. Instead, various indirect techniques that correlate well with measured $\dot{V}O_2$ are used to guide exercise intensity. These methods include heart rate measurement, the lactate threshold, or rating of perceived exertion. All can be used to set exercise intensity between 50% and 85% of $\dot{V}O_2$ max. Because of its limited use in training for sport performance, discussion concerning rating of perceived exertion is deferred to chapter 14.

The two primary heart-rate-based methods include the *straight percentage method* and the *heart rate reserve method*. Recall that heart rate and $\dot{V}O_2$ bear a linear relationship: the greater the $\dot{V}O_2$ or exercise intensity, the higher the heart rate (figure 12.4).

The easiest of the two primary heart-rate-based methods is the straight percentage method. In this technique, exercise training heart rate is calculated as a percentage of maximal heart rate, usually between 60% and 90% of maximum. Maximum heart rate can either be directly measured during peak effort on an exercise test, or estimated using the simple formula $220 - \text{age}$.*[167] Why, you might ask, do we set our target heart rate (THR) between 60% and 90% of heart rate max? As figure 12.4 shows, although the rela-

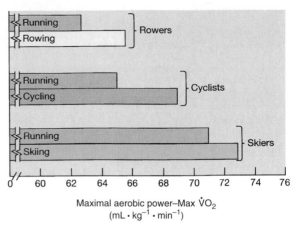

Figure 12.2

The max $\dot{V}O_2$ of three different groups of athletes—rowers, cyclists, and skiers—was determined while they ran on a treadmill and while they performed their specific sport activity. The max $\dot{V}O_2$ was higher when performing the specific sport activity than when running.

(Data from Stromme et al.[157])

tionship between $\dot{V}O_2$ and heart rate is linear, *it is not a one-to-one relationship.* In this case a THR between 60% and 90% of maximum corresponds to a $\dot{V}O_2$ that is between 50% and 85% of maximum. Table 12.1 provides examples of THR ranges computed using the straight percent method in both a 25-year-old and a 75-year-old person.

A second heart-rate-based method for guiding exercise intensity involves the heart rate reserve method. This method was developed by Karvonen[100] and requires that a heart rate reserve first be calculated. **Heart rate reserve** is simply the difference between the resting heart rate and the maximal or peak heart rate. It is an expression of the increase in heart rate that occurs above rest at maximal effort.

For example, suppose your resting heart rate was 65 beats per min and your maximal or peak heart rate was 200 beats per min. Your heart rate reserve would equal 135 beats per min. Alternately, how about a 50-year-old patient who has an elevated resting heart rate of 100 beats per min four weeks after having undergone coronary artery bypass surgery. This is not an uncommon finding among such patients, and given a peak heart rate of—let's say 165 beats per min—his heart rate reserve would be 65 beats per min.

After heart rate reserve has been determined, the THR can be calculated. *This is accomplished by computing a percentage of heart rate reserve—usually between 50% and 85%—and then adding this to the resting heart rate.* Putting all this together and using a 75% level, the formula for computing THR via the heart rate reserve method is as follows:

THR = (peak heart rate − resting heart rate)

× 0.75 + resting heart rate

---

*An alternate method for predicting maximum heart rate is: $210 - (0.65 \times \text{age})$.

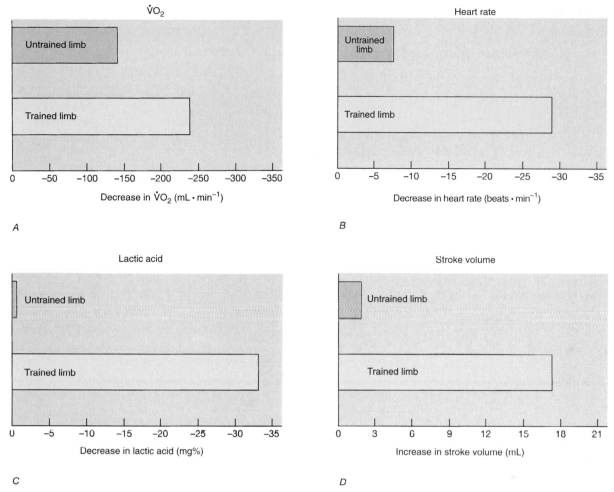

Figure 12.3

Training effects are specific to the muscle groups used during the training program. The magnitude of the posttraining changes were always greater when the exercise was performed with the trained rather than with the untrained muscle groups (limbs).

(Based on data from Fox et al.[57])

A comparison of the two heart-rate-based methods is shown in table 12.1. Note that regardless of the peak heart rate (195 b · min⁻¹ or 145 b · min⁻¹), the difference in THR computed using straight percentage versus heart rate reserve is greatest at the lower end.

Besides heart-rate-based methods, there is another way to guide exercise intensity during endurance training. This approach is based on the *blood lactate threshold.* Recall from chapter 7 that lactate threshold is identified as that point during exercise where a non-linear increase in blood lactate occurs. Since lactic acid results from anaerobic glycolysis within the skeletal muscles, it contributes to blood lactate concentration. The methods used to determine blood lactate threshold are briefly described as follows.

1. When using the *blood lactate threshold method,* a graph plotting measured blood lactate concentration against exercise (e.g., swimming, running) velocity is first constructed (see chapter 7, figure 7.9). That point during exercise where there is a disproportionate increase in blood lactate concentration is termed the lactate threshold. For some athletes, but certainly not all, this value will fall around a blood lactate concentration of 3 to 4 mmol · L⁻¹. Depending on their goals and progress, the athletes then train at a heart rate (or pace) that is just below, at, or just above their blood lactate threshold.

2. Also recall from chapter 7 (page 182) that measuring gas exchange during exercise allows us to estimate lactate threshold (or **anaerobic threshold**).[167] Briefly, carbon dioxide production ($\dot{V}CO_2$) is plotted as a function of $\dot{V}O_2$ in order to identify that point during exercise where the slope of the line exceeds 1.00. Using the V-slope method, endurance athletes then train just below, at, or just above the heart rate or exercise velocity that approximated lactate threshold.

12.1

Exercise intensity for athletic training using two heart-rate-based methods

	Peak heart rate (b · min^{-1})	Resting heart rate (b · min^{-1})	Exercise intensity		Computed exercise training heart rate (b · min^{-1})	
			Lower limit	Upper limit	Lower limit	Upper limit
Subject 1 (Age = 25 years)						
% of Peak*	195	—	70%	90%	137	176
Heart-rate reserve†	195	70	65%	85%	151	176
Subject 2 (Age = 75 years)						
% of Peak*	145	—	70%	90%	102	131
Heart-rate reserve†	145	70	65%	85%	119	134

*Exercise training heart rate computed as follows: lower limit = peak heart rate × 0.7
upper limit = peak heart rate × 0.9

†Exercise training heart rate computed as follows: lower limit = (peak heart rate − resting heart rate) × 0.65 + resting heart rate
upper limit = (peak heart rate − resting heart rate) × 0.85 + resting heart rate

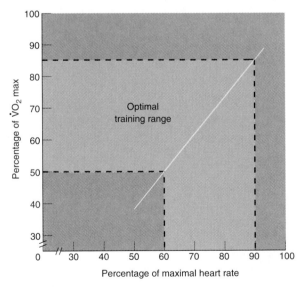

Figure 12.4

Using the straight percentage of peak heart rate method, an exercise heart rate of 60% to 90% of maximum is roughly equivalent to 50% to 85% of $\dot{V}O_2$ max. Within this optimal training range, the stimulus placed on the cardiorespiratory system and skeletal muscles is sufficient to cause adaptive responses.

The physiological difference between heart-rate-based methods and the lactate method lies, somewhat, in the different systems being stressed. For example, with heart-rate-based methods, training intensity is judged mainly by the degree of stress placed on the cardiorespiratory system. Conversely, the lactate threshold method guides exercise intensity based on the degree of stress placed on the metabolic system(s) within the skeletal muscles. On an individual basis, a given degree of stress placed on one system does not guarantee the same degree of stress placed on the other system.

Which method, then, should be used? First, either of the two heart rate methods is easier to use, at least initially, than lactate threshold methods. From a practical standpoint, this certainly is an advantage. Also, when the blood lactate threshold method is used to determine training intensity, the corresponding heart rate will be approximately 85% to 90% of maximum.[104] Alternately, at an exercise heart rate equivalent to 80% of maximum, only 55% of the subjects (table 12.2) will be working at or above their anaerobic threshold.[101] Therefore, to ensure adequate cardiorespiratory and metabolic stress during the endurance training of athletes, heart rate during exercise should be 85% of maximum or greater. An equivalent value using the heart rate reserve method would be obtained if using 80% to 85% of heart rate reserve.

Many studies have shown that with interval or continuous types of training programs, the intensity of the training sessions is of paramount importance in guaranteeing maximal gains in fitness.[6,48,53,114,146] Figure 12.5A shows that as the intensity of the training program is increased, the improvement in max $\dot{V}O_2$ is increased. It also points out that the improvement in max $\dot{V}O_2$ is greater in females than in males at the same relative intensity. The reason for this is not entirely clear. One possible explanation might be that

table 12.2

Percentage of subjects at or above lactate/anaerobic threshold while exercising at different percentages of the maximal heart rate and the maximal heart rate reserve[*]

Percentage of subjects at or above lactate/anaerobic threshold	Exercise heart rate based on percentage of:	
	Maximal heart rate	Heart rate reserve
0	60	40
3	70	55
55	80	70
75	85	80
100	> 90	85

[*]Based on data from Katch et al.[101] and Kindermann et al.[104]

gains in max $\dot{V}O_2$ are inversely related to initial max $\dot{V}O_2$ levels (figure 12.5B).[57,110,138] This means that the lower the initial max $\dot{V}O_2$, the greater the improvement with training. However, differences in improvement in max $\dot{V}O_2$ between males and females being trained at the same relative intensity are not due to the lower initial max $\dot{V}O_2$ of females alone (figure 12.5A). For now we can say that females respond to training as well as, if not better than, males do.

A final point about intensity of exercise: keep in mind that intensity is relative—that is, what is hard for one individual may be easy for another. This is why an individual's training intensity is established as either a percentage of his or her peak heart rate or is based on his or her own measured lactate threshold. It is inappropriate to simply set all persons, especially competitive athletes, on a team at the same absolute training heart rate or pace.

Determining Frequency and Duration of Aerobic Training

Most of the information concerning the influence of training frequency and duration on training effects has come from studies conducted over relatively short periods of time.[54,66,93,110,133] Duration can refer to both the length of a training program (number of weeks or months) and/or the length of a single training session (number of minutes or hours). Generally, the more frequent and the longer (weeks or months) the endurance training program is, the greater will be the fitness benefits.

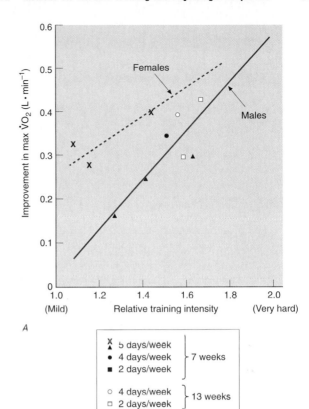

A

X ▲	5 days/week	
●	4 days/week	7 weeks
■	2 days/week	
○	4 days/week	13 weeks
□	2 days/week	

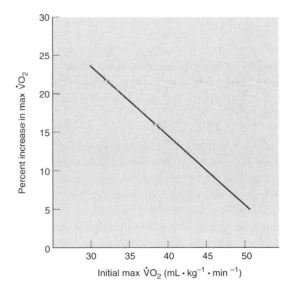

B

Figure 12.5

(*A*) The intensity of the training sessions is of paramount importance in guaranteeing maximal gains in fitness. In this case, as the intensity of the training program is increased from mild (1.0 units) to very hard (2.0 units), the improvement in max $\dot{V}O_2$ is likewise increased. Also, across various intensities, the improvement in max $\dot{V}O_2$ is greater in females than in males at the same relative intensity. (*B*) The gains in max $\dot{V}O_2$ are inversely related to the initial max $\dot{V}O_2$ levels, regardless of the intensity of the training program. Specifically, the lower the initial max $\dot{V}O_2$, the greater the relative improvement with training.

(*Based on data from Fox et al.[53,54] and Cohen and Fox.[26]*)

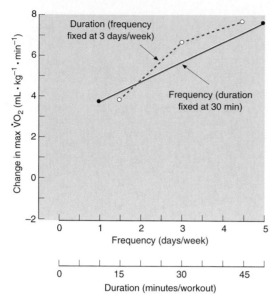

Figure 12.6

Interaction between frequency and duration of training and gains in max $\dot{V}O_2$. For example, a program conducted 1 day per week for 30 minutes resulted in a gain in max $\dot{V}O_2$ comparable to a program conducted 3 days per week for 15 minutes each workout.

(Based on data from Milesis et al.[123] and Gettman et al.[66])

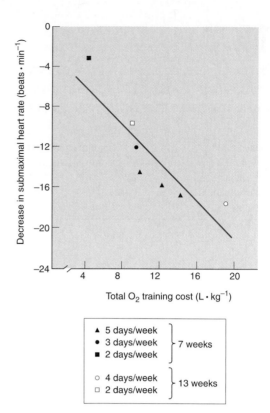

▲ 5 days/week		
● 3 days/week	}	7 weeks
■ 2 days/week		
○ 4 days/week	}	13 weeks
□ 2 days/week		

Figure 12.7

One of the most prominent effects of training frequency and duration is an exercise bradycardia (decreased submaximal-exercise heart rate). The more frequent and intense the training program (expressed as total oxygen cost during training), the greater the decrease in submaximal heart rate.

(Based on data from Fox et al.[54])

A recommended training frequency for endurance programs would be between three and five days per week. However, some sports may require training frequencies of six to seven days per week to optimize skill or technique acquisition.

The influence of frequency and duration on aerobic fitness is shown in figure 12.6. The changes in max $\dot{V}O_2$ induced by walking/running programs of 30 minutes duration for one, three, or five days per week are compared with the changes in max $\dot{V}O_2$ elicited by walking/running programs performed three days per week for 15, 30, or 45 minutes per session. All programs, regardless of duration or frequency, were conducted over a 20-week period and were of equal intensities (88% of the maximum heart rate reserve). What figure 12.6 shows is that frequency and duration of training programs can be "traded off" to produce comparable training effects, provided the same intensity is used over the same number of weeks.

One of the most observed changes related to frequency and duration involves submaximal exercise heart rate. This is illustrated in figure 12.7, where the combined effects of frequency and duration of the training program (expressed on the horizontal axis as *total oxygen cost of training*) are compared to change in heart rate during submaximal exercise. As shown, the greater the oxygen cost of training, the greater the decrease in heart rate during submaximal exercise.

A question often raised concerning training frequency is, do multiple daily workouts lead to greater fitness and performance gains? This question is of particular importance to track and swimming coaches, some of whom advocate two and even three workouts per day. From both a physiologic and a performance standpoint, presently there is no conclusive scientific evidence that multiple daily workouts (two or three per day) lead to greater gains in fitness or performance.[29,126,168]

A summary of the factors involved in the overload principle as applied to aerobic (endurance) training programs is given in table 12.3.

Training Phases

In chapter 11, we discussed much of what is presently known about the off-season, preseason and in-season training programs of various athletes (p. 276). However, we should consider one additional point at this time.

Across a variety of sports at the high school, college, and professional levels, the concept of **tapering** before a big meet or competition is often employed. Several studies, mostly involving runners and swimmers, have shown that

12.3

General guidelines for determining intensity, frequency, and duration of training for an aerobic (endurance-type) sport

Training factor	Guideline
Intensity	Using the straight percent method, heart rate computed at 85% to 90% of peak Using the heart rate reserve method, heart rate computed at 80% to 85% of heart-rate reserve Heart rate that is just below, at, or just above heart rate measured at lactate threshold
Frequency	4 to 6 days per week
Sessions per day	1 (maybe 2)
Minimum	8 weeks
Duration per session	Fast, 25-minute work bouts, with 5 minutes of slow work in between slow, continuous work bout of 30 minutes to 1 hour or more

decreasing training duration by ∼ 80% to 90% some 5 days to 3 weeks[88] before athletic competition is associated with an approximate 3% improvement in athletic performance.[29,87,95,147] This reduction in training duration during the taper may or may not be accompanied by an associated increase in training intensity.

A unique study by Houmard and associates[88] looked at the effects of *training mode* and an 85% reduction in training volume—conducted over seven days—on running performance. One group of runners continued to run during taper; a second group of runners rode a stationary cycle (instead of running) during taper; and the final group of runners maintained their training volume and served as controls. The use of the stationary cycle was meant to test the hypothesis that cycling would improve muscular power and therefore further enhance the benefits of tapering. As figure 12.8 indicates, the run taper group experienced a beneficial 3% reduction in 5 km run time following the taper. However, contrary to their initial hypothesis, there was no additional reduction in 5 km run time among the cycle taper group. In fact, there was no difference in performance after taper between the cycle taper group and the no taper (control) group. This study, therefore, suggested that the use of nonweight-bearing exercise (i.e., cycling) during the taper can maintain, but does not enhance, performance. The fact that it maintained run performance during the taper is of importance. Why? Because for athletes trying to care for an injury while at the same time prepare for an upcoming competition, a cycle taper allows for nonweight-bearing recovery without sacrificing performance.

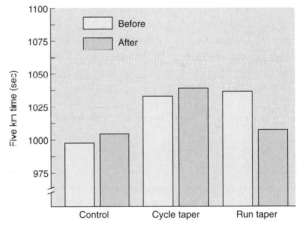

Figure 12.8

The effects of a seven-day taper on 5-km run time. No improvement in performance was observed for the group that did not undergo taper (control) or the group that cycled as their mode of exercise during taper. Note, however, the ∼3% decrease in run time after taper in the run taper group.

(Used with permission from Houmard et al.[88])

Warm-Up and Cool-Down Exercises

The physiological rationale behind the use of proper warm-up and cool-down activities are described on pages 278–279. Part of that discussion includes the important role that active (versus rest) recovery plays in removing lactate from the blood. Based on this information, it would seem that

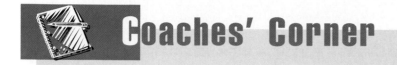

For some athletes, performance during competition is often better (or worse) than what we, as exercise scientists, are able to predict based on measurements made in the laboratory. One reason for the discrepancy between what we measure in the laboratory and what we see on the field has to do with how we go about our laboratory testing. For instance, the pattern of how power is generated during a treadmill running test is markedly different from how power is generated during a soccer match or ice hockey game. Therefore, part of the science of coaching involves being sure that the improvements measured during field or laboratory tests accurately reflect gains made in competition.

To illustrate, 20 professional soccer players from the Danish National League were subjected to various laboratory tests.[9] These tests included intermittent running to exhaustion (felt to be a good measure of soccer specific endurance capacity), muscle biopsies for enzymes and structure, and blood lactate and max $\dot{V}O_2$ measurements during treadmill running. Subjects also completed a unique 16.5 min high- and low-intensity interval field test involving the different forms of locomotion (side-stepping, backwards running, forwards running) used in soccer. The authors found that traditional laboratory tests, such as max $\dot{V}O_2$, blood lactate during submaximal running, and muscle biopsy,

were poor methods for predicting soccer-specific endurance capacity. However, performance during the high- and low-intensity interval field test was strongly associated with endurance capacity and therefore represented a more sensitive and realistic method to test endurance capacity among soccer players.

Foster and associates[50] took the above concept one step further and modified testing so that the pattern of how power output was generated during laboratory assessment mimicked that experienced during actual competition. In their study, four male and four female athletes (ice skaters, cyclists, triathletes) completed both a 5 km simulated time trial on a modified racing bicycle and a graded exercise test using a standard cycle ergometer. Results showed that max $\dot{V}O_2$ was 6% higher, peak heart rate was 5% higher, and blood lactate was 24% higher during the 5 km time trial versus the standard cycle ergometer. The take-home message is, how we test our athletes (the protocol we select) and what we use to test them (the equipment we use) influences the results we obtain during testing.

The science of coaching, therefore, must involve not only our ability to quantify changes in an athlete's performance over time, but it must do so in a manner that best simulates athletic competition.

---

active recovery is the preferred method of recovery. However, this is not always the case. According to a study by Choi and co-workers,[25] although blood lactate concentration at 10 minutes and 30 minutes after intense exercise was indeed lower with active versus passive recovery, at one hour after exercise any observable difference had disappeared. More importantly, at one hour after exercise muscle glycogen level was actually higher with passive than with active recovery.

This dichotomy between improved lactate removal with active recovery versus greater muscle glycogen resynthesis with passive recovery carries practical implications. Specifically, the type of recovery we choose will depend, in part, on whether or not another bout of activity (multibout activities) is to be performed soon after completing the last one. If another bout of intense aerobic activity is to be conducted within the next hour, then an active recovery period should be used to remove lactate during cool down. If, on the other hand, the highest possible level of muscle glyco-

gen is needed and the next "glycogen-demanding" match is not scheduled to begin for at least one hour, then a passive recovery period, such as slow walking, might be employed. This will allow sufficient time to both clear muscle lactate and to enhance glycogen resynthesis. This information might best be applied to tournament play, such as that with soccer, tennis, basketball or wrestling.

Training Methods for Aerobic Performance

Before plunging into the various methods of developing improved endurance performance, it is essential that we pause for a moment and review the big picture relative to aerobic power or fitness. Recall that the physiological capacities needed to perform aerobic or endurance sports involve the cardiorespiratory system, the metabolic capacities of the skeletal muscles, and neuromuscular function. Specifically,

table 12.4

Training practices typical of national and elite-class runners, swimmers, and cyclists

	Volume of training	Aerobic training	Anaerobic training	Training at race pace or faster	Seasonal variations
Runners	80–100 miles/wk	1–3 hr runs	Fartlek or longer intervals 1–2 times/wk	1 time/wk	• Greatest training volume achieved during off-season and preseason • Peak 1–2 times/yr
Swimmers	7,000–15,000 meters/day*	Frequent, longer intervals with very short rest periods	At least 1–2 shorter distance interval sets/day (approximately 500–1,000 meters)	Generally performed only during 2–3 week taper period or 1–2 times/wk during month prior to taper	• Peak 2 times/yr • Shortened off-season (2–3 weeks/yr)
Cyclists	350–500 miles/wk	2–6 hr rides are common	Interval work or Fartlek 1 time/wk	Time trial usually 1 time/wk or every other week	• Mileage increased as season progresses • May peak several times/yr

*The daily volume of training needed by elite swimmers is somewhat controversial, when compared to competitive swimmers who are national class or less. It appears that elite swimmers can handle and need more training volume to attain peak performance. Table developed courtesy of Dr. Jonathan Ehrman.

the body operates as an integrated system that, when optimized through training, can sustain an enormous power output over an extended period of time.

Coyle,[31] Sjodin and Svedenhag,[151] and Pate and Branch[131] all recognized this interplay between organ systems when they discussed the integration of the various factors that contribute to endurance performance. Several of the broader factors they cited that influence performance include *resistance to movement, velocity at lactate threshold, performance* $\dot{V}O_2$, *economy of movement, primary fuel supply,* and $\dot{V}O_2$ *max.* Most all of these factors are, themselves, influenced by other components operating at the organ system or cellular level. The message, therefore, is that a superior $\dot{V}O_2$ max, in and of itself, does not guarantee success in endurance performance—other factors are involved, and training strategies should be developed accordingly.

Like anaerobic training practices, various methods exist that promote the development of endurance performance.[131] They include long-duration, moderate-intensity training; moderate-duration, high-intensity training; and short-duration, very high-intensity training. These methods and the Fartlek training method are discussed below and incorporated into table 12.4. We conclude this section discussing a topic of contemporary interest: *cross-training.*

Long-Duration, Moderate-Intensity Training

This method of endurance training involves 30 min to 2 hr or more of continuous exercise (running, cycling, Nordic skiing, swimming), usually performed over relatively long distances. This is perhaps the most common element in contemporary endurance training programs and is sometimes referred to as LSD (long, slow distance).[33] The pace will vary from athlete to athlete. For example, for running the pace might be 8 min per mile for an inexperienced athlete and less than 6 min per mile for the international class competitor. However, no matter what the pace or the sport, the intensity of exercise generally increases heart rate to 75% to 85% of maximum or about 60% to 70% of max $\dot{V}O_2$. For most athletes this pace is below lactate threshold, and as a result, it is slower than race pace.

Moderate-Duration, High-Intensity Training

In this method of endurance training, often referred to as *pace* or **tempo training,** exercise intensity is set very near an athlete's lactate threshold—at heart rates that approach

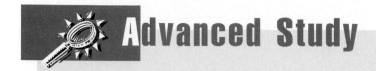

Resistance to movement (drag) affects performance. For example, while road cycling at 40 km · hr^{-1}, over 80% of the power generated by the athlete is used to overcome drag caused by equipment and athlete. As a result, the more aerodynamic both the equipment (bicycle, helmet) and the athlete can become, the less drag that results and the faster the performance.

For example, consider the cyclist who won the 1995 pursuit race world championship using a riding position where his head was positioned far in front of (and below) the handlebars of his bicycle. His arms were tucked under his chest. Upon review, the International Cycling Union declared that this position was too dangerous, and as a result, it was banned from use during competition.

Less dangerous and fully accepted among governing sport organizations is the concept of reducing drag through the practice of drafting. In this technique athletes take turns leading and following one another to save energy. As the lead athlete encounters the full impact of resistance to movement (and expends more energy), the second (third and fourth) athlete(s) drafts in his or her less turbulent windstream. This allows those athletes following the lead athlete to "rest" for a bit without having to sacrifice pace. While in the lead position, the athlete willingly works harder, knowing that he or she too will soon be in the draft position. The net effect is that a faster pace is intentionally set by the lead athlete, increasing the overall pace for the event.

Most studies on the effects of drafting have been conducted using ice speed skaters and cyclists. However, in 1993 Bilodeau and associates[17] studied three pairs (matched for $\dot{V}O_2$ max) of cross-country skiers asked to ski around a 1 km course. Athletes in each pair took turns skiing in the lead and in the draft positions, and the distance between skiers was maintained at 2.5 m. Not surprisingly, average heart rate for athletes skiing in the draft position was 9 beats lower than while skiing in the lead position. Results also showed that the lowest heart rates were achieved when smaller skiers drafted behind larger skiers.

The observed influence of drag is less noticeable when sports are performed at slower (e.g., running, race walking) versus faster (e.g., skating, cycling) velocities. Fedel and coworkers demonstrated this during a study of 12 male in-line skaters asked to skate first in the upright (torso near vertical) and then the bent (torso near horizontal) positions.[49] Each skater conducted trials at both 22.5 km · h^{-1} and 27.4 km · h^{-1}. During steady-state skating at the slower velocity of 22.5 km · h^{-1}, no differences were observed for heart rate or $\dot{V}O_2$ when comparing the upright and bent positions. However, when asked to skate at 27.4 km · h^{-1} the mean increases in heart rate and $\dot{V}O_2$ were 12 b · min^{-1} and 7.3 mL · kg^{-1} · min^{-1} greater, respectively, while skating in the upright versus the bent position. When skating at the slower velocity any difference in wind resistance because of body position was negligible, with respect to influencing cardiorespiratory response. However, skating at the faster velocity provided a wind resistance or drag that influenced cardiorespiratory response when changes in body position (upright versus horizontal) occurred.

The idea of having the athlete make himself (or his equipment) as aerodynamic as possible applies to swimmers as well (i.e., hydrodynamics). Drag (from water) is very important during competition, to the extent that some swimmers move over and swim as close to the lane line as possible to "surf" off the wake of a nearby competitor.

85% to 90% of maximum. Exercise is generally still continuous in nature (30 to 60 min) but duration is shortened because of the increased intensity. If exercise intensity is increased even further, so that the athlete is working just above lactate threshold, then duration is shortened to 4 min to 10 min. This type of training is referred to as either *repetition training* or *aerobic interval training*. The approach is similar to interval training but differs in that (1) the length of the work interval is longer and (2) the degree of recovery between repetitions is shorter. The main objective of aerobic interval training is to improve tolerance to racing *at* lactate threshold. Among athletes who have "plateaued" rel-

ative to further improvements in max $\dot{V}O_2$, this method may be effective for improving $\dot{V}O_2$ at lactate threshold and/or economy of movement.

Short-Duration, Very High-Intensity Training

This method of training involves a modification of interval training; in fact it is often called **interval sprinting.** Using running as an example, the athlete might alternately sprint 50 m then jog 60 m for distances of up to 3 to 4 continuous miles. Because of fatigue setting in after the first few sprints, the athlete will not be able to run subsequent sprints at top speed. This factor, plus the relatively long distances covered per training session (up to 4.5 km), makes this type of training system suitable for the development of the aerobic system. Both runners and cyclists often incorporate hills into this type of training.

Speed Play or Fartlek Training

Fartlek (a Swedish word meaning "speed play") **training** is said to be the forerunner of the interval-training system. However, neither the work nor the relief intervals are precisely timed, and all exercise is performed continuously. It involves alternating fast and slow exercise over natural terrain. Fartlek training is used by swimmers, runners, and cyclists and should only be used once every week or so. Such a program predominately leads to improvements in aerobic capacity, but improvement in anaerobic ability can be expected as well. An example of a training schedule for a runner using the Fartlek method is as follows:[32]

1. Warm up by running easily for 5 to 10 minutes.
2. Run at a fast, steady speed over a distance of 1.2 to 2 km.
3. Walk rapidly for 5 minutes.
4. Practice easy running, broken by sprints of 60 to 70 m, repeating until fatigue becomes evident.
5. Run easily, injecting 3 to 4 swift steps occasionally.
6. Run at full speed uphill for 150 to 175 m.
7. Run at a fast pace for 1 minute.
8. Finish the routine by running 1 to 5 laps around a 400 m track, depending on the distance run in competition.

Cross-Training

The concept of **cross-training** is not new. For decades, if not longer, athletes have realized that performance can be maintained and recovery from injury speeded along if an alternate mode of work is adopted for a period of time. However, it is only within the past 2 decades, mostly since the popularization of the triathalon and other multisport events among the general public, that the concept of cross-training has been applied so widely.

Although there appears to be no scientific agreement as to a definition of cross-training, the one we favor involves *the transfer of training effects gained in one mode of training to another*[159]—for example, the use of swim training in place of running to influence running performance. Included in this definition are those athletes who add a second mode of exercise to their existing training regimen, such as swim and run training on running performance. A second definition of cross-training, one heralded by Houmard and associates,[88] is *the practice of changing one's mode of activity to either facilitate recovery from injury or to lessen the likelihood of overtraining.* This evokes the concept of "keeping fit when injured."

A practical application of the first definition involves having the athlete choose an alternate form of endurance training (e.g., cycling in place of running), one meant to minimize the risk of injury while at the same time maintaining or further improving cardiorespiratory fitness. Such a practice can be used during the off-season and can involve either muscularly similar tasks (in-line skating in place of ice speed skating[35]) or muscularly dissimilar activities (aerobic dance in place of running[64]). Alternately, during the preseason, athletes might combine two sports—for example running and cycling—to further enhance training volume and subsequent athletic performance. Let's now look at two separate studies that address the concept of cross-training.

In the first study,[51] 30 equally trained runners (10 males, 20 females) were randomized to one of three different groups. The first group increased their running volume by 10%, the second group also increased their training volume by 10% but did so by swimming, and the third group served as a control group and did not increase their weekly running mileage. The investigators found that enhanced training volume via either running or swimming had no effect on max $\dot{V}O_2$ during treadmill running. More importantly, of the three groups, only the two groups who underwent enhanced training showed any improvement in a two-mile timed run trial. A 3% improvement was observed in two-mile run time among those in the enhanced running group, and a 1.5% improvement was observed among those in the swim cross-training group.

Mutton and coworkers[127] studied the effects of running four days per week for five weeks versus combined cycle/run training (two days cycling and two days running) on max $\dot{V}O_2$ and running performance. As figure 12.9 indicates, run training and cycle/run training demonstrated somewhat equal increases in max $\dot{V}O_2$ using either treadmill or cycle ergometer testing. Similar improvements (7% and 8%) were observed in 5 km run times as well.

The above-mentioned studies demonstrate that cross-training can enhance training volume and/or successfully involve an alternate training modality. At the same time it can maintain or possibly improve aerobic performance. We must point out, however, that despite the wide-spread claims as to the success of cross-training, very few actual scientific studies specifically address the issue. An excellent review of the cross-training topic is provided by Tanaka.[159] At minimum, cross-training appears to be an appropriate supplement to maintain endurance performance during periods of recovery or rehabilitation.

Before leaving the topic of cross-training we hope that the attentive reader has pondered about a somewhat obvious question—specifically, the contradictory approach cross-training may represent relative to the principle of specificity of training. Haven't we learned that the cardiorespiratory, neuromuscular, and skeletal muscle gains

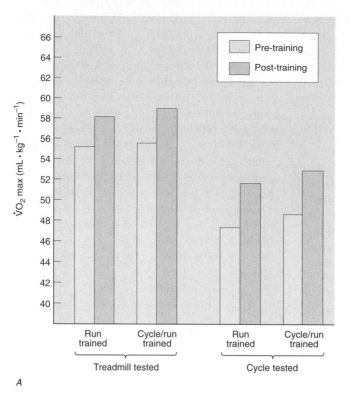

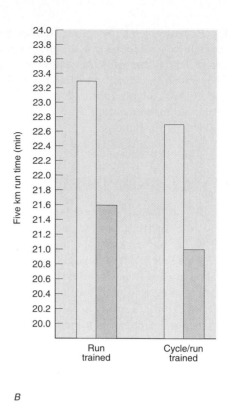

A

B

Figure 12.9

Effects of run training and cross-training (cycle/run) on (*A*) max $\dot{V}O_2$ during treadmill and cycle training, and (*B*) 5-km timed run trials.

(Based on data from Mutton et al.[127])

made through endurance training are specific for the activity of choice? The answer is an unequivocal yes! Therefore, the "take-home message" here is that the adaptations induced through cross-training never exceed those induced by sport-specific training. This concept is especially true among highly trained athletes.

Physiological Effects of Aerobic Training

For our purposes, the effects of endurance training can be studied most easily by classifying the changes as follows: (1) those occurring within the skeletal muscle and (2) those occurring *systemically*—that is, those affecting the circulatory and respiratory systems. Throughout this text we address various other changes that occur with training, such as those concerned with body composition (chapter 16), blood lipids (chapter 14), blood pressure (chapter 9), and heat acclimatization (chapter 19). Finally, except where noted, readers can assume that the adaptations we discuss secondary to endurance training occur similarly among males and females.

Aerobic Training and the Skeletal Muscle

Although much research continues to occur at the subcellular and molecular levels, the effects of physical training on skeletal muscle histology* and general biochemistry is now well defined. Several of these adaptations are discussed in this section.

Biochemical Changes

The "metabolic mill" found within skeletal muscle undergoes fabulous changes in response to exercise training. All of these adaptations lead to an improved ability to generate ATP.

1. *Increased Myoglobin Content.* **Myoglobin**'s main function is in aiding the intracellular movement (delivery) of oxygen from the cell membrane to the mitochondria where it is consumed. The myoglobin content of skeletal muscle has been shown to be substantially increased following endurance training,[124]

---

*Histology is the microscopic study of the structure, function, and composition of the tissues.

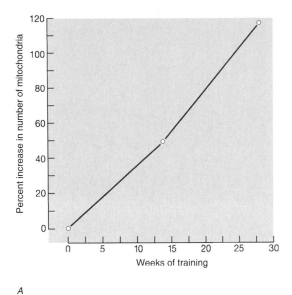

A

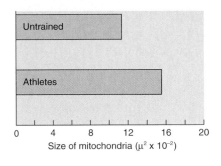

B

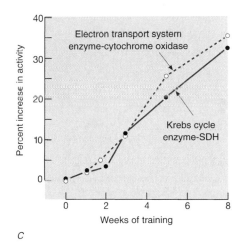

C

Figure 12.10

Major subcellular adaptations that contribute to the muscle cells' increased capacity to oxidize carbohydrate following training are an increased (*A*) number and (*B*) size of muscle mitochondria, and (*C*) an increased level of activity of the enzymes involved in the Krebs Cycle (e.g., succinate dehydrogenase, or SDH) and electron transport system (cytochrome oxidase).

(Data in A and B from Kiessling et al.[103]; data in C from Henriksson and Reitman.[78])

possibly by as much as 75% to 80%. This response is specific because myoglobin increases only in those muscles involved in the training program. Hickson[81] has shown, in studies with rats, that myoglobin increases are associated with the frequency of training. With exercise at two days, four days, and six days per week, myoglobin levels increased 14%, 18%, and 26%, respectively.

2. *Improved Oxidation of Carbohydrate (Glycogen).*
   Training increases the capacity of skeletal muscle to completely break down glycogen in the presence of oxygen to CO_2, H_2O, and ATP. The two major subcellular adaptations that contribute to the muscle cells' ability to accomplish this are (1) increases in the number, size, and membrane surface area of skeletal muscle mitochondria;[28,70,84] and (2) an increase in the level of activity and/or concentration of the enzymes involved in the Krebs Cycle and the electron transport system.[11,13,34,68,84]

Generally, the number of mitochondria per myofibril is less in females than in males.[28,86] Regardless, several studies[70,84,86] show an increase in the number and the size of mitochondria following training. For example, as shown in figure 12.10*A*, a 120% increase in the number of mitochondria in the vastus lateralis muscle was observed following a 28-week, 5-days-per-week training program of distance running and calisthenics. The increase in mitochondrial size (figure 12.10*B*) is not as large as the increase in number, averaging in humans between 14% and 40% greater in athletes versus nonathletes.[86,103] This too, is likely a specific response, occurring only in those muscle fibers involved in the training program.

Recall from chapter 2 that the many metabolic reactions involved in the Krebs Cycle and electron transport system are controlled by the presence of specific enzymes. A dramatic increase among these

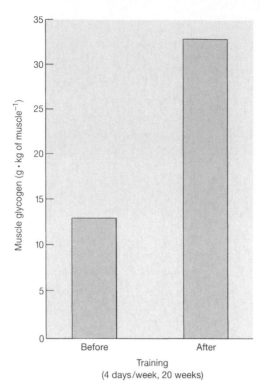

Figure 12.11

Human skeletal muscle normally contains between 13 and 15 grams of glycogen per kilogram of muscle. After training, this amount has been shown to increase as much as 2.5 times.

(Based on data from Gollnick et al.[68])

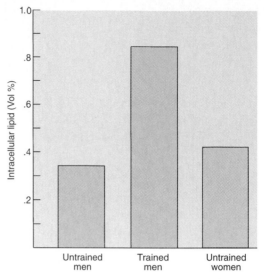

Figure 12.12

Intramuscular fat stores have been found to be as much as $1\frac{1}{2}$ times greater in endurance-trained, male athletes compared with their untrained counterparts. Intramuscular fat stores between untrained men and women are similar.

(Based on data from Hoppeler et al.[86])

enzymes occurs secondary to training, meaning that more ATP can be produced in the presence of oxygen. The activity of the aerobic enzymes in rat skeletal muscle have been shown to double following a 12-week, 5-days-per-week training program.[84] In humans, as shown in figure 12.10C, the increase in just 8 weeks of training approaches 40%.[78]

Aside from the increased ability of muscle to oxidize glycogen, there is also an increase in the amount of glycogen stored in the muscle following training.[68,69] As stated in chapter 2, human skeletal muscle normally contains between 13 and 15 grams of glycogen per kilogram of muscle. After training, this amount has been shown to increase 2.5 times[68] (figure 12.11). This increase in glycogen storage is due, in part, to the fact that training causes increased activity of the enzymes responsible for glycogen synthesis and breakdown (glycogen cycle enzymes).[160]

3. *Improved Oxidation of Fat.* Like glycogen, the breakdown (oxidation) of fat to CO_2, H_2O, and ATP is increased following training.[67,124,128] Because fat serves as a major source of fuel for skeletal muscle during endurance exercise, an increased capacity to oxidize fat is a definite advantage in increasing endurance. Actually, at a given submaximal work load, the trained person oxidizes more fat and less carbohydrate than does the untrained person.[67,79,94,141] During heavy but submaximal exercise, a greater fat oxidation would mean less glycogen depletion, less lactic acid accumulation, and less muscular fatigue.[34]

The increase in the muscles' capacity to oxidize fat following endurance training is related to three factors. First, increases in muscle triglyceride stores have been demonstrated in humans following endurance training (figure 12.12).[86,160] Specifically, fat stores within the skeletal muscle cell were $1\frac{1}{2}$ times greater in endurance-trained male athletes compared with their untrained counterparts. Intramuscular fat stores between untrained men and women were the same.

Second, previous studies indicate that increased availability of fats to the skeletal muscle can have a positive effect on endurance performance.[19,27,83] This response leads to a glycogen-sparing effect, which results from greater fat oxidation. Third, there is an increase in the enzymes responsible to break down the large fat molecules prior to their entry into both the beta-oxidation pathway and the Krebs Cycle. This includes increases in the enzymes that work within these two metabolic pathways.[13]

Changes in Type I and Type II Muscle Fibers

With endurance training the overall aerobic potential of skeletal muscle is increased equally in both Type I and Type II fibers.[8,69] This means that the inherent differences in

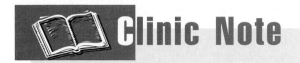

Clinic Note

Exercise and Heart Failure

Patients with heart failure have a reduced (weakened) pumping capacity of the heart (ejection fraction usually < 35%), a reduced peak heart rate, and an overactive sympathetic nervous system (as evidenced by increases in resting heart rate and plasma norepinephrine). Additionally, these patients often show symptoms of fatigue during even mild to moderate exertion. The cause of their exercise intolerance seems to be several fold. For example, peak cardiac output to and peak blood flow within the skeletal muscles are reduced during exercise, both of which contribute to a reduced transport of oxygen to the skeletal muscles.

When compared to age-matched healthy controls, patients with heart failure also show abnormalities of the skeletal muscle fibers.[119,158] Specifically, and somewhat surprisingly, the percentage of Type I fibers (slow oxidative) is reduced, and there is an increase in Type II fibers—mostly Type IIB (fast glycolytic). Additionally, there are reductions in capillary density, mitochondrial volume, and the oxidative enzymes of the Krebs Cycle. As you might surmise, such changes limit the ability of these patients to utilize oxygen and to sustain endurance type activities.

The mechanism(s) responsible for the histologic and biochemical changes stated above are not entirely known. Perhaps it is caused by the reduced blood flow within the skeletal muscle or by alterations in the firing pattern of the motor neuron that innervates the muscle fibers. Additionally, most of these skeletal muscle changes might simply be the result of the inactive lifestyle which many of these patients are forced to lead.

In any event, the good news is that several investigators have shown that moderate, regular exercise can reverse the exercise intolerance that these patients experience.[75,102] When combined with maximal medical therapy, exercise training can lead to a decrease in resting heart rate, a decrease in blood catecholamine levels, and a 15% to 30% increase in max $\dot{V}O_2$. Such an increase is partly caused by improvement in cardiac output (heart rate and stroke volume), and improvements within the skeletal muscle have been shown as well. The latter includes increases in mitochondrial density and aerobic enzyme activity. In clinical practice, the therapeutic role of exercise training in this special patient population is becoming more commonplace, helping them lead more comfortable and symptom-free lives.

---

oxidative capacity between the fiber types is not altered by training. In other words, the Type I fiber has a higher aerobic capacity than the Type II fiber, both before and after endurance training.

Additionally, among both male and female endurance athletes, Type I fibers occupy a greater area of the muscle than do Type II fibers.[28,69] The converse is true for anaerobically trained athletes, such as shot putters and sprinters. This information implies a selective hypertrophy dependent on the kind of training and/or sports activities performed by the athletes.

Finally, among healthy persons, most evidence suggests that there is no interconversion of Type I and Type II fibers as a result of aerobic training. With aerobic training, however, there can be a gradual conversion of Type IIB (fast glycolytic) to Type IIA (fast oxidative glycolytic) fibers without gross changes in the ratio between Type I and Type II fibers. In one study, subjects trained for eight weeks on a bicycle working at 81% of their aerobic capacity. Following training, Type IIA fibers were observed to have increased from 65% to 75% of all Type II fibers. The percentage of Type I (slow-oxidative) fibers remained the same as before.[2]

Interestingly, prolonged (up to 20 years) exposure to endurance training does not appear to impact fiber composition. In a study of 28 highly trained distance runners assessed in 1973 and then again in 1992, increases in the percentage of Type I fibers occurred most often among those subjects who either discontinued their training regimen or continued their training habits at lesser amounts for fitness purposes only.[163] A group of men that remained highly trained—especially those initially characterized by a high percentage (> 70% to 80%) of Type I fibers—showed no change at follow-up testing some 20 years later. It appears, therefore, that the percentage of Type I fibers is increased from young adulthood to middle age, especially among those persons who do not initially display a relatively high (< 70%) percentage of fibers. A summary of changes that result within the skeletal muscle secondary to aerobic training is given in table 12.5.

Cardiorespiratory (Systemic) Changes

The cardiorespiratory (systemic) changes induced by training include those that affect mainly the oxygen transport system. As pointed out in chapter 9, the oxygen transport system involves many circulatory, respiratory, and

12.5

Biochemical changes in skeletal muscle induced by endurance physical training

Aerobic changes

Increased myoglobin content
Increased oxidation of glycogen
    Increased number and size of mitochondria
    Increased activities of Krebs Cycle and electron
        transport system enzymes
    Increased muscular stores of glycogen
Increased oxidation of fat
    Increased muscular stores of triglycerides
    Increased availability of fats as fuels
    Increased activity of enzymes involved in fatty acid
        activation, transport, and oxidation

Relative changes in Type I and Type II muscle fibers

Increased aerobic capacity equal in both fiber types
Selective hypertrophy:
    Type I—endurance training
No fiber type conversion

tissue-level factors, all working together for one common goal—to deliver oxygen to the working muscles. First, we will discuss changes that are observable under resting conditions, and then we will outline the systemic changes that are evident during submaximal and maximal exercise.

Changes at Rest

There are six main changes resulting from training that are apparent at rest: (1) an increased heart size (cardiac hypertrophy), (2) a decreased heart rate, (3) an increased stroke volume, (4) little or no change in resting lung measures, (5) an increased blood volume and hemoglobin, and (6) an increased capillary density and hypertrophy of skeletal muscle.

1. *Increased Heart Size.* As discussed in chapter 11 (page 289), the overall size of the heart is generally greater (hypertrophy) among athletes than nonathletes.[36,41,65,116,134,136,143,144,156,164,165,172] And, using echocardiography, we know that the increase in heart size is caused by an increase in the size of the cavity of the ventricles and/or an increase in the thickness of the ventricular wall.

    a. The cardiac hypertrophy of endurance athletes (e.g., distance runners, swimmers, and field hockey players) is usually characterized by a *large ventricular cavity* and a *normal thickness* of the ventricular wall. This means that the volume of blood that fills the ventricle during diastole is also larger. We will soon see that this effect

causes the stroke volume capabilities of the endurance athlete to be greater than those of both the anaerobically trained athlete and the nonathlete. Using two-dimensional echocardiography, figure 12.13 clearly shows the difference in left ventricular cavity size when comparing an endurance-trained athlete to a normal healthy control. Be aware, however, that the "enlarged" heart observed in the athlete does not exceed the upper limit for a normal sized heart (5.6 cm).

    b. The cardiac hypertrophy of nonendurance athletes—that is, athletes engaged in anaerobic activities such as wrestling and short-distance sprinting—is generally characterized by a *normal-sized ventricular cavity* and a *thicker ventricular wall*. Therefore, although the magnitude of the cardiac hypertrophy in these athletes is the same as in endurance athletes, their stroke volume capabilities are similar to those of nonathletes.

    The different types of cardiac hypertrophy resulting from physical training are shown in figure 12.14.

    Just how does training influence whether or not the heart experiences an increase in ventricular cavity size or an increase in ventricular wall thickness? The answer appears to be related to the type of mechanical stress placed on the heart. For example, training for endurance activities usually requires prolonged bouts of exercise during which the cardiac output is sustained at higher levels.[56] This type of stimuli is called *volume overload*. On the other hand, athletes who participate in brief but powerful activities, such as wrestling and putting the shot, intermittently subject themselves to marked elevations of arterial blood pressure. In this case the stimulus is termed *pressure overload*.

    Remember that the response of the left ventricular (cavity size or wall thickness) to physical training is variable.[43,61,155] If an increase in heart size is not observed, one must question whether the imposed training stimulus was of sufficient intensity and/or duration to elicit the changes expected. Literally, months, if not years, of training may be required before the changes described above become evident.

2. *Decreased Heart Rate.* The decrease in resting heart rate or bradycardia (heart rate < 60 beats · min⁻¹) that often results from training is:

    a. most evident among cross-sectional studies where athletes are compared to nonactive persons (figure 12.15*A*)

    b. less evident but still clearly observable among nonactive persons who undergo a training program, and

    c. least distinct when athletes previously studied in the trained state are subsequently studied in the untrained state.[59]

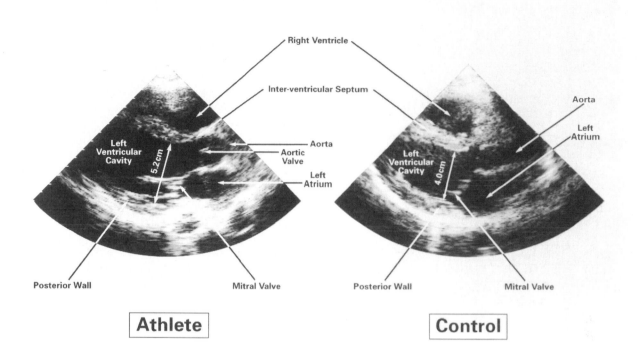

Right Ventricle

Inter-ventricular Septum

Aorta

Left Atrium

Left Ventricular Cavity

5.2cm

Aorta

Aortic Valve

Left Atrium

Posterior Wall

Mitral Valve

Left Ventricular Cavity

4.0cm

Posterior Wall

Mitral Valve

Athlete

Control

Figure 12.13

Two-dimensional echocardiographs of a 28-year-old male competitive cyclist (athlete) and a 27-year-old nonexercising medical resident (control). Note the larger left ventricular end-diastolic cavity in the athlete (5.2 cm) versus the control (4 cm). In both cases the size of the left ventricular cavity is within normal limits (< 5.6 cm). Both measures were made at the tip of the mitral valve.

Photo courtesy of Dr. John Schairer.

We've also learned that:

a. the extent of the training bradycardia is related to the duration (maybe years) of intensive training, and

b. the magnitude of the decrease in resting heart rate produced by training is greater when the initial level of fitness is lower

What causes this training bradycardia at rest? Recall (p. 253) that the heart is regulated by the two components of the autonomic nervous system: (1) the sympathetic nerves, which, when stimulated, increase heart rate; and (2) the vagus (parasympathetic) nerves, which lead to a decrease in rate when stimulated. With this type of dual neural input, the heart rate can be decreased by increased parasympathetic (vagal) tone, decreased sympathetic tone, or a combination of these. Existing evidence supports all three theories[59,90,150,154,162,170]; however, since it is the parasympathetic nervous system that predominantly regulates heart rate at rest, it's no wonder that the training-induced bradycardia is mostly due to increased vagal tone.[148,154]

Before moving on, another factor that must be introduced when discussing training-induced bradycardia is the *intrinsic rate of the atrial pacemaker* or S-A node.[7,150,152] (See further discussion on the S-A node in chapter 9, p. 217). If the intrinsic rate of the S-A is reset (decreased) with exercise training, then the heart rate would beat slower, independently of the influences of the autonomic nervous system. Such slowing of the S-A node could be caused by (1) an increased level of acetylcholine (the parasympathetic neurotransmitter) found in atrial tissue following exercise training;[7] (2) a decreased sensitivity of cardiac tissue (i.e., the beta$_1$ receptors) to *catecholamines* (which are a class of chemicals that includes dopamine, epinephrine, and norepinephrine); or (3) a mechanical effect related to a training-induced change in cardiac dimensions (cavity size or wall thickness). Any effect exercise training

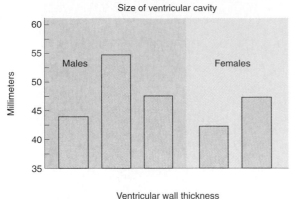

Size of ventricular cavity

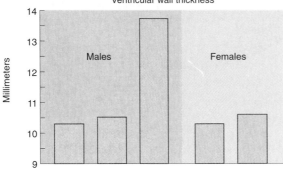

Ventricular wall thickness

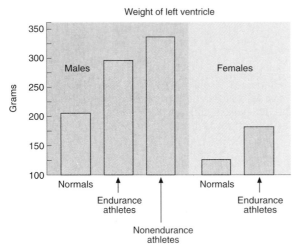

Weight of left ventricle

Figure 12.14

The cardiac hypertrophy of endurance athletes is characterized by a large ventricular cavity with a normal thickness of the wall. On the other hand, the cardiac hypertrophy of nonendurance athletes is characterized by a thicker ventricular wall with a normal-sized ventricular cavity.

(Male data from Morganroth et al.[125]; female data from Zeldis et al.[172])

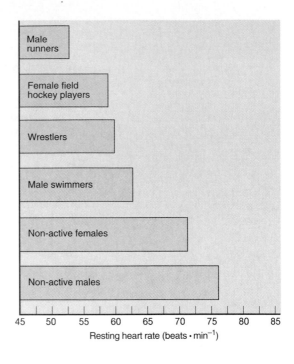

A

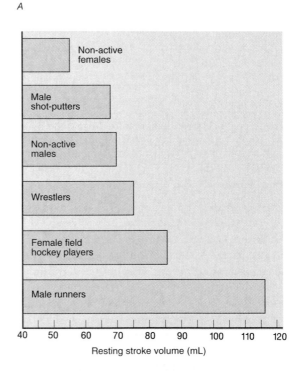

B

Figure 12.15

(*A*) Training induces a resting bradycardia (a decreased heart rate). (*B*) Training induces an increased resting stroke volume. The magnitude of the bradycardia is generally the same in endurance and nonendurance athletes, but the increase in stroke volume is most pronounced in endurance athletes.

(Male data from Morganroth et al.[125]; female data from Zeldis et al.[172])

table 12.6

Normal values of hemoglobin (Hgb), blood volume (Bv), and heart volume (Hv) for trained and untrained men and women[*]

Subjects	Mean age (yr)	Hgb (g)	Hgb (g · kg^{-1})	Hgb concentration (g · 100 mL^{-1} blood)	Bv (L)	Bv (mL · kg^{-1})	Hv (mL)	Hv (mL · kg^{-1})
Untrained								
Females	37.6	555	8.5	13.6	4.07	62.1	560	8.5
Males	24.0	805	11.6	15.3	5.25	75.0	785	11.2
Trained								
Females	26.0	800	12.5	14.1	5.67	88.6	790	12.3
Males	36.0	995	13.7	15.1	6.58	90.1	930	12.7

[*]Based on data from Kjellberg et al.[105,106]

may have on the intrinsic rate of the S-A node does not appear to occur with relatively short duration programs (weeks to months) and is more likely associated with years of elite-level training.[115,148,154]

3. *Increased Stroke Volume.* Because resting cardiac output is approximately the same for trained and nontrained subjects, it is easy to see (recall $\dot{Q} = SV \times HR$) why the resting stroke volume of trained athletes is higher than that of their nonathletic counterparts (figure. 12.15*B*).[14,125] Specifically, consistent with the lower resting heart rate that occurs in trained versus untrained athletes, resting stroke volume must be greater if cardiac output is to be similar between the two groups. This increase in stroke volume is most pronounced in endurance athletes because, as explained previously, these athletes generally have an increased ventricular cavity (allowing more blood to fill the ventricle during diastole). Another factor contributing to the exercise training-induced increase in resting stroke volume may be an associated increase in myocardial contractility.[41,122,144] An increase in contractility could be related to increases in ATPase activity within the heart muscle[15,16,145] and/or to enhanced interaction of the cellular contractile elements (due to enhanced extracellular calcium availability).[10,161]

The greater resting stroke volume is felt by many to be the best indicator of the trained versus the untrained state. Such a stroke volume requires a long-term training program (years), which explains why when previously untrained subjects train for only weeks to several months, an increased resting stroke volume may not be observed.[43]

4. *Little or No Change in Resting Lung Measures.* Minute ventilation (liters of air exhaled per min) is generally

unchanged at rest following exercise training. And, despite what you might think, endurance training has little effect on resting lung volumes (chapter 7). Overall, **total lung capacity** is generally unchanged or may be increased slightly, while there is a small increase in vital capacity and a slight decrease in **residual volume.** At best, only a poor relationship exists between improvement in athletic performance and whatever changes might occur in lung volumes.

5. *Increased Blood Volume and Hemoglobin.* Total blood volume and the total amount of hemoglobin are both increased with endurance training.[105,106,128] An example of these changes among males and females is given in table 12.6. Both parameters are important to the oxygen transport system and are closely correlated with max $\dot{V}O_2$.[4,5] In addition, the increase in blood volume represents an *early* adaptive response to exercise training. Green et al.[72] showed a 12% increase in blood volume after only three days of training (two hours of stationary cycling per day at 65% of max $\dot{V}O_2$).

Students should note that *hemoglobin concentration* does not usually change with training (table 12.6). It may, in fact, decrease slightly. For example, the average hemoglobin concentration for males is ~15 g · 100 mL^{-1} of blood. In a group of highly trained endurance runners, the average hemoglobin concentration was only 14.3 g · 100 mL^{-1} of blood.[44]

6. *Increased Capillary Density and Hypertrophy of Skeletal Muscle.* Capillary density refers to the number of capillaries that surround a skeletal muscle fiber. Long-term endurance training almost always leads to an increased capillary density.[1,3,21,80,91] This effect is shown in figure 12.16*A* and *B*, which also indicates that the muscle fibers

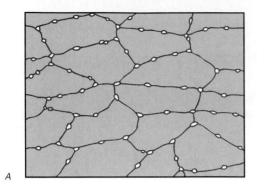

A

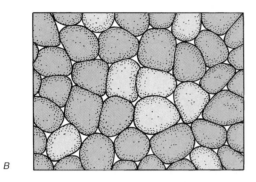

B

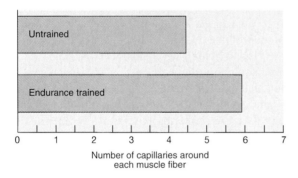

C

Figure 12.16

Training results in hypertrophy of skeletal muscle and increased capillary density. The muscle fibers of the highly trained endurance athlete (A) are 30% larger than the fibers of the untrained subject (B). Additionally, endurance training results in a greater number of capillaries around each muscle fiber (C).

(Data in A and B from Hermansen and Wachtlova[80]; data in C from Brodal et al.[21])

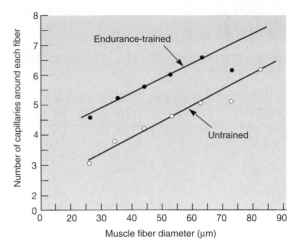

A

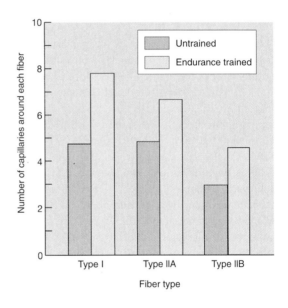

B

Figure 12.17

The number of capillaries surrounding each skeletal muscle fiber is related to: (A) the size or diameter of the muscle fiber (the larger the diameter, the greater the number of capillaries); and (B) the fiber type or number of mitochondria per muscle fiber. Type I fibers generally have more mitochondria than Type II fibers.

(Data in A from Brodal et al.[21]; data in B from Inger.[91])

of highly trained endurance athletes (max $\dot{V}O_2$ = 71.4 mL · kg^{-1} · min^{-1}) are larger (~30%) than those of a group of age-matched untrained subjects (max $\dot{V}O_2$ = 50.2 mL · kg^{-1} · min^{-1}). Among the athletes, each muscle fiber was surrounded on aver-

age by 5.9 capillaries. This differed from the untrained subjects, where capillary density was only 4.4 capillaries per fiber (figure 12.16C). The supply of oxygen and other nutrients to—and the removal of waste products from—the muscle is enhanced because of the exercise training-induced increase in capillary density.

Skeletal muscle capillary density is related to two factors: (1) the size or diameter of the muscle fiber[21,91] and (2) the fiber type or number of mitochondria per muscle fiber.[1,3,91] The relationship between fiber diameter and capillary density is shown in figure 12.17A. This association holds for both trained and untrained subjects. Relative to fiber type, Type I fibers have more mitochondria than do Type II fibers. Therefore, the number of capillaries surrounding Type I fibers is generally greater than Type IIA fibers and almost always greater than Type IIB fibers. This is especially true for endurance-trained subjects (figure 12.17B).

A summary of the changes induced by physical training at rest is given in table 12.7.

Changes during Submaximal Exercise

Following chronic exposure to endurance training, several important changes occur during steady-state, submaximal exercise. These major changes apply uniformly to males and females; they are discussed here and also presented graphically in figure 12.18.

1. *No Change or Slight Decrease in Oxygen Consumption.* The $\dot{V}O_2$ at a given submaximal work load is unchanged[54] or slightly lower[43,57] following participation in a regular endurance-training regimen. The decrease results from an increase in mechanical efficiency (skill) and is most pronounced when comparing highly trained athletes to untrained individuals.

2. *Decrease in Muscle Glycogen Usage (Glycogen Sparing).* During prolonged submaximal exercise at a given work rate or $\dot{V}O_2$, the amount of muscle glycogen utilized is less following training.[93,138] This effect is sometimes referred to as **glycogen sparing** and is probably related to the muscles' increased ability to use (oxidize) free fatty acids as a metabolic fuel, which is due to some of the biochemical alterations (i.e., an increase in oxidative enzymes) discussed previously. As the oxidation of fatty acids improves, both glycogen usage and lactic acid production are reduced—leading to an increase in sustained submaximal work effort.[71]

3. *Decrease in Lactate Accumulation.* Training is associated with a decrease in the accumulation of blood lactate while exercising at a standardized submaximal exercise level.[43,52,57] This is an important change because most exertion, including that performed during training sessions and competitive events, is generally submaximal in nature.

table 12.7

Changes at rest induced by endurance training

Cardiac hypertrophy
Increased size of ventricular cavity (endurance athletes)

Decreased heart rate
Increased parasympathetic (vagal) tone
Decreased sympathetic influence
Decreased intrinsic rate of the sino-atrial node

Increased stroke volume
Cardiac hypertrophy
Likely increase in myocardial contractility

No change in minute ventilation or total lung capacity
Little, if any, increase in vital capacity with little, if any, decrease in residual volume

Increased blood volume and total hemoglobin

Increased skeletal muscle capillary density and hypertrophy

The physiological mechanisms responsible for the training-induced decrease in lactate accumulation during submaximal exercise are not entirely known. However, there are several possibilities:

a. A smaller oxygen deficit incurred at the beginning of exercise, due to a faster adjustment of oxygen uptake relative to energy demands. Such a training effect has been shown to occur.[23,74,82]

b. A greater use of the lactate produced during exercise as a fuel source for energy (produced via the Cori cycle, page 413).

c. As mentioned previously, exercise training increases the number and size of muscle mitochondria as well as the level or concentration of the enzymes involved with fatty acid oxidation, the Krebs Cycle, and the electron transport system. The net result is an improved ability of the skeletal muscle to utilize fatty acids[55] and to operate aerobically during prolonged exercise—versus having to rely sooner on anaerobic glycolysis to generate ATP. This does not necessarily mean that less oxygen is required by the cell; instead, the cell is now simply able to better use what is delivered to it. This increased reliance on aerobic metabolism versus anaerobic glycolysis leads to less lactate production during exercise performed at a standardized work rate. (Remember, lactic acid results from the incomplete breakdown of glycogen or glucose.) This concept is shown in figure 12.19.

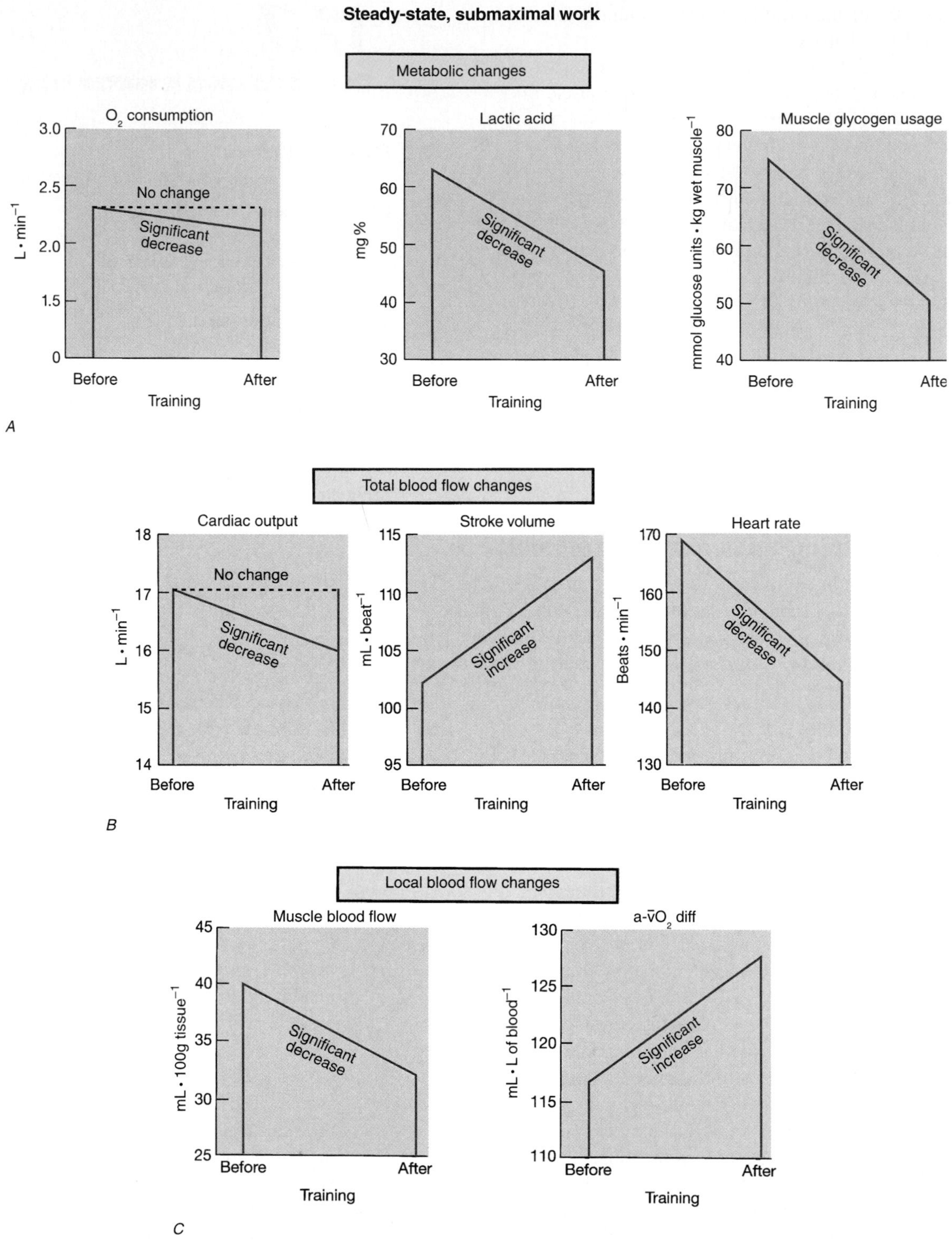

Steady-state, submaximal work

Metabolic changes

A

Total blood flow changes

B

Local blood flow changes

C

Figure 12.18

Following training, important changes occur in the functioning of the oxygen transport and related systems during submaximal work. These include no change or slight decrease in oxygen consumption, decreased lactic acid production, decreased muscle glycogen usage, no change or slight decrease in cardiac output, increased stroke volume, decreased heart rate; and a decreased blood flow per kilogram of working muscle.

(Based on data from Ekblom et al,[43] Frick et al.,[60] Grimby et al.,[73] and Karlsson et al.[99])

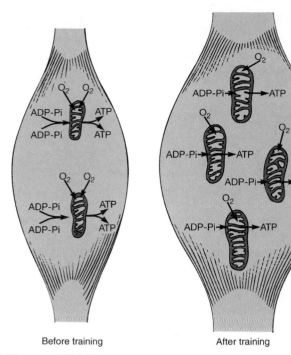

Before training   After training

Figure 12.19

After training there is an increase in the number and the size of mitochondria. With more mitochondria, the oxygen as well as the ADP and Pi required *per* mitochondrion will be less for a given submaxial exercise load after training as compared to before training. This in turn leads to less reliance on anaerobic glycolysis for ATP production as well as an improved ability to operate aerobically. The end result is a slower production of lactic acid in the cell.

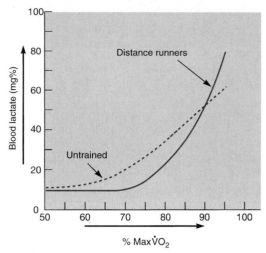

Figure 12.20

The lactate threshold (the work intensity at which lactic acid begins to accumulate) is around 60% of the max $\dot{V}O_2$ in untrained subjects, but about 75% of the max $\dot{V}O_2$ in trained distance runners.

4. *Increase in Performance Velocity/Lactate Threshold.* Competitive endurance athletes (e.g., runners, rowers) must not only have a highly developed maximal aerobic power (max $\dot{V}O_2$), but they must also be able to sustain a submaximal pace (performance $\dot{V}O_2$ or performance velocity) that is equal to or slightly faster than the pace associated with a sustained accumulation of lactate in the blood (pace at lactate threshold).[30,31,98] In fact, among elite athletes, as further increases in max $\dot{V}O_2$ become more and more difficult to achieve, continued improvements in performance velocity or pace at lactate threshold can occur over time. Specifically, with proper training, the pace where muscle anaerobic glycolysis becomes more involved can be increased so that overall performance, albeit submaximal, is increased. A summary of this concept is shown in figure 12.20.

5. *No Change or Slight Decrease in Cardiac Output.* During submaximal exercise at a given work rate or $\dot{V}O_2$, the cardiac output of trained subjects is either unchanged or slightly lower than that of untrained subjects. The reason for this discrepancy is not fully known, but it may be related to the type, intensity, and duration of the training programs involved.

6. *Increase in Stroke Volume.* One of the most dramatic changes that occurs as a result of endurance training is that stroke volume is increased at a standardized level of submaximal work.[14,57,60,140,155] Just like increased stroke volume at rest, this exercise effect is related mainly to changes in preload and to the increased size of the ventricular cavity (and possibly to increased myocardial contractility). Stated simply, the greater the amount of blood filling the cavity, the greater will be the stroke volume. And remember that one of the most important components of the oxygen transport system is stroke volume.

7. *Decrease in Heart Rate.* Perhaps the most consistent change associated with training is an exercise training-induced decrease in heart rate during submaximal exercise.[43,53,60,117,166,170] This decrease is most apparent when nonathletic subjects are compared to highly trained athletes. A slower beating heart is more efficient, and requires less oxygen than a faster beating heart working at the same cardiac output.[12]

This decrease in heart rate during submaximal exercise following endurance training is thought to be caused by modifications within the heart muscle and/or the autonomic nervous system. For example, indirect evidence for a general decrease in sympathetic tone during exercise is shown in figure 12.21. During the first two or three weeks of training, the reduction in heart rate parallels the decreases in plasma norepinephrine and epinephrine. However, with further training the plasma catecholamines tend to level off, yet exercise heart rate continues to fall. This suggests that other factors, such as an increased

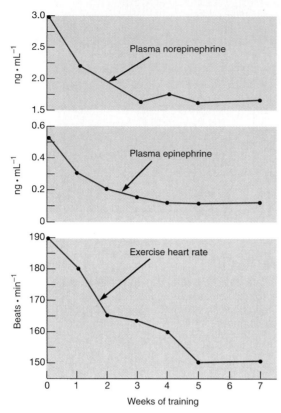

Figure 12.21

During the first two or three weeks of training, the reduction in heart rate during standardized submaximal exercise parallels the decreases in plasma catecholamine (norephinephrine and epinephrine) levels. However, with further training the catecholamines tend to level off, yet heart rate continues to fall.

(Based on data from Winder et al.[170])

parasympathetic (vagal) tone, a slowing of the intrinsic rate of the S-A node, or (more likely) a decrease in sympathetic tone to the myocardium itself might also be involved. Evidence exists for each of these possibilities.[45]

8. *Decrease in Muscle Blood Flow per Kilogram of Active Muscle.* Contrary to what you might think, blood flow per kilogram of working muscle is lower in trained than in untrained individuals at the same absolute submaximal work load.[73,107,155] This results, in part, from the increase in capillarization that occurs. The working muscles compensate for the lower blood flow in the trained state by extracting (and utilizing) more of the oxygen that is available. This is evidenced by a greater arterial mixed venous oxygen difference (a-$\overline{v}O_2$ diff) and may also be related to the biochemical changes mentioned previously.

The exercise training-induced decrease in blood flow to the active muscles during submaximal

exercise means that more blood is now available for nonexercising tissues, such as the skin. During exercise in the heat, this would be an advantage with respect to heat elimination. A summary of the changes induced by training during submaximal exercise is given in table 12.8.

Changes during Maximal Exercise

Physical training greatly increases maximal working capacity. Some of the physiological changes that contribute to this improvement are depicted in figure 12.22.

1. *Increase in Maximal Aerobic Power (max $\dot{V}O_2$).* The increase in max $\dot{V}O_2$ from exercise training has been studied extensively, and there is little doubt that it is increased among both males and females.[6,40,43,47,53,61,63,77,78,118,121,140,169] The magnitude of the increase can vary based on training volume, type of training program, mode of activity, and initial fitness level. In general, an average improvement of between 5% and 25% can be anticipated for college-age men or women following 8 to 12 weeks of training. Among sedentary persons and persons with chronic diseases, the increase in

---

table 12.8

12.8

Exercise training-induced changes during submaximal exercise

No change or slight decrease in $\dot{V}O_2$

Decrease in muscle glycogen usage
    Increase in fatty acid oxidation

Decrease in lactic acid lactate accumulation
    Increase in fatty acid oxidation
    Decrease in oxygen deficit
    Increase in use of lactate as metabolic fuel
    Increase in number and size of mitochondria

Increase in performance velocity/lactate threshold

No change or slight decrease in cardiac output

Increase in stroke volume
    Cardiac hypertrophy
    No change or increase in myocardial contractility

Decrease in heart rate
    Increase in vagal tone
    Decrease in general and cardiac sympathetic tone
    Decrease in intrinsic sino-atrial rate

Decrease in blood flow per kg of active muscle
    Increase in oxygen extraction by muscles

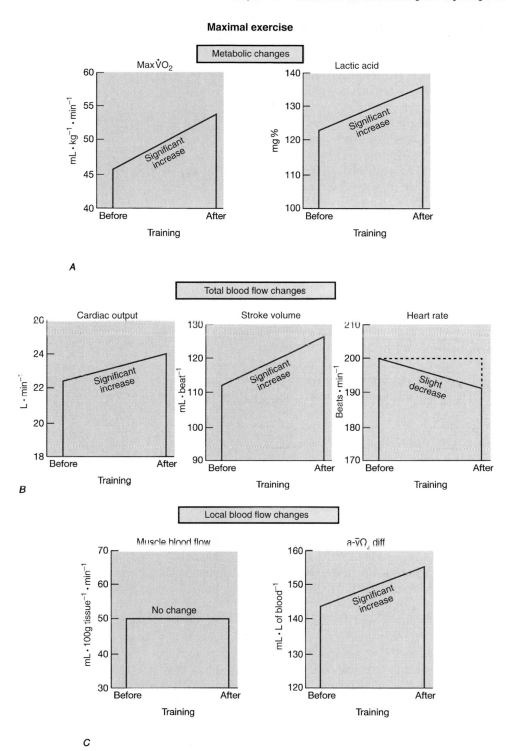

Figure 12.22

Following training, important changes occur in the functioning of the oxygen transport and related systems during maximal work. These include the following: increased max $\dot{V}O_2$, increased lactic acid production, increased cardiac output, increased stroke volume, no change or slight decrease in heart rate, no change in muscle blood flow per kilogram of working muscle, and an increased a-$\bar{v}O_2$ diff.

(Based on data from Ekblom et al.[44] and Grimby et al.[73])

max $\dot{V}O_2$ with training can be as high as 35%. When gain in max $\dot{V}O_2$ is expressed in mL of O_2 per kg of body weight per min, the values achieved for males and females are quite similar (figure 12.23). However, because the initial max $\dot{V}O_2$ of females is generally lower than males, the percent increase in max $\dot{V}O_2$ is greater among females (figure 12.23).

To appreciate those factors that, when altered, contribute to the increase in $\dot{V}O_2$ max, we must first recall that $\dot{V}O_2$ is our overall measure of the body's ability to transport and utilize oxygen (chapters 4 and 9). It reflects the integration of various tissues, organs, and organ systems. Rearranging the Fick equation:

$$\dot{V}O_2 \text{ max} = \text{heart rate} \times \text{stroke volume} \times \text{a-}\overline{v}O_2 \text{ diff}$$

we can see that increases in max $\dot{V}O_2$ are brought about by two main changes: (1) an increased O_2 delivery to the working muscles (cardiac output), and (2) an increased O_2 extraction from the blood by the skeletal muscles (a-$\overline{v}O_2$ diff). Changes in stroke volume and a-$\overline{v}O_2$ diff represent the primary factors responsible for the increase in max $\dot{V}O_2$ with training.[42,43,155] This concept is shown in table 12.9.

A logical question to ask at this time is, *Which factor(s) limit max $\dot{V}O_2$—the transport of oxygen to the skeletal muscles or the ability of the skeletal muscles to extract oxygen from the blood and utilize it?* The answer is not entirely clear, partly because an individual's maximal ability to transport and utilize oxygen represents a severe challenge to a multitude of integrated bodily functions. A failure in any one could prevent full utilization of oxygen; however, present information suggests that, for most persons, peak cardiac output (i.e., stroke volume) is the limiting factor.[142]

Among some elite athletes it appears that respiratory function may represent a potential limitation. Specifically, during heavy exercise the lung is unable to fully oxygenate the returning venous blood; therefore, the net effect is arterial desaturation.[96] One important reason for this arterial desaturation during extreme exercise in elite athletes is that as the greatly increased blood flow speeds the transit of red blood cells through the pulmonary capillaries, the time needed to achieve equilibrium between alveolar and arterial oxygen tensions is insufficient.

2. *Increase in Cardiac Output.* Maximal cardiac output increases with training, and the magnitude of the change is similar to that of the max $\dot{V}O_2$ (figure 12.24A). The mechanism responsible for the increase in cardiac output is explained below. As would be expected, maximal cardiac output is greatest in highly trained endurance athletes.[44]

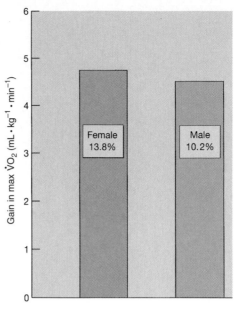

Figure 12.23

The increase in max $\dot{V}O_2$ is similar in females and males following identical programs of training. Expressed in mL · kg^{-1} · min^{-1}, the gain in max $\dot{V}O_2$ is the same; however, because the initial max $\dot{V}O_2$ of the females was lower, the percent increase was larger for the females.

(Based on data from Fox et al.[54] and Romero.[135])

3. *Increase in Stroke Volume.* The increase in maximal stroke volume resulting from training is related to the left ventricular chamber enlargement described earlier as well as to changes in preload, afterload, and possibly, myocardial contractility. A larger ventricular volume allows for a greater output of blood with each beat. The increase in preload is related to the increase in total blood volume and possibly to an increase in the distensibility of the ventricles (ability of the chambers to accept blood). An exercise training-induced reduction of afterload is also known to occur at peak exercise—making it easier for the left ventricle to eject blood into the aorta. The decrease in afterload is likely caused by (1) a training-induced increase in the vasculature in and around skeletal muscle cells and (2) a decrease in arteriolar tone.

The single most important feature that distinguishes the endurance athlete who has been training for several years from the person who has been training for only a few months is the magnitude of the stroke volume.[44,138] In other words, as shown in figure 12.24B, stroke volume is a major determinant of cardiac output and thus directly impacts max $\dot{V}O_2$.

4. *No Change or Slight Decrease in Heart Rate.* The maximal attainable heart rate is usually unchanged or

12.9

table

Cross-sectional comparison of variables that contribute to aerobic capacity in untrained and trained persons and in elite athletes

	Max $\dot{V}O_2$ (L · min^{-1})	=	HR*$_{max}$ (b · min^{-1})	×	SV*$_{max}$ (mL)	×	a-$\bar{v}O_2$ diff (mL · L^{-1})
Untrained	2.8		196		104		137
Trained	3.5		195		124		143
Elite athlete	5.6		193		187		156

*Peak cardiac output (HR × SV) is 20.3 L · min^{-1}, 24.2 L · m^{-1}, and 36.0 L · min^{-1} for the untrained, trained, and elite athlete, respectively. Based on data from Ekblom et al.,[43] Ekblom and Hermansen,[44] and Saltin et al.[141]

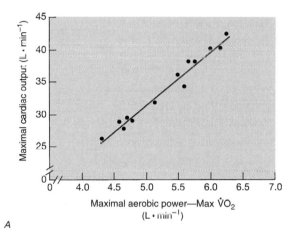

A

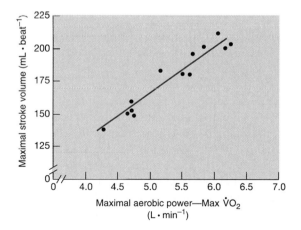

B

Figure 12.24

(*A*) The maximal attainable cardiac output and the max $\dot{V}O_2$ are directly related; the former is a factor in determining the latter. (*B*) The maximal attainable stroke volume is a major determinant of the magnitude of the cardiac output and thus the max $\dot{V}O_2$.

(Based on data from Ekblom and Hermansen.[44])

decreases slightly following training. Although the decrease in maximal heart rate is particularly evident among endurance-trained athletes,[139] short-term training of previously sedentary subjects can also cause a slight but significant decrease in maximal heart rate.[43,53,54] The mechanism(s) responsible for this possible decrease in maximal heart rate with training are not well understood. Probable reasons include (1) an increased left ventricular cavity or chamber size, (2) a decreased sympathetic drive, and (3) a decreased intrinsic rate of the S-A node.

5. *Increase in Maximal Minute Ventilation.* Although minute ventilation is unchanged at rest, it is increased during maximal exercise. The increase in maximal minute ventilation results from increases in both maximal tidal volume and breathing frequency. Young, untrained, healthy persons may achieve peak exercise values approaching 120 L · min^{-1}, while patients with heart disease may achieve peak values of 60 to 80 L · min^{-1}. In both cases an approximate 15% to 25% increase in maximal minute ventilation can be achieved through training.

Competitive athletes may achieve a maximal minute ventilation well over 180 to 200 L · min^{-1}. Generally, except for certain elite athletes, pulmonary function is not a limiting factor for max $\dot{V}O_2$. Therefore, the increase in maximal ventilation should be considered secondary to the increase in max $\dot{V}O_2$.

6. *Greater Pulmonary Diffusion Capacity.* When compared to nonathletes, athletes tend to have larger pulmonary diffusion capacities at rest and during submaximal and maximal exercise. This is particularly true for endurance athletes (see chapter 8, figure 8.6). Part of the reason for the increase may be an exercise training-induced increase in pulmonary blood flow, which means that more blood is brought into the lungs for gas exchange at the level of the alveoli. And recall from the previous discussion that maximal minute

ventilation is also increased with training. The sum effect is that pulmonary diffusion is increased with training.

7. *Increase in Lactate Accumulation.* One of the biochemical changes induced by training is an increase in blood lactate levels achieved during exhaustive maximal work. This may be caused by a learning effect on the part of athletes who voluntarily push themselves harder at the end of exercise and/or by an increase in anaerobic glycolytic capacity.

8. *No Change in Muscle Blood Flow per Kilogram of Muscle.* Surprisingly, during maximal exercise, blood flow *per kilogram of muscle* is no different when comparing a trained versus untrained individual.[73] This does not mean that the blood flow to the body's entire working muscle mass is unchanged after training. In fact, with training, blood flow to the total working musculature is indeed greater during maximal work.[140] How can this apparent contradiction be resolved? The answer lies in the fact that the total muscle mass required to perform the work is also greater. In other words, the exercise training-induced increase in blood flow is distributed over an exercise training-induced increase in muscle mass, thus keeping blood flow per kilogram of muscle relatively unchanged.[138]

A summary of the changes induced by physical training during maximal work is given in table 12.10.

Changes in Connective Tissues

The connective tissues include bone, ligaments and tendons, and joints and cartilage.

1. *Changes in Bone.* Bone formation and breakdown is a dynamic process, often referred to as "remodeling." Bone is deposited by cells called *osteoblasts,* and bone resorption is achieved by cells called *osteoclasts.* Bone tissue, much like muscle, adapts in response to the functional forces acting upon it. And, the changes produced in the bone by physical training are related to the intensity of the training program.[18] For example, in growing animals exposed to low-intensity programs, there is either no effect or a stimulating effect on the growth of bone length and girth. On the other hand, in growing animals exposed to high-intensity programs, bone growth (length and girth) is inhibited. Other changes in bone resulting from training may involve increases in bone enzyme activity, increased breaking strength, and in some cases (e.g., following weight training) bone hypertrophy.

2. *Changes in Bone Mineral Content/Density.* Bone mineralization results from calcium phosphate deposition in a protein matrix synthesized by

table 12.10

Changes during maximal exercise induced by endurance-type training

Increase in V̇O₂ max
  Increase in total blood flow (cardiac output)
  Increase in oxygen extraction by muscles

Increase in cardiac output
  Increase in stroke volume

Increase in stroke volume
  Cardiac hypertrophy (ventricular cavity)
  No change or increase in myocardial contractility
  Increase in blood volume
  Decrease in afterload

No change or slight decrease in heart rate
  Increase in ventricular cavity
  Decrease in sympathetic drive
  Decrease in intrinsic rate of S-A node

Increase in minute ventilation
  Increase in tidal volume
  Increase in breathing frequency

Greater pulmonary diffusion capacity

Increase in lactic acid lactate accumulation
  Increase in glycolytic enzyme activities (capacities)

No change in blood flow per kilogram of working muscle
  Blood flow distributed over larger muscle mass

osteoblasts. Osteoporosis, a serious health problem characterized by a low bone mineral content and a low bone mineral density, is a disease associated with great disability in the U.S. (more than one million disease-related fractures annually). It is a disease that is most common in postmenopausal females. The maximization of bone mass early in life (before age 30), through a calcium-rich diet and weight-bearing exercise, is felt to reduce the risk for osteoporosis and related fractures later in life. Relative to exercise training, the beneficial mechanical load or stress that weight-bearing activities impose on bone (which lead to improved bone mineral density) is site-specific. In other words, the site where increased bone mineral density occurs corresponds to the type of activity employed. For example, basketball players demonstrate greater bone mineral density of the femur than do swimmers.[112] And upper-limb bone mineral density is greater among weight lifters than among runners.[76]

3. *Changes in Ligaments and Tendons.* Physical training has been shown to increase the breaking strength of

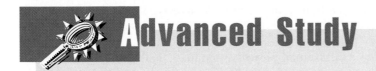

Advanced Study

Loss of Bone Mass in Space

When humans are exposed to a microgravity environment (i.e., spaceflight), a myriad of physiological changes take place. Two such changes are a reduction in bone mineral content/density and a negative calcium balance (calcium loss by the body is greater than calcium intake). However, the study of these problems is complicated in humans because of the limited number of flights that occur and the limited availability of bone samples (i.e., astronauts willing to undergo bone biopsies). In lieu of human studies, the study of animals in space is of particular interest. In this case, the rhesus monkey is considered a good model of human bone and calcium metabolism.

Zerath et al.[173] recently reported their study of two male rhesus monkeys exposed to a 11.5-day mission sponsored by Russia during which diet, fluids, light-dark cycles and atmosphere were all maintained. Testing conducted before and after the mission included a bone biopsy (0.5 cm) of the anterior part of the iliac crest. When compared to preflight data, the postflight biopsy revealed an ~ 20% decrease in bone mass in each of the two monkeys. Additionally, whole body bone mineral content also appeared to be reduced.

Present data indicates that osteoclast activity (resorption of bone) is increased during the first few hours of exposure to microgravity. This may account, in part, for the decrease in bone mass. Additionally, it has been shown that osteoblast activity (bone formation) is inhibited during spaceflight. This would also contribute to the reduced bone mass.

The exact mechanisms responsible for the microgravity-related decrease in bone mass is unknown. Possible explanations might include altered in-flight metabolism resulting from weightlessness and/or a decrease in physical activity, hormonal changes caused by stress (e.g., cortisol), or hormonal changes during space flight. In any event, countermeasures, such as appropriate nutrition combined with in-flight exercise, do not appear to be particularly effective in preventing the decrease in bone mass. Clearly, additional research is needed in this area as humans strive to extend the amount of time they live and work in a microgravity environment.

---

both ligaments and tendons. In addition, the strength of ligamentous and tendinous attachments to bone (junction strength) have been shown to increase following training. This may be interpreted to mean that greater stresses can be sustained and thus there is less chance of injury.

4. *Changes in Joints and Cartilage.* Perhaps the most consistent training-induced change in joints and cartilage is an increase in the thickness of load-bearing cartilage. Unfortunately, the significance of this effect during exercise or with respect to arthritis is not known.

Other Factors Influencing Training and Training Effects

The effects of training are influenced by many factors. At the beginning of this chapter we described how specificity of training and the intensity, duration, and frequency of exercise can influence physiologic changes. We conclude this

chapter discussing three other factors that can influence training adaptations: specifically, genetic limitations, the effects of menstruation among females, and training state.

Genetic Limitations

The saying "Great athletes are born, not made" leads us into our discussion that even with the best possible training program, improvement in physiological and functional capacities is determined, in part, by genetic make-up. Before pursuing the influence of heredity on changes in max $\dot{V}O_2$ caused by endurance training, we must first discuss the role of heredity in determining max $\dot{V}O_2$ in untrained persons. Earlier studies involving monozygous (identical) and dizygous (fraternal) twins suggested that the heritability level may account for 50% or more of max $\dot{V}O_2$.[108,109] These estimates, however, may have been overinflated—influenced by the small number of subjects studied and the difficulty in distinguishing shared common environmental effects from shared genetic effects. Although data on the heritability of max $\dot{V}O_2$ in untrained subjects are not yet conclusive, most recent data suggests that the heritability level is more likely 25% or less—once age, gender, body mass, and body composition are accounted for.[20] Specific variables which have been implicated in the connection between heredity and aerobic performance include cardiac dimension, maximal oxygen pulse (considered to be an estimate of stroke volume), and skeletal muscle fiber-type proportion/enzyme activity.

Given this, one might surmise that inheritance makes only a minor contribution to aerobic power. And in fact this may be true relative to the max $\dot{V}O_2$ in sedentary persons. The more important issue, however, is to what extent heredity influences the *magnitude of changes* that occur secondary to endurance training. We know for a fact that several factors that contribute to improved aerobic performance (e.g., stroke volume and skeletal muscle oxidative enzymes) are improved through training. We also know that it is not uncommon for a training program to produce only small changes in aerobic capacity for some participants (low responders), while others exposed to the same regimen experience a dramatic effect (high responders). Such differences cannot be accounted for by age, gender, and/or initial fitness level alone.

Relative to changes in aerobic power, what then causes the individual variability that occurs from one subject to another following training? Although data in this area is just emerging, Bouchard et al. suggest that yet undetermined genetic characteristics play an important role.[20] For example, in a study of 46 sedentary male subjects who underwent 12 or 20 weeks of endurance training, the increase in max $\dot{V}O_2$ ranged from 0.06 to 1.03 L · min^{-1}.[38] This wide range in response to exercise training between individuals was statistically related to variations in mitochondrial DNA among the subjects. The authors concluded, therefore, that such variations may contribute to the gains achieved in max $\dot{V}O_2$ subsequent to exercise training.

All in all, it seems true that great athletes are, in part, born and not made. However, just like their less genetically endowed counterparts, the level of success or performance they enjoy will only be achieved through personal commitment to a long-term, well-planned training regimen. And the issue of genetic endowment likely becomes even less important when discussing skill-specific sports such as golf, archery, and fencing.

Training and Competition during Menstruation

The affect of menstruation on athletic performance is quite varied, with some studies reporting as low as 8% of the female athletes experiencing a negative effect, while other studies reporting upwards of 35%.[4,46,92,111,171] And, although less common, some athletes have reported a better performance during menstruation.

Of those athletes who report poorer performances during menstruation, a large percentage are usually in-

volved in the more endurance-type activities (e.g., tennis players and rowers). Athletic performance during menstruation is generally less affected among volleyball players, basketball players, swimmers, and gymnasts versus endurance athletes, but it still can be "below normal." Performances by track-and-field athletes, especially sprinters, may be the least affected.[46] Gold-medal performances during menstruation have been reported in swimming and track and field.[97]

From a physiological standpoint, metabolic and cardiovascular responses at rest, during submaximal exercise, and during maximal exercise are not systematically affected during different phases of the menstrual cycle.[37,58,120] An example of this is shown in figure 12.25. In these studies, metabolic and cardiovascular responses were determined at rest and during exercise on eight trained female athletes and nine untrained females during the following three phases of the menstrual cycle: (1) seven days after ovulation (premenstrual phase), (2) three days after the onset of bleeding (menstrual phase), and (3) thirteen days after the onset of bleeding (postmenstrual phase). As can be seen, none of the responses, either at rest or during exercise, was significantly affected by the different phases of the cycle.

Ultimately, whether female athletes should train and/or compete during their menstrual flow (menses) is an individual matter. Previous opinion among some in the medical community opposed sport participation during menses—this included swimming while menstruating. However, research has since been determined that during menstruation there is no bacterial contamination of the water in the pool and no sign of increased bacterial infections of the reproductive organs of the swimmers.[5,137]

From the preceding information, it is appropriate that female athletes be allowed to train and compete in any sport during menstruation—provided they know through experience that no unpleasant symptoms will occur and that their performance will not be greatly affected. With the level of competition in modern sport, the athlete cannot afford missing three or four days of practice. In fact, for the majority of competitive athletes, the thought of missing training is not even considered. Additionally, it is equally reasonable to expect that no female athlete should be forced or ordered to train or compete during menstruation if, by doing so, she feels uncomfortable during this time.

Training State

Several important questions remain about training: (1) How fast are the benefits gained from training lost once training is stopped? (2) How can the benefits gained from training be best maintained? (3) Does prior training facilitate the magnitude and speed of regaining the training effects (retraining)? (4) What constitutes overtraining? The following information should help answer these questions.

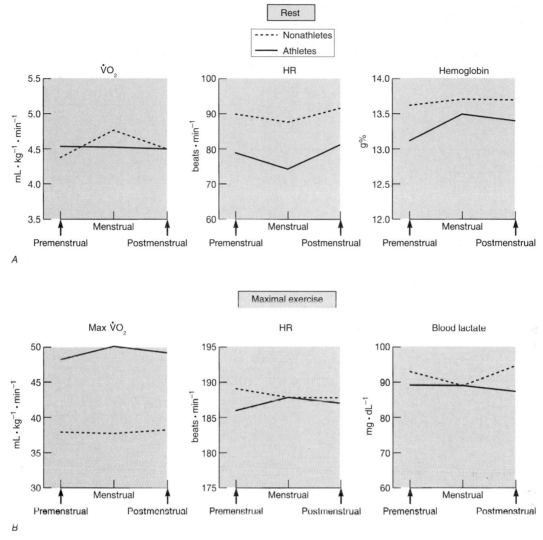

Figure 12.25

Metabolic and cardiovascular responses, (*A*) at rest and, (*B*) during maximal exercise, are not systematically affected during the premenstrual phase (7 days after ovulation), the menstrual phase (3 days after the onset of bleeding), and the postmenstrual phase (13 days after the onset of bleeding) of the menstrual cycle.

(Based on data from Fox et al.[58] and Martin.[120])

Detraining

Among both males and females, numerous studies have shown that most of the metabolic and cardiorespiratory benefits gained through exercise training are lost within a relatively short period of time after training is stopped.[39,41,62,63,78,129,130,140,153] Two of these studies are worth describing in greater detail. In the first project (figure 12.26*A*–*C*), two active, somewhat trained college-age subjects and three sedentary students underwent a variety of measurements before and after 20 days of bed rest. The same measurements were taken for a third time after the subjects completed approximately eight weeks of regular exercise training. As demonstrated, decreases in maximal $\dot{V}O_2$, cardiac output, and stroke volume occurred with bed rest—with the observed changes being generally more pronounced among the two more highly trained subjects. Note

also that the negative effects of prolonged bed rest were subsequently reversed via retraining—a topic we will explore later. A similar **detraining** response has been demonstrated for characteristics unique to skeletal muscle (e.g., enzymes).[78]

In the second study, Ehsani et al.[41] assessed six competitive cross-country runners just before and at several time points after having stopped their training regimen. Prior to detraining, these athletes had been running 60 to 70 miles per week. As table 12.11 indicates, dramatic decreases in left ventricular characteristics (i.e., mass, internal dimension, posterior wall thickness, and end diastolic volume) were noted within just 4 to 7 days after stopping exercise. The time course of these changes are somewhat staggering, given the fact that many of the changes likely took months, if not years, to develop.

table 12.11

Maximal oxygen consumption and left ventricular characteristics among runners undergoing three weeks of detraining

	Prior to Detraining	Detraining			
		Day 4	Week 1	Week 2	Week 3
Max $\dot{V}O_2$ (mL · kg^{-1} · min^{-1})	62.3	—	56.4	57.2	56.7
Mass (g · m^{-2})	109.5	92.7	80.2	70.2	67.1
Internal dimension (cm)	5.1	4.9	4.7	4.7	4.6
Posterior wall thickness (mm)	10.7	9.6	9.0	8.2	8.0
End diastolic volume (mL · m^{-2})	64.5	61.9	56.7	55.2	53.8

Data from Ehsani et al.[41]

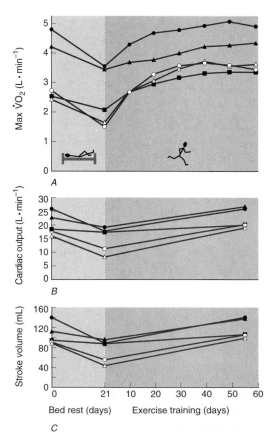

Figure 12.26

Changes in max $\dot{V}O_2$ (*A*), cardiac output (*B*), and stroke volume (*C*) in two trained and three untrained subjects who underwent 20 days of bed rest and approximately eight weeks of regular exercise training.

(*Adapted from Saltin et al.*[140])

Maintenance

One way to effectively maintain the benefits gained from training would be to vigorously train on a regular basis throughout the year. Except for possibly the elite athlete, such an approach is impractical and undesirable. Instead, a number of beneficial training effects can be *maintained* for several months with reduced training frequencies.

For example, with interval training, a reduction in training frequency but not intensity can effectively maintain one's max $\dot{V}O_2$. As shown in figure 12.27*A*, reducing the training frequency among females from three to two days per week completely maintains the max $\dot{V}O_2$ for at least 10 weeks.[129] On the other hand, a reduction in training frequency from three to only one day per week retards, but does not totally prevent, a decline in max $\dot{V}O_2$ (~ 7%). Similar findings on male subjects have also been reported.[22,24]

Another important training adaptation that can be maintained is the ability to perform a given submaximal work load with less accumulation of lactic acid. As shown in figure 12.27*B*, this effect can be maintained for up to 16 weeks. Yet in this case, all that is needed is just one maintenance workout per week—as long as the workout is the same as that used during the final week of the regular training program. Note that the lower lactic acid accumulation cannot be maintained with a maintenance program conducted only once every two weeks.

Retraining

Popular belief once held that the training effects one achieved via endurance training could be increased if the athlete had previously undergone a training and detraining

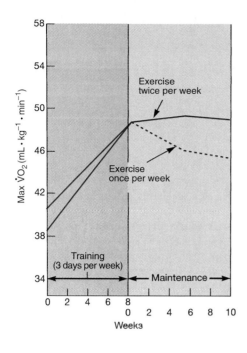

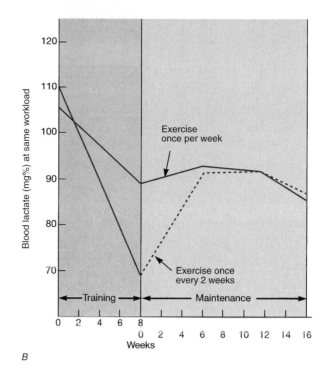

A   B

Figure 12.27

(*A*) The gains in max V̇O₂ following a 3-day-per-week interval training program can be completely maintained with a maintenance program of the same intensity but with a frequency of only 2 days per week. A 1-day-per-week program retards, but does not totally prevent, a decline in max V̇O₂. (*B*) One of the most important benefits retained by a maintenance training program is the ability to perform a given submaximal work load with less accumulation of lactic acid. This effect can be maintained by exercise once per week.

(Data in A from Otto[129] and Otto et al.[130]; data in B from Chaloupka.[24])

period. Scientific studies, however, do not support this concept.[89,132] The effects of retraining on max V̇O₂ are shown in figure 12.28. In this study, previously untrained female subjects were trained on a bicycle ergometer two days per week for seven weeks. At the end of training, their max V̇O₂ was increased by 13.8% on the average. This was followed by a seven-week period of detraining, during which time max V̇O₂ declined to within 3% of pretraining values. The subjects then retrained for seven weeks, with the magnitude and rate of increase of max V̇O₂ being quite similar to that induced by the initial training period. Thus, there was no indication of a positive transfer from one training period to the other.

Beyond studies on the untrained, nonathletic subject, what about the elite athlete who is forced into brief periods of inactivity as a result of minor injuries? A partial answer to this question is shown in figure 12.29. In this study,[89] six male competitive runners were used as subjects and specific variables were tested at the peak of their training (day zero in figure 12.29), after only 15 days of detraining,* and after

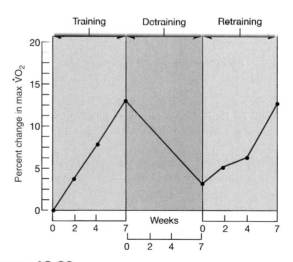

Figure 12.28

At the end of the training, the max V̇O₂ of a group of female students was increased by 13.8% on the average. After a 7-week period of detraining, the average max V̇O₂ was decreased to within 3% of the pretraining value. Following another 7 weeks of training, the average max V̇O₂ increased to the same extent and at the same rate as in the initial training period. Thus there was no indication of a beneficial or positive transfer from one training period to the other.

(Based on data from Pedersen and Jorgensen.[132])

---

*For the first seven days of detraining, a walking plaster cast was placed on the right leg, immobilizing the muscles of the calf. For the final eight days of detraining, the subjects performed routine daily activities, except no strenuous physical activity was performed.

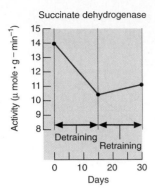

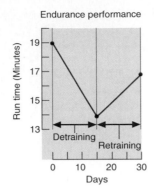

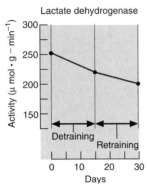

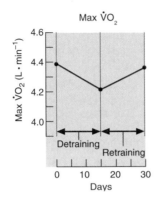

Figure 12.29

Six male competitive runners were tested at the peak of their training (day zero), after 15 days of detraining, and after 15 days of retraining. Significant decreases in muscle enzyme activity (succinate dehydrogenase and lactic dehydrogenase), endurance performance, and max $\dot{V}O_2$ were induced during the 15 days of detraining. Fifteen days of retraining did not return all the variables to their previous levels. These results suggest that brief layoffs among trained athletes can significantly decrease performance.

(Based on data for Houston et al.[89])

15 days of retraining. Significant decreases in muscle aerobic enzyme activity (succinate dehydrogenase and lactic dehydrogenase), endurance performance, and max $\dot{V}O_2$ were induced during the 15 days of detraining. Of equal importance is that a 15-day retraining period did not return all of these variables to their previous levels. This confirms that prior training does not, in itself, positively influence the gains made through a subsequent retraining period. It also points out that a relatively brief layoff by highly trained athletes can significantly decrease performance.

Overtraining

Although the concept of **overtraining** has received increased research attention over the past 15 years, it is by no means a contemporary problem. Overtraining can occur when high volume and/or high intensity training is combined with inadequate recovery periods between workouts. It means that there is an imbalance between training and recovery. Another term sometimes given to overtraining is

12.12

Signs and symptoms that may indicate overtraining

1. Physical performance
   - loss in muscle strength
   - loss in coordination
   - decrease in maximal aerobic capacity

2. Biologic function
   - increased (or decreased) resting heart rate (or blood pressure) relative to baseline values
   - increased oxygen uptake, heart rate, and blood lactate during standardized submaximal exercise
   - decrease or no change in body mass
   - muscle tenderness
   - increased risk for infection

3. Mood state
   - easily fatigued
   - loss of appetite
   - possible sleep disturbances

Adapted in part from Lehmann et al.[113]

staleness. However, some researchers and coaches use this word only if fatigue, psychologic changes, and/or loss of performance accompany the unwanted physiologic changes that are indicative of overtraining (e.g., increased resting or submaximal heart rate). Observable manifestations of long-term overtraining are given in table 12.12.

Part of the recent research endeavors in the area of overtraining have included establishing markers by which to monitor whether an athlete is in fact overtrained and to assess their recovery if necessary. Hooper and coworkers conducted a longitudinal study whereby they measured a wide range of parameters in 14 male and female elite Australian swimmers over a six-month season.[85] All of the athletes were asked to keep detailed training logs of various parameters designed to rate "well-being." Some of these parameters included quality of sleep, fatigue, causes of stress, and muscle soreness. Three of the swimmers (all females) were, at one time during the season, classified as "stale" based upon performance fall-off and prolonged high levels of fatigue. In all three of these athletes, the comments/ratings made in their training logs coincided with them being classified as "stale." Comments such as "washed out," "feeling sluggish," and "can't get going" were noted. In the end, the authors felt that self-assessment logs on the part of the athletes represented a unique and cost-effective method to monitor for overtraining.

It seems obvious that every reasonable attempt should be made, on the part of both the coach and the athlete, to avoid overtraining. Strategies to accomplish this might include proper nutrition, adequate rest/recovery, monitoring training load, and varying exercise intensity. A driving force behind this is the fact that once an athlete becomes overtrained, it may take weeks or even months to fully recover. As long as many athletes continue to be obsessed with training and performance, overtraining will remain a potential problem. The problem is also confounded by the vast individual variability that exists relative to how athletes respond to an intense exercise training regimen. As a result, the identification, monitoring, and recovery from overtraining are not easily predictable.

Finally, for both sport psychologists and exercise physiologists, overtraining is a difficult problem to research and study. Most athletes are unwilling to subject themselves to a longitudinal study that imposes the level of training needed to manifest the signs and symptoms of the disorder. Therefore, much of the research conducted on the topic is either cross-sectional or the work of a coach who has research interests in this area.

Summary

Improving aerobic or endurance performance involves exercise training-induced adaptations of the skeletal muscle, cardiorespiratory system, and neuromuscular function. Generally, the training effects are specific to the type of training program used—for example, running versus bicycling, sprint versus endurance, and trained versus untrained limb. Also, the greater the intensity, frequency, and duration of the individualized training program, the greater will be the improvement in most functions. Intensity can be guided by heart rate-based methods or lactate threshold.

Training programs can be long-duration, moderate-intensity; moderate-duration, high-intensity (pace or tempo training); short-duration, very high-intensity (interval sprinting); fartlek; or cross-training in design.

Changes in skeletal muscle secondary to aerobic training include:

1. Biochemical changes
   a. Increased myoglobin content
   b. Improved oxidation of carbohydrate (glycogen)
   c. Improved oxidation of fat
2. Changes within Type I and Type II muscle fibers

Systemic (oxygen transport system) changes induced by training include the following:

1. At rest
   a. Cardiac hypertrophy
   b. Decreased heart rate
   c. Increased stroke volume
   d. No change in minute ventilation
   e. Increased blood volume and hemoglobin
   f. Increased skeletal muscle capillary density and hypertrophy
2. During submaximal exercise
   a. No change or slight decrease in $\dot{V}O_2$
   b. Decrease in muscle glycogen usage
   c. Decrease in lactate accumulation
   d. Increase in performance velocity/lactate threshold
   e. No change or slight decrease in cardiac output
   f. Increase in stroke volume
   g. Decrease in heart rate
   h. Lower blood flow per kilogram of active muscle
3. During maximal exercise
   a. Increase in max $\dot{V}O_2$
   b. Increase in cardiac output
   c. Increase in stroke volume
   d. No change or slight decrease in heart rate
   e. Increase in minute ventilation
   f. Greater pulmonary diffusion capacity
   g. Increase in lactate accumulation
   h. No change in blood flow per kilogram of muscle

Genetic limitations can also influence the magnitude of the change in max $\dot{V}O_2$ with training. Differences between individuals exposed to the same training regimen may be mediated through such factors as stroke volume and skeletal muscle adaptations.

Most of the beneficial effects of training return to pretraining levels within four to eight weeks of detraining. Some training benefits, such as an increased max $\dot{V}O_2$ and a decreased lactic acid production during submaximal exercise, can be maintained for several months with maintenance programs consisting of one or more likely two days of exercise per week.

Contrary to popular belief, prior training does not hasten the rate or increase the magnitude of training benefits gained from subsequent training programs. Brief detraining periods by competitive athletes, such as those caused by minor injuries, can significantly decrease performance. Overtraining represents an individualized response to an imbalance between training volume and recovery. It is characterized by a decrease in performance and fatigue.

Questions

1. Compare and contrast heart rate-based methods and the lactate threshold method as techniques used to guide exercise training intensity. Include in your answer which is simpler to use and what tissues, organs, or organ systems are "targeted" with each method.
2. In what situation might a passive recovery period be the preferred method of recovery, as compared to an active recovery method? Give the scientific rationale to support your answer.

3. Compare and contrast the usefulness of cross-training relative to recovery from injury and specificity of training.

4. How does an exercise training-induced increase in myoglobin concentration enhance the aerobic system?

5. To what extent, if any, is there interconversion of skeletal muscle fiber types with endurance training? Explain your answer.

6. Discuss the major subcellular adaptations that contribute to the muscle cell's increased ability to oxidize carbohydrate and fat following training.

7. Discuss the major *systemic* changes resulting from training that are apparent at rest.

8. What are the major differences between cardiac hypertrophy in endurance and nonendurance athletes?

9. What physiological mechanisms are responsible for the resting bradycardia induced by training?

10. List the changes in the oxygen transport system following training that are evidenced during steady-state submaximal exercise.

11. What mechanisms may be responsible for a decreased blood lactate accumulation during submaximal work following training?

12. What limits max $\dot{V}O_2$ in most persons?

13. Explain why in some elite athletes respiratory function may limit max $\dot{V}O_2$.

14. Describe any differences between male and female athletes relative to gains made in absolute and relative max $\dot{V}O_2$ following a similar training regimen.

15. In what manner does heredity influence training effects?

16. Discuss the time course of the decrease in most training benefits during detraining.

17. Explain how brief periods of detraining-retraining affect performance.

References

1. Andersen, P. 1975. Capillary density in skeletal muscle of man. *Acta Physiol Scand.* 95:203–205.

2. Andersen, P., and J. Henriksson. 1977. Training induced changes in the subgroups of human type II skeletal muscle fibres. *Acta Physiol Scand.* 99:123–125.

3. ———. 1977. Capillary supply of the quadriceps femoris muscle of man: adaptive response to exercise. *J Physiol.* 270:677–690.

4. Åstrand, P. O. 1952. *Experimental Studies of Physical Working Capacity in Relation to Sex and Age.* Copenhagen: Ejnar Munksgaard.

5. Åstrand, P. O., B. Eriksson, I. Nylander, L. Engstrom, P. Karlbert, B. Saltin and C. Thoren. 1963. Girl swimmers. *Acta Paediat.* (suppl):147

6. Atomi, Y., K. Ito, H. Iwasaki, and M. Miyashita. 1978. Effects of intensity and frequency of training on aerobic work capacity of young females. *J Sports Med.* 18(1):3–9.

7. Badeer, H. S. 1975. Resting bradycardia of exercise training: a concept based on currently available data. In Roy, P.-E., and G. Rona (eds.), *The Metabolism of Contraction.* Baltimore: University Park Press, pp. 553–560.

8. Baldwin, K., G. Klinerfuss, R. Terjung, and J. Holloszy. 1972. Respiratory capacity of white, red, and intermediate muscle: adaptive response to exercise. *Am J Physiol.* 222:373–378.

9. Bangsbo, J., and F. Lindquist. 1992. Comparison of various exercise tests with endurance performance during soccer in professional players. *Int J Sports Med.* 13(2):125–132.

10. Barnard, R. J. 1975. Long-term effects of exercise on cardiac function. In Wilmore, J. H., and J. F. Keough, (eds.), *Exercise and Sport Sciences Reviews.* New York: Academic Press, pp. 113–133.

11. Barnard, R., R. V. Edgerton, and J. Peter. 1970. Effects of exercise on skeletal muscle. I: Biochemical and histological properties. *J Appl Physiol.* 28:762–766.

12. Barnard, R. J., R. MacAlpin, A. A. Kattus, and G. D. Buckberg. 1977. Effect of training on myocardial oxygen supply/demand balance. *Circulation.* 56(2):289–291.

13. Benzi, G., P. Panceri, M. DeBernardi, R. Villa, E. Arcelli, L. d'Angelo, E. Arrigoni, and F. Berte. 1975. Mitochondrial enzymatic adaptation of skeletal muscle to endurance training. *J Appl Physiol.* 38(4):565–569.

14. Bevegard, S., A. Holmgren, and B. Jonsson. 1963. Circulatory studies in well-trained athletes at rest and during heavy exercise, with special reference to stroke volume and the influence of body position. *Acta Physiol Scand.* 57:26–50.

15. Bhan, A. K., A. Malhotra, and J. Scheuer. 1975. Biochemical adaptations in cardiac muscle: effects of physical training on sulfhydryl groups on myosin. *J Mol Cellular Cardiol.* 7:435–442.

16. Bhan, A. K., and J. Scheuer. 1975. Effects of physical training on cardiac myosin ATPase activity. *Am J Physiol.* 28:1178–1182.

17. Bilodeau, B., B. Roy and M. R. Boulay. 1994. Effect of drafting on heart rate in cross-country skiing. *Med Sci Sports Exerc.* 26(5):637–641.

18. Booth, F. W., and E. W. Gould. 1975. Effects of training and disuse on connective tissue. In Wilmore, J. H., and J. E. Keough (eds.), *Exercise and Sport Sciences Reviews.* New York: Academic Press, pp. 83–112.

19. Borensztajn, J., M. Rone, S. Babirak, J. McGarr, and L. Oscai. 1975. Effects of exercise on lipoprotein lipase activity in rat heart and skeletal muscle. *Am J Physiol.* 29:394–397.

20. Bouchard, C., F. Dionne, J.-A. Simoneau, and M. R. Boulay. 1992. Genetics of aerobic and anaerobic performance. In J. O. Hollosy (ed.), *Exercise and Sport Sciences Reviews,* vol. 20. Baltimore: Williams & Wilkins, pp. 339–368.

21. Brodal, P., F. Inger, and L. Hermansen. 1977. Capillary supply of skeletal muscle fibers in untrained and endurance-trained men. *Am J Physiol.* 232(6):H705–H712.

22. Brynteson, P., and W. Sinning. 1973. The effects of training frequencies on the retention of cardiovascular fitness. *Med Sci Sports.* 5(1):29–33.

23. Cerretelli, P., D. Pendergast, W. C. Paganelli, and D. W. Rennie. 1979. Effects of specific muscle training on $\dot{V}O_2$ response and early blood lactate. *J Appl Physiol.* 47(4):761–769.

24. Chaloupka, E. 1972. *The Physiological Effects of Two Maintenance Programs Following Eight Weeks of Interval Training.* Doctoral dissertation: The Ohio State University, Columbus, OH.

25. Choi, D., K. J. Cole, B. H. Goodpaster, W. J. Fink, and D. L. Costill. 1994. Effect of passive and active recovery on the resynthesis of muscle glycogen. *Med Sci Sports Exerc.* 26(8):992–996.

26. Cohen, K., and E. L. Fox. 1970. Intensity and distance of interval training programs and metabolic changes in females. Unpublished manuscript.

27. Costill, D. L., E. Coyle, G. Dalsky, W. Evans, W. Fink, and D. Hoppes. 1977. Effects of elevated plasma FFA and insulin on muscle glycogen usage during exercise. *J Appl Physiol.* 43(4):695–699.

28. Costill, D. L., J. Daniels, W. Evans, W. Fink, G. Krahenbuhl, and B. Saltin. 1976. Skeletal muscle enzymes and fiber composition in male and female track athletes. *J Appl Physiol.* 40(2):149–154.

29. Costill, D. L., R. Thomas, R. A. Robergs, D. Pascoe, C. Lambert, S. Barr, and W. J. Fink. 1991. Adaptations to swimming training: influence of training volume. *Med Sci Sports Exerc.* 23(3):371–377.

30. Costill, D. L., H. Thomason, and E. Roberts. 1973. Fractional utilization of the aerobic capacity during distance running. *Med Sci Sports.* 5(4):248–252.

31. Coyle, E. F. 1995. Integration of the physiological factors determining endurance performance ability. In J. O. Hollosy (ed.), *Exercise and Sport Sciences Reviews,* vol. 23. Baltimore: Williams & Wilkins, pp. 25–63.

32. Cretzmeyer, F., L. Alley, and C. Tipton. 1974. *Track and Field Athletics,* 8th ed. St. Louis: C. V. Mosby.

33. Daniels, J., R. Fitts, and G. Sheehan. 1978. *Conditioning for Distance Running.* New York: John Wiley.

34. Davies, K. J. A., L. Packer, and G. A. Brooks. 1981. Biochemical adaptation of mitochondria, muscle, and whole-animal respiration to endurance training. *Arch Biochem Biophys.* 209:539–554.

35. DeBoer, R. W., E. Vos, W. Hutter, G. deGroot and G. J. van Ingen Schenau. 1987. Physiological and biomechanical comparison of roller skating and speed skating on ice. *Eur J Appl Physiol.* 56:562–569.

36. DeMaria, A. N., A. Neuman, G. Lee, W. Fowler, and D. T. Mason. 1978. Alterations in ventricular mass and performance induced by exercise training in man evaluated by echocardiography. *Circulation.* 57:237–244.

37. De Souza, M. J., M. S. Maguire, K. R. Rubin, and C. M. Maresh. 1990. Effects of menstrual phase and ammenorrhea on exercise performance in runners. *Med Sci Sports Exerc.* 22(5):575–580.

38. Dionne, F. T., L. Turcotte, M. C. Thibault, M. B. Boulay, J. S. Skinner, and C. Bouchard. 1991. Mitochondrial DNA sequence polymorphism, VO_2 max and response to endurance training. *Med Sci Sports Exerc.* 23(2):177–185.

39. Drinkwater, B., and S. Horvath. 1972. Detraining effects on young women. *Med Sci Sports.* 4:91–95.

40. Edwards, A. 1974. The effects of training at pre-determined heart rate levels for sedentary college women. *Med Sci Sports.* 6:14–19.

41. Ehsani, A. A., J. M. Hagberg, and R. C. Hickson. 1978. Rapid changes in left ventricular dimensions and mass in response to physical conditioning and deconditioning. *Am J Cardiol.* 42:52–56.

42. Ekblom, B. 1969. Effect of physical training on the oxygen transport system in man. *Acta Physiol Scand.* (suppl)328:1–45.

43. Ekblom, B., P. Åstrand, B. Saltin, J. Stenberg, and B. Wallstrom. 1968. Effect of training on circulatory response to exercise. *J Appl Physiol.* 24(4):518–528.

44. Ekblom, B., and L. Hermansen. 1968. Cardiac output in athletes. *J Appl Physiol.* 25(5):619–625.

45. Ekblom, B., A. Kilbom, and J. Soltysiak. 1973. Physical training, bradycardia and autonomic nervous system. *J Clin Lab Invest.* 32:251–256.

46. Erdelyi, G. 1962. Gynecological survey of female athletes. *J Sports Med.* 2:174–179.

47. Eriksson, B. O., I. Engstrom, P. Karlberg, A. Lunden, B. Saltin, and C. Thorne. 1978. Long-term effect of previous swim-training in girls, a 10-year follow-up of the "Girl Swimmers." *Acta Paediat Scand.* 67:285–292.

48. Faria, I. 1970. Cardiovascular response to exercise as influenced by training of various intensities. *Res Q.* 41:44–50.

49. Fedel, F. J., S. J. Keteyian, C. A. Brawner, C. R. C. Marks, M. J. Hakim, and T. Kataoka. 1995. Cardiorespiratory responses during exercise in competitive in-line skaters. *Med Sci Sports Exerc.* 27(5):682–687.

50. Foster, C., M. A. Green, A. C. Snyder, and N. N. Thompson. 1993. Physiological responses during simulated competition. *Med Sci Sports Exerc.* 25(7):877–882.

51. Foster, C., L. L. Hector, R. Welsh, M. Schrager, M. A. Green, and A. C. Snyder. 1995. Effects of specific versus cross-training on running performance. *Eur J Appl Physiol.* 70:367–372.

52. Fox, E. L. 1975. Differences in metabolic alterations with sprint versus interval training programs. In Howald, H., and J. Poortmans (eds.), *Metabolic Adaptation to Prolonged Physical Exercise.* Basel, Switzerland: Birkhauser Verlag, pp. 119–126.

53. Fox, E., R. Bartels, C. Billings, D. K. Mathews, R. Bason, and D. Webb. 1973. Intensity and distance on interval training programs and changes in aerobic power. *Med Sci Sports.* 5(1):18–22.

54. Fox, E., R. Bartels, C. Billings, R. O'Brien, R. Bason, and D. K. Mathews. 1975. Frequency and duration of interval training programs and changes in aerobic power. *J Appl Physiol.* 38(3):481–484.

55. Fox, E. L., R. L. Bartels, J. Klinzing, and K. Ragg. 1977. Metabolic responses to interval training programs of high and low power output. *Med Sci Sports.* 9(3):191–196.

56. Fox, E. L., and D. L. Costill. 1972. Estimated cardiorespiratory responses during marathon running. *Arch Environ Health.* 24:315–324.

57. Fox, E., D. McKenzie, and K. Cohen. 1975. Specificity of training: metabolic and circulatory responses. *Med Sci Sports.* 7(1):83.

58. Fox, E. L., F. L. Martin, and R. L. Bartels. 1977. Metabolic and cardiorespiratory responses to exercise during the menstrual cycle in trained and untrained subjects. *Med Sci Sports.* 9(1):70.

59. Frick, M., R. Elovainio, and T. Somer. 1967. The mechanism of bradycardia evoked by physical training. *Cardiologia.* 51:46–54.

60. Frick, M., A. Konttinen, and S. Sarajas. 1963. Effects of physical training on circulation at rest and during exercise. *Am J Cardiol.* 12:142–147.

61. Frick, M., A. Sjogren, J. Persasalo, and S. Pajunen. 1970. Cardiovascular dimensions and moderate physical training in young men. *J Appl Physiol.* 29(4):452–455.

62. Friman, G. 1979. Effect of clinical bed rest for seven days on physical performance. *Acta Med Scand.* 205(5):389–393.

63. Fringer, M. N., and G. A. Stull. 1974. Changes in cardiorespiratory parameters during periods of training and detraining in young adult females. *Med Sci Sports.* 6(1):20–25.

64. Garber, C. E., J. S. McKinney, and R. A. Carlton. 1992. Is aerobic dance an effective alternative to walk-jog exercise training? *J Sports Med Phys Fitness.* 32:136–141.

65. George, K. P., L. A. Wolfe, G. W. Burggraf, and R. Norman. 1995. Electrocardiographic and echocardiographic characteristics of female athletes. *Med Sci Sports Exerc.* 27(10):1362–1370.

66. Gettman, L. R., M. L. Pollock, J. L. Durstine, A. Ward, J. Ayres, and A. C. Linnerud. 1976. Physiological responses of men to 1, 3, and 5 day per week training programs. *Res Q.* 47(4):638–646.

67. Gollnick, P. D. 1977. Free fatty acid turnover and the availability of substrates as a limiting factor in prolonged exercise. *Ann NY Acad Sci.* 301:64–71.

68. Gollnick, P., R. Armstrong, B. Saltin, C. Saubert, W. Sembrowich, and R. Shepherd. 1973. Effect of training on enzyme activity and fiber composition of human skeletal muscle. *J Appl Physiol.* 34(1):107–111.

69. Gollnick, P., R. Armstrong, C. Saubert, K. Piehl, and B. Saltin. 1972. Enzyme activity and fiber composition in skeletal muscle of untrained and trained men. *J Appl Physiol.* 33(3):312–319.

70. Gollnick, P., and D. King. 1969. Effects of exercise and training on mitochondria of rat skeletal muscle. *Am J Physiol.* 216:1502–1509.

71. Gollnick, P. D., and B. Saltin. 1982. Significance of skeletal muscle oxidative enzyme enhancement with endurance training. *Clin Physiol.* 2:1–12.

72. Green, H. J., L. L. Jones, and D. C. Painter. 1990. Effects of short-term training on cardiac function during prolonged exercise. *Med Sci Sports Exerc.* 22(4):488–493.

73. Grimby, G., E. Haggendal, and B. Saltin. 1967. Local xenon 133 clearance from the quadriceps muscle during exercise in man. *J Appl Physiol.* 22(2):305–310.

74. Hagberg, J. M., R. C. Hickson, A. A. Ehsani, and J. O. Hollosy.

1980. Faster adjustment to and recovery from submaximal exercise in the trained state. *J Appl Physiol.* 48(2):218–224.

75. Hambrecht, R., J. Niebauer, E. Fiehn, et al. 1995. Physical training in patients with stable chronic heart failure: effects on cardiorespiratory fitness and ultrastructural abnormalities of leg muscles. *JACC.* 25:1239–1249.

76. Hamdy, R. C., J. S. Anderson, K. E. Whalen, and L. M. Harvill. 1994. Regional differences in bone density of young men involved in different exercises. *Med Sci Sports Exerc.* 26(7):884–888.

77. Hanson, J., and W, Nedde. 1974. Long-term physical training effect in sedentary females. *J Appl Physiol.* 37:112–116.

78. Henricksson, J., and J. S. Reitman. 1977. Time course of changes in human skeletal muscle succinate dehydrogenase and cytochrome oxidase activities and maximal oxygen uptake with physical activity and inactivity. *Acta Physiol Scand.* 99:91–97.

79. Hermansen, L., E. Hultman, and B. Saltin. 1967. Muscle glycogen during prolonged severe exercise. *Acta Physiol Scand.* 71:129–139.

80. Hermansen, L., and M. Wachtlova. 1971. Capillary density of skeletal muscle in well trained and untrained men. *J Appl Physiol.* 30(6):860–863.

81. Hickson, R. C. 1981. Skeletal muscle cytochrome c and myoglobin, endurance, and frequency of training. *J Appl Physiol.* 51:746–749.

82. Hickson, R. C., H. A. Bomze, and J. O. Holloszy. 1978. Faster adjustment of O_2 uptake to the energy requirement of exercise in the trained state. *J Appl Physiol.* 44(6):877–881.

83. Hickson, R. C., M. J. Rennie, R. K. Conlee, W. W. Winder, and J. O. Holloszy. 1977. Effects of increased plasma fatty acids on glycogen utilization and endurance. *J Appl Physiol.* 43:829–833.

84. Holloszy, J. 1967. Effects of exercise on mitochondrial oxygen uptake and respiratory enzyme activity in skeletal muscle. *J Biol Chem.* 242:2278–2282.

85. Hooper, S. L., L. T. MacKinnon, A. Howard, R. D. Gordon, and A. W. Bachmann. 1995. Markers for monitoring overtraining and recovery. *Med Sci Sports Exerc.* 27(1):106–112.

86. Hoppeler, H., P. Luthi, H. Claassen, E. R. Weibel, and H. Howald. 1973. The ultrastructure of the normal human skeletal muscle: a morphometric analysis on untrained men, women, and well-trained orienteers. *Pflugers Arch.* 344:217–232.

87. Houmard, J. A. 1991. Impact of reduced training on performance in endurance athletes. *Sports Med.* 12:380–393.

88. Houmard, J. A., B. K. Scott, C. L. Justice and T. C. Chenier. 1994. The effects of taper on performance in distance runners. *Med Sci Sports Exerc.* 26(5):624–631.

89. Houston, M. E., H. Bentzen, and H. Larsen. 1979. Interrelationships between skeletal muscle adaptations and performance as studied by detraining and retraining. *Acta Physiol Scand.* 105:163–170.

90. Hughson, R. L., J. R. Sutton, J. D. Fitzgerald, and N. L. Jones. 1977. Reduction of intrinsic sinoatrial frequency and norepinephrine response of the exercised rat. *Can J Physiol Pharmacol.* 55:813–820.

91. Inger, F. 1979. Capillary supply and mitochondrial content of different skeletal muscle fiber types in untrained and endurance trained men: a histochemical and ultrastructural study. *Eur J Appl Physiol.* 40:197–209.

92. Ingman, O. 1952. Menstruation in Finnish top class sportswomen. In *Sports Medicine International Symposium of the Medicine and Physiology of Sports and Athletes.* Helsinki: Finnish Association of Sports Medicine.

93. Jackson, J., B. Sharkey, and L. Johnston. 1968. Cardiorespiratory adaptations to training at specified frequencies. *Res Q.* 39:295–300.

94. Jansson, E., and L. Kaijer. 1977. Muscle adaptation to extreme endurance training in man. *Acta Physiol Scand.* 100:315–324.

95. Johns, R. A., J. A. Houmard, R. W. Kobe, et al. 1992. Effects of taper on swim power, stroke distance and performance. *Med Sci Sports Exerc.* 24:1141–1146.

96. Johnson, B. D., and J. A. Dempsey. 1991. Demand versus capacity in the aging pulmonary system. In J. O. Holloszy (ed.), *Exercise and Sport Sciences Reviews,* vol. 19. Baltimore: Williams & Wilkins, pp. 171–210.

97. Jokl, E. 1956. Some clinical data on women athletes. *J Assoc Physical Mental Rehab.* 10(2):48–49.

98. Joyner, M. J. 1993. Physiological limiting factors and distance running: influence of gender and age on record performance. In J. O. Holloszy (ed.), *Exercise and Sport Sciences Reviews,* vol. 21. Baltimore: Williams & Wilkins, pp. 103–133.

99. Karlsson, J., L.-O. Nordesjo, and B. Saltin. 1974. Muscle glycogen utilization during exercise after physical training. *Acta Physiol Scand.* 90:210–217.

100. Karvonen, M., E. Kentala, and O. Mustala. 1957. The effects of training on heart rate: a longitudinal study. *Ann Med Exper Biol Fenn.* 35:307–315.

101. Katch, V., A. Weltman, S. Sady, and P. Freedson. 1978. Validity of the relative per cent concept for equating training intensity. *Eur J Appl Physiol.* 39:219–227.

102. Keteyian, S. J., A. B. Levine, C. A. Brawner, et al. 1996. A randomized controlled trial of exercise training in patients with heart failure. *Ann Intern Med.* 124:1051–1057.

103. Kiessling, K., K. Piehl, and C. Lundquist. 1971. Effect of physical training on ultrastructural features in human skeletal muscle. In Pernow, B., and B. Saltin (eds.), *Muscle Metabolism during Exercise.* New York: Plenum Press, pp. 97–101.

104. Kinderman, W., G. Simon, and J Keul. 1979. The significance of the aerobic-anaerobic transition for determination of work load intensities during endurance training. *Eur J Appl Physiol.* 42:25–34.

105. Kjellberg, S., U. Rudhe, and T. Sjostrand. 1949. Increase of the amount of hemoglobin and blood volume in connection with physical training. *Acta Physiol Scand.* 19:146–151.

106. ———. 1949. The amount of hemoglobin and the blood volume in relation to the pulse rate and cardiac volume during rest. *Acta Physiol Scand.* 19:136–145.

107. Klassen, G., G. Andrew, and M. Becklake. 1970. Effect of training on total and regional blood flow and metabolism in paddlers. *J Appl Physiol.* 28(4):397–406.

108. Klissouras, V. 1971. Heritability of adaptive variation. J Appl Physiol. 31(3):338–344.

109. Klissouras, V., F. Pirnay, and J. Petit. 1973. Adaptation to maximal effort: genetics and age. *J Appl Physiol.* 35(2):288–293.

110. Knuttgen, H., L. Nordesjo, B. Ollander, and B. Saltin. 1973. Physical conditioning through interval training with young male adults. *Med Sci Sports.* 5:220–226.

111. Kral, J., and E. Markalous. 1937. The influence of menstruation on sports performance. In Mallwitz, A. (ed.), *Proceedings of the 2nd International Congress on Sports Medicine.* Leipzig: Theime.

112. Lee, E. J., K. A. Long, W. L. Risser, H. B. W. Poindexter, W. E. Gibbons, and J. Goldzieher. 1995. Variations in bone status of contralateral and regional sites in young athletic women. *Med Sci Sports Exerc.* 27(10):1354–1361.

113. Lehmann, M., C. Foster, and J. Keul. 1993. Overtraining in endurance athletes: a brief review. *Med Sci Sports Exerc.* 25(7):854–862.

114. Lesmes, G. R., E. L. Fox, C. Stevens, and R. Otto. 1978. Metabolic responses of females to high intensity interval training of different frequencies. *Med Sci Sports.* 10(4):124, 229–232.

115. Lewis, S., P. Thompson, N. Areskog, et al. 1980. Endurance training and heart rate control studied by combined parasympathetic and beta-adrenergic blockade. *Int J Sports Med.* 1:42–49.

116. Longhurst, J. C., A. R. Kelley, W. J. Gonyea, and J. H. Mitchell. 1980. Echocardiographic left ventricular masses in distance runners and weight lifters. *J Appl Physiol.* 48(1):154–162.

117. McKenzie, D. C., E. L. Fox, and K. Cohen. 1978. Specificity of metabolic and circulatory responses to arm or leg interval training. *Eur J Appl Physiol.* 39:241–248.

118. McNab, R., P. Conger, and P. Taylor. 1969. Differences in maximal

and submaximal work capacity in men and women. *J Appl Physiol.* 27:644–648.

119. Mancini, D. M., G. Walter, N. Reichek, R. Lenkinski, K. K. McCully, and J. L. Mullen. 1992. Contribution of skeletal muscle atrophy to exercise intolerance and altered muscle metabolism in heart failure. *Circulation.* 85:1364–1373.

120. Martin, F. L. 1976. *Effects of the Menstrual Cycle on Metabolic and Cardiorespiratory Responses.* Doctoral dissertation: The Ohio State University, Columbus, OH.

121. Massicotti, D. R., G. Avon, and G. Corrivean. 1979. Comparative effects of aerobic training on men and women. *J Sports Med.* 19(1):23–32.

122. Michielli, D. W., R. A. Stein, N. Krasnow, J. R. Diamond, and B. Horwitz. 1979. Effects of exercise training on ventricular dimensions at rest and during exercise. *Med Sci Sports.* 11(1):82.

123. Milesis, C., M. L. Pollock, M. D. Bah, J. J. Ayres, A. Ward, and A. C. Linnerud. 1976. Effects of different durations of physical training on cardiorespiratory function, body composition, and serum lipids. *Res Q.* 47(4):716–725.

124. Molé, P., L. Oscai, and J. O. Holloszy. 1971. Adaptation of muscle to exercise: increase in levels of palmityl CoA synthetase, carnitine palmityltransferase, and palmityl CoA dehydrogenase, and in the capacity to oxidize fatty acid. *J Clin Invest.* 50:2323–2330.

125. Morganroth, J., B. Maron, W. Henry, and S. Epstein. 1975. Comparative left ventricular dimensions in trained athletes. *Ann Intern Med.* 82:521–524.

126. Mostardi, R., R. Gandee, and T. Campbell. 1975. Multiple daily training and improvement in aerobic power. *Med Sci Sports.* 7(1):82.

127. Mutton, D. L., S. F. Loy, D. M. Rogers, G. J. Holland, W. J. Vincent, and M. Heng. 1993. Effect of run vs combined cycle/run training on VO$_2$ max and running performance. *Med Sci Sports Exerc.* 25(12):1393–1397.

128. Oscai, L., R. Williams, and B. Hertig. 1968. Effect of exercise on blood volume. *J Appl Physiol.* 24(5):622–624.

129. Otto, R. M. 1977. *Metabolic Responses of Young Women to Training and Maintenance/Detraining.* Doctoral dissertation: The Ohio State University, Columbus, OH.

130. Otto, R. M., E. L. Fox, and C. J. Stevens. 1978. Metabolic responses of young women to training and maintenance/detraining. *Med Sci Sports.* 10(1):52.

131. Pate, R. R., and J. D. Branch. 1992. Training for endurance sport. *Med Sci Sports Exerc.* 24(9 Suppl):S340–S343.

132. Pedersen, P., and J. Jorgensen. 1978. Maximal oxygen uptake in young women with training, inactivity, and retraining. *Med Sci Sports.* 10(4):233–237.

133. Pollock, M., T. Cureton, and L. Greninger. 1969. Effects of frequency of training on working capacity, cardiovascular function, and body composition of adult men. *Med Sci Sports.* 1(2):70–74.

134. Roeske, W. R., R. A. O'Rourke, A. Klein, G. Leopold, and J. Karliner. 1975. Noninvasive evaluation of ventricular hypertrophy in professional athletes. *Circulation.* 53:286–292.

135. Romero, L. 1970. *The Effects of an Interval Training Program on Selected Physiological Variables in Women.* Master's Thesis: The Ohio State University, Columbus OH.

136. Rubal, B. J., J. Rosentswieg, and B. Hamerly. 1981. Echocardiographic examination of women collegiate softball champions. *Med Sci Sports Exerc.* 13:176–179.

137. Ryan, A. 1975. Gynecological considerations. *J Phys Educ Res.* 46(10):40–44.

138. Saltin, B. 1969. Physiological effects of physical training. *Med Sci Sports.* 1(1):50–56.

139. Saltin, B., and P.-O. Åstrand. 1967. Maximal oxygen uptake in athletes. *J Appl Physiol.* 23:353–358.

140. Saltin, B., G. Blomqvist, J. Mitchell, R. Johnson, K. Wildenthal, and C. Chapman. 1968. Response to exercise after bed rest and after training. *Circulation.* 38 (suppl 7):1–78.

141. Saltin, B., L. Hartley, A. Kilbom, and I. Åstrand. 1969. Physical training in sedentary middle-aged and older men. II: Oxygen uptake, heart rate and blood lactate concentrations at submaximal and maximal exercise. *Scand J Clin Invest.* 24:323–334.

142. Saltin, B., and S. Strange. 1992. Maximal oxygen uptake: old and new arguments for cardiovascular limitation. *Med Sci Sports Exerc.* 24(1):30–37.

143. Schairer, J. R., S. J. Keteyian, J. W. Henry, and P. D. Stein. 1993. Left ventricular wall tension and stress during exercise in athletes and sedentary men. *Am J Cardiol.* 71:1095–1098.

144. Schairer, J. R., P. D. Stein, S. J. Keteyian, F. Fedel, J. Ehrman, M. Alam, J. W. Henry, and T. Shaw. 1992. Left ventricular response to submaximal exercise in endurance trained athletes and sedentary adults. *Am J Cardiol.* 70:930–933.

145. Scheuer, J., S. Penpargkul, and A. K. Bhan. 1974. Experimental observations on the effects of physical training upon intrinsic cardiac physiology and biochemistry. *Am J Cardiol.* 33:744–751.

146. Sharkey, B., and J. Holleman. 1967. Cardiorespiratory adaptations to training at specified intensities. *Res Q.* 38:698–704.

147. Shepley, B., J. D. MacDougall, N. Cipriano, J. R. Sutton, M. A. Tarnopolsky, and G. Coates. 1984. Physiologic effects of tapering in highly trained athletes. *J Appl Physiol.* 57:1668–1673.

148. Shi, X., G. H. J. Stevens, B. H. Foresman, S. A. Stern, and P. B. Raven. 1995. Autonomic nervous system control of the heart: endurance exercise training. *Med Sci Sports Exerc.* 27(10):1406–1413.

149. Shields, C., F. E. Whitney, and V. D. Zomar. 1984. Exercise performance of professional football players. *Am J Sports Med.* 12(6):455–459.

150. Sigvardsson, K., E. Svanfeldt, and A. Kilbom. 1977. Role of the adrenergic nervous system development of training-induced bradycardia. *Acta Physiol Scand.* 101:481–488.

151. Sjodin, B., and J. Svendenhag. 1985. Applied physiology of marathon running. *Sports Med.* 2:83–99.

152. Smith, D. C., and A. El-Hage. 1978. Effect of exercise training on the chronotropic response of isolated rat atria to atropine. *Experientia.* 34(8):1027–1028.

153. Smith, D. P., and F. W. Stransky. 1976. The effect of training and detraining on the body composition and cardiovascular response of young women to exercise. *J Sports Med.* 16:112–120.

154. Smith, M. L., D. L. Hudson, H. M. Graitzer, and P. B. Raven. 1989. Exercise training bradycardia: the role of autonomic balance. *Med Sci Sports Exerc.* 21(1):40–44.

155. Smith, M. L., and J. H. Mitchell. 1993. Cardiorespiratory adaptations to exercise training. In *ACSM's Resource Manual for Guidelines for Exercise Testing and Prescription,* 2d ed. Philadelphia: Lea & Febiger, pp 75–81.

156. Snoeckx, L. H., E. H. Abeling, J. A. C. Lanbreghts, J. J. F. Smitz, F. T. J. Verstappen, and R. S. Reneman. 1982. Echocardiographic dimensions in athletes relative to their training programs. *Med Sci Sports Exerc.* 14:428–434.

157. Stromme, S. B., F. Ingjer, and I. D. Meen. 1977. Assessment of maximal aerobic power in specifically trained athletes. *J Appl Physiol.* 42(6):833–837.

158. Sullivan, M. J., H. J. Green, and F. R. Cobb. 1990. Skeletal muscle biochemistry and histology in ambulatory patients with long-term heart failure. *Circulation.* 81:518–527.

159. Tanaka, H. 1994. Effects of cross-training. *Sports Med.* 18(5)330–339.

160. Taylor, A. W. 1975. The effects of exercise and training on the activities of human skeletal muscle glycogen cycle enzymes. In Howald, H., and J. R. Poortmans (eds.), *Metabolic Adaptation to Prolonged Physical Exercise.* Basel, Switzerland: Birkhauser Verlag, pp. 451–462.

161. Tibbits, G., B. J. Koziol, N. K. Roberts, K. M. Baldwin, and R. J. Barnard. 1978. Adaptation of the rat myocardium to endurance training. *J Appl Physiol.* 44(1):85–89.

162. Tipton, C., R. J. Barnard, and K. T. Tcheng. 1969. Resting heart rate investigations with trained and nontrained hypophysectomized rats. *J Appl Physiol.* 26(5):585–588.

163. Trappe, S. W., D. L. Costill, W. J. Fink, and D. R. Pearson. 1995. Skeletal muscle characteristics among distance runners: a 20-year follow-up study. *J Appl Physiol.* 78(3):823–829.

164. Turpeinen, A. K., J. T. Kuikka, E. Vanninen, P. Vainio, R. Vanninen, H. Litmanen, V. A. Koivisto, K. Bergstrom, and M. I. J. Usitupa. 1996. Athletic heart: a metabolic, anatomical, and functional study. *Med Sci Sports Exerc.* 28:33–40.

165. Underwood, R. H., and J. L. Schwade. 1977. Non-invasive analysis of cardiac function of elite distance runners echocardiography, vectorcardiography, and cardiac intervals. *Ann NY Acad Sci.* 301:297–309.

166. Van Handel, P. J., D. L. Costill, and L. H. Getchell. 1976. Central circulatory adaptations to physical training. *Res Q.* 47(4):815–823.

167. Wasserman, K., J. E. Hansen, D. Y. Sue, B. J. Whipp, and R. Casaburi. 1994. *Principles of Exercise Testing and Interpretation,* 2d ed. Philadelphia: Lea and Febiger.

168. Watt, E., E. Buskirk, and B. Plotnicki. 1973. A comparison of single vs. multiple daily training regimens: some physiological considerations. *Res Q.* 44(1):119–123.

169. Wilmore, J. H., J. Davis, R. O'Brien, P. Vodak, G. Walder, and E. Amsterdam. 1975. A comparative investigation of bicycling, tennis, and jogging as modes for altering cardiovascular endurance capacity. *Med Sci Sports.* 7(1):83.

170. Winder, W. W., J. M. Hagberg, R. C. Hickson, A. A. Ehsani, and J. A. McLane. 1978. Time course of sympathoadrenal adaptation to endurance exercise training in man. *J Appl Physiol.* 45(3):370–374.

171. Zaharieva, E. 1965. Survey of sportswomen at the Tokyo Olympics. *J Sports Med.* 5:215–219.

172. Zeldis, S. M., J. Morganroth, and S. Rubler. 1978. Cardiac hypertrophy in response to dynamic conditioning in female athletes. *J Appl Physiol.* 44(6):849–852.

173. Zerath, E., V. Novikov, A. Leblanc et al. 1996. Effects of spaceflight on bone mineralization in the rhesus monkey. *J Appl Physiol.* 81:194–200.

Selected Readings

American College of Sports Medicine. 1995. *Guidelines for Exercise Testing and Prescription,* 5th ed. Philadelphia: Lea and Febiger.

Costill, D. L., R. Thomas, R. A. Robergs, D. Pascoe, C. Lambert, S. Barr, and W. J. Fink. 1991. Adaptations to swimming training: influence of training volume. *Med Sci Sports Exerc.* 23(3):371–377.

Daniels, J. T., R. A. Yarbrough, and C. Foster. 1978. Changes in max VO$_2$ and running performance with training. *Eur J Appl Physiol.* 39:249–254.

Kearney, J. T. 1996. Training the Olympic athlete. *Sci American.* June:52–63.

Mazzeo, R. S. 1991. Catecholamine responses to acute and chronic exercise. *Med Sci Sports Exerc.* 23(7):839–845.

Paavolainen, L., K. Hakkinen, and H. Rusko. 1991. Effects of explosive type strength training on physical performance characteristics in cross-country skiers. *Eur J Appl Physiol.* 62:251–255.

Rundell, K. W. 1996. Effects of drafting during short-track speed skating. *Med Sci Sports Exerc.* 29(6):765–771.

Tabata, I., Y. Atomi, H. Kanehisa, and M. Miyashita. 1990. Effect of high-intensity training on isokinetic muscle power. *Eur J Appl Physiol.* 60:254–258.

Tipton, C. M., and A. C. Vailas. 1990. Bone and connective tissue adaptations to physical activity. In Bouchard, C., R. J. Shephard, T. Stephens, J. R. Sutton, and B. D. McPherson (eds.), *Exercise, Fitness, and Health.* Champaign, IL: Human Kinetics, pp. 331–344.

Wells, C. L. 1991. *Women, Sport and Performance: A Physiological Perspective.* Champaign, IL: Human Kinetics Publishers

Wolfe, L. A., D. A. Cunningham, P. A. Rechnitzer, and P. H. Nichol. 1979. Effects of endurance training on left ventricular dimensions in healthy men. *J Appl Physiol.* 47(1):207–212.

13

Development of Muscular Strength, Endurance, and Flexibility

This chapter investigates the concepts involved in the development of muscular strength and endurance-training programs and discusses joint flexibility as it relates to physical performance. Coaches, physical educators, clinicians, and trainers have always had an interest in muscular strength, endurance, and flexibility. Such interest has frequently centered on the following questions:

1. What is the most effective way in which strength, endurance, and flexibility may be gained?
2. What is the mechanism of "biological stimulation" that drives increases in muscle strength and cross-sectional area?
3. What physiological and biochemical changes do muscles undergo when they increase in strength and endurance?
4. Does strength development result in more rapid muscular contractions and therefore in increased power output for the individual?
5. Do weight-training programs and flexibility exercises positively affect sports performance?
6. Do people of all ages and both genders respond in a similar manner to strength and flexibility training regimens?
7. How long will these gains last?

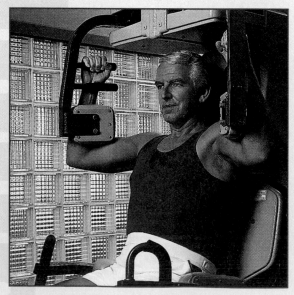

Weight-Training Programs

Flexibility

Summary

The major concepts to be learned from this chapter are as follows:

- When a muscle shortens while lifting a constant load, the tension developed over a range of motion depends on the length of the muscle, the angle of pull of the muscle on the skeleton, and the speed of shortening.
- Muscular strength and endurance can be significantly improved with properly planned weight resistance exercise programs.
- Increases in strength and endurance are accompanied by such physiological changes as increased muscle size (hypertrophy), small biochemical alterations, and adaptations within the nervous system.
- The physiological principle on which strength and endurance development depend is called the overload principle.
- Acute muscular soreness is caused by lack of adequate blood flow (ischemia), whereas delayed muscular soreness is probably caused by disruption of the connective tissues.
- The greatest improvement in skill performance caused by weight training-induced gains in muscle strength and endurance occur when training regimens include the muscle groups and simulate the movement patterns used during the skill.
- The "specificity" of progressive-resistance exercise programs relates to choices of type of training (e.g., static versus dynamic), joint angles used (isometric), and speed of contractions (isokinetic).
- Flexibility, the range of motion about a joint, is related to health, and to some extent, to athletic performance.

Weight-Training Programs

In this chapter, we will concentrate on the various kinds of weight-training and progressive-resistance exercise (PRE) programs that have been used for the development of muscular strength and endurance. We will start with some basic definitions and will then proceed to a discussion of the physiological changes induced by such programs. Finally, we will attempt to answer some of the questions posed earlier, relating strength and endurance to physical performance.

Muscular Strength: Definition and Types of Contractions

Muscular strength may be defined as the force or tension a muscle or, more correctly, a muscle group can exert against a resistance in one maximal effort. There are four basic types of muscular contraction: isotonic, isometric, eccentric, and isokinetic (table 13.1).

Isotonic Contraction

Isotonic contraction is one of the most familiar types of contraction. It is sometimes referred to as a **concentric contraction** or a **dynamic contraction.** Concentric simply means that a muscle shortens during contraction. Actually, the term dynamic contraction is more accurate, because isotonic literally means same or constant (*iso*) tension (*tonic*). In other words, an isotonic contraction supposedly is one that produces the same amount of tension while shortening as it overcomes a constant resistance. However, this is not true for intact muscles, because the tension exerted by a muscle as it shortens is affected by several important factors, three of which are (1) the initial length of the muscle fibers, (2) the angle of pull of the muscle on the bony skeleton, and (3) the speed of shortening. Speed of shortening is affected by the percentage of distribution of Type I and Type II fibers within a given muscle which was discussed previously (p. 150). Therefore, we will discuss only the first two factors here.

1. *Muscle Length-Tension Relationships.* As shown in figure 13.1, an isolated muscle can exert its maximal force or tension while in a stretched position. The range of peak tension is slightly greater than the resting length of the muscle as it would be positioned in the body. As the muscle shortens, less tension can be exerted. For instance, at about 60% of its resting length, the amount of tension that a muscle can exert approaches zero. The physiological reason for this is explained in figure 13.2 as follows: with excessive shortening (figure 13.2A), there is an overlap of actin filaments such that the filament from one side

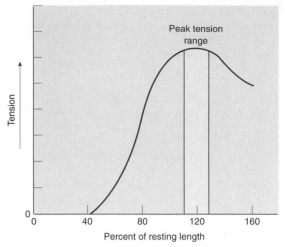

Figure 13.1

Relationship between tension developed during contraction and muscle length in an isolated muscle. Outside the body, the muscle is strongest at slightly greater than resting length.

interferes with the coupling potential of the cross-bridges on the other side. Because there are fewer cross-bridges "pulling" on the actin filaments, less tension can be developed. In figure 13.2*B* the length of the muscle (sarcomere)[66] is optimal so that all cross-bridges can connect with the actin filaments, and maximal tension can be developed. In figure 13.2*C* the sarcomere is stretched to such an extent that the actin filaments are pulled completely out of the range of the cross-bridges. Consequently, the bridges cannot connect, and no tension can be developed.

2. *Angle of Pull of Muscle.* From the previous discussion, we might conclude that a person can lift the heaviest load when the muscle is at its resting stretched length. However, this is not true, because the intact mechanical system with which we lift objects involves the use of both muscles for force and the use of bones for levers. It is the arrangement of the muscles and bones together that determines the final effect. Such an effect is shown in figure 13.3, which depicts the force or tension exerted by various intact muscle groups throughout their range of joint motion. If we let the joint angle represent the angle of pull of the muscle on the bone to which it is attached,* we see that for the elbow (forearm) flexor muscles, for instance, the strongest force is exerted between joint angles of 100 and 140 degrees (180 degrees is complete extension). At a joint angle of 180 degrees (the position of resting stretch), the

---

*The joint angle generally, but not always, accurately reflects the angle of pull of the muscle on the bone.

13.1

Summary of the types of muscular contraction

Type of contraction	Definition
Dynamic, isotonic, or concentric	The muscle shortens with varying tension while lifting a constant load.
Isometric or static	Tension develops but there is no change in the length of the muscle.
Eccentric	The muscle lengthens while contracting (developing tension).
Isokinetic	The tension developed by the muscle while shortening at constant speed is maximal over the full range of motion.

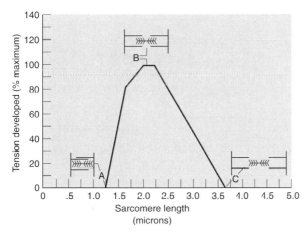

Figure 13.2

Relationship between the length of a sarcomere and the tension developed. *A*. With excessive shortening, there is an overlap of actin filaments such that the filament from one side interferes with the coupling potential of the cross-bridges on the other side, and little tension is developed. *B*. The length of the sarcomere is optimal, and all cross-bridges connect with the actin filaments, producing maximal tension. *C*. The sarcomere is stretched so that the actin filaments are beyond the range of the cross-bridges, and no tension is developed.

muscle group can exert only 64 pounds (29 kg) of force. The same thing can be seen of the other muscle groups in the figure. Note the great variability in the shapes of the curves for different muscle groups.

The preceding information has some applications to weight-training programs. First, remember that a dynamic (isotonic) contraction is one in which the muscle shortens while lifting a *constant* resistance, with the muscular tension varying somewhat over the full range of joint motion. Second, the tension required of a muscle to lift an object must be greater than the weight of the object. It follows then that the heaviest constant weight that can be lifted through a full range of joint motion can be no heavier than the weight that can be lifted at the weakest point of the muscle. As an ex-

ample, look at figure 13.3 again. Notice that the weakest point of the forearm flexor muscles through a range of motion between 40 and 180 degrees is 48 pounds pulled at 40 degrees. Therefore, the heaviest load that can be lifted over that range of forearm flexion is 48 pounds. When this is done, it is easy to see from figure 13.4 that the muscle is maximally contracted only at the joint angle of 40 degrees, or at its weakest point. At its strongest point (115 to 120 degrees), the muscle is contracted to only 53% of its maximum.

This same concept applies to other muscle groups, as is also shown in figure 13.4. The knee flexor muscle group, for instance, is taxed to only 25% of its maximum at joint angles between 140 and 180 degrees. This is a definite disadvantage with respect to strength-training programs that involve only isotonic contractions using constant loads, such as lifting free weights (e.g., barbells).

Recognizing this problem, manufacturers of weight-training equipment have developed machines to compensate for this disadvantage in weight training while lifting constant loads. One of these manufacturers (Nautilus/Sports Medical Industries) uses an odd-shaped cam (figure 13.5*A*) to compensate for the variations in muscular tension at different joint angles. It does this by changing the lever (moment) arm of the machine so that the load varies accordingly. This variation in load provides for maximal or at least near maximal muscular tension throughout the full range of joint motion. Other manufacturers (e.g., Universal Gym, Hammer Home Gym) have also developed variable resistance machines that provide for production of near maximal isotonic tension over a range of motion.

Isometric Contraction

The term *isometric* literally means same or constant (*iso*) length (*metric*). In other words, **isometric contraction** (or action) occurs when tension is developed, but there is no change in the external length of the muscle. The muscle does not shorten because the external resistance against which the muscle is pulling is greater than the maximal

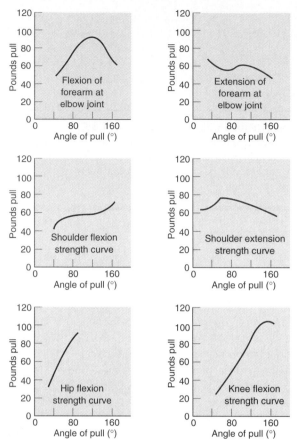

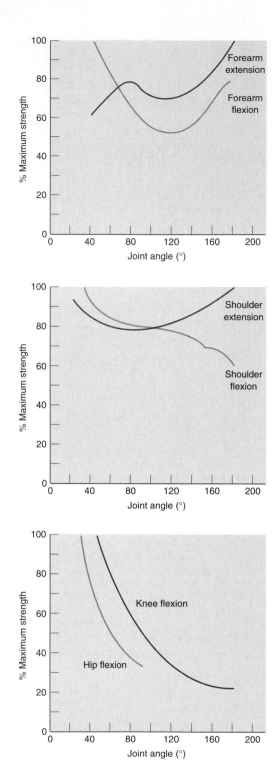

Figure 13.3

Relationship between tension (pounds pull) developed during contraction and angle of pull of the muscle (as indicated by joint angle) on the bone to which it is attached. In this case, strength is not always greatest at resting length (180°). For example, the elbow flexor muscles are strongest between 100° and 140°.

tension (internal force) the muscle can generate. Observe the use of the term pull rather than push. Although it is true that you may attempt to push a heavy, immovable object, the isometric force is always applied by muscles "pulling" on the bones. Another term used for isometric contraction (although isometric is accurate in its literal derivation) is **static contraction.**

Eccentric Contraction

Eccentric contraction (or action) refers to the lengthening of a muscle during contraction (i.e., during the development of active tension). A good example of an eccentric action is as follows: Flexing your elbow, have someone try to extend your forearm by pulling down on your wrist. At the same time, resist the pull by attempting to flex your elbow. As your forearm is extended, the elbow flexor muscles will lengthen while contracting. This, by definition, is an eccentric contraction. Eccentric contractions are used in resisting

Figure 13.4

When lifting a constant load through a range of joint motion (isotonic contraction), the muscle is maximally contracted only at its weakest point in the range.

gravity, such as walking down a hill or down steps. They also are often used in wrestling where one competitor will resist the efforts of the other to forcefully move their arm or leg but eventually may lose out in the struggle.

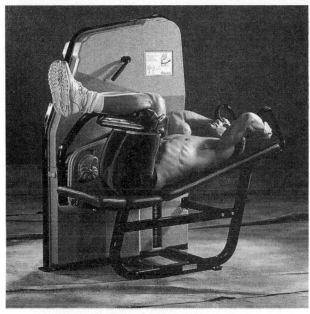

A

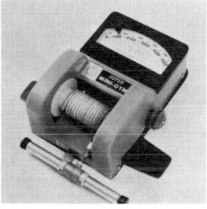

B

Figure 13.5

Strength training machines that provide partial accommodating resistance through different mechanisms. *A.* The Nautilus hip and back machine. A cam compensates for the variations in muscular force at different joint angles by changing the lever (moment) arm; as a result, the muscles exert maximal or near maximal force throughout the full range of motion. The Mini-Gym, *B,* uses a centrifugal clutch as the speed governor.

(Courtesy, Nautilus Sports/Medical Industries, DeLand, Florida and MGI Strength/Fitness, Independence, MO.)

Isokinetic Contraction

During an **isokinetic contraction,** the tension developed by the muscle as it shortens at constant (*iso*) speed (*kinetic*) is *maximal* at all joint angles over the full range of motion. Such contractions are common during sports performances; a good example is the arm stroke during freestyle swim-

ming. The application of full tension in either a sports performance setting or during clinical or laboratory testing is, of course, dependent on the motivation level of the performer.

Although isokinetic and isotonic contractions are both concentric (i.e., involve shortening), the two are not identical. As just mentioned, maximal tension can be developed throughout the full range of motion during isokinetic contractions but not during isotonic contractions. In addition, in an isotonic contraction the speed of movement is not controlled and may be relatively slow. This is something of a limitation, for as mentioned in an earlier chapter, it is more and more apparent that muscular power (i.e., both strength and speed of contraction) is a major success factor in many athletic performances.

To perform a controlled isokinetic contraction, special equipment is required (figure 13.6). The equipment contains a speed governor so that the speed of movement is constant no matter how much tension is produced in the contracting muscles. Therefore, if one attempts to make the movement as quickly as possible, the tension generated by the muscles will be maximal throughout the full range of motion, but the speed of movement will be constant. This feature, which is unique to truly isokinetic apparatus (figure 13.6*B*), is called **accommodating resistance.** The movement speed on many isokinetic devices can be preset and can vary between 0 and approximately 300 degrees of motion per second. Many movement speeds during actual athletic performances exceed 200 degrees per second. Most of the isokinetic machines also have devices for readout that record either force or torque. Some also simultaneously record joint angles so the points of low- and high-force outputs throughout the range of limb movement can be identified. This is a particular advantage, because a readout provides for scientific evaluation and research and can serve as a training monitor during actual training and injury rehabilitation sessions.

There also are strength-training machines that provide partial accommodating resistance (figures 13.5, 13.6*A*). Most of them operate on the principle of hydraulics i.e., forced oil displacement through an adjustable orifice in a closed cylinder similar to a car's shock absorber. The greater the force applied to the system, the greater the resistance offered by the oil as it is squeezed from one chamber to another. The difference between this and isokinetics, in the strictest sense of the word, is that the hydraulic machines can be pushed and pulled at somewhat different rates of speed depending on the strength of the user. This is in contrast to the fully accommodating resistance of the true isokinetic machines where the apparatus moves only at a fixed, preset speed, regardless of the amount of force applied against it.

The strength of intact muscle groups can be measured in a variety of ways. The techniques and apparatus parallel the different types of contractions (i.e., isometric, isotonic, eccentric, and isokinetic). The three latter test modes are called dynamic because they involve movement, whereas

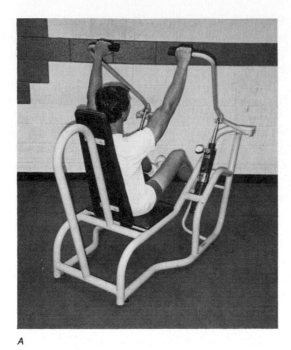

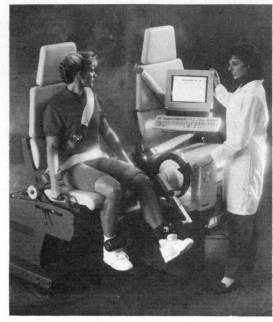

A   B

Figure 13.6

Near-isokinetic strength training and testing equipment. The Hydra-Fitness chest press machine, *A,* uses a hydraulic oil displacement system to provide partial accommodating resistance. The Cybex test machine, *B,* uses electric servo-braking to provide nearly complete accommodating resistance so that the muscles shorten at constant speed and can be maximally loaded throughout the full range of motion.

(Courtesy Hydra-Fitness Industries, Belton, TX, and Cybex, Division of Lumex, Inc., Ronkonkoma, NY.)

isometric tests are frequently called static tests. Examples of static tests are those that use a cable tensiometer or electronic force transducer (strain gauge) attached in series with an immoveable linkage system. Maximum force is measured at joint angles that approximate the most favorable angle for a given muscle group and joint. Isokinetic tests are usually conducted at different speed settings on equipment where a zero speed setting can also be used to measure static strength at different joint angles. Isotonic tests often involve repeated trials at lifting free or machine weights (figure 13.7) to determine the maximum weight that can be lifted one time. This is called **one repetition maximum** or **1 RM.** Because of its simplicity and control over shifts in body position, the bench press 1 RM test using either free or machine weights is a popular test of isotonic strength. Similar tests can be conducted for other muscle groups and the results used to initiate weight-training programs, usually at 80% to 90% of 1 RM. Tests of eccentric strength require special apparatus to measure dynamic force during muscle elongation. Each testing method has its advantages and disadvantages. A comparison of isometric, isotonic, and isokinetic methods of testing the strength of knee and elbow flexor and extensor muscles of the same subjects yielded similar results. The average correlation among the three testing modes was quite high, $r = 0.78$, suggesting that a similar phenomenon termed maximal voluntary strength was being measured.[92]

From both a theoretical and practical viewpoint, isokinetic contractions and, therefore, isokinetic measurements and training programs appear to be most suited for improving muscular strength and endurance for athletic performances. Further details of such programs and their effects will be discussed later in this chapter.

Muscular Endurance Defined

As with strength, there are four kinds of local muscular endurance depending on which of the four types of contraction are used. Local **muscular endurance** is usually defined as the ability or capacity of a muscle group to perform repeated contractions (isotonic, isokinetic, or eccentric) against a load or to sustain a contraction (isometric) for an extended period of time. Dynamic endurance tests may be of the *absolute* or *fixed load* type where all subjects are required to lift a common amount of weight—say 50 lb—at a set cadence until they can no longer keep up the pace. This is in contrast to *relative load* endurance tests where subjects are assigned a fixed percentage of their maximum strength, say 20% to 50% of 1 RM or of peak isometric tension. They are then timed for their ability to endure a given lifting cadence in dynamic tests, or to sustain a predetermined level of static force in isometric tests. Interestingly, women often outperform men on these static and dynamic relative load

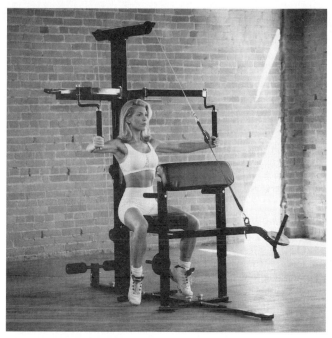

A

Figure 13.7

Strength training machines that utilize pulleys and weight stacks to promote safety and some change in leverage. The Hammer Home Gym, *A*, utilizes a unique leverage system so multiple lifts can be performed using light weights on the same small frame. The Cybex seated chest press machine, *B*, is an example of a special machine that is fully dedicated to a specific exercise.

(Courtesy Hammer Home Gym, Ann Arbor, MI, and Cybex, Division of Lumex, Inc., Ronkonkoma, NY.).

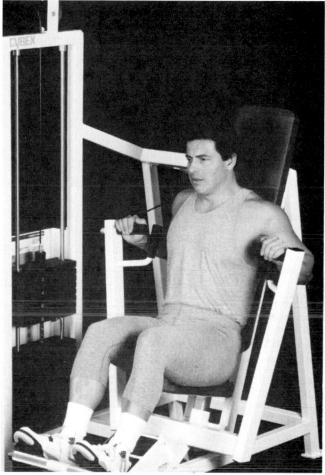

B

endurance tests, especially at the lower load assignment percentages.[119]

Muscular endurance may also be defined as the opposite of muscular fatigue (i.e., a muscle that fatigues rapidly has a low endurance capacity and vice versa). Some of the factors that contribute to local muscular fatigue, including the influence of Type I and Type II fiber distribution, were discussed in an earlier chapter (p. 158) and should be reviewed now. In this chapter we will limit our discussion as to how local muscular endurance can be increased through weight-resistance training programs.

Physiological Changes Accompanying Increased Strength

Muscular exercise is such a common experience that the more striking effects are evident to all. One need go no farther than the school playground to hear the familiar challenge, "Show us your muscle." Indeed, muscle enlargement with a corresponding increase in strength is a commonly observed phenomenon (it was first shown scientifically as early as 1897).[124] However, Jones[89] points out that the strength of an individual muscle depends on a number of factors in addition to its cross-sectional area (CSA)—such as, (1) the extent to which the muscle can be activated by voluntary effort, (2) the overall length of the muscle and the position in which it is used, (3) the fiber type composition, and (4) the velocity at which the movement takes place.

Jones et al.[90] have also identified three phases that commonly make up the strength training adaptation process. Phase one is a period of rapid improvement in lifting ability resulting from a learning process—i.e., a correct sequence for lifting, which is laid down in the CNS as a motor pattern. There is little or no real increase in size or strength of individual muscles but the trainee may feel "stronger." Phase two is a period where there is an increase in strength of individual muscle fibers but no accompanying increase in cross-sectional area (CSA). This could be the result of increased neural activation or some change in muscle fibers or connective tissue, but the mechanism is not clear. Phase three is a period after some weeks of training where there is a slow but steady increase in both size and strength of exercised muscles. This latter phase may not

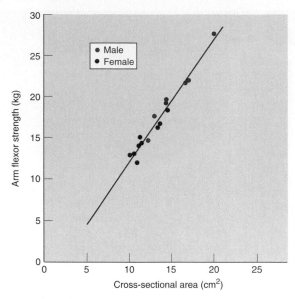

Figure 13.8

Relationship between the strength of the arm flexor muscles and their cross-sectional area. Notice that the relationship is the same for both males and females.

(Based on data from Ikai and Fukunaga.[83])

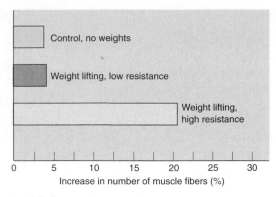

Figure 13.9

Effects of longitudinal fiber splitting on number of muscle fibers. A 20% increase in the number of muscle fibers was found in cats following a 5-day-per-week, 34-week-long program of weight lifting. Note that the fiber splitting is apparently intensity related in that it occurred only after a high-resistance program.

(Based on data from Gonyea.[65])

occur until after 12 weeks in some trainees, with possible contributing mechanisms mentioned in the following discussion. Studies suggest that high forces in the muscle may induce some form of damage that promotes hypertrophy, possibly through division of satellite cells and their incorporation into existing muscle fibers.[89]

Hypertrophy

The enlargement of muscle that results from weight-training programs is mainly due to an increase in the cross-sectional area of the individual muscle fibers. This increase in fiber diameter is called **hypertrophy;** a reduction in size is called **atrophy.** In untrained muscle, the fibers vary considerably in diameter. The objective of a strengthening exercise program is to bring the smaller muscle fibers up to the size of the larger ones. Rarely does hypertrophy of the once smaller fibers exceed the cross-sectional area of the previously existing larger ones. The relationship between the strength of a muscle and its cross-sectional area is shown in figure 13.8. Notice that it is the same for men and women.

Hypertrophy of individual muscle fibers is attributable to one or more of the following changes:[62]

1. Increased number and size of myofibrils per muscle fiber.[63,67,112]
2. Increased total amount of contractile protein,[67,113] particularly in the myosin filament.[131]
3. Increased capillary density per fiber.
4. Increased amounts and strength of connective, tendinous, and ligamentous tissues.[166,167]

The changes that contribute most to hypertrophy following weight-training programs are probably the first three listed. Although an increased number of capillaries per fiber (number 3) is likely to be more closely associated with increased muscular endurance, five weeks of intense strength training caused capillary endothelial cells to swell by 23%.[22]

The finding of **longitudinal fiber splitting** in chronically exercised (weight lifting) animals[48,64,65,79] is an interesting phenomenon and deserves further comment. For nearly 85 years, the increased size of a muscle, as a result of weight training, has been attributed solely to an increase in the diameter of the muscle fibers already present (hypertrophy) and not to an increase in the number of fibers (**hyperplasia**). Observation of fiber splitting, of course, casts some doubt on earlier theories about increases in muscle size. For example, studies were reported, figure 13.9,[64,65] in which a 20% increase in the number of fibers was found in cats following a 5-day-per-week, 34-week-long program of weight lifting. Fiber splitting, in this case, was apparently intensity related in that it occurred only after a high-resistance program. Also, although fiber splitting has been shown in several different animals (e.g., rats and cats), it has not as yet been shown to occur in humans following weight-training programs.[112]

Hypertrophy and Testosterone Levels

It is a popular belief that a large muscle mass and hypertrophy resulting from weight-training programs are related to high levels of the male hormone **testosterone.** This is particularly true regarding the so-called masculinizing effect of weight training in females. Although these ideas may be popular, they are not supported by scientific fact. For example, correlations among serum testosterone, body composition, and muscular strength were all nonsignificant in both high school and college men and women.[52] In another study,[75] it was concluded that chronic androgen (testosterone) levels do not change significantly in adult men or women during the course of weight-lifting programs. Although blood levels of testosterone are elevated following single bouts of maximal exercise,[56,157] including weight lifting,[52] no physiological changes occur as a result.

Because the preceding studies were conducted only on adults, the question may be raised as to whether there is a difference in the response of pre- and postpubescent children to strength-training programs. In this case, the presence of testosterone in the blood might lead to a different or more profound physiological response. Study of this issue[172] found that among prepubescent boys, no consistent pattern of strength change was noted following a weight-training program. On the other hand, in postpubescent boys there were significant increases in strength in all muscles tested. These results suggest that the presence of testosterone may at least be a prerequisite for promoting strength gains and that weight-training programs for the purpose of increasing muscular strength in prepubescent children are not effective. Obviously, more research along these lines is required.

Biochemical and Muscle Fiber Compositional Changes

The following biochemical and fiber compositional changes in skeletal muscle have been shown to occur following weight-training programs:

1. Increases in concentrations of muscle creatine (by 39%), phosphocreatine (by 22%), ATP (by 18%), and glycogen (by 66%).[114]
2. Increase[32,94] or no change[32,165] in glycolytic enzyme activities (phosphofructokinase, or PFK; lactate dehydrogenase, or LDH; muscle phosphorylase; and hexokinase).
3. Little or no consistent change in the activity of ATP turnover enzymes, such as myokinase and creatine phosphokinase.[32,94,165]
4. Small but significant increases in aerobic Krebs Cycle enzyme activities (e.g., malate dehydrogenase, or MDH; succinic dehydrogenase, or SDH).[32,94]
5. No interconversion of Type I and Type II fibers.[32,45,165]
6. A decrease in the volume (density) of mitochondria due to increases in size of the myofibrils and the sarcoplasmic volume.[113]
7. A selective hypertrophy of Type II fibers as evidenced by an increase in the Type II:Type I fiber area ratio[32,45,165] and a retardation of their loss.[137]
8. A shift in percentage of Type IIB to Type IIA fibers from both strength and endurance training programs.[96]

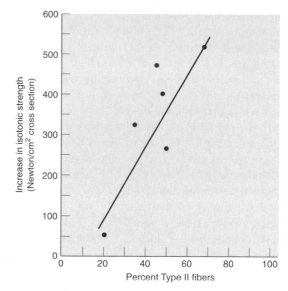

Figure 13.10

The increase in isotonic strength per unit of muscle cross-sectional area is positively correlated with the percentage of distribution of Type II muscle fibers.

(Based on data from Dons et al[45])

Two major conclusions seem warranted based on the previous changes. First, the biochemical changes are small and to some extent inconsistent. Therefore, it is highly likely that other changes are mostly responsible for improved muscle function following weight training. Although these other changes have not been precisely identified, they probably involve adaptations within the nervous system,[141] including changes in the recruitment pattern[164] and synchronization[120] of motor units.

Second, it appears that a high percentage of distribution of Type II fibers is a prerequisite for maximal gains from strength-training programs. This is suggested by the selective hypertrophy of Type II fibers, which reflects their preferential use during the strength-training exercises. In addition, as shown in figure 13.10, the increase in isotonic strength per unit of muscle cross-sectional area is positively correlated with the percentage of Type II fibers.[45] This relationship may also help explain why the individual response to training varies considerably, and why there is a lack of consistency in the weight-training literature regarding the relative effects of different training programs.[45]

Stimulus for Strength and Endurance Gains

What causes a muscle to increase in strength and endurance? We have already indicated that certain physiological and biochemical changes are somewhat associated with an increased capacity of the muscle to exert maximal force as well as to exert submaximal force over an extended period of time. Additionally, we know that chronic stress or use of the muscles, as would be the case with regularly scheduled weight-training programs, is the ultimate stimulus for increased levels of strength and endurance. This translates into the presence of high forces within the muscles on a regular and frequent basis as the biological stimulus.

Two other specific stresses that have been investigated are hypoxia and fatigue. Strength training at an altitude of 5050 m (called chronic hypobaric hypoxia) results in less of an increase in isometric strength and cross-sectional area than does training at sea-level.[127] Studies have suggested that hypoxic conditions may reduce work-induced skeletal muscle hypertrophy by inhibiting the rate of protein synthesis. This would make it more difficult to increase muscle mass if one trained at altitude. It also calls into question the importance of hypoxia as a mechanistic explanation for skeletal muscle adaptation. The case for fatigue being an important stimulus is stronger. Allowing no rest between lifts results in more of an increase in dynamic strength (56.3% versus 41.2%) than allowing 30 sec of rest between lifts.[138] These findings indicate that strength trainees should perform lifts without resting between reps and sets so that fatigue will contribute to the overall strength training stimulus.

All the changes described thus far can be said to have occurred in the muscle tissue itself. What about the nervous system? Is it not true that within the body, a muscle voluntarily contracts through the control of the central nervous system? This fact, coupled with the belief that early "strength" gains reflect the laying down of new motor programs, point to the importance of the nervous system. This learning process appears to be very specific—i.e., lifting weights produces better weight lifters but not necessarily better sprinters.[90] There also is some evidence to suggest that changes in the central nervous system act as stimuli for gains in both strength and endurance. A good example of this was mentioned in the discussion of the Golgi tendon organ (p. 119), where we said that the breaking point of strength testing could very well be limited by the inhibiting influence of these proprioceptor.

Another example is given by well documented stories of extraordinary feats of muscular strength and endurance. These feats usually occur under exceptional circumstances, such as frightening or life-and-death situations. Nevertheless, they may be interpreted to mean that under normal circumstances, strength and endurance are *inhibited* by the central nervous system.[84] Such feats could be explained on the basis that normally it is not possible, because of central nervous system inhibitions, to activate all the motor units available within a muscle or muscle group. Under extreme circumstances, such inhibitions would be removed and thus all motor units activated. A reduction in central nervous system inhibition with concomitant increases in strength and endurance might also seem to be a reasonable change that could be "learned" through weight-training programs. The effects of this learning could be reflected in a combination of neural reflex facilitation and removal of reflex-mediated inhibition of motor neurons at the spinal cord level. Each change would result in an expansion of the recruitable motor neuron pool. Such expansion would translate into increases in maximum strength performance independent of any changes in the muscles themselves.

There are other data to support the notion that early changes during strength training programs are occurring within the nervous system. Jones[89] explains that "over a period of 2 to 3 months the major benefit of training is to improve the skill with which the training exercise is carried out." Even subjects accustomed to strength training show a significant increase in neural activation (as indicated by integrated, electromyographic, or EMG, measures) that correlates with strength increases during early periods of more intense training.[71] Kraemer, et al., in their excellent review, concluded that the time course of the development of the neuromuscular system with strength training is dominated in the early phase by neural factors. These neural changes are accompanied by only modest changes in contractile proteins, and it is not until a later adaptation phase that changes in the contractile unit begins to contribute most to improvements in performance capabilities. They suggest that several factors can affect this pattern of adaptation. Namely, functional capabilities of the individual, age, nutritional status, and behavioral factors (e.g. sleep, health habits).[95]

Weight Training and Body Composition Changes

For the average college-age male and female, body composition changes following a weight-training program will consist of (1) little or no change in total body weight, (2) significant losses of relative and absolute body fat, and (3) a significant gain in lean body weight (presumably muscle mass). For example, 5 weeks of one-leg isokinetic strength training produced the following changes in ten middle-aged females: increases in thigh muscle thickness, relative number of Type II fibers, and relative area of Type IIB fibers, and a decrease of subcutaneous adipose tissue.[98] The fat changes were determined by ultrasound and skinfold caliper measurements. Because fat cell size did not change, the decrease in thickness of the subcutaneous fat layer was due to geometrical factors related to hypertrophy of the underlying muscles. These findings were therefore not viewed as evidence in support of the concept of "spot fat reduction" or local emptying of fat depots in the areas of exercising muscles.[98] More is said about these changes in chapter 16.

The Overload Principle

The physiological principle on which strength and endurance development depends is known as the **overload principle.** This principle states simply that the strength, endurance, and hypertrophy of a muscle will increase only when the muscle performs for a given period of time at near its maximal strength and endurance capacity (i.e., against work loads that are above those normally encountered). As early as 1919, Lange[100] expressed in the scientific literature the first views on the relationship between muscle hypertrophy and the overload phenomenon:

> Only when a muscle performs with greatest power, i.e., through the overcoming of greater resistance in a unit of time than before, would its functional cross section need to increase. . . . If, however, the muscle performance is increased merely by working against the same resistance as before for a longer time, no increase in the contractile substance is necessary.

One of the first experimental demonstrations in humans of the overload principle was made by Hellebrandt and Houtz in 1956.[74] Some of their results are shown in figure 13.11. The gains in strength and endurance are most pronounced when the muscle is exercised in the overload zone (i.e., with resistances far above those normally encountered). Underload, in this case, refers to resistances below those normally encountered by the muscle.

The overload principle, when applied to weight-training programs, means that the resistance against which the muscle works should be increased throughout the course of the program as the muscle gains in strength and endurance. For this reason, the original version of the overload principle, as first stated by Lange, has been modified to what we now call the principle of **progressive-resistance exercise (PRE).** In fact there is some preference for this term to describe all types of resistance-training methods including devices that can be stretched or compressed, calisthenics that are progressive, as well as various types of weight training.

A unique study of chronic overload training among eleven international caliber jumpers and throwers has been reported.[20] They wore weighted vests equal to 13% of their body weight all day except while sleeping. After a three-week period of overload the subjects showed significant improvements in vertical jumping ability from a squat position and also for a 15-second endurance test period. These improvements were lost within 4 weeks after removal of the vests.[20]

Specificity of Weight Training

Experience has taught successful coaches that to increase the performance of their athletes, a specific training program must be planned for each athlete. This is referred to as **specificity of training.** In other words, the training programs must be relevant to the demands of the event for which the athlete is being trained. Such demands include (1) the predominant energy system(s) involved and (2) the movement patterns and the specific muscle groups involved. The first demand is discussed in more detail in chapter 11

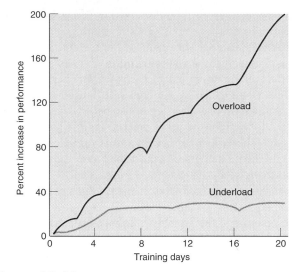

Figure 13.11

The overload principle. Gains in strength and endurance are most pronounced when the muscle is exercised in the overload zone (i.e., with resistances above those normally encountered by the muscle).

(Based on data from Hellebrandt and Houtz.[74])

(p. 270). The second demand means that gains in strength and endurance will improve skill performance to the greatest extent when the training program consists of progressive-resistance exercises that include the muscle groups and simulate the movement patterns most often used during the actual execution of that skill. For example, weight-training exercises for improvement in swimming the breast stroke should focus on those muscles and their movement patterns associated with the breast stroke. Likewise, performing strength-training exercises in a posture (e.g., supine vs. upright) that more closely matches the movements they are attempting to facilitate is an important aspect of training specificity. This may be due to an enhanced neural input to the musculature that is posture-specific.[178]

The specificity of weight training is demonstrable in other ways. You will recall from chapter 6 that Type II fibers are preferentially recruited for sprintlike activities, including weight lifting, and Type I fibers for endurance exercises. To maximally improve performance in either of these activities, training must be specific to increasing the functional capabilities of the respective fiber types. The information presented earlier on fiber type and the force-velocity curve (p. 156) bears this out. Also, strength training has been shown to be somewhat specific to the joint angle at which the muscle group is trained.[10,57,108] In other words, a muscle group trained, for example, at a joint angle of 115 degrees will not necessarily show increased strength at other joint angles. Specificity is further evidenced by the fact that isometric programs will increase isometric strength more than they will isotonic strength and vice versa.[14,47] The importance of specificity of training speed as it translates to performance power will be discussed in the section on isokinetic training.

A further aspect of specificity of weight training and exercise is the matter of **cross training** or **transfer of training** effects to other regions of the body. The basic question is whether strengthening the legs will transfer to the arms and shoulders so that these areas also become stronger. Will continuing to train the arms protect against losses in leg strength? There is some evidence that leg exercise influences the EMG activity of arm biceps muscles so they appear as though they also had been contracting.[180] This would support the existence of an electrophysiological transfer effect. There is less evidence that exercising with one region of the body (e.g., the arms) can promote retention of training effects derived from training a different region (e.g., the legs).[130] Any strength gains by transfer effects would likely be small so it is appropriate to think of PRE training benefits as being specific to body regions and not generally transferable.

Finally, there is some evidence that simultaneously training (dual-mode) for strength and muscular endurance will interfere with strength development.[77,96] In one study there was a reduced increase in performance measures when strength and endurance training were combined, and only subjects who trained specifically for strength showed improvements in power output. It was concluded that dual-mode training attenuates the expected performance improvements and physiological adaptations that ordinarily accompany single-mode training.[96] In another study three exercise groups comprised of adult males and females were used: a strength-training group that weight trained 30 to 40 minutes per day, 5 days per week; an aerobic endurance-training group that rode stationary bicycle ergometers for 40 minutes per day, 6 days per week; and a combination strength and endurance group that did both workouts each day. After 10 weeks the strength group showed no improvement in $\dot{V}O_2$ max and the aerobic endurance group showed no improvement in strength. The combination group showed improvements in $\dot{V}O_2$ max at 10 weeks and in strength up to the seventh week. Thereafter strength gains leveled off and actually declined during the ninth and tenth weeks.

In the above study, simultaneously training for both muscle strength and aerobic endurance eventually reduced somewhat the subjects' capacity to develop strength, but did not affect their ability to improve their $\dot{V}O_2$ max—~20%. Similar improvements in $\dot{V}O_2$ max (i.e., 25%) have been shown for young female subjects who ran 45 minutes per day, 3 days per week over 24 weeks.[85] Contrary to these findings, others have shown that combined training has produced improvements in both strength and $\dot{V}O_2$ peak measures.[110] Differences between studies may be because a conventional three-day-per-week strength and endurance training program was used rather than a higher intensity regime. These findings have important implications when working with clients who have only a limited time for training and are interested in improving both their aerobic endurance and strength at the same time.

Other studies have been conducted to determine the effects of selected training combinations in terms of their specificity. For example, combining heavy (80% to 120% of 1RM) concentric and eccentric training over a 16-week period produced significant increases in maximal isometric force of leg extensor muscles.[72] Increases in strength were accompanied by increases in vertical jump heights and mechanical parameters indicative of improved muscle function—e.g., increased positive force during fast dynamic contraction was correlated with reduced time to produce a given submaximal isometric force. There also are some indications that strength training along with flexibility training inhibits gains in shoulder abduction range of motion.[61] Finally, findings from a recent study of rats[144] indicates that combining cardiorespiratory endurance training with strength training may add some protection for tendons and ligaments—i.e., some lower intensity repetitive muscle contractions may prevent strengthened muscles from damaging connective tissues.

Two questions frequently raised in discussions of training specificity are (1) how transferable is strength that is gained from one type of muscle contraction to another type of muscle contraction? and (2) do increases in strength result in a diminished ability to perform submaximal tasks? It appears that transferability is limited. For example, increases in 10-RM strength gained through either single- or multiple-joint isotonic training is not transferable to isometric or isokinetic movements or to rate of torque development.[150] With regard to any negative effect of strength gains, neither upper (23%) or lower (37%) extremity strength increases brought about by training 3 days per week over 16 weeks produced any performance deficits.[78] These findings suggest that improvements in strength approaching 40% have no negative effect on the performance of submaximal exercise tasks.

Specificity of training is obviously important and should be taken into account when planning a weight-training program whether it is meant to improve athletic or recreational performance. For optimal results appropriate choices of training mode (type of training) should be made, such as static versus dynamic. If isometric training is practiced, the most appropriate joint angles should be selected. Likewise, if isokinetic training is considered to have the greatest specificity, then thought should be given to the best speed to use during practice contractions. Arguments also have been made for specificity as it relates to the strength testing of muscle groups in different regions of the body. Limb muscles should be tested dynamically (isotonic or isokinetic) because they are involved in rapid movements. Trunk muscles, on the other hand, might best be tested using static tests because their major roles are stabilization and maintenance of posture.[156]

Muscular Soreness

At one time or another, all of us have experienced muscular soreness, particularly with weight-training programs. Generally, two types of muscle soreness are recognized: (1) acute soreness and (2) delayed soreness.

Acute Soreness

Acute muscular soreness and pain that, as its name implies, occurs *during* and *immediately following* the exercise period is thought to be associated with a lack of adequate blood flow (**ischemia**) to the active muscles. Perhaps the most conclusive scientific evidence pointing to ischemia as the primary cause was gathered more than 40 years ago.[46] Some of these data are presented in figure 13.12. In *A* a sustained isometric contraction of the finger flexor muscles was performed at the same time that the circulation to those muscles was occluded. Notice how the pain (soreness) increased not only during the contraction period but also for nearly a minute after the contraction was stopped, and while the circulation remained occluded. When blood flow was restored, the muscle pain decreased rather rapidly. In *B* the same kind of experiment was conducted but with the circulation to the active muscles left intact. Under these conditions, muscle pain followed fairly well the intensity of the contraction. For example, the pain increased to maximum when the intensity of the contraction was maximal, then declined slowly along with contraction intensity.

From the preceding experiments, the following conclusions concerning acute muscular soreness were made:

1. Muscular pain during contractions occurs when the tension generated is great enough to occlude blood flow to the active muscles (ischemia).
2. Because of the ischemia, metabolic waste products, such as lactic acid and potassium, cannot be removed and thus accumulate to the point of stimulating the pain receptors located in the muscles.
3. The pain continues until either the intensity of the contraction is reduced or the contraction ceases altogether—restoring blood flow so that accumulated waste products can be removed.

Delayed Muscular Soreness

Acute soreness, although often an annoyance, does not pose much of a problem because it is short-lived and is soon alleviated when exercise is discontinued. The more serious problem is **delayed onset muscular soreness (DOMS),** which is the pain and soreness that occurs 24 to 48 hours after exercise sessions have stopped.

Experiments designed to induce delayed muscular soreness,[93,160] have found that the degree of DOMS is related to the type of muscle contraction performed. In one experiment, muscle soreness was induced with weight-

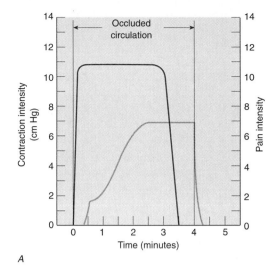

A

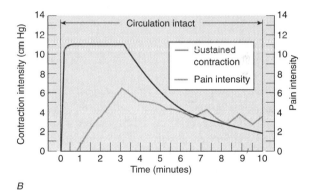

B

Figure 13.12

Acute muscular soreness and muscle ischemia. *A.* A sustained isometric contraction of the finger flexor muscles was performed at the same time that the circulation to those muscles was occluded (ischemia). The pain (soreness) increased during and was maintained after the contraction period than decreased when blood flow was restored. *B.* The same experiments as in *A* but with the circulation to the active muscles intact. Muscular pain followed fairly well the intensity of the contraction.

(Based on data from Dorpat and Holmes.[46])

lifting exercises as follows: male and female subjects performed two sets of exhaustive contractions of the elbow flexor muscles with barbells. During eccentric contractions, the barbell was only actively lowered, whereas during isotonic contractions, it was only actively raised. During isometric contractions, the barbell was held stationary. As shown in figure 13.13, muscle soreness was found to be most pronounced following eccentric contractions and was least pronounced following isotonic contractions. The soreness following isometric contractions was only slightly greater than that following isotonic contractions, but it was still considerably below that found after eccentric contractions. Also, in all cases the soreness was delayed, the greatest delay being 24 to 48 hours after exercise.

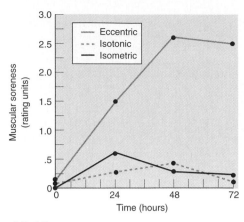

Figure 13.13

Delayed muscle soreness is most pronounced following eccentric contractions and is least pronounced following isotonic and isometric contractions.

(Based on data from Talag.[160])

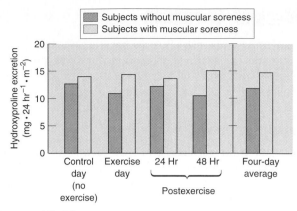

Figure 13.14

Hydroxyproline excretion was higher on the exercise day and after 24 and, particularly, 48 hours after exercise in subjects who had muscular soreness than in those who did not. These results suggest that delayed muscular soreness is most likely due to disruption of the connective tissue elements in the muscles and tendons.

(Based on data from Abraham.[1])

Although not presented in figure 13.13, this experiment also showed that muscular strength decreased appreciably following eccentric contractions and remained depressed throughout the duration of the soreness period. No significant decrease in strength was noted during the soreness period following isotonic or isometric contractions. Finally, little or no delayed muscle soreness was noted following isokinetic contractions, nor was there any decrease in strength.

What causes delayed muscular soreness and how can it be avoided? The exact cause (or causes) of delayed onset muscle soreness are not known. However, three different theories have been advanced.

1. *The Torn Tissue Theory.*[81] This theory proposes that tissue damage, such as the tearing of muscle fibers, could explain muscle soreness.
2. *The Spasm Theory.*[42,44] In this theory, three stages of action are suggested: (a) exercise causes ischemia within the active muscle, (b) ischemia leads to the accumulation of an unknown "pain substance" (or P substance) that stimulates the pain nerve endings in the muscle, and (c) the pain brings about a reflex muscle spasm that causes further ischemia, and the entire cycle is repeated.
3. *The Connective Tissue Theory.*[8,93] This theory suggests that the connective tissues, including the tendons, are damaged during contraction, thus causing muscular pain.

Some current studies support the torn tissue theory. Serum creatine kinase (CK), a cellular enzyme whose presence in the blood indicates muscle cell disruption, was found to be elevated twofold above baseline eight hours af-

ter older male subjects (50 to 69 years of age) engaged in a heavy resistance strength-training program.[82] Conversely, there was much less of an increase in CK among these subjects at the same absolute and relative resistance loading following 16 weeks of training. Interestingly, increases in CK activity were not accompanied by reports of muscle soreness, which was only occasionally reported at the beginning of training and was almost nonexistent after training. It was concluded that middle-aged and older men can safely participate in a total body strength-training program that is intense enough to produce substantial increases in muscle strength and hypertrophy without it promoting muscle soreness or significant cell disruption.[82] The comparative effect of electromyostimulation (EMS) versus concentric contractions on damage to muscle fibers has been studied using plasma CK and lactate dehydrogenase (LDH) as markers. Muscle soreness was greatest in the EMS subjects, with peak soreness occurring on the second day after contractions. Peak soreness coincided with significant increases in CK and LDH enzymes, suggesting that electrical stimulation causes more myofiber membrane damage than does a similar amount of voluntary strength-training exercise.[123]

Other studies designed specifically to investigate these theories[1,2] concluded that delayed muscular soreness is most likely related to disruption of the connective tissue elements in the muscles and tendons. Some of the results of these studies are shown in figure 13.14. One of the products from the damage and breakdown of connective tissue is a substance called *hydroxyproline,* which appears in the urine. Therefore, urinary excretion of hydroxyproline was monitored in subjects over several days as follows: on a control day when no exercise was performed, on an exercise day during which some of the subjects experienced muscular soreness and some did not, and 24 and 48 hours following exercise. Among subjects who experienced muscle soreness, hydroxyproline excretion was higher on the exercise day, after 24 hours and, particularly, after 48 hours, when compared to subjects who were not sore. In addition, a more detailed analysis of the data showed a significant correlation between the day of maximal hydroxyproline excretion and the day when the subjects reported their greatest soreness.

The connective tissue theory appears consistent with the findings mentioned earlier of greatest soreness following eccentric contractions.[93,158] Recall that during eccentric contractions, the muscle lengthens under tension thus stretching the connective tissue components associated with both the tendons and the muscle fibers. In contrast, during concentric contractions (isotonic and isokinetic), the majority of stretch is put on the connective tissues associated with tendons. Furthermore, the tension developed during maximal eccentric contractions is greater than that possible during other types of contractions. This greater tension could possibly cause more damage to the connective tissues.

The following suggestions have been made to prevent muscle soreness:

1. Stretching appears to help not only the prevention of soreness but also the relief of it when present.[43] However, stretching exercises should be performed without bouncing or jerking, because this may further damage the connective tissues. More about stretching exercises is presented later in this chapter.
2. A gradual progression in the intensity of exercise usually helps in reducing the possibility of excessive muscular soreness. Such a progression in a weight-training program involves using relatively light weights at the start of the program and then gradually increasing the load as gains in strength are made.
3. It has been proposed that ingestion of 100 mg · day^{-1} of vitamin C (about twice the daily recommended dosage) for a period of 30 days will prevent or at least reduce subsequent muscle soreness.[153] However, the efficacy of consuming vitamin C (ascorbic acid) has not been established through scientific experimentation.

Strength and Endurance Programs

Because there are four basic kinds of muscular contraction (see table 13.1), it is not surprising to find that there are also four basic types of strength and endurance programs, each structured around one of the basic contractions. In answering some of the questions posed earlier, we will consider each type of program. A fifth type of training program that combines a prestretch of muscle-tendon units followed by an isotonic contraction also will be considered. This combination program is called **plyometrics.**

Isotonic Programs

One of the first isotonic progressive-resistance programs advocated was that of DeLorme and Watkins in 1948.[39,40] In setting forth their method of exercises for maximal development of strength, they first established the idea of a **repetition maximum (RM).** A repetition maximum is the maximal load that a muscle group can lift over a given number of repetitions before fatiguing. In their program they used a 10-repetition maximum (10 RM), in other words, the maximal load that can be lifted 10 times. For each muscle group to be trained, the exercise program consisted of a total of 30 repetitions per training session divided into three *sets* of 10 repetitions each as follows:

Set 1 = 10 repetitions at a load of ½ 10 RM*
Set 2 = 10 repetitions at a load of ¾ 10 RM
Set 3 = 10 repetitions at a load of 10 RM

A set is the number of repetitions performed consecutively without resting (in this case, one set = 10 repetitions). From day to day the subject tries to increase the number of repetitions while maintaining the same resistance load. When more than 10 repetitions are possible, the load is increased to a new 10 RM load. The most important part of this program is set 3 (i.e., 10 repetitions at the full 10 RM load). This represents the greatest resistance for the muscle group. Variations in sets 1 and 2 do not affect the results appreciably.

DeLorme and Watkins also recommended a training frequency of four consecutive days per week and found that five days per week was the heaviest schedule that could be employed without developing serious signs of delayed recovery. These findings have been verified in that training three, four, or five days per week produced significantly greater gains in 1 RM bench-press performances than did training only one or two days per week.[60] Some caution in generalizing these results may be warranted because the subjects performed 18 sets of 1 RM during each workout. This can be viewed as an unusually large number of sets. In fact, when 3 sets of 6 to 8 RM were studied, subjects made similar strength gains lifting two days as opposed to three days per week.[68] It is now common practice to recommend that PRE training be performed three or four days per week on alternate rather than consecutive days.

Further research was conducted later concerning the optimum number of sets and repetitions that would most effectively increase strength.[12,14,15,17,18]

These studies employed programs with a training frequency of 3 days per week over a duration of 8 to 12 weeks. Some of the results are shown in figure 13.15. The greatest improvement in strength is obtained from 3 sets, each with a 6 RM load.[15] Generally, the optimal number of repetitions

---

*If the 10 RM load were 100 pounds, a ½ 10 RM load would equal 50 pounds.

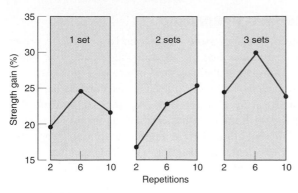

Figure 13.15

Strength gains resulting from isotonic weight-training programs consisting of various sets and repetitions. All programs were performed 3 days per week for 12 weeks. When different numbers of sets are combined with different repetition maximum (RM) loads, several equivalent programs for strength can be developed.

(Based on data from Berger.[15])

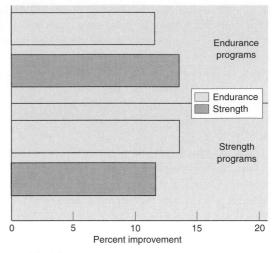

Figure 13.16

Both muscular strength and endurance were developed equally from either a low-repetition, high-load program (so-called strength program) or a high-repetition, low-load program (so-called endurance program).

(Based on data from Clarke and Stull[28] and Stull and Clarke.[155])

maximum lies somewhere between three and nine.[17,179] When different numbers of sets are combined with different RM loads, several equivalent programs for strength can be developed.[11] This is apparent when comparing the mean strength gains from the various programs shown in figure 13.15.

We can conclude that there is no *single* combination of sets and repetitions that yields optimal strength gains for everyone. Although there is some disagreement regarding the details of a strength-training program, there is one agreement in principle: *If you want to develop strength, use progressive resistance exercises in the overload zone.*

So far we have discussed only isotonic weight-training programs that have been shown to improve strength. What about muscular endurance? The "old rule"—strength = low repetitions and high loads, and endurance = high repetitions and low loads—appears still to be valid; but it needs first to be clarified and second to be extended. Clarification involves the term *low load.* We must remember that the progressive overload principle is also a requisite for improvement of muscular endurance. Prolonged repetitions of "underloaded" muscles (figure 13.11) have little effect on endurance.[74]

Extension of the rule is based on the fact that both strength and endurance have been shown to be equally developed from either a low-repetition and high-load program or a high-repetition and low-load program.[28,38,155] This can be seen in figure 13.16. In this case, both the so-called endurance and strength programs consisted of three training sessions per week for 6 or 7 weeks. Each training session of the "endurance" program[28] consisted of elbow flexion at a rate of 40 repetitions per minute with a load of 11 pounds until exhaustion was reached. The strength program[155] con-

sisted of arm curls performed according to the DeLorme-Watkins progression outlined on page 353. However, this progression involved a total of 30 repetitions and as such may not be considered as a low-repetition program. Especially since 20 of the 30 repetitions were completed using less than 100% of 10 RM loads—i.e., somewhat like muscular endurance training. In support of this argument, it was later found that isotonic strength could be improved significantly more with a weight-training program involving 12 repetitions of an 80% maximum load than with 20 repetitions of a 50% maximum load.[45] Isotonic endurance, on the other hand, increased significantly more in the latter program.

These findings were verified by reports that maximum strength gains of 20% over 9 weeks resulted from lifting 3 sets of 6 to 8 RM, 3 days per week.[6] Surprisingly, this high-resistance, low-repetition training yielded similar improvements in absolute-load endurance compared with the medium-resistance, medium-repetitions (2 sets, 30 to 40 RM) and low-resistance, high-repetition (1 set, 100 to 150 RM) training. The medium- and low-resistance groups excelled on relative-load endurance tests with 22 and 28% gains whereas the high-resistance training group decreased by 7% after training.

One point that can be made from these findings is that maximal strength gains are achieved in a more economical way by higher intensity, lower repetition techniques.[155] Likewise, it is apparent that maximal gains in absolute endurance are also derived from those strength-type regimens rather than vice versa. Said differently, endurance accompanies strength better than strength accompanies endurance. Because strength, power, and absolute endurance are needed more than relative-load endurance in sports, it makes sense that competitive athletes train for strength using high resistance and low repetitions. This is not to say that other factors such as safety and subject limitations would not indicate the preferential use of lower intensity, higher repetition programs for middle-age and older subjects or among patients in rehabilitation programs.

Isometric Programs

Similar to what DeLorme and Watkins did for isotonic programs, Hettinger and Müller[76] in 1953 provided the impetus for the scientific inquiry into and establishment of isometric resistance-training programs. Their original studies revealed that maximal strength could be increased at a rate of about 5% per week merely by isometrically contracting a muscle group for 6 seconds at $\frac{2}{3}$ maximal tension once a day for five days per week. Strength gain was unaffected by increasing either the tension (even to maximum) or the number and duration of the contractions. Such findings revolutionized the entire concept of strength-training programs.

Their findings concerning strength development and the amount of tension and number and duration of isometric contractions stimulated a great deal of further research both in Europe and in the United States.[23] The results of these studies proved to be inconsistent. Some findings confirmed Hettinger and Müller's original results;[124,133] others did not.[7,106,126,175] Most interestingly, one of the latter studies was done by Müller himself.[126] This time his results showed that maximal isometric strength could be developed best by training five days per week, with each training session consisting of 5 to 10 maximal contractions held for 5 seconds each. More recent research[142] indicates that continuous, longer (4 sets of 1 rep at 30 sec, 1 min rest between sets) isometric contractions at 70% maximum voluntary contraction (MVC) are more effective in increasing the isometric strength of the left leg muscles than a shorter, intermittent (4 sets × 10 reps × 3 sec, 2 sec rest between reps, 2 min rest between sets) program for the right leg. The possible difference in adaptive stimulus may be the greater changes in phosphate metabolites and pH measured for the leg that performed longer contractions.[142]

Again, we see that several types of isometric training programs will yield substantial strength gains. There does not seem to be just one program that will be best for everyone. Probably the program outlined by Müller in his last study and reported previously should provide almost everyone with satisfactory results. In addition, it is generally agreed that muscular endurance can be increased through isometric exercises.[26,29,30,134] However, once again the design of such a program varies considerably. For example, when isometric exercises are used in a rehabilitation program, they may follow the application of heat treatments. It is of interest that 20 minutes of diathermy heat has been reported to cause an initial decrease in static strength measures followed by an increase 30 minutes after the heat is removed.[25]

At least two factors related to isometric training programs need to be mentioned at this time. First, we said earlier that the development of strength and endurance is specific to the joint angle at which the muscle group is trained.[108] This, of course, implicates isometric training in particular because of its static nature. Thus, if strength and endurance are desired at different joint angles, the isometric exercises must be performed at all specified joint angles.

The second factor deals with the changes in blood pressure that accompany weight-training exercises. Most muscular contractions and, in particular, isometric contractions involve what is called a **Valsalva maneuver.** A Valsalva maneuver means making an expiratory effort with the glottis* closed. Because air cannot escape, intrathoracic pressure increases appreciably (even to the point where it can cause the venae cavae, which return blood to the heart, to collapse). This increase in intrathoracic pressure, along with a myriad of other factors, causes systolic and diastolic blood pressures to increase beyond values normally seen during exercise in which a Valsalva maneuver does not occur. Even though the Valsalva maneuver can be avoided by exhaling during a sustained isometric contraction, many clinicians advise against isometrics as an activity for the recovering heart patient. Moderate PRE under proper supervision is allowable in these patients as long as the Valsalva maneuver is avoided.

Evidence for the specificity of isometric versus dynamic training exists from a unique study of intact adductor pollicus (thumb) muscles of human subjects. After 3 months of comparable isometric (10 daily 5-second contractions) or dynamic (100 daily 0.5-second lifts) training, the subject's ulnar nerves were stimulated using supramaximal electrical stimulation. One of the advantages of this type of stimulation is that all muscle fibers are made to contract and the variable effects of subject motivation are removed. Isometric training produced greater improvements in maximal tetanic tension whereas dynamic training produced greater increases in the peak rate of tension development. Once again it is clear that, generally, static strength can be increased best by isometric training and dynamic strength best by dynamic training.

Finally, the relative-load endurance time is known to be much decreased for both static and dynamic exercise when loads exceed 15% to 20% of **maximum voluntary contraction (MVC)** levels.[69] Such a decrease relates to the occlusion of blood flow to working muscles. If the dynamic exercise is performed slowly, there is not much difference in static and dynamic fatigue curves because the occlusion of blood flow is similar. However, with both faster dynamic contractions and intermittent isometric contractions (i.e., contract, relax, contract) endurance times are enhanced.[69]

---

*The glottis is the space or opening between the vocal cords.

Blood flow is not reduced during low-level static contractions, such as 5% of MVC for 1 hour, because muscles can receive adequate blood flow.[148,149]

Eccentric Programs

Weight-training programs structured around eccentric contractions are not common. Furthermore, they have not been adopted for use by coaches. What little information is available concerning eccentric programs indicates that although strength gains can be made through such programs,[101] by comparison with other programs they are not any more effective.[88,145] In fact, a recent study[152] indicates that although 35% greater weights were used in eccentric training, concentric training produced larger increases in isometric strength with no significant differences in isokinetic strength. The authors suggested that metabolic cost, and not high forces alone, provide part of the stimulus for strength gains and muscle hypertrophy during high-resistance training.

As mentioned earlier, delayed muscular soreness is greatest following eccentric contractions, a definite disadvantage to competitive athletes. The use of eccentric training is, however, advocated in therapy and rehabilitation.[135] Also there is more recent evidence that the specific benefit of longer term eccentric training is remarkable. Eight weeks of eccentric training on a modified bicycle ergometer produced only slight improvements in dynamic concentric muscle strength but an enormous 375% improvement in eccentric work capacity.[55] After training there was little evidence of soreness and disruption of myofibrillar materials that had been caused by single maximal bouts of eccentric exercise prior to training. It appears that the tissues adapt to repeated bouts of eccentric training just as they do for other modes of training. These and future findings may cause coaches and trainers to look more closely at the potential benefits of eccentric training for events such as gymnastics and wrestling, especially if concerns over muscular soreness can be overcome.

Isokinetic Programs

These are the newest type of weight-training programs. Because of this, numerous research studies have been conducted using such programs.[33,53,86,105,121,122,161] In theory, isokinetic exercises should lead to the greatest improvement in muscular performance. For example, as mentioned earlier, isokinetic exercises permit development of maximal muscular tension throughout the full range of joint movement. In other words, a greater number of motor units are activated. As a result, greater demands (greater overload) than were previously possible can be placed on the muscles being exercised.

One should remember, however, that a high level of *motivation* on the part of the athlete in training or the subject being tested is a key essential when isokinetic procedures are used. After all, the apparatus will move at a preset speed even if submaximal efforts are applied. By way of

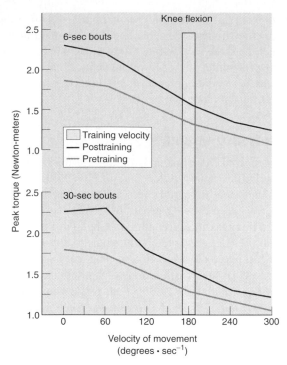

Figure 13.17

Gains in isokinetic strength (knee flexion) following a 7-week, 4-day-per-week training program in which one leg was trained using 6-second bouts of work and the other 30-second bouts. The magnitude of the increase in strength was the same for each leg, and each program produced a "speed specificity" in that maximal gains in strength were made at velocities of movement equal to or slower than the training velocity of 180 degrees per second.

(Based on data from Lesmes et al.[105])

example, such a lack of motivation on the part of nonathletes during initial testing may partially explain why they outperformed athletes on certain all-out isokinetic endurance tests.[129] In a word, if you "sandbag" early on, it is easy to look good during later tests. This matter of motivation during all testing is also a concern to clinicians who use isokinetic testing to monitor postinjury or postsurgical progress.[73]

Examples of the strength gains possible with isokinetic training programs are given in figures 13.17 and 13.18. In figure 13.17, the isokinetic strength gains are shown following a 7-week, 4-day-per-week training program in which the subjects performed maximal extensions and flexions of the knee at a constant velocity of 180 degrees per second. One leg was trained with a 6-second work bout repeated 10 times, with 114 seconds of rest between each work bout. The other leg was trained with a 30-second work bout repeated two times with 20 minutes of rest between bouts. Three important points to notice are as follows:

1. The increase in strength for knee flexion (and extension, although not shown in fig. 13.17) was the same in the leg trained with 6-second bouts of work as the one trained with 30-second bouts.

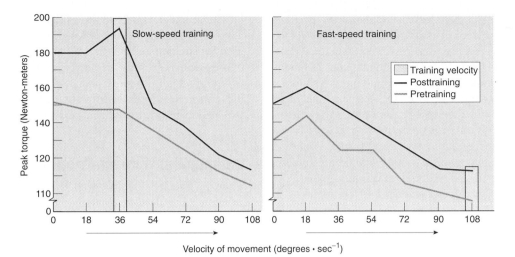

Figure 13.18

Gains in isokinetic strength (knee extension) following a 6-week, 3-day-per-week training program consisting of a 2-minute period of knee extensions and flexions either at a slow speed (36 degrees per second) or fast speed (108 degrees per second) of movement. Note that speed specificity (i.e., maximal increases in strength occurring only at speeds of movement equal to or slower than the training velocity).

(Based on data from Moffroid and Whipple.[121])

2. Each leg was trained exactly 60 seconds per day, four days per week for a total of seven weeks. Therefore, the total training time was only 4 minutes per week × 7 weeks = 28 minutes for the entire program. This suggests that large volumes of training are not necessary to improve muscular strength using isokinetic contractions.

3. Each of the training programs produced similar gains in strength at velocities of movement equal to or slower, but not faster, than the training velocity of 180 degrees per second. This "speed specificity" is of practical value to athletes, as it suggests that athletic strength training should take place at speeds approximating or exceeding those used during their actual sport.

The results presented in figure 13.18 agree very well with the findings just described. The isokinetic training program used in this case consisted of a continuous 2-minute period of repeated knee extensions and flexions either at a constant slow speed of 36 degrees per second or at a constant fast speed of 108 degrees · sec⁻¹. The subjects exercised three days per week for a total of six weeks. Again note the speed specificity (i.e., the improvement in knee extensor strength occurring only at speeds of movement equal to or slower than the training velocity). Although not shown in figure 13.18, the speed specificity principle was also found to hold true for improvement in muscular endurance. In other words, training at a fast speed increased muscular endurance at fast speeds more than slow-speed training increased muscular endurance at slow speeds.[121] Likewise, slow-speed cardiorespiratory training (50 rpm) on a bicycle

ergometer has been shown to only improve slow-speed isokinetic strength measures.[159] And competitive collegiate bike riders who completed a six-week high-intensity aerobic interval training program (cadence = 70 to 80 rpm, ~210 degrees · sec⁻¹ at knee) showed gains in isokinetic leg strength but only at slower contraction speeds.[116]

The total training time of the program used in figure 13.18 was 6 minutes per week × 6 weeks = 36 minutes. The strength gains are comparable in magnitude (percentage) to those obtained from the 28-minute program, again emphasizing that volume of training may not be necessary with isokinetic contractions. These basic findings have been verified and refined for college-age male[37] and female[3] subjects and for adolescent male subjects.[151] Fast-speed training produced the greatest improvements in isokinetic strength, power, and endurance as well as for field tests including the vertical jump, standing broad jump, and 40-yard dash. High-speed training apparently has a limited transfer effect toward static endurance performance at 20% of maximum voluntary contraction.[143] It does produce significant gains in power for moving light to medium loads whereas slow-velocity isokinetic training has been shown to produce added power for moving heavy loads.[91] There is also limited evidence that power outputs may be improved by high-speed isokinetic training at performance speeds faster than those used in training.[91] These findings contradict earlier indications that significant gains are made only at or below the speeds used for training. Future research will likely resolve this discrepancy.

Some interesting similarities and differences exist between isokinetic and isotonic or isometric test results. For example, there is little or no correlation between isokinetic peak strength and isokinetic relative endurance.[9] This lack of relationship is based, of course, on the assumption that subjects are highly motivated to perform continuous repetitions at an all-out effort to a predetermined point of fatigue, say 75% of maximum torque.* These findings are similar to isotonic or static relative-load endurance tests where the motivational levels of the subjects also enters into consideration. One major difference for isokinetic tests is that peak knee extension torques have been found to occur at a speed of 96 degrees per second rather than at an isometric speed setting of 0 degrees per second (no movement). This has led to the suggestion that the force-velocity curves for in-vivo human muscles are not the same as those for isolated animal muscles.[132]

Numerous coaches have adopted the isokinetic idea and have developed specific weight-training programs structured entirely around isokinetic contractions. For example, swimmers contract their arm muscles isokinetically when pulling through the water; therefore, it is important that their weight-training programs on land also be isokinetically oriented.[34,35,36,171] Another specific advantage of isokinetic training for swimmers may relate to an increase in functional capacity of skeletal muscle without undue hypertrophy.[33]

Although for a different muscle group, a study of subjects who maximally contracted their plantar flexor muscles in a continuous series of 200 isokinetic contractions may have relevance here. Measures of their torque, work, and power all decreased rapidly during the first 70 contractions but then leveled off to a steady-state performance the rest of the way.[58] How this pattern of reduced and then maintained endurance performance might be favorably altered with optimal isokinetic training is an intriguing thought. How much might the period of reduced performance be reduced?

Still another application of isokinetic training relates to a search for the best way to strengthen muscles of runners so as to reduce unwanted pronation during the heel strike phase.[53] The amount of pronation is determined from a biomechanical analysis of videotaped running on a treadmill. Isokinetic training included three sets of eight concentric and eccentric contractions at 20, 90, and 180 degrees per second for both ankle inversion and eversion muscle groups. Compared to exercises commonly used in ankle rehabilitation, isokinetic training was superior. The study concluded that pronation can more effectively be decreased by an isokinetic strength training program for the inversion and eversion muscles. This allows for less rear foot motion during running.[53]

Special equipment is needed for isokinetic exercises when such equipment is used in the clinical testing, reha-

bilitation, and research settings. Equipment manufacturers have developed numerous isokinetic machines that may be used for strength and endurance development in specific activities such as swimming, running, throwing, shot put, volleyball, football, jumping, and kicking. Still other companies have developed various pieces of equipment for isokinetic strength assessment and injury rehabilitation.

Comparison among Programs

Thus far we have considered the changes in muscular strength and endurance brought about as a result of each of the programs separately. Which program is the best? Again, there is no simple answer to the question. There are research design problems associated with equating the various programs in such a way that the only differing factor is the type of contraction. Further complications result because of specificity. In an attempt to answer the question, some results from comparative studies are presented in figure 13.19. Figure 13.19A presents a comparison of strength gains resulting from various isotonic programs and one type of isometric program.[12] The exact designs of the isotonic programs are given in the figure. The isometric program consisted of two maximal contractions held for 6 to 8 seconds; each contraction was at a different joint angle. The subjects were college-age men; the training frequency and duration were three days per week and 12 weeks, respectively, for all programs. Only one isotonic program was superior to the isometric program. By the same token, the isometric program was superior to only one isotonic program. In other words, the two types of programs are quite comparable in this case.

Figure 13.19B provides a comparison of isokinetic, isotonic, and isometric programs.[161] The subjects in this study were patients with varying degrees of rehabilitative problems. The training frequency and duration were four days per week and eight weeks, respectively. The programs were consistent with normal clinical programs (e.g., the isotonic program followed the DeLorme-Watkins technique). In this case, it is easy to conclude that the isokinetic program was clearly superior to the other programs in both strength and endurance gains.

A survey of studies comparing isotonic and isometric training programs has been conducted by Clarke[30] and is summarized as follows:

1. Motivation is generally superior with isotonic exercises, as they are self-testing in nature. Conversely, isometrics may be performed anywhere, whereas some isotonics may place considerable demands on available space and require special equipment.
2. Both isometric and isotonic forms of exercise improve muscular strength. Most studies do not favor one method over another; however, greater gains have been reported for trainees using the isotonic form.

---

*The product of force and the perpendicular distance from the line of action of the force to the axis of rotation (SI unit: Newton-meter).

3. Muscular endurance is developed more effectively through isotonic exercise than through isometric exercise. Recovery from muscular fatigue is faster after isotonic exercise than after isometric exercise.
4. Isometric training at one point in the range of joint motion develops strength significantly at that point but not at other positions. Isotonic exercises produce a more uniform development of strength.

Getting back to the problem of the best program, one has to ask the question, Best for what? For the physical educator the answer might be designing a weight-training program for students or a particular group in the community. For the coach, it most likely will involve designing a program that will improve performance of a particular athletic skill. Finally, the physical therapist might construct a program aimed at rehabilitating a sport-related injury. These programs will of course be different. However, all of them can best be designed by considering (1) the overload principle, (2) the specificity of training, and (3) the availability of equipment.

Interested readers are encouraged to review the article, "A Hypothetical Model for Strength Training."[154] This article includes a discussion of the concept of "periodization," which means that strength-training workouts are matched to the athlete's season so that peak strength is attained at the most appropriate time (see also chapter 11). A basic tenet of periodization is a shift from low-load, high-repetition training during the early season preparation phase to high-load, low-repetition training during the late season competition phase. It is of interest that a stimulus for this work was the observation that competitive weight lifters rarely use the 3 set, 6 RM method for year-round training.

A summary of the advantages and disadvantages of isokinetic, isometric, and isotonic weight-training programs is presented in table 13.2. The type of muscular training with the best overall rating is the isokinetic program.

Circuit Training

A different kind of training program that may also be effective in improving strength and in preparing athletes for competition is *circuit training*. This type of program consists of a number of "stations" where a given exercise is performed, usually within a specified time. Once the exercise is completed at one station, the trainee moves to the next station, performing another exercise also within a prescribed time period. The circuit is completed once all stations have been visited.

The exercises at the various stations consist mainly of weight-resistance exercises, but running, swimming, cycling, calisthenics, and stretching exercises may also be included. Circuit training, therefore, may be designed to increase muscular endurance, flexibility, and—if running, swimming, or cycling are involved—to increase cardiorespiratory endurance as well.

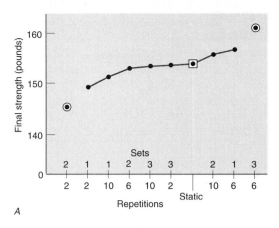

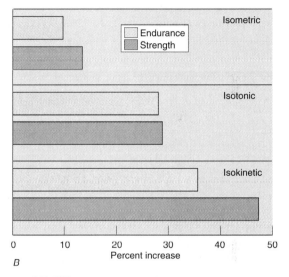

Figure 13.19

Comparison of different weight-training programs. *A.* Comparison of strength gains resulting from various isotonic programs and one isometric program. All programs were performed 3 days per week for 12 weeks. Only one isotonic program (circled dot to the right) was superior to the isometric program, and the isometric program was superior to only one isotonic program (circled dot at left). *B.* Comparison of isokinetic, isotonic, and isometric programs. All programs were performed 4 days per week for 8 weeks. The isokinetic program was superior to the other programs in both strength and endurance gains.

(Data in A from Berger,[13] data in B from Thistle et al.[161])

The circuit should include exercises that will develop the particular capabilities required in the sport for which the athlete is training. For example, circuits that consist mainly of weight-resistance exercises are good for sports in which muscular strength is a major factor and cardiorespiratory endurance a minor factor—sports such as gymnastics, wrestling, swimming sprints, running sprints, competitive weight lifting, and football. The weight-resistance exercises should, of course, emphasize development of those muscles most used in the performance of the particular sport.

table

13.2

Summary of advantages and disadvantages of the three most common types of resistance training programs

Criterion	Comparative rating		
	Isokinetic	Isometric	Isotonic
Rate of strength gain	Excellent	Poor	Good
Rate of endurance gain	Excellent	Poor	Good
Strength gain over range of motion	Excellent	Poor	Good
Time per training session	Good	Excellent	Poor
Expense	Poor	Excellent	Good
Ease of performance	Good	Excellent	Poor
Ease of progress assessment	Poor	Good	Excellent
Adaptability to specific movement patterns	Excellent	Poor	Good
Least possibility of muscle soreness	Excellent	Good	Poor
Least possibility of injury	Excellent	Good	Poor
Skill improvement	Excellent	Poor	Good

Regardless for which sports the circuits are designed, they should consist of between 6 and 15 stations, requiring a total time of between 5 and 20 minutes to complete. Usually, each circuit is performed several times in one training session. Only 15 to 20 seconds rest should be allowed between stations. For the weight resistance stations, the load should be adjusted so that the working muscles are noticeably fatigued after performing as many repetitions as possible (say 6 to 12) within a designated time period (e.g., 30 seconds). This load should be increased periodically to ensure progressive overload. In addition, the sequence of exercises should be arranged so that no two consecutive stations consist of exercises involving the same muscle groups. For example, alternate exercises for arms, legs, and trunk, and between flexor and extensor muscle groups. Training frequency should be three days per week, with a duration of at least six weeks.

As previously mentioned, circuit training may be designed to increase muscular strength and power, muscular endurance, flexibility, and, to a limited extent, cardiorespiratory endurance. However, the physiological effects depend to a large extent on the type of circuit that is set up. For example, circuits consisting only of weight-resistance exercises produce substantial gains in strength but only minimal gains in cardiorespiratory endurance.[4,59,177]

Although an increase in cardiorespiratory endurance can and does result from circuit training, especially when cardiorespiratory activities are included in the stations, the magnitude of the increase is generally not as great as that from training programs consisting entirely of running, swimming, or cycling. This is somewhat puzzling, because heart rates during circuit weight training have been shown to be substantially elevated (above 138 beats · min^{-1}) throughout

completion of the circuit.[4,59] (An elevated heart rate is one criterion for realizing a cardiovascular training effect; for more on this, see chapters 11 and 12.) One possible explanation is that during weight training, a reduction in muscle blood flow caused by high levels of intramuscular pressure results in a lessened stimulus for biochemical and vascular adaptations at the local muscular level.[4] More importantly, although heart rate is reasonably elevated, $\dot{V}O_2$ is not—usually falling below 55% of maximum, a level generally believed to be necessary to stimulate changes in the aerobic system.

From the rather limited research thus far available, one may conclude that circuit training is an effective training technique for altering muscular strength and endurance, and, to a limited extent, flexibility and cardiorespiratory endurance. The use of circuit training, particularly for off-season programs, therefore, may be recommended for athletes whose sports require high levels of muscular strength, power, and endurance and lower levels of cardiorespiratory endurance.[177]

Weight Training and Sports Performance

Several of the questions asked at the beginning of this chapter were concerned with strength development and increases in speed of contraction and sports performance. Although a few studies suggest little or no improvement in speed of contraction, most show that strengthening exercises do indeed increase both speed and power of contraction.[16,27,117,182] Incidentally, the fact that speed of contraction is improved by strength training provides evidence that the term *muscle-bound* has no scientific merit. In addition, research generally demonstrates that specific sports skills, such as speed in running, swimming, throwing, speed and force of offensive football charge, and jumping, all can be improved significantly through weight-training programs.[24,162,163]

In a review of the research completed on strength development and motor and/or sports improvement, Clarke[31] reached the following conclusions:

1. Both isometric and isotonic forms of strength training can produce improvements in many motor and sports performances. Although the evidence is at times conflicting, it is generally accepted that progressive weight-training programs are superior.
2. Some studies did not provide adequate overload in applying both isometric and isotonic strength training. In general, exercises confined to single static contractions of short duration or isotonic efforts limited to a single bout were not effective in developing either strength or motor skills. Strenuous resistance exercises of either form are needed for best results.
3. Fear of muscle-bound effects from weight training may be laid to rest. The majority of studies show that speed of movement may be enhanced rather than retarded as a consequence of strength development.
4. Exercise programs designed to strengthen muscles primarily involved in a particular sport can be used as supplements to regular practice to effectively improve an athlete's skills and motor fitness.

Earlier we mentioned that a fifth type of strength training, plyometrics, would be discussed. This method of training primarily has been used by track-and-field jumpers, volleyball and basketball players, gymnasts, and other athletes who must project their bodies upward against the force of gravity. Currently, there are efforts to apply the basic plyometrics training concepts to other competitive and recreational sports, such as, baseball and skiing. A basic example of plyometric training would be athletes who drop down from a platform, land on the balls of their feet, and as their body weight is settling down through their heels, force themselves to explosively jump back onto the platform. The controlled settling of body weight puts an eccentric load on the calf muscles and Achilles tendons and induces a stretch on the muscle-tendon unit. One effect of this is the storage of energy in the elastic components. A second effect is the prestretch that operates on the stretch receptors (muscle spindles) located within the calf muscles. The prestretch results in afferent impulses being sent via reflex pathways to facilitate the calf muscle motor neurons located in the spinal cord. Theoretically, the explosive muscular power should be enhanced because it is a combination of stored energy and recruitment of facilitated motor neurons and their associated motor units.

Although the clear benefits of this training over and above those derived from isotonic, isokinetic, or more conventional methods needs additional documentation, there are three main potential advantages. First, the athletes may learn to better time their voluntary muscle contractions to match up with any release of stored elastic energy. Timing could mean everything here. Second, more forceful muscle contractions because of prestretch facilitation may allow a greater adaptive stimulus to promote strength gains. Third, the exercises are a natural form of training for jumpers and others who might apply the prestretch principle. Also the plyometric drills can be designed to be progressive in intensity, duration, and frequency as the athlete improves.

Retention of Strength and Endurance

Once desired strength and endurance levels have been attained with a weight-training program, how do we retain them? Do we have to continue with the same type of weight-training program for an indefinite time? The answer to the last question is no. Let's see why.

It is generally agreed that strength and endurance, once developed, subside at slower rates than they were developed. As shown in figure 13.20A, strength gained during a 3-week isotonic training program consisting of 3 sets at a 6 RM load, 3 days per week, was not lost during a subsequent 6-week period of no training (detraining). Second, strength was further improved during a subsequent 6-week training program involving only one set at a 1 RM load performed once a week.[13] Other studies using both isotonic and isometric programs have confirmed these results.[115,124,134,136] In another study, 45% of the strength gained from a 12-week program was still retained after 1 year.[115]

In figure 13.20B, the retention of muscular endurance is shown. The training program consisted of 3 sessions per week for 8 weeks, with each session comprising an exhausting bout of elbow flexions at a work rate of 40 repetitions per minute against a 5-kg load. Endurance was lost most rapidly during the first few weeks of the detraining period. However, after 12 weeks of detraining, the loss of endurance had stabilized and 70% of that gained was still retained.

This information emphasizes that the most difficult phase of the weight-training program is the development of strength and endurance. Once this has been accomplished, they are relatively easy to retain. As little exercise as once per week or once every two weeks will maintain strength and endurance, provided maximal contractions are used. Specific examples of weight-training programs for various sports activities are provided by Bowers and Fox.[21]

Special Training Considerations

Side Benefits of Strength Training

Strength and endurance training has recently found its way into a wide variety[107,109] of areas and applications—often with important side benefits to participants. We will review

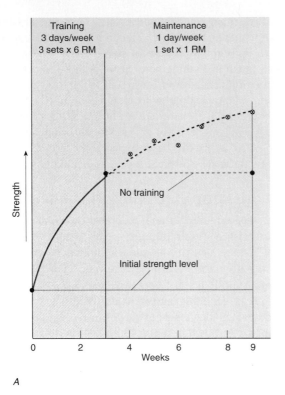

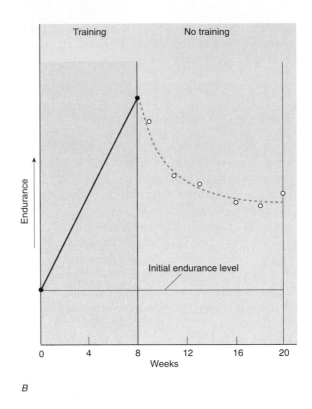

A

B

Figure 13.20

Retention of strength and endurance. *A.* The strength gained during a 3-day-per-week, 3-week isotonic training program (three sets of 6 RM) was not lost during a subsequent 6-week period of no training (dotted line); and strength was further improved during a subsequent 6-week training program involving only one set at a 1 RM load performed once a week. *B.* Retention of muscular endurance. The program was performed 3 days per week for 8 weeks with each session consisting of an exhausting bout of elbow flexions at a work rate of 40 repetitions per minute against an 11-pound load. Although endurance was lost most rapidly during the first few weeks of the detraining (no training) period, after 12 weeks of no training, 70% of the endurance gained was still retained.

(Data in A from Berger,[17] data in B from Syster and Stull[158] and Waldman and Stull.[173])

a few results to highlight recent applications of strength training. For example, the dietary intake of adult women was judged to be improved as a result of their participation in a strength training program.[170] Also, older women (mean age of 67 years) who strength trained three times per week for 16 weeks at 67% of 1 RM showed increases in strength and muscle area and a decrease in intra-abdominal adipose tissue.[168] Elderly women (age range of 76 to 78 years) who participated in 18 weeks of intensive strength training increased leg muscle mass and decreased intramuscular fat, as measured by computed tomography.[146] The femoral neck bone density (determined via dual energy X-ray absorptiometry or DEXA) of older men (mean age of 61 years) increased by 2.8% as a result of 16 weeks of strength training.[139] Patients with recent-onset inflammatory arthritis benefited from participation in a 6-month experimental progressive dynamic strength training program in that their maximal muscle strength significantly improved, along with less increase in joint erosive changes.[70] Eccentric knee extension training proved to be more beneficial than concentric training in strengthening the injured leg of stroke patients.[49,50] And finally, patients who have suffered a heart attack and then participated in eight weeks of combined strength and aerobic training displayed more improvement in peak $\dot{V}O_2$, exercise time, and submaximal perceived exertion than did similar patients who participated in only aerobic training.[181]

Response of the Elderly to Strength Training

The population of the U.S. is truly "aging." This rapid increase in the proportion of older citizens has led to an upsurge in all aspects of gerontological research: including the benefits of strength training. We will review a few selected studies to give a feel for this research. Tseng, et al.[169] define the aging-associated muscle wasting as a progressive neuromuscular syndrome that lowers the quality of life because the elderly cannot lift loads (decreased strength) or perform activities of daily living (decreased endurance). This condition of muscle wasting, called **sarcopenia,** results in lower basal metabolic rate, weakness, reduced activity levels, decreased bone density, and low calorie needs.[51] For many older patients, exercise represents the safest, least expensive means to offset or reverse sarcopenia and thereby maintain long-term independence.[51]

Postmenopausal women (mean age of 60 years) who performed progressive resistance exercises at 80% or more of 1 RM twice weekly for 12 months showed their greatest strength gains in the first three months but continued to improve over the entire year.[125] Similar age males (50 to 69 years) who practiced heavy resistance strength training for 16 weeks increased their strength by 43% and mid-thigh cross-sectional area (CSA) by 7.2%.[82] Elderly males and females (60 to 80 years of age) who strength trained at 50% to 80% 1 RM over 42 weeks displayed a 65% improvement in strength and a 5.5% increase in CSA as contrasted to control subjects.[111]

Both short and long duration isometric contractions were equally effective in increasing quadriceps strength by ~ 50% after 6 months of training in elderly men and women subjects (average age of 72 years).[176] An 18-week strength training program proved more effective than an endurance training program in increasing quadriceps muscle lean tissue CSA and in decreasing intramuscular fat in 76 to 78 year old women.[147] Measures of knee extension strength were greater in elderly women athletes (66 to 85 years of age) and were related more to cardiorespiratory endurance training distance during the prior year and less intramuscular fat than to either quadriceps CSA or lean tissue area.[147] Finally, 10 frail, institutionalized volunteers (average age of 90 ± 1 years of age) participated in eight weeks of high-intensity resistance training with very impressive average strength increases of 174%.[54] Truly remarkable, wouldn't you agree?

Flexibility

Along with strength and endurance, flexibility is also an important component of muscular performance. In studying flexibility, we will concentrate our discussion around four topics: (1) definitions, (2) structural limits to flexibility, (3) development of flexibility, and (4) flexibility and performance. A review concerning the physiology of flexibility has been written by Holland.[80]

Definition of Flexibility

Two kinds of flexibility, *static* and *dynamic,* have been described.[42]

Static Flexibility

The *range of motion about a joint* is defined as **static flexibility.** Static flexibility can be measured most reliably with an instrument called a flexometer.[104] As shown in figure 13.21, it has a weighted 360-degree dial and a weighted pointer that are independently controlled by gravity. While in use, the flexometer is strapped to the segment being

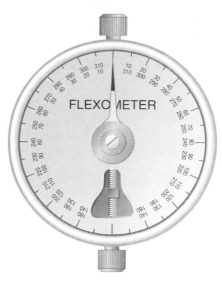

Figure 13.21

The Leighton flexometer.

(Figure from Measurement in Physical Education, Fourth Edition, by Donald K. Mathews,[118] copyright © 1973 by Saunders College Publishing, reprinted by permission of the publisher.)

tested. The dial is locked at one extreme position (e.g., full extension of the elbow), and the limb is moved to the opposing extreme limit (full flexion). The reading of the pointer on the dial is the arc through which the entire movement has taken place. It is called static flexibility because when the dial is actually read, there is no joint motion.

Dynamic Flexibility

Dynamic flexibility is defined as the *opposition or resistance of a joint to motion.* In other words, it is concerned with the forces that oppose movement over any range rather than the range itself. This type of flexibility is more difficult to measure and as such has been given little attention in physical education and athletics.

Structural Limits to Flexibility

The structural limits to flexibility are (1) bone, (2) muscle, (3) ligaments and other structures associated with the joint capsule, (4) tendons and other connective tissues, and (5) skin. Limitations by bony structures are confined to certain joints, for example, the hinge-type joint, such as the elbow. However, in all the joints, including the hinge, the so-called soft tissues (e.g., ligaments, cartilage, etc.) provide the major limitation to the range of joint movement.

The relative importance of the soft tissues with respect to limiting flexibility is given in table 13.3. These particular data were obtained from the wrist joints of cats, but they are applicable to humans.[87] The joint capsule and associated connective tissues plus the muscle itself provide the majority of resistance to flexibility. The values were

13.3

Relative contribution of soft-tissue structures to joint resistance*

Structure	Resistance to flexibility (percentage of total)
1. Joint capsule	47
2. Muscle	41
3. Tendon	10
4. Skin	2

*Based on data from Johns and Wright[87]

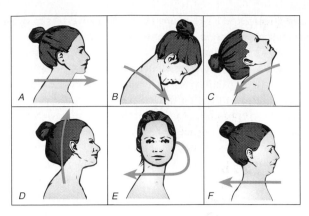

Figure 13.22

Neck stretches. Five common static positions used to stretch the neck muscles are shown. *A*, neutral position with head forward. *B*, forward flexion. *C*, backward extension. *D*, sideward (lateral) flexion. *E*, rotation. *F*, chin tucked back. Caution should be used to not overdo the backward extension exercise. The chin-tuck is especially important to counteract the head forward position common with aging (see *A*).

obtained from the mid-range of joint motion. At the extremes of joint motion, the tendons have a more limiting effect. Because flexibility can be modified through exercise, so also can these soft-tissue limitations. The reason for this, at least in part, is related to the *elastic* nature of some of the tissues.

Development of Flexibility

Flexibility is significant in performing certain skills. Also, recent advances in physical medicine and rehabilitation indicate that flexibility is important to general health and physical fitness. For example, flexibility exercises have been successfully prescribed for relief of dysmenorrhea, general neuromuscular tension, and low back pains.[19,97] For athletes, if they maintain a satisfactory degree of flexibility, they may be less susceptible to certain muscular injuries.

Types of Exercise

The best exercise to use for flexibility are the so-called stretching exercises. A number of these are shown in figures 13.22 through 13.31. Many variations, which involve similar joints and muscle groups, can also be used. A book on stretching exercises for various sports has been published.[5]

Methods of Stretching

Stretching exercises can be performed in one of three ways: (1) statically, (2) *ballistically*,[41,175] and (3) *contract-relax*.[140,174] Static stretching involves stretching without bouncing or forcing, then holding the final stretched position for a given amount of time. Ballistic stretching involves bouncing or active movements. The final stretched position is not held. Contract-relax (C-R) stretching involves stretching to the limits of motion, doing a static contraction against

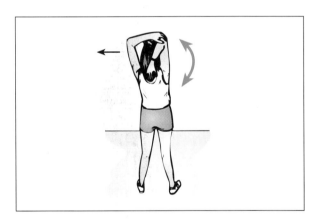

Figure 13.23

Arm triceps and shoulder stretch. A common exercise for stretching the triceps of the arms and some muscles acting on the shoulder. Note that the opposite hand is used to provide a pulling force at the elbow of the arm being stretched. This is called "active" stretching as opposed to "passive" stretching where a therapist or partner would apply the force.

opposition for a few seconds, relaxing and stretching further. This also has been called **proprioceptive neuromuscular facilitation** or the **PNF** method. Although all three types of stretching will improve flexibility, the static method might be preferred because (1) there is less danger of tissue damage, (2) the energy requirement is less, and (3) there is prevention and/or relief from muscular distress and soreness.[41,43] The ballistic method is least preferred.

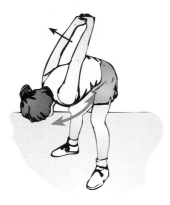

Figure 13.24

Shoulders and arms biceps stretch. This exercise stretches the biceps of the arms and some additional rotator muscles of the shoulders. Note that the hands are grasping one another and are being forced upward while the head is held up and the back is arched. The legs can be bent at the knees but if they are kept straight, a modest amount of stretch is also placed on the hamstring muscles on the back of the thighs.

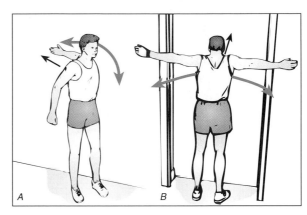

Figure 13.25

Chest and arms biceps stretch. *A,* an outstretched hand is placed flat against a wall and the trunk is rotated away from the wall so stretch is felt at the chest and upper arm. A corner also works well for stretching one side at a time. *B,* to stretch both sides at once, use an open door frame and attempt to lean forward with arms outstretched to contact the door frame at shoulder level.

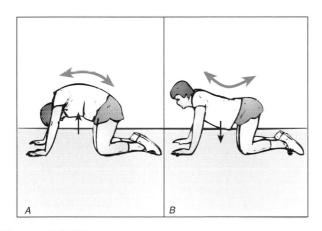

Figure 13.26

Back arch and sway stretch. This excellent exercise is sometimes called the cat and camel. *A,* it emphasizes flexion (arch position) and *B,* extension (sway position) of the entire spine while in a wide-base position with less body weight loaded on the spine. Part of a series of exercises known as the Williams exercises, which are used to prevent chronic low-back pain or to rehabilitate from its debilitating effects.

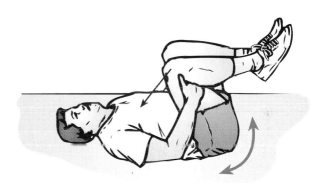

Figure 13.27

Low-back lumbar stretch. This simple exercise where one or both knees are pulled toward the chest and held is very effective in alleviating the pain related to muscle spasms and tight connective tissues in the lower back. Note the position of the hands below the knees, their pulling action, and also the bent knees. In this position, less stretch is being placed on the hamstrings and more stretch on the buttocks and lower lumbar back region.

In static stretching and the C-R method, the Golgi tendon organs (p. 119) are stretched, resulting in *inhibition* of contraction or, in other words, in relaxation of the muscles involved in the stretch. As a result, the stretch is greater and less painful. With ballistic stretching, the bouncing and jerking cause activation of the muscle spindles, which in turn causes *contraction* of the muscles under stretch. In this case the stretching is actually hindered and can be more painful.

Design of the Program

The frequency and duration of the static program should be two to five days per week for 15 to 30 minutes each day. Within five weeks, improvement should be noted.[41] The stretched position should be held for longer periods as the program progresses. For example, at first hold the position for 10 to 15 seconds, then after several sessions increase the holding time by five seconds up to 30 seconds. Start by

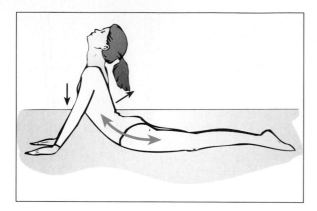

Figure 13.28

Abdominal stretch. Sometimes called a press-up because either the elbows (at first) or hands (later) can be used to press against the floor. The extensor muscles all along the spine are also used to lift the chest off the floor and this strengthens them. This exercise should be used with caution, if at all, by persons who have chronic low back pain or muscle spasms. Their lower backs require stretching exercises like those shown in figures 13.26 and 13.27.

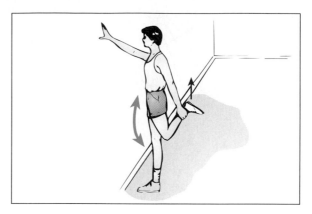

Figure 13.29

Thigh quadriceps stretch. A common exercise used for stretching out the large muscles on the front of the thigh. Some people may not be able to grab their ankle and pull their heel toward their buttocks as shown. In the beginning they may need to grab their stocking or pantsleg or wrap a towel across their ankle and pull on it. Note the use of a wall for stability.

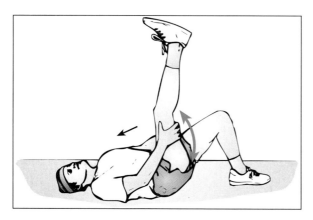

Figure 13.30

Thigh hamstrings stretch. This exercise places the muscles on the back of the thigh under stretch. Note that the leg being stretched is held straight while the other leg is in a bent-knee position. This is important since the hamstring muscles cross over both the hip and knee joints, i.e., to stretch them well, the leg must be straight. A towel can be pulled against the shoe sole to keep the leg straight. It is recommended for chronic low-back pain due to shortened hamstrings.

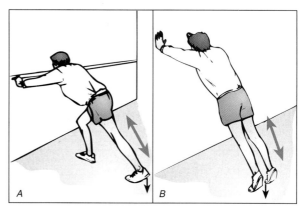

Figure 13.31

Calf Achilles stretch. A common exercise used to stretch out the muscles on the back of the lower leg. *A,* this example shows one leg in a straightened position so that the heel is about 3 inches off the floor. Body weight is then shifted backward and down so the heel is driven toward the floor and the muscles of the triceps surae are stretched. *B,* another method involves leaning against a wall with outstretched arms and moving away until the heels come off the floor. Shift weight to stretch both at once.

performing each exercise three times, then progress to four reps. These general guidelines are based on a program that would include ten different stretching exercises.

Although static stretching programs are recommended from the standpoint of safety and minimization of soreness, the C-R programs appear to be superior for improving flexibility. For example, shoulder, trunk, and hamstring muscle areas were compared in college men who had trained three days per week over six weeks using static, ballistic, or PNF methods.[140] Only the PNF group had flexibility increases greater than the control subjects. Similar findings have been

published for plantar flexor, hip adductor, and hip extensor muscle areas.[174] Such findings may result in a future progressive shift toward more widespread use of C-R or PNF methods.

Flexibility and Performance

Earlier, we mentioned that flexibility aids the performance of certain skills. Figure 13.32 presents flexion and extension flexibility measurements (with the **flexometer**) of seven

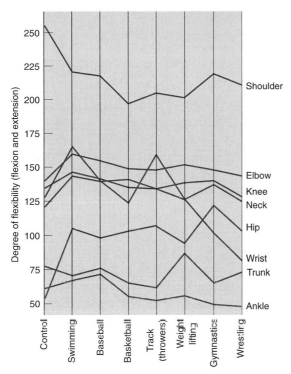

Figure 13.32

Flexion and extension flexibility measures of seven different athletic groups. For further information, see text.

(Based on data from Leighton.[103,104])

different athletic groups.[102,103] The following factors concerning flexibility are evident from the figure.

Specificity of Flexibility

The range of motion about a joint is specific in two ways. First, there is a tendency toward a specific pattern of flexibility and selected sporting events. For example, shot-putters and discus throwers have greater flexibility in the wrist than do wrestlers. Second, flexibility is joint-specific. In other words, a high degree of flexibility in one joint does not necessarily indicate a high flexibility in other joints. For example, gymnasts can be seen to have above-average flexibility in the hip but are below average in the ankle.

Stability versus Flexibility

Certain joints are structurally very weak. As a result, they are prone to injury. The shoulder is one of these joints. The reason is that the glenoid fossa of the scapula, into which the head of the humerus fits, is very shallow. Its main stability is provided by the surrounding musculature. You will notice that shoulder flexibility in all of the athletic groups shown in figure 13.32 is below controls. This probably reflects an increased muscular strength, which in this case limits flexibility. However, in most other joints, flexibility is at least average or above in those athletes for whom

strength is especially important (throwers, weight lifters, gymnasts, and wrestlers). This further refutes the concept of being "muscle-bound."

Excessive flexibility is often indicative of proneness to injury, particularly in contact sports. Thus, flexibility measurements might prove to be a useful screening tool for young prospective football players.[128]

Warm Up, Cool Down, and Flexibility

The performance of stretching or warm-up exercises that increase flexibility probably can prevent serious injury during subsequent athletic competition. Also, stretching exercises are excellent as part of a warm-down or cool-down program.

As mentioned in chapter 11, some distinction should be made here between the static stretching exercises and warm-up calisthenics (e.g., jumping jacks, squat-thrusts, bridging, arm circles, running in place). The former might emphasize enhancing the range of motion of joints, whereas the latter might emphasize overall readiness to engage in competition. The main effects derived from dynamic calisthenics, which may involve ballistic movements and bouncing actions, are threefold: (1) an increase in body temperature leading to light sweating, (2) a general sense of body readiness such that the "kinks" are out, and (3) exposure of joints, muscles, tendons, and connective tissues to ballistic stretching loads under more controlled conditions. It is these types of sudden loads that will be experienced once competition is begun, for which static stretching alone may not do an adequate job of preparing the athlete.

Summary

Muscular strength is the force that a muscle or muscle group can exert against a resistance in one maximal effort. There are four types of muscular contraction: isotonic, isometric, eccentric, and isokinetic.

With isotonic contractions (muscle shortening while lifting a constant load), the tension developed over the range of motion is related to (1) the length of the muscle fibers, (2) the angle of pull of the muscle on the bony skeleton, and (3) the speed of shortening. As a result, the tension developed during the lifting of a constant load varies over the full range of joint motion with the muscle stressed maximally only at its weakest point in the range. This is in contrast to an isokinetic contraction in which the tension developed by the muscle as it shortens at constant speed is maximal at all joint angles.

An isometric contraction is one in which tension is developed but there is no change in the external length of the muscle. An eccentric contraction refers to the lengthening of a muscle during contraction.

Local muscular endurance is usually defined as the ability of a muscle group to perform repeated contractions (either isotonic, isokinetic, or eccentric) against a load or to sustain a contraction (isometric) for an extended period of time. However, muscular endurance may also be defined as the opposite of muscular fatigue.

Physiological changes that accompany increased strength are as follows:

1. Hypertrophy—an increase in the size of the muscle due to an increased size of muscle fibers (mainly Type II) and myofibrils, an increased total amount of protein, an increased number of capillaries, and increased amounts of connective, tendinous, and ligamentous tissues.
2. Biochemical changes—including increased concentrations of creatine, phosphocreatine, ATP, and glycogen and a decreased volume of mitochondria, but only small changes in anaerobic and aerobic enzyme activities.
3. Adaptations within the nervous system—including changes in recruitment pattern and synchronization of motor units.

The physiological principle on which strength and endurance development depends is called the overload principle. It states that strength and endurance increase only when a muscle performs at near its maximal capacity. With weight-training programs, the resistance against which the muscle works should be increased periodically as gains in strength are made. This is the principle of progressive-resistance exercises, or PRE.

Weight training is specific in that gains in strength and muscular endurance improve skill performance to the greatest extent when the training program consists of exercises that include the muscle groups and simulate the movement patterns used during the skill. Also, strength training is specific to the joint angle at which the muscle is trained (isometrics) and to the type of contraction used.

There are two types of muscular soreness—acute and delayed. Acute soreness is due to muscle ischemia (lack of adequate blood flow). Delayed soreness (onset 24 to 48 hours after exercise) could be due to torn muscle tissue or muscle spasms but is more likely due to disruption of the connective tissues, including the tendons. There is no known prevention or cure for soreness; however, stretching exercises may relieve it when present and may sometimes prevent or delay its onset. Delayed muscular soreness is greatest following eccentric contractions and is least following isokinetic contractions.

With isotonic strength programs, there is no single combination of sets (number of repetitions performed consecutively) and repetition maximums (maximal load that can be lifted a given number of repetitions before fatiguing) that yields optimal strength gains. However, most programs should include between one and three sets with repetition maximums between three and nine. Although improvement in strength and muscular endurance are generally greater with low repetitions and high resistances than with high repetitions and low resistances, equal increases in strength and endurance have been found with either program.

Isometric programs can significantly increase strength by training 5 days per week, with each training session consisting of 5 to 10 maximal contractions held for 5 seconds each. Isometric endurance can also be improved, but the design of such a program varies considerably.

Eccentric exercise programs, in comparison with isotonic and isometric programs, are not any more effective in developing strength and endurance. They may excel, however, in developing eccentric contraction strength.

Isokinetic programs are speed specific (i.e., they cause maximal gains in strength and endurance at velocities of movement equal to or slower, but usually not faster, than the training velocity). Gains in isokinetic strength and endurance can be made with programs consisting of as little exercise as 1 minute per day, 4 days per week, for 7 weeks (total time = 28 minutes). In theory and in comparison with other programs, isokinetic programs should lead to the greatest improvement in muscular performance. Once gained, strength and endurance are retained for relatively long periods of time.

Circuit training consists of a number of stations where a given weight-lifting exercise is performed within a specified time. It, too, is an effective training technique for improving muscular strength, muscular endurance, and to a lesser extent, flexibility and cardiovascular endurance.

Although a few studies suggest little or no improvement in speed of contraction, most show that weight-training programs do increase both speed and power of contraction. Specific sports skills can also be significantly improved through weight-training programs.

Flexibility, the range of motion about a joint, is related to health, and, to some extent, to athletic performance. Regularly scheduled programs involving stretching exercises (2 to 5 days per week, 15 to 30 minutes per day) will improve flexibility within a few weeks.

Questions

1. Define strength and the following types of contractions: (a) isotonic, (b) isometric, (c) eccentric, and (d) isokinetic.
2. Identify the factors that affect the tension of a muscle undergoing an isotonic contraction in the body, and explain how they affect them.
3. Define muscular endurance.
4. What structural and biochemical changes are brought about within a muscle as a consequence of a weight-training program?
5. What stimulates gains in strength and endurance?

6. Explain the overload principle. How are the overload principle and progressive resistance related?
7. Give several examples of the specificity of weight training.
8. What causes muscular soreness, and how can it be relieved or prevented?
9. Describe how you would structure a weight-training program around (a) isotonic exercises, (b) isometric exercises, and (c) isokinetic exercises.
10. Compare the effectiveness of the previous programs.
11. Define circuit training and describe how you would design such a program.
12. How does weight training affect sports performance?
13. How can strength and endurance be retained and/or maintained?
14. What are the structural limitations to flexibility?
15. How can flexibility be gained, and why is it important to health and physical performance?

References

1. Abraham, W. M. 1979. Exercise-induced muscle soreness. *Physician Sportsmed.* 7(10):57–60.
2. ———. 1977. Factors in delayed muscle soreness. *Med Sci Sports.* 9(1):11–20.
3. Adeyanju, K., T. R. Crews, and W. J. Meadors. 1983. Effects of two speeds of isokinetic training on muscle strength, power, and endurance. *J Sports Med.* 23:352–356.
4. Allen, T. E., R. J. Byrd, and D. P. Smith. 1976. Hemodynamic consequences of circuit weight training. *Res Q.* 47(3):299–306.
5. Anderson, R. A. 1975. *Stretching.* P.O. Box 2734, Fullerton, CA 92633.
6. Anderson, T., and J. T. Kearney. 1982. Effects of three resistance training programs on muscular strength and absolute and relative endurance. *Res Q Exerc Sport.* 53(1):1–7.
7. Asa, M. 1959. *The Effects of Isometric Exercise on the Strength of Skeletal Muscle.* Doctoral Dissertation, Springfield College.
8. Asmussen, E. 1956. Observations on experimental muscle soreness. *Acta Rheumatologica Scand.* 1:109–116.
9. Barnes, W. S. 1980. The relationship between maximum isokinetic strength and isokinetic endurance. *Res Q Exerc Sport.* 51(4):714–717.
10. Belka, D. 1968. Comparison of dynamic, static, and combination training on dominant wrist flexor muscles. *Res Q.* 39:244–250.
11. Berger, R. 1963. Comparative effects of three weight training programs. *Res Q.* 34:396–398.
12. ———. 1963. Comparison between static training and various dynamic training programs. *Res Q.* 34:131–135.
13. ———. 1965. Comparison of the effect of various weight training loads on strength. *Res Q.* 36:141–146.
14. ———. 1962. Comparison of static and dynamic strength increases. *Res Q.* 33:329–333.
15. ———. 1962. Effect of varied weight training programs on strength. *Res Q.* 33:168–181.
16. ———. 1963. Effects of dynamic and static training on vertical jumping ability. *Res Q.* 34:419–424.
17. ———. 1962. Optimum repetitions for the development of strength. *Res Q.* 33:334–338.
18. Berger, R., and B. Hardage. 1967. Effect of maximum loads for each of ten repetitions on strength improvement. *Res Q.* 38:715–718.
19. Billing, H., and E. Loewendahl. 1949. *Mobilization of the Human Body.* Palo Alto, CA: Stanford University Press.
20. Bosco, C., S. Zanon, H. Rusko, A. DalMonte, P. Bellotti, F. Latteri, N. Candeloro, E. Azzaro, R. Pozzo, and S. Bonomi. 1984. The influence of extra load on the mechanical behavior of skeletal muscle. *Eur J Appl Physiol.* 53:149–154.
21. Bowers, R. W., and E. L. Fox. 1992. *Sports Physiology.* Dubuque, IA: Wm. C. Brown Communications.
22. Brzank, K. D., and K. S. Piepers. 1986. Effect of intensive, strength-building exercise training on the fine structure of human skeletal muscle capillaries. *Anat Anz.* 161:243–248.
23. Byrd, R., and W. Hills. 1971. Strength, endurance, and blood flow responses to isometric training. *Res Q.* 42:357–361.
24. Campbell, R. 1962. Effects of supplemental weight training on the physical fitness of athletic squads. *Res Q.* 33:343–348.
25. Chastain, P. B. May 1978. The effect of deep heat on isometric strength. *Phys Ther.* 58(5):543–546.
26. Clarke, D. 1973. Adaptations in strength and muscular endurance resulting from exercise. In Wilmore, J. (ed.), *Exercise and Sport Sciences Reviews,* vol. 1. New York: Academic Press, pp. 73–102.
27. Clarke, D., and F. Henry. 1961. Neuromuscular specificity and increased speed from strength development. *Res Q.* 32:315–325.
28. Clarke, D., and G. Stull. 1970. Endurance training as a determinant of strength and fatigability. *Res Q.* 41:19–26.
29. Clarke, H. (ed.) Jan. 1974. Development of muscular strength and endurance. *Phys Fit Res Digest.* Series 4, No. 1.
30. ———. Jul. 1971. Isometric versus isotonic exercises. *Phys Fit Res Digest.* Series 1, no. 1.
31. ———. Oct. 1974. Strength development and motor-sports improvement. *Phys Fit Res Digest.* Series 4, no. 4.
32. Costill, D. L., E. F. Coyle, W. F. Fink, G. R. Lesmes, and F. A. Witzmann. 1979. Adaptations in skeletal muscle following strength training. *J Appl Physiol.* 46(1):96–99.
33. Cote, C., J-A. Simoneau, P. Lagasse, M. Boulay, M-C. Thibault, M. Marcotte, and C. Bouchard. 1988. Isokinetic strength training protocols: do they induce skeletal muscle fiber hypertrophy? *Arch Phys Med Rehab.* 69:281–285.
34. Counsilman, J. Feb. 1972. Isokinetic exercise. *Athletic J.* 52(6).
35. ———. 1969. Isokinetic exercise: a new concept in strength building. *Swimming World.* 10:4.
36. ———. 1971. New approach to strength building. *Scholastic Coach.*
37. Coyle, E. F., D. C. Feiring, T. C. Rotkis, R. W. Cote III, F. B. Roby, W. Lee, and J. H. Wilmore. 1981. Specificity of power improvements through slow and fast isokinetic training. *J Appl Physiol: Respirat Environ Exerc Physiol.* 51(6):1437–1442.
38. DeLateur, B., J. Lehmann, and W. Fordyce. 1968. A test of the DeLorme axiom. *Arch Phys Med Rehab.* 49:245–248.
39. DeLorme, T., and A. Watkins. 1951. *Progressive Resistance Exercise.* New York: Appleton-Century-Crofts.
40. ———. 1948. Techniques of progressive resistance exercise. *Arch Phys Med Rehab.* 29:263–273.
41. DeVries, H. 1962. Evaluation of static stretching procedures for improvement of flexibility. *Res Q.* 33:222–229.
42. ———. 1980. *Physiology of Exercise for Physical Education and Athletics,* 3rd ed. Dubuque, IA: W. C. Brown.
43. ———. 1961. Prevention of muscular distress after exercise. *Res Q.* 32:468–479.
44. ———. 1966. Quantitative electromyographic investigation of the spasm theory of muscle pain. *Am J Phys Med.* 45:119–134.
45. Dons, B., K. Bollerup, F. Bonde-Petersen, and S. Hancke. 1979. The effects of weight-lifting exercise related to muscle fiber composition and muscle cross-sectional area in humans. *Eur J Appl Physiol.* 40:95–106.
46. Dorpat, T. L., and T. H. Holmes. 1955. Mechanisms of skeletal muscle pain and fatigue. *Arch Neurol Psych.* 74:628–640.
47. Duchateau, J., and K. Hainaut. 1984. Isometric or dynamic training: differential effects of mechanical properties of a human muscle. *J Appl Physiol: Respirat Environ Exerc Physiol.* 56(2):296–301.

48. Edgerton, V. 1970. Morphology and histochemistry of the soleus muscle from normal and exercised rats. *Am J Anat.* 127:81–88.

49. Engardt, M. 1994. Rising and sitting down in stroke patients. Auditory feedback and dynamic strength training to enhance symmetrical body weight distribution. *Scand J Rehabil Med Suppl.* 31:1–57.

50. Engardt, M., E. Knutsson, M. Jonsson, and M. Sternhag. 1995. Dynamic muscle strength training in stroke patients: effects of knee extension torque, electromyographic activity, and motor function. *Arch Phys Med Rehabil.* 76:419–425.

51. Evans, W. J. 1996. Reversing sarcopenia: how weight training can build strength and vitality. *Geriatrics.* 51:46–47.

52. Fahey, T. D., R. Rolph, P. Moungmee, J. Nagel, and S. Mortara. 1976. Serum testosterone, body composition, and strength of young adults. *Med Sci Sports.* 8(1):31–34.

53. Feltner, M. E., H. S. MacRae, P. G. MacRae, N. S. Turner, C. A. Hartman, M. L. Summers, and M. D. Welch. 1994. Strength training effects on rearfoot motion in running. *Med Sci Sports Exerc.* 26:1021–1027.

54. Fiatarone, M. A., E. C. Marks, N. D. Ryan, C. N. Meredith, L. A. Lipsitz, and W. J. Evans. 1990. High-intensity strength training in nonagenarians. Effects on skeletal muscle. *JAMA.* 263:3029–3034.

55. Friden, J., J. Seger, M. Sjöström, and B. Ekblom. 1983. Adaptive response in human skeletal muscle subjected to prolonged eccentric training. *Int J Sports Med.* 4:177–183.

56. Galbo, H., L. Hummer, I. B. Petersen, N. J. Christensen, and N. Bie. 1977. Thyroid and testicular hormone responses to graded and prolonged exercise in man. *Eur J Appl Physiol.* 36:101–106.

57. Gardner, G. 1963. Specificity of strength changes of the exercised and nonexercised limb following isometric training. *Res Q.* 34:98–101.

58. Gerdle, B., and M. Langstrom. 1987. Repeated isokinetic plantar flexions at different angular velocities. *Acta Physiol Scand.* 130:495–500.

59. Gettman, L. R., J. J. Ayres, M. L. Pollock, and A. Jackson. 1978. The effect of circuit weight training on strength, cardiorespiratory function, and body composition of adult men. *Med Sci Sports.* 10(3):171–176.

60. Gillam, G. M. 1981. Effects of frequency of weight training on muscle strength enhancement. *J Sports Med.* 21:432–436.

61. Girouard, C. K., and B. F. Hurley. 1995. Does strength training inhibit gains in range of motion from flexibility training in older adults? *Med Sci Sports Exerc.* 27:1444–1449.

62. Goldberg, A., J. Etlinger, D. Goldspink, and C. Jablecki. 1975. Mechanism of work-induced hypertrophy of skeletal muscle. *Med Sci Sports.* 7(3):185–198.

63. Goldspink, G. 1964. The combined effects of exercise and reduced food intake on skeletal muscle fibers. *J Cell Comp Physiol.* 63:209–216.

64. Gonyea, W. J. 1980. The role of exercise in inducing skeletal muscle fiber number. *J Appl Physiol.* 48(3):421–426.

65. Gonyea, W. J., G. C. Ericson, and F. Bonde-Petersen. 1977. Skeletal muscle fiber splitting induced by weightlifting exercise in cats. *Acta Physiol Scand.* 99:105–109.

66. Gordon, A. M., A. F. Huxley, and F. J. Julian. 1966. Variation in isometric tension with sarcomere length in vertebrate muscle fibers. *J Physiol* (London). 184:170–192.

67. Gordon, E. 1967. Anatomical and biochemical adaptations of muscle to different exercises. *JAMA.* 201:755–758.

68. Gregory, L. W. 1981. Some observations on strength training and assessment. *J Sports Med.* 21:130–137.

69. Hagberg, M. 1981. Muscular endurance and surface electromyogram in isometric and dynamic exercise. *J Appl Physiol: Respirat Environ Exerc Physiol.* 51(1):1–7.

70. Hakkinen, A., K. Hakkinen, and P. Hannonen. 1994. Effects of strength training on neuromuscular function and disease activity in patients with recent-onset inflammatory arthritis. *Scand J Rheumatol.* 23:23–42.

71. Hakkinen, K., M. Alen, and P. V. Komi. 1985. Changes in isometric force- and relaxation-time, electromyographic and muscle fibre characteristics of human skeletal muscle during strength training and detraining. *Acta Physiol Scand.* 125:573–585.

72. Hakkinen, K., and P. V. Komi. 1983. Alterations of mechanical characteristics of human skeletal muscle during strength training. *Eur J Appl Physiol.* 50:161–172.

73. Harter, R. A., L. R. Osternig, and L. W. Standifer. 1990. Isokinetic evaluation of quadriceps and hamstrings symmetry following anterior cruciate ligament reconstruction. *Arch Phys Med Rehab.* 71:456–468.

74. Hellebrandt, F., and S. Houtz. 1956. Mechanisms of muscle training in man: experimental demonstration of the overload principle. *Phys Ther Rev.* 36:371–383.

75. Hetrick, G. A., and J. H. Wilmore. 1979. Androgen levels and muscle hypertrophy during an eight week weight training program for men/women. *Med Sci Sports.* 11(1):102.

76. Hettinger, T., and E. Müller. 1953. Muskelleistung und Muskeltraining. *Arbeitsphysiol.* 15:111–126.

77. Hickson, R. C. 1980. Interference of strength development by simultaneously training for strength and endurance. *Eur J Appl Physiol.* 45:255–263.

78. Hickson, R. C., K. Hidaka, and C. Foster. 1994. Skeletal muscle fiber type, resistance training, and strength-related performance. *Med Sci Sports Exerc.* 26:593–598.

79. Ho, K., R. Roy, J. Taylor, W. Heusner, W. Van Huss, and R. Carrow. 1977. Muscle fiber splitting with weightlifting exercise. *Med Sci Sports.* 9(1):65.

80. Holland, G. 1968. The physiology of flexibility: a review of the literature. *Kinesiology Review,* pp. 49–62.

81. Hough, T. 1902. Ergographic studies in muscular soreness. *Am J Physiol.* 7:76–92.

82. Hurley, B. F., R. A. Redmond, R. E. Pratley, M. S. Trueth, M. A. Rogers, and A. P. Goldberg. 1995. Effects of strength training on muscle hypertrophy and muscle cell disruption in older men. *Int J Sports Med.* 16:378–384.

83. Ikai, M., and T. Fukunaga. 1968. Calculation of muscle strength per unit cross-sectional area of human muscle by means of ultrasonic measurements. *Int Z Angew Physiol.* 26:26–32.

84. Ikai, M., and A. Steinhaus. 1961. Some factors modifying the expression of human strength. *J Appl Physiol.* 16:157–163.

85. Ingjer, F. 1979. Effects of endurance training on muscle fibre ATPase activity, capillary supply and mitochondrial content in man. *J Physiol.* 294:419–432.

86. Johansson, C., R. Lorentzon, and A. R. Fugl-Meyer. 1989. Isokinetic muscular performance of the quadriceps in elite ice hockey players. *Am J Sports Med.* 17:30–34.

87. Johns, R., and V. Wright. 1962. Relative importance of various tissues in joint stiffness. *J Appl Physiol.* 17:824–828.

88. Johnson, B. L., W. Adamczyk, K. O. Tennoe, and S. B. Stromme. 1976. A comparison of concentric and eccentric muscle training. *Med Sci Sports.* 8(1):35–38.

89. Jones, D. A. 1992. Strength of skeletal muscle and the effects of training. *Br Med Bull.* 48:592–604.

90. Jones, D. A., O. M. Rutherford, and D. F. Parker. 1989. Physiological changes in skeletal muscle as a result of strength training. *Q J Exp Physiol.* 74:233–256.

91. Kanehisa, H., and M. Miyashita. 1983. Effect of isometric and isokinetic muscle training on static strength and dynamic power. *Eur J Appl Physiol.* 50:365–371.

92. Knapik, J. J., J. E. Wright, R. H. Mawdsley, and R. H. Braun. 1983. Isokinetic, isometric and isotonic strength relationships. *Arch Phys Med Rehab.* 64:77–80.

93. Komi, P. V., and E. R. Buskirk. 1972. The effect of eccentric and concentric muscle activity on tension and electrical activity of human muscle. *Ergonomics.* 15:417–434.

94. Komi, P. V., J. T. Viitasalo, R. Rauramaa, and V. Vihko. 1978.

Effect of isometric strength training on mechanical, electrical, and metabolic aspects of muscle function. *Eur J Appl Physiol.* 40:45–55.

95. Kraemer, W. J., S. J. Fleck, and W. J. Evans. 1996. Strength and power training: physiological mechanisms of adaptation. *Exerc Sport Sci Rev.* 24:363–397.

96. Kraemer, W. J., J. F. Patton, S. E. Gordon, E. A. Harman, M. R. Deschenes, K. Reynolds, R. U. Newton, N. T. Triplett, and J. E. Dziados. 1995. Compatibility of high-intensity strength and endurance training on hormonal and skeletal muscle adaptations. *J Appl Physiol.* 78:976–989.

97. Kraus, H., and W. Raab. 1961. *Hypokinetic Disease.* Springfield, IL: Charles C. Thomas.

98. Krotkiewski, M., A. Aniansson, G. Grimby, P. Björntorp, and L. Sjöström. 1979. The effect of unilateral isokinetic strength training on local adipose and muscle tissue morphology, thickness, and enzymes. *Eur J Appl Physiol.* 42:271–281.

99. Lamb, D. R. 1984. *Physiology of Exercise,* 2nd ed. New York: Macmillan.

100. Lange, L. 1919. *Uber funktionelle Anpassung.* Berlin: Springer Verlag.

101. Laycoe, R., and R. Marteniuk. 1971. Learning and tension as factors in static strength gains produced by static and eccentric training. *Res Q.* 42:299–306.

102. Leighton, J. 1957. Flexibility characteristics of four specialized skill groups of college athletes. *Arch Phys Med Rehab.* 38:24–28.

103. ———. 1957. Flexibility characteristics of three specialized skill groups of champion athletes. *Arch Phys Med Rehab.* 38:580–583.

104. ———. 1955. Instrument and technic for measurement of range of joint motion. *Arch Phys Med Rehab.* 36:571–578.

105. Lesmes, G. R., D. L. Costill, E. F. Coyle, and W. J. Fink. 1978. Muscle strength and power changes during maximal isokinetic training. *Med Sci Sports.* 10(4):266–269.

106. Liberson, W., and M. Asa. 1959. Further studies of brief isometric exercises. *Arch Phys Med Rehab.* 40:330–336.

107. Lieber, R. L., P. D. Silva, and D. M. Daniel. 1996. Equal effectiveness of electrical and volitional strength training for quadriceps femoris muscles after anterior cruciate ligament surgery. *J Orthop Res.* 14:131–138.

108. Lindh, M. 1979. Increase of muscle strength from isometric quadriceps exercises at different knee angles. *Scand J Rehab Med.* 11:33–36.

109. Lukaski, H. C., W. W. Bolunchuk, W. A. Siders, and D. B. Milne. 1996. Chromium supplementation and resistance training: effects on body composition, strength, and trace element status of men. *Am J Clin Nutr.* 63:954–965.

110. McCarthy, J. P., J. C. Agre, B. K. Graf, M. A. Pozniak, and A. C. Vailas. 1995. Compatibility of adaptive responses with combining strength and endurance training. *Med Sci Sports Exerc.* 27:429–436.

111. McCartney, N. A. L. Hicks, J. Martin, and C. E. Webber. 1995. Long-term resistance training in the elderly: effects on dynamic strength, exercise capacity, muscle, and bone. *J Gerontol A Biol Sci Med Sci.* 50:B97–104.

112. MacDougall, J. D., D. G. Sale, G. Elder, and J. R. Sutton. 1976. Ultrastructural properties of human skeletal muscle following heavy resistance training and immobilization. *Med Sci Sports.* 8(1):72.

113. MacDougall, J. D., D. G. Sale, J. R. Moroz, G. C. B. Elder, J. R. Sutton and H. Howald. 1979. Mitochondrial volume density in human skeletal muscle following heavy resistance training. *Med Sci Sports.* 11(2):164–166.

114. MacDougall, J. D., G. R. Ward, D. G. Sale, and J. R. Sutton. 1977. Biochemical adaptation of human skeletal muscle to heavy resistance training and immobilization. *J Appl Physiol.* 43(4):700–703.

115. McMorris, R., and E. Elkins. 1954. A study of production and evaluation of muscular hypertrophy. *Arch Phys Med Rehab.* 35:420–426.

116. Martin, D. T., J. C. Scifres, S. D. Zimmerman, and J. G. Wilkinson. 1994. Effects of interval training and a taper on cycling performance and isokinetic leg strength. *Int J Sports Med.* 15:485–491.

117. Masley, J., A. Hairabedian, and D. Donaldson. 1952. Weight training in relation to strength, speed and coordination. *Res Q.* 24:308–315.

118. Mathews, D. 1973. *Measurement in Physical Education,* 4th ed. Philadelphia: W. B. Saunders.

119. Maughan, R. J., M. Harmon, J. B. Leiper, D. Sale, and A. Delman. 1986. Endurance capacity of untrained males and females in isometric and dynamic muscular contractions. *Eur J Appl Physiol.* 55:395–400.

120. Milner-Brown, H. S., R. B. Stein, and R. G. Lee. 1975. Synchronization of human motor units: possible roles of exercise and supraspinal reflexes. *Electroenceph Clin Neurophysiol.* 38:245–254.

121. Moffroid, M. T., and R. H. Whipple. 1970. Specificity of speed and exercise. *J Am Phys Ther Assoc.* 50:1699–1704.

122. Moffroid, M., R. Whipple, J. Hofkosh, E. Lowman, and H. Thistle. 1968. A study of isokinetic exercise. *Phys Ther.* 49:735–746.

123. Moreau, D., P. Dubots, V. Boggio, J. C. Guilland, and G. Cometti. 1995. Effects of electromyostimulation and strength training on muscle soreness, muscle damage and sympathetic activation. *J Sports Sci.* 13.95–100.

124. Morehouse, C. 1967. Development and maintenance of isometric strength of subjects with diverse initial strengths. *Res Q.* 38:449–456.

125. Morganti, C. M., M. E. Nelson, M. A. Fiatarone, G. E. Dallal, C. D. Economos, B. M. Crawford, and W. J. Evans. 1995. Strength improvements with 1 yr of progressive resistance training in older women. *Med Sci Sports Exerc.* 27:906–912.

126. Müller, E., and W. Rohmert. 1963. Die Geschwindigkeit der Muskelkraft-Zunahme bei isometrischem Training. *Arbeitsphysiol.* 19:403–419.

127. Narici, M. V., and B. Kayser. 1995. Hypertrophic response of human skeletal muscle to strength training in hypoxia and normoxia. *Eur J Appl Physiol.* 70:213–219.

128. Nicholas, J. A. 1970. Injuries to knee ligaments. Relationship to looseness and tightness in football players. *JAMA.* 212:2236–2239.

129. Nicholas, J. J., L. R. Robinson, A. Logan, and R. Robertson. 1989. Isokinetic testing in young nonathletic able-bodied subjects. *Arch Phys Med Rehab.* 70:210–213.

130. Pate, R. R., R. D. Huges, J. V. Chandler, and J. L. Ratliffe. 1978. Effects of arm training on retention of training effects derived from leg training. *Med Sci Sports.* 10(2):71–74.

131. Penman, K. 1969. Ultrastructural changes in human striated muscle using three methods of training. *Res Q.* 40:764–772.

132. Perrine, J. J., and V. R. Edgerton. 1978. Muscle force-velocity and power-velocity relationships under isokinetic loading. *Med Sci Sports.* 10(3):159–166.

133. Rarick, G., and G. Larsen. 1958. Observations on frequency and intensity of isometric muscular effort in developing static muscular strength in post-pubescent males. *Res Q.* 29:333–341.

134. Rasch, P. 1971. Isometric exercise and gains of muscle strength. In Shephard, R. (ed.), *Frontiers of Fitness.* Springfield, IL: Charles C Thomas, chapter 5.

135. ———. 1974. The present status of negative (eccentric) exercise: a review. *Am Corr Ther J.* 28:77.

136. Rasch, P., and L. Morehouse. 1957. Effect of static and dynamic exercises on muscular strength and hypertrophy. *J Appl Physiol.* 11:29–34.

137. Rissanen, A., H. Kalimo, and H. Alaranta. 1995. Effect of intensive training on the isokinetic strength and structure of lumbar muscles in patients with chronic low back pain. *Spine.* 20:333–340.

138. Rooney, K. J., R. D. Herbert, and R. J. Balnave. 1994. Fatigue

contributes to the strength training stimulus. *Med Sci Sports Exerc.* 26:1160–1164.

139. Ryan, A. S., M. S. Trueth, M. A. Rubin, J. P. Miller, B. J. Nicklas, D. M. Landis, R. E. Pratley, C. R. Libanati, C. M. Gundberg, and B. F. Hurley. 1994. Effects of strength training on bone mineral density: hormonal and bone turnover relationships. *J Appl Physiol.* 77:1678–1684.

140. Sady, S. P., M. Wortman, and D. Blanke. 1982. Flexibility training: ballistic, static or proprioceptive neuromuscular facilitation? *Arch Phys Med Rehab.* 63:261–263.

141. Sale, D. G., J. D. MacDougall, A. R. M. Upton, and A. J. McComas. 1979. Effect of strength training upon motoneuron excitability in man. *Med Sci Sports.* 11(1):76.

142. Schott, J., K. McCully, and O. M. Rutherford. 1995. The role of metabolites in strength training. II. Short versus long isometric contractions. *Eur J Appl Physiol.* 71:337–341.

143. Seaborne, D., and A. W. Taylor. 1984. The effect of speed of isokinetic exercise on training transfer to isometric strength in the quadriceps muscle. *J Sports Med.* 24:183–188.

144. Simonsen, E. B., Klitgaard, H., and F. Bojsen-Moller. 1995. The influence of strength training, swim training and ageing on the Achilles tendon and m. soleus of the rat. *J Sports Sci.* 13:291–295.

145. Singh, M., and P. Karpovich. 1967. Effect of eccentric training of agonists on antagonistic muscles. *J Appl Physiol.* 23:742–745.

146. Sipila, S., and H. Suominen. 1995. Effects of strength and endurance training on thigh and leg muscle mass and composition in elderly women. *J Appl Physiol.* 78:334–340.

147. Sipila, S., and H. Suominen. 1994. Knee extension strength and walking speed in relation to quadriceps muscle composition and training in elderly women. *Clin Physiol.* 14:433–442.

148. Sjogaard, G. 1988. Muscle energy metabolism and electrolyte shifts during low-level prolonged static contraction in man. *Acta Physiol Scand.* 134:181–187.

149. Sjogaard, G., B. Kiens, K. Jorgenson, and B. Saltin. 1986. Intramuscular pressure, EMG and blood flow during low-level prolonged static contraction in man. *Acta Physiol Scand.* 128:475–484.

150. Sleivert, G. G., R. D. Backus, and H. A. Wenger. 1995. The influence of a strength-sprint training sequence or multi-joint power output. *Med Sci Sports Exerc.* 27:1655–1665.

151. Smith, M. J., and P. Melton. 1981. Isokinetic versus isotonic variable-resistance training. *Am J Sports Med.* 9:275–279.

152. Smith, R. C., and O. M. Rutherford. 1995. The role of metabolites in strength training. I. A comparison of eccentric and concentric contractions. *Eur J Appl Physiol.* 71:332–336.

153. Staton, W. M. 1952. The influence of ascorbic acid in minimizing post-exercise soreness in young men. *Res Q.* 23:356–360.

154. Stone, M. H., H. O'Bryant, and J. Garhammer. 1981. A hypothetical model for strength training. *J Sports Med.* 21:342–351.

155. Stull, G., and D. Clarke. 1970. High-resistance, low-repetition training as a determiner of strength and fatigability. *Res Q.* 41:189–193.

156. Sunnegardh, J., L-E. Bratteby, L-O. Nordesjo, and B. Nordgren. 1988. Isometric and isokinetic muscle strength, anthropometry, and physical activity in 8 and 13 year old Swedish children. *Eur J Appl Physiol.* 58:291–297.

157. Sutton, J. R., M. J. Colemean, J. Casey, and L. Lazarus. 1973. Androgen responses during physical exercise. *Br Med J.* 1:520–522.

158. Syster, B., and G. Stull. 1970. Muscular endurance retention as a function of length of detraining. *Res Q.* 41:105–109.

159. Tabata, I., Y. Atomi, H. Kanehisa, and M. Miyashita. 1990. Effect of high-intensity endurance training on isokinetic muscle power. *Eur J Appl Physiol.* 60:254–258.

160. Talag, T. S. 1973. Residual muscular soreness as influenced by concentric, eccentric, and static contractions. *Res Q.* 44(4):458–469.

161. Thistle, H., H. Hislop, M. Moffroid, and E. Lowman. 1967. Isokinetic contraction: a new concept of resistive exercise. *Arch Phys Med Rehab.* 48:279–282.

162. Thompson, C., and E. Martin. 1965. Weight training and baseball throwing speed. *J Assoc Phys Ment Rehab.* 19:194.

163. Thompson, H., and G. Stull. 1959. Effects of various training programs on speed of swimming. *Res Q.* 30:479–485.

164. Thorstensson, A. 1977. Muscle strength, fibre types, and enzyme activities in man. *Acta Physiol Scand.* (suppl. 443).

165. Thorstensson, A., B. Hultin, W. von Döbeln, and J. Karlsson. 1976. Effect of strength training on enzyme activities and fibre characteristics in human skeletal muscle. *Acta Physiol Scand.* 96:392–398.

166. Tipton, C. M., R. K. Martin, R. D. Matthes, and R. A. Carey. 1975. Hydroxyproline concentrations in ligaments from trained and nontrained rats. In Howald, H., and J. R. Poortmans (eds.), *Metabolic Adaptation to Prolonged Physical Exercise.* Basel, Switzerland: Birkhüser Verlag, pp. 262–267.

167. Tipton, C. M., R. D. Matthes, J. A. Maynard, and R. A. Carey. 1975. The influence of physical activity on ligaments and tendons. *Med Sci Sports.* 7(3):165–175.

168. Treuth, M. S., G. R. Hunter, T. Kekes-Szabo, R. L. Weinsier, M. I. Goran, and L. Berland. 1995. Reduction in intra-abdominal adipose tissue after strength training in older women. *J Appl Physiol.* 78:1425–1431.

169. Tseng, B. S., D. R. Marsh, M. T. Hamilton, and F. W. Booth. 1995. Strength and aerobic training attenuate muscle wasting and improve resistance to the development of disability with aging. *J Gerontol A Biol Sci Med Sci.* 50 Spec No:113–119.

170. Tucker, L. A., K. Harris, and J. R. Martin. 1996. Participation in a strength training program leads to improved dietary intake in adult women. *J Am Diet Assoc.* 96:388–390.

171. Van Oteghen, S. Oct. 1974. Isokinetic conditioning for women. *Scholastic Coach.*

172. Vrijens, J. 1978. Muscle strength development in the pre- and post-pubescent age. *Med Sport* (Basel). 11:152–158.

173. Waldman, R., and G. Stull. 1969. Effects of various periods of inactivity on retention of newly acquired levels of muscular endurance. *Res Q.* 40:393–401.

174. Wallin, D., B. Ekblom, R. Grahn, and T. Nordenborg. 1985. Improvement of muscle flexibility: a comparison between two techniques. *Am J Sports Med.* 13:263–268.

175. Walters, C., C. Stewart, and J. LeClaire. 1960. Effect of short bouts of isometric and isotonic contractions on muscular strength and endurance. *Am J Phys Med.* 39:131–141.

176. Welsh, L., and O. M. Rutherford. 1996. Effects of isometric strength training on quadriceps muscle properties in over 55 year olds. *Eur J Appl Physiol.* 72:219–223.

177. Wilmore, J. H., R. B. Parr, R. N. Girandola, P. Ward, P. A. Vodak, T. J. Barstow, T. V. Pipes, G. T. Romero, and P. Leslie. 1978. Physiological alterations consequent to circuit weight training. *Med Sci Sports.* 10(2):79–84.

178. Wilson, G. J., A. J. Murphy, and A. Walshe. 1996. The specificity of strength training: the effect of posture. *Eur J Appl Physiol.* 73:346–352.

179. Withers, R. 1970. Effect of varied weight-training loads on the strength of university freshmen. *Res Q.* 41:110–114.

180. Wolf, E., A. Blank, M. Shochina, and B. Gonen. 1984. Effect of exercise of the lower limbs on the non-exercised biceps brachii muscle. *Am J Phys Med.* 63:113–121.

181. Yamasaki, H., S. Yamada, K. Tanabe, N. Osada, M. Nakayama, H. Itoh, and M. Murayama. Effects of weight training on muscle strength and exercise capacity in patients after myocardial infarction. *J Cardiol.* 26:341–347.

182. Zorbas, W., and P. Karpovich. 1951. The effect of weight lifting upon the speed of muscular contractions. *Res Q.* 22:145–148.

Selected Readings

Booth, F. W., and D. B. Thomason. 1991. Molecular and cellular adaptation of muscle in response to exercise: perspective of various models. *Physiol Rev.* 71:541–585.

Fleck, S. J., and W. J. Kraemer. 1987. *Designing Resistance Training Programs.* Champaign, IL: Human Kinetics.

Hickson, R. C., and J. R. Marone. 1993. Exercise and inhibition of glucocorticoid-induced muscle atrophy. *Exer Sport Sci Rev.* 21:135–168.

Komi, P. (ed.). 1992. *Strength and Power in Sports. The Encyclopaedia of Sports Medicine.* Oxford, England: Blackwell.

Kraemer, W. J., S. J. Fleck, and W. J. Evans. 1996. Strength and power training: Physiological mechanisms of adaptation. *Exer Sport Sci Rev.* 24:363–397.

14
Physical Activity and Health

Only since the early 1990s has physical activity and exercise been formally recognized as playing an integral role in health improvement and disease management. Such recognition is associated with two important issues. First and foremost, it acknowledges the overwhelming scientific evidence linking regular physical activity with both the primary and secondary prevention* of disease. It is precisely this information that is presented in this chapter. In fact, you may find that the material covered in this chapter is the most meaningful information that you take with you from this entire book. Regardless of whether you ever enter an exercise physiology-related career in the future, the discussion that follows will benefit not only you but your family and friends as well.

Second, the increased recognition that physical activity and exercise now experience relative to health management is due, in part, to decades of hard work by countless exercise physiologists,† cardiologists, epidemiologists, behavioralists, public health officials, and many other men and women of science.[101] Much of their work, and the work of others, culminated in the 1996 publication, *Physical Activity and Health: A Report of the Surgeon General*[118]—truly a landmark document.

Relative to this chapter, we will focus our discussion on (1) an overview of the public health impact of physical inactivity, (2) how much exercise is needed to prevent and treat disease, (3) physical activity and other health-related issues, (4) physical activity in children/adolescents and older adults, and (5) female-specific issues. Clearly, our emphasis will not be on the athlete; instead we will direct our

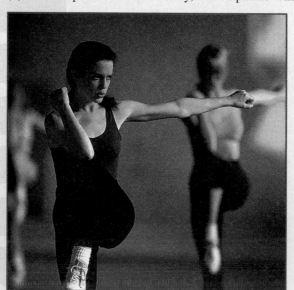

attention toward the individual who may simply wish to be in better shape and contribute to his or her health through regular physical activity.

We will begin with what is now one of the most important areas of exercise physiology: the role of physical activity and health—your health, the health of those around you, and the health of our nation as a whole.

---

*Primary prevention refers to the use of a strategy or treatment intended to prevent or decrease the likelihood of the first occurrence of a disease-related event. Secondary prevention means the treatment being used is intended to decrease the likelihood of a second event.
†An exercise physiologist working in research or teaching has almost always completed a doctoral degree that involved coursework/training in medicine, physiology, physical education, kinesiology, exercise science, epidemiology, and/or biochemistry.

The major concepts to be learned from this chapter are as follows:

- Over the past decade physical inactivity has been increasingly recognized as a major public health problem. Approximately one-quarter of all U.S. residents are inactive during times of leisure.
- Physical inactivity is a major contributing factor for all-cause mortality, cardiovascular disease, certain cancers, and Type II diabetes.
- Atherosclerosis is a disease that causes a narrowing of the lumen of an artery with cholesterol and other substances, and contributes to deaths from coronary heart disease and stroke.
- Cigarette smoking, physical inactivity, high blood pressure, and elevated total cholesterol all represent major, independent risk factors* that lead to the development of atherosclerosis.
- The present public health recommendation for the minimal dose of physical activity is that all Americans should accumulate a minimum of 30 minutes of moderate physical activity on most and preferably all days of the week.
- In addition to cardiovascular disease and stroke, other physiologic states and health disorders such as diabetes, blood clotting and fibrinolysis, blood lipids, immunology, and mental health also are influenced by regular physical activity.
- At both ends of the human life span, children/adolescents and older adults, physical activity can be enjoyed.
- High-volume exercise training can influence, somewhat, both menarche and menstruation.
- Generally, there are no negative effects of moderate, regular physical activity on pregnancy, childbirth, or fetal development. In fact, some evidence exists suggesting that exercise during pregnancy results in less perceived discomforts during later pregnancy, less weight gain, and a shorter period of labor.

*A risk factor is a medical condition or habit that is associated with an increased risk or danger of developing a specific health problem in the future. Risk factors can be lifestyle-related—for example, not wearing one's seatbelt increases one's risk for greater trauma during an automobile accident—or non-modifiable, such as increasing age and the development of coronary artery disease.

Physical Activity and Public Health: An Overview

Take a good look around. We're surrounded by labor-saving devices designed to make our lives easier. Need the garage door open? Push a button! Time to cut the lawn? Adjust the seat and turn the key! Want to change the channel? Just aim and push!

Although some of the technological advances border on the frivolous, for the most part they have made our lives simpler and easier. Such progress, however, has not occurred without a cost. In making our lives safer and more comfortable, we have removed an all too important ingredient for good health: daily physical activity. So just how bad is the current problem?

The Magnitude of the Problem

To answer this question we draw your attention to table 14.1, which presents the prevalence of *no leisure time physical activity (LTPA)* among the U.S. population aged 20 years and older. Before looking at specific population subgroups, note that the overall prevalence of *no LTPA* is ~ 22%. This value is consistent with the 24% figure reported from the National Health Interview Survey.[118] Taken together, these surveys indicate that about one-quarter of U.S. adults are sedentary during times of leisure.

Table 14.1 also shows that the prevalence of no LTPA is greater among females than males and is greater among blacks and Mexican Americans than among whites. In fact, almost *50%* of Mexican American females are sedentary! Relative to physical activity habits and age, among both males and females the rate of no LTPA increases as age increases (table 14.1). With advancing age, females consistently have higher rates of no LTPA than do males. Among adolescents, the overall frequency of no LTPA is ~ 10%, again being higher in females than in males (14% vs. 7%).[118]

The prevalence of persons who do regularly engage in light to moderate leisure time physical activity five or more times per week for at least 30 minutes ranges between 20% and 24%.[118] This dose or level of physical activity was surveyed because it is considered sufficient to promote good health and prevent disease. Given these figures, we can now determine that the prevalence of persons engaged in leisure time physical activity on an *irregular basis* (or at levels less than sufficient to promote heath improvement) is between 54% and 58%.

So, you might ask, if current levels of physical activity are not so good, how does this compare to previous years? Is the situation getting worse or better? First, in the United States and in other industrialized nations, the availability of leisure time has increased over the past 30 to 50 years. And as you might have guessed, between the mid-1960s and the mid-1980s, regular participation in LTPA rose in the U.S. Such an increase was most evident in the 1970s, being more pronounced among females than males and among older persons than younger persons. Unfortunately, however, there has been little improvement in the percentage of persons engaging in LTPA since the mid-1980s to present. As a nation, we have plateaued at ~ 22% to 24%, despite growing public awareness about the health benefits of physical activity, an increase in the number of fitness facilities available in the community and at work sites, and a marked increase in the type of exercise equipment available for in-home use. Later in this chapter we will discuss possible reasons and barriers that seem to impact the number of persons regularly participating in LTPA.

Health vs. Fitness

Throughout this chapter we will use the words *physical activity* and *exercise* somewhat interchangeably. Physical activity means, just as the name implies, being physically active to the extent that there is a significant increase in energy expenditure during work, routine activities of daily living, or leisure. Conversely, exercise is a subtype of physical activity, usually performed during leisure time and with the intention of improving one's physical fitness.* It usually involves a specific, planned routine of bodily movements. For example, going to an aerobic dance class after work or school is certainly a form of physical activity, but we subclassify it as exercise because it is performed in addition to routine daily activities—and with the intention of improving health or fitness. This differs from a postal worker who walks a delivery route each day and is considered to have an occupation that is quite physically active. In this case it is part of his or her normal occupation. Regardless of how you want to define it, *the take-home message here is that behind all this movement (physical activity or exercise), is one common denominator: the expenditure of energy (kcal).*

It may help to think about physical activity, exercise, and human performance as operating along a spectrum (figure 14.1). To the far right we find the elite endurance athlete, an individual who spends an enormous amount of time and energy (kcal) trying to improve his or her ability to perform. Hours of training each week may mean the difference between first and second place during competition. These individuals possess high levels of fitness (bottom curve) and have, along the way, derived the majority of the health benefits (top curve) achievable through exercise.

To the far left of the spectrum exists the sedentary or inactive individual who, from a public health point of view,

---

*There are many different types of physical fitness, yet for our purposes here we are referring to cardiorespiratory or aerobic fitness—the ability of the body to transport and utilize oxygen. This type of fitness is associated with a lower mortality from chronic diseases.

14.1

table

Prevalence (per 100) or percentage of No Leisure Time Physical Activity (LTPA) among the U.S. population aged 20 years or older, 1988–1991, National Health and Nutrition Examination Survey III*

Population group	Overall	20–29	30–39	40–49	Age (y) 50–59	60–69	70–79	> 80
Total	22	—	—	—	—	—	—	—
Male	17	13	14	16	18	17	23	40
Female	27	17	24	26	30	30	44	62
Non-Hispanic White								
Male	13	—	—	—	—	—	—	—
Female	23	—	—	—	—	—	—	—
Non-Hispanic Black								
Male	24	—	—	—	—	—	—	—
Female	40	—	—	—	—	—	—	—
Mexican American								
Male	33	—	—	—	—	—	—	—
Female	46	—	—	—	—	—	—	—

*Based on data from Crespo et al.[34]; sample size = 9,488.

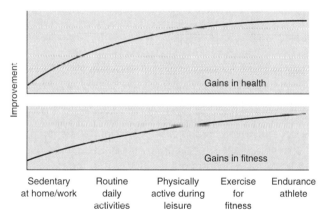

Figure 14.1

Physical activity, exercise, and human performance operate along a spectrum. Increasing one's energy expenditure (moving from left to right) provides gains in both health and fitness.

is at highest risk of developing disease such as heart disease, certain cancers, and diabetes. These persons also possess the lowest fitness levels. As figure 14.1 shows, increasing daily caloric expenditure (moving from left to right along the spectrum) improves health, in that the more active one becomes the greater the gains in health (or the lower the risk for certain diseases). In addition to gains in health, they experience fitness benefits as well. Note, however, that the majority of the health benefits occurred when the once sedentary person began to regularly engage in activity. So

high-dose exercise such as marathon running means that these people often choose to do so because they enjoy the competition or desire a higher levels of fitness. This is not to say that additional health benefits are not conferred when moving from moderately fit to highly fit,[67,90] just not to the same magnitude when compared to the once sedentary person who becomes regularly active. The bottom line here is that not everyone needs to become a highly fit person to achieve the majority of the health benefits derived from being physically active.

Before leaving this topic of health vs. fitness, we need to discuss one final important point: specifically, a high level of fitness through regular exercise does not make one immune to disease. Yes, regular exercise confers health benefits, but if achieved without concern for other risk factors, it provides no guarantee of longevity. Therefore, the regular walker, cyclist, swimmer, or runner who has an elevated cholesterol but chooses not to follow a proper low-fat diet or take a prescribed medication to lower blood cholesterol is not immune from having a heart attack or stroke. Yes, his/her risk of having such a problem is lower than if he/she were not exercising,[19] but exercise alone does not confer immunity from disease. Simply put, good fitness does not mean that a person is indeed enjoying optimal health!

Healthy People 2000 Objectives

Over a three-year period in the late 1980s scientists, public health officials, and educators held countless meetings to establish broad public health objectives for the year 2000

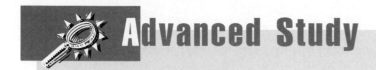

Advanced Study

U.S. Surgeon General's Report

On July 11, 1996, the Department of Health and Human Services of the United States released the *Surgeon General's Report on Physical Activity and Health.*[118] This 259-page document states that people can substantially improve their health and quality of life by including moderate amounts of physical activity in their daily lives. The report also emphasizes the message that physical activity need not be of vigorous intensity for it to improve health, although additional benefits can be achieved by further increases in intensity of activity among people who are already physical active.

The Surgeon General's report brought together epidemiologists, exercise scientists, and health professionals to review and discuss the impact of physical activity on heart disease, diabetes, certain cancers, depression, bone disease, and various other disorders. The consensus was that physical activity performed most days of the week improves health in the following ways:

1. Reduces the risk of dying prematurely
2. Reduces the risk of dying from heart disease
3. Reduces the risk of developing diabetes
4. Reduces the risk of developing high blood pressure—a major risk factor for heart disease and cerebrovascular disease
5. Helps to reduce high blood pressure among people who already suffer from this condition
6. Reduces the risk of developing colon cancer
7. Reduces the feelings of depression and anxiety and promotes psychological well-being
8. Helps to control body weight
9. Helps to build and maintain healthy bones, muscles, and joints
10. Helps older adults to become stronger and better able to move without the risk of falling

The experts who wrote the report concluded that physical inactivity is a serious, nationwide problem. Several national surveys confirm that approximately one of four Americans do not engage in any leisure-time physical activity.

Daily physical education classes for high school students dropped from 42% in 1991 to 25% in 1995. More importantly, only 19% of all high school students are physically active for 20 minutes or more during the physical education class itself. Physical activity decreases as adolescents become older, and female adolescents are less likely to engage in physical activity than male.

People who are usually inactive can improve their health and well-being by becoming even moderately active on a regular basis. Moderate amounts of physical activity can be achieved in a variety of ways. The amount of activity is a function of duration, intensity, and frequency. Activities range from the less vigorous activities (e.g., vacuuming, gardening, slow walking) that will require longer duration, to more vigorous activities such as jogging, running, rope jumping, snow shoveling, and stair walking that will require less time. Dancing, water aerobics, and raking leaves represent good examples of moderate activities that should be performed for 30 minutes. Overall, people should select activities that they enjoy and that fit into their daily lives.

The Surgeon General's report suggests that schools, work sites, health care providers, federal and non-federal agencies, and community-based groups work together to bring about an increase in the number of persons who are physically active.

Source: Courtesy of Dr. Carlos Crespo, National Heart, Lung, and Blood Institute.

---

and beyond. Their efforts culminated in a 692-page document titled *Healthy People 2000: National Health Promotion and Disease Prevention Objectives.*[117] Although the Federal Government facilitated the development of the report, the objectives it provides do not represent federal standards or requirements. Instead, they are to be viewed as guidelines that a variety of agencies and organizations should work toward—both individually and, whenever possible, through collaborative efforts.

In the *Healthy People 2000* report, more than 20 health priority areas are discussed such as nutrition, tobacco, can-

cer, and environmental health. Table 14.2 lists the original 12 *Healthy People 2000* objectives for one of the priority areas: physical activity and fitness. A thirteenth objective was added during a midcourse review published in 1995.[116] Note that the objectives are organized into three types: those meant to reduce death and disability *(Health Status),* those meant to reduce risks to health *(Risk Reduction),* and those meant to increase accessibility and quality of preventive services *(Services and Protection).* Using heart disease as an example, objective 1.1 calls for a reduction in coronary heart disease mortality to no more than 100 per

14.2

Healthy People 2000 Physical Activity and Fitness Objectives

Health status

1.1 Reduce coronary heart disease deaths to no more than 100 per 100,000 people.
1.2 Reduce overweight prevalence to no more than 20% among people aged 20 and older and to no more than 15% among adolescents aged 12–19.
1.3 Increase to at least 30% the proportion of people who regularly engage in light to moderate physical activity for at least 30 minutes per day.

Risk reduction

1.4 Increase to at least 20% the proportion of people aged 18 and older and to at least 75% the proportion of people aged 6–17 who engage in vigorous physical activity that promotes cardiorespiratory fitness 3 or more days per week for 20 or more minutes.
1.5 Reduce to no more than 15% the proportion of people who engage in no leisure time physical activity.
1.6 Increase to at least 40% the proportion of people who perform physical activities that enhance muscular strength/endurance and flexibility.
1.7 Increase to at least 50% the proportion of overweight people aged 12 and older who have adopted sound dietary practices combined with regular physical activity to attain an appropriate body weight.

Service and protection objectives

1.8 Increase to at least 50% the proportion of people in 1st–12th grade who participate in daily school physical education.
1.9 Increase to at least 50% the proportion of school physical education class time that students spend being physically active in lifetime activities.
1.10 Increase the proportion of worksites offering employer-sponsored physical activity and fitness programs.*
1.11 Increase community accessibility to physical activity and fitness facilities (e.g., hiking/fitness trails, swimming pools, open park/recreation space).
1.12 Increase to at least 50% the proportion of primary care providers who assess and counsel their patients regarding physical activity practices.

Health status

1.13 Reduce to no more than 90 per 1,000 people those people aged 65 and older who have difficulty performing two or more personal care activities (e.g., bathing, dressing), thereby preserving their independence.

*Targets vary according to the number of employees per work site.

100,000 people by the year 2000. Glance ahead to table 14.3 for just a moment and note that deaths due to heart disease in 1994 exceeded 140 per 100,000. This 1994 rate is down considerably from the rate in 1979 of 200 deaths per 100,000 persons. Obviously, however, there is still room for improvement.

The Economic Benefits of Physical Activity

Controlling soaring health-care costs is an issue that has received much discussion over the past five to ten years. Medicare and other governmental agencies admonish doc-

tors and hospitals about treatment costs, while at the same time the health-care facilities point a "guilty" finger at both the pharmaceutical companies and at governmental regulations. By the year 2000, health care costs in the U.S. will approach, if not exceed, $1 trillion per year.[51] One way to cut costs is to improve how health care is delivered (the treatment side of the equation). This means lowering the cost of the service without sacrificing, and maybe improving, quality of service. Another way to reduce costs is by preventing health problems before they arise. Enter physical activity!

A recent review of the economic benefits of physical activity reported that as a result of physical activity or a work-site fitness program, as much as $3.4 dollars can be

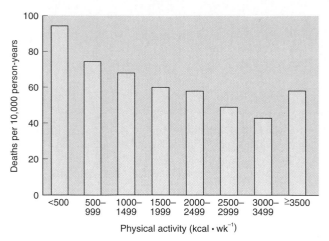

Figure 14.2

All-cause mortality and weekly energy expenditure among Harvard alumni.

Based on data from Paffenbarger, et al.[94]

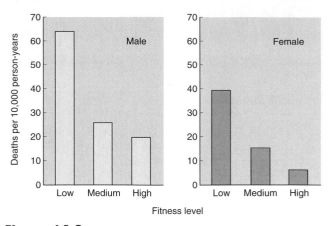

Figure 14.3

All-cause mortality among males and females over an 8-year follow-up period according to fitness level at baseline.

Based on data from Blair et al.[19]

saved for every dollar that is spent to promote or implement physical activity.[51] This is quite a return on one's investment, especially if you are the employer trying to lower health-care premiums in your company. The economic benefits usually present themselves as less absenteeism at work, lower medical costs, or reduced expenses from disability.

Conducting research aimed at assessing the dollars saved because of physical activity is difficult. Well-controlled scientific experiments are complicated by many factors, not the least of which is the ethical problem of asking a control group to remain sedentary (i.e., place themselves at higher risk for disease), while researchers observe how many dollars are saved over time in another group of subjects randomly assigned to a regular exercise regimen. Considering all the evidence to date, which often involves observational research, it was concluded that physical activity is economically beneficial.[51]

The Public Health Burden of Physical Inactivity

According to physical activity advocate Dr. Steven Blair, physical inactivity represents "one of our nation's most pressing health problems."[16] What, specifically, are the health consequences resulting from physical inactivity?

Overall Mortality

Although the number of population studies intended to relate physical activity/fitness to overall or all-cause mortality are few, there are two research groups that have done much to advance our knowledge in this area. The first group is led by Dr. Ralph Paffenbarger and the work he and his coworkers have accomplished via the Harvard Alumni Study.

In a study of 16,936 males entering college between 1916 and 1950 and then followed after graduation, 1,413 alumni died between 1962 and 1978.[94] They found that death rates were inversely related to total kcal expended per week (figure 14.2). Note, however, that a substantial drop in mortality occurred with relatively moderate levels of activity (greater than 1,000 kcal · week[−1]). Interestingly, death later in life was not related to participation in varsity athletics during college, meaning regular physical activity throughout life was more important. By age 80, the amount of additional life attributable to adequate exercise vs. a sedentary lifestyle was one to two more years. Using the same database, Lee et al.[71] showed that engaging in vigorous activity (greater than 6 METs) rather than nonvigorous activity (less than 6 METs) was associated with lower all-cause mortality.

The second research group that deserves mention is led by Dr. Blair and his colleagues at the Institute for Aerobics Research in Dallas, TX. In 1989 they reported their findings on 10,224 males and 3,120 females followed for 8 years after undergoing baseline exercise testing.[22] As figure 14.3 shows, subsequent death due to all-causes was higher in the low fitness groups when compared to both the moderate fitness or high fitness groups. In fact, notice the dramatic decrease in mortality when comparing low fit to moderately fit people. This again suggests that a relatively moderate dose of regular physical activity is all that is needed to markedly lower mortality.

Of possibly equal importance, subsequent work by Blair et al., showed that changing one's physical fitness level altered future mortality. Specifically, least fit males who changed their lifestyle and improved their fitness through exercise experienced a 44% reduction in future all-cause mortality over a five-year period, when compared to men who remained unfit.[21]

14.3

Ten leading causes of death (United States, 1994)

Cause of death	Deaths per 100,000 population*	Potential life lost†
Heart disease	140.4	3.3
Cancers	131.5	4.3
Accidents and other unintentional injuries	30.3	2.6
Stroke	26.5	0.6
Chronic lung disease	21.0	0.4
Human immunodeficiency virus	15.4	1.5
Pneumonia and influenza	13.0	0.3
Diabetes	12.9	0.4
Suicide	11.2	1.0
Homicide	10.3	—
All causes	507.4	—

*Age-adjusted rate.
†In millions of years, based on average remaining years of life up to age 75.
Data from Monthly Vital Statistics Report, vol. 45, no. 3, September 30, 1996.

Looked at collectively, findings from both research groups indicate that all-cause mortality is lowered by moderate physical activity; however, greater gains appear to be conferred with the achievement of even higher fitness levels. The benefits discussed here relative to physical activity appear to hold up regardless of whether other risk factors are present.[19,20]

Disease-Specific Mortality

Table 14.3 lists the 10 leading causes of death among persons living in the U.S. Which of these do you feel are caused, at least in part, by a lifestyle of improper behavioral habits? Which of those that you identified include physical inactivity as a risk factor? At the very least, coronary heart disease, certain forms of cancer (colon cancer), and diabetes have been linked to physical inactivity.[96,100] Although definitive evidence is not yet available, it may also be true that cerebrovascular accidents (e.g., stroke) are associated with a sedentary existence.[118,122] Physical inactivity or a lower level of cardiorespiratory fitness are related to the risk of developing hypertension (high blood pressure),[17,122] which is a primary risk factor for stroke.

Present estimates are that as many as 250,000 deaths each year are attributable to a lack of regular physical activity,[54,75] which is ~ 12% of all deaths. Assuming not everyone asked to will become physically active, if just 50% of the once sedentary people become irregularly active and 50% of the irregularly active people become regularly active, there would be an almost 3% reduction in overall mortality each year from heart disease, colon cancer, and diabetes alone. This equates to ~ 70 thousand lives saved each year.[99]

Now let's look at table 14.3 in a different way. We see that the majority of people in the U.S. die one of two ways: either cancers or cardiovascular diseases (all heart diseases combined with stroke). Summed together, cancers and cardiovascular diseases account for almost 59% of all deaths in our country. Relative to cardiovascular diseases, the underlying problem is often atherosclerosis, which leads to ischemic heart disease (e.g., heart attacks) and strokes. A 1997 study analyzing the factors that accounted for the favorable decrease in deaths due to heart disease between 1980 and 1990 suggested that more than 50% of the reduction was attributed to primary and secondary preventive efforts aimed at risk factor modification.[60] The balance was due to advances in interventional care (e.g., "balloon" angioplasty), emergency care, and medical therapies.

Obviously, no one can live forever; what we are most interested in is reducing the risk of premature death. Using public health jargon for a moment, this is referred to as *years of potential life lost*—in this case, before the age of 75 years. As table 14.3 indicates, heart disease, cancer, and automobile and unintentional injuries are associated with much premature death. As a population, millions of years of potential life are lost each year in this manner.

Atherosclerosis

Atherosclerosis is a slow, progressive disease involving the narrowing of the lumen of arteries. This narrowing is in turn caused by fatty substances, calcium, collagen, and other

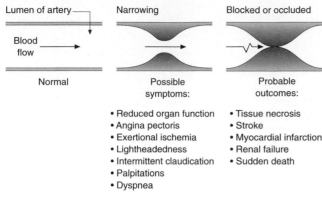

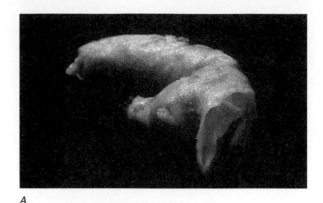

A

Figure 14.4

The narrowing of the lumen of an artery by atherosclerosis is progressive. Narrowing may produce warning symptoms as shown. In an advanced stage, the blood flow through the artery can be completely blocked, often from a blood clot, resulting in permanent tissue organ damage or even death.

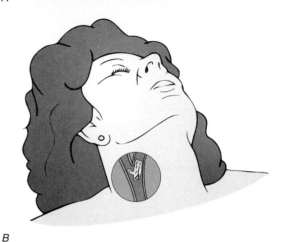

B

Figure 14.5

This plug of placque (A), nearly an inch long, was surgically removed from the branching point of a carotid artery (B). Despite the size of the obstruction, the stroke patient survived.

cellular materials being deposited as a plaque-like material on the inside wall of the arteries. Besides the narrowing effect, the arteries so afflicted also become somewhat stiff or hardened; thus, the term *hardening of the arteries.* As shown in figure 14.4, the narrowing is progressive and, based on where it is located, may produce a variety of symptoms. Portions of the arterial system where branching occurs are more prone to plaque deposition than others. As shown in figure 14.5, the branch point of the carotid artery represents a common site of atherosclerotic plaque formation.

Although atherosclerosis leads to a progressive narrowing of the artery lumen, the action most often responsible for sudden or acute cardiovascular events (e.g., a heart attack) is plaque thrombosis (i.e., clot formation). Approximately 30% of the time the thrombus is simply superimposed on top of the plaque, extending into and occluding an already narrowed artery. More commonly, thrombus formation is caused by plaque fissuring, tearing, or rupturing. A tear usually occurs along areas of the plaque that are structurally weak, and in doing so, allows blood to move into the inside of the plaques where it comes in contact with substances that strongly stimulate clot formation. A clot that forms can be quickly sealed—so there is only limited additional growth of the plaque—or the thrombus can grow out into the lumen itself and completely occlude it. Always remember that the atherosclerotic process is dynamic!

Relative to the heart, two events that result from thrombi formation within the coronary arteries are unstable angina (i.e., chest pain or discomfort) or a heart attack. Concerning the latter, heart muscle that was once supplied with oxygen via the blood now goes without it and dies. This is why a heart attack is called a myocardial infarction—*myocardial* meaning *heart* and *infarction* meaning *death to tissue.* The severity of the event is determined by the exact location of the blockage within the artery. For ex-

ample, as shown in figure 14.6, if it is toward the end of the artery, then the heart attack may not be too severe because the amount of heart tissue involved would be minimal. However, if the blockage is more toward the beginning of the artery, the amount of tissue involved would be large and the heart attack severe.

A current, standard treatment that is effective among persons who are experiencing a heart attack is the administration of various drugs meant to dissolve a thrombosis—the so-called thrombolytics or "clot busters." The sooner this type of medication can be given to a patient with an evolving heart attack, the better—such that time to delivery of the medication literally means how many cardiac muscle cells are saved. This time-dependent relationship represents the rationale behind the public health message that encourages people to go to an emergency room right away if they suspect a heart attack, versus trying to wait it out to see if the pain goes away.

Because plaque development from atherosclerosis is a relatively slow-developing disease, it is generally thought of as an "old age" disease. However, this is not necessarily true. For example, autopsies performed on American

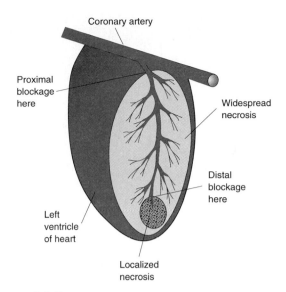

Coronary artery

Proximal
blockage
here

Widespread
necrosis

Distal
blockage
here

Left
ventricle
of heart

Localized
necrosis

Figure 14.6

A heart attack occurs when the blood flow through a coronary artery is blocked. If the blockage is toward the distal end of the artery, the heart attack may not be too severe because the amount of heart tissue involved would be localized. However, if the block is more toward the beginning (proximal) part of the artery, the amount of tissue involved would be large and the heart attack more severe.

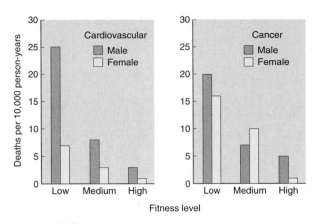

Figure 14.7

Disease-specific mortality among males and females over an 8-year follow-up period according to fitness level at baseline.
Based on data from Blair et al.[19]

soldiers killed in the Korean and Vietnam wars, most of who were less than 30 years old, revealed moderately advanced stages of atherosclerosis in the majority of these men.[43,77] The beginning stages of atherosclerosis have even been found in children less than 5 years of age,[62] and 62% of children between the ages of 7 and 12 years have been found to have at least one coronary artery disease risk factor.[52,126]

Risk Factors Associated with Heart Attack

Previously we stated that regular physical activity or exercise lessens the likelihood for a variety of health problems, including having a heart attack. Thus, one risk factor for having a heart attack is physical inactivity or sedentary living. Using data again from Blair et al,[22] we find that among both males and females, deaths from cardiovascular disease are lower among persons classified as moderately fit or highly fit, when compared to persons with a lower fitness level (figure 14.7). The possible biologic mechanisms by which physical activity lowers cardiovascular mortality rates include the following:[58,118]

1. Increased electrical stability of the myocardium (e.g., decreased catecholamines at rest and during exercise, increased ventricular fibrillation threshold);
2. Decreased myocardial work and O_2 demand (e.g., decreased heart rate and blood pressure at rest and during exercise);

3. Increased myocardial function (e.g., increased myocardial contractility); and
4. Maintained myocardial oxygen supply (e.g., delayed progression of atherosclerosis from decreased adiposity and increased high-density lipoprotein cholesterol).

Well, in addition to physical inactivity, what are some of the other known risk factors associated with having a heart attack? The most commonly identified are as follows: (1) age, (2) heredity, (3) obesity (body weight), (4) tobacco smoking, (5) diabetes, (6) high blood cholesterol levels, (7) high blood pressure, (8) male gender, and (9) stress. Several of these are linked to lifestyle choices (e.g., tobacco smoking, obesity, blood pressure, and blood cholesterol levels), while others are not (e.g., gender, age, and heredity). Up until age 50, the death rate due to heart disease is several times greater in males than females. However, after *menopause* (cessation of menstruation), heart disease rates among women increases markedly, such that they almost catch up to males by age 60 years. The protective effect from heart disease observed in premenopausal women may be caused by endogenous estrogens, which drop after menopause.[102] Also, the exact way that heredity plays a role in heart attack is not known. Clearly, persons with parents or siblings who suffered a heart attack or sudden death before the age of 55 are at increased risk for having a heart attack. However, one should always question whether it is family genes that are placing a person at increased risk or improper lifestyle habits such as poor eating, physical inactivity, and smoking that were passed along? In other words, parents who themselves are inactive tend to have children who are also inactive. These inactive children, then, grow up to become inactive adults.

While each of the ten cardiovascular risk factors are important, four of them (called the "big four") are especially important and are classified as major risk factors

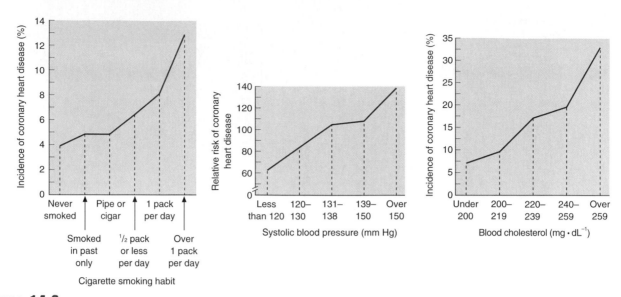

Figure 14.8

Incidence (smoking, blood cholesterol) or relative risk (systolic blood pressure) of coronary heart disease in relation to coronary risk factor. For each risk factor, likelihood of the disease increases as the "problem" worsens.

Based on data from the American Heart Association[8] and Loviglio.[74]

because of their strong, independent relationship to the future likelihood of developing the disease. The big four risk factors are physical inactivity, cigarette smoking, high blood pressure, and elevated total blood cholesterol level. It's worth noting here that up until the early 1990s, there were only the "big three" risk factors for heart disease—until the American Heart Association and the Centers for Disease Control and Prevention recognized physical inactivity as the fourth major risk factor for cardiovascular disease.

TOBACCO SMOKING. The more cigarettes smoked per day and the longer one smokes, the greater the risk of coronary heart disease (and lung cancer). As shown in figure 14.8, a more than one-pack-a-day smoker has over twice the risk of heart attack compared to the nonsmoker.

The exact physiological link between smoking and the development of atherosclerosis is not known. However, it is thought that cigarette smoking may, via carbon monoxide and other identified agents in smoke, injury the inner artery wall and contribute to atherosclerosis and/or initiate the development of small blood clots.

HIGH BLOOD PRESSURE (**HYPERTENSION**). Although many people believe that diastolic blood pressure is associated with a greater risk than systolic blood pressure for the development of heart disease, both are independently and strongly related. As shown in figure 14.8, an individual with a systolic blood pressure of more than 150 mm Hg has over twice the risk of developing coronary heart disease than does someone with a pressure below 120 mm Hg. Generally, the lower the blood pressure, the better, but values below a systolic reading of 140 mm Hg and below a diastolic reading of 90 mm Hg are usually not treated by medications.[28] The means by which hypertension induces atherosclerosis

are not clear. It may be that altered blood flow characteristics injures the inner artery wall, contributing to the development of plaque formation. Treatment strategies for patients with hypertension include medications, achievement of ideal body weight, reducing alcohol and dietary sodium intake as needed, and regular, moderate exercise (chapter 9, p. 241).

BLOOD CHOLESTEROL (LIPID) LEVELS. Dietary lipids or fats are perhaps one of the most important lifestyle agents responsible for severe atherosclerosis in industrially developed parts of the world. In America, the diet is typically very rich in animal product foods containing saturated fat and cholesterol (see chapter 15, p. 413 for definition of saturated fats). Dietary saturated fats, even more so than dietary cholesterol, are known to increase blood cholesterol levels—which is related to the incidence of coronary heart disease. Such a relationship is shown in figure 14.8. The likelihood of coronary heart disease in a person with a total blood cholesterol of over 259 mg% is nearly five times that of a person with a total blood cholesterol under 200 mg%. Presently, ~ 52% of adult Americans have a cholesterol level above 200 mg · dL^{-1}.

The various blood cholesterol values used to guide treatment strategies in the *primary prevention* setting (adults without evidence of coronary heart disease) are shown in table 14.4.[119] Notice that in addition to the measurement of total cholesterol, *lipoprotein* cholesterols (HDL and LDL) are also included in the stated treatment strategies.

Lipoproteins are high-molecular weight particles comprised of water insoluble lipids (primarily triglycerides and cholesterol esters) and proteins (apoprotein). The majority of plasma lipids are packaged and transported in these struc-

14.4

Classification and follow-up strategies for patients without evidence of coronary heart disease (National Cholesterol Education Program Adult Treatment Panel II 1993 Guidelines)

Total cholesterol ($mg \cdot dL^{-1}$)	Risk classification	Low HDL cholesterol ($< 35\ mg \cdot dL^{-1}$)	Follow-up strategies
< 200	Desirable	No	Provide risk-reduction materials and repeat total cholesterol and HDL cholesterol within 5 years.
		Yes	Provide information on risk factor reduction; re-evaluate in 1 to 2 years.
200–239	Borderline high	No	If one risk factor present, provide risk reduction materials and re-evaluate in 1 to 2 years. If two or more other risk factors present, do lipoprotein analysis.*
		Yes	Do lipoprotein analysis.*
≥ 240	High	No	Do lipoprotein analysis.*
		Yes	Do lipoprotein analysis.*

*Further action (diet, exercise, and/or medications) guided by LDL cholesterol. LDL cholesterol $< 130\ mg \cdot dL^{-1}$ − desirable; $130–159\ mg \cdot dL^{-1}$ = borderline high risk; $> 130\ mg \cdot dL^{-1}$ = high risk.

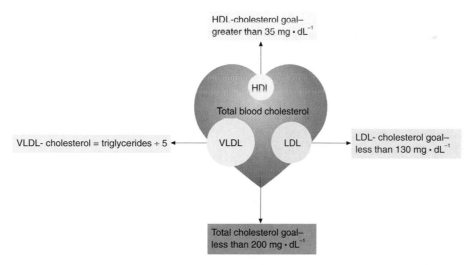

Figure 14.9
Graphic representation of the various liproproteins and total cholesterol based on primary prevention guidelines.[119]

tures. Three major classes of lipoprotein carriers found in the blood are: low-density lipoprotein (LDL), high-density lipoprotein (HDL), and very low-density lipoprotein (VLDL). These relationships are depicted in figure 14.9, using primary prevention guidelines. Not shown in table 14.4 is the treatment strategy for patients *with* evidence of coronary heart disease *(secondary prevention)*. Therapy (diet and medication) in these patients is meant to achieve an **LDL cholesterol** less than or equal to $100\ mg \cdot dL^{-1}$.

Measuring total blood cholesterol can be accomplished via either a simple finger-stick method, such as that often used at shopping malls, worksites, and health fairs, or by drawing a sufficiently sized venous blood sample following a twelve hour fast. The latter is performed when obtaining a *lipoprotein profile,* which includes LDL cholesterol, **HDL cholesterol,** and triglycerides. In this profile, LDL cholesterol is computed using the formula (when triglycerides are less than 400 mg · dL^{-1}):

$$LDL = total\ cholesterol - HDL - (triglycerides \div 5)$$

For example, in a person with a total cholesterol of 270 mg · dL^{-1}, an HDL cholesterol of 45 mg · dL^{-1}, and a triglyceride level of 250 mg · dL^{-1}, estimated LDL cholesterol would be 175 mg · dL^{-1}.

LDL, or the so-called "bad cholesterol", typically contains 60% to 70% of the total serum cholesterol and is directly associated with the risk of coronary heart disease. One function of LDL cholesterol is to supply cholesterol to cells for the synthesis of cell membranes and steroid hormones. However, exposure of LDL to endothelial cells (the cells that make up the inner-most lining of arteries) can result in its oxidation (i.e., removal of electrons). This can lead to the accumulation of cholesterol esters within the macrophages and smooth muscle cells located in an arterial wall—and to the formation of an atherosclerotic plaque. In the primary prevention setting, achieving an LDL cholesterol less than 130 mg · dL^{-1} is desirable,[119] although some preventive-minded persons aim for values below 100 mg · dL^{-1}.

HDL, or the so-called "good cholesterol", normally contains 20% to 30% of the total cholesterol, and values equal to or greater than 60 mg · dL^{-1} have a negative or inverse relationship with heart disease (decreased risk for coronary heart disease). An HDL cholesterol below 35 mg · dL^{-1} is defined as low and constitutes a major risk factor for coronary heart disease. Initially, HDL particles do not enter circulation as fully mature particles, in that they are devoid of cholesterol. Subsequently, they perform a scavenger function, acquiring unesterified cholesterol originating from cell membranes during cell renewal or death. Accumulation of cholesterol in this manner results in the enlargement of the cholesterol particle, from HDL$_3$ to HDL$_2$. This, in turn, increases the cholesterol carrying capacity of HDL, driving the process termed *reverse cholesterol transport*—returning cholesterol from the peripheral tissues to the liver for excretion into the bile.

The principal component of VLDL is triglycerides, another blood fat whose ability to predict future coronary heart disease is much less straightforward when compared to cholesterol. The Expert Panel on the Detection, Evaluation and Treatment of High Blood Cholesterol in Adults classifies a triglyceride level below 200 mg · dL^{-1} as normal.[119] However, many preventive-minded clinicians recommend values below 120 mg · dL^{-1}.

Given the above, a low total cholesterol level, with low LDL and VLDL fractions and a high HDL fraction, represents a healthy profile with respect to blood lipids. The effects of exercise training on the various blood lipids are reviewed later in this chapter.

INFLUENCE OF MULTIPLE RISK FACTORS. Having just one of the above-mentioned risk factors increases future likeli-

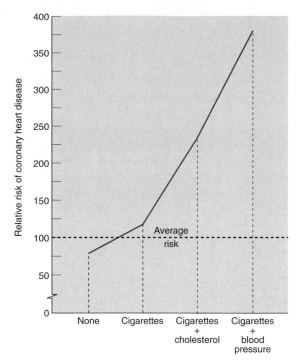

Figure 14.10

Exponential increase in relative risk of coronary heart disease when two of the four major risk factors are present. If three of the major risk factors are present, the danger of a heart attack is increased even further.

(Based on data from the American Heart Association.[8])

hood for coronary heart disease. To make matters worse, the presence of two or more risk factors increases risk that much more (figure 14.10). If three of the four major risk factors are present, the danger of a heart attack approaches five times that when none are present!

Cerebrovascular Accident—Stroke

To function, brain cells must have a continuous and ample supply of oxygen-rich blood, which, if completely stopped, causes the cells to die (i.e., stroke, cerebral infarction). The result of a stroke is usually *hemiparesis* (paralysis of one side of the body). It also may result in *aphasia* (loss of the power of expression or understanding communications) or in loss of memory. The effects may be slight or severe, temporary or permanent—depending on which brain cells have been damaged and on how widespread the damage is.

A leading cause of stroke is a clot blocking an already atherosclerotic artery that supplies blood to a section of the brain. This condition is called **cerebral thrombosis** and accounts for ~ 70% of all strokes. Just like patients suffering an acute heart attack, thrombolytic therapy can be successful in treating these patients; however, treatment must be started within 2 to 3 hours after the onset of symptoms.[86]

Stroke also occurs when an artery bursts, flooding the surrounding tissue with blood. This is called a *subarachnoid* or *cerebral hemorrhage.* Cells once nourished by the artery are deprived of blood and cannot function. A cerebral hemorrhage is more likely to occur when a person suffers from a combination of atherosclerosis and high blood pressure. For example, if you are a 45-year-old male who smokes cigarettes and has high blood cholesterol and high blood pressure, your risk of a stroke is more than ten times that of a male of the same age with none of these risk factors. Hemorrhage of an artery in the brain may also be caused by a burst *aneurysm.* Aneurysms are blood-filled pouches that balloon out from a weak spot in the artery wall and are often associated with high blood pressure.

Physical Inactivity—A Risk Factor for Cancer

Cigarette smoking and chronic alcohol abuse represent two self-imposed lifestyle habits that are well linked to cancer. However, during the past 15 years, physical inactivity has emerged as yet another risk factor for certain cancers. This connection between physical activity and cancer prevention may be hard for some to appreciate, because the data on this issue has been inconsistent and is difficult to interpret since cancer represents not one disease but many distinct, site-specific diseases.

Scan back to figure 14.7 and note that just like cardiovascular disease, level of fitness is related to death from all-cancers among both males and females. And, just like cardiovascular disease, it appears that significant improvements in lowering cancer mortality can be achieved with relatively moderate-dose physical activity—moving from the low fit to moderately fit groups. However, this relationship does not hold true for all cancers. To better understand this, we divide the cancer by site: colon, rectal, prostate, estrogen-dependent type (breast, ovarian, endometrial), and other (e.g. lung, pancreatic).

Of the various cancers mentioned above, the most studied and the one with the clearest inverse relationship between physical activity and incidence of disease is colon cancer.[70,122] Generally, comparing both occupational and leisure-time activities, sedentary males and females are at a nearly 1½ to 2-fold increased risk for colon cancer when compared to their active counterparts.[70] Although the mechanism(s) responsible for this relationship has not been specifically identified, one postulated reason is that regular exercise shortens intestinal transit time, which decreases the amount of time carcinogenic substances are in the fecal stream and in contact with intestinal/colonic tissue. In a 1995 review by Lee,[70] she stated that 25 of 33 papers published on the topic of physical activity and colon cancer found that a beneficial relationship existed.

In contrast to colon cancer, evidence that physical activity is inversely related to the incidence of all other site-specific cancers is less convincing and less studied. Of the ten epidemiologic studies that have looked at prostrate cancer, only five have shown a beneficial effect from physical activity.[70] One proposed mechanism is that changes in hormones from physical activity lessens the risk. Alternately, three studies have actually shown a harmful, direct effect, in that increased physical activity placed males at an even greater risk for this cancer. Clearly, more research is needed in this area.

Relative to breast cancer, the timing of physical activity may be important. Specifically, athletics during adolescence both delays the age when **menarche** appears (beginning of **menstruation**) and leads to shorter menstrual cycles. Additionally, after menarche, strenuous physical activity may lead to ovulatory dysfunction, a shortened luteal phase, and/or **amenorrhea.** Looked at together, both factors favorably lower estrogen exposure.[64] Another possible mechanism, more so among postmenopausal females than premenopausal females, may be through the important role that regular physical activity has in the achievement and maintenance of low levels of body fat. Obesity is known to be associated with a reduction in the number of protein carriers (i.e., sex-hormone binding globulin) responsible to bind and transport estradiol. Free estradiol, the most active form of endogenous estrogen, plays an important role in the development of breast tumors. When sex-hormone binding globulin levels are low, because of obesity, more free estradiol is present to interact with target tissues.

Frisch et al.[50] assessed the prevalence of breast cancer in more than 5,398 females, of which 2,622 participated in collegiate athletics between 1925 and 1981. These athletes were compared to a random sample of matched nonathletes. A higher percentage of former athletes reported they were currently exercising. Comparing the prevalence of breast cancer between the two groups, the nonathletes experienced almost 1.9 times the risk of developing cancer than did the former athletes.

For all other cancers, data is even more sparse. While one or two studies may show a beneficial relationship between physical activity and endometrial cancer or testicular cancer, others do not. In addition, no evidence exists supporting physical activity lowering risk for rectal, lung, or pancreatic cancers. It appears, therefore, that relative to certain types of cancer (colon and possibly breast* or prostate), physical activity represents another modifiable lifestyle habit that, in addition to not smoking and limiting alcohol use, can be used to influence mortality.

How Much Exercise Is Enough?

In chapters 11 and 12 we discussed the components of the exercise prescription relative to the competitive athlete. You will find that although similarities can be found between the prescription of exercise for improved human performance

---

*For additional recent evidence supporting the beneficial relationship between physical activity and a reduced risk of breast cancer, see Thune et al., cited in the Selected Readings section at the end of this chapter.

table

14.5

Comparison of exercise prescription guidelines for health vs. human performance reasons

	Guideline	
Training factor	**Health***	**Aerobic Sport Performance**
Frequency	Daily	5–7 per week
Intensity	Moderate, 50%–70% of maximal heart rate	85%–95% of maximal heart rate
Time (duration)	≥ 30 minutes	30 minutes to 1 hour
Type (specificity)	Rhythmical use of large muscle groups per personal choice	Sport-specific activity (i.e., swimming for swimmers)

*Target goal is 150 kcal · day^{-1} (1,000 kcal · week^{-1}).

and the prescription of exercise for improved health, differences do exist (table 14.5). Specifically, training for improved sport performance usually involves higher intensity sessions conducted daily if not, sometimes, twice daily. An acronym commonly used to help remember the components of an exercise prescription is FITT, which stands for *F*requency, *I*ntensity, *T*ime (or duration), and *T*ype of activity.

Not listed in table 14.5 is the issue of progression, which is also important—especially among previously sedentary persons who are just beginning an exercise or physical activity regimen. Progressively increasing dose of activity helps limit activity related injuries and leads to attainment of achievable goals, the latter of which enhances self-efficacy.

Medical Evaluation

Before prescribing an exercise program, one must, at the very least, consider whether the person they are counseling should receive some type of screening or medical evaluation prior to engaging in exercise. The extent of any evaluation partly depends on how vigorous the intended program will be and the health status of the person they are counseling. For example, if a 49-year-old premenopausal, previously sedentary, and otherwise healthy female wishes to start a simple program of mild to moderate walking, the extent of her medical evaluation, if any, should be limited and should not represent a barrier to getting started. Conversely, a slightly overweight, sedentary 45-year-old male who has high blood pressure and wishes to play in an adult ice hockey league should have a thorough medical evaluation prior to beginning. The latter example depicts an individual

at higher risk for having a medical problem during exercise, based on the various risks he possess in his lifestyle and on the intense type of activity he has chosen.

If a medical evaluation is indicated, then one or more of the following procedures might be included:[3]

1. A comprehensive medical history questionnaire or review;
2. A physical examination, to include resting systolic and diastolic blood pressure;
3. Blood analysis for fasting blood sugar, total cholesterol and triglyceride determinations;
4. A twelve-lead resting electrocardiogram (ECG); and
5. A symptom-limited graded exercise "stress" test with ECG monitoring.

The American College of Sports Medicine has published guidelines to identify who should undergo an exercise stress test before beginning an exercise program and who should not.[3] Generally, apparently healthy persons and persons who are without symptoms and have one or fewer risk factors for coronary artery disease do not need an exercise test prior to becoming moderately active. The protocols and methods associated with graded exercise tests, along with interpretation of the data obtained from such tests, were discussed in chapters 4 and 9.

Dose of Physical Activity

Similar to a medication that is prescribed to treat a certain illness or disease, exercise is increasingly prescribed as a treatment modality. When prescribing exercise, issues such as (1) effectiveness of treatment, (2) safety, (3) optimal dose tolerated without harmful side effects (e.g., an injury), and

(4) achievable benefit expected within the general population are all important to consider. To better appreciate how it came to be that physical activity is now formally viewed as an important weapon in the primary and secondary prevention of disease, it is helpful to first review what types of expert statements have been made about exercise in the past.

Between the 1970s and the early 1990s, more than 10 separate sets of recommendations or papers were published by expert panels relative to exercise among the U.S. population.[118] One position statement that provided a basis for many subsequent reports was the 1978 statement by the American College of Sports Medicine (ACSM),[6] which can be summarized as follows:

- frequency of training: 3–5 days per week

- intensity of training: 60%–90% of maximum heart rate or 50%–85% of $\dot{V}O_2$ max

- time or duration of training: 15–60 min per session

- type or mode of training: rhythmical and aerobic use of large muscle groups

Such a dose of exercise was known to be sufficient to promote improvement in cardiorespiratory fitness and body composition. However, in that statement, like other reports of that time period, no mention was made about the health implications of physical activity.

In 1990 the ACSM slightly modified its 1978 statement, such that duration of training was changed from 15–60 min to 20–60 min per session.[5] In that statement, the health benefits of physical activity were mentioned; however, no definitive dose or prescriptive guidelines were given. In the end, the 1990 statement was again aimed at improving cardiorespiratory fitness and body composition, with an added intention of enhancing muscular strength and endurance.

It was not until 1994 that experts from the ACSM and the Centers for Disease Control and Prevention, after having completed an extensive review of the scientific literature, made a formal statement concerning physical activity and health.[96] It was then that the exercise for fitness paradigm was shifted to include exercise for health. Although the specifics of the statement vary slightly from one authoritative body to another, the current public health recommendation can be summarized as follows:

All children and adults should accumulate a minimum of 30 minutes of moderate physical activity on most and preferably all days of the week.[10,90,96,118]

Compare the statements made by the ACSM in 1978 and 1990 to this one. Clear differences exist relative to the frequency (3–5 days per week vs. preferably daily) and intensity of activity (60%–90% of maximum heart rate vs. moderate). Don't be misled, however. The exercise recommendation for health does not invalidate or replace prior exercise statements meant to develop cardiorespiratory

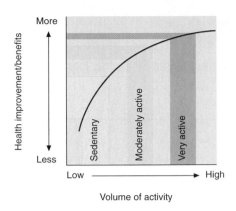

Figure 14.11

Dose-response curve between volume of activity and derived health benefit. The lower the initial activity status, the greater is the derived health benefit, given an increase in physical activity.

fitness.[5,9] The public health statement simply expands the opportunity for Americans to be more active for health reasons alone.

A primary aim of the statement is that sedentary people accumulate 30 min of moderate physical activity most days of the week, where *moderate activity* is defined as ~ 1,000 kcal or more per week.[58,72,94,95,96,118] Doing so will allow them to fall on an optimal (steep) portion of the dose-response curve, where increasing physical activity levels to moderate and beyond result in further gains in health (figure 14.11). Note that although the greatest gains are achieved when once sedentary persons engage in moderate activity, additional but smaller gains are achievable for both moderately active persons who become more active, and already active persons who become even more active.[22,90,94,99] Obviously, there is some diminishing return, in that the more active one becomes, the less dramatic is the increase in health-related benefits, but the message is quite clear: physical activity provides, in a dose-dependent fashion, health benefits. Clearly, much more work is needed to refine this curve relative to specific diseases and conditions.

With this in mind, persons prescribing exercise for health-promotion and disease-prevention reasons can do so by adjusting duration and intensity such that caloric expenditure during leisure time is ~ 150 kcal per day (1,000 kcal per week). This means that a mild activity, such as walking 4.8 km · h^{-1} (3 miles · hr^{-1}), which expends ~ 4.3 kcal per min, needs to be performed for 35 min. Conversely, in place of walking we can substitute a 6 to 7 kcal per min activity, such as square dancing, that is performed for 20 to 25 min. Hopefully you get the picture: the higher the intensity of the activity, the shorter the duration, and vice versa. Specifically, the recommended 150 kcal of physical activity can be achieved through a variety of activities performed at different intensities and durations. This will allow activities to be changed from day to day if desired, helping satisfy the goals and interests of the participating individual. Table

table

14.6

Examples of activities (or exercise) that can be used to achieve a moderate dose of physical activity*

Activity	Intensity/duration
	Less vigorous/more time
Washing and waxing a car for 45–60 minutes	
Vacuuming (light) for 50 minutes	
Playing volleyball for 45 minutes	
Gardening for 30–45 minutes	
Wheeling self in wheelchair for 30–40 minutes	
Walking 1¾ miles in 35 minutes (3 mph)	
Basketball (shooting baskets) for 30 minutes	
Bicycling 5 miles in 30 minutes	
Pushing a stroller 1½ miles in 30 minutes	
Raking leaves for 30 minutes	
Walking 2 miles in 30 minutes (4mph)	
Water aerobics for 30 minutes	
Mowing lawn, walking with power mower for 28 minutes	
Golf, pulling clubs for 25 minutes	
Square dancing for 20–25 minutes	
Basketball (playing a game) for 15–20 minutes	
Bicycling 4 miles in 15 minutes	
Shoveling snow for 15 minutes	
Stairwalking for 15 minutes	
	More vigorous/less time

Modified from *Physical Activity and Health: A Report of the Surgeon General, At a Glance.*
*Equivalent to approximately 150 kcal of energy.

14.6 lists a variety of activities, performed at different durations and intensities, all of which provide the minimum daily dose of physical activity. Some of the activities listed can be classified as exercise, while others simply represent common daily activities that involve physical effort.

Intermittent (Accumulated) vs. Continuous Activity

Several of the expert statements addressing exercise or physical activity during the past 3 years included the advice of *accumulating* 30 minutes of moderate physical activity throughout the day.[90,96,118] This differs from the long-held view of having to perform one continuous 30 minute bout of activity. The new language suggests that, with respect to health improvement, the body is not very finicky about how the calories are expended over the course of a day, just as long as they are expended at a moderate intensity or higher.

With this new model of accumulated activity, the sedentary persons hopefully becomes "more willing" to be active, knowing that they can now combine shorter duration actions such as climbing flights of stairs, parking in the back of a parking lot, or going for 10 min walks during lunchtime. We must point out that the lower time limit defining what is an acceptable "short bout" of activity is not well-defined. Present suggestions include at least 5 or more minutes[56] and eight to ten minutes or more.[96]

After having read this, you may still be asking whether the stimulus provided through accumulated moderate activity is indeed sufficient to cause improvement in one's health? Well, the answer to that question appears to be yes, as discussed in papers by Haskell[57,58] and Pate et al.[96] Using a practical example, the health benefits appear to be similar whether a person cuts her lawn for 50 continuous min using a walk-behind power mower or cuts the same lawn in five 10-minute segments spaced out over the day. Without going into great detail, suffice to say that the concept of intermittent (accumulated) vs. continuous activity is difficult for many students, and for some exercise professionals, to appreciate. It may help to keep in mind that the intent is to improve health vs. optimizing maximal gains in cardiorespiratory fitness.

The concept of having more U.S. residents become involved in physical activity throughout the day, either accumulated or continuous, is exemplified in the Activity Pyramid shown in figure 14.12. Developed to compliment

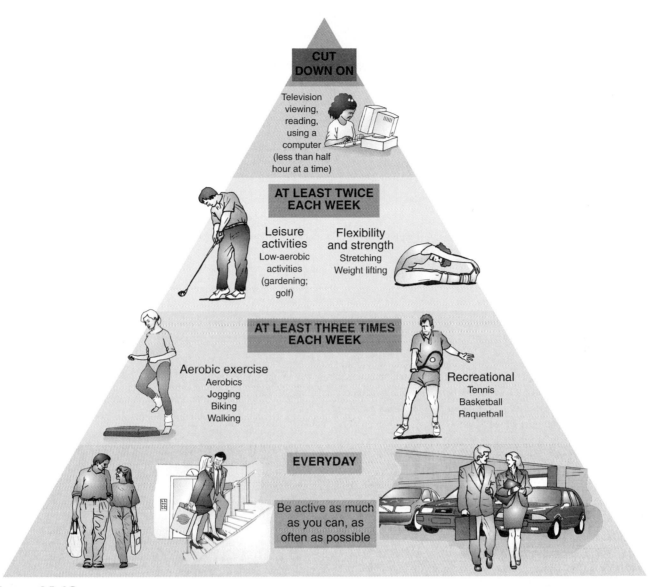

CUT DOWN ON

Television viewing, reading, using a computer (less than half hour at a time)

AT LEAST TWICE EACH WEEK

Leisure activities
Low-aerobic activities (gardening; golf)

Flexibility and strength
Stretching
Weight lifting

AT LEAST THREE TIMES EACH WEEK

Aerobic exercise
Aerobics
Jogging
Biking
Walking

Recreational
Tennis
Basketball
Raquetball

EVERYDAY

Be active as much as you can, as often as possible

Figure 14.12

Every adult American should accumulate 30 min or more of moderate physical activity most days of the week. This Physical Activity Pyramid depicts this guideline (base of pyramid), while suggesting limiting physical inactivity (top of pyramid).

the Food Guide Pyramid (figure 15.6, page 424), the Activity Pyramid can be applied to inactive, irregularly active, and active individuals alike. It encourages fun, supports a person's involvement in a variety of activities, and places an emphasis on doing some activity each day (base of pyramid) vs. a lifestyle of inactivity (top of pyramid).

Intensity of Exercise

No pain, no gain! Right? Wrong! Despite the widespread media attention over the past three years promoting the health benefits of moderate physical activity, many Americans still think "if it doesn't hurt, then it isn't helpful." Nothing could be farther from the truth.

We learned in chapters 11 and 12 that exercise intensity can be guided using heart-rate-based techniques such as the straight percent of peak heart rate method or the heart-rate reserve method. These methods can be used not only in elite athletes but in the general population interested in improved health and fitness as well. However, as pointed out earlier, the level of exercise intensity one prescribes does differ when coaching athletes vs. counseling nonathletic populations. Among elite endurance athletes, training intensity may approach 90% of measured peak heart rate, compared to a more moderate intensity of 50% to 70% of maximum among persons interested in health improvement.[10] Obviously, the latter group of individuals can train harder if in the future they desire a greater level of fitness.

14.7

Estimated peak heart rates and exercise training heart rates by age for normal persons*

	Age (years)				
	21–30	**31–40**	**41–50**	**51–60**	**61–70**
Estimated peak HR	195	185	175	165	155
Training HR at 70% $0.70(HR_{max} - 75) + 75$	159	152	145	138	131
Training HR at 60% $0.60(HR_{max} - 75) + 75$	147	141	135	129	123
Training HR at 50% $0.50(HR_{max} - 75) + 75$	135	130	125	120	115

*Computed using the heart rate reserve method, using a resting heart rate of 75 beats $\cdot$ min^{-1}; HR = heart rate.

Typical peak heart rates and exercise training heart rates at specific intensities across different age groups are given in table 14.7. (Recall from chapter 12 that peak or maximal heart rate can be estimated as 220 − age). You also need to know that the expected range or deviation around an estimated peak heart rate is ± 10 b $\cdot$ min^{-1}. This means if a 50-year-old person's HR max was estimated to be 170 b $\cdot$ min^{-1}, we are confident that his or her known true or measured peak heart rate would be between 160 and 180 b $\cdot$ min^{-1}. The imprecision associated with estimating peak heart rate does not greatly influence the exercise prescription but it is does support the direct measurement of peak heart rate when possible. Also, when using heart-rate-based methods to prescribe exercise intensity, it is common practice that it be prescribed using a target heart rate range (THRR) or zone. Figure 14.13 shows a range of 50% to 70% using the heart rate reserve method for subjects of various ages with a resting heart rate of 75 b $\cdot$ min^{-1}.

Before concluding our discussion of exercise intensity we must recognize the difficulty that some exercise specialists, trainers, and clinicians experience when prescribing exercise using heart-rate-based methods. In some people time does not permit the teaching of pulse taking, while in others certain disease states or medications render pulse taking less accurate. In these instances we can use a scale named after the man who popularized it, the Borg Rating of Perceived Exertion (RPE) scale.[24] This scale (table 14.8) has been tested in a variety of healthy and patient populations and represents a valid means to prescribe exercise intensity because of its co-existing relationship to heart rate and $\dot{V}O_2$ during exercise testing or training. It involves simply asking the patient or client to rate overall (not just legs or breathing) body exertion or fatigue, using a scale of 6 to 20. A value of six is equated with minimal exertion, such as

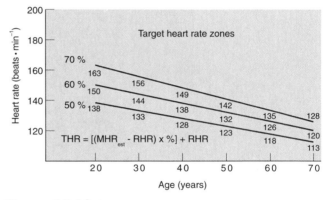

Figure 14.13
Target heart rate (THR) zone for different age subjects using heart-rate reserve method set at 50%, 60%, and 70%. Maximum heart rate (MHR_{est}) = 220–age and a resting heart rate (RHR) = 75 beats per minute.

resting in a chair, and a value of 20 is described as all-out maximal exhaustion. During exercise testing RPE can also be used to assess whether or not a maximal or near-maximal effort was achieved.

Relative to exercise intensity during training, an RPE of 11 to 12 is equivalent to moderate work and a heart rate approximating 50% to 69% of peak (or a $\dot{V}O_2$ approximating 45% to 59% of maximum; see table 14.9). In absolute terms, this corresponds to activities roughly between 3 to 5 METs,* although slightly lower MET activities may be appropriate for persons greater than 65 years and higher MET

---

*Metabolic equivalents expressed as multiples of resting energy expenditure; see chapter 4.

14.8

The Borg Rating of Perceived Exertion scale[24]

6	
7	very, very light
8	
9	very light
10	
11	fairly light
12	
13	somewhat hard
14	
15	hard
16	
17	very hard
18	
19	very, very hard
20	

activities for persons less than 35 years. Training at a higher RPE (13 to 15) is associated with training at a greater percentage of one's maximum heart rate or $\dot{V}O_2$ (table 14.9). Doing so will provide additional gains in fitness and some additional gains in health as well.

Another subjective method sometimes used to help "roughly" guide exercise intensity is called the Talk Test. Simply, clients or patients are asked to exercise at a pace or intensity that still allows them to comfortably carry on a conversation with another person. Preliminary work with the Talk-Test method in our laboratory involving healthy sedentary adults (6 females, 12 males) and outdoor and indoor track walking showed that up to 50% of subjects trained at an intensity that exceeded 85% of max $\dot{V}O_2$.[26] A subsequent study using stationary exercise equipment (treadmill, dual-action cycle) and 15 sedentary adults (9 females, 6 males) found the Talk-Test method resulted in a training intensity approximating 72% of max $\dot{V}O_2$ during dual-action cycling and 65% of max $\dot{V}O_2$ during treadmill walking.[36] Although the second study appeared more promising, looked at together both studies suggest that the Talk-Test method may produce an exercise intensity that is initially too strenuous for sedentary persons just starting a moderate activity program for health reasons.

Spellman and co-workers conducted a unique study where they first observed 29 habitual walkers using an unseen observer; and then treadmill tested the subjects to determine the $\dot{V}O_2$ achieved while walking at their usual training pace.[109] They found that the walkers self-selected an average exercise pace of 52% of $\dot{V}O_2$ max (range = 36 to 79%), which was equal to an average energy expenditure of 1127 kcal · week^{-1}—a dose of activity associated with improvement in health and longevity.

Determinants and Barriers to Physical Activity

A myriad of physiological, behavioral, and psychosocial variables are related to physical activity. Common reasons for not exercising include lack of time, personal safety, sedentary family or social environment, confounding medical problems, perceptions of body weight/image, self efficacy, and others.[56,83,96]

Depending on the population being studied and duration of follow up, current estimates are that as low as 20% to more than 60% of those people who start an exercise program eventually stop![118] Reasons associated with dropping out include cigarette smoking, level of enjoyment, injury, the time of day when exercise is planned, age, gender, job type (blue collar less likely to comply than white collar), and level of education.[93,96,118] For persons who experience a heart problem and then enter a cardiac rehabilitation program, lack of routine exercise habits prior to the illness is associated with noncompliance to their home exercise program after finishing the program.[37]

Given the somewhat bleak outlook we've described, what strategies are available to us to assist with developing a more active nation? Let's begin by saying that many theories have been proposed detailing how people best learn or adopt new behaviors. One good model that has been applied to physical activity is the transtheoretical model,[100] which conceptualizes 5 stages of behavioral change that operate along a continuum. These stages are precontemplation, contemplation, preparation, action, and maintenance. People can, over time, move back and forth from one stage to another. Adapting three of these stages to physical activity, *precontemplators* realize that a change is needed, but are not willing to consider doing so (e.g., "I have no desire to start an exercise program"). *Contemplators* know they need to be active but may not have the skills, knowledge, or incentive to do so (i.e., "I want to, but I just don't have the time to exercise"). *Actives* are doing something, and it may be sufficient to promote health benefits or it may require a bit of further counseling (e.g., "I walk two or three times a week"). Two behavioral strategies that may prove useful with respect to improving long-term compliance are:

1. Self-monitoring, which means use of record keeping techniques such as exercise diaries/logs or personal calendars to document frequency and duration of activity. Heart rate, perceived exertion, and symptoms can also be monitored.

2. Social support, which involves both *perceived* and *actual* support from the family/social network the person operates within. *Perceived* support means that the person trying to become more active receives verbal and nonverbal cues from those around him that they support his intentions. Perceived support often helps the person who is contemplating or just starting an exercise program. *Actual* support means that the

table 14.9

Classification of exercise intensity for endurance-type activities

| Intensity | Relative intensity | | |
	%$\dot{V}O_2$ max	% Peak heart rate	RPE*
Very light	< 25	< 30	< 9
Light	25–44	30–49	9–10
Moderate	45–59	50–69	11–12
Hard	60–84	70–89	13–16
Very hard	≥ 85	≥ 90	> 16
Maximal†	100	100	20

Modified from *Physical Activity and Health: A Report of the Surgeon General.*[118]
*Borg Rating of Perceived Exertion scale, 6–20.
†Maximal values are mean values achieved during maximal exercise by healthy adults.

actions and behaviors of other persons support an individual's desire to be active. For example, he has a partner or friend who actually goes for walks with him. Group exercise classes can provide this type of support.

The message you need to take with you here is that it's easy to prescribe exercise and follow an individual's progress over time if she is interested and motivated to exercise, but what is your success rate among inactive persons who come across with the attitude, "I dare you to help me"? Here lies your biggest challenge! And remember, these are the people—the ones who are likely inactive or irregularly active to begin with—who will benefit the most from becoming more active. So when prescribing exercise, it may prove worthwhile to think less about teaching intensity, duration, and frequency and begin with identifying both a person's readiness to change and some solutions to the barriers they'll encounter along the way. Doing so will likely enhance long-term compliance.

Risks of Exercise and Physical Activity

The idea of dying during exercise evokes the image of someone suddenly collapsing while engaged in vigorous activity. Such an event often receives much media attention and raises questions about whether the benefits associated with being habitually active outweigh the short-term risks of sudden death during a bout of physical activity.[63]

Let's begin by first examining the underlying reasons why people suddenly die during exercise. Using autopsy data, sudden death during exercise generally falls into one of two categories: those resulting from ischemic heart disease (i.e., atherosclerosis) and those resulting from other causes.[63] Among persons older than 35 years of age, coronary atherosclerosis is the underlying cause of death ~ 75% to 80% of the time.[63] In many of these cases, ischemia from atherosclerosis triggers a lethal irregular heart rhythm or arrhythmia.

The second cause of sudden death during exercise is much more common (> 85%) in persons less than 35 years of age and is related to abnormalities that were either present at birth or were acquired somewhat independent of a person's lifestyle habits. Examples include abnormal ventricular chamber size or wall thickness, aortic rupture, and anomalies of the coronary arteries. One study analyzed 134 of the sudden cardiac deaths that occurred in *young competitive athletes* between 1985 and 1995 and found that among the deceased, the median age was 17 years (range = 12 to 40 years), 120 (90%) were male, 70 (52%) were white, 121 (90%) occurred during or immediately following training or competition, 115 (86%) had a standard preparticipation medical evaluation, 47 (35%) involved basketball, and 45 (34%) involved football.[82]

In the general population, the risk of sudden death during exercise is ~ 1 per every 100,000 person-hours of exercise.[9,63] This rate is greater than the rate of sudden death during periods of rest or nonexertion, indicating that physical activity is associated with a transient increase in risk of sudden death.[84,107] It is important to note, however, that the average risk of sudden death during exercise, although small to begin with (~ 1 per 100,000 person-hours of exercise), is higher in persons who are ordinarily sedentary and lower in persons who are habitually active.[84,107] Therefore, the small, transient increased risk of sudden death during or immediately following exercise, which is lower in regularly active persons than in inactive persons, is far outweighed by the favorable benefits and lower overall risk derived from being habitually active.

Exercise Training and Other Health-Related Issues

So far in this chapter we have mostly discussed the role of exercise and physical activity in the primary prevention of all-cause mortality and disease-specific mortality (i.e., cardiovascular disease and cancer). Additionally, in several other places throughout this text we discuss the role of exercise training in treating a variety of health disorders. In chapter 9 we addressed the role of exercise training as a means to facilitate recovery among patients who suffered a heart attack (page 236) or those with hypertension (page 241). Similarly, in chapter 12 (page 311) we discussed the use of exercise as a means to reverse the overactive sympathetic nervous system and the exercise intolerance that are so characteristic of patients with heart failure. Chapter 7 reviewed the efficacy of pulmonary rehabilitation in patients with obstructive lung disease (page 177), and chapter 16 discusses the important role that exercise plays in a proper weight management program—one meant for either health maintenance or athletic performance. In each disorder, exercise training was shown to improve functional capacity, enhance physiological response, modify risk, increase health related quality of life, and/or improve survival. In the section that follows, we explore how exercise therapy impacts five other health-related issues.

Diabetes Mellitus

Diabetes is a disorder associated with the inability of cell membranes to efficiently take up glucose into the cell. As a result, blood glucose levels become elevated (hyperglycemia) if left untreated. There are two types of diabetes: one caused by the absence of insulin production by the pancreas, which is often referred to as *Type I* (also called juvenile-onset or insulin-dependent diabetes mellitus); the other, caused by resistance of peripheral tissues (e.g., skeletal muscles) to insulin-stimulated glucose uptake, is known as

Type II (maturity-onset or noninsulin-dependent diabetes mellitus). People with Type I diabetes usually develop the disorder before age 30 and must inject insulin on a daily basis as part of their treatment. Patients with Type II diabetes generally acquire the condition later in life. Risk factors for developing Type II are excess body weight, the presence of a family history of diabetes, and a history of mild to moderate hypertension.[18] Although a multitude of physiologic changes occur as a result of either form of the disease, treatment historically has focused on diet and drug therapy. However, moderate exercise training continues to make inroads into the clinical care of these patients as a means to improve functional capacity and lower associated risks.

Type I

The management of blood glucose in Type I patients generally represents a bigger challenge for the clinician than do Type II patients. Although some Type I patients achieve improved control of blood glucose and lessened daily insulin requirements as a result of exercise training, this is not always the case. Despite the varied response among patients with Type I diabetes to exercise, the American Diabetes Association encourages them to engage in moderate activity because of its potential to improve cardiovascular fitness and psychological well-being.[7] Those with Type I diabetes must keep in mind, however, that physical exercise is not without risks. Hypo- and hyperglycemia, ketosis, silent myocardial ischemia, worsening of retinal problems, and lower-extremity injury all represent potential complications.[120] Given the varied response to training among patients with Type I diabetes, it is difficult to provide uniform recommendations that apply to all patients. Clearly, a thorough medical evaluation to assess pre-exercise risk, achieving adequate control prior to initiating a program, and engaging in aerobic-type activities are all important. Table 14.10 provides some broad, general guidelines to be considered for Type I (and Type II) patients.

Type II

Approximately 13 million Americans have Type II diabetes, half of whom are not yet diagnosed. In these people an exercise program represents an appropriate adjunct to nutrition and/or drug therapy—one meant to improve glycemic control, reduce certain cardiovascular risk factors, and enhance psychological well-being.[7] Regular exercise improves cell membrane insulin sensitivity and glucose transport across the cell membrane, and it lowers plasma insulin levels. For those persons at risk of developing the disease, such as people with hypertension or those who are obese, regular exercise has a protective effect.[18]

Following a pre-exercise medical evaluation designed to uncover previously undiagnosed hypertension, neuropathy, retinopathy, or ischemic heart disease, an exercise prescription for these patients should include the following:[7,106]

14.10

General exercise guidelines in patients with diabetes

1.   Use proper footwear to avoid friction-related skin injuries (i.e., blisters). Inspect feet daily and after exercise.

2.   Avoid/limit exercise during periods of poor metabolic control.

3.   Frequency of exercise can range from 4 to 7 days per week. Once exercise habits have been established, maintaining a regular regimen (week to week and month to month) is important.

4.   Longer duration, less intense exercise is preferred. Patients with Type II diabetes should maximize caloric expenditure if overweight.

5.   Self-monitor blood glucose, especially when beginning an exercise program.

6.   Adequate serum glucose concentrations are considered to be $< 160 \text{ mg} \cdot dL^{-1}$. Patients with values between 200 to 400 $\text{mg} \cdot dL^{-1}$ likely require clinical supervision during exercise. Exercise should be withheld in patients with values $> 400 \text{ mg} \cdot dL^{-1}$, and these patients should seek follow-up medical care.

7.   Rotate and inject insulin into muscles that will not be experiencing a dramatic increase in metabolic activity during exercise (e.g., abdominal group during walking).

8.   Increase pre-exercise carbohydrate intake and/or decrease insulin dose as needed over time as guided by post-exercise blood glucose values.

9   Drink plenty of fluids and use caution when exercising in hot/humid weather.

Adapted from ACSM[3] and American Diabetes Association.[7]

1.   Intensity = 50% to 70% of max $\dot{V}O_2$ or 60% to 85% of maximum heart rate
2.   Time = 20 to 60 minutes
3.   Frequency = 4 to 7 days per week
4.   Type = walking and other types of low-intensity, high-compliance exercise are preferred to enhance reduction of body fat and minimize injury; high-intensity activities that excessively raise blood pressure (e.g., resistance training while holding breath) should be avoided

Blood Clotting and Fibrinolytic Activity

As mentioned in our discussion of atherosclerosis, the formation of a blood clot is called a *thrombus*. If the thrombi forms inside an artery supplying the heart or brain and occludes blood flow, it results in a heart attack or stroke, respectively. If part of a thrombi formed in a vessel breaks off and "floats" downstream and occludes the same or another vessel, it is called an *embolus*.

The clotting of blood involves a complicated cascade of chemical reactions involving platelets, coagulation factors, fibrinolysis, and the vessel wall. The initiation of a thrombus is triggered by damaged or traumatized tissue, a good example of which is an atherosclerotic artery. The atherosclerotic plaque is rough and can fracture, providing ample opportunities to initiate the clotting mechanism. If either

the time required for clotting and/or the time required to dissolve a clot (referred to as *fibrinolysis*) is altered, the rate and number of blood clots formed is also altered. Obviously, an agent or therapy that both slows the rate of clot formation and enhances fibrinolytic activity would be ideal with respect to reducing the risk of heart attack or stroke.

The effects of exercise training on coagulation and fibrinolysis are not well understood. In a cross-sectional study comparing lean marathon runners to more sedentary individuals, Ferguson et al.[47] found no difference between groups relative to platelet aggregation (which leads to clot formation) at rest or during maximal exercise. Conversely, other studies have reported a favorable effect from exercise training on coagulation.[25] A similar cloudy picture also exists for fibrinolysis, in that some studies substantiate the beneficial effects of exercise training, while others do not.[25,32,40,113] Overall, the balance of research suggests that exercise training probably slows coagulation rate and increases fibrinolytic activity.[58] However, additional studies on this topic using modern, specific assays and standardized techniques of measurement is warranted.

Blood Cholesterol (Lipid) Levels

Although reducing total fat and substituting unsaturated fat for saturated fat are effective strategies to improve lipid profiles in many people, exercise training may also be helpful.

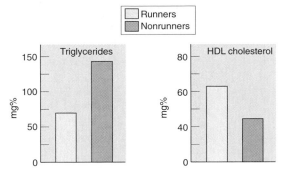

Figure 14.14

Chronic exercise training causes a decrease in triglyceride concentration and an increase in high-density lipoprotein (HDL-cholesterol) concentration in both men and women. In this study, the subjects were active men, ages 35 to 49 years, who averaged 39 miles of running per week.

(Based on data from Wood et al.[128])

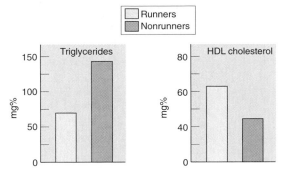

However, despite popular belief to the contrary, chronic exercise does not beneficially affect all of the various blood lipids. For starters, unless the exercise regimen has been associated with loss of body fat or improved dietary habits, exercise by itself does not lower total blood cholesterol or LDL (bad) cholesterol.[42] This is an important point to remember.

On the other hand, HDL cholesterol, the subfraction that has a protective inverse relationship to heart disease, can be beneficially influenced by habitual aerobic exercise. Figure 14.14 presents the results from a study where active men between the ages of 35 and 49, who were running an average of 39 miles · week^{-1}, were compared to nonexercisers of the same age who served as the control group. Although limited by the cross-sectional design of this study, the runners had an HDL cholesterol above 60 mg · dL^{-1}, almost 50% higher than the sedentary control group.[128] Notice that blood triglycerides were also lower in the trained group versus the untrained group. Unlike cholesterol, triglycerides represent a potential fuel source for the skeletal muscles, and elevated values can often be reduced if exercise bouts are repeated on a regular basis.[42] The extent of any reduction appears dependent on pretraining concentration and the volume of exercise completed over the course of the training regimen.

Returning to HDL cholesterol, there are inconsistencies in the literature relative to exercise training and results observed from various studies. Such inconsistencies, however, can be explained by a number of extraneous variables such as length of training regimen, pretraining HDL level, smoking status, dietary habits, changes in body weight, and variability associated with HDL measures. To evaluate the affect of aerobic exercise on HDL cholesterol concentration, changes in this variable are frequently compared to weekly caloric expenditure. Generally, an individual needs to increase his or her energy expenditure by 1000 or more kcal · week^{-1} (equivalent to walking or jogging ∼ 16 km · week^{-1}), before HDL is positively affected. However, it may require several months of training at this level before increases in HDL cholesterol are observed. In addition to total energy expenditure, cross-sectional data suggests that the number of additional kilometers run per week is associated with a quantifiable increase in HDL cholesterol[124,125]— specifically, an increase of 0.136 and 0.133 mg · dL^{-1} for every additional kilometer run per week in males and females, respectively.

A number of physiological mechanisms may be responsible for the training-induced improvement in HDL cholesterol. These include both an increase in muscle capillary density and an increase in skeletal muscle lipoprotein lipase activity (LPLA). The latter, LPLA, is located in capillary endothelium and is responsible for the catabolism of triglyceride-rich lipoproteins and for the conversion of the smaller HDL$_3$ cholesterol to the larger HDL$_2$ cholesterol. Higher levels of LPLA following exercise training may be responsible for increasing the formation of HDL cholesterol. In addition, hepatic triglyceride lipase activity (HTGLA) is lower in trained athletes. HTGLA is responsible for the conversion of HDL$_2$ cholesterol to HDL$_3$ cholesterol and for the catabolism of HDL cholesterol. These changes within the liver may prolong the survival of HDL cholesterol and, therefore, increase HDL cholesterol concentration within the body.

Immunology

The body's **immune system** is basically a system of surveillance, and "errors" in the system appear to have two dominating complications: infection and cancer.[29] As you can imagine, some of these complications can be life-threatening. To assist you with understanding how exercise or physical activity might interact with the immune system, we must first provide an overview of the system itself. To do this we summarize two excellent reviews by Calabrese[29] and Smith.[108]

The immune system can be viewed as a compartmentalized system, some of which involves cells that have developed from the thymus gland (T lymphocytes) or the bone marrow (B lymphocytes). T lymphocytes are primarily responsible to provide protection from a variety of pathogens (e.g., viruses and bacteria) and parasites. They can also secrete *cytokines,* which possess strong anticancer effects. B lymphocytes produce antibody and can be identified by the presence of immunoglobulin molecules on their surfaces and by B-cell-specific antigens. Antibody provides defense against a variety of infectious agents. Combined, T and B lymphocytes represent *adaptive* or *specific* responses within the immune system designed to recognize nonself (from self) molecules on an infectious agent or an infected host cell.

In addition, there are other cells and cell products that operate as part of a *nonspecific* or *innate* arm of the immune system. The first is known as a natural killer (NK) cell,

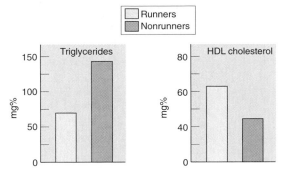

capable of spontaneously killing a wide range of unwanted targets such as tumors and viral agents. The second is the phagocytes (e.g., neutrophils, macrophages), which serve to not only trigger the immune response but also perform phagocytosis (scavenger) and phagocytic killer functions. Third, to support all of the above is a series of more than 20 proteins capable of producing inflammation and cellular lysis. Acting in concert, these immune system components serve as potent regulators of the human immune response.

The response of the immune system to a singe, acute bout of exercise is profound, and these changes are nicely reviewed by Nieman.[87] However, over the past 10 to 15 years an ever-increasing amount of research has focused on the relationship between *chronic* exercise training and the beneficial or harmful changes that may occur in the human immune system. Current thinking is that there is a dual response of the immune system to training.[76] Specifically, the immune system is stimulated (or unchanged) by regular, moderate exercise, whereas the same system may be impaired when repetitive, intense exercise is involved. This concept is depicted in figure 14.15 and highlights why elite athletes may be at risk for increased susceptibility to illness.[76,87,112]

For the coach or athletic trainer interested in keeping their athletes healthy, developing a balance between rest/recovery and training, optimizing diet, managing outside stresses and the stress of competition, and gathering additional knowledge about what aspects of training (e.g., intensity of exercise) influence susceptibility to infection are all important.[76,87] In the public health arena (the downward phase of the J-shaped curve in figure 14.15), a population at lower risk for developing cancer and infections from moderate exercise represents less illness, less time lost at school and work, and less utilization of health care resources. Finally, for patients with diseases that are known to affect the immune system (e.g., human immunodeficiency virus, or HIV), exercise therapy may not only enhance quality of life and the ability to perform daily activities but may possibly enhance components of the immune system as well.

The mechanism(s) by which exercise assists with lessening susceptibility to infection is not completely understood. Possible explanations include (1) creating an environment that is hostile to invading pathogens, such as the increase in core temperature that accompanies exercise; (2) developing a more favorable balance between the immune system, the body's response to stress, and the release of neurohormones/endocrines (e.g., cortisol, epinephrine); (3) exercise-induced reductions of body fat; and (4) favorable alterations in the components of the immune system itself. Studies by Nieman et al.,[89] and Christ et al.,[112] both showed increases in natural killer cells with a moderate aerobic program of 3 to 5 times per week for 15 to 16 weeks. The first of these two studies showed a more than 50% increase in natural killer cell cytotoxic activity. A cross-sectional study conducted by Nieman et al.[88] showed that

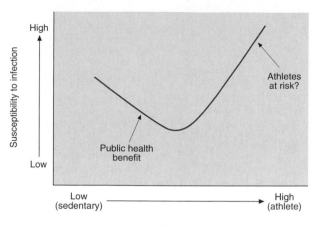

Figure 14.15

Exercise training influences susceptibility to infection in a dual-response fashion. Moderate, regular exercise decreases likelihood for infection, whereas repetitive, intense exercise may place athletes at increased risk for infection.

marathon runners who completed at least seven prior marathons and had been training for marathons for at least the past four years also had significantly greater natural killer cell cytotoxic activity when compared to age-matched sedentary controls. However, no differences were noted between groups for lymphocytes or phagocytes. Finally, LaPerriere et al.[68] showed that when homosexual males were informed during the fifth week of a 10-week training study that they tested positive for HIV serostatus, no decline in natural killer cell status was observed, which was much different from what occurred among homosexual males randomized to a no exercise control group when they were also told they tested HIV positive. In that study, exercise training not only improved the cardiorespiratory fitness of the subjects but it also lessened the immunologic response to a strong stressor. Additionally, HIV patients in the exercise group showed significant improvement in "helper" cell (CD-4) counts after training, a component of the immune system that is compromised in these patients over time. Clearly, much more work needs to be completed in the field of exercise immunology, a subspecialty area within the discipline of exercise physiology that has public health, human performance, and clinical ramifications.

Mental Health

Mental disorders represent an important public health problem in the U.S. For example, ~ 4% of adults are characterized as having a major depressive disorder, a condition associated with the ninth leading cause of death among Americans: suicide (table 14.3). In studies of physical activity on mental health, the most frequently assessed outcomes include anxiety, depression, and Health-Related Quality of Life (e.g., self-esteem, self-efficacy).

As reviewed in the 1996 Surgeon General's Report on Physical Activity and Health, the literature supports a beneficial effect of physical activity on relieving symptoms of depression and anxiety, improving mood state, and enhancing Health-Related Quality of Life.[118] Mondin et al. conducted an interesting detraining experiment involving 10 (4 female, 6 male) volunteers who regularly exercised 6 to 7 $d \cdot week^{-1}$. Exercise was withheld for just three days and follow-up testing on day four already revealed increases in mood disturbance, anxiety, tension, and depression.[85] These changes were reversed when exercise was resumed.

Two possible biologic mechanisms contributing to the exercise-induced changes in mental health include (1) a decrease in muscle tension or (2) the influence of endogenous opiates. The latter includes a group of chemicals called the "β-endorphins", agents produced by the central nervous system during times of stress and/or physical activity.[59] These chemicals have a wide range of physiologic activity including pain inhibition, cardiovascular (blood pressure) effects, appetite modulation, and behavioral and mood effects.

Under resting conditions blood β-endorphin levels are low, but during exercise at intensities exceeding 60% of $\dot{V}O_2$ max, elevated levels of this endogenous opiate are observed—peaking approximately 15 minutes after exercise is stopped.[59] This exercise/post-exercise increase in β-endorphins is felt, by some, to be linked to the "endorphin calm" or "runner's high" described in habitually active persons.[61] These findings are not conclusive, however, because the euphoric mood state associated with exercise still persists somewhat after the effect of β-endorphins are blocked by an agent called Naloxone.

The effects of exercise on other mental-health issues such as sleep and eating disorders, schizophrenia, substance abuse disorders, and personality disorders is not well studied. A comprehensive review of the effects of exercise on sleep physiology and habits by O'Connor and Youngstedt[91] suggests that (1) regular exercise more than two times per week is associated with less daytime sleepiness and (2) that sleep duration and rapid eye movement periods may be influenced by the timing of the exercise (morning vs. evening). The authors raise a voice of caution because it really is too early to make definitive statements about the effects of exercise on sleep. They call for additional rigorous research—especially in light of the attractiveness of using a low-cost, low-risk therapy such as exercise to treat health problems caused by inadequate sleep.

Exercise at Both Ends of the Human Life Span

As our population continues to grow older, more and more research is being focused on exercise throughout the human life span. Although such a topic is deserving of a text by itself, we will focus our attention on the two extremes.

Specifically, children/adolescents between 5 and 19 years of age and older adults greater than 60 years. By no means do we infer that the population between 20 and 60 years of age is not important. On the contrary, much of the research and discussion found within this text was based on such people. Instead, this section deals with the less-often-discussed interactions between exercise and the growing youth and exercise and the aging adult.

Children and Adolescents

Anyone who has watched the Olympic games would likely have noticed the participation of some very young athletes in events such as gymnastics and swimming. Without question, however, these elite athletes are not representative of today's youth. In fact, the physical fitness of today's children/adolescents as a whole is a concern.[4] The primary responsibility to address this issue likely rests with both the schools and parents. At present, ~ 40% of all school-age children participate in daily physical education[117,118]— a value that is 10% below our stated objective for the year 2000 (see table 14.2, objective 1.8). At the same time, continued curricular emphasis must be placed not only on team sports but on individually performed, health-promoting leisure activities as well.

Having said all this, the important role that parents play cannot to be overlooked. Presenting themselves as a physically active role model to their children plays an integral role in fostering their child's interest in physical activity now and in the future. Not including time spent playing video and computer games, children spend almost three hours watching television each day!

In normal children and adolescents, peak $\dot{V}O_2$ increases with growth and maturation,[12] leveling off around 14 years of age in females and sometime after 16 years of age in males. Previously sedentary children and adolescents who become involved with cardiorespiratory activities improve their max $\dot{V}O_2$ in a manner that is physiologically similar to adults (see chapter 12). There appear to be no long-term detrimental cardiorespiratory side effects with competitive endurance training in young athletes. However, like adults, proper training techniques, adequate rest/recovery periods, and proper nutritional habits should be followed to achieve sound performances and to avoid overtraining.

Relative to sport participation and training, there appear to be no consistent adverse effects on attained stature (height) or rate of growth in stature.[78] However, cautions have been raised relative to epiphyseal plate (growth plate) maturation. The growth plate represents the location along long bones (e.g., tibia) where bone growth occurs. In normal maturation, once growth has stopped, the epiphyseal plate is replaced by cartilage during adulthood. Present concerns are that various extremes of physical activity may lead to injury or premature growth plate closure among adolescents.[105] Concerning injury, there are two types of epiphyseal injury that you need to be aware of. The first is an epiphysitis that develops from overuse, such as baseball thrower's elbow (i.e., medial epicondyle of the humerus) or jumper's knee (i.e., tibial tubercle). A second injury to the epiphysis, less common than the first, is a contact-induced fracture across the growth plate that leads to disruption of normal growth. As mentioned, premature growth plate closure is also a concern, possibly caused by constant forces and trauma resulting from heavy endurance training or heavy resistance training. The actual scientific evidence confirming the existence of this problem is rare, but given the importance of the problem should it occur, a somewhat conservative course of action by coaches, parents, team physician, and trainers appears warranted. This includes ensuring that young competing athletes pay special attention to proper training habits and safety.[2]

Older Adults

Before proceeding, there is an often-spoken myth surrounding the aging process that should be discussed. It's the idea that it is normal for a person to get out of shape; lose muscular strength/flexibility; and experience increases in blood pressure, body weight, and cholesterol with advancing age. Although these changes may be typical of what happens to the aging adult in our society, they are by no means normal or an absolute consequence of the aging process. The typical aging process can, in fact, be slowed— if not reversed—through regular exercise.

Without question, there is a clear decrease in cardiorespiratory fitness with age. A good rule of thumb is an approximate 10% to 15% decrease in aerobic power for every decade of life.[115] However, a greater loss in aerobic capacity is more often observed in sedentary persons than in active individuals. Loss of aerobic capacity in highly trained persons may be as low as 5% to 7% per decade.[115] Reasons responsible for the loss of aerobic capacity with age include a decrease in cardiac output caused by an age-associated decrease in peak heart rate,[92,114] a possible decrease in stroke volume,[92] and a decrease in peak arterio-mixed venous oxygen difference.[92] The age-related decrease in peak heart rate occurs at a rate of approximately one beat per year, after age 25.[4]

And not only is the decline in aerobic capacity blunted by regular exercise training, but gas kinetics during early exercise are altered as well. Babcock et al. studied eight older men (72 years old) and found that 6 months of vigorous cycle training resulted in a 21% increase in $\dot{V}O_2$ max (21.7 mL $\cdot$ kg^{-1} $\cdot$ min^{-1} to 26.2 mL $\cdot$ kg^{-1} $\cdot$ min^{-1}) and significantly faster kinetics of gas exchange and ventilation.[15]

In addition to age-related declines in cardiorespiratory fitness, skeletal muscle in males and females is also affected by aging. Specifically, there is loss of muscle size

(atrophy), strength, capillarization, and Type II fibers.[11,69] Exercise training, however, has been shown to reverse these changes.[23,30] Resistance training has been shown to increase muscle protein synthesis among 63 to 66 year old persons.[129] Finally, typical age-related changes in autonomic function,[104] pulmonary function,[53] and glucose transport and glycogen transport[31] all appear to be favorably reversed/slowed by exercise training. Therefore, despite the popularized myth that the aging process is associated with loss of physiologic function with age, many of these changes can be reversed and/or blunted through proper aerobic and resistance training programs.

Female-Specific Issues and Physical Activity

Two "normal" conditions that alter physiology in the absence of disease are exercise and pregnancy. In this section we review the interaction between exercise and pregnancy. Our discussion is separated into two parts: (1) menstruation; and (2) pregnancy, injuries to the breasts and reproductive organs, and the developing fetus.

Menstruation

Relative to physical activity and the menstrual cycle, the primary focus here is on the development of either an irregular pattern (oligomenorrhea) or cessation extending beyond 90 days (amenorrhea). *Primary amenorrhea* is defined as the delay of menarche beyond 16 years of age, whereas *secondary amenorrhea* is the absence of menstruation in women who have been previously menstrual.[73]

Age of Menarche

The age at which menstruation begins (*menarche*) is generally higher in the female athlete than in her nonathletic counterpart. For example, as shown in figure 14.16 both high-school and college athletes attained menarche later than nonathletes, and the various groups of national and Olympic athletes attained menarche significantly later than the high-school and college athletes. These results clearly indicate a relationship between delayed (or later developing) menarche and advancing levels of competition.[81]

Given the fact that menarche is later in most highly skilled female athletes, two questions arise: (1) what causes the late menarche and (2) what is its significance? Regarding the cause, studies have shown[27] that exercise causes an increase in *prolactin,* one of the hormones secreted by the pituitary gland and responsible for readying the breasts for nursing (lactation). In the adolescent athlete, this could create what is referred to as a "prolactin impregnation" on the maturing ovary, an effect sufficient to delay further maturation of the ovary by another hormone called *follicle-stimulating hormone.* This in turn could result in delayed menarche

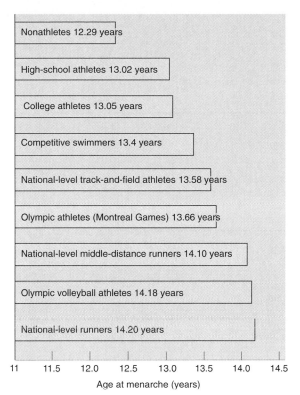

Figure 14.16

The age at which menstruation begins (menarche) is significantly higher in the female athlete than in her nonathletic counterpart.

(Based on data from Feicht et al.,[46] Malina er al.,[79] Stager et al.,[111] and Wakat and Sweeney.[121])

or in a transient amenorrheic (absence of the menses) condition somewhat similar to the one observed in the nursing mother. Other factors must also be considered, such as a genetic component, nutritional status, and family size.[80]

The later attainment of menarche has two main significances—one dealing with health (estrogen-dependent cancers) and the other with sports.[79,81] Relative to the first issue, we mentioned earlier in this chapter that a delay in menarche may favorably lower future risk for breast cancer by decreasing the total number of ovulatory cycles—which means less estrogen exposure to tissues over the life span.[65]

In some respects, the later menarche and maturation are more suitable for successful athletic performance. For example, the later-maturing female has longer legs, narrower hips, less weight per unit of height, and less relative body fat than does her earlier-maturing counterpart. Conversely, in swimming, earlier rather than later maturation may be more beneficial because greater strength and body fat, which follow menarche, would tend to enhance performance.

The mean age of menarche in the United States has been reported at ~13 years, with a standard deviation of ~1.2 years. This means that, statistically, 95% of all girls reach menarche by 15.3 years and 99% achieve menarche by 16 years. None of the athletic groups depicted in Figure 14.16 had a mean value outside this normal distribution. The onset of menarche is not considered late unless a young female remains premenarchal past 16 years of age.[65,130]

Exercise and Menstrual Disorders

Research over the past 20 years has shown that chronic exercise can influence menstrual function, however, the frequency of the problem may not be what we first thought. Female athletes who appear to be the most susceptible are those involved in high-intensity training and competition, such as in long-distance running, gymnastics, swimming, and professional ballet dancing.[38,39,46,55] For example, 34% of female distance runners training more than 48 km · week^{-1} developed *amenorrhea* (a cessation of menstruation) during their training and competitive seasons,[38,39] which is much higher than the 2% to 4% prevalence estimates among nonexercising females. However, because of potential bias introduced when using voluntary questionnaires assessing self-reported menstrual status, the frequency of exercise-associated amenorrhea is felt to be less than what was once thought.[35]

The exact cause of amenorrhea in exercising females is not known. It may be related to intensity of training, training volume, and/or nutritional deficiencies. This could mean that the amenorrhea is caused by the training itself (weekly mileage),[46] by the stress of competition, or by some other factors related to chronic exercise training—such as the stress of being a student-athlete.[55] The lower body fat stores of many female athletes, particularly of long-distance runners and gymnasts, could also contribute.[48,49,110,121] However, there is probably no single amount of body fat loss—and no particlar amount of training, for that matter—that will induce amenorrhea in every female. Instead, each female probably has a different threshold for amenorrhea, which may be related to any of the previously mentioned factors.[39]

The question of bone loss in amenorrheic athletes represents a foremost concern; this is especially true if one understands that most clinicians do not have ready access to the instrumentation needed to detect loss of bone.[35] This problem can be made worse if the athlete also demonstrates poor eating habits or an eating disorder that results in an inadequate calcium intake. Presently, managing bone loss in these athletes through the possible use of estrogen therapy is controversial.

Additionally, the issue of what happens to amenorrhea once exercise training is stopped also deserves attention. As might be expected, the complete answer to this question is not yet available. However, one study involving young female swimmers[45] showed that once competition and training are stopped, the menses resume a normal pattern, and the childbearing functions of the female are normal in every respect. Presumably, this would apply to other sport athletes as well.

14.11

Physiologic adaptations at rest resulting from pregnancy

Cardiovascular

↑ in resting cardiac output by as much as 50%
↑ in circulating blood volume
↑ in left ventricular end-diastolic size
↑ in resting heart rate and stroke volume
↑ in uterine blood flow

Pulmonary

↑ in minute ventilation causing a slight decrease in arterial PCO_2
↑ in tidal volume
↔ in vital capacity

Other

↑ in $\dot{V}O_2$ at rest, approaching 30% above nonpregnant values in the third trimester
↑ in the hormones estrogen and relaxin
↑ in total body weight of 10–14 kg
↑ in resting energy expenditure of approximately 150 kcal · day^{-1} during the first trimester, and of approximately 350 kcal · day^{-1} during the second and third trimesters.

Dysmenorrhea (painful menstruation) is probably neither aggravated nor cured by exercise participation. If anything, it may be less common in those women who are physically active than in those who are not.[44,103,131]

Menopause

Menopause is associated with numerous physiologic changes and with an increased risk for cardiovascular disease. It is also associated with a reduced energy expenditure during rest and physical activity, an accelerated loss of fat-free mass, and an increased central adiposity.[98] The mean age for menopause in the U.S. is 51 years, and although more is becoming known about the effects of exercise on aging, until recently little was known about the influence of menopause on aerobic capacity (max $\dot{V}O_2$). Wells et al.[123] assessed 49 endurance trained female runners between the ages 35 and 70 years and observed that although max $\dot{V}O_2$ decreased with increasing age, the decline in $\dot{V}O_2$ was not influenced (accelerated or blunted) by menopause status.

Pregnancy, Injuries to the Breasts and Reproductive Organs, and the Developing Fetus

Historically, there have been misunderstandings about the effects of exercise participation on pregnancy and about injuries caused to the breasts and reproductive organs.

Although many questions still remain, fortunately we know much more now than we did 20 years ago.

Pregnancy and Childbirth

Pregnancy induces profound alterations in maternal anatomy and physiology at rest. These include cardiovascular, respiratory, metabolic, thermoregulatory and biomechanical changes. Many of these changes are summarized in table 14.11, the magnitude of which may vary over the course of the pregnancy.

Several investigations have been conducted addressing whether or not exercise during pregnancy enhances delivery, creates complications, or has no effect. In general, female athletes and persons who exercise tend to have fewer pregnancy- and childbirth-related complications than do nonexercising women.[13,44,112,127,131] This may include a shorter period of labor, less weight gain, fewer cesarean sections, fewer spontaneous abortions, and less perceived discomforts during later pregnancy.

Concerning the continuation of exercise and changes in aerobic capacity during pregnancy, we present a case study,[41] detailing the max $\dot{V}O_2$ of a female tested before, during, and after pregnancy. The subject began a training program following her first pregnancy and was studied through a second pregnancy 14 months after the first. The results are shown in figure 14.17. Although the max $\dot{V}O_2$ fell dramatically during the first trimester of pregnancy (0.48 L · min^{-1}), there was a partial recovery (0.25 L · min^{-1})

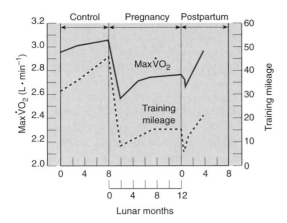

Figure 14.17

The max $\dot{V}O_2$ before (control), during, and after (postpartum) pregnancy. Max $\dot{V}O_2$ fell sharply during the first trimester and recovered during the remainder of the pregnancy. This was probably a function of the training mileage, which also fell. Max $\dot{V}O_2$ returned to control values after pregnancy.

(Based on data from Dressendorfer.[41])

through the remainder of the pregnancy. This was probably a function of the training mileage, which decreased from about 50 miles per week to about 5 to 7 miles per week. After the first 3 months of the pregnancy, the subject was able to continue running about 15 miles per week up to a few days before delivery. Finally, max $\dot{V}O_2$ returned to control values after parturition (postpartum), as running mileage increased.

Injuries to the Breast and Reproductive Organs

Actually, injuries to the reproductive organs are less frequent and less severe in the female than in the male athlete. The most common injury in the female is to the breasts. Females should use breast protectors in sports where body contact is likely.

Injuries to the female genital organs, though rare, are usually confined to minor contusions and lacerations of the external genitalia.[103] The internal organs (i.e., the uterus, fallopian tubes, and ovaries) are extremely well protected by virtue of their position deep within the bony pelvis. Although rare, serious injury to these organs can occur, such as that caused by the forceful entry of water into the vagina following a fall in water skiing.[97] In this regard, rubber wet suits should be worn by females when water skiing.

The Developing Fetus

Our efforts thus far have focused on the mother, her activity during pregnancy, and pregnancy outcomes. Well, what effect does exercise have on the developing fetus? This question is equally important and worthy of an answer.

We know that a reduction in infant birth weight of ~ 300 to 350 g is not unexpected among very active pregnant females, caused mostly by a decrease in subcutaneous fat.[1,127] However, in and of itself, this does not appear to be harmful to the newborn. Alternately, during moderate exercise, blood norepinephrine levels increase, overall visceral-splanchnic blood flow diminishes by ~ 50%, and fetal temperature increases somewhat. These changes raise the issue that diminished uterine blood flow and/or intrauterine hyperthermia might negatively impact normal fetal development, especially if they were to occur during the first trimester. In the developing fetus, ~ 15% of heat loss occurs through the uterine wall, with the balance via utero-placental circulation.[66] Fortunately, maternal thermoregulatory changes occur during exercise which facilitate heat loss.[66,127] Interestingly, these thermal protective changes appear to be less effective during maternal infection.[66]

Vigorous maternal exercise increases fetal heart rate by 5 to 20 beats · min[-1], and in rare instances a fetal brady-cardia may occur soon after maternal maximal exercise.[1,127] To this end, submaximal exercise is most often preferred.

Developing an Exercise Program

The American College of Obstetricians and Gynecologists have issued recommendations for exercise in pregnancy and postpartum.[1] Highlights from this statement are given here:

1. Regular, mild-to-moderate exercise (at least three times per week) is preferable to irregular activity and can provide health benefits. No data supports limiting exercise intensity or target heart rate to prevent potential adverse effects, unless risk factors for adverse maternal or fetal outcome are known to exist.
2. Women should avoid exercise in the supine position after the first trimester of pregnancy. Such a position is associated with a decreased cardiac output in most women.
3. Women should be encouraged to modify exercise intensity according to maternal symptoms (nausea, vomiting, balance). They should stop excising when fatigued and not exercise to exhaustion. Non-weight-bearing exercise (cycling or swimming) will minimize the risk of injury and facilitate continued exercise throughout pregnancy.
4. Any type of exercise that risks loss of balance or abdominal trauma should be avoided.
5. Women who exercise in the first trimester should ensure proper heat dissipation via adequate hydration, appropriate clothing, and choice of environmental conditions.

A woman should discuss with a clinician her interest to initiate or continue an exercise program once she suspects that she is pregnant. Exercise is contraindicated in some women, supporting further the need for a medical evaluation.

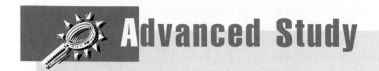

At the 38th annual meeting of the American College of Sports Medicine in Orlando, Florida, distinguished physician and physiologist Per-Olof Åstrand presented the J. B. Wolffe Memorial Lecture. The title of his talk was "Why Exercise?"[14] The material that follows represents brief excerpts from the very end of his lecture, when Dr. Åstrand addressed, in a unique fashion, the evolutionary aspects of humankind and physical activity. Keep in mind that these words were spoken by an individual who, quite possibly, has done more over the past 40 or so years for the advancement of physical activity and exercise physiology than any other one person.

"The hominid *Australopithecus* can be traced back ~ 4 million years. Approximately 2 million years ago he gave way to true *Homo* individuals (*Homo habilis,* then later on *Homo erectus*). Hunting and foraging for food and other necessities in the wilds were a condition of human life during those times. Evolutionary changes in the genetic code that made survival of the hominids possible were promoted. Major adaptations for this survival included habitual physical activity, including endurance and peak effort alternated with periods of rest and socialization. Now, after a brief 10,000 years as an agrarian (farming and agriculture) culture, we have in some privileged societies ended up in an urbanized, highly technologic society dominated by a sedentary lifestyle. The latter has occurred mostly within this century alone, literally the last 100 years.

Without experience and scientific backups, we are now facing a new phase in human history. Insights into our biological heritage may help us to modify our current lifestyle in a positive way. It is an important and urgent challenge to teach and promote regular physical activity from childhood up to old age to promote successful aging and an optimal lifestyle. It is a risk factor to quickly change from the lifestyle of hunter-gatherer to one of an urban high-technologist. Close to 99% of the existence of the *hominid/homo* species has been dominated by outdoor activities. We, *Homo sapiens,* are now exposed to an enormous experiment—one without a control group."

Summary

Approximately one-fourth of the U.S. population aged 20 years and older are sedentary during times of leisure. Among specific subpopulations such as black or Hispanic females, no leisure time physical activity approaches 50%!

In 1996 the U.S. Surgeon General released a report on physical activity and health. One of the issues addressed in this report is the public health burden of physical inactivity. Present estimates are that as many as 250,000 deaths each year are attributable to a lack of regular physical activity. Various researchers have shown that moving from sedentary or low-fit to moderately fit greatly lowers all-cause and disease specific mortality (coronary heart disease and cancers).

The major cause of coronary heart disease and stroke is atherosclerosis, a disease that causes a narrowing of the lumen of the coronary and other arteries. When a coronary artery is completely blocked, the heart tissue normally supplied with blood from that artery dies, and a heart attack is said to have occurred. Similarly, a blockage in a cerebral artery leads to a stroke. In both cases, a blood clot or thrombi often forms in conjunction with the underlying atherosclerotic lesion to completely occlude the artery.

Risk factors associated with coronary heart disease include: (1) age, (2) heredity, (3) obesity, (4) tobacco smoking, (5) lack of exercise, (6) high blood cholesterol (lipid) levels, (7) high blood pressure (hypertension), (8) male gender, (9) diabetes, and (10) stress. The big four risk factors are cigarette smoking, high blood pressure, lack of exercise, and high blood levels of cholesterol.

Guidelines for total cholesterol levels as set by the National Cholesterol Education Program are: under 200 mg · dL^{-1} equals "desirable," from 200 to 239 mg · dL^{-1} equals "borderline high," and over 240 mg · dL^{-1} equals "high." Persons with borderline high and high levels are treated with dietary therapy and should also have their LDL cholesterol estimated. An LDL level less than 130 mg · dL^{-1} is "desirable." Dietary treatment alone and/or in combination with drug treatment is recommended for lowering these factors.

Prior to the early 1990s, authoritative statements about the recommended quality and quantity of exercise were meant to improve cardiorespiratory fitness. Training frequency was set at 3 to 5 days per week, with intensity at 60% to 90% of maximum heart rate and 15 to 60 minutes per session. Exercise intensity can be guided by (1) heart-rate-based methods, such as the straight percent method or heart rate reserve, or (2) rating of perceived exertion. In the mid-1990s several authoritative bodies provided statements aimed at improving public health, such that all Americans should now strive to accumulative 30 minutes of moderate activity most days of the week.

Physical activity plays an important role in a variety of other health-related issues such as diabetes, blood clotting and fibrinolysis, blood lipids, immunology, and mental health. Additionally, except in extreme training conditions, where growth plate injury or premature closure is of concern, physical activity does not negatively impact maturation in the developing child/adolescent. If anything, current physical habits among youth is a concern, and reversing this problem likely will involve greater efforts on the part of both the parents and the schools.

Previously sedentary, older adults can also benefits from a program of regular physical activity. Several studies have shown that exercise reverses or delays the changes in the cardiorespiratory fitness, pulmonary function, and skeletal muscle function that are usually attributable to getting older.

Mild exercise does not appear to have a significant adverse effect on menstrual disorders. However, heavy intensive training has been found to induce amenorrhea (cessation of menstruation) in some athletes, particularly in long-distance runners and gymnasts. The amenorrhea is temporary and uncomplicated and disappears on cessation of heavy training.

Complications of pregnancy and childbirth appear to be fewer in female athletes than in nonathletes. Pregnancy per se does not adversely affect athletic participation or exercise performance and vice versa. Following childbirth, performance returns to previous levels. Equally as important, physical activity during pregnancy does not appear to endanger the developing fetus.

Questions

1. Compare and contrast exercise vs. physical activity.
2. Compare and contrast the achievement of health vs. fitness relative to increasing the mount of physical activity one engages in on a regular basis.
3. State three causes of death that are associated with leading a sedentary lifestyle.
4. Discuss the death rate from cardiovascular disease compared with all other deaths.
5. Define and discuss atherosclerosis relative to myocardial or cerebral ischemia/infarct. Include in your answer the contributory role of thrombosis.
6. Discuss how each of the "big four" risk factors might contribute to the development of coronary heart disease?
7. What levels of blood total cholesterol has the National Cholesterol Education Program (NCEP) used to indicate "desirable," "borderline high," and "high"?
8. A 53-year-old female has a total cholesterol of $215 \text{ mg} \cdot dL^{-1}$, an HDL cholesterol of $51 \text{ mg} \cdot dL^{-1}$, and a triglyceride level of $200 \text{ mg} \cdot dL^{-1}$. Using the formula provided in this chapter, estimate her LDL cholesterol. Also, is this value considered desirable, borderline high, or high?

9. What threshold amount of additional physical activity (in $kcal \cdot day^{-1}$) should be expended to promote the health benefit derived from such a strategy?
10. Compare and contrast intermittent (accumulated) vs. continuous physical activity relative to achieving health benefits.
11. Does an acute bout of exercise increase one's risk of sudden death vs. sitting in a chair? If yes, is this risk greater in active or nonactive people? And, how does any increase in risk that might occur compare to the benefits derived from regular physical activity?
12. What broad guidelines do you need to consider when prescribing exercise in a patient with Type II diabetes?
13. Your 42-year-old uncle just informed you that during his annual exam with his physician he was told that his total cholesterol is high at $252 \text{ mg} \cdot dL^{-1}$. He has come to you to see what he should do to rectify this problem. Outline and provide the rationale for your response.
14. How does regular exercise impact changes in the cardiovascular and skeletal muscle systems that often occur with aging?
15. What are the effects of training on menarche and menstruation?
16. Does exercise training during pregnancy provide any beneficial or negative consequences relative to labor and delivery? What are the effects of exercise on the developing fetus?

References

1. American College of Obstetricians and Gynecologists. 1994. Exercise during pregnancy and the postpartum period. *ACOG Technical Bulletin.* No. 189:1–6.
2. American College of Sports Medicine. 1993. Current comment on the prevention of sports injuries of children and adolescents. *Med Sci Sports Exerc.* 25(suppl.):1–7
3. American College of Sports Medicine. 1995. *Guidelines for Exercise Testing and Prescription,* 5th ed. Philadelphia: Lea and Febiger. pp. 95–97.
4. American College of Sports Medicine. 1988. Physical fitness in children and youth. *Med Sci Sports Exerc.* 20:422–423.
5. American College of Sports Medicine. 1990. The recommended quantity and quality of exercise for developing and maintaining cardiorespiratory and muscular fitness in healthy adults. *Med Sci Sports Exerc.* 22:265–274.
6. American College of Sports Medicine. 1978. The recommended quantity and quality of exercise for developing and maintaining fitness in healthy adults. *Med Sci Sports.* 10(3):vii–x.
7. American Dietetic Association. 1997. Diabetes mellitus and exercise. *Diabetes Care.* 20(suppl.):S51.
8. American Heart Association. 1977. *Heart Facts—1978.* Dallas, TX.
9. American Heart Association. 1992. Statement on exercise: benefits and recommendations for physical activity programs for all Americans. *Circulation.* 86:340–344.
10. American Heart Association. 1996. Statement on exercise: benefits and recommendations for physical activity programs for all Americans. *Circulation.* 94:857–862.
11. Aniansson, A., G. Grimby, M. Hedberg, and M. Krotkiewski. 1981. Muscle morphology, enzyme activity and muscle strength in elderly men and women. *Clin Physiol.* 1:73–86.

12. Armstrong, N., and J. R. Welsman. 1994. Assessment and interpretation of aerobic fitness in children and adolescents. *Exercise and Sports Sciences Reviews.* 22:435–476.

13. Artal, R., A. R. Wiswell, and B. Drinkwater (eds). 1990. *Exercise in Pregnancy.* Baltimore: Williams and Wilkins

14. Åstrand, P. O. 1992. Why exercise? *Med Sci Sports Exerc.* 24:153–162.

15. Babock, M. A., D. H. Paterson, and D. A. Cunningham. 1994. Effects of aerobic endurance training on gas exchange kinetics of older men. *Med Sci Sports Exerc.* 26:447–452.

16. Blair, S. N. 1996. Physical inactivity: the public health challenge. *Sports Med Bulletin.* 31:3.

17. Blair, S. N., N. N. Goodyear, L. W. Gibbons, and K. H. Cooper. 1984. Physical fitness and incidence of hypertension in healthy normotensive men and women. *JAMA.* 252:487–490.

18. Blair, S. N., E. Horton, A. S. Leon, I-M. Lee, B. L. Drinkwater, R. K. Dishman, M. Mackey, and M. L. Kienholz. 1996. Physcial activity, nutrition, and chronic disease. *Med Sci Sports Exerc.* 28:335–349.

19. Blair, S. N., J. B. Kampert, H. W. Kohl, C. E. Barlow, C. A. Macera, R. S. Paffenbarger, and L. W. Gibbons. 1996. Influences of cardiorespiratory fitness and other precursors on cardiovascular disease and all-cause mortality in men and women. *JAMA.* 276:205–210.

20. Blair, S. N., W. H. Kohl, C. E Barlow, and L. W. Gibbons. 1991. Physical fitness and all-cause mortality in hypertensive men. *Annals of Med.* 23:307–312.

21. Blair, S. N., H. W. Kohl, C. E. Barlow, R. S. Paffenbarger, L. W. Gibbons, and C. A. Macera. 1995. Changes in physical fitness and all-cause mortality. *JAMA.* 273:1093–1098.

22. Blair, S. N., H. W. Kohl, R. S. Paffenbarger, D. G. Clark, K. H. Cooper, and L. W. Gibbons. 1989. Physical fitness and all-cause mortality. *JAMA.* 262:2395–2401.

23. Booth, F. W., S. H. Weeden, and B. S. Tseng. 1994. Effect of aging on human skeletal muscle and motor function. *Med Sci Sports Exerc.* 26:556–560.

24. Borg, G., 1978. Subjective effort in relation to physical performance and working capacity. In H. J. Pick, H. W. Liebowitz, J. E. Singer, A. Steinschneider, and H. Stevenson (eds.), *Psychology: From Research to Practice.* New York: Plenum, pp. 333–361.

25. Bourey, R. E., and S. A. Santoro. 1988. Interactions of exercise, coagulation, platelets, and fibrinolysis—a brief review. *Med Sci Sports Exerc.* 20:439–446.

26. Brawner, C. A., S. J. Keteyian, and T. E. Czaplicki. 1995. A method of guiding exercise intensity: the talk test. *Med Sci Sports Exerc.* 27(No. 5, suppl.):S241.

27. Brisson, G. R., M. A. Volle, M. Desharnais, D. DeCarnfel, and A. Audet. 1979. Exercise-induced blood prolactin responses and sports habits in young women. *Med Sci Sports.* 11(1):91.

28. Burt, V. T., P. Whelton, E. J. Roccella, C. Brown, J. A. Cutler, M. Higgins, M. J. Horans, and D. I. Labarthe. 1995. Prevalence of hypertension in the U.S. adult population. *Hypertension.* 25:305–313.

29. Calabrese, L.H. 1990. Exercise, immunity, cancer and infection. In C. Bouchard, et al. (eds.), *Exercise, Fitness and Health: A Consensus of Current Knowledge,* Champaign, IL: Human Kinetics. pp. 567–571.

30. Cartee, G. D. 1994. Aging skeletal muscle: response to exercise. *Exercise and Sports Sciences Reviews.* 22:91–120.

31. Cartee, G. D. 1994. Influence of age on skeletal muscle glucose transport and glycogen metabolism. *Med Sci Sports Exerc.* 26:577–585.

32. Chandler, W. L., R. S. Schwartz, J. R. Stratton, and M. V. Vitiello. 1996. Effects of endurance training on the circadian rhythm of fibrinolysis in men and women. *Med Sci Sports Exerc.* 28:647–655.

33. Christ, D. M., L. T. Mackinnon, R. F. Thompson, H. A. Atterbom, and P. A. Egan. 1989. Physical exercise increases natural cellular-mediated tumor cytotoxicity in elderly women. *Gerontology.* 35:66–71.

34. Crespo, C. J., J. Keteyian, G. W. Heath, and C. T. Sempos. 1996. Leisure time physical activity among U.S. adults. *Arch Intern Med.* 156:93–98.

35. Cumming, D. C. 1990. Discussion: reproduction: exercise-related adaptations and the health of women and men. In C. Bouchard, et al. (eds.), *Exercise, Fitness and Health: A Consensus of Current Knowledge,* Champaign, IL: Human Kinetics. pp 677–685.

36. Czaplicki, T. E., S. J. Keteyian, C. A. Brawner, and M. A. Weingarten. 1997. Guiding exercise training intensity on a treadmill and dual-action bike using the talk test. *Med Sci Sports Exerc.* 29(No. 5, suppl.):S70.

37. Czaplicki, T. E., S. J. Keteyian, F. J. Fedel, D. M. Williams, and A. Kiel. 1995. Non-compliance after cardiac rehabilitation. *Med Sci Sports Exerc.* 27(No. 5, suppl.):S33.

38. Dale, E., D. H. Gerlach, D. E. Martin, and C. R. Alexander. 1979. Physical fitness profiles and reproductive physiology of the female distance runner. *Phys Sportsmed.* 7(1):83–95.

39. Dale, E., D. H. Gerlach, and A. L. Wilhite. 1979. Menstrual dysfunction in distance runners. *Obstet Gynecol.* 54(1):47–53.

40. De Paz, J. A., J. Lasierra, J. G. Villa, et al. 1992. Changes in the fibrinolytic system associated with physical conditioning. *Eur J Appl Physiol.* 65:388–393.

41. Dressendorfer, R. H. 1978. Physical training during pregnancy and lactation. *Phys Sportsmed.* 6(2):74–75,78,80.

42. Durstine, J. L., and W. L. Haskell. 1994. Effects of exercise training on plasma lipids and liporproteins. *Exercise and Sports Sciences Reviews.* 22:477–521.

43. Enos, W. F., R. H. Holmes, and J. Beyer. 1953. Coronary disease among United States soldiers killed in action in Korea. *JAMA.* 152:1090–1093

44. Erdelyi, G. 1962. Gynecological survey of female athletes. *J Sports Med.* 2:174–179.

45. Eriksson, B. O., I. Engstrom, P. Karlberg, A. Lunden, B. Saltin, and C. Thorne. 1978. Long-term effect of previous swim-training in girls, a 10-year follow-up of the "Girl Swimmers." *Acta Paediat Scand.* 67:285–292.

46. Feicht, C. B., T. S. Johnson, B. J. Martin, K. E. Sparks, and W. W. Wagner. 1978. Secondary amenorrhea in athletes. *Lancet.* 2(8100):1145–1146

47. Ferguson, E. W., L. L. Berner, G. R. Banta, J. Yu-Yahiro, and E. B. Schoomaker. 1987. Effects of exercise and conditioning on clotting and fibrinolytic activity in men. *J Appl Physiol.* 62:1416–1421.

48. Frisch, R. E. 1977. Fatness and the onset and maintenance of menstrual cycles. *Res Reprod.* 9:1.

49. Frisch, R. E., and J. W. McArthur. 1974. Menstrual cycles: fatness as a determinant of minimum weight for height necessary for this maintenance or onset. *Science.* 185:949–951.

50. Frisch, R. E., G. Wyshak, N. L. Albright, et al. 1985. Lower prevelance of breast cancers and cancers of the reproductive system among college athletes compared to non-athletes. *British J Cancer.* 52:885–891.

51. Gettman, L. R. 1996. Economic benefits of physical activity. *Physical Activity and Fitness Research Digest.* 2:1–6.

52. Gilliam, T. B., V. L. Katch, W. Thorland, and A. Weltman. 1977. Prevalence of coronary heart disease risk factors in active children, 7 to 12 years of age. *Med Sci Sports.* 9(1):21–25

53. Hagberg, J. M., J. E. Yerg, and D. R. Seals. 1988. Pulmonary function in young and older athletes and untrained men. *J Appl Physiol.* 65:101–105.

54. Hahn, R. A., S. M. Teutsch, R. B. Rothenberg, and J. S. Marks. 1986. Excess deaths from nine chronic diseases in the United States. *JAMA.* 264:2654–2659.

55. Harris, D. 1978. Quoted in: Secondary amenorrhea linked to stress. *Phys Sportsmed.* 6(10):24.

56. Harris, M. B. 1990. Feeling fat: motivations, knowledge, and attitudes of overweight women and men. *Psych Reports.* 67:1191–1202.

57. Haskell, W. L. 1994. Health consequences of physical activity: understanding and challenges regarding dose-response. *Med Sci Sports Exerc.* 26:649–660.

58. Haskell, W. L. 1995. Physical activity in the prevention and management of coronary heart disease. *Physical Activity and Fitness Research Digest.* 2:1–8.

59. Hoffman, P., I. H. Jonsdottir, and P. Thorén. 1996. Activation of different opioid systems by muscle activity and exercise. *News Physiol Sci.* 11:223–228.

60. Hunink, M. G., M., L. Goldman, A. N. A. Tosteson, et al. 1997. The recent decline in mortality from coronary heart disease, 1980–1990. *JAMA.* 277:535–542.

61. Janal, M. N., E. W. D. Colt, W. C. Clark, and M. Glusman. 1984. Pain sensitivity, mood and plasma endocrine levels in man following long-distance running: effects of naloxone. *Pain.* 19:13–25.

62. Kannel, W. B., and T. R. Dawber. 1972. Atherosclerosis as a pediatric problem. *J Pediatrics.* 80:544–554

63. Kohl, H. W., K. E. Powell, N. F. Gordon, S. N. Blair, and R. S. Paffenbarger. 1992. Physical activity, physical fitness, and sudden cardiac death. *Epidemiologic Rev.* 14:37–58.

64. Kramer, M. M., and C. L. Wells. 1996. Does physical activity reduce risk of estrogen-dependent cancer in women? *Med Sci Sports Exerc.* 28:322–334.

65. Kustin, J., and R. W. Rebar. 1987. Menstrual disorders in the adolescent age group. *Prim Care.* 14:139–166.

66. Laburn, H. P. 1996. How does the fetus cope with thermal challenge? News Physiol Sci. 11:96–100.

67. Lakka, T. A., J. M. Venëläinen, R. Rauramaa, et al. 1994. Relation of leisure-time physical activity and cardiorespiratory fitness to the risk of acute myocardial infarction in men. *N Engl J Med.* 330:1549–1554.

68. LaPerriere, A., M. H. Antoni, N Schneiderman, et al. 1990. Exercise intervention attenuates emotional distress and natural killer cell decrements following notification of positive serologic status for HIV-1. *Biofeedback Self-Regul.* 15:229–242.

69. Larsson, L., B. Sjödin, J. Larsson. 1978. Histochemical and biochemical changes in human skeletal muscle with age in sedentary males, age 22–65 years. *Acta Physiol Scan.* 103:31–39

70. Lee, I-M. 1995. Physical activity and cancer. *Physical Activity and Fitness Research Digest.* 2:1–8.

71. Lee, I-M., C. Hsieh, and R. S. Paffenbarger. 1995. Exercise intensity and longevity in men. *JAMA.* 1995:1179–1184.

72. Leon, A. S., J. Connett, D. R. Jacobs, and R. Rauramaa. 1987. Leisure-time physical activity levels and risk of coronary heart disease and death: the multiple risk factor intervention trial. *JAMA.* 258:2388–2395.

73. Loucks, A. B., and S. M. Horvath. 1985. Athletic amenorrhea: a review. *Med Sci Sports Exerc.* 17(1):56–72.

74. Loviglio, L. 1978. What's your risk: A layman's guide to cardiovascular disease. *Bostonia* (Boston University Alumni Magazine). 52:1

75. McGinnis, J. M., and W. H. Foege. 1993. Actual causes of death in the United States. *JAMA.* 270:2207–2212.

76. Mackinnon, L. T. 1994. Current challenges and future expectations in exercise immunology: back to the future. *Med Sci Sports Exerc.* 26:191–194.

77. McNamara, J. J., M. A. Molot, J. F. Stremple, and R. T. Cutting. 1971. Coronary artery disease in combat casualties in Vietnam. *JAMA.* 216:1185–1187

78. Malina, R. M. 1994. Physical activity and training: effects on stature and the adolescent growth spurt. *Med Sci Sports Exerc.* 26:759–766.

79. Malina, R., A. Harper, H. Avent, and D. Campbell. 1973. Age at menarche in athletes and non-athletes. *Med Sci Sports.* 5(1):11–13.

80. Malina, R. M., P. T. Katzmarzyk, C. M. Bonci, et al. 1997. Family size and age at menarche in athletes. *Med Sci Sports Exerc.* 29:99–106.

81. Malina, R. M., W. W. Spirduso, C. Tate, and A. M. Baylor. 1978. Age at menarche and selected menstrual characteristics in athletes at different competitive levels and in different sports. *Med Sci Sports.* 10(3):218–222

82. Maron, B. J., J. Shirani, L. C. Poliac, et al. 1996. Sudden death in young competitive athletes. *JAMA.* 276:199–204.

83. Martin, J. E., and D. M. Duppert. 1982. Exercise applications and promotion in behavioral medicine. *J Consult Clin Psychol.* 50:1004–1017.

84. Mittleman, M. A., M. Maclure, G. H. Tofler, et al. 1993. Triggering of acute myocardial infarction by heavy physical exertion. *N Engl J Med.* 329:1677–1683.

85. Mondin, G. W., W. P. Morgan, P. N. Piering, et al. 1996. Psychological consequences of exercise deprivation in habitual exercisers. *Med Sci Sports Exerc.* 28:1199–1203.

86. National Institute of Neurological Disorders and Stroke rt-PA Stroke Study Group. 1995. Tissue plasminogen activator for acute ischemic stroke. *N Engl J Med.* 333:1581–1587.

87. Nieman, D. C. 1994. Exercise, upper respiratory tract infection, and the immune system. *Med Sci Sports Exerc.* 26:128–139.

88. Nieman, D. C., K. S. Buckley, D. A. Henson, et al. 1995. Immune function in marathon runners versus sedentary controls. *Med Sci Sports Exerc.* 27:986–992.

89. Nieman, D. C., S. L. Nehlsen-Cannarella, P. A. Markoff, et al. 1990. The effects of moderate exercise training on natural killer cells and acute upper respiratory tract infections. *Int J Sports Med.* 11:467–473.

90. NIH Consensus Development Panel on Phyical activity and Cardiovascular Health. 1995. Physical activity and cardiovascular health. *JAMA.* 276:241–246.

91. O'Connor, P. W., and S. D. Youngstedt. 1995. Influence of exercise on human sleep. In J. O. Hollosy (ed.), *Exercise and Sport Sciences Reviews,* vol. 23. Baltimore: Williams & Wilkins, pp. 105–134.

92. Ogawa, T., R. J. Spina, W. H. Martin, et al. 1992. Effects of aging, sex, and physical training on cardiovascular responses to exercise. *Circulation.* 86:494–503.

93. Oldridge, N. B., B. Ragowski, and M. Gottlieb. 1992. Use of outpatient cardiac rehabilitation services. *J Cardiopulmonary Rehabil.* 12:55–31.

94. Paffenbarger, R. S., R. T. Hyde, A. L. Wing, and C. Hsieh. 1986. Physical activity, all-cause mortality, and longevity of college alumni. *N Engl J Med.* 314:605–613.

95. Paffenbarger, R. S., R. T. Hyde, A. L. Wing, et al. 1993. The association of changes in physical activity level and other lifestyle characteristics with mortality among men. *N Engl J Med.* 328:538–545.

96. Pate, R. R., M. Pratt, S. N. Blair, et al. 1995. Physical activity and public health. *JAMA.* 273:402–407.

97. Pfanner, D. 1964. Salpingitis and water-skiing. *Med J Australia.* 1:320.

98. Poehlman, E. T., M. J. Toth, and A. W. Gardner. 1995. Changes in energy balance and body composition at menopause: a controlled longitudinal study. *Ann Intern Med.* 123:673–675.

99. Powell, K. E., and S. N. Blair. 1994. The public health burdens of sedentary living habits: theoretical but realisitic estimates. *Med Sci Sports Exerc.* 26:851–856.

100. Prochaska, J. O., and C. C. DiClemente. 1983. Stages and processes of self-change in smoking: toward an integrative model of change. *J Consult Clin Psych.* 51:390–395.

101. Raven, P. B., and W. G. Squires. 1989. What is science? *Med Sci Sports Exerc.* 21:351–352.

102. Ross, R. 1994. Factors influencing atherosclerosis. In Schlant, R. C., and R. W. Alexander (eds), *Hurst's The Heart (8th ed).* New York: McGraw-Hill. pp. 989–1008.

103. Ryan, A. 1975. Gynecological consideration. *J Phys Educ Res.* 46(10):40–44.

104. Seals, D. S., J. A. Taylor, A. V. Ng, and M. D. Esler. 1994. Exercise and aging: autonomic control of the circulation. *Med Sci Sports Exerc.* 26:568–576.

105. Shephard, R. J. 1993. Physiologic changes over the years. *ACSM's Resource Manual for Guidelines for Exercise Testing and Prescription, 2d ed.* Philadelphia:Lea & Febiger. pp. 397–408.

106. Sherman, W. M., and A. Albright. 1992. Exercise and Type II diabetes. *Sports Science Exchange.* 4:number 37.

107. Siscovick, D. S., N. E. Weiss, R. H. Fletcher, and T. Lasky. 1984. The incidence of primary cardiac arrest during vigorous exercise. *N Engl J Med.* 311:874–877.

108. Smith, J. A. 1995. Guidelines, standards, and perspectives in exercise immunology. *Med Sci Sports Exerc.* 27:497–506.

109. Spellman, C. C., R. R. Pate, C. A. Macera, and D. S. Ward. 1993. Self-selected exercise intensity of habitual walkers. *Med Sci Sports Exerc.* 25:1174–1179.

110. Speroff, L., and D. Redwine. 1980. Exercise and menstrual function. *Phys Sportsmed.* 8(5):42–52.

111. Stager, J. M., D. Robershaw, and E. Miescher. 1984. Delayed menarche in swimmers in relation to age at onset of training and athletic performance. 16:550–555.

112. Sternfeld, B., C. P. Quesenberry, B. Eskenazi, and L. A. Newman. 1995. Exercise during pregananacy and pregnancy outcome. *Med Sci Sports Exerc.* 27:634–640.

113. Stratton, J. R., W. L. Chandler, R. S. Schwartz, et al. 1991. Effects of physical conditioning on fibrinolytic variables and fibrinogen in young and old healthy adults. *Circulation.* 83:1692–1697.

114. Stratton, J. R., W. C. Levy, M. D. Cerqueira, et al. 1994. Cardiovascular response to exercise, effects of aging and exercise training in healthy men. *Circulation.* 89:1648–1655.

115. Trappe, S. W., D. L. Costill, M. D. Vukovich, et al. 1996. Aging among elite distance runners: a 22-year longitudinal study. *J Appl Physiol.* 80:285–290.

116. U.S. Department of Health and Human Services. 1995. Healthy people 2000: midcourse review and 1995 revisions. Washington, D.C.: Public Health Service.

117. U.S. Department of Health and Human Services. 1990. Healthy people 2000: national health promotion and disease prevention objectives, full report, with commentary. Washington, D.C.: Public Health Service. DHHS Publication No. (PHS) 88-50210.

118. U.S. Department of Health and Human Services. 1996. Physical activity and health: a report of the Surgeon General. Atlanta: National Center for Chronic Disease Prevention and Health Promotion.

119. U.S. Department of Health and Human Services. 1993. Second report of the expert panel on detection, evaluation, and treatment of high blood cholesterol in adults. Washington, D.C.: Public Health Service, National Institutes of Health. NIH Publication No. 93-3096.

120. Vitug, A., S. Schneider, and N. Ruderman. 1988. Exercise and Type I diabetes mellitus. *Exercise and Sports Sciences Reviews.* 16:285–304

121. Wakat, D. K., and K. A. Sweeney. 1979. Etiology of athletic amenorrhea in cross-country runners. *Med Sci Sports.* 11(1):91.

122. Wells, C. L. 1996. Physical activity and women's health. *Physical Activity and Fitness Research Digest.* 2:1–6.

123. Wells, C. L., M. A. Boorman, and D. M. Riggs. 1992. Effect of age and menopausal status on cardiorespiratory fitness in masters women runners. *Med Sci Sports Exerc.* 24:1147–1154.

124. Williams, P. T. 1996. High-density lipoprotein cholesterol and other risk factors for coronary heart disease in female runners. *N Engl J Med.* 334:1298–1303.

125. Williams, P. T., P. D. Wood, W. L. Haskell et al. 1982. The effects of running mileage and duration on plasma lipoprotein levels. *JAMA.* 247:2674–2679.

126. Wilmore, J. H., and J. J. McNamara. 1974. Prevalence of coronary heart disease risk factors in boys 8 to 12 years of age. *J Pediatrics.* 84:527–533.

127. Wolfe, L. A., I. K. M. Brenner, and M. F. Mottola. 1994. Maternal exercise, fetal well-being, and pregnancy outcome. *Exercise and Sports Sciences Reviews.* 22:145–194.

128. Wood, P. D., W. Haskell, H. Klein, S. Lewis, M. P. Stern, and J. W. Farquhar. 1976. The distribution of plasma lipoprotein in middle-aged male runners. *Metabolism.* 25(11):1249–1257.

129. Yarasheski, K. E., J. J. Zachwieja, and D. M. Bier. 1993. Acute effects of resistance exercise on muscle protein synthesis rate in young and elderly men and women. *Am J Physiol.* 265 (*Endocrinol Metab.* 28):E210–E214.

130. Zacharias, L. W., W. M. Rand, and R. J. Wurtman. 1976. A prospective study of sexual development and growth in American girls: the statistics of menarche. *Obstet Gynecol Surv.* 31:325–337.

131. Zaharieva, E. 1965. Survey of sportswomen at the Tokyo Olympics. *J Sports Med.* 5:215–219.

Selected Readings

American College of Sports Medicine. 1997. *ACSM's Exercise Management for Persons with Chronic Diseases and Disabilities.* Champaign, IL: Human Kinetics.

American Dietetic Association. 1997. Position of the American Dietetic Association: weight managment. *J Am Dietetic Assoc.* 97:71–74.

Brown, D. R. 1990. Exercise, fitness, and mental health. In C. Bouchard, et al. (eds.), *Exercise, Fitness and Health: A Consensus of Current Knowledge,* Champaign, IL: Human Kinetics. pp. 607–626.

Katzel, L. I., E. R. Bleeker, E. G. Colman, et al. 1995. Effects of weight loss vs. aerobic exercise training on risk factors for coronary artery disease in healthy, obese, middle-aged and older men. *JAMA.* 274:1915–1921.

Lee, I-M, and R. S. Paffenbarger. 1996. Do physical activity and physical fitness avert premature mortality? Exercise and Sports Sciences Reviews. 24:135–171.

Nieman, D. C. 1997. Immune response to heavy exertion. *J Appl Physiol.* 82:1385–1394.

Thune, I., T Brenn, E. Lund, and M. Gaard. 1997. Physical activity and the risk of breast cancer. *New Eng J Med.* 336:1269–1275.

Vranic, M., and D. Wasserman. 1990. Exercise, fitness, and diabetes. In C. Bouchard, et al. (eds.), *Exercise, Fitness and Health: A Consensus of Current Knowledge,* Champaign, IL: Human Kinetics. pp. 467–490.

section 5

Nutrition and Body Weight Control

In section 5 we will highlight the relationships among nutrition, body composition, weight control, and exercise performance. The importance of these relationships is made obvious by the fact that good nutrition is essential to not only proper growth and development but to successful athletic performance as well. Too often coaches and athletes alike think of good nutrition only during the season of their sport. As we will learn in this section, good nutritional habits are critical throughout the year to achieve both athletic success and a lifetime of fitness and well-being.

To start this section, we first discuss the relationship between nutrition and exercise performance (chapter 15) and then move on to exercise, obesity, and weight control (chapter 16). Chapter 15 includes a thorough discussion of the nutritional issues surrounding pre-event, during event, and post-event food practices. Chapter 16 includes a healthy discussion about the many—some new and some not so new—methods or techniques available for assessing body composition. Being able to quantify the two primary body compartments (fat-free tissue and body fat) provides insight that applies not only to athletic performance and exercise science but to clinical issues as well.

Basic to the understanding of obesity and nutrition are the principles of weight management. These principles apply to the nonathlete as well as to the athlete, but for different reasons. The nonathlete most always is concerned with the problem of obesity, whereas the athlete is often concerned with gaining muscle mass or fat-free weight. Along these same lines is the increased prevalence of obesity among U.S. school children—which is troublesome because a child who is overweight and practices poor eating habits is likely to grow up to be an overweight adult with equally poor eating habits. In any case, the dos and don'ts associated with proper weight management must be learned and thoroughly understood by the clinician, athletic trainer, physical educator, or coach.

Without question, over the past five years much has been learned about what constitutes good nutrition, ideal body composition, and sound weight management principles. A great deal of this information is contained in the material that follows. Let's dig in.

The following chapters are contained within this section:

15

Nutrition and Exercise Performance

Let there be no mistake—this is a textbook on exercise physiology! In the scope of this book, however, we must also focus on the important relationship between exercise performance and nutrition. In fact, human performance improves with wise nutrition and crumbles with nutritive deficiency.[3] And, although it seems obvious that any athlete would do all he or she could to practice good nutrition so as to maximize performance, this is not always the case. Fortunately, many coaches now recognize that the consumption of junk food, poor eating practices, and an unbalanced diet can all adversely affect exercise performance.[22]

Confounding the issue further is the willingness of many athletes to "experiment" with techniques (dietary supplements, training practices, and drugs) that claim improved performance. E. C. Percy was aware of this when he stated: "The competitive athlete is by nature superstitious, impressionable, faddish, gullible, and extremely susceptible to suggestions. He or she is prepared to experiment with any material which has been recommended as having the potential ability of improving their performance . . ."*

As a nation we consume too much fat, protein, and fast foods; eat too little fiber, fruits, and vegetables; and believe that vitamin and mineral supplements serve as a dietary "safety net." Our mission, 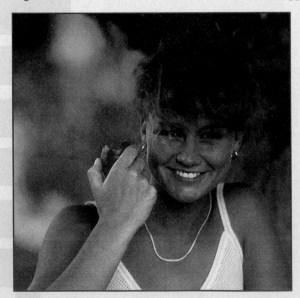 therefore, is to help you sift through the "sea of misinformation" in hopes that you will pass onto others the practice of good nutrition relative to physical activity and performance. We will draw you into several contemporary and controversial topics, such as antioxidants, sport drinks, and vegetarian practices. The science in these and other areas is changing rapidly, dictating that students be well-versed and able to interpret new findings and research.

---

*Presented as part of the J. B. Wolffe Memorial Lecture at the 25th annual meeting of the American College of Sports Medicine in Washington, D.C., May 1978.[67]

Nutrients

Food Requirements and Habits

Summary

The major concepts to be learned from this chapter are as follows:

- Carbohydrates, fats, proteins, vitamins, minerals, and water are essential to the diet.
- Carbohydrates, fats, and proteins are referred to as energy nutrients because they are used as food fuels for metabolism.
- The protein requirement during heavy exercise and training is only moderately increased in adults and can usually be met by the average U.S. diet.
- Vitamins are parts of enzymes or coenzymes that are vital for metabolism. However, vitamin and mineral supplementation above the recommended daily allowances does not increase exercise performance.
- The athletes' food requirements are generally the same as for the nonathlete, except that more calories in the form of carbohydrates are needed.
- Carbohydrates should be the major constituent of the pregame meal and should be consumed 2.5 to 6 hours before exercise or competition. During prolonged exercise, replacement fluids with carbohydrate concentrations between 4% and 8% should be consumed to spare glycogen use and stabilize blood sugar. Replenishment of carbohydrates should begin soon after exercise is stopped.
- Endurance performance is positively correlated with the amount of glycogen stored in the working muscles. Muscle glycogen storage can be greatly increased by several diet and/or exercise procedures.
- Although high-fat diets and meals may theoretically spare carbohydrate stores and prolong endurance performance, this methodology is not advocated.

Nutrients

The nutrients are the chemicals our bodies must have to sustain life and they fall into six categories: (1) water, (2) carbohydrates, (3) fats, (4) proteins, (5) vitamins, and (6) minerals. All six nutrients are found in most foods and water is by far the most abundant. Carbohydrates, fats, and proteins are the only sources of useful food energy; hence, they are called the **energy nutrients.** Since vitamins contain carbon (i.e., are organic) they too have energy. However, they are not "used" by the body in a manner that allows for the release of energy. Instead, vitamins play a regulatory or metabolic role in every single cell of the body. Devoid of carbon, minerals and water are the inorganic nutrients. Finally, despite the fact that alcohol contains carbon and therefore energy, it is not considered a nutrient.

   The body can make some nutrients from others. For example, some amino acids (parts of protein) can be converted to carbohydrate. The body can also make most of its fats (except linoleic acid and alpha-linolenic acid) using the chemicals "on board." Those nutrients that cannot be manufactured by the body or that are manufactured at a pace that is slower than the body's needs are referred to as **essential nutrients.** Carbohydrates, linoleic acid, alpha-linolenic acid, several proteins, most vitamins and minerals, and water all represent essential nutrients.

Carbohydrates

Structure of Carbohydrates

Simple sugars and complex carbohydrates are chemical compounds that comprise the nutritional group referred to as **carbohydrates.** All carbohydrates contain atoms of carbon (C), hydrogen (H), and oxygen (O). The distinguishing structural feature of carbohydrates is that there are two hydrogen atoms per atom of oxygen. For example, the chemical formula of glucose and fructose is the same ($C_6H_{12}O_6$); however, they differ because of the different arrangement of atoms within each molecule (figure 15.1).

   Two of the sugars, glucose and fructose, are referred to as **monosaccharides.** Galactose is also a monosaccharide; however, it never exists by itself in nature and instead is always found bonded to something else. When two monosaccharides are bonded together, they form a **disaccharide.** The three disaccharides are *sucrose* (glucose + fructose), *maltose* (glucose + glucose), and *lactose* (glucose + galactose). The monosaccharides and disaccharides are known as simple sugars. The complex carbohydrates or **polysaccharides** are starch, glycogen, and the fibers (e.g., cellulose). They may contain numerous (1000 or more) glucose molecules bonded or linked together. Plants store sugar in the form of starch, whereas animals (i.e., humans) can store a limited amount of sugar as glycogen in both the liver and the skeletal muscles. Starch and glycogen can be

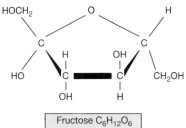

Figure 15.1

The simple sugars, glucose and fructose, have the same chemical formula, $C_6H_{12}O_6$; however, they are different because of the different arrangement of the same atoms within each molecule.

used by the body for energy production; fiber cannot. Disaccharides and polysaccharides are broken down through digestion—which starts in the mouth and finishes in the small intestine—to monosaccharides before being absorbed. Fibers (discussed later in this chapter) are derived only from plants, yet they generally pass through the body's digestive system without being broken down.

Deriving Energy from Carbohydrates

Recall from chapter 2 that there are six forms of energy, and each can be converted from one form to the other (e.g., chemical energy to heat energy). We know that energy is supplied to us through the foods we eat; therefore, the key is understanding how this energy is converted to ATP. This conversion must take place because ATP is the only chemical used by the body to perform physiological functions and work.

   The monosaccharides are absorbed by the small intestine and travel to the liver where they are converted to glucose. Glucose is then either stored in the liver as glycogen or released into the blood. Blood glucose can then be taken up and used by the cells or, if needed, stored as intramuscular glycogen. These two forms of carbohydrates (glucose and glycogen) serve as major fuels that enter the cellular metabolic processes through anaerobic or aerobic glycolysis. Through these pathways, the carbohydrates we eat result in ATP. Remember, the only difference between these two pathways is whether or not sufficient oxygen is being supplied during an activity to inhibit the accumulation of lactic acid by diverting pyruvic acid to the aerobic pathways (see chapter 2).

Blood glucose levels are maintained mainly through the glycogen stored in the liver. For example, when blood glucose is low, or during prolonged exercise when skeletal muscles are using it as a fuel substrate, glycogen from the liver is broken down to glucose by a process called **glycogenolysis.** The hormones that facilitate this process originate from the pancreas (*glucagon*) and the adrenal medulla (epinephrine). The end result is an increase or the maintenance of blood glucose. Just the opposite occurs when blood glucose is high, such as after a meal. Glucose is taken up by the tissues with the help of a hormone called *insulin*, which is also released by the pancreas. When taken up by the liver, glucose can either be used for metabolism or it can be converted to glycogen through a process referred to as **glycogenesis.** If converted to glycogen, it is stored right there in the liver. Similarly, glucose taken up by skeletal muscles that is not used for metabolic purposes can be stored as muscle glycogen. If liver and muscle glycogen stores are filled, excess glucose can be converted by **adipose (fat)** cells to fat as stored energy. The net result is that blood glucose level is brought back down to normal as the body stores the excess. By the way, storing energy in the form of fat versus glycogen is quite effective. Adipose cells are 80% fat and 20% water and protein. In contrast, approximately 2.6 grams of water are stored for every 1 gram of glycogen. Think of the weight gain due to water that would occur if we stored all our energy found in fat as glycogen.

Once glucose enters the cell it is not directly released back into the bloodstream. As such, muscle glycogen stores do not contribute directly to the maintenance of the blood glucose level. However, blood glucose levels can be indirectly affected by muscle glycogen metabolism. Specifically, when anaerobic glycolysis occurs within the muscles, some of the lactic acid formed diffuses into the blood. From there some of it is carried to the liver, where it is converted back to glucose and:

1. Dumped back into the blood as blood glucose
2. Used by the liver as a metabolic fuel
3. Converted to glycogen and stored as liver glycogen

The process of combining two molecules of lactic acid to form glucose occurs within the Cori cycle. Additionally, during both exercise and recovery, the Cori cycle also serves to help remove lactic acid from the blood.

Food Sources of Carbohydrates

In the United States people consume less complex carbohydrates today than they did in the early 1900s. The typical diet of a person now living in America includes approximately 50% of calories from carbohydrates (24% complex carbohydrates and 26% from mono- and disaccharides). A reasonable goal is increasing our calories from carbohydrate to 55% to 60%, with 45% from complex carbohydrates and 10% to 15% from mono- and disaccharides.[90] As a general rule, the higher caloric requirements among athletes involved in endurance training and events should be met by increasing to 60% to 70% the calories from carbohydrates.[90] The primary source of complex carbohydrates in the United States and Canada is bread. Some other common food sources of carbohydrates are legumes (peas and beans), grain (wheat, rice, oats, barley, corn) products such as pasta and waffles, dried fruits, fresh fruits, honey, sugar, and potatoes.

Fats and Oils

Thirty four percent to 38% of the total energy intake in the U.S. is derived from fat![90] In Canada, this number is a bit higher, about 42%. Unquestionably, eating a large quantity of fat contributes to excessive obesity, certain cancers, and cardiovascular diseases. Most health professionals and health agencies recommend that dietary fat not exceed 30% of total energy intake, with a ratio of 10%:10%:10% for saturated:monounsaturated:polyunsaturated fatty acids.

Structure of Lipids

You probably know *lipids* as fats and oils. In fact, when we discuss lipids in the foods we eat, we use the terms *fats* and *oils*. However, when we discuss these substances in the body, we use the term **lipids.** The **fatty acid** is the common lipid in the body. Like carbohydrates, fatty acids contain atoms of carbon, hydrogen, and oxygen. Its basic structure is a long chain of carbon atoms bonded to hydrogen atoms. Although there are numerous fatty acids, three of the more common are *stearic acid, oleic acid,* and *palmitic acid.* Two fatty acids, *linoleic acid* and *alpha-linolenic acid,* cannot be manufactured by the body. Therefore, they are called essential fatty acids.

A fatty acid whose carbon atoms are saturated with hydrogen atoms is referred to as a **saturated fatty acid** (figure 15.2). If, however, a fatty acid has one double bond between any two carbon atoms, and subsequently has two less hydrogen atoms, then it is referred to as monounsaturated fatty acid. Oleic acid is an example of a monounsaturated fatty acid. Finally, if along the carbon chain two or more of the bonds between carbon atoms are double bonds, then the fatty acid is **polyunsaturated** (figure 15.2).

Where the double bond occurs along the carbon chain can influence the physiologic effect of the unsaturated fatty acid. For instance, if the first double bond is between the third and fourth carbon atoms, it is referred to as an omega-3 fatty acid. If the first double bond is between the sixth and seventh carbon acids, it is referred to as an omega-6 fatty acid.

The consumption of foods rich in omega-3 fatty acids (marine fat, such as salmon, tuna, sardines, seal, and whale)

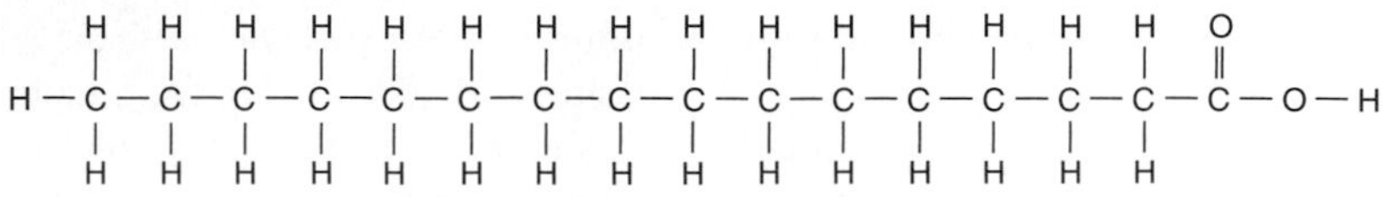

Saturated fatty acid
Palmitic acid $C_{16}H_{32}O_2$

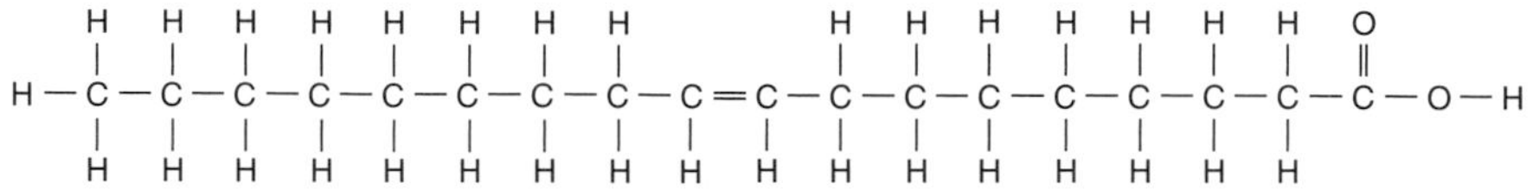

Monounsaturated fatty acid
Oleic acid $C_{18}H_{34}O_2$

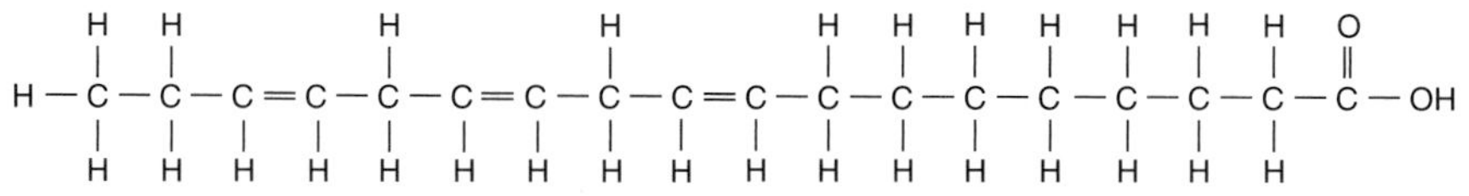

Polyunsaturated fatty acid
Alpha-linoleic acid $C_{18}H_{30}O_2$

Figure 15.2

The chemical structure of a saturated fatty acid, a monounsaturated fatty acid, and a polyunsaturated fatty acid. Fatty acids contain long chains of carbon atoms (C) linked together with hydrogen atoms (H) and oxygen atoms (O) also linked to the carbon atoms.

are associated with a lower incidence of heart disease. For example, Greenland Eskimos obtain 40% of their kcal intake from omega-3 fatty acids but have one-tenth the risk of heart attacks of Danes, who eat much less fish and other marine foods.[90] How is this accomplished? First, omega-3 fatty acids decrease the "stickiness" of platelets, the blood elements responsible for blood clotting. Individuals with platelets that are more prone to clot formation, such as those of a smoker, are believed to play a role in occluding already narrowed arteries that supply blood to the heart. The net result is an increased risk for heart attack. A second possible mechanism by which omega-3 fatty acids lower heart disease rates is that it helps lower blood cholesterol levels. With the above benefits, it's no wonder that many Americans buy and consume fish oil capsules. However, doing so also not only provides extra calories but it can also lead to serious health problems (e.g., increased tendency for bleeding, excessive vitamin D intake). A more realistic approach would be to include the consumption of fish (salmon, herring, Atlantic halibut, tuna) in one's normal diet at least

2 or 3 times per week. Also, when oils are called for in cooking, use canola oil or soybean oil, since these products also provide appreciable amounts of omega-3 fatty acids.

The main lipids in the body are **triglycerides, phospholipids** and **cholesterol.** Triglycerides consist of one molecule of a compound called glycerol bonded to three molecules of fatty acids. Triglycerides are stored in the adipose cells (adipocytes) located throughout the body and within the skeletal muscles. Cholesterol is structured quite differently than a triglyceride and is, in fact, classified as a sterol. It forms part of some hormones (estrogen, testosterone), forms the bile acids used in digestion, and is incorporated into cell membranes.

Deriving Energy from Lipids

Fatty acids represent the predominant fuel source to aerobically manufacture ATP while at rest and during light to moderate activity. Cholesterol, because of its sterol structure, cannot be used as a fuel source by the body. As a con-

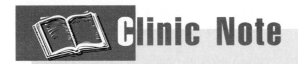

The nondigestible part of a plant is called fiber. Some fibers, like cellulose, hemicellulose, or pectin, are carbohydrates with chemical bonds (beta bonds) that cannot be split apart by the body. Lignin (wheat, cabbage, pears) represents a noncarbohydrate dietary fiber (an alcohol derivative).

There are two types of fiber: soluble and insoluble. Soluble fibers are those that either dissolve or swell when put in water. Insoluble fibers do not. No evidence exists to suggest that the consumption of either type of fiber improves athletic performance. However, much direct and correlational evidence indicates that fiber does have important health benefits, and the benefits appear related to the type of fiber consumed. For example, water soluble fibers (e.g., gum from oat bran) have been shown to reduce blood cholesterol levels.[90] Insoluble fibers such as bran (e.g., wheat fiber) helps soften the stool within the digestive tract and may protect the colon from cancer and diverticulosis (weakened areas within the intestinal wall). A recent

prospective study involving over 45,000 U.S. male health professionals[74] reported that as the amount of total fiber intake increased in the diet, there was a corresponding decrease in heart attacks. The beneficial effect was most evident among subjects with a total dietary fiber intake approaching 29 $g \cdot d^{-1}$. Interestingly, of the different food sources of fiber, the fiber found in cold breakfast cereals seemed to have the most profound impact.

There seems to be widespread consensus that the American diet is generally deficient in fiber. At present, we consume approximately 12 to 16 grams of dietary fiber per day. Although there are complications associated with consuming too much fiber, present recommendations are that Americans increase their total dietary fiber intake to 20 to 35 $g \cdot d^{-1}$ (10 to 13 $g \cdot 1000$ $kcal^{-1} \cdot d^{-1}$). The U.S. Department of Agriculture recommends 25 to 30 $g \cdot d^{-1}$. Persons increasing their fiber intake should do so slowly, over several weeks, with an associated increase in water intake.

---

sequence, a person with an elevated total cholesterol level cannot lower it through exercise alone.

Before fatty acids are metabolized, they must first be split off from the triglyceride molecule through a process called lipolysis. This is accomplished by the enzyme hormone-sensitive lipase, which is present in abundance in adipocytes and greatly influenced by epinephrine and norepinephrine. During exercise, free fatty acid concentration in the blood may increase eightfold. Once having entered the skeletal muscle, fatty acids are then activated at the expense of 1 ATP. Then, through the process of beta-oxidation (see page 32), two-carbon compounds (acyl groups) are split off to become acetyl CoA for entry into the Krebs Cycle.

Food Sources of Fatty Acids

As mentioned earlier, most persons living in the U.S. consume too much total fat. Much of this excess dietary fat is saturated fat, which is also a problem because it leads to high blood cholesterol levels and cardiovascular disease. Animal fats (found in beef, pork, and whole milk products), fats that are solid at room temperature (butter, lard), and certain plants oils (coconut, palm kernel) are high in saturated fats. Examples of foods that are rich in monounsaturated fats are olive oil and canola oil. These fatty acids gen-

erally have no effect on blood cholesterol levels. Examples of foods rich in polyunsaturated fats are soybean, sunflower, and corn oils.

Proteins

Protein has a wide variety of physiological functions that are considered essential to health and physical performance. Although the role of protein in providing energy has not been considered important for most forms of muscular activity, it is becoming increasingly clear that protein catabolism is increased in endurance activity (greater than 60 minutes) and may contribute between 4% and 10% of the energy needs.[12,28,56] This issue will be explored in more detail later.

Structure of Proteins

Proteins are more complex and larger than either carbohydrate or fat molecules. In addition to carbon, hydrogen, and oxygen, proteins contain nitrogen; some also contain sulfur, phosphorus, or iron. Proteins are the building blocks of tissue, and as such, form a vital part of the nucleus and membrane of all cells. In addition, all enzymes found in the body are proteins.

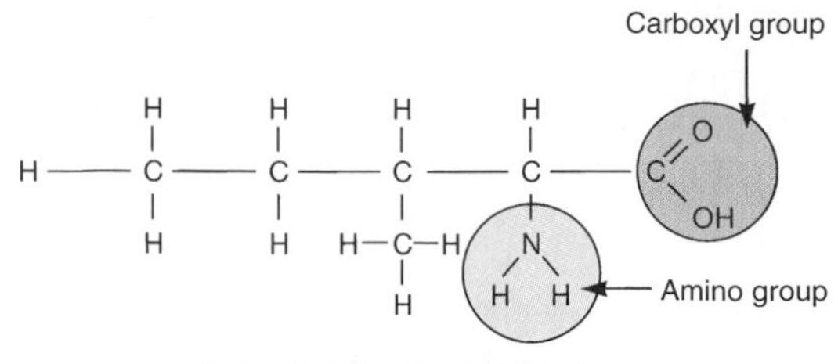

The amino acid isoleucine

Figure 15.3

The chemical structure of the amino acid isoleucine. The nitrogen component of amino acids (NH_2) is referred to as an amino group whereas the COOH component is called a carboxyl group.

The basic structural units of proteins are **amino acids.** In proteins, the amino acids are chemically bonded into long chains by what are referred to as *peptide linkages.* There are 20 different kinds of amino acids in the body. The structure of one of these is given in figure 15.3. The nitrogen component of the amino acid (NH_2) is referred to as an *amino radical* or *group.* This chemical group plus the *carboxyl group* (COOH) distinguishes amino acids from other compounds containing the same atoms. Of the 20 known amino acids, 10 are referred to as essential amino acids and 10 as nonessential amino acids. The essential amino acids cannot be synthesized within the body—or they cannot be synthesized fast enough. The 10 essential amino acids are arginine (more so during periods of growth), histidine (children only), isoleucine, leucine, lysine, methionine, phenylalanine, threonine, tryptophan, and valine.

The nonessential amino acids are equally as important as the essential amino acids but are so named because they may be synthesized in the body as well as provided in the food we eat. Some nonessential amino acids include alanine, aspartic acid, cysteine, glutamic acid, glutamine, glycine, proline, serine, and tyrosine.

General Protein Requirement

The normal recommended dietary allowance (RDA)* for protein in the United States for healthy males or females 19 years old and older is 0.8 g · kg of body weight^{-1} · d^{-1}. For younger people and pregnant lactating women, this value is increased. In Canada the corresponding values is differentiated by gender at 0.84 g · kg^{-1} · d^{-1} for adult males, and 0.75 g · kg^{-1} · d^{-1} for adult females.

To compute your own protein allowance for the day, first convert your *ideal*† body weight in pounds to kilograms (1 pound = 2.2 kg). Then, multiply this value by 0.8. For example, the daily protein requirement of a person who

should weigh 75 kg (165 pounds) would be 75 kg × 0.8 g · kg^{-1} = 60 g (2.1 oz). Compare this amount (60 g) to the average American male who consumes about 105 g · d^{-1} and the average American female who consumes about 65 g · d^{-1}.[90] In fact, a single meal of 5 ounces of chicken, 8 ounces of skim milk, one slice of bread, and one-half cup of vegetables provides 56 g of protein. In a country where ~16% of our calories come from protein, it should come as no surprise to learn that our daily protein intake is more than sufficient. When amino acids are oversupplied, the body has no place to store them. It removes and excretes the amine group and then converts the remainder of the molecule to glucose, glycogen, or fat (as stored energy).

Protein Requirement during Heavy Exercise Training

Earlier studies, most of which were contrary to what many coaches and athletes believed at the time, indicated that the protein requirement during heavy exercise is not significantly increased in adults.[21,27,69,71,72] The daily requirements for protein among athletes now range between 0.94 and 1.5 g · kg^{-1},[42,43,80] which is greater than the 0.8 g · kg^{-1} mentioned above. And, some experts recommend an even higher intake for endurance athletes (1.2 to 2 g · kg^{-1} · d^{-1} and strength-training athletes (1.3 to 1.8 g · kg^{-1} · d^{-1}).[4,13,43,44,55,80] Generally, most athletes can obtain these protein needs without making major changes, if any, in their dietary habits.[33,42,90] Some researchers have suggested a protein intake greater than 2.0 to 2.5 g · kg^{-1} · d^{-1}.[80] However, further substantiation of this recommendation has not been provided.

With respect to persons initiating a heavy resistance weight training regimen, extra protein is not required because the major fuels that provide the calories to perform such an activity are phosphocreatine and carbohydrate. Theoretically, extra protein is required for the synthesis of new muscle tissue, which is most needed during the initial phases of weight training and muscle gain.[43] Once this is accomplished and the major increase in muscle mass has stabilized, protein intake need not exceed 1.5 g · kg^{-1} · d^{-1}. Relative to "hurrying along" the promotion of muscle growth through the consumption of excessive quantities of protein in pill or powder form, more protein intake is not better. What may be important, however, is the timing of when protein is consumed. Consider the study by Chandler and colleagues, where nine experienced male weight lifters were asked to eat a carbohydrate and protein supplement (versus water only) immediately after a standardized resistance-training workout. They showed that the consumption of carbohydrates and protein at this time created an environment favorable for muscle growth,[15] compared to the water-only condition. Specifically, increases in the plasma concentrations of both *growth hormone* and *insulin* were observed—two hormones known to possess *anabolic* (muscle-building) characteristics.

---

*Recommended dietary allowances for the various nutrients are intended to meet the needs of almost all healthy people and are based on age and gender. These allowances were established in 1989 by the National Research Council.
†Ideal body weight is used instead of actual body weight because the amino acids are needed for fat-free tissue not for the fat cells.

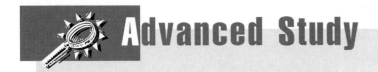

Advanced Study

Nitrogen Balance

The daily allowance for protein of 0.8 g · kg^{-1} is meant to ensure a healthy protein balance (protein intake equals or just exceeds protein loss). To monitor protein balance, such as during weight loss programs involving severe caloric restriction, we usually measure **nitrogen balance.** This means that the nitrogen-in must equal or slightly exceed nitrogen-out.

Why assess nitrogen? Because it is easier to track nitrogen intake and loss than it is to track protein intake and loss. Since nitrogen makes up about 16% of the weight of protein, we can assess nitrogen intake by dividing grams of protein consumed in a day by 6.25

(the reciprocal of 16%). This value is then compared to, and should equal or exceed, the grams of nitrogen lost, as measured in the urine (as urea) over a matched 24-hour period. Although nitrogen is also lost from the skin, hair, nails and feces, the combined amount from these sources is generally felt to be negligible. A negative nitrogen balance means more proteins are being broken down than are being built up, which, if left unchanged, will effect tissue growth and maintenance, immune-system function, fluid balance, and several other bodily functions.

Because protein requirement is computed based on body mass, the formula automatically provides for greater protein intake as muscle mass increases. For example, an active male football player who weighs 115 kg (253 pounds) would have a daily protein requirement of 104 to 173 g (based on a daily allowance of 0.9 to 1.5 g · kg^{-1} · day^{-1}). If his daily caloric requirement were 4500 kcal, a well-balanced diet containing 12% to 15% of calories from protein should be more than sufficient, providing him with 135 to 169 g of protein.*

There are two athletic groups that might require some manipulation of normal dietary patterns to achieve their daily protein requirements. The first group includes wrestlers. In this instance their absolute protein needs are not increased but, given the fact that wrestlers often restrict calories to "make weight," they need to be sure that they consume foods that are protein-dense. A second group consists of athletes who have elevated protein needs because of special physiologic states; these include pregnancy, adolescence, or lactation.[13,57]

Deriving Energy from Protein during Prolonged Exercise

Without question, the metabolism of protein during exercise is complex. Generally, during endurance exercise there is an approximate 20% to 50% decrease in the rate of protein synthesis and an increase in the rate of protein breakdown

in both the liver and the skeletal muscles.[41] The above responses are likely regulated by the exercise related increases in glucagon that occurs. Because the body's free amino acid pool is small, the amount catabolized for energy predominately comes from the liver or the skeletal muscle. In skeletal muscles the degradation of protein is isolated to the non-contractile proteins, which comprise approximately 35% of the total proteins.

In 1925 Cathcart suggested that physical activity increases, "if only in small degree," the metabolism of protein[14] Except for this, the role of protein metabolism as a means to produce ATP during exercise was mostly ignored until the early 1980s. At that time investigators again began discussing the limited but potentially important contribution of protein to total exercise energy expenditure.[28,41,57,61,90] The contribution that protein makes to energy is approximately 2% to 5% of kcal at rest and 4% to 15% of kcal during exercise. However, because some endurance athletes train for prolonged periods (1 to 2 hours) each day, the total protein amount can become quite significant.

It may turn out, however, that the metabolism of protein during exercise is a very individual matter, because such a process is related to several factors. Among these factors are exercise intensity, duration, and modality, as well as training environment, level of protein and energy intake, and the age and gender of the individual.[13,41]

Deriving energy from amino acids involves removal of the amino group (deamination). This leaves a product (alpha keto acid) that is changed further before it enters the Krebs Cycle to produce energy in a manner similar to carbohydrates and fatty acids. Additionally, 18 amino acids have been identified as glucogenic (can be converted to glucose or glycogen), with leucine, isoleucine, and valine being the most readily available and able to be metabolized in

---

*Using 12% (or 0.12), we compute the following: 4500 kcal · d^{-1} × 0.12 = 540 kcal · d^{-1} from protein. Then, at 4 kcal · g^{-1} of protein, we get 135 grams of protein per day (540 ÷ 4 = 135). Using 15% (or 0.15), we get 675 kcal · d^{-1} (4500 × 0.15) from protein or 169 g of protein per day (675 ÷ 4 = 169).

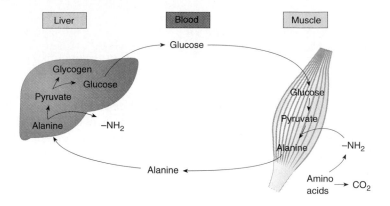

Figure 15.4

The glucose-alanine cycle provides a small amount of energy for muscular contraction during prolonged work. Amino acid breakdown provides an amino group (NH_2) that interacts with pyruvate to form alanine. Alanine is transferred to the liver where it can be converted to pyruvate then glycogen and glucose. Glucose is then transported to the working muscle where it can be utilized as an energy substrate.

the muscles. For example, the $-NH_2$ radical split off from leucine combines with pyruvic acid to form alanine. Alanine is transferred from the muscle, via circulation, to the liver where it is deaminated to form urea and pyruvic acid. The pyruvic acid is then converted to liver glycogen and glucose. The glucose can then be recirculated to the working muscle to provide energy for muscular contraction. A small amount of energy is made available from protein during exercise through this process, which is called the **glucose-alanine cycle** (figure 15.4).

Food Sources of Proteins

Without question, the foods that are richest in essential amino acids are animal products and milk. In North America more than 60% of our protein comes from animal products. Contrast this to Africa and East Asia, where approximately 25% of the consumed protein comes from animal products. Plant proteins contain some but not many of the essential amino acids. Therefore, to meet one's protein needs through plants requires not only more, but also a wide variety of vegetables. Common sources of protein are tuna packed in water, skinless poultry, fish, lean beef, skim milk, low-fat cheeses, nuts, legumes, and grains.

Vitamins and Minerals

Read carefully this joint statement from the American and Canadian Dietetic Associations:[4]

> Vitamins and minerals serve an important role in the metabolism of lipids, carbohydrates, and proteins and in muscle function. Although physical activity increases the need for some vitamins and minerals, this increased requirement typically can be met by consuming a balanced high-carbohydrate, moderate-protein, low-fat diet. Individuals at risk for low vitamin/mineral intake are those who consume a low-calorie diet.

Compare this statement to the fact that billions of dollars are spent each year on vitamin and mineral supplements. In fact, nearly 80% of all U.S. residents buy vitamin and mineral supplements, and up to 85% of competitive/elite athletes use them on a regular basis. Although athletes feel that vitamin and mineral supplements improve their performance, little support is found within the scientific literature with respect to such claims.[4,67,77,90] *The message is clear, supplementing one's diet with vitamins and minerals to levels above the RDA does not increase physical performance.* The "authorities" who recommend vitamin supplements to athletes usually do so only on theoretical grounds (since they are essential for proper bodily function—more must be better). As you read through the following material, keep in mind that the RDA (and more) is easily met for most all vitamin and minerals through a *varied and well-balanced diet* designed to meet the increased caloric needs of exercise and sport.

Vitamins serve as parts of enzymes or coenzymes that are essential for life. Thus, although vitamins do not in themselves yield energy; they are nutrients. Vitamins are classified as **water-soluble** or **fat-soluble.** The water-soluble vitamins are *vitamin C (ascorbic acid)* and the *B-complex vitamins.* They are not stored in the body and therefore must be constantly supplied in the diet. Because they are not stored, when taken in excess (above what is required), they will be passed through in the urine. For example, the RDA for vitamin C among adult men and women is 60 mg $\cdot$ day^{-1}, an amount that is easily obtained through diet alone (one medium orange contains 80 mg). Therefore, the consumption of 1000 mg of vitamin C in supplement or pill form means that more than 900 mg pass right through the body and are excreted. If, perhaps, additional vitamin C is needed because of increased physical activity, then as the athlete increases his calorie intake to meet metabolic requirements, so too is his intake of vitamin C.

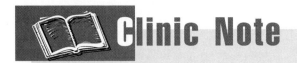

Clinic Note

Vegans

What comes to mind when we say protein? Did you say meat? Maybe beef? In America it is common for us to associate protein with red meat and animal products. However, some persons (1% to 2%) eat no animal products (a **vegan**) or eat eggs, dairy products and plant foods only (a lacto-ovo vegetarian). In fact, many elite athletes have who are vegans or vegetarians have shown us that the consumption of animal products is not essential for optimal athletic performance.

Regardless of the reason behind one's dietary habits, eating no animal protein versus including some animal products makes a great deal of difference in nutritional planning. The difference is related to the fact that foods of animal origin are excellent sources of protein, iron, zinc, calcium, riboflavin, vitamin D and vitamin B-12. Therefore, the strict vegan must carefully plan his or her dietary intake to ensure that a wide variety of foods are included. Since lacto-ovo vegetarians consume some dairy products, this helps greatly with respect to ensuring the adequate intake of some but not all of the above stated nutrients.

With respect to the vegan and amino acid intake, a real effort must be made to eat grains and legumes to obtain good quality protein. Doing so means that the essential amino acids that are deficient in the legumes (e.g., beans) are made up for through the consumption of grains (e.g., wheat or barley). In this way the two foods complement one another. A potential limitation of a vegan diet is highlighted in the following research study.

Taurine, a free amino acid abundant in humans, is found almost exclusively in foods of animal origin. Laidlaw and associates assessed the dietary, plasma, and urinary taurine levels of 11 male vegans at a Seventh-Day Adventist college.[53] These individuals reported having no regular animal products (meat, dairy, or eggs) for at least four years. When compared to 14 nonvegetarian control subjects, an inadequate intake of taurine and zinc was detected in the vegan group. Also, both plasma taurine levels and urinary taurine output were lower in the vegan group than in controls. The clinical significance of a reduced dietary taurine intake and a reduced plasma taurine level among vegans is not known. However, the difficulty associated with consuming certain nutrients while following a vegan diet is clear.

The fat-soluble *vitamins—A, D, E, and K—* are stored in the body, principally in the liver but also in fatty tissue. Although this means that these vitamins need not be supplied each day, it also means that excessive accumulations can cause toxic effects. A deficiency of either the water-soluble or fat-soluble vitamins can lead to serious illness, chronic disease, and even death. However, deficiencies, particularly in the United States and Canada, are very rare. Although most fats, carbohydrates, and protein foods contain vitamins, some of the richest sources are green leafy vegetables, whole and enriched grains, skim or low-fat milk products, nuts and seeds, lean meats, poultry, and citrus fruits.

Minerals are inorganic compounds found in the body that are vital to proper bodily function. Minerals are categorized based on the amount we need per day. Generally, if we need 100 mg or more per day, it is called a major mineral. *The major minerals include calcium, chloride, magnesium, phosphorus, potassium, sodium, and sulfur.* Minerals required in the diet in amounts less than 100 mg per day are called trace minerals. *Some of the trace minerals are copper, fluoride, iodide, iron, manganese, selenium, and zinc.*

Mineral deficiencies are generally uncommon today in the United States. Plant foods are good sources for many of the trace minerals; however, animal products (especially seafood) represent the best sources of most minerals. A vegan diet (no animal products) requires that one choose a variety of plant foods that provide a good source of minerals. Minerals are more concentrated in animal products than in plant products because as animals eat plants year after year, minerals from the plants become concentrated in the animal's tissues. With respect to iodine, it is artificially added to table salt and yields "iodized" salt.

Calcium

Calcium is the most abundant mineral found in the body. Approximately 99% of the body's calcium is found in bone and teeth. Calcium also plays an important role in blood clotting, muscle function, nerve transmission, normal heart activity, and activation of several metabolic enzymes. The RDA for calcium for both males and females is greatest between the ages of 11 and 24 years (1200 mg $\cdot$ d^{-1}). The RDA for ages 1 to 10 and for ages 25 and older is 800 mg $\cdot$ d^{-1}. When amenorrhea is present, the consumption of

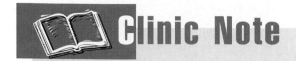

Clinic Note

Antioxidants

The **antioxidants**—what a question mark they represent for public health in America! The most noted nutritional antioxidants are vitamin E (alpha tocopherol,), vitamin C (ascorbic acid), and beta carotene (a vitamin A precursor). The reason for all the notoriety, epidemiologic studies link the ingestion of these substances (particularly alpha tocopherol and beta carotene) to lower rates of heart disease and certain cancers.

The mechanism by which antioxidants likely accomplish this is through the detoxification of potentially damaging free radicals. Free radicals are molecules or ions containing an unpaired electron (radical) and are capable of existing independently (free). Some of these free radicals are produced during long-duration, strenuous (exhaustive) exercise at levels that overwhelm the body's normal ability to detoxify the reactive agents.[50,76] The increased presence of these reactive agents during strenuous exercise appears to be associated with increases in oxygen consumption and catecholamines. On the other hand, moderate and regular physical training seems to favorably modify the body's normal physiological antioxidant defenses.

In some cells free radicals represent a strategic mechanism that contributes to our well-being, such as the phagocytic destruction of invading micro-organism. In other instances their presence is not so helpful. For example, the "oxidation" of LDL cholesterol appears to play a role in the initiation and/or progression of atherosclerotic plaque development or its rupture. Theoretically, and with some supportive laboratory evidence, antioxidants prevent or limit the oxidation of LDL cholesterol.[49,90]

The question here is whether or not a well-nourished person would benefit from consuming antioxidant supplements. The difficulty in answering this question is that most all of the studies to date which relate the use of antioxidants with lower disease rates are epidemiological. As a result, it is difficult to draw a definitive cause-and-effect relationship. Unbiased and reliable statements about the effectiveness of antioxidants can only be obtained from large scale randomized trials. To date, only four such trials involving more than 1,000 subjects have been completed—three of which showed no correlation between using antioxidant supplementation and preventing certain cancers.[48] Recently, a fourth randomized study of 2,000 heart patients in England showed that the risk of future nonfatal heart attacks among patients taking 400 or 800 units of vitamin E daily was only 23% that of patients in the control group taking a placebo (no vitamin E).[83]

Given the above, most authorities are calling for more research data before the routine consumption of antioxidants are recommended as a pill supplement.[49,50,76,90] Fortunately, such studies are presently in progress. Quitting smoking, obtaining ideal body weight, engaging in regular physical activity, and practicing dietary habits that both limit saturated fat intake and ensure five servings of fruits and vegetables each day appear to be the prudent course at present.

---

calcium at 1.2 times the RDA is recommended.[4] Adolescent girls and women are more likely to have a calcium intake below the RDA than others.[17]

Bone, as a living, dynamic tissue, is constantly being "remodeled" throughout life. Maximal bone density is achieved among most people by age 30. However, a lifetime of a low calcium intake may contribute to a gradual demineralization and weakening of bone tissue. Osteoporosis, a disease more common in postmenopausal women and one that is characterized by a decrease in bone density, is related to calcium intake, estrogen level, alcohol and caffeine intake, and the amount and type of physical activity. Achieving the RDA for calcium, in combination with regular weight-bearing activities, promotes calcium deposition to the bone and reduces the risk of developing osteoporosis.[4,17]

Rarely, some young, amenorrheic female athletes may even exhibit the early stages of osteoporosis, a bone mineral density equivalent to that of a 70 year old women. A combination of a high sweat rate (calcium is excreted in sweat) during chronic endurance exercise and a low calcium intake (through a restricted calorie diet) contribute to such a problem.[82] Myburgh and associates found lower lumbar and femoral bone mineral densities and lower calcium and dairy product intakes among 25 female athletes with stress fractures of the lower limbs as compared to age-matched controls.[63] Female athletes can also report amenorrhea or dysmenorrhea, thus making them a high risk group because of reduced levels of bone-protecting estrogen.[13]

Sources for calcium include skim milk (2 cups per day provides 500 mg), green leafy vegetables, low-fat cheeses, turnip greens, and citrus fruits. However, only about 20% to 40% of ingested calcium is absorbed by the body. Some commercially available supplements and antacids also provide calcium, although the absorption rate in these products may not be as high as that found in calcium-rich foods.

Iron

Iron is an important mineral in the diet of both the female and male athlete.[17,18,31,54,61,70] It is an essential constituent of hemoglobin, myoglobin, and several enzymes in the metabolic pathways (e.g., cytochromes of electron transport system). An anemia (i.e., hemoglobin concentration is reduced) caused by iron deficiency contributes to diminished performance, especially among endurance athletes. Clark[16] identified groups of individuals who may be susceptible to iron deficiency, such as (1) menstruating women, (2) dieters, (3) endurance athletes, (4) those who do not eat red meat, and (5) lacto-ovo vegetarians.

The RDA for iron is 15 mg for females age 11 to 50 years; 12 mg for males age 11 to 18 years; and 10 mg for all other age groups. The higher RDA for women between 11 and 50 years of age is meant to account for menstrual blood loss. On average, males consume 17 mg of iron per day, and females consume 12 mg per day, or approximately 5 to 6 mg of iron per 1000 kcal of food. Thus athletes who restrict food intake for weight-control purposes—such as dancers, wrestlers, ice skaters, and gymnasts—are generally more prone to an iron deficiency.

Many athletes are often "judged" as slightly anemic because they tend to have a lower blood hemoglobin concentration than their sedentary counterparts. In this instance, however, the anemia usually turns out to be a "false anemia," which is caused by the ~15% increase in plasma volume that occurs as a result of exercise training.[17,32] This increase in plasma volume dilutes the red blood cells and thus the hemoglobin concentration (hemodilution).

Iron deficiency (serum ferritin level <20 ng $\cdot$ ml^{-1}) in the absence of a true anemia (hemoglobin concentration: <13 g $\cdot$ dl^{-1} for males; <12 g $\cdot$ dl^{-1} for females) may or may not effect performance. A recent study by LeManca and Haymes[54] involving 10 female athletes without anemia but with iron deficiency showed a quite small (4%) but significant increase in max $\dot{V}O_2$ following an eight week treatment plan comprised of daily iron supplements. Submaximal endurance time to exhaustion was also improved, and plasma ferritin concentration was returned to normal. Generally, however, other research has not shown an improvement in performance among athletes with depleted iron stores in the absence of a true anemia.[32]

In contrast, even a mild *true anemia resulting from iron deficiency* clearly limits exercise performance. Recall that hemoglobin's ability to combine with oxygen (in the lung) and transport it (to the skeletal muscles) is related to its iron (heme) component (p. 203). It makes sense, therefore, that factors that negatively effect plasma hemoglobin concentration also limit endurance performance.

Although the primary reason behind the body's depletion of iron stores (and a low serum ferritin level) is inadequate iron intake, it may also be caused by physical activity. Examples include "footstrike hemolysis," which can result in the destruction of red cells when the heel forcefully strikes the ground during running; gastrointestinal bleeding; and, possibly, sweating. Sweat contains ~0.4 mg of iron per liter. Thus, depending on sweat rate, some endurance athletes may lose 0.8 to 1.2 mg $\cdot$ d^{-1} via sweating alone. Waller and Haymes[89] recently compared nine male and nine female athletes to assess differences in sweat iron loss during 60 minutes of exercise. Sweat iron concentration was not different between males and females; however, whole body iron loss from sweat was two times greater in males due, in part, to a greater sweat rate.

Should athletes take an iron supplement? Not really. By first pursuing dietary/cooking habits that include the following, it is possible to achieve adequate iron intake and absorption.[16,91]

1. Include foods that are rich in vitamin C. Vitamin C helps the body absorb iron.
2. Include breads, cereals, and pastas that have been "fortified," "enriched," or have iron listed among the ingredients.
3. Avoid drinking tea or coffee at meal time. The tannins found in tea and the tannin-like substances found in coffee can reduce iron absorption.
4. Eat lean red meats and the dark meat of chicken and turkey.
5. If taking both calcium and iron supplements, be sure to take nutrients at least three hours apart. Calcium supplements, especially amounts >300 mg, can decrease iron absorption.
6. When cooking acidic foods, such as tomato sauce, use iron cookware because some of the iron from the pan is taken up by the food.

In our foods iron is present in several different forms. Iron that is part of the hemoglobin or myoglobin molecule in animal meat is called heme iron. This type is absorbed more than twice as efficiently as elemental iron (nonheme iron). Nonheme iron is also present in animal products as well as in vegetables and grains. Consuming heme iron along with nonheme iron increases the absorption of nonheme iron. Ultimately, however, the most important factor influencing iron absorption is the body's need for it.

Although an iron supplement has not been shown to definitely improve performance in persons without anemia, it is indicated for most athletes who have anemia resulting from an iron deficiency.[32,66] This may include some females who experience extra iron loss during menstruation.[93] Note that this does not mean that all female athletes should ingest an iron supplement—rather only those who are iron deficient and/or anemic. Although studies of physically trained females have shown significant decreases in serum iron or iron stores,[11,31,52] consistent alterations in serum iron levels, hemoglobin concentration, or iron-binding capacity have not been observed.[100] A first indication of a

table 15.1

Comparison of energy nutrients and fiber content among the daily typical American diet, a preferred (more healthy) diet, and a diet for an endurance training athlete

Nutrient	Typical Diet*		Preferred Diet*		Endurance Athlete's Diet†	
	(% of total kcal)	(grams)	(% of total kcal)	(grams)	(% of total kcal)	(grams)
Carbohydrate	50%	300	60%	360	70%	963
Simple	26%	156	15%	90	20%	275
Complex	24%	144	45%	270	50%	688
Fiber	—	12–16	—	20–35	—	20–35
Fat	35%–38%	93–101	28%–30%	75–80	17%–18%	103–110
Saturated	15%	40	10%	27	7%–8%	42–49
Others	20%–23%	53–61	18%–20%	48–53	10%	61
Protein	12%–15%	72–90	10%–12%	60–72	12%–13%	165–178

*Based on a 2400 kcal · d^{-1} diet.
†Based on a 5500 kcal · d^{-1} diet.

problem in iron stores may be a reduced aerobic capacity.[13,66] If iron deficiency is suspected by the athlete or coach, a medical examination is needed to confirm the condition. If confirmed, therapy should be initiated and monitored.

Other Trace Minerals

As the name implies, large quantities of the trace minerals are not required in our diet. Except for zinc[64,90] and possibly chromium,[90] most persons living in the U.S. achieve their RDA or adequate daily estimate of the trace minerals through their normal dietary habits. This includes most athletes, who, as they increase their caloric intake in response to the increased energy demand of their activity, experience an associated increase in the trace minerals. The RDA for zinc is 12 mg · d^{-1} and 15 mg · d^{-1} for females and males age 11 and older, respectively. The daily zinc intake among the general U.S. population is estimated to be 9 mg for females and 15 mg for males. Notice the discrepancy among females between the RDA for zinc and the estimated dietary intake.

As you might guess, some athletes exhibit a deficiency in some of the trace nutrients.[29,30] Such a finding may result from how a trace mineral is metabolized, absorbed, or lost (urine, sweat) as a consequence of exercise. These include athletes who restrict caloric intake for sport-specific purposes (e.g., gymnasts, wrestlers) and others regularly involved in endurance events associated with very high sweat rates.[64] Clearly, much more research is needed in this area. However, the best approach for both athletes and persons in the general population is, again, a well-balanced diet that provides trace minerals from a variety of sources. This includes lean red meats, skim milk and skim milk products, skinless poultry, seafood, grains, legumes, and green vegetables.

Food Requirements and Habits

The current and suggested relative contributions for each of the energy nutrients are summarized in table 15.1. The total amount of energy a person requires is directly related to:

1. Periods of rapid growth
2. Age
3. Physical activity
4. Body size

During the rapid growing years (10 to 22 years for boys and 10 to 18 years for girls), there is a gradual increase in the minimal daily food requirements. This increase is more pronounced in males than in females (table 15.2). As we become older, however, our daily energy needs decrease (figure 15.5). The biggest difference in food requirements for the athlete versus the nonathlete is the total number of calories consumed—with the athlete requiring more. This is accomplished by increasing the relative contribution of carbohydrates to 60% to 70% of calories consumed[4,44] (table 15.1).

15.2
table

Median weight, height and energy intake per the recommended dietary allowances established in 1989 by the National Research Council

	Age	Weight		Height	
	(yr)	(lb)	(kg)	(in.)	kcal · d^{-1}
Males	7–10	62	28	52	2000
	11–14	99	45	62	2500
	15–18	145	66	69	3000
	19–24	160	72	70	2900
Females	7–10	62	28	52	2000
	11–14	101	46	62	2200
	15–18	120	55	64	2200
	19–24	128	58	65	2200

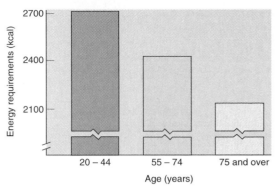

Figure 15.5

Daily energy requirements for men ages 20 years and older.

(Based on data from McGandy, et al.[60])

Selecting Foods

Exactly, how does one go about eating "a well-balanced diet from a variety of foods?" Well, the answer is quite simple and it applies to both the general population and the athlete alike—it is called the *Food Guide Pyramid*! Developed in 1991 by the U.S. Department of Agriculture and the U.S. Department of Health and Human Services,[86] the Food Guide Pyramid (figure 15.6) represents an effective visual outline of how much to eat from each of the five food groups. The pyramid's message is "Bottoms Up"! Specifically, to eat a healthy diet Americans need to choose the majority of their foods from the bottom two levels of the pyramid. Conversely, they should decrease their intake of dietary fat by choosing less often those foods from the top two levels of the pyramid. Some ultra or heavy endurance athletes may need to increase even further their intake of carbohydrates. This is accomplished by simply choosing even more foods from the base of the pyramid.

Snack Foods and Fast Foods

In the 1960s and 1970s much research was undertaken to evaluate the spacing between and number of meals eaten per day. Some studies suggested that eating fewer and larger meals (e.g., 2 to 3 per day) impaired the body's normal physiology[34,35,87,97,98] or led to weight gain, while others did not.[10,36,59,85,87,99] It appears that eating more than three meals per day either has no effect or provides a beneficial effect on metabolism. Additionally, very active persons, such as the athlete[4] requiring 5,000 to 6,000 kcal · d^{-1}, or the triathlete[94] who may consume up to 10,000 kcal · d^{-1},

simply cannot consume all the food they need to in 2 to 3 meals.[45] Therefore, extra meals or healthful snacks are a "mathematical" must (table 15.3). A list of both **fast foods** and more healthful snacks is shown in table 15.4. Generally, a healthier snack represents one that provides < 5 g of fat per serving.

Eating before Exercise: The Pregame Meal

Proper nutrition, as emphasized throughout this chapter, is an ongoing and year-round task. No foods consumed just prior to competition will lead to "super" aerobic or anaerobic performance.

What then should the pregame meal consist of? To answer this question we must recall which energy nutrients are predominately used for fuel during exercise as well as understand the differences in the rate of digestion among the various nutrients. With respect to rates of digestion—in order from fastest to slowest—they are simple carbohydrates (sugars), complex carbohydrates, protein, and fat. The bottom line: athletes should consume 300 to 1400 kcal from a meal consisting of 50 to 300 grams of carbohydrate, <15% to 20% kcal from fat, and a very modest amount of protein, 2.5 to 6 hours prior to an endurance event.[4,20,44,45,80,90] Such a meal is easily digested and will supply the carbohydrates needed to "top off" glycogen stores in both the skeletal muscles and the liver. Foods to avoid include those known to produce intestinal gas (legumes and other foods rich in fiber) and highly seasoned foods. Because of individual differences among athletes, the timing and composition of the pregame meal should be modified according to the needs of the individual. Doing so will help avoid gastrointestinal distress during exercise.

For those athletes prone to experiencing gastrointestinal distress (nausea, cramps, diarrhea, indigestion) before and soon after starting competition, a moderate liquid pregame meal might be considered. Such a meal offers

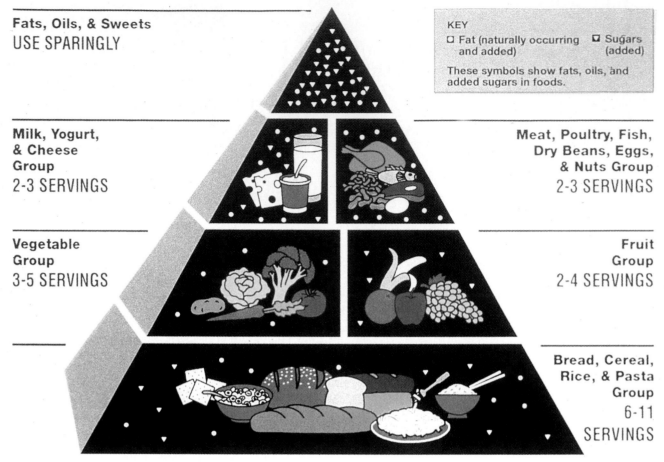

Fats, Oils, & Sweets
USE SPARINGLY

KEY
□ Fat (naturally occurring   ▽ Sugars
    and added)   (added)

These symbols show fats, oils, and
added sugars in foods.

**Milk, Yogurt,
& Cheese
Group**
2-3 SERVINGS

**Meat, Poultry, Fish,
Dry Beans, Eggs,
& Nuts Group**
2-3 SERVINGS

**Vegetable
Group**
3-5 SERVINGS

**Fruit
Group**
2-4 SERVINGS

**Bread, Cereal,
Rice, & Pasta
Group**
6-11
SERVINGS

Figure 15.6
The Food Guide Pyramid—emphasizing the consumption of foods from the lower two levels of the pyramid.
Source: U.S. Department of Agriculture and U.S. Department of Health and Human Services.[86]

15.3

**Distribution of calories from meals and snacks
for an athlete who consumes 5,000 kcal · d⁻¹**

	kcal	% of daily total
First breakfast	1050	21
Second breakfast	700	14
Lunch	1350	27
Dinner	1150	23
Two snacks	750	15

satiety (desire to eat is diminished), assists with hydration, is more easily digested, and does not hinder performance.[38,39] Various commercially prepared liquid formulas are available in a variety of flavors, yet these too may require a bit of trial and error before finding one that provides

the nutrients required while at the same limiting stomach upset. A word of advice to coaches and athletes: the practice of changing a pregame meal (from solid to liquid or from 6 hours to 3 hours before event) should be introduced and modified slowly over the course of the preseason and/or early season. It is unwise to adjust pre-event plans to such an extent when one is preparing for end-of-the-season meets or events. Finally, some athletes may not tolerate eating any foods prior to competition; these individuals should then consume a meal similar to that stated above the evening before. Examples of carbohydrate-rich food servings include spaghetti (1 cup), a bagel, two low-fat or nonfat muffins, pita bread (1½ slices), and breakfast cereal (¾ cup) with nonfat milk (1½ cup). Each of the above contains approximately 30 grams of carbohydrates.

Ingestion of Large Amounts of Glucose (Sugar) before Exercise

The ingestion of large amounts (50 to 200 grams) of carbohydrates (hard candy, juice) just 30 to 60 minutes before competition was previously thought to adversely affect per-

15.4

Carbohydrate and fat content of various fast foods and healthier* snacks

	Total kcal	Fat (g)	Fat (% of kcal)	Carbohydrate (g)	Carbohydrate (% of kcal)
Breads and Cereal					
Bagel	163	< 2	8	31	76
Cereal (1 cup) with skim milk (1 cup)	175	2	10	28	63
Pancake (1; 4″ diameter)	60	2	30	9	60
Pretzels (1 ounce)	112	1	8	23	82
Waffle (medium)	245	13	48	26	42
Fruits					
Apple (1)	90	< 1	5	21	94
Banana (1)	116	< 1	4	27	92
Cranberry juice (1 cup)	144	< 1	2	36	98
Grape juice	154	< 1	1	38	95
Grapes (1 cup)	114	< 1	7	28	90
Raisins (2/3 cup)	296	< 1	1	71	96
Meats, Poultry, and Nuts					
Grilled chicken sandwich (plain, with bun)	290	7	22	35	48
Hot dog (with bun)	242	15	55	18	30
McDonald's hamburger	260	10	35	31	48
McDonald's Big Mac	560	32	51	43	31
Nuts (3 tablespoons)	155	13	75	5	13
Roast beef sandwich	346	14	36	33	38
Taco Bell's mexican pizza	575	37	58	40	28
Milk and Milk Products					
Carnation Instant Breakfast with skim milk	216	< 1	1	36	67
Dairy Queen sundae	319	10	28	53	66
Lowfat frozen yogurt (1 cup)	216	2	8	42	78
McDonald's low-fat shake	320	2	6	66	82
Desserts and Other Foods					
Angel food cake (1 slice)	126	< 1	1	29	92
Brownie	105	5	43	15	57
Cupcake	130	5	35	21	66
Fig Newton (1)	53	< 1	16	11	80
Layer cake (with frosting)	268	11	37	40	60
Microwave light popcorn (1 cup)	28	1	32	4	58
Nutri-Grain Bar	140	4	26	26	74
Pie (1 slice)	323	14	39	49	60
Pizza Hut Thin 'n Crispy pizza (cheese, 1 slice)	199	9	41	19	38
Popcorn (1 cup, in oil)	40	2	45	5	50
Potato chips (1 ounce)	139	9	60	15	43
Soda (16 oz.)	202	0	0	51	100

*Less than 5 grams of fat per serving.

Source: Data from Jean A. T. Pennington, IB, *Bowers & Church's Food Values of Portions Commonly Used,* 16th edition, 1994, Lippincott, and Nutritions IV™,

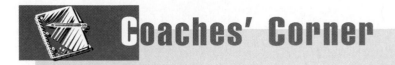

In 1992, the American College of Sports Medicine convened an expert panel to address an area of growing concern in sports medicine—the Female Athlete Triad. The Triad represents a group of disorders observed in adolescent and young adult female athletes, which includes disordered eating, osteoporosis, and amenorrhea.[96] By themselves, each disorder is worrisome and potentially disabling. When observed in combination, the outcome can be devastating.

With respect to eating disorders, the two most common eating disorders are **anorexia nervosa** and bulimia nervosa.[90] A pressure to maintain a coach-prescribed or self-prescribed weight puts the female athlete at risk for these disorders. The frequency of anorexia nervosa (anorexia implies loss of appetite) in the general population is estimated at 1% in girls between the ages of 12 and 18 years. It is less common among adult women and rare among African-American women. Men too can exhibit this disorder, but they represent only 5% of reported cases. Fifty percent of persons with this disorder recover in 6 months; the rest simply exist with the disease. About 3% to 8% of persons with anorexia nervosa die prematurely. The prevalence of bulimia nervosa (bulimia means "great hunger") has been difficult to determine, but present estimates are that 3% to 9% of adolescent and college-age women suffer from it. Health problems associated with this disorder include demineralization of teeth (due to repeated vomiting), increased infections, stomach and esophageal ulcers and tears, and hypokalemia.

At the elite level, potentially all adolescent and some adult female athletes are at risk. Male athletes (e.g., boxers, jockeys) may also be affected, but less research has been reported in this area. Additionally, athletes within certain sports are at an even greater risk than others. For example, 522 of all 603 elite Norwegian female athletes (age 12 to 35 years) were recently screened and 117 (22%) were classified as "at risk" for an eating disorder.[84] Using a follow-up interview/clinical examination, 92 of the 117 athletes were classified with anorexia nervosa, bulimia nervosa, or athletica nervosa. The latter represents a subclinical but still serious eating disorder specific to athletes. In this study the prevalence of eating disorders was higher among athletes participating in sports that emphasized a lean appearance (diving, figure skating, gymnastics) or obtaining a specific weight (judo, karate). Trigger factors associated with the onset of eating disorders included prolonged periods of dieting, frequent weight fluctuations, a sudden increase in training volume, and traumatic events such as an injury or loss of a coach.

Treating the incidence of these disorders, and the disorders themselves, requires a multidimensional approach. Widespread education of the athletes' coaches, parents, and trainers about the "trigger factors" and consequences has already begun and must continue. Additionally, further research and action is needed to develop coordinated treatment strategies between athlete, parent, physician, and coach. Such strategies should reduce preoccupation with food and body weight, improve eating habits, increase body weight, and restore menstrual function.[90]

---

formance because of an exaggerated release of insulin by the pancreas. Over a 30 to 60 minute time period, such a release leads to a fall in blood sugar and, much to the dismay of the endurance athlete, can force the body to call upon muscle glycogen sooner as a metabolic fuel during exercise.[24,37] We know now that this practice does not usually cause premature fatigue or decrease performance among most athletes, especially if they have eaten a meal within the past several hours and perform an adequate warm up.[40,58,95] However, since some athletes may be sensitive to the insulin surge as described above, individuals should first experiment with pre-event (30 to 60 min) carbohydrate feeding during practice or an early season meet to see if it adversely or positively impacts performance. In any event, if a person wishes to consume glucose or sugar 30 to 60 min-utes before exercise, it would be best to use a carbohydrate concentration that is similar to what is recommended during exercise (see below).

Eating during Exercise/Competition: Replacement of Sugar and Water

Let us not forget that the most important nutrient to consume during exercise is water (chapter 19). For events lasting greater than 30 minutes, every attempt should be made to consume water at a pace equal to water loss. In fact, even it is prudent to consume 250 mL to 500 mL of water about 1.5 to 2 hr before exercise.[2,90] Doing so promotes adequate hydration and allows sufficient time for excretion of any excess.

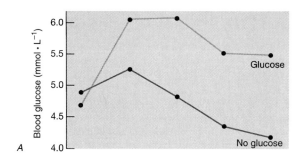

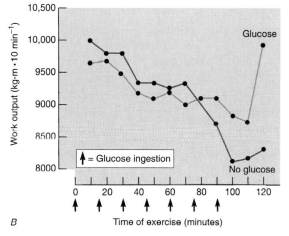

Figure 15.7

A. Ingestion of some liquid glucose during prolonged physical exercise will help spare muscle glycogen and delay or prevent hypoglycemia or low blood sugar levels. This in turn helps reduce and/or delay fatigue as demonstrated by an 11% greater work output during the last 30 minutes of exercise, B.

(Based on data of Ivy et al.[48])

For endurance events that are longer than 60 to 90 minutes, it is generally agreed that adding flavoring (e.g., grape) and carbohydrates to the fluid is beneficial because not only do carbohydrates and flavoring improve palatability and therefore fluid intake,[92] but the carbohydrates also help spare muscle glycogen and delay or prevent hypoglycemia (low blood-sugar levels).[1,19,23,48,68,88] Both the glycogen-sparing effect and the deterrent effect on hypoglycemia help reduce and/or delay fatigue. An example of this is shown in figure 15.7. The subjects in this study[45] were orally given 12.5 g of liquid glucose every 15 minutes for the first 90 minutes of a two-hour exercise period using a cycle ergometer. As is indicated in figure 15.7A, blood glucose was maintained at much higher levels when glucose was consumed than when no glucose was given. The total work performed during the two-hour ride was not much different between trials until the last 30 minutes of exercise (figure 15.7B).

Current recommendations for carbohydrate ingestion during exercise are related to the volume of fluid ingested. When drinking 600 to 1200 mL · hr^{-1}, a volume associated

with a gastric emptying rate that is comfortable for most people,[26] the carbohydrate concentration of the drink can range between 4% to 8%.[2,20,44,90] This approach supplies the 30 to 60 g of carbohydrates that are needed per hour,[2,4,90] which is consistent with the approximate rate of glucose metabolism during exercise (up to 1 g · min^{-1}). Table 15.5 shows how a variety of commercially available sport drinks stack up to the American College of Sports Medicine guideline for the replacement of carbohydrates during exercise. The inclusion of sodium (125 to 175 mg · 250 mL^{-1} of water) in the fluid may also enhance palatability, promote fluid retention, and assist with the prevention of hyponatremia due to the excessive consumption of fluids. Sodium, however, has little effect on enhancing the intestinal absorption of water.[2]

The nature of the carbohydrate in the drink can be glucose, sucrose, or a complex carbohydrate (maltodextrin). Fructose does not appear to have the same effect on enhancing performance and may lead to intestinal disturbance in some athletes.[20] Additionally, an interesting study conducted by Mason and colleagues in Australia compared liquid versus solid carbohydrate feedings during two hours of exercise at 65% of V̇O$_2$ max.[62] Carbohydrate (25 g) was ingested at 30, 60, and 90 min of exercise, via either 500 mL of a 5% (5 g · 100 mL^{-1}) liquid supplement or as a food bar eaten (chewed well) along with 500 mL of water. Results indicated that both the liquid and solid forms of carbohydrate produced similar heart rate, V̇O$_2$, blood glucose, and blood insulin responses during the two hours of exercise.

Table 15.6 is provided to assist the athlete or coach with knowing just how many g of carbohydrates are consumed, when a desired amount of fluid is ingested *every 15 minutes* using a carbohydrate concentration of between 4% and 8%. For example, if the day is hot, sweat rate is high, and a 3 hour event is anticipated, then a needed water intake of 1200 mL · hr^{-1} (300 mL every 15 min) would require a 4% to 5% drink and provide 48 to 60 g of carbohydrates. Alternately, on cooler days and/or during shorter events of 60 min to 90 min, a needed water intake of 600 mL · hr^{-1} (150 mL every 15 min) might involve a 7% to 8% drink to provide 42 g to 48 g of carbohydrates. Both methods will promote a glycogen-sparing effect and delay or prevent hypoglycemia. However, since most athletes like to spend as little time as possible drinking during competition, the smaller volume (150 mL) is most often appreciated.

Consuming a drink with a concentration >10% carbohydrates results in the net movement of fluid into the intestinal lumen because of the high osmolality of the solution. The fluid entering the lumen came from the vascular system and extracellular space. The end result: the potential to worsen the effects of dehydration.[2]

Eating after Exercise/Competition

Many athletes find that eating a meal right after having exercised is unsettling. Despite this, a concerted effort should be made to replenish carbohydrates and water. Not only will

15.5

Comparison of nutrient content (per 8 oz. or 240 mL serving) of various sport drinks and other drinks to the American College of Sports Medicine guidelines for fluid replacement during exercise[2]

Beverage	Energy (kcal)	Carbohydrate (g)	Carbohydrate %	Sodium (mg)	Potassium (mg)	Carbohydrate Ingredient
American College of Sports Medicine Position Statement	40–76	10–19	4–6%	*	*	Sucrose, glucose and other complex carbohydrates
Allsport® Pepsico	70	19	8%	55	55	High-fructose corn syrup
Coca-Cola®	103	27	11%	6	0	High-fructose corn syrup, sucrose
Diet soft drinks	1	0	0%	2–8	18–100	None
Endura® Meta Genics, Inc.	60	15	6%	46	80	Glucose polymers, fructose
Exceed® Weider Health & Fitness	70	17	7%	50	45	Glucose polymers, fructose
Gatorade® Thirst Quencher The Gatorade Co.	50	14	6%	110	30	Sucrose, glucose, fructose
Orange Juice	104	25	10%	6	436	Fructose, sucrose, glucose
Powerade® Coca-Cola	70	19	8%	55	30	High-fructose corn syrup, glucose polymers (maltodextrins)
Quickick® Quickick	67	16	7%	100	23	High-fructose corn syrup
Water	0	0	0	Low	Low	None

*No guideline given.
Reprinted by permission of Robert Murray, The Quaker Oats Company, Barrington, IL.

this help with rehydration and the maintenance of blood glucose, but it is essential if the athlete plans to vigorously exercise the next day.

Both liver glycogen and skeletal muscle glycogen stores are nearly fully depleted after an endurance event, such as the marathon. However, given adequate carbohydrate consumption (650 to 900 g), both sites can be fully replenished in a 24-hour period.[4,79] As part of this process, it appears that the muscle glycogen stores are preferentially replenished over liver glycogen stores.[79]

If the athlete intends to exercise vigorously or compete the next day, then the timing and amount of carbohydrate ingestion become very important. Generally, up to 600 g of easily digestible carbohydrate should be consumed over the 4 to 6 hours immediately following an event.[4] Specifically, ingestion of 0.5 to 1.5 $g \cdot kg^{-1}$ of body weight should begin one hour after a glycogen depleting event and be repeated at two-hour intervals. This promotes the resynthesis of muscle glycogen at a much faster rate than if the athlete had waited for one or two hours before starting.[45,79,80]

table 15.6

The amount of carbohydrates injested based on desired fluid intake and carbohydrate concentration of the drink

Carbohydrate concentration	Grams of carbohydrates consumed per hour at various fluid intakes			
(g · 100 mL^{-1})*	150 mL · 15 min^{-1}	200 mL · 15 min^{-1}	250 mL · 15 min^{-1}	300 mL · 15 min^{-1}
4%	—	32	40	48
5%	30	40	50	60
6%	36	48	60	—
7%	42	56	—	—
8%	48	—	—	—

*For example, 4 g · 100 mL^{-1} of water = 4%.

Muscle glycogen synthesis is improved even further if replenishment is begun immediately after finishing exercise and repeated at two-hour intervals. The message is clear: to quickly re-establish muscle glycogen, carbohydrate ingestion should start as soon as possible after exercise is finished.

With respect to the type of carbohydrate consumed, the rate of muscle glycogen synthesis is enhanced when using sucrose or glucose (versus fructose).[45] Several commercially available sport drinks containing a higher (10% to 20%) concentrations of carbohydrates are available and may prove useful at this time. There is, however, no difference if an equal amount of carbohydrate is consumed in a liquid versus a solid form.[73] Finally, glycogen resynthesis in the skeletal muscles appears to be attenuated when the muscle was previously exercised in an eccentric versus concentric manner.[25]

Can Diet Affect Performance?

Hopefully, by now, it is clear that carbohydrates play an important role in endurance exercise performance. Diets lacking in carbohydrates negatively effect work performance.[5,7,46] One study (figure 15.8) administered three different diets to men who were then asked to exercise to exhaustion on a bicycle ergometer. Time to exhaustion on a normal (mixed) diet was 114 minutes, whereas on a high-carbohydrate diet men did not stop until after 167 minutes. Not surprisingly, while on the low-carbohydrate diet (high-protein, high-fat diet) exhaustion was reached after only 57

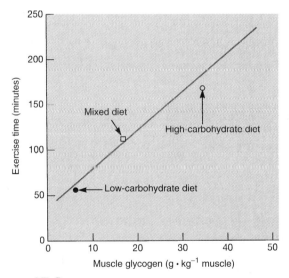

Figure 15.8

Effects of a mixed diet, a low-carbohydrate diet, and a high-carbohydrate diet on the initial glycogen content of the quadriceps femoris muscle and the duration of exercise on a bicycle ergometer; the higher the initial muscle glycogen content, the longer the duration of exercise.

(Based on data from Bergström et al.[7])

minutes of exercise. Therefore, an almost threefold increase in exercise time was evident when comparing the low-carbohydrate diet to the high-carbohydrate diet. In agreement with the above data was the fact that glycogen content of the quadriceps femoris muscle (obtained via skeletal muscle needle biopsy) prior to exercise was 17.5 g · kg^{-1}

15.7

Food choices suitable for a high carbohydrate diet

Breakfast

Cold cereal (1½ cup)
Oatmeal (1½ cup)
Pancakes
2–4 slices of whole wheat toast
1 oz. low-fat cheese
Low-fat yogurt

Low-fat/nonfat muffin
Banana, strawberries, other fruit
½ cup juice
Skim milk
Bagel with nonfat cream cheese

Lunch or Dinner

4 oz. grilled chicken (without skin) or
   turkey breast sandwich with bun
3–4 oz. lean hamburger (ground sirloin) or
   lean roast beef
2 tortillas with beans, lettuce, tomatoes,
   and salsa
Rice (brown, white, wild)
Legumes (garbanzo beans, kidney beans)
Tuna in water, with or without nonfat salad
   dressing
Pasta (1½ cup)
Cornbread

Pita bread
2 slices of whole wheat bread or roll
Baked potato with low-fat cottage cheese
Salad with nonfat dressing
½ cup applesauce
Vegetable/lentil soup
Low-fat yogurt
Assorted fresh fruits and vegetables
Sherbert
Fat-free frozen yogurt
Skim milk
Oatmeal/raisin cookies

---

of wet muscle while on the mixed diet, 35.1 g · kg^{-1} of wet muscle when following the high-carbohydrate diet, and only 6.3 g · kg^{-1} of wet muscle while following the low-carbohydrate diet.

Muscle Glycogen-Loading or Carbohydrate-Loading

The amount of glycogen resynthesized in skeletal muscle can be increased to values much higher than normal by manipulating an athlete's diet and/or training regimen.[7,8,9,46,47,51,65,75,78] For most athletes such an approach—called carbohydrate loading—has an advantageous effect on performance. The practice of carbohydrate loading is effective for continuous events lasting 90 to 120 minutes or longer or for shorter-duration (10 to 30 min), continuous events that are repeated several times in a 24-hour period (e.g., 24-hour relay). Why these events? Because muscle glycogen stores do not limit one-time high-intensity, short-duration events. A brief description of each of three methods used to carbohydrate load are listed below.

1. The first and now most common method involves dietary manipulation only. Endurance athletes who, after eating their usual diet of 350 to 500 g of carbohydrate per day, then consume a high-carbohydrate diet (600 g or more per day) for three or four days prior to competition. This approach can increase glycogen stores from approximately 20 g to around 35 g · kg^{-1} of muscle. If the athlete has an usual diet that already exceeds 600 g · d^{-1} (likely 60% to 65% of total kcal), carbohydrate intake should be calculated at a greater percentage (70% to 75%) of total kcal and consumed at that higher level. Food choices suitable for a high-carbohydrate diet are shown in table 15.7. During the high-carbohydrate diet period no exhausting exercise should be performed.

2. A second and less common procedure for carbohydrate loading combines exercise and diet. Starting four to five days prior to competition, glycogen stores in the muscles are first depleted over a one to two-day period using strenuous, longer duration (60 min tapering to 40 min) exercise. During this time the athlete consumes a normal diet (350 to 500 g of carbohydrates). They then follow with a high-carbohydrate diet for three days, during which no exhaustive exercise is performed. This has been shown to increase glycogen stores to approximately 40 g · kg^{-1} of muscle (figure 15.9).

3. The least common (and least enjoyed) method for carbohydrate loading involves exercise and two

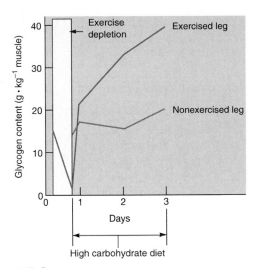

Figure 15.9

In this study, subjects pedaled a cycle ergometer with one leg to exhaustion to deplete muscle glycogen content while the other leg rested. Subjects then consumed a high-carbohydrate diet for three days. Note that glycogen content increased markedly in the leg previously emptied of its glycogen content.

(Based on data from Bergström and Hultman.[9])

special diets. Strenuous exercise is again started six days prior to competition to deplete glycogen stores over a three-day period. During this time, the athlete follows a diet very low in carbohydrates and high in fat and protein. This is followed by three days of light or no exercise along with a diet high in carbohydrates. Literally starved for glycogen, the muscles supercompensate at levels approaching $45 \text{ g} \cdot \text{kg}^{-1}$ of muscle.

Several cautions should be observed when attempting carbohydrate loading:

1. Of the procedures described above, the first (diet alone) is clearly the one that is now in widespread use among endurance athletes. It provides quite satisfactory increases in muscle glycogen, with few athlete-related complaints. For obvious reasons, the third method is the most difficult to follow—*and it often results in feelings of fatigue, nausea, and irritability among athletes.* Although this method may provide a higher level of muscle glycogen than the first method, it should only be used, if at all, for more important competitions. In fact, most athletes feel the associated dietary manipulations are just too cumbersome, and the exhaustive training represents a window for injury.

2. Whichever procedure is used, carbohydrate loading is associated with water being stored in the skeletal muscles. For example, increasing muscle glycogen stores from $15 \text{ g} \cdot \text{kg}^{-1}$ of muscle to $40 \text{ g} \cdot \text{kg}^{-1}$ of

muscle in a person with 20 kg of muscle, increases glycogen in the body by 500 g or 0.5 kg [$(40 \text{ g} \cdot \text{kg}^{-1} - 15 \text{ g} \cdot \text{kg}^{-1}) \times 20$ kg of muscle]. Along with this there is a 1.3 kg increase in body weight because of water (2.6 g of water stored for every 1 g of glycogen $\times$ 500 g of glycogen). The total increase in weight is 1.8 kg. For some athletes, this may be enough to create a feeling of heaviness or stiffness that initially hinders rather than helps performance.

3. On very rare occasions there have been clinical reports of myoglobinuria (myoglobin in the urine) in athletes who persistently use carbohydrate loading.[6]

4. Most importantly, athletes considering carbohydrate loading should do so with advanced planning. The use of practices, scrimmages, or early season meets to experience its effect on performance and to modify the approach accordingly is advised.

A summary of the three glycogen-loading procedures is shown in figure 15.10. As mentioned above, the simplest procedure (procedure 1) is now favored among endurance-trained athletes. Procedure 2 and especially procedure 3 have fallen into disfavor because of shortcomings associated with the depletion phase.

Fat Loading

You should recall that fat, too, is an important fuel that is used during the performance of endurance exercise. Indeed, the proportion of the energy expended from the oxidation of fat is related to exercise duration and intensity. In theory, making fat more available for oxidation during higher intensity endurance exercise (fat loading) could help delay fatigue via a carbohydrate sparing effect. This hypothesis is plausible and, in fact, some data supports such an effort.[13,81] For example, in one study[24] seven men were analyzed during 30 minutes of treadmill exercise to determine the effects of increased availability of blood-borne free fatty acids on the utilization of muscle glycogen. The fatty acids were made available by first having the subjects consume a "fatty" meal 4.5 to 5 hours before the exercise was to begin. Then, 30 minutes prior to exercise, heparin, an anticoagulant, was injected into a vein in the forearm to promote the breakdown of the blood triglycerides to free fatty acids. The results are shown in figure 15.11. As you can see, more fat and less muscle glycogen was used when a fatty meal preceded the 30-minute exercise period than when no fatty meal was consumed.

It is important to note that the above study does not apply to the typical exercise training setting or competition. Clearly, intravenous heparin is not part of standard pre-race planning and preparation. Despite a resurgence in the popularity of this method among misinformed yet well-intentioned athletes, fat loading has not been proven as a means to optimize human performance.[81] A diet that is largely carbohydrates remains preferred.

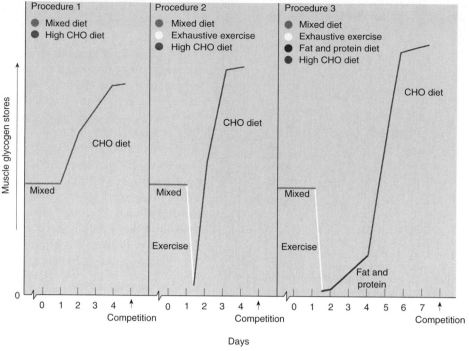

Figure 15.10

Summary of muscle glycogen-loading procedures. CHO = carbohydrates.

Source: Data from B. Saltin and L. Hermansen, "Glycogen Stores and Prolonged Severe Exercise" in G. Blix, Ed., Symposia of the Swedish Nutrition Foundation V, Nutrition and Physical Activity, 1967, Almquist & Wiksell International, Stockholm, Sweden.

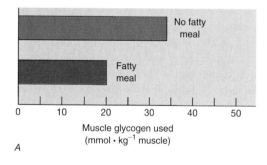

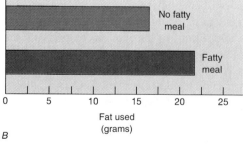

Figure 15.11

Effects of a fatty meal on fat and muscle glycogen usage. Less muscle glycogen (A) and more fat (B) were used when a fatty meal preceded the 30 minute exercise period than when no fatty meal was consumed. As a result, muscle glycogen is spared, fatigue is delayed, and endurance prolonged.

(Based on data from Costill et al.[24])

Summary

Carbohydrates, fats, proteins, vitamins, minerals, and water are essential to the diet. Carbohydrates, fats, and proteins are called the energy nutrients because they are used as food fuels during metabolism. Monosaccharides and disaccharides represent simple carbohydrates, and polysaccharides (glycogen, starch) represent complex carbohydrates. Glycogen (stored in the liver and skeletal muscles) and blood glucose are the two forms of carbohydrate food fuels. Excess carbohydrate intake is stored as a lipid.

Lipids are found in the body as triglycerides, phospholipids, and cholesterol. Triglycerides are stored in the skeletal muscles and in the fat cells (adipocyte) and are made up of glycerol and three fatty acids (FA). When the carbon atoms of FA are chemically saturated with hydrogen atoms, it is referred to as a saturated fatty acid; when they are not, it is referred to as an unsaturated fatty acid.

Proteins play a more limited role as a food fuel, contributing between 5% and 15% of total kcal during endurance activities. Proteins consist of various combinations of amino acids and are the building blocks of tissue. There are twenty different amino acids in the body, 10 of which are referred to as essential amino acids.

Essential amino acids cannot be synthesized by the body and as a result, their only source is through the diet. Contrary to popular belief, the protein requirement during heavy exercise training, or the initial muscle development phase that occurs with resistance weight training, is only moderately increased in adults (from 0.8 g · kg^{-1} of body weight to 1.8 g · kg^{-1} of body weight). This increase can usually be met by the average U.S. diet.

Vitamins are essential parts of enzymes or coenzymes that are vital to normal metabolism. The water soluble vitamins (C and B complex) need to be constantly supplied in the diet. The fat soluble vitamins (A, D, E, and K) are stored in the body. Vitamin supplementation above the recommended dietary allowance does not increase exercise performance.

Deficiencies of either the major or trace minerals are generally uncommon in the U.S. and Canada. The only minerals that may need supplementation, for both health and performance reasons, are calcium and iron. This is of special concern among young females involved in endurance training or elite level competition—especially those with amenorrhea.

The biggest difference in food requirements for the athlete versus the nonathlete is the total number of calories consumed; the athlete needs more. The Food Guide Pyramid published in 1991 is meant to assist individuals with selecting a diet that is high in complex carbohydrates and low in fat. Athletes who require a large daily caloric intake may need to eat five or six meals per day.

Carbohydrates should be the major constituent of the pregame meal and should be consumed no later than 2½ to 6 hours before competition. Doing so will help ensure that glycogen levels are "topped off" prior to competition. Liquid meals for some athletes are suitable as the pregame meal and may help lessen gastrointestinal distress. Fats and spicy foods should be excluded from the pregame meal. Large amounts of sugar in liquid and solid form should be avoided 30 to 45 minutes before exercise is to begin. Drinks containing 4 to 8 grams per 100 mL of liquid can be consumed both immediately prior to and during exercise. The consumption of such a drink helps prevent low blood-sugar levels (hypoglycemia) and dehydration, and it delays fatigue.

Immediately after exercise, carbohydrate ingestion, even in the liquid form (20% carbohydrate replacement drink), should be started—especially for persons who are scheduled to compete the next day. Doing so will ensure that glycogen stores in both liver and the skeletal muscles are replenished.

Endurance performance can be enhanced by increasing muscle glycogen stores via various manipulations of diet and/or exercise. The one approach that is most common among endurance athletes and is associated with less pre-event fatigue and irritability involves eating a mixed diet (350 to 450 g of carbohydrates · d^{-1}) up to three days prior to competition. Athletes then eat a high carbohydrate diet (600 g or more) for the final three days. Greater gains in muscle glycogen can be attained by further depleting the muscles of glycogen over a three-day period, via both a low-carbohydrate and high-fat/protein diet and strenuous exercise. This is then followed by eating a high-carbohydrate diet and engaging in light or no exercise for the two to three days leading up to competition. This method, however, is associated with symptoms that are not well tolerated by many athletes.

Fat loading, or the procedure of consuming a high-fat diet prior to competition, is theoretically designed to spare carbohydrate use and delay fatigue. Good scientific evidence does not overwhelmingly support this practice among athletes.

Questions

1. Describe the nutrient composition of the current American diet and contrast it to a more healthful diet. Is there a difference between the latter and the diet of an endurance athlete? Explain.
2. What are the energy nutrients? Broadly describe how the chemical structure for these nutrients are similar and different.
3. What is the difference between saturated fat, a monounsaturated fat, and a polyunsaturated fat?
4. Using the Food Guide Pyramid, explain how you would instruct high school athletes about what choices should be made for a general dietary plan that is well balanced. Include any special comments you might wish to make to females or vegetarians in the group.
5. To this same group of athletes, what are your suggestions about what foods (and the timing thereof) should be included in the pre-game meal for endurance activities? How about the power athletes, such as the football players and shot putters?
6. State the three disorders that, according to the American College of Sports Medicine, comprise the female athlete triad. Compare and contrast anorexia nervosa and bulimia nervosa. Characterize the type of athlete that is at risk for these problems.
7. What would you tell an endurance athlete concerning the intake of fluids (including carbohydrate concentration) before and during competition?
8. Following competition, should one's diet be modified? Explain.
9. Athletes participating in what types of sports might benefit from carbohydrate loading? Explain. Compare and contrast the strengths and shortcomings associated with the three methods of improving muscle glycogen stores via changes in diet and/or exercise.

10. Your friend is a member of the university basketball team, and during the off-season he is going to embark on a heavy weight-lifting and endurance-training program. He plans to begin consuming 25% of his calories from fat, 50% of his calories from carbohydrates, and the balance from protein. Do you agree or disagree with this plan? Support your answer.

References

1. Ahlborg, G., and P. Felig. 1976. Influence of glucose ingestion on fuel-hormone response during prolonged exercise. *J Appl Physiol.* 41(5):683–688.

2. American College of Sports Medicine Position Stand. 1996. Exercise and fluid replacement. *Med Sci Sports Exerc.* 28(1):i–vii.

3. American Dietetic Association. 1987. Position stand on nutrition for physical fitness and athletic performance for adults. *J Am Diet Assoc.* 87:933–939.

4. American Dietetic Association and the Canadian Dietetic Association. 1993. Position stand on nutrition for physical fitness and athletic performance for adults. *J Am Diet Assoc.* 93(6):691–696.

5. Åstrand, P.-O. 1968. Diet and athletic performance. *Fed Proc.* 26:1772, 1967; *Nutr Today.* 3(2):9.

6. Bank, W. J. 1977. Myoglobinuria in marathon runners: possible relationships to carbohydrate and lipid metabolism. *Ann NY Acad Sci.* 301:942–948.

7. Bergström, J., L. Hermansen, E. Hultman, and B. Saltin. 1967. Diet, muscle glycogen and physical performance. *Acta Physiol Scand.* 71:140–150.

8. Bergström, J., and E. Hultman. 1966. Muscle glycogen synthesis after exercise: an enhancing factor localized to the muscle cells in man. *Nature.* 210(5033):309–310.

9. ———. 1972. Nutrition for maximal sports performance. *JAMA.* 221(9):999–1006.

10. Bortz, W. M., A. Wroldsen, B. Issekutz, and K. Rodahl. 1966. Weight loss and frequency of feeding. *N Engl J Med.* 274:376–379.

11. Bottiger, L. E., A. Nyberg, I. Astrand, and P. O. Astrand. 1971. Iron administration to healthy, physically very active students. *Nord Med.* 85:396–398.

12. Brotherhood, J. 1984. Nutrition and sports performance. *Sports Med.* 1:350–389.

13. Burke, L., and R. Read. 1989. Sports nutrition. Approaching the nineties. *Sports Med.* 8:80–100.

14. Cathcart, E. P. 1925. The influence of muscle work on protein metabolism. *Physiol Rev.* 5:225–243.

15. Chandler, R. M., H. K. Byrne, J. G. Patterson, and J. L. Ivy. 1994. Dietary supplements affect the anabolic hormones after weight-training exercise. *J Appl Physiol.* 76(2):839–845.

16. Clark, N. 1985. Increasing dietary iron. *Phys Sportsmed.* 13(1):131–132.

17. Clarkson, P. M., and E. M. Haymes. 1995. Exercise and mineral status of athletes: calcium, magnesium, phosphorus, and iron. *Med Sci Sports Exerc.* 27(6):831–843.

18. Clement, D. B., and R. C. Asmundson. 1982. Nutritional intake and hematological parameters in endurance runners. *Phys Sportsmed.* 10(32):37–43.

19. Coggan, A. 1991. Carbohydrate ingestion during prolonged exercise: effects on metabolism and performance. *Exer Sport Sc Rev.* 19:1–40.

20. Coggan, A. R., and S. C. Swanson. 1992. Nutritional manipulations before and during endurance exercise: effects on performance. *Med Sci Sports Exerc.* 24(9-Suppl):S324–S330.

21. Consolazio, C. F., H. L. Johnson, R. Q. Nelson, J. G. Dramise, and J. H. Skala. 1975. Protein metabolism of intensive physical training in the young adult. *Am J Clin Nutr.* 28:29–35.

22. Corley, G., M. Demarest-Litchford, and T. Bazzarre. 1990. Nutrition knowledge and dietary practices of college coaches. *J Am Diet Assoc.* 90:705–709.

23. Costill, D. L., A. Bennett, G. Branam, and D. Eddy. 1973. Glucose ingestion at rest and during prolonged exercise. *J Appl Physiol.* 34:764–769.

24. Costill, D. L., E. Coyle, G. Dalsky, W. Evans, W. Fink, and D. Hoopes. 1977. Effects of elevated plasma FFA and insulin on muscle glycogen usage during exercise. *J Appl Physiol.* 43(4):695–699.

25. Costill, D. L., D. D. Pascoe, W. J. Fink, R. A. Roberts, and S. I. Barr. 1990. Impaired muscle glycogen resynthesis after eccentric exercise. *J Appl Physiol.* 69:46–50.

26. Coyle, E. F., and S. J. Montain. 1992. Benefits of fluid replacement with carbohydrate during exercise. *Med Sci Sports Exerc.* 24(9-Suppl):S324–S330.

27. Darling, R. C., R. E. Johnson, G. C. Pitts, R. C. Consolazio, and P. F. Robinson. 1955. Effects of variations in dietary protein on the physical well-being of men doing manual work. *J Nutr.* 28:273–281.

28. Dohm, G. L., G. J. Kasperak, E. B. Tapscott, and H. A. Barakat. 1985. Protein metabolism during endurance exercise. *Fed Proc.* 44(2):348–352.

29. Dressendorfer, R. H., and R. Sockolov. 1980. Hypozincemia in runners. *Physician Sportsmed.* 8:4, 97–100, 1980.

30. Duester, P. A., S. B. Kyle, P. B. Moser, et al. 1986. Nutritional survey of highly trained women runners. *Am J Clin Nutr.* 45:954–962, 1986.

31. Ehn, L., B. Carlmark, and S. Hoglund. 1984. Iron status in athletes involved in intense physical activity. *Med Sci Sports Exerc.* 12(1):61–64.

32. Eichner, E. R. 1992. Sports anemia, iron supplements, and blood doping. *Med Sci Sports Exerc.* 24:9(Suppl):S315–S318.

33. Elliot, D. L., and L. Goldberg. 1985. Nutrition and exercise. *Med Clin North Am.* 69(1):71–82.

34. Fabry, P., J. Fodar, Z. Hejl, T. Braun, and K. Zvolankova. 1964. The frequency of meals: its relation to overweight, hypercholesterolemia, and decreased glucose-tolerance. *Lancet.* Sept. 19, pp. 614–615.

35. Fabry, P., and J. Tepperman. 1970. Meal frequency-a possible factor in human pathology. *Am J Clin Nutr.* 23:1059–1068.

36. Finkelstein, B., and B. A. Fryer. 1971. Meal frequency and weight reduction of young women. *Am J Clin Nutr.* 24:465–468.

37. Foster, C., D. L. Costill, and W. J. Fink. 1979. Effects of pre-exercise feedings on endurance performance. *Med Sci Sports.* 11(1):1–5.

38. Fox, E. L., J. Keller, R. Bartels, V. Vivian, J. Chase, D. Delio, E. Burke, and M. Toner. 1979. Multiple daily exercise: solid vs. liquid diets. *Med Sci Sports.* 11(1):102.

39. Girandola, R. N., R. Bulbulian, A. Hecker, and R. Wiswell. 1979. Effects of liquid and solid meals and time of feeding on VO_2 max. *Med Sci Sports.* 11(1):101.

40. Gleeson, M., R. J. Maughan, and P. L. Greenhaff. 1986. Comparison of the effects of pre-exercise feeding of glucose, glycerol, and placebo on endurance and fuel homeostasis in man. *Eur J Appl Physiol.* 55:6645–6653.

41. Graham, T. E., J. W. E. Rush, and D. A. MacLean. 1995. Skeletal muscle amino acid metabolism and ammonia production during exercise. In Hargreaves, M.(ed), *Exercise Metabolism.* Champaign, IL: Human Kinetics.

42. Grandjean, A. 1989. Macronutrient intake of U.S. athletes compared with the general population and recommendations made for athletes. *Am J Clin Nutr.* 49:1070–1076.

43. Hickson, J. F. 1994. Research directions in protein nutrition for athletes. In Wolinsky, I. and J. F. Hickson (eds): *Nutrition in Exercise and Sport,* 2d ed. Boca Baton, FL: CRC Press.

44. Hoffman, C. J., and E. Coleman. 1991. An eating plan and update on recommended dietary practices for the endurance athlete. *J Am Diet Assoc.* 91:325–330.

45. Houtkooper, L. 1992. Food selection for endurance sports. *Med Sci Sports Exerc.* 24(9-suppl.):S349–S359.

46. Hultman, E. 1967. Studies on muscle metabolism of glycogen and active phosphate in man with special reference to exercise and diet. *Scand J Clin Invest.* 19(Suppl 94):1–63.

47. Hultman, E., and J. Bergström. 1967. Muscle glycogen synthesis in relation to diet studied in normal subjects. *Acta Med Scand.* 182:109–117.

48. Ivy, J. L., D. L. Costill, W. J. Fink, and R. W. Lower. 1979. Influence of caffeine and carbohydrate feedings on endurance performance. *Med. Sci Sports.* 11(1):6–11.

49. Jha, P., M. Flather, E. Lonn, M. Farkouh, and S. Yusuf. 1995. The antioxidant vitamins and cardiovascular disease. Ann Intern Med. 123:860–872.

50. Kanter, M. M., and M. H. Williams. 1995. Antioxidants, carnite, and choline as putative ergogenic aids. *International Journal of Sport Nutrition.* 5(suppl.):S120.

51. Karlsson, J., and B. Saltin. 1971. Diet, muscle glycogen and endurance performance. *J Appl Physiol.* 31(2):203–206.

52. Kilbom, A. 1971. Physical training in women. *Scand J Clin Lab Invest.* 28(suppl.):119.

53. Laidlaw, S. A., T. D. Schultz, J. T. Cecchino, and J. D. Kopple. 1988. Plasma and urine taurine levels in vegans. *Am J Clin Nutr.* 47:660–663.

54. LaManca, J. J., and E. M. Haymes. 1993. Effects of iron supplementation on $VO_{2\,max}$, endurance, and blood lactate in women. *Med Sci Sports Exerc.* 25(12):1386–1392.

55. Lemon, P. W. R. 1995. Do athletes need more dietary protein and amino acids? *International Journal of Sport Nutrition.* 5(suppl):S39–S61.

56. Lemon, P. W. R., and N. J. Nagle. 1981. Effects of exercise on protein and amino acid metabolism. *Med Sci Sports Exerc.* 13(3):141–149.

57. Lemon, P., K. Yarasheski, and D. Dolny. 1984. The importance of protein for athletes. *Sports Med.* 1:474–484.

58. Liebman, M. and J. F. Wilkinson. 1994. Carbohydrate metabolism and exercise. In Wolinsky, I. and J.F. Hickson (eds.), *Nutrition in Exercise and Sport,* 2d ed. Boca Raton: CRC Press.

59. Macdonald, I., B. L. Coles, J. Brice, and M. H. Jourdan. 1970. The influence of frequency of sucrose intake on serum lipid, protein and carbohydrate levels. *Br J Nutr.* 24:413–423.

60. McGandy, R. B., C. H. Barrows, Jr., A Spanias, et al. 1966. Nutrient intake and energy expenditures in men of different ages. *J Geront.* 21(4):581–587.

61. Martin, D. E., D. H. Vroon, D. F. May, and S. P. Pilbeam. 1986. Physiological changes in elite male distance runners training for Olympic competition. *Phys Sportsmed.* 14(1):152–171.

62. Mason, W. L., G. McConell, and M Hargreaves. 1993. Carbohydrate ingestion during exercise: liquid vs solid feedings. *Med Sci Sports Exerc.* 25(8):966–969.

63. Myburgh, K. H., J. Hutchins, A. B. Fataar, S. F. Hough, and T. D. Noakes. 1990. Low bone density is an etiologic factor for stress fractures in athletes. *Ann Intern Med.* 113:754–759.

64. Newhouse, I. J., D. B. Clement, and C. Lai. 1993. Effects of iron supplementation and discontinuation on serum copper, zinc, calcium, and magnesium levels in women. *Med Sci Sports Exerc.* 25(5):562–571.

65. *Nutrition for the Athlete.* 1971. American Association for Health, Physical Education and Recreation, Washington, D.C.

66. Pate, R. R., M. Maguire, and J. Van Wyk. 1979. Dietary iron supplementation in women athletes. *Phys Sportsmed.* 7(9):81–89.

67. Percy, E. C. 1978. Ergogenic aids in athletics. *Med Sci Sports.* 10(4):298–303.

68. Pirnay, F., M. Lacroix, F. Mosora, A. Luyckx, and P. Lefebvre. 1977. Glucose oxidation during prolonged exercise evaluated with naturally labeled (13C) glucose. *J Appl Physiol.* 43(2):258–261.

69. Pitts, G. C., F. C. Consolazio, and R. E. Johnson. 1944. Dietary protein and physical fitness in temperate and hot environments. *Am J Physiol.* 27:497–508.

70. Plowman, S. A., and P. C. McSwegin. 1981. The effects of iron supplementation in female cross-country runners. *J Sports Med Phys Fit.* 21:407–416.

71. Rasch, P. J. 1960. Protein and the athlete. *Phys Educ.* 17(4):143–144.

72. Rasch, P. J., and W. R. Pierson. 1962. Effect of a protein dietary supplement on muscular strength and hypertrophy. *Am J Clin Nutr.* 11:530–532.

73. Reed, M. J., J. T. Broznick, N. C. Lee, and J. L. Ivy. 1989. Muscle glycogen storage postexercise: effect of mode of carbohydrate administration. *J Appl Physiol.* 66:720–726.

74. Rimm, E. B., A. Ascherio, E. Giovannucci, D. Spiegelman, M. J. Stampfer, and W. C. Willett. 1996. Vegetable, fruit, and cereal fiber intake and risk of coronary heart disease among men. *JAMA.* 275(6):447–451.

75. Saltin, B., and L. Hermansen. 1967. Glycogen stores and prolonged severe exercise. In Blix, G. (ed.), *Nutrition and Physical Activity.* Uppsala, Sweden: Almqvist and Weksells.

76. Sen, C. K. 1995. Oxidants and antioxidants in exercise. *J. Appl Physiol.* 79(3):675–686.

77. Sharman, I. M., M. G. Down, and R. N. Sen. 1971. The effects of vitamin E on physiological function and athletic performance in adolescent swimmers. *Br J Nutr.* 26:265–276.

78. Sherman, W. M. 1983. Carbohydrates, muscle glycogen, and muscle glycogen supercompensation. In Williams, M., (ed.), *Ergogenic Aids in Sport.* Champaign, IL: Human Kinetics, pp. 3–26.

79. Sherman, W. M. 1992. Recovery form endurance exercise. *Med Sci Sports Exerc.* 24(9-Suppl):S336–S339.

80. Sherman, W. M., and E. W. Maglischo. 1991. Minimizing chronic athletic fatigue among swimmers: special emphasis on nutrition. *Sports Science Exchange.* 4(35).

81. Sherman, W. M., and N. Leenders. 1995. Fat loading: the next magic bullet? *International Journal of Sport Nutrition.* 5-suppl.:S1–S12.

82. Snow-Harter, C., and R. Marcus. 1991. Exercise, bone mineral density, and osteoporosis. *Exer Sport Sc Rev.* 19:351–388.

83. Stephens, N. G., A. Parsons, P. M. Schofield, F. Kelly, K. Cheeseman, M. J. Mitchinson, and M. J. Brown. 1996. Randomised controlled trial of Vitamin E in patients with coronary disease: Cambridge Heart Antioxidant Study (CHAOS). *Lancet.* 347:781–786.

84. Sundgot-Borgen, J. 1994. Risk and trigger factors for the development of eating disorders in female elite athletes. *Med Sci Sports Exerc.* 26(4):414–419.

85. Swindells, Y. E., S. A. Holmes, and M. F. Robinson. 1968. The metabolic response of young women to changes in the frequency of meals. *Br J Nutr.* 22:667–680.

86. United States Department of Agriculture and United States Department of Health and Human Services. 1995. *Nutrition and Your Health: Dietary Guidelines for Americans,* 4th ed.

87. Wadhwa, P. S., E. A. Young, K. Schmidt, C. E. Elson, and D. J. Pringle. 1973. Metabolic consequences of feeding frequency in man. *Am J Clin Nutr.* 26:823–830.

88. Wahren, J. 1977. Glucose turnover during exercise in man. *Ann NY Acad Sci.* 301:45–55.

89. Waller, M. F., and E. M. Haymes. 1996. The effects of heat and exercise on sweat iron loss. *Med Sci Sports Exerc.* 28(2):197–203.

90. Wardlaw, G. M., and P. M. Insel. 1996. *Perspectives in Nutrition,* 3rd ed. St. Louis: Mosby-Year Book Inc.

91. Whiting S. J. 1994. The inhibitory effect of dietary calcium on iron bioavailability: a cause for concern? *Nutrition Reviews.* 53:77

92. Wilk, B., and O. Bar-Or. 1996. Effect of drink flavor and NACL on voluntary drinking and hydration in boys exercising in the heat. *J Appl Physiol.* 80:1112–1117.

93. Wirth, J. C., T. G. Lohman, J. P. Avallone, T. Shire, and R. A. Boileau. 1978. The effects of physical training on serum iron levels of college-age women. *Med Sci Sports Exerc.* 10(3):223–226.

94 Worme, J., T. Doubt, A. Sighn, C. Ryan, F. Moses, and P. Deuster. 1990. Dietary patterns, gastrointestinal complaints, and nutrition knowledge of recreational triathletes. *Am J Clin Nutr.* 51:690–697.

95. Wright, D. A., W. M. Sherman, and A. R. Dernbach. 1991. Carbohydrate feedings before, during, or in combination improve cycling endurance performance. *J Appl Physiol.* 71:1082-1088.

96. Yeager, K. K., R. Agostini, A. Nattiv, and B. Drinkwater. 1993. The female athlete triad: disorder eating, amenorrhea, osteoporosis. *Med Sci Sports Exerc.* 25(7):775–777.

97. Young, C. M., D. L. Frankel, S. S. Scanlan, V. Simko, and L. Lutwak. 1971. Frequency of feeding, weight reduction and nutrient utilization. *J Am Diet Assoc.* 59:473–480.

98. Young, C. M., L. F. Hutter, S. S. Scanlon, C. E. Rand, L. Lutwak, and V. Simko. 1972. Metabolic effects of meal frequency on normal young men. *J Am Diet Assoc.* 61:391–398.

99. Young, C. M., S. S. Scanlon, C. M. Topping, V. Simko, and L. Lutwak. 1971. Frequency of feeding, weight reduction, and body composition. *J Am Diet Assoc.* 59:466–472.

100. Zaharieva, E. 1965. Survey of sportwomen at the Tokyo Olympics. *J Sports Med.* 5:215–219.

Selected Readings

Ahlborg, B., J. Bergström, L. Ekelund, and E. Hultman. 1967. Muscle glycogen and muscle electrolytes during prolonged physical exercise. *Acta Physiol Scand.* 70:129–142.

Benardot, D. Sports Nutrition, *A Guide for the Professional Working with Active People,* 2d ed. Chicago: The American Dietetic Association.

Bergström, J., and E. Hultman. 1967. A study of the glycogen metabolism during exercise in man. *Scand J Clin Invest.* 19:218–228.

Bergström, J., and E. Hultman. 1967. Synthesis of muscle glycogen in man after glucose and fructose infusion. *Acta Med Scand.* 182:93–107.

Guyton, A. C. and J. E. Hall. 1996. *Textbook of Medical Physiology,* 9th ed. Philadelphia: W. B. Saunders Co.

Hamilton, E. M. and E. N. Whitney 1994. *Nutrition Concepts and Controversies,* 6th ed. St. Paul: West Publishing Co.

Hultman, E. 1967. Muscle glycogen in man determined in needle biopsy specimens. Method and normal values. *Scand J Clin Invest.* 19:209–217.

Klesges, R. C., K. D. Ward, M. L. Shelton, et al. 1996. Changes in bone mineral content in male athletes. *JAMA.* 276:226–230.

16

Exercise, Body Composition, and Weight Control

Whether we are active as athletes, interested in physical fitness and wellness, or are inactive, we have an interest in body composition. Athletes, in a variety of sports, may have different objectives when it comes to weight control and proper body composition. For some, gaining weight (preferably muscle mass) is the goal; for others, "looking slim" or "making weight" is a goal.

The nonathlete may have a simple concern: avoiding obesity. In this regard, James[67] has cautioned that overweight and obesity have an underestimated impact on public health and therefore on national economic costs. He states further that unless governments are willing to make needed changes to enhance physical activity and alter food quality, our societies are doomed to escalating obesity rates. An ominous message, to say the least! Common to this concern, however, is an inadequate knowledge base concerning nutrition and obesity. In this chapter, we will examine concepts related to (1) body composition, (2) the relationship of body composition to exercise performance, and (3) principles involved in body weight control. Included in this latter category will be the estimation of minimal wrestling weights for high-school and college wrestlers.

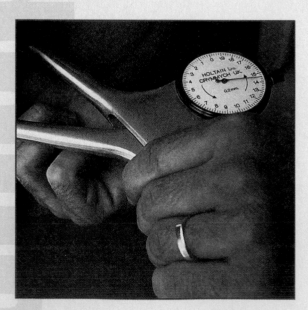

Body Composition

Body Weight Control

Exercise and Training Effects

Summary

The major concepts to be learned from this chapter are as follows:

- Body composition is significantly related to physical activity.
- Endomorphy (fat component), mesomorphy (muscle component), and ectomorphy (lean component) describe the somatotype or body build of a person. Each of us has a degree of all three components.
- Athletes and other active people tend to have higher mesomorphic and ectomorphic components and a lower endomorphic component than do nonathletes or sedentary individuals.
- Lack of exercise and excessive caloric intake are the primary causes of obesity in all age groups.
- The degree of obesity is dependent on the fat content of each fat cell and on the total number of fat cells.
- Total body fat can be estimated by measuring the specific gravity of the body through underwater weighing and by measuring skinfold thicknesses to estimate body density.
- Energy balance means consuming the same amount of energy through food intake as is being expended for resting metabolism plus activity.
- When more energy is consumed than expended (positive energy balance), body weight is gained. When less energy is consumed than expended (negative energy balance), body weight is lost.
- Making weight in wrestling is a potentially hazardous practice that can be made considerably safer by predicting with anthropometric measures each wrestler's minimal wrestling weight.

Body Composition

When we think of body composition as related to exercise, we generally think in terms of body fat assessments by various means. However, another method involves the assessment of body physique by means of the somatotype. We will first discuss somatotyping, and then explore the world of body composition.

Somatotypes

Somatotype deals with the body type or physical classification of the human body. The terms *endomorph, mesomorph,* and *ectomorph* are used to describe a person in terms of his or her somatotype. These descriptive methods have a research application[20,21,23,25,55,116] and are associated with their chief proponents, Sheldon and Heath-Carter. According to Sheldon, included in these three body components are the following characteristics.[110]

Endomorphy

The first component is **endomorphy** and is characterized by roundness and softness of the body. In ordinary language, endomorphy is the "fatness" component of the body. Anteroposterior diameters as well as lateral diameters tend toward equality in the head, neck, trunk, and limbs. Features of this component are a predominance of abdomen over thorax, high square shoulders, and short neck. There is a smoothness of contours throughout, with no muscle relief.

Mesomorphy

The second component is **mesomorphy** and is characterized by a square body with hard, rugged, and prominent musculation. The bones are large and legs, trunks, and arms are usually heavily muscled throughout. Outstanding characteristics of this type are forearm thickness and heavy wrists, hands, and fingers. The thorax is large and the waist is relatively slender. Shoulders are broad, the trunk is usually upright, and the trapezius and deltoid muscles are quite massive. The abdominal muscles are prominent and thick. The skin appears coarse and acquires a deep tan readily, retaining it for a long time. Many athletes have a large degree of this component [123]and consequently a greater predisposition toward coronary artery disease.[91]

Ectomorphy

The third component, **ectomorphy,** includes as predominant characteristics linearity, fragility, and delicacy of body. This is the leanness component. The bones are small and the muscles thin. Shoulder droop is seen consistently in the ectomorph. The limbs are relatively long and the trunk short; however, this does not necessarily mean that the individual is tall. The abdomen and the lumbar curve are flat, whereas the thoracic curve is relatively sharp and elevated. The shoulders are mostly narrow and lacking in muscle relief. There is no bulging of muscle at any point on the physique. The shoulder girdle lacks muscular support and padding, and the scapulae tend to wing out posteriorly.

Body Fat: Concepts and Assessment

For many people, the somatotype method just described may help classify physical appearance. However, "what we are made of" goes beyond both first appearance and what we see in the mirror. It may help to think of the body as being made up of various compartments (e.g., bone, muscle, fat); and quantifying these compartments has much to do with both health and performance.

Although most of us have a general understanding of the concept of body fat, the search for practical and valid methods of accurately assessing body fat remains a challenge.[78] This is true not only in sports medicine, exercise physiology, epidemiology, growth and development, but in human biology, nutrition, physical education, and physical and occupational therapy as well. Knowing the percent body fat of an individual has many applications. One of the more important for most people is the percentage body fat at which weight maintenance occurs.[37]

All readily available methods for assessing body composition are based on certain assumptions and thus are estimates of the actual percentage of body fat. This fact, plus information concerning performance and percent body fat, should make a coach, teacher, fitness director, or other health professional very cautious when interpreting body composition data to athletes, students, or clients. A particular result is indeed an estimate and, as such, has a predicted range within which the body fat of an individual will be found. For example, if an athlete is assessed via hydrostatic weighing (using a measured residual volume) and is told that the percent body composition equals 15.0% fat, the athlete needs to realize that the true percent fat may be between 13.8% and 16.2%. Reliance on a single figure is misleading.

Physically active people possess considerably less total body fat than their inactive contemporaries. Table 16.1 contains a sampling of the results from a number of studies reporting percentage of fat among male and female athletes.

Before proceeding, we need to understand some basic terms.

1. *Body Density.* **Density** (D) is the mass (M) of a substance per unit of volume (V).

$$D = \frac{M}{V}$$

   In humans, density is influenced by the densities of various components of the human anatomy and physiology, such as bone and mineral content, total

Table 16.1

Percent body fat among athletes*

Sport	Male	Female
Track and field		
Runners	6.3–7.5	15.2–19.2
Discus and javelin	16.3	25.0
Shotput	16.5–19.6	28.0
Sprinters	—	19.3
Weight lifting (general)	9.8	—
Power	15.6	—
Olympic	12.2	—
Body building	8.4	—
Wrestlers	5.0–10.7	—
Swimmers	5.0–8.5	26.3
Skiers	7.4	—
Baseball	11.8–14.2	—
Football (general)	13.9	—
Defensive backs	9.6–11.5	—
Offensive backs	9.4–12.4	—
Linebackers	13.4–14.0	—
Quarterbacks and kickers	14.4	—
Offensive linemen	15.6–19.1	—
Defensive linemen	18.2–18.5	—
Gymnasts	4.6	9.6–23.8
Jockeys	14.1	—
Ice hockey	15.1	—
Basketball	9.7	20.8–26.9
Volleyball	—	25.3
Tennis	15.2	—
Nonathletes	16.8	25.5

*Compiled from various sources by Wilmore et al.[143]

body water, and total body fat stores. In general, the fat-free component is assumed to have a density of 1.100 g/cm³, whereas the fat mass is considered to have a density of about 0.90 g/cm³.

2. *Fat-Free Body (FFB).* The weight of all tissues in the body minus the extractable fat.[18]

3. *Lean Body Mass (LBM).* **Lean body mass** includes the essential lipids and the FFB mass it has a density and water content somewhat less than FFB mass.[77] The constant of 1.100 g/cm³ is based on the FFB compartment. Lean body mass really represents a slightly larger compartment than the FFB mass.

4. *Two-Compartment Model.* For our discussion, the body is considered to have two compartments: the FFB compartment and the fat compartment. This concept is used in assessing body composition via either hydrostatic weighing or skinfold methods.

5. *Percent Body Fat.* The proportion of the total body weight that is fat tissue expressed as a percentage. It is an expression of relative body fat.

$$\% \text{ Body fat} = \frac{(\text{Total body weight} - \text{Fat-free weight})}{\text{Total body weight}} \times 100$$

6. *Absolute Body Fat.* The absolute weight of body fat expressed either in kilograms or pounds.

Assessment Methods for Body Composition

A variety of methods exist for assessing body composition,[27,68] some of which are beyond the technical and financial means of most programs and facilities.[119] Such methods include magnetic resonance imaging (MRI),[56] computed tomography,[2] potassium-40 counting, ultrasound imaging,[56] total body electrical conductivity (TOBEC),[108] isotope dilution (tritiated or deuterated water),[36] computer-assisted axial tomography (CAT),[46] and thermography (figure 16.1). While all of these methods are subject to considerable between and within subject variation, the MRI gives body composition values most similar to those obtained by underwater weighing.[32] Underwater or hydrostatic weighing will be explained later but it is mentioned here as a "gold standard" for estimating body composition against which the above methods are often compared.

Other methods that are accessible to a broad base of practitioners in the health and fitness professions include bioelectrical impedance analysis (BIA),[22] hydrostatic (underwater) weighing, and skinfold and/or anthropometric methods. The ratio of body weight to stature, referred to as **body mass index (BMI),** is also often used to assess health risk. BMI is calculated by dividing body weight in kg by height in meters squared—i.e., $BMI = BW(kg) \div Ht(m^2)$. The relationship between BMI and fat as a percentage of body weight is approximately linear.[87] Although different cutoffs have been used, if BMI is greater than 30, a person is judged to be obese.

BIA uses a small portable instrument that measures whole body electrical resistance to a weak current passed through the body. The resistance is assessed by placement of two electrodes each (source and receiving) on the right wrist and right ankle.[7] BIA is highly reliable[7,54]—that is, the results are reproducible. However, certain assumptions must be made with this method, including: (1) that the body has a homogeneous composition, (2) that each segment has a fixed cross-sectional area, and (3) that there is a uniform current-density distribution. These assumptions are not met with the human body.

Other factors that affect the measurement of impedance include: (1) consistency of positioning of the electrodes, (2) closeness of the electrodes (makes measures on

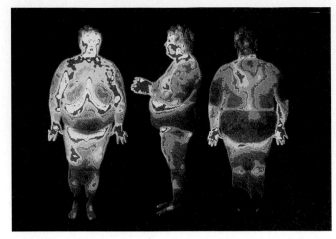

Figure 16.1

Thermogram of an obese woman shown in three different views. Note layering of adipose tissue and differences in regional heat production, shown in red.

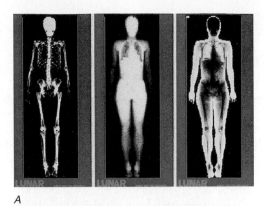

A

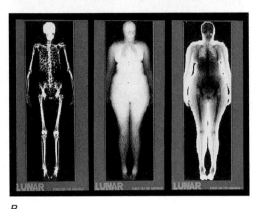

B

Figure 16.2

Dual energy X-ray absorptiometry (DEXA) images of (*A*) a normal weight woman and (*B*) an obese woman.

children difficult), (3) hydration level of the subject (dehydrated or overhydrated), (4) body position, and (5) ambient air and skin temperature, among others. Concern over measurement errors when BIA is used for body composition analysis led to the formation of an expert panel to evaluate the appropriateness of the procedure.[9] The panel concluded that BIA can be a useful technique for body composition in healthy individuals, even with mild-to-moderate obesity if disturbances of body water distribution are not prominent. Others[64] have argued that BIA is most appropriate for estimating adiposity of groups in epidemiologic and field studies but has only limited accuracy for estimating body composition in individuals.

In summary, BIA continues to show promise, especially for conducting group surveys, but needs further refinement for meaningful applications to a broad base of individuals on the basis of age, gender, ethnic background, and fitness levels.

Advances in CAT and MRI methods now allow for accurate estimates of whole body skeletal muscle and fat components and should allow for resolution of many of the confusing issues related to our better understanding of body composition.[58] Laskey[75] has reviewed the advantages and limitations of a new high-tech method called dual-energy X-ray absorptiometry (DEXA). DEXA machines are manufactured by companies with the names of Lunar, Hologic, and Norland. They all generate X-rays at two different energies and make use of the differential attenuation of the X-ray beam at these two energies to calculate the bone mineral content and soft tissue composition within a whole body scan (figure 16.2). This allows for estimations of fat and fat-free tissues for the whole body or subregions like the arms, legs, and trunk. While DEXA is currently used to assess osteoporosis risk and to monitor the effects of therapy, it cannot be regarded as a new "gold standard" for body composition analysis.[75]

Measurement of Body Density: Hydrostatic (Underwater) Weighing

Hydrostatic weighing results in a measure of body density and is based on the principle of Archimedes. Archimedes' principle states that an object submerged in water is buoyed by a "force" that equals the volume of water displaced. The *volume* of water displaced equals the *weight* of water displaced by the object immersed in the water (e.g., 1 liter of water displaced equals 1 kilogram of weight).

$$\text{Density} = \frac{\text{Weight of object in air}}{\text{Weight of water displaced}}$$

How do we get from the weight of water displaced to the volume of water displaced? The *weight of water,* in grams, is converted to *volume* by dividing by its density (g/cm^3).* Thus, by weighing a person on land, immersing the individual in water, and recording the weight of the submersed person, the density (D) of that person can be determined (see figure 16.3). The denominator in the following equation represents, then, the volume displaced.

$$D = \frac{\text{Wt in air}}{\text{Wt in air} - \text{Wt in water}}$$

*The density of water at 30 C is 0.99567 g/cm^3.

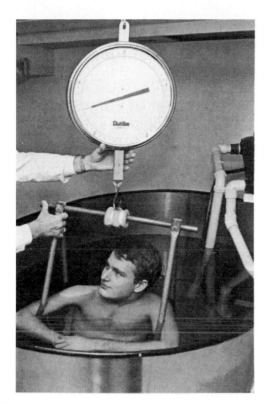
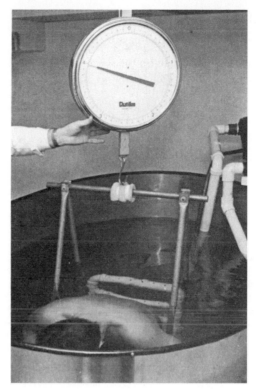

Figure 16.3

Underwater weighing for measuring body density. One could measure either the weight of the water displaced by the body or the weight of the body when completely submerged.

(Photo by Cliffton Boutelle, News and Information Service, Bowling Green State University.)

This equation now has to be modified slightly to account for air in the lungs, gastrointestinal gas, and the density of water.

Air in the Lungs

Standard practice is to perform a forced expiration and breath hold so that the lungs contain only the **residual volume (RV)**. Residual volume may be estimated by multiplying the vital capacity (corrected to BTPS; see appendix C) by the constant 0.24 for males or 0.28 for females.[139] These values will be approximately 1300 mL and 1000 mL for males and females, respectively. Although these approximations can be used, a more precise measure of residual volume is available involving an oxygen dilution technique.[144]

For individuals uncomfortable with head submersion, the head may remain out of the water and a full inhalation performed. This method has been reported to give similar results for body density when compared with head submersion and exhalation method.[29,125,137]

Intestinal Gas

Although the volume of intestinal gas is not readily measurable, it has been estimated to be approximately 100 mL.[49]

Density of Water

The density of water varies with its temperature, as shown in table 16.2.

table 16.2

Density (D) of water (g/cm³) at various temperatures (°C)

T (°C)	D (g/cm³)	T (°C)	D (g/cm³)
25	0.99707	31	0.99535
26	679	32	503
27	651	33	470
28	623	34	438
29	595	35	406
30	567	36	374

The final form of the equation is

$$D_b = \frac{W_a}{K - (V_R + 100)}$$

Where:

D_b = body density (g/cm³)
W_a = weight in air in grams
K = weight in air (W_a, g) minus weight in water (W_w, g) divided by the density of water (g/cm³) at the weighing temperature (What will the calculated units be for K? Think about it before looking at the following sample problem.)

RV = residual volume in cm^3

100 = estimate of gastrointestinal gas in cm^3

Adam Kicker, a candidate for the soccer team, wanted to know his body density. The following data were collected:

Subject: male

Weight (W_a): 90 kg (198 lb)

Weight submerged in water (W_w): 4 kg (8.8 lb)

Vital capacity (V_c BTPS): 6000 cm^3 (or mL)

Density of water at 32°C (D_{H_2O}): 0.9951 g/cm^3 (or g/mL)

Gastrointestinal gas volume (V_g): 100 cm^3 (or mL)

Step 1. Find residual volume (RV).

RV = Vital capacity × 0.24
    = 6000 cm^3 × 0.24
RV = 1440 cm^3

(Note: We are estimating RV by using the multiplier for males.)

Step 2. Calculate K:

$$K = \frac{Wa - Ww)}{D_{H_2O}}$$

$$K = \frac{(90,000 \text{ g} - 4,000 \text{ g})}{0.9951 \text{ g/cm}^3}$$

$$K = \frac{86,000 \text{ g}}{0.9951 \text{ g/cm}^3}$$

K = 86,423 cm^3

(Note 1: The g units cancel, and we are left with cm^3, a volume unit.)

(*Note 2:* The units may be left as kg, but then you must remember that the density of water will be in kg·L^{-1} and the residual volume must be converted to liters: 1440 cm^3 = 1.440 L.)

Step 3. Coming back to the original equation, we can simply "plug in" the measured and calculated values.

$$D_b = \frac{W_a}{K - (V_R + 100)}$$

$$D_b = \frac{90,000 \text{ g}}{86,423 - (1440 + 100) \text{ cm}^3} \text{ or } \frac{90,000}{84,883}$$

D$_b$ = 1.060 g/cm^3

What have we accomplished so far in this calculation process? We have estimated the whole body density of our subject. Actually, the estimation of body density by means of hydrostatic weighing is very accurate.[78] The process of converting density to relative body fat (percent body fat) introduces further unavoidable error. Recall that we said earlier that the FFB had an assumed density of 1.100 g/cm^3. Biologically, FFB density may vary depending on age, gender, ethnic origin, fitness level, variability in water content, bone density, body mineral content, and potassium content. Also technical errors may be committed during the measurement process. Misreading the scale during hydrostatic weighing (figure 16.3) and error in estimating or measuring residual volume are two examples. Procedurally, all subjects should void the bladder prior to assessment.

Before converting our calculated body density from hydrostatic weighing to percent body fat, let us examine another popular method for estimating body density skinfolding procedures.

Measurement of Body Density: Skinfold Measurements

Body density estimates may be reasonably made based on measurement of subcutaneous fat as reflected by skinfold thickness. Such measurements, which are relatively uncomplicated, have been adopted by physicians, trainers, coaches, and physical educators as a means of assessing the body composition of various persons, including athletes. Such measurements are taken with an instrument called a *skinfold caliper.*[*] Well over 150 equations using both anthropometric (combinations of girth and circumference measures, age, stature, weight) and skinfold measures have been developed over the past 80 years or so. Most of these equations are specific to the populations from which they were derived.[52,72,90,112,141,142]

Generalized Equations

As mentioned above, the development of skinfold equations for estimating either body density or percent body fat has been popular for several decades. Two contemporary formulas will be presented at this time. These equations appear to be good estimators of body density. The two equations presented are called *generalized equations* and have broad application in the population. They take into account both skinfold thickness and age. There is one equation for each gender.

The first equation, for women, may be used for nonathletic individuals.[66] The second equation, called Jackson-Pollock (JP), for males,[65] incorporates three skinfold sites and can be applied to athletes and nonathletes.[†] We will present other equations later in this chapter for application to specific athletic groups—namely, wrestlers and women gymnasts.

The Jackson-Pollock-Ward (JPW) generalized equation for estimating body density for *females* is[66]

$$D_b = 1.099421 - 0.0009929 (X_1) + 0.0000023 (X_1)^2 - 0.0001392 (X_2)$$

Where:

D_b = body density in grams per cubic centimeter (g/cm^3)
X_1 = sum of triceps, iliac crest, and midthigh skinfolds, in millimeters
X_2 = age to the nearest year

---

[*]Several manufacturers of skinfold calipers are available. Two such instruments are the Lange caliper and the Harpenden caliper.

[†]In references 65 and 66 the authors have presented a "family" of equations based on 3, 4, and 7 skinfold sites for both men and women, each of comparable application. Convenience versus a slightly improved accuracy dictate one's choice. Tables are also presented where sums of skinfolds and age can be directly converted to a percent body fat value.

The Jackson-Pollock (JP) generalized equation for estimating body density in *males* is[65]

$$D_b = 1.10938 - 0.0008267 (X_1) + 0.0000016 (X_1)^2 - 0.0002574 (X_2)$$

Where:

X_1 = sum of chest, abdominal, and midthigh skinfolds, in millimeters
X_2 = age to the nearest year

Calculating Percent Body Fat

Up to this point, we have presented some procedures and equations for *estimating body density*. The practical application for these calculations is, of course, in converting them to relative body fat (percent body fat). Two commonly used equations for converting density to body fat will be demonstrated: the Siri equation[114] (based on the assumption that density of the FFB is 1.100 g/cm^3) and the Brozek equation[17,18] (based on the chemical composition of "reference man"). Each of the conversions is widely accepted but is applied to specific density equations. For example, the JPW and JP skinfold equations presented above are converted to percent body fat via the Siri equation. The Brozek equation is often used in converting densities derived from hydrostatic weighing. In any case, when making any body composition evaluations, make certain that your applications are consistent with the published information. Except for fat values *"0% fat" and over 30%, both equations give similar results.*[78,80] At these extremes they give more divergent results and more caution should be used when interpreting the results to clients or students.

Hydrostatic Weighing

Remember Adam Kicker from the hydrostatic weighing exercise? His $D_b = 1.060$ g/cm^3. Applying the Brozek equation we can find percent body fat as follows:

$$\% \text{ Fat} = \frac{457}{D_b} - 414.2$$

$$\% \text{ Fat} = \frac{457}{1.060} - 414.2$$

$$\% \text{ Fat} = 431.1 - 414.2 = \textbf{16.9}$$

Applying the Siri equation:

$$\% \text{ Fat} = \frac{495}{D_b} - 450$$

$$\% \text{ Fat} = \frac{495}{1.060} - 450$$

$$\% \text{ Fat} = 467 - 450 = \textbf{17}$$

The two estimates for percent body fat are very close.

Skinfold Equations

We need some data for estimating percent body fat from the skinfold equations. First let us do an example for a female and then one for a male.

Example 1. A 20-year-old female has the following skinfold measurements:

Triceps skinfold	= 12 mm
Iliac crest skinfold	= 20 mm
Midthigh skinfold	= 25 mm
Sum of skinfolds	= $\overline{\textbf{57 mm}}$

Applying the JPW equation for women:

$$D_b = 1.099421 - 0.0009929 (X_1) + 0.0000023 (X_1)^2 - 0.0001392 (X_2)$$

$$D_b = 1.099421 - 0.0009929 (\textbf{57}) + 0.0000023 (\textbf{57} \times \textbf{57}) - 0.0001392 (\textbf{20})$$

$$D_b = 1.099421 - 0.056595 + 0.007473 - 0.002784$$

$$\textbf{D}_b = \textbf{1.047515}$$

The next step is to translate density into a percent body fat using the Siri equation.

$$\% \text{ Body fat} = \frac{495}{D_b} - 450$$

$$\% \text{ Body fat} = \frac{495}{1.0475} - 450$$

$$\% \textbf{ Body fat} = 472.6 - 450 = \textbf{22.6}$$

Example 2. A 23-year-old male has the following skinfold measurements:

Chest skinfold	= 6 mm
Abdominal skinfold	= 25 mm
Midthigh skinfold	= 19 mm
Sum of skinfolds	= $\overline{\textbf{50 mm}}$

Applying the JP equation for men:

$$D_b = 1.10938 - 0.0008267 (X_1) + 0.0000016 (X_1)^2 - 0.0002574 (X_2)$$

$$D_b = 1.10938 - 0.0008267 (\textbf{50}) + 0.0000016 (\textbf{50} \times \textbf{50}) - 0.0002574 (\textbf{23})$$

$$D_b = 1.10938 - 0.041335 + 0.0040 - 0.00592$$

$$\textbf{D}_b = \textbf{1.066125}$$

Then apply the percent body fat formula by Siri.

$$\% \text{ Fat} = \frac{495}{D_b} - 450$$

$$\% \text{ Fat} = \frac{495}{1.066} - 450$$

$$\% \textbf{ Body Fat} = 464.4 - 450 = \textbf{14.4}$$

Interpretation of Results

What do these results mean? Recall at the beginning of this section we gave a caution concerning the interpretation of body fat calculations. Measurement error and biological variability are great enough that we cannot interpret precisely enough to give an exact value. The true value for percent body fat lies within a given range of values. The statistic that quantifies the range of values is called a standard error of the estimate and represents a range where there is a 68% probability for the true value to be located. Let us examine the effects on interpretation for the calculations we have just made.

Hydrostatic Weighing

The results for hydrostatic weighing depend, in part, on whether the residual volume (RV) was measured or estimated.[104] When RV is measured, the range for the true value may be plus or minus (±) 1.2% body fat, or 17 ± 1.2%. In other words, Adam Kicker's percent body fat would lie between 15.8% and 18.2% if we had used measured residual volume.

Because we estimated residual volume from vital capacity, it is possible that the true value for Adam's body fat would lie within 17 ± 3.9% body fat of the estimated value, or between 13.1% and 20.9% body fat (quite a range).

Skinfold Methods

Different equations will obviously have variable standard errors of the estimate. The JPW and JP equations are reported to have about a ± 3.5% body fat value.[104] From Example 1 the reported body fat of 23.2% would fall between 19.8% and 26.7%.

In an athletic population, if a coach wanted one athlete with a body fat of 23% to achieve 20%, it is entirely possible that the athlete is already at that level of body fat.

What Is a Desirable Body Composition?

As you might guess, the answer to this question is not simple. However, a panel of recognized experts in the study of body composition have given us some guidelines, which are presented in table 16.3. These guidelines generally relate to individuals from the late teen years into advanced adult years.

What Is a Desirable Body Weight?

How does knowing your desirable body composition translate into a recommended weight? First, it is important to think in terms of a weight range rather than a single value. Referring to table 16.3, determine your desired classification to establish a reasonable weight. A reasonable goal would be to achieve "optimal fitness." That means attaining a percent body fat, for males, between 12% and 18%. What, then, would the corresponding weight range be? The equations necessary to answer this question are now presented.

table 16.3

Suggested guidelines for body composition for sport, health, and fitness*

Classification	Men	Women
Essential fat	1 to 5%	3 to 8%
Most athletes	5 to 13%	12 to 22%
Optimal health	10 to 25%	18 to 30%
Optimal fitness	12 to 18%	16 to 25%
Borderline obesity	22 to 27%	30 to 34%

*Modified from a roundtable discussion.[106] Data from Food and Nutrition Board: *Recommended Dietary Allowances,* 7th ed. Washington, D.C., National Academy of Sciences, 1968. Modified from Table 80, Hathaway and Ford, 1960, "Heights and Weights of Adults in the U.S.", *Home Economics Research Report No. 10.* ARS, USDA.

Process:

1. Calculate the *fat weight:*

$$FW = BW \times F_f$$

2. From 1 above, calculate the *fat-free weight:*

$$FFW = BW - FW$$

3. Calculate the desired target weight:

$$TW = \frac{FFW}{(1 - F_x)}$$

The above equations (1, 2, and 3) can be combined to provide a single equation for reporting a recommended target weight as follows:

$$TW = \frac{BW\,(1 - F_f)}{(1 - F_x)}$$

Where:

  FW = fat weight
  BW = measured body weight
   F_f = fractional (decimal) expression of the percent body fat
FFW = fat-free weight or lean body weight
  TW = desired target weight
   F_x = fractional expression of the target percent body fat

Assume that Dexter Fittmann wants to become physically fit and, as part of his preprogram evaluation, has been given a body composition assessment with the following results:

Current weight: 200 lb (90.7 kg)

Percent fat: 27%

16.4

Suggested weights for heights of college men and women

Height (In.)†	Men Normal	Men Obese	Women Normal	Women Obese
60			109 ± 9	> 136
62			115 ± 9	> 144
64	133 ± 11	> 166	122 ± 10	> 152
66	142 ± 11	> 177	129 ± 10	> 161
68	151 ± 14	> 189	136 ± 10	> 170
70	159 ± 14	> 199	144 ± 11	> 180
72	167 ± 15	> 209	152 ± 12	> 190
74	175 ± 15	> 219		
76	182 ± 16	> 228		

Median weight (Lbs)†

†Measurements—nude.

± refers to weight range between 25th and 75th percentile of each height category. For example, 50% of the women sampled at 60 inches weighed between 100 and 118 lbs.

Height: 70 in (178 cm)

Age: 27

Goal: to achieve "optimal fitness" for body composition (12 to 18% body fat)

What weight range would we recommend?

Step 1. FW = BW × F_f
         FW = 200 × 0.27 = **54 lb**

Step 2. FFW = BW − FW
         FFW = 200 − 54 = **146 lb**

Step 3. This is a two-part process, because we want to give a range for the target weight.

A. Target weight at 12% fat

$$TW = \frac{FFW}{(1 - F_x)}$$

$$TW = \frac{146}{(1 - 0.12)} = \frac{146}{0.88} = 166 \text{ lb}$$

B. Target weight at 18% fat

$$TW = \frac{FFW}{(1 - F_x)}$$

$$TW = \frac{146}{(1 - 0.18)} = \frac{146}{0.82} = 178 \text{ lb}$$

Dexter must lose between 22 and 34 lb of his 54 lb of body fat to achieve the recommended 12% to 18% body fat. Also, it is not necessary that he lose 34 pounds of body fat. That is merely the lower end of the recommended range.

Body Weight Control

In discussing body weight control, we will start with a few words about obesity, then present guidelines for losing fat weight and gaining lean or fat-free weight, and then address some concerns in sport and "making weight."

Obesity

An unvarnished tale states, "most people become obese because of *physical inactivity*."[85] Such is true for teenagers as well as adults. A study in California revealed that 14% of high-school seniors (boys and girls) were obese. The need for physical education in elementary, junior, and senior high schools can be substantiated on this verity alone.

Obesity is related to a number of diseases including diabetes, coronary heart disease, psychological disturbances, kidney disease, hypertension, stroke, liver ailments, and biomechanical ailments (particularly, back and foot problems). As a consequence, life expectancy is significantly reduced among the obese population. Excessive obesity may result in as high as 100% increase in mortality over that which might be expected!

What Is Obesity?

Authorities generally concur that the normal body weight attained between the ages of 25 and 30 years of age should not be exceeded throughout life. Table 16.4 contains

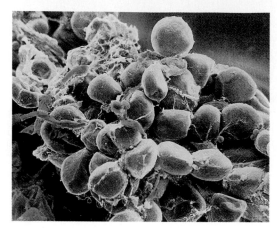

Figure 16.4

Colored scanning electron micrograph (SEM) of adipocytes or fat storage cells (yellow).

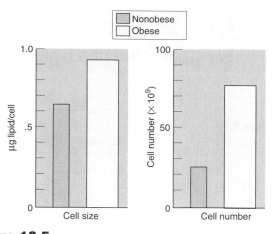

Figure 16.5

Obese people have a larger number of fat cells (right), which contain a greater volume of lipids (left), than their lean counterparts.

(Based on data from Hirsch and Knittle.[60])

suggested weights based on a sample of college men and women. This table serves as a means of estimating a reasonable body weight when body fat is unknown. A weight in excess of 15% of that regarded as normal would be considered tending toward obesity, whereas 25% above normal would be truly obese. Since these figures do not take into account measured body fat they are not, alone, currently considered to be an adequate indicator of one's obesity status.

Buskirk,[19] in addressing the question "Who is fat?" states that obesity is difficult to define in quantitative terms. Obesity refers to the above-average amount of fat contained in the body, this in turn being dependent on the lipid content of each fat cell and on the total number of fat cells. But assessment of fat cell number and size is an expensive clinical procedure that also does not tell the entire story. So what methods should be used? In addition to body weight, an evaluation for obesity should include measures of body composition, dietary quality, energy expenditure, risk factor status, and body image.[133]

For example, a BMI greater than 30 (Appendix E) is often considered to indicate obesity.[5] A high waist to hip circumference (WHC) ratio also is used as an indicator of intra-abdominal or "central" fat distribution. This pattern of fat distribution carries more risk for disease than a low WHC ratio which indicates a "peripheral" fat distribution and less risk for metabolic disorders.[5,83] The WHC ratio, however, may work better as a prediction measure for men than for women, where total body fat represents a more complex regulation.[132]

Imaging techniques such as computerized tomography and magnetic resonance imaging have been recommended as the optimal techniques available for the measurement of visceral fat.[131] All of this represents a major shift in emphasis toward measuring visceral fat and a bet-

ter understanding of the metabolic-related risk factors in the obese. This has led to the suggestions that a major contribution of exercise to obesity may be through the use of low intensity programs to develop "metabolic fitness" in a less strenuous, safer and more interesting way—i.e., less boring than traditional aerobic endurance training programs.[10]

Adipocytes (figure 16.4), or fat cells, increase in number (hyperplasia) through early adolescence. They also increase in size (hypertrophy). Lack of exercise and overeating may stimulate their formation. Obesity, then, is a combination of the number of adipocytes and their lipid content.[126] Obese people have a larger number of fat cells that contain a greater volume of lipids than their lean counterparts (figure 16.5). In adults, with changes in body weight over a 3- to 4-month period of about 20 pounds, it appears that most of the increase is due to increased storage in existing adipocytes. Whereas, if continued weight gain is allowed, there appears to be a trigger mechanism wherein hyperplasia occurs. As a consequence, health professionals and physical educators should seriously consider that:

1. Prevention of obesity results in greater success than treatment. This is particularly true during preadolescence. Evidence suggests that overeating during this period may cause adipocyte hyperplasia (an increase in the number of fat cells), thus cultivating the garden in which obesity may grow and bloom.
2. Exercise keeps total body fat content low and may reduce the rate at which adipose cells accumulate.
3. If a given food intake does not allow weight reduction, then physical activity must be increased for a negative energy balance to occur.

4. Activities must be selected requiring long-term energy expenditure but at the same time within the physical and skill capabilities of the individual.

5. Living habits are developed early, and so the sooner control programs are initiated, the better.

Energy Balance and Weight Control

The quantity of food required by an individual above that which is necessary for body maintenance and growth depends on the amount of physical activity that he or she experiences. Just as an automobile traveling 60 miles each day requires more gasoline than one traveling 30 miles per day, a person walking 20 miles a day requires more food than a person walking 2 miles each day. For body weight to remain constant, food intake must equal energy needs. If, in fact, too much food is consumed, we will gain weight or be in what is referred to as a **positive energy balance.** On the other hand, if our energy needs exceed that produced by the food we eat, a **negative energy balance** occurs. In this case, the body consumes its own fat, and then protein, with a concomitant loss in body weight.

To understand our daily energy needs, we must have some concept of our daily energy expenditure. Components that make up our daily energy expenditure include (1) basal energy expenditure (BEE);[104] (2) the energy cost of general activities (GA), such as eating, walking, sitting, or reading; and (3) the energy cost of exercise (EX), or

$$\text{daily caloric need} = \text{BEE} + \text{GA} + \text{EX}$$

To determine each one of these, study the following procedures:

1. Ross and Jackson[104] present equations for estimating basal energy expenditure, *in calories,* that takes into account age, gender, height, and weight.

   A. For males:

   $$\text{BEE} = 66 + (13.7 \times \text{Wt}) + (5 \times \text{Ht}) - (6.9 \times \text{A})$$

   B. For females:

   $$\text{BEE} = 665 + (9.6 \times \text{Wt}) + (1.7 \times \text{Ht}) - (4.7 \times \text{A})$$

   Where:

   > Wt = Weight in kilograms (kg)
   > Ht = Height in centimeters (cm)
   > A = Age in years

2. Estimate the energy cost for activity.

   A. General activity: multiply BEE by 20%.

   $$\text{GA} = \text{BEE} \times 0.2$$

3. Determine the energy cost of exercise by referring to table 16.5. The energy expenditure for a variety of activities is reported in both kcal/lb of body weight/min ($\text{kcal} \cdot \text{lb}^{-1} \cdot \text{min}^{-1}$) and in kcal/kg of body weight/minute ($\text{kcal} \cdot \text{kg}^{-1} \cdot \text{min}^{-1}$). This allows you to calculate the energy cost of an activity based on your body weight and the actual time spent in activity.

$$\text{EX} = (\text{kcal} \cdot \text{lb}^{-1} \cdot \text{min}^{-1})\ (\text{Wt})\ (\text{min of activity})$$

Application: Remember Dexter Fittmann who wanted to start an exercise program (p. 446)? One of his goals was to achieve a weight of 178 lb. We can estimate Dexter's daily caloric need to maintain his current weight of 200 lb (90.7 kg) without regular exercise in the following way:

Current weight: 200 lb (90.7 kg)

Percent fat: 27%

Age: 27 years

Height: 70 in (178 cm)

kcal needed per day = BEE + GA
BEE = 66 + (13.7 × Wt in kg) + (5 × Ht in cm)
$$(6.9 \times \text{age in yr})$$
= 66 + (13.7 × 90.7 kg) + (5 × 178 cm)
$$(6.9 \times 27)$$
BEE = 66 + 1243 + 890 − 186 = **2013 kcal**
GA = BEE × 0.2 = 2013 × 0.2 = **403 kcal**
BEE + GA = 2416 kcal per day

(This is what Dexter must consume daily to maintain his current weight at 200 lb.)

To achieve a weight loss of 22 pounds, Dexter would have to have a total caloric deficit of 77,000 kcal (3500 $\text{kcal} \cdot \text{lb}^{-1}$ of fat × 22 lb). How long will it take him to achieve this goal? First, he should reduce his caloric intake by about 500 kcal per day,* and then he should select a physical activity that he enjoys and start an exercise program. Let us assume that he selects jogging, and after starting slowly and gradually building his time for jogging to ½ hour over a 3- to 4-week period, he is jogging at a pace of 8.5 minutes per mile, five times per week. How great is the negative energy balance?

1. Dietary control that reduces total caloric intake 500 calories per day gives him a caloric deficit of 3500 $\text{kcal} \cdot \text{wk}^{-1}$ (500 $\text{kcal} \cdot \text{d}^{-1}$ × 7 days).

2. Exercise: Table 16.5 shows that jogging at a pace of 8.5 $\text{min} \cdot \text{mile}^{-1}$ provides an energy expenditure of 0.09 $\text{kcal} \cdot \text{lb}^{-1} \cdot \text{min}^{-1}$, or

$$\text{EX} = (0.09\ \text{kcal} \cdot \text{lb}^{-1} \cdot \text{min}^{-1}) \times (200\ \text{lb}) \times (30\ \text{min})$$
EX = 540 kcal/run or **2700 kcal · week⁻¹** (i.e., 5 days × 540 kcal)

Therefore, through a combination of activity and dietary control, Dexter would have a weekly caloric deficit of

---

*In general, a diet should not go below about 1200 kcal for males and 1100 kcal for females unless under close supervision by a physician who understands nutrition or a registered dietitian.

table 16.5

Estimated energy cost for various physical activities expressed as kcal · lb^{-1} · min^{-1} and kcal · kg^{-1} · min^{-1}*

Activity	kcal · lb^{-1}· min^{-1}	kcal · kg^{-1}· min^{-1}	Activity	kcal · lb^{-1}· min^{-1}	kcal · kg^{-1}· min^{-1}
Aerobic dance			Rope jumping	0.060	0.132
Moderate	0.075	0.165	Rowing (vigorous)	0.090	0.198
Vigorous	0.095	0.209	Running		
Archery	0.030	0.066	11.0 min/mi	0.070	0.154
Badminton			8.5 min/mi	0.090	0.198
Recreational	0.380	0.084	7.0 min/mi	0.102	0.225
Competition	0.065	0.143	6.0 min/mi	0.114	0.251
Baseball	0.310	0.068	Deep water treading	0.100	0.221
Basketball			Skating (moderate)	0.038	0.084
Moderate	0.380	0.084	Skiing		
Competition	0.065	0.143	Downhill	0.060	0.132
Bowling	0.030	0.066	X-country (5 mph)	0.078	0.172
Calisthenics	0.033	0.073	Soccer	0.059	0.130
Cycling			Strength training	0.050	0.110
5.5 mph	0.033	0.073	Swimming†		
10.0 mph	0.050	0.110	20 yds/min	0.031	0.068
13.0 mph	0.071	0.157	25 yds/min	0.040	0.088
Dance			45 yds/min	0.057	0.126
Moderate	0.030	0.066	50 yds/min	0.070	0.154
Vigorous	0.055	0.121	Table tennis	0.030	0.066
Field hockey	0.061	0.134	Tennis		
Football	0.060	0.132	Moderate	0.045	0.099
Golf	0.030	0.066	Competitive	0.064	0.141
Gymnastics			Volleyball	0.030	0.066
Light	0.030	0.066	Walking		
Heavy	0.056	0.123	4.5 mph	0.045	0.099
Handball	0.064	0.141	Shallow pool	0.090	0.198
Hiking	0.040	0.088	Water aerobics		
Judo/Karate	0.086	0.190	Moderate	0.080	0.176
Marching (fast)	0.064	0.142	Vigorous	0.100	0.221
Racquetball	0.065	0.143	Wrestling	0.085	0.187

*Modified from Hoeger.[61]
†See Table 16.6 for more information.

6200 kcal. This would theoretically result in a weight loss of about 1¾ lb per week (6200 ÷ 3500). How long would it take him to achieve a 22 lb weight loss? A 34 lb weight loss?* What would be his caloric need to maintain weight at 178 pounds (80.7 kg) with the same exercise of jogging 30 minutes, 5 days each week?†

Let us examine table 16.5, which contains a listing of a number of activities with their caloric expenditures ex-

pressed as kcal · kg^{-1} · min^{-1} or kcal · lb^{-1} · min^{-1}. The advantage for expressing energy output in these terms is that (1) the weight of the individual is taken into account and (2) energy output can be determined for the actual amount of time spent in the activity. By knowing the energy cost of activity in these terms, we can more judiciously plan our diets to maintain proper energy balance and thus body weight control.

For example, suppose you had a goal to expend about 2000 kcal per week in activity. Using the data from Dexter Fittmann, jogging at a pace of 8.5 minutes per mile for 30 minutes four times per week (120 minutes per week) will yield an energy output of 2160 kcal (540 kcal · d^{-1} × 4

---

*About 12 to 13 weeks (22 wk/1.75 lb · wk^{-1}); about 19 to 20 weeks (34 wk/1.75 lb · wk^{-1}).
†Caloric need = [66 + (13.7 × 80.7) + (5 × 178) − 6.9 × 27)] × 1.2 + 540 = 2790 kcal.

days). If the activity of choice is walking rather than jogging, how many minutes per week would have to be spent in walking? The energy expenditure from table 16.5 is 0.045 kcal · lb^{-1} · min^{-1} (at 4.5 mph—a brisk walking pace!). Remember Dexter weighs 200 lb at this point. Therefore:

$$\text{kcal} \cdot \text{min}^{-1} = (0.045 \text{ kcal} \cdot \text{lb}^{-1} \cdot \text{min}^{-1}) \times 200 \text{ lb}$$
$$\text{kcal} \cdot \text{min}^{-1} = 9$$

Minutes per week = 2160 kcal/9 kcal · min^{-1}
Minutes per week = 240

Let us summarize the above information. If your goal is to expend a given number of calories per week in conjunction with a weight-loss program, you may choose a variety of activities. However, there is at least one trade off with each choice. In our example, if Dexter chooses jogging, he will need to exercise 120 minutes per week to expend 2160 calories. If he chooses brisk walking, he would need approximately 240 minutes per week or 4 one-hour sessions.

These data are for energy expenditure approximations and depend on a number of factors, including the physical condition of the person, his or her degree of skill, and the degree of effort employed. For example, table 16.4 estimates recreational tennis at 0.045 kcal · lb^{-1} · min^{-1}, whereas competitive tennis is estimated at 0.064 kcal · lb^{-1} · min^{-1}. A novice might spend considerable time walking after balls, whereas the expert engages in vigorous rallies. The same would be true for golf. Terrain, skill, and body weight are also important considerations related to the energy cost of the activity. Usually, it costs you more in the rough than on the fairway—in more ways than one!

Swimming provides an extreme example of the importance of skill as one determinant of energy cost of activity. Table 16.6 contains information on differences in energy cost for swimming one mile for both men and women of various skill levels. There is variability not only between skill levels and gender (women are more efficient) but also within a gender and skill level (e.g., competitive women show a range of approximately 115 to 230 calories per mile).

Negative Energy Balance and Weight Loss

The average daily caloric requirement for young adult nonathletic males is about 2900 kcal, and that for young adult nonathletic females is about 2100 kcal (includes light activity). If the daily caloric expenditure from all sources for the young male was 2900 kcal, then his body weight would remain constant. However, if he were to engage in an hour of activity without changing his caloric intake, he could be expending between 300 to 800 kcal more than he takes in; his body weight would decrease. As pointed out above, the magnitude of the decrease may be calculated in terms of how long it would take one pound of pure fat, which contains about 3500 kcal, to be lost. In this example,

table 16.6

Energy cost in calories for swimming one mile as influenced by gender and skill level*

Skill Level	Women (kcal · mi^{-1})	Men (kcal · mi^{-1})
Competitive	115–230	231–308
Skilled	231–270	309–385
Average	271–308	386–462
Unskilled	309–385	463–617

*Modified from Holmer.[63] From N. J. Smith, *Food for Sport*. Copyright © 1976 Bull Publishing Co., Palo Alto, CA. Reprinted with permission from Bull Publishing Company.

it could take 4½ to 11½ days for a pound of fat to be lost (3500/300 = 11½ and 3500/800 = 4½).

For highly active male and female athletes, the daily caloric requirements might be as high as 4000 to 5000 kcal and 3000 to 4500 kcal, respectively. Although these might appear to be excessively high, remember that athletes' daily energy expenditures are also high (e.g., running a 26.2 mile marathon requires about 2500 to 2800 kcal).

Positive Energy Balance and Weight Gain

If our average man from the preceding example were consuming 3500 kcal and expending only 3000 kcal, then he would be in positive energy balance (500 kcal) and would gain body weight. The question to answer is whether he would gain fat weight or fat-free weight. If he were not engaged in an exercise program, the weight gain would be mainly in the form of stored fat.[39] In this case, it would require an excess caloric intake of 3500 kcal to gain one pound of fat. With a +500 kcal balance per day, this would take about seven days.

On the other hand, if an exercise program (strength training) is undertaken at the same time during positive energy balance, the weight gain would be mainly in the form of lean (muscle) weight or fat-free weight. In this case, it requires about 2500 kcal of excess intake to gain one pound of lean or fat-free weight. Assuming the same +500 kcal positive energy balance per day as before, this would take five days.

Figure 16.6 summarizes the relationship of food consumption and energy expenditure (energy balance) to body weight control. Although this model is simplistic and may not represent all the factors that might be considered in energy balance equations, it does accurately represent the concept of energy balance. This describes most people, such that overeating produces fatness, whereas semistarvation

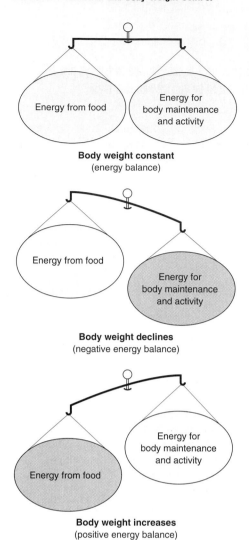

Body weight constant
(energy balance)

Body weight declines
(negative energy balance)

Body weight increases
(positive energy balance)

Figure 16.6
Relationship of food consumption, energy expenditure, and body weight.

and malnutrition produce decreases in body fat and body cell mass.[111] Some factors that are not considered in the most basic forms of the energy balance equations are differences in muscle tone, very small differences in basal energy requirements, prolonged effects of exercise on resting caloric expenditure, and individual differences in the thermic effect of food.[148] The eventual inclusion of these and other factors will yield energy balance equations that are more precise in a scientific sense but may not prove to be more useful in clinical applications.

Guidelines for Losing Body Fat

Although male athletes who have an estimated body fat of less than 7% and female athletes of less than 12% should not be concerned about losing fat (except under medical advisement), many nonathletes and other athletes will find it

necessary to shed body fat. For athletes, this is especially true at the beginning of the season. At the same time, these "overfat" athletes may want to gain, or at least maintain, their fat-free weight. The following guidelines should be helpful in achieving these goals:

1. Remember, it requires an excess expenditure of 3500 kcal to lose one pound of body fat.
2. It is recommended that the caloric deficit not exceed 500 to 1500 kcal · day⁻¹. This is equivalent to a loss of 1 to 3 pounds of fat per week. It is essential to estimate daily or weekly caloric intake and expenditure. This is most readily accomplished with a registered dietitian and/or a qualified exercise physiologist.
3. The caloric deficit should represent both an increased expenditure of energy through physical activity and a controlled, reduced caloric intake. A caloric deficit that is solely the result of diet restriction will also cause fat-free weight loss.
4. For most active athletes, the lower limit of a restricted diet is a 1800 to 2000 kcal intake per day. Caloric reductions below this level should be medically supervised. An example of a 2000-kcal diet is presented in table 16.7. All the essential nutrients are provided in amounts adequate for most athletes.

Guidelines for Gaining Fat-Free Weight

For most people, gaining weight is easy. Unfortunately, the gain is mostly in body fat, which can lead to health problems. Ideally, increases in weight should reflect gains in fat-free weight. Such gains are often desired by athletes, because fat-free weight is generally associated with athletic performance. However, for many athletes, gaining or at least maintaining fat-free weight during the long, difficult season is a real problem. One way of handling this problem is to follow the guidelines for gaining fat-free weight presented as follows:

1. As previously mentioned, to gain weight, caloric intake must be greater than caloric expenditure. To gain one pound of fat-free weight (muscle), an excess intake of about 2500 kcal is required. An excess of this size should not be consumed in one day but, rather, spread over several days.
2. The daily caloric intake should not exceed expenditure by more than 1000 to 1500 kcal. On the basis of 5 diet days per week, this would mean a gain of 2 to 3 pounds per week. This would represent a very ambitious program and would require a very intensive weight-training program.
3. An estimate of how many calories are being taken in and how many are being expended daily or weekly should be made through a diet recall procedure. This is not easy, but it can be done with the help of the

table 16.7

Example of a low-calorie (2000 kcal) diet in five meals*

Breakfast	Snack
½ cup orange juice 1 soft-boiled egg 1 slice whole wheat toast 2 tsp. margarine 1 glass skim milk or other beverage Total kcal: 345	1 banana Total kcal: 100

Lunch	Snack

1 hamburger (3 oz.) on
    a roll with relish
½ sliced tomato
1 glass skim milk
1 medium apple
Total kcal: 510
	1 carton fruit-flavored
	    yogurt
	1 cup grape juice
	
	Total kcal: 385

Dinner	

1 serving of baked
    chicken marengo
    (½ breast)
¾ cup rice
5–6 Brussels sprouts
1 bowl of green salad
    with French dressing
1 small piece
    gingerbread
1 cup skim milk or other
    low-cal beverage
Total kcal: 660
	Daily total kcal: 2000

*From Smith.[115]

athlete's parents and perhaps the home economics teacher or school dietitian.

4. Calories needed to maintain weight must be added to excess intake for an accurate picture of the diet of an athlete on a weight-gain plan. In this regard, an intake of 4000 kcal · day^{-1} is a realistic diet for young male athletes, because their average daily caloric expenditure may be about 3000 kcal.

5. To ensure that the excess calories will be laid down primarily as muscle, a vigorous training program, particularly of weight training, should be undertaken during the high-caloric diet period. The skinfold measures mentioned earlier can be used to determine whether any excess fat is being added.

Examples of programs of weight gain and weight reduction are given in table 16.8.

Making Weight in Wrestling

The Committee on Medical Aspects of Sports of the American Medical Association has posed several questions relevant to the wrestling community:[24]

1. What are the hazards of indiscriminate and excessive weight reduction?
2. How much weight can a wrestler lose safely?
3. What are defensible means of losing weight?
4. What weigh-in plan would best serve the purpose intended?

In the following discussion, we will attempt to address many of these issues. The committee also states that the amount of weight that a wrestler can safely lose should be related to his *most effective* weight level (the weight level that yields his best performance) rather than the lowest possible weight that the wrestler thinks he can achieve. It is difficult to define scientifically the limits of safe weight control. Argument is in favor of a good pre-participation medical examination and weight determination 6 to 8 weeks prior to the start of the season. Such a plan involves the weight history, which allows the physician, parents, and coach a more valid judgment regarding how much weight an athlete can safely lose.

Wrestlers who "cut weight" often deny themselves the very nutrients they need for maintaining strength and endurance. Cutting weight by restricting water intake for prolonged periods of time can have deleterious effects on performance as well. Wrestling is one of the few sports where the athlete will purposely reduce his performance capacity just prior to competition![98] A recent study on collegiate wrestlers evaluated strength, aerobic power, and anaerobic power following a 36-hour period of **dehydration** for weight loss.[136] The athletes lost an average of 3.3 kg (4.9% of body weight). On retesting, the athletes were found to have deteriorated in upper body strength, aerobic power (endurance), anaerobic power (explosiveness), and lactate threshold. During bouts of acute, forced dehydration the athlete is not losing body fat; he is losing athletic performance.

The wrestler uses a combination of food restriction, liquid deprivation, and other dehydration methods, such as working in rubberized suits, induced vomiting, and ingestion of laxatives to lose weight. These practices have not changed significantly from earlier times.[117]

The American College of Sports Medicine in its Position Stand on Weight Loss in Wrestlers[4] concluded that the simple and combined effects of these practices are generally associated with (1) a reduction in muscular strength; (2) a de-crease in work performance times (the athlete cannot work as long); (3) lower plasma and blood volumes; (4) a reduction in cardiac functioning during submaximal work conditions; (5) a lower oxygen consumption, especially when food restriction is a critical part of the weight-reduction plan; (6) an impairment of thermoregulatory processes; (7) a decrease in renal blood flow and in the volume of fluid being filtered by the kidney; (8) a depletion of liver glycogen stores; and (9) an increase in the amount of electrolytes being lost from the body. Some studies have shown that weight losses caused by dehydration of 3% or more result in diminished athletic performance. Prolonged semistarvation diets, unbalanced dets, and excessive sweating combined with dehydration may cause severe harm to the athlete.

The amount of weight that a wrestler can safely lose should be related to his effective *weight level* (the weight level that yields his best performance) rather than to the lowest weight, according to the Committee on the Medical Aspects of Sports.

The committee is quick to emphasize that there is no alternative to:[24]

1. a balanced diet at a sustaining caloric level
2. adequate fluid intake
3. high-energy output for attaining and maintaining an effective competitive weight

Finally, the committee suggests that the weight of the wrestling candidates can best be assessed through a natural approach:[24]

1. Educate youth who are interested in athletics regarding the importance of periodic medical examinations and the advantages of a general, year-round conditioning program for cardiovascular-pulmonary endurance, muscular fitness, and nutritional readiness.
2. Building on this orientation, assist any aspiring wrestler in an intensive conditioning program related to the demands of wrestling for at least four weeks—preferably six—without emphasis on weight level.
3. At the end of this period and without altering his daily training routine, take his weight in a prebreakfast, postmicturition state.
4. Consider this weight his minimal effective weight for competition as well as for certification.
5. Educate the wrestler and his parents in the concept of defensible weight control to avert fluctuation from his effective weight level.

The Iowa Studies

Tipton and colleagues have performed extensive studies concerning the effect of weight loss in high-school wrestlers. One study shows that:[127]

1. A large number of young athletes lose an excessive amount of weight in a relatively short period of time. This holds true for all classes below 175 lb. The lightest lose the highest percentage (about 10%) of body weight during a 17-day period (figure 16.7).
2. The majority of weight loss occurs immediately preceding the date of certification.

table

16.8

Examples of fat-free weight (FFW) gain and fat reduction programs

Athlete	Present body composition
Football player	Total body weight: 200 pounds Fat: 10% FFW: 180 pounds
Field hockey player	Total body weight: 127 pounds Fat: 25% FFW: 95 pounds

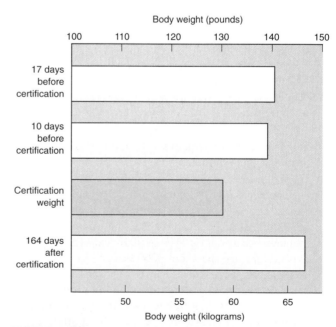

Figure 16.7

During a 17-day period, 6.8 pounds or 4.9% of the body weight was lost, most of which occurred during the last 10 days. An average increase of 13.6 pounds above the certification weight occurred at the end of the season.

16.8

table

(Continued)

| | Means of achieving goal | | |
Daily caloric intake	Daily caloric expenditure	Difference between intake and expenditure	Goal (after 3 months)
6000 kcal	4940 kcal, including calories spent in training*	6000 – 4940 = 1060 kcal *excess*	Total body weight: 225 pounds Fat: 8% FFW: 207 pounds
2000 kcal; see Table 16.7	3000 kcal, including calories spent in training†	3000 – 2000 = 1000 kcal *deficit* (500 from restricted diet, 500 from exercise)	Total body weight: 112 pounds Fat: 15% FFW: 95 pounds

*Training for the football player interested in gaining fat-free weight might include repeated 40-yard sprints (2 days per week) and weight-resistance training (3 days per week).

†Training for the field hockey player interested in losing body fat might include jogging 3 miles per day, calisthenics, and weight-resistance training (2 days per week).

3. Weight-loss methods were suggested by either coach or teammate.
4. Of the 835 boys measured, the average percentage of fat is 8%, whereas the state finalists (n = 224) had a 4% to 6% body-fat content.

Tipton has been particularly concerned with the lack of professional supervision dealing with the method or amount of weight that an athlete should lose. He recommends a body weight containing 7% fat (not less than 5% without medical supervision) and one that does not exceed 7% loss of the initial weight. Ideally, one would predict minimum weight at the beginning of the school year; then under professional guidance, a proper and gradual weight reduction could take place. Relying on the judgment of experienced coaches is not effective in determining minimum weight for wrestlers. An informed judgment as to the effective minimum weight for a particular athlete must be made on various measures, which may include underwater weighing, prediction by anthropometric methods, or prediction by skinfold methods.

Predicting Minimal Weight Values for Wrestlers

Research by Tcheng and Tipton[122] resulted in an equation that allows prediction of minimal weight values. The original work has been revalidated and a slightly modified formula has been developed.[89] Several anthropometric measurements are obtained six to eight weeks before the start of the wrestling season. The minimal weight is computed and the result then used as a screening device, along with the physician's judgment concerning the proper minimal weight for the particular high-school wrestler.

Anthropometrical Measurements

The following **anthropometric measurements** (see figure 16.8) are necessary for predicting minimal weights in wrestlers:

1. *Chest Diameter.* Subject stands with both hands on the crests of the ilium. Calipers are placed in the axillary region with ends placed on the second or third rib. At the end of the expiration, the measurement is obtained.
2. *Chest Depth.* Subject stands with right hand behind head. One end of the caliper is placed on the tip of the xiphoid process while the other end is placed over the vertebrae of the twelfth rib. Measurement is taken at the end of the expiration.
3. *Wrist Diameter.* Distance between the styloid processes of the radius and ulna is measured on the right wrist.

Data from the preceding anthropometric measures may then be substituted in "model II" of the Tcheng-Tipton formula, as follows:

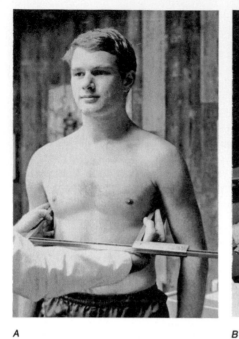
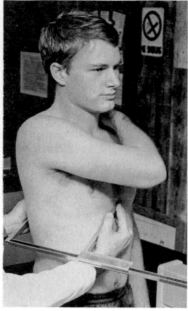
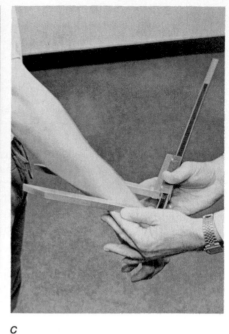

A   B   C

Figure 16.8

Measurements required for predicting minimal wrestling weight for high-school males. *A,* Chest diameter; *B,* chest depth; and *C,* wrist diameter.

(Photos by Cliffton Boutelle, News and Information Service, Bowling Green State University.)

Model II Tcheng-Tipton Equation

Minimal weight = 1.65 × height in inches

+ 0.49 × current weight in lbs

+ 1.81 × chest diameter in cm

+ 1.35 × chest depth in cm

+ 6.70 × right wrist diameter in cm

− 156.56 (a constant)

The result is reported, then, as the predicted minimal weight for the wrestler.

As an example of how to use the equation, a young aspiring wrestler was measured at the beginning of the wrestling season with the following results:

Weight = 160 lb
Height = 68 in
Chest diameter = 25.4 cm
Chest depth = 18.5 cm
Right wrist diameter = 5.8 cm

Minimal Weight (Tcheng-Tipton Model II)

Minimal weight	= 1.65 × ht	= 1.65 × 68	= 112.2
	+ 0.49 × wt	= 0.49 × 160	= 78.4
	+ 1.81 × ch. dia.	= 1.81 × 25.4	= 45.97
	+ 1.35 × ch. depth	= 1.35 × 18.5	= 24.98
	+ 6.70 × wrist dia.	= 6.70 × 5.8	= 38.86
			= 300.41
			− 156.56

Calculated minimal weight = 143.85

The young athlete's predicted minimal weight equals 143.85 (or 144) lbs. Weighing 160 lb some 8 weeks prior to the season, the absolute maximum this wrestler should be allowed to lose would be 16 pounds. A systematic weight-reduction program, in consultation with a physician and/or a dietician, could be incorporated where the wrestler, through dietary controls and vigorous exercise, could lose 1.5 to 2.0 pounds per week.

The Midwest Wrestling Study

A recent study by a group of investigators at five midwestern universities has proposed new equations for predicting minimal weight for high-school wrestlers.[124] The study investigated the use of approximately thirty anthropometric measurements including circumferences, diameters, and skinfolds as well as age, height, and weight. The conclusion to the study identified five possible equations for estimating body density, from which percent body fat may be calculated. One of those equations, by Lohman, is presented here as an example. The Lohman equation is presented because it uses familiar skinfold sites.

$$D_b = 1.0982 - (0.000815)(X) + (0.00000084)(X^2)$$

where: D_b = body density
X = sum of the triceps, subscapular, and abdominal skinfolds

To recommend a reasonable body weight for a high-school wrestler, the three skinfolds must be measured, along with the athlete's body weight, approximately *6 to 8 weeks prior* to the start of the wrestling season (that is, prior to the time that the wrestler starts to "cut weight").

Example: A 16-year-old wrestling candidate, Matt Bouts, is assessed in early September with these results:

Weight: 146 lbs   Skinfolds: Triceps = 6 mm
Subscapular = 9 mm
Abdominal = 15 mm
Sum of the skinfolds = $\overline{30}$ mm

Apply the equation of Lohman:

D_b = 1.0982 − (0.000815) (**30**) + (0.00000084) (**30** × **30**)
D_b = 1.0982 − 0.02445 + 0.000756
D_b = 1.07451

Using the Brozek conversion for percent body fat (p. 445), we see the following results:

$$\% \text{ Fat} = \frac{457}{D_b} - 414.2$$

$$\% \text{ Fat} - \frac{457}{1.07451} - 414.2$$

$$\% \text{ Fat} = 425.3 - 414.2 = \textbf{11.1}$$

Based on this result, Matt's fat-free body weight would be calculated as follows (p. 446):

$$\textbf{FFW} = \textbf{(TBW)} \times \textbf{(1.00 − F_f)}$$

Where:

FFW = fat-free body weight
TBW = total body weight
F_f = decimal expression of the percent body fat

FFW = (**146**) × (1.00 − **0.111**)
FFW = (146) × (0.889)
FFW = **129.8** lbs.

For a 5% fat level divide the FFW by 0.95, and for a 7% level divide the FFW by 0.93.

Thus, Matt's weight at 5% and 7% body fat would be as follows:

TBW at 5% = 129.8/0.95 = **137 lbs**
TBW at 7% = 129.8/0.93 = **140 lbs**

Interpretation and action: in accordance with the American College of Sports Medicine guidelines, Matt could lose some body fat to reach a lower weight.

Matt Bouts would have a relatively simple task of losing between 6 and 9 pounds of body fat over 6 to 8 weeks prior to starting the wrestling season. The goal is to have the wrestler training at a body weight that would allow him to be within 3 pounds of his weight class at all times during the season.

ACSM Guidelines for Weight Loss in Wrestlers

The American College of Sports Medicine (ACSM) suggests that the potential health hazard created by the procedures that are used by wrestlers to "make weight" can be eliminated if state and national organizations will incorporate the following guidelines.[4]

1. Assess the body composition of each wrestler several weeks in advance of the competitive season. Individuals with a fat content less than 5% of their certified body weight should receive medical clearance before being allowed to compete.
2. Emphasize the fact that the daily caloric requirements of wrestlers should be obtained from a balanced diet and determined on the basis of age, body surface area, growth, and physical activity levels. The minimal caloric needs of wrestlers in high schools and colleges should range from 1700 to 2500 kcal · day^{-1}; therefore, it is the responsibility of coaches, school officials, physicians, and parents to discourage wrestlers from securing less than their minimal needs without prior medical approval.
3. Discourage the practice of fluid deprivation and dehydration. This can be accomplished by:
   (a) Educating the coaches and wrestlers [so that they are aware of] to the physiological consequences and medical complications that can occur as a result of these practices.
   (b) Prohibiting the single or combined use of rubber suits, steam rooms, hot boxes, saunas, laxatives, and diuretics to "make weight."
   (c) Scheduling weigh-ins just prior to competition.
   (d) Scheduling more official weigh-ins between team matches.
4. Permit more participants per team to compete in those weight classes (119 to 151 lb) which have the highest percentages of wrestlers certified for competition.
5. Standardize regulations concerning the eligibility rules at championship tournaments so that individuals can participate only in those weight classes in which they had the highest frequencies of matches throughout the season.
6. Encourage local and county organizations to systematically collect data on the hydration state of wrestlers and its relationship to growth and development.

Women Gymnasts

Another group of athletes who are constantly aware of attaining a minimum body weight are female gymnasts. However, the reasons for attaining a minimum weight are different than for wrestlers. First, the appearance and presentation of the gymnast is taken into account by judges in the sport. Second, the gymnast must be able to control the body during free exercise, balance beam, uneven parallel bars, and vaulting performances.

As with wrestling, gymnastics is a highly anaerobic activity and, although the intensity of exercise is high, the duration is short. The opportunity to burn large quantities of calories is minimized in both practice and competition. As

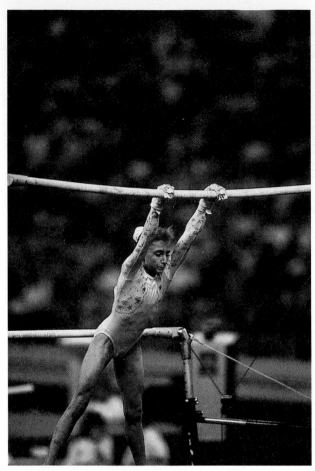

Figure 16.9

Photo of international-level competitive woman gymnast whose body fat percentage would be very low.

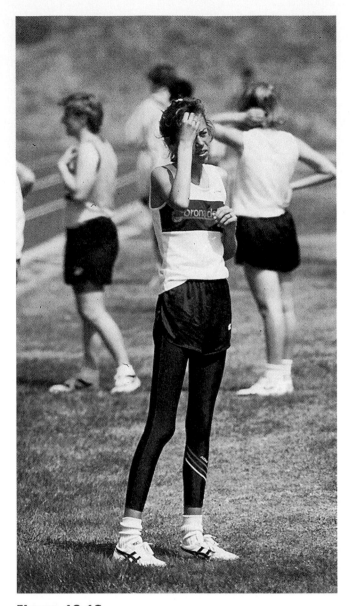

Figure 16.10

Photograph of a woman runner showing the near "anorexic" appearance that some of these dedicated athletes attain. This condition of extreme thinness is often accompanied by amenorrhea and symptoms of osteoporosis.

a consequence, women gymnasts resort to bizarre behaviors, similar to wrestlers, to achieve a low body weight. In one study a survey concerning nutritional habits of collegiate women gymnasts reported that all athletes were actively attempting to diet.[103] Of the gymnasts studied, 62% were using at least one form of pathogenic weight control practice, including self-induced vomiting, diet pills, fasting, diuretics, fluid restriction, and laxatives. These practices are identical to those practiced by anorexia nervosa patients[88] and have led to the death of at least one elite-level woman gymnast.

What can the gymnast do to control body weight in a healthy manner? Year-round management of body weight is important and emphasizing aerobic activity in the off-season helps to maintain a desired weight. A controlled, balanced diet is essential. Finally, having a body composition assessment performed helps give a realistic assessment of body composition. Hydrostatic weighing is the method of choice for determining body density but, in lieu of that, the four-site equation of Jackson, Pollock, and Ward may be used with female gymnasts.[66,113] Sinning[113] has examined

the validity of using this equation with gymnasts and other athletes. The following skinfold sites are measured for application to the equation below: triceps, abdominal, iliac crest, and midthigh (see figure 16.11).

Example: A 20-year-old female has the following skinfolds:

$$\begin{array}{rl}
\text{Triceps skinfold} & = 12 \text{ mm} \\
\text{Abdominal skinfold} & = 23 \text{ mm} \\
\text{Iliac crest skinfold} & = 20 \text{ mm} \\
\text{Midthigh skinfold} & = \underline{25 \text{ mm}} \\
\textbf{Sum of skinfolds} & = \overline{\textbf{80 mm}}
\end{array}$$

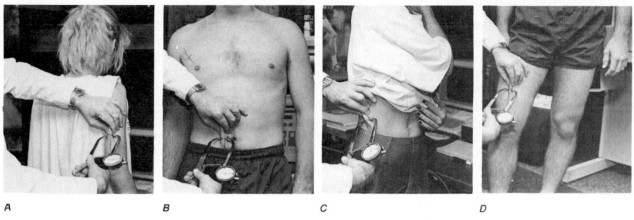

A　　　　　　B　　　　　　C　　　　　　D

Figure 16.11 A–D.

Skinfold sites for estimating body density in women gymnasts using the Jackson-Pollock-Ward equation for four skinfolds.[65]

Note: Although two of the demonstrated skinfold sites are on a male, they are valid for a female.

Applying the JPW four-site equation for women gymnasts:

$$D_b = 1.096095 - 0.0006952 (X_1) + 0.0000011 (X_1)^2 - 0.0000714 (X_2)$$

Where:

$$X_1 = \text{sum of four skinfolds}$$
$$X_2 = \text{age}$$
$$D_b = 1.096095 - 0.0006952 (\textbf{80}) + 0.0000011$$
$$(\textbf{80} \times \textbf{80}) - 0.0000714 (\textbf{20})$$
$$D_b = 1.096095 - 0.055616 + 0.00704 - 0.001428$$
$$\textbf{D}_b = 1.046091 \text{ or } \textbf{1.0461}$$

The next step is to translate density into a percent body fat using the Siri equation.

$$\% \text{ Body fat} = \frac{495}{D_b} - 450$$
$$\% \text{ Body fat} = \frac{495}{1.0461} - 450$$
$$\textbf{\% Body fat} = 473.2 - 450 = \textbf{23.2}$$

As with wrestling, education of both the athlete and the coach is essential, not only in gymnastics, but in all sports.[15]

Summary of Body Composition Assessment Processes

We have presented several alternatives for evaluating body composition for athletes and others in a variety of settings. Each of the methods presented is only as good as the skill of the test administrator in making the measurements. Therefore, prior to making the measurements, the coach, trainer, or exercise specialist must be trained in identifying and measuring the various sites. Wrestling and women's gymnastics represent special cases where care must be taken in translating the results of assessment processes. The Wisconsin Interscholastic Athletic Association is currently developing a program for both training coaches to measure body composition and providing sound dietary advice.*

Exercise and Training Effects

In this section we will review some research findings as they pertain to several subtopics in the general area of body composition and weight control. Namely, we will concentrate on the effects of exercise, either acute bouts or short-term activity programs, the effects of longer-term training, the differences that exist between groups of athletes, and some findings related to children and older adults. To begin, the reader is referred to reviews on the measurement of body composition in clinical settings[96] and future directions for body composition research in sports and exercise programs.[140] Recent studies strongly support the notion that low energy expenditure at rest or during physical activity can facilitate rapid weight gain in susceptible individuals.[99] They also indicate that an individual's physical activity level can be a strong determinant of the level of body weight and body fatness at which a steady-state of true energy balance is attained.[59] Wood[145] reiterates this important point in saying "there is persuasive evidence that much obesity is due to underexercising rather than overeating."

As indicated earlier, there is a definite place for exercise and an increased expenditure of energy in activities of daily living as part of programs to assist people to lose

---

*For information concerning "The Wrestler's Diet" and the "Wisconsin Wrestling Minimum Weight Project," write to Wisconsin Interscholastic Athletic Association, 41 Park Ridge Drive, P.O. Box 267, Madison, WI 54481.

weight[42] and to maintain weight loss. Grubbs[51] has reviewed the comparative benefits of different exercise intensities, durations, frequencies, and modalities as related to body weight control. The exercise should be of long duration and of low to moderate intensity so as to maximize energy expenditure and promote a negative caloric "balance."[45] That is, the activities should be aerobic in nature, should be performed frequently and should promote the liberation and metabolism of the person's own stored fat energy sources. For maximal effect, the selected activities should be combined with a diet low in fat.[129] Remember that exercise alone can produce a modest gain of lean body mass (LBM) and loss of fat in weight-stable individuals.[40]

The programmed activities must be safe and take into consideration some specific concerns and precautions related to obese and overweight persons.[41,43] The effects of aerobic exercise such as walking and jogging have been found to be reliable and directly related to energy expenditure.[31] Exercise is of benefit to overweight persons even if it does not make them lean and is recommended as an important part of weight-control programs.[13] That is to say, the multitude of positive, beneficial "side effects" that accompany participation in exercise sessions during an overall weight-loss program tend to more than compensate for the arguments that it takes a lot of exercise to "burn off a pound of fat."

Exercise Classes

Aerobic dancing at an intensity of 70% of maximum heart rate for 30 minutes during the first week and progressing to 90 minutes by the thirteenth week produced only small reductions in the body weights of previously sedentary female college students.[70] Estimations of percent body fat decreased more predictably and dramatically, but it did not matter whether the students danced two or three times per week, the same effects were seen. A second study reports contradictory results in that a 10-week period of aerobic dance classes (3 classes per week, 45 minutes per class) failed to produce any reductions in either body weight or percent fat.[130] The training intensity was not reported but was adequate to produce improvements in cardiorespiratory measurements. The underlying reason for the failure of this aerobic dance activity to produce reductions in percent body fat was not apparent, but the short duration of the study has been suggested. This argument is countered by the report that male physical education students who exercised at various team games and sports for 20 to 30 hours per week were heavier and had higher body fat percentages at the end of a three-year period of study.[134]

Reductions in body fat and body weight have been reported for participants who have engaged in a variety of other activities. For example, participants in a 4-week, intensive Alpine climbing expedition lost both body fat and lean body mass.[6] Likewise, six sedentary obese men, ages 19 to 31, lost a significant amount of body weight and fat during the completion of 16 weeks of vigorous walking 90 minutes per day, 5 days per week, on a treadmill at speeds up to 3.2 mph on a 10% grade.[76] It was estimated that they expended about 1100 kcal per session or about 88,000 kcal during the experimental period. This would be equivalent to 25 lbs of fat. The subjects actually lost an average of 11.5 lbs (5.7 kg). So, by any rough accounting of caloric balance, it is apparent that no attempt was being made to "influence their diet." When there is no attempt to control dietary intakes, exercise-induced reductions in body weight and body fat are not closely related to exercise intensity[120] (cycle ergometer, 45 min $\cdot$ d^{-1}, 5 d $\cdot$ wk^{-1}, 12 weeks, 540 kgm $\cdot$ min^{-1} versus 900 kpm $\cdot$ min^{-1}), or duration[128] (jogging 1.6 km, 3.2 km, or 4.8 km, 3 d $\cdot$ wk^{-1}, 85% HRmax, 12 weeks). Finally, exercising in cool water (17 to 22° C, bicycle ergometer, 5 times per week, 30% to 40% of maximum oxygen consumption, 8 weeks) was well tolerated by obese women but did not reduce their body weight, body fat, fat-free body weight, or caloric intake.[109] The best way to effectively lose body fat is to combine a regular, steady exercise program and dietary control.

Training Programs

The effects of exercise in supervised and unsupervised training programs have been studied. These results are more consistent because subjects in all cases lost body weight and body fat and showed reductions in skinfolds in studies where these important measurements were made. For example, sixteen young female swimmers (mean age 15.8 years) decreased their percentage of body fat from 21.9% to 19.8% during 7 weeks of training where they swam an average of 12,806 yards per week and worked out an average of 4 days per week.[118] Fat percentage losses were a bit greater, 17.3% to 14.6%, for thirteen sedentary male subjects (mean age 24.3 years) who participated in a 20-week aerobic training program (bicycle ergometer, 40 to 45 minutes per session, 4 to 5 times per week, progressing from 60% to 85% of heart rate range).[26] The sum of seven skinfolds was significantly reduced with most of the reductions occurring in trunk rather than extremity measures. This latter finding was interpreted to mean that exercise-induced fat losses are not due to a preferential depletion of subcutaneous fat layers. Similar losses in body fat from 25.8% down to 23.2% occurred in twenty-two women runners (mean age 28.4 years, range 23 to 37) who increased their running by 30 miles per week over a 4- to 7-month period.[105] These reductions in body fat were accompanied by small increases in lean body weight from 42.3 to 43.0 kg.

Estimations of percent body fat of eighty-seven male and fifty-seven female army trainees were made using four skinfold measurements and the regression equations of Durnin and Wormsley.[92] After 7 weeks of basic training, the estimated body fat had decreased by 11% in males (from

16.3% to 14.5%) and 7% in females (28.2% to 26.2%). The fat losses were greatest in personnel who had the highest starting levels (i.e., those who had the most to lose). A contrasting study of the effects of marathon-run training on young men (mean age 21.7 years) who started with relatively low body fat percentages of 13.4% has been reported.[69] The subjects participated in a 16-week special training program where they ran 50 to 70 miles per week to prepare them to run a certified marathon. Their body fat dropped to 10.8% and the sum of six skinfolds decreased from 70.1 to 52.6 mm. It was concluded that transition from moderate to extreme endurance training levels in normal young men is accompanied by significant reductions in body fat.

Finally, a study of lean and obese middle-aged female subjects who participated together in a supervised, 12-week aerobic training program has been reported.[44] The program was structured along ACSM guidelines (walking-jogging 15 to 25 minutes, 4 days per week, 75% max $\dot{V}O_2$). Normal-weight subjects decreased their body fat from 24.7% to 23.9%, obese subjects reduced from 38.0% to 36.2%, and the sum of ten skinfolds decreased significantly in both groups. This moderate-intensity physical conditioning program affected both obese and leaner women in a similar fashion. An 18-month follow-up of a subsample of these subjects indicated that they regained body weight and body fat to pretraining levels.[82] Because only half of the well-intentioned subjects were exercising on their own, it was concluded that the majority of middle-aged women who have participated in supervised walk-jog conditioning interventions will regress to their preprogram levels of fitness and fatness when left to exercise ad libitum ("take it as you will"). This is the principal reason why good exercise leaders always will be in demand.

Health/Disease Implications

Obesity is a major health problem for both adult and adolescent populations of the United States and has implications for a variety of diseases.[53] At the same time, lifestyle choices leading to weight loss can have a favorable impact in preventing or alleviating certain chronic diseases that are relatable to obesity—i.e., coronary heart disease, stroke, and diabetes.[121] Both the duration and magnitude of an individual's obesity increases their risk for developing diabetes[14] as does the accumulation of visceral fat deposits.[11] Indexes associated with high metabolic disease risk in obese persons often return to normal with appropriate physical activities, dietary habits, and a small weight loss even when body weight and percentage body fat remain above recommended amounts.[1] Likewise, increased blood pressure correlates closely with excess body weight and can be reduced by weight loss, often by the initiation of a regular physical exercise regimen.[81]

Although most dieters strive to achieve "ideal" body weight, achieving a modest weight loss goal as low as 5%

may be adequate to attain improved health and emotional benefits.[12] Brownell[16] has reviewed studies on the effects of repeated weight cycling or "yo-yo" dieting and has found no consistent demonstration that this practice makes subsequent weight loss more difficult or regaining weight more rapid. This is not as originally believed but is supported by data that body composition is not altered by weight cycling resulting from an annual hunger cycle in rural African people.[97] This finding also holds for moderately obese British women who underwent three cycles of weight loss and regain through very low-calorie diets.[97]

The secretion of growth hormone and the mass and distribution of body fat are linked through a complex series of interactions. In fact, the obese state may, in some cases, reflect a defect in growth hormone release which can be reversed by weight loss.[48] Yarasheski[147] has reviewed the effects of GH on body composition but mainly as it relates to muscle mass and strength. Among healthy adults, GH secretion relates in a negative manner to the amount of abdominal obesity—i.e., with more abdominal fat, less GH secretion.[71]

Sports-Specific Responses

Body composition differences among athletes who compete in different sports has been an area of research interest for several decades. These efforts are driven by questions such as which athletes have the lowest body fat percentages and which have the highest, which athletes have the greatest amount of lean muscle mass and how does this contribute to their performance, and how do "average" performers compare with elite athletes? The review by Wilmore[140] covers these questions well and includes height, weight, and body fat percentages for twenty different sports, from twenty different reports published since 1980. Fat percentage levels ranged from 4.6 and 5.0 for male gymnasts and wrestlers up to 26% and 28% for some female swimmers, basketball players, and discus or shot-putters. The lowest values for female athletes were between 9.6% and 11% for gymnasts and pentathlon competitors.

Since this report, a variety of other athletes have been described including Nigerian female athletes by sport,[84] and elite American athletes by sport.[38] The latter report is based on 528 male and 298 female athletes participating in twenty-six and fifteen different Olympic events. Generally speaking, participants in sports where their body weight is supported have higher percent fat values (canoe and kayak—males 13%, females 22%) than athletes who have to meet a weight class (boxing or wrestling—males 7% to 8%), perform very anaerobically (100 and 200 meters—males 6%, females 14%), or perform extremely aerobically (marathon—males 6%). The athletes with the highest lean body masses were participants in sports where body size is a definite advantage (basketball—males 84 kg, females 55 kg; volleyball—males 75 kg, females 58 kg).

Other reports of body fat exist for rugby union or club players[8] (11% to 18% depending on position), female ballet and modern dancers[28] (18% to 26%), speed skaters[95] (non-Olympic 8.1%, Olympic 6.8%), college football players by position[138] (defensive backs 7.3%, offensive linemen 14.8%), and 9- to 12-year-old experienced wrestlers[107] (controls 20%, wrestlers 13%). Lean body mass has been measured in thirty middle-aged male marathon runners who were found to be slightly taller and lighter in weight than a comparison group.[3] More importantly, their total body calcium and potassium levels were higher, which supports the concept that rigorous exercise prevents the involuntary loss of skeletal and lean body mass. Finally, high-school basketball officials have been reported to be overweight with average body densities of 1.047 and 22% body fat levels.[62]

Children and Fatness

Another topic we will address is that of children, including their body composition and changes that occur during the process of growth. It is well known that obese children often become obese adults, that dramatic changes in body composition and fatness can occur during the peripubertal years, and that some children are at risk for disease. Further labeling of these children as obese and recommending weight control therapy may do more harm than good, especially since it is not always clear whether or not they are experiencing an adverse impact to their overall health.[101]

Our current understanding of children's overweight and obesity is limited because there have been relatively few studies of total energy expenditure and macronutrient intake in children.[50] Other limitations to our understanding relate to the best choice of assessment methods to be used with this special age group. A movement away from the two-compartment (fat and fat-free body) system to newer methodologies that allow a better understanding of muscle and bone changes with training has been suggested.[79] Arguments also have been made that BMI is a preferred method to use with children in that BMI patterns reflect real changes in body shape and indicate later development.[102]

Part of the problem with childhood fatness might relate to differences between the perceptions that obese and slim children have of physical education and other school activities.[146] Obese children evaluate endurance activities more negatively and flexibility-coordination activities more positively than slim children.

Girls at an age of 8.75 years have a higher percentage of body fat than boys, 24.3% (range 14.7% to 41.6%) versus 20.1% (range 11.7% to 34.3%).[74] Fatness levels in girls cannot be related to longitudinal activity scores obtained from the age of 6 months, whereas there is a negative correlation between activity scores of boys at age 3 and 4 years and their fatness levels at age 8. Percent fat levels in obese

adolescents (mean 12.7 years, range 10 to 16 years) are higher for girls (42.2%) than for boys (39.3%).[73] Physical work capacities determined at a selected heart rate of 170 b · min^{-1} (PWC$_{170}$) are not related to percent body fat in male youths between the ages of 15 and 19 years.[135] Finally, Meredith has alerted us that there may be differences in the body weight and other somatic dimensions of rural compared with urban children in different countries of the world.[86]

Aging and Fatness

Currently, there is much interest in the matter of aging, the aging process, and the influence of exercise on older populations. Durnin[30] has addressed the topic of body composition and energy expenditure in elderly people (defined as being 60 to 75 years of age). Changes in body mass and body composition accompany aging, making measurement of these components much more variable.[47] These changes also reduce the total energy expenditure[93] and the need for a large food intake. The body, however, retains its ability to regulate energy balance during periods of over- and under-eating[100] so excess nutrient intake contributes to fatness.

Height is known to decrease by as much as 5 to 7 cm between the ages of 30 and 70 years for some groups, with larger reductions in industrial communities and among less privileged socioeconomic classes. There is additional evidence that the skeletal mass and the mineral content of the skeleton decrease and the fat mass of the body increases in elderly people. There also is a change in the ratio of fat between the subcutaneous layers and adipose tissue deposits on the trunk of the body, with more of the fat being deposited in the deeper regions in older people.

Basal metabolic rate measures are lower in older persons, but much of this might be due to the shifts in lean to fat components, which favor a lowered metabolic rate. The body composition of most elderly people will be more influenced by differences in energy expenditure related to their leisure time activity levels than to whether they still work at a sedentary job. Other considerations include whether they suffer from degenerative diseases of the cardiorespiratory or bone and joint systems, which makes it uncomfortable or even painful for them to be more active. They also may have experienced a reduction in the mechanical efficiency of their limbs or in control over their balance, which occurs more often with aging. For the stay-at-home mother, physical activity around the home may become progressively less after the children are raised. This means that her energy expenditure starts to decrease at age 45 to 50, and falls proportionally more than that of a man up to the age of 70 years. She is especially vulnerable to weight gain and obesity around the time of menopause.[57]

Durnin[30] suggests that it might be more important to emphasize what the levels of physical activity and energy expenditure of elderly persons ought to be rather than to spend more time in assessing what they currently are. He suggests that we should "actively" encourage physical activity in the elderly, which, in turn, will be accompanied by an increase in their energy expenditure and a decrease in fatness, and at the same time promote the need to ingest adequate amounts of essential dietary nutrients. In essence, the elderly should strive for an activity-driven metabolic system that is truly in a harmonious balance.

Numerous studies have emphasized the capacity of older men and women to adapt to regularly performed "aerobic" exercise with consistent improvements in functional capacity.[33] Other studies indicate that progressive resistance training produces improvements in strength, muscle size, and skeletal muscular function and reduces the loss of muscle mass associated with **sarcopenia**.[35] Evans[34] suggests that the positive changes in body composition that occur with exercise, and especially with resistance training, may not only prevent sarcopenia but also a wide array of associated abnormalities. Further, there is no pharmacological intervention that holds a greater promise of improving health and promoting independence in the elderly than exercise. Poehlman[94] cautions that aerobic exercise might be counterproductive to stimulating fat loss if older subjects become less active during the remainder of the day. This may make resistance training the exercise of choice since it helps to both preserve fat-free mass and raise resting metabolic rate. This combination of adaptations results in a more predictable oxidation of whole body fat.

Summary

Endomorph, mesomorph, and ectomorph are the terms employed in describing the somatotype or body type of a person. Endomorph refers to fat; mesomorph to muscle; and ectomorph to a body that is lean. Each of us has a degree of all three body-type components. Athletes and other active people tend to have higher mesomorphic and ectomorphic components than do nonathletes or sedentary individuals.

Fat content of the body is significantly associated with physical activity. Athletes and other active people are less obese than sedentary individuals. Lack of exercise with overeating is the prime cause of obesity in all age groups. Obesity refers to the above-average amount of fat contained in the body, which in turn is dependent on the lipid (fat) content of each adipocyte (fat cell) and on the total number of fat cells. The prevention of obesity through regular exercises and proper diet is more successful than is the treatment for it.

Two methods are commonly employed in estimating fat content of the body: (1) measuring the density of the person and (2) measuring skinfolds to estimate body density. The density of the body can be measured by hydrostatic (underwater) weighing. This is the most accurate, readily available method for estimating body density, but it is also difficult from a technical standpoint. Estimates of body density from skinfold measures are less accurate and more specific than underwater weighing but are a less difficult and more practical method. Body fat can be estimated from body density measures using one of two equations: (1) Brozek, percent fat = (457/body density) − 414.2, or (2) Siri, percent body fat = (495/body density) − 450.

Energy balance means consuming the same amount of energy through food intake as is being expended by activity. When more energy is consumed than expended, the person is said to be in a positive energy balance and body weight is gained. When less energy is consumed than expended, the person is said to be in a negative energy balance and body weight is lost. The weight gained may be in the form of fat or fat-free (lean or muscle) weight. The latter is possible when a person is in a positive energy balance while participating in an exercise program.

Considerable attention is being given to the serious malpractices associated with "making weight" in wrestling. This is particularly true for high-school wrestlers. Various methods are available that give a reasonable estimate for minimum weight for the young wrestler. Women gymnasts also represent a special challenge in body weight control and nutrition education.

Questions

1. Define endomorphy, mesomorphy, and ectomorphy.
2. How do the somatotypes of marathon runners compare with those of football players, according to Carter?
3. Would you consider that female and male somatotypes in comparable sport events are similar?
4. Explain how the difference in track performance between men and women might be partially attributed to the body's fat content.
5. Illustrate how density determinations are used to compute body fat.
6. Calculate the body density (JPW equation) of a 21-year-old female who has the following skinfold measurements: triceps = 13mm, iliac crest = 19mm, midthigh = 29mm. (Answer below.*)
7. Compute the percentage of fat, using both the Brozek and Siri formulas, of a person whose body density equals 1.0456 g/cm³.
8. Explain and give an example of a person in a positive energy balance.

*Answer: About 20.6%.

9. Explain and give an example of a person in a negative energy balance.
10. The Committee on the Medical Aspect of Sports suggests that the weight of a wrestler can best be assessed through a natural approach. What are some of their suggestions?
11. What are the results of Tipton's studies dealing with weight loss among high-school wrestlers?
12. What procedures might be used in predicting minimal weight values for high-school wrestlers?
13. According to the American College of Sports Medicine, how can the hazards of weight loss in wrestlers be eliminated?

References

1. Abernathy, R. P., and D. R. Black. 1996. Healthy body weights: an alternative perspective. *Am J Clin Nutr.* 63 (3 suppl.):448S–451S.
2. Abrams, H. L., and B. J. McNeil. 1978. Medical implications of computed tomography ("CAT scanning"). *N Eng J Med.* 298:255.
3. Aloia, J. F., S. H. Cohn, C. Babu, C. Abesamis, N. Kalici, and K. Ellis. 1978. Skeletal mass and body composition in marathon runners. *Metabolism.* 27(12):1793–1796.
4. American College of Sports Medicine. 1996. Position stand on weight loss in wrestlers. *Med Sci Sports Exer.* 28(2): xi–xii.
5. Ashwell, M. 1994. Obesity in men and women. *Int J Obes Relat Metab Disord.* 18 (suppl.1):S1–7.
6. Baker, S. J. 1980. An intensive alpine climbing expedition and its influence on some anthropometric measurements. *Br J Sports Med.* 14(2,3):126–130.
7. Baumgartner, R. N., W. C. Chumlea, and A. F. Roche. 1990. Bioelectric impedance for body composition. In Pandolf, K. (ed.), *Exercise and Sports Science Reviews,* vol 18 (American College of Sports Medicine). Baltimore: Williams and Wilkins, pp. 193–224.
8. Bell, W. 1980. Body composition and maximal aerobic power of rugby union forwards. *J Sports Med.* 20:447–451.
9. Bioelectrical impedance analysis in body composition measurement: National Institutes of Health Technology Assessment Conference Statement. 1996. *Am J Clin Nutr.* 64(3 suppl.): 524S–532S.
10. Bjorntorp, P. 1995. Evolution of the understanding of the role of exercise in obesity and its complications. *Int J Obes Relat Metab Disord.* 19 (Suppl.4): S1–4.
11. Bjorntorp, P. 1992. Regional fat distribution—implications for type II diabetes. *Int J Obes Relat Metab Disord.* (16 suppl.)4:S19–27.
12. Blackburn, G. 1995. Effect of degree of weight loss on health benefits. *Obes Res.* (3 suppl.) 2:211s–216s.
13. Blair, S. N. 1993. Evidence for success of exercise in weight loss and control. *Ann Intern Med.* 119(7 pt 2):702–706.
14. Bray, G. A. 1992. Obesity increases risk for diabetes. *Int J Obes Relat Metab Disord.* (16 suppl.)4:S13–17.
15. Briggs, G. M., and D. H. Calloway. 1984. *Bogert's Nutrition and Physical Fitness,* 9th ed. Philadelphia: W. B. Saunders.
16. Brownell, K. D., and J. Rodin. 1994. Medical, metabolic, and psychological effects of weight cycling. *Arch Intern Med.* 154(12):1325–1330.
17. Brozek, J. 1959 (January). Techniques for measuring body composition. Natick, MA: Quartermaster Research and Engineering Center (A.D.*286506*), p. 95.
18. Brozek, J., F. Grande, J. Anderson, and A. Keys. 1963. Densitometric analysis of body composition: revision of some quantitative assumptions. *Ann NY Acad Sci.* 110:113–140.
19. Buskirk, E. R. 1974. Obesity: a brief overview with emphasis on exercise. *Fed Proc.* 33(8):1948–1951.
20. Carter, J., and B. Heath. 1971. Somatotype methodology and kinesiology research. *Kinesiol Rev.* 10–19.
21. Carter, J., and W. Phillips. 1969. Structural changes in exercising middle-aged males during a 2-year period. *J Appl Physiol.* 27(6):787–794.
22. Chumlea, W. C., and S. S. Guo. 1994. Bioelectrical impedance and body composition: present status and future directions [see comments] *Nutr Rev.* 52(4):123–131.
23. Churchill, E., J. McConville, L. Laubach, and R. White. 1971 (December). Anthropometry of U.S. Army Aviators—1970. Technical Report 72-52-CE. Natick, MA: United States Army Natick Laboratories.
24. Committee on Medical Aspects of Sports. 1967. Wrestling and weight control. *JAMA.* 201(7):131–133.
25. DeGaray, A., L. Levine, and J. Carter (eds.). 1974. *Genetic and Anthropological Studies of Olympic Athletes.* New York: Academic Press, p. 55.
26. Depres, J. P., C. Bouchard, A. Tremblay, R. Savard, and M. Marcotte. 1985. Effects of aerobic training on fat distribution in male subjects. *Med Sci Sports Exerc.* 17(1):113–118.
27. Deurenberg, P., and Y. Schutz. 1995. Body composition: overview of methods and future directions of research. *Ann Nutr Metab.* 39(6):325–333.
28. Dolgener, F. A., T. C. Spasoff, and W. E. St. John. 1980. Body build and body composition of high ability female dancers. *Res Q Exer Sport.* 51(4):599–607.
29. Donnelly, J. E., T. E. Brown, R. G. Israel, S. Smith-Sintek, K. F. O'Brien, and B. Caslavka. 1988. Hydrostatic weighing without head submersion: description of a method. *Med Sci Sports Exerc.* 20(1):66–69.
30. Durnin, J. V. G. A. 1983. Body composition and energy expenditure in elderly people. *Biblthca Nutri Dieta.* 33:16–30.
31. Epstein, L. H., and R. R. Wing. 1980. Aerobic exercise and weight. *Addictive Behaviors.* 5:371–388.
32. Estimating body fat in lean and obese women. 1992. *Nutr Rev.* 50(3):80–81.
33. Evans, W. J. 1995. Effects of exercise on body composition and functional capacity of the elderly.
34. Evans, W. J., and W. W. Campbell. 1993. Sarcopenia and age-related changes in body composition and functional capacity. *J Nutr.* 123(2 suppl.):465–468.
35. Fielding, R. A. 1995. The role of progressive resistance training and nutrition in the preservation of lean body mass in the elderly. *J Am Coll Nutr.* 14(6):587–594.
36. Finberg, L. 1985. Clinical assessment of total body water. In Roche, A. F. (ed.), *Body Composition Assessments in Youth and Adults.* Columbus, OH: Ross Laboratories, pp. 22–23.
37. Flatt, J. P. 1995. Body composition, respiratory quotient, and weight maintenance. *Am J Clin Nutr.* 62(5 suppl.):1107S–1117S.
38. Fleck, S. J. 1983. Body composition of elite American athletes. *Am J Sports Med.* 11(6):398–421.
39. Forbes, G. B. 1985. Body composition as affected by physical activity and nutrition. *Fed Proc.* 44:343–347.
40. Forbes, G. B. 1992. Exercise and lean weight: the influence of body weight [see comments] *Nutr Rev.* 50(6):157–161.
41. Foss, M. L. 1984. Exercise concerns and precautions for the obese. In Storlie, J., and H. A. Jordan (eds.), *Nutrition and Exercise in Obesity Management.* New York: Spectrum Publications.
42. Foss, M. L. 1981. Exercise prescription and training programs for obese subjects. In Bjorntorp, P., M. Cairella, and A. N. Howard (eds.), *Recent Advances in Obesity Research: III.* London: John Libbey.
43. Foss, M. L., and D. A. Strehle. 1984. Exercise testing and training for the obese. In Storlie, J., and H. A. Jordan (eds.), *Nutrition and Exercise in Obesity Management.* New York: Spectrum Publications.
44. Franklin, B., E. Buskirk, J. Hodgson, H. Gahagan, J. Kollias, and J. Mendez. 1979. Effects of physical conditioning on

cardiorespiratory function, body composition and serum lipids in relatively normal-weight and obese middle-aged women. *Int J Obesity.* 3:97–100.

45. Franklin, B., and M. Rubenfire. 1980. Losing weight through exercise. *JAMA.* 244(4):377–379.

46. Fuller, M. F., P. A. Fowler, G. McNeill, and M. A. Foster. 1994. Imaging techniques for the assessment of body composition. *J Nutr.* 124(8 suppl.):1546S–1550S.

47. Fuller, N. J., M. B. Sawyer, M. A. Laskey, P. Paxton, and M. Elia. 1996. Prediction of body composition in elderly men over 75 years of age. *Ann Hum Biol.* 23(2):127–147.

48. Gertner, J. M. 1992. Growth hormone actions on fat distribution and metabolism. *Horm Res.* (38 suppl.)2:41–43.

49. Goldman, R. F., and E. R. Buskirk. 1961. Body volume measurement by underwater weighing. In Brozek, J. (ed.), *Techniques for Measuring Body Composition.* Washington, D.C.: National Academy of Sciences, National Research Council, pp. 78–89.

50. Goran, M. I., R. Figueroa, A. McGloin, V. Nguyen, M. S. Treuth, and T. R. Nagy. 1995. Obesity in children: recent advances in energy metabolism and body composition. *Obes Res.* 3(3):277–289.

51. Grubbs, L. 1993. The critical role of exercise in weight control. *Nurse Pract.* 18(4):20–22, 25–26, 29.

52. Hall, L. K. 1977. *Anthropometric Estimations of Body Density of Women Athletes in Selected Athletic Activities.* Doctoral dissertation: The Ohio State University, Columbus, OH.

53. Harris, R. B. 1993. Factors influencing body weight regulation. *Dig Dis.* 11(3):133–145.

54. Hartman, C., R. W. Bowers, and N. Y. Liu. 1988. Relationship between bio-resistance body composition analyzer and hydrostatic weighing methods for body composition. *Med Sci Sports Exerc.* 20:S20.

55. Heath, B., and J. Carter. 1967. A modified somatotype method. *Am J Phys Anthropol.* 27(1):57–74.

56. Heymsfield, S. B. 1985. Clinical assessment of lean tissues: future directions. In Roche, A. F. (ed.), *Body Composition Assessment in Youths and Adults.* Columbus, OH: Ross Laboratories, pp. 53–58.

57. Heymsfield, S. B., D. Gallagher, E. T. Poehlman, C. Wolper, K. Nonas, D. Nelson, and Z. M. Wang. 1994. Menopausal changes in body composition and energy expenditure. *Exp Gerontol.* 29(3–4):377–389.

58. Heymsfield, S. B., D. Gallagher, M. Visser, C. Nunez, and Z. M. Wang. 1995. Measurement of skeletal muscle: laboratory and epidemiological methods. *J Gerontol A Biol Sci Med Sci.* 50 spec no:23–29.

59. Hill, J. O., and R. Commerford. 1996. Physical activity, fat balance, and energy balance. *Int J Sport Nutr.* 6(2):80–92.

60. Hirsch, J., and J. L. Knittle. 1970. Cellularity of obese and nonobese human adipose tissue. *Fed Proc.* 29(4):1516–1521.

61. Hoeger, W. W. K. *Principles and labs for physical fitness and wellness.* Englewood, CO: Morton Publishing, p. 44.

62. Holland, J. C., and R. B. Cherry. 1979. Aerobic capacity, body composition, and heart rate response curves of high school basketball officials. *J Sports Med.* 19:63–72.

63. Holmer, I. 1979. Physiology of swimming man. In Hutton, R. S., and D. I. Miller (eds.), *Exercise and Sports Sciences Reviews,* vol. 7. The Franklin Press (American College of Sports Medicine Series), pp. 87–124.

64. Houtkooper, L. B., T. G. Lohman, S. B. Going, and W. H. Howell. 1996. Why bioelectrical impedance analysis should be used for estimating adiposity. *Am J Clin Nutr.* 64 (3 suppl.):436S–448S.

65. Jackson, A. S., and M. L. Pollock. 1978. Generalized equations for predicting body density of men. *Br J Nutr.* 40:497–504.

66. Jackson, A. S., M. L. Pollock, and A. Ward. 1980. Generalized equations for predicting body density of women. *Med Sci Sports Exerc.* 12(3):175–182.

67. James, W. P. A public health approach to the problem of obesity. *Int J Obes Relat Metab Disord.* (19 suppl.)3:S37–45.

68. Jebb, S. A., and M. Elia. 1993. Techniques for the measurement of body composition: a practical guide. *Int J Obes Relat Metab Disord.* 17(11):611–621.

69. Johnson, G. O., W. G. Thorland, J. M. Crabbe, R. Dienstbier, and T. Fagot. 1982. Effects of a 16-week marathon training program on normal college males. *J Sports Med.* 22:224–230.

70. Johnson, S., K. Berg, and R. Latin. 1984. The effect of training frequency of aerobic dance on oxygen uptake, body composition and personality. *J Sports Med.* 24:290.

71. Jorgensen, J. O., N. Vahl, T. B. Hansen, S. Fisker, C. Hagen, and J. S. Christiansen. 1996. Influence of growth hormone and androgens on body composition in adults. *Horm Res.* 45(1–2):94–98.

72. Katch, F. I., and W. D. McArdle. 1973. Prediction of body density from simple anthropometric measurements in college-age men and women. *Hum Biol.* 45:445–454.

73. Katch, V., A. Rocchini, D. Becque, C. Marks, and K. Moorehead. 1985. Basal metabolism of obese adolescents: age, gender and body composition effects. *Int J Obesity.* 9:69–76.

74. Ku, L. C., L. R. Shapiro, P. B. Crawford, and R. L. Huenemann. 1981. Body composition and physical activity in 8-year-old children. *Am J Clin Nutr.* 24:2770–2775.

75. Laskey, M. A. 1996. Dual energy X ray absorptiometry and body composition. *Nutrition.* 12(1):45–51.

76. Leon, A. S., J. Conrad, D. B. Hunninghake, and R. Serfass. 1979. Effects of a vigorous walking program on body composition, and carbohydrate and lipid metabolism of obese young men. *Am J Clin Nutr.* 32:1776–1787.

77. Lohman, T. G. 1986. Applicability of body composition techniques and constants for children and youth. In Pandolf, K. (ed.), *Exercise and Sports Science Reviews,* vol 14. (American College of Sports Medicine). New York: Macmillan Publishing, pp. 325–358.

78. Lohman, T. G. 1982. Body composition methodology in sports medicine. *Phys Sports Med.* 10(12):47–58.

79. Lohman, T. G. 1992. Exercise training and body composition in childhood. *Can J Sport Sci.* 17(4):284–287.

80. Lohman, T. G. 1981. Skinfolds and body density and their relation to body fatness: a review. *Hum Biol.* 53(2):181–225.

81. McCarron, D. A., and M. E. Reusser. 1996. Body weight and blood pressure regulation. *Am J Clin Nutr.* 63(3 suppl.):423S–425S.

82. MacKeen, P. G., B. A. Franklin, W. C. Nicholas, and E. Buskirk. 1983. Body composition, physical work capacity and physical activity habits at 18-month follow-up of middle-aged women participating in an exercise intervention program. *Internat J Obesity.* 7:61–71.

83. Marin, P., and P. Bjorntorp. 1993. Endocrine-metabolic pattern and adipose tissue distribution. *Horm Res.* (39 suppl.)3:81–85.

84. Mathur, D. N., and S. O. Salokun. 1985. Body composition of successful Nigerian female athletes. *J Sports Med.* 25:27–31.

85. Mayer, J. 1968. *Overweight: Causes, Cost, and Control.* Englewood Cliffs, NJ: Prentice-Hall.

86. Meredith, H. V. 1979. Comparative findings on body size of children and youths living at urban centers and in rural areas. *Growth.* 43:95–104.

87. Norgan, N. G. Population differences in body composition in relation to the body mass index. *Eur J Clin Nutr.* (48 suppl.)3: S10–25.

88. Obarzanek, E., M. D. Lesem, and D. C. Jimerson. 1994. Resting metabolic rate of anorexia nervosa patients during weight gain. *Am J Clin Nutr.* 60(5):666–675.

89. Opplinger, R. A., and C. M. Tipton. 1988. Iowa wrestling study: cross validation of the Tcheng-Tipton minimal wrestling weight prediction formulas for high school wrestlers. *Med Sci Sports Exerc.* 20(3):310–316.

90. Parizkova, J. 1961. Total body fat and skinfold thickness in children. *Metabolism.* 10:794–801.

91. Parnell, R. 1959. Etiology of coronary heart disease. *Br Med J.* 1:232.

92. Patton, J. F., W. L. Daniels, and J. A. Vogel. 1980. Aerobic power and body fat of men and women during army basic training. *Aviat Space Environ Med.* 51(5):492–496.

93. Poehlman, E. T. 1993. Regulation of energy expenditure in aging humans. *J Am Geriatr Soc.* 41(5):552–559.

94. Poehlman, E. T., M. J. Toth, and T. Fonong. 1995. Exercise, substrate utilization and energy requirements in the elderly. *Int J Obes Relat Metab Disord.* (19 suppl.)4:S93–96.

95. Pollack, M. L., C. Foster, J. Anholm, J. Hare, P. Farrell, M. Maksud, and A. S. Jackson. 1982. Body composition of Olympic speed skating candidates. *Res Q Exer Sport.* 53(2):150–155.

96. Pollack, M. L., D. H. Schmidt, and A. S. Jackson. 1980. Measurement of cardiorespiratory fitness and body composition in the clinical setting. *Comp Ther.* 6(9):12–27.

97. Prentice, A. M., S. A. Jebb, G. R. Goldberg, W. A. Coward, P. R. Murgatroyd, S. D. Poppitt, and T. J. Cole. 1992. Effects of weight cycling on body composition [see comments] *Am J Clin Nutr.* 56(1 suppl.)209S–216S.

98. Ribisl, P. 1974. When wrestlers shed pounds quickly. *Phys Sports Med.* 2(7):30–35.

99. Roberts, S. B. 1995. Abnormalities of energy expenditure and the development of obesity. *Obes Res.* (3 suppl.)2:155s–163s.

100. Roberts, S. B., P. Fuss, W. J. Evans, M. B. Heyman, and V. R. Young. 1993. Energy expenditure, aging and body composition. *J Nutr.* 123(2 suppl.)474–480.

101. Robinson, T. N. 1993. Defining obesity in children and adolescents: clinical approaches. *Crit Rev Food Sci Nutr.* 33(4–5):313–320.

102. Rolland-Cachera, M. F. 1993. Body composition during adolescence: methods, limitations and determinants. *Horm Res.* (39 suppl.)3:25–40.

103. Rosen, L. W., and D. O. Hough. 1976. Pathogenic weight control behavior of female college gymnasts. *Phys Sports Med.* 16(9):141–146.

104. Ross, R. M., and J. S. Jackson. 1990. *Exercise Concepts, Calculations, and Computer Applications.* Dubuque, IA: Brown & Benchmark.

105. Rotkis, T., T. W. Boyden, R. W. Pamenter, P. Stanforth, and J. Wilmore. 1981. High density lipoprotein cholesterol and body composition of female runners. *Metabolism.* 30(10):994–995.

106. Roundtable discussion. 1986. Body composition. *Phys Sports Med.* 14(3):144–162.

107. Sady, S. P., W. H. Thomson, M. Savage, and M. Petratis. 1982. The body composition and physical dimension of 9- to 12-year old experienced wrestlers. *Med Sci Sports Exerc.* 14(3):244–248.

108. Segal, K. R. et al. 1985. Estimation of human body composition by electrical impedance methods: a comparative study. *J Appl Physiol.* 58:1565–1571.

109. Sheldahl, L. M., E. R. Buskirk, J. L. Loomis, J. L. Hodgson, and J. Mendez. 1982. Effects of exercise in cool water on body weight loss. *Int J Obesity.* 6:29–42.

110. Sheldon, W. 1954. *Atlas of Men.* New York: Harper and Brothers.

111. Shizgal, H. M. 1981. The effect of malnutrition on body composition. *Surg Gynecol Obstet.* 152:22–26.

112. Sinning, W. E. 1978. Anthropometric estimation of body density, fat, and lean body weight in women gymnasts. *Med Sci Sports.* 10(4):243–249.

113. Sinning, W. E. 1984. Validity of "generalized" equations for body composition analysis in women. *Res Quart Exerc Sport.* 55(2):153–160.

114. Siri, W. E. 1961. Body composition from fluid spaces and density: analysis of methods. In Brozek, J., and A. Henschel (eds.), *Techniques for Measuring Body Composition.* Washington, D.C.: National Academy of Sciences, National Research Council, pp. 223–244.

115. Smith, N. J. 1989. *Food for Sport.* Palo Alto: Bull Publishing.

116. Sodhi, H. S. 1980. A study of morphology and body composition on Indian basketball players. *J Sports Med.* 20:413–422.

117. Steen, S. N., and K. D. Brownell. 1990. Patterns of weight loss and regain in wrestlers: has the tradition changed? *Med Sci Sports Exerc.* 22(6):762–768.

118. Stransky, A. W., R. J. Mickelson, C. van Fleet, and R. Davis. 1979. Effects of a swimming training regimen on hematological, cardiorespiratory and body composition changes in young females. *J Sports Med.* 19:347–354.

119. Sutcliffe, J. F. 1996. A review of in vivo experimental methods to determine the composition of the human body. *Phys. Med Biol.* 41(5):791–833.

120. Swenson, E. J., and R. K. Conlee. 1979. Effects of exercise intensity on body composition in adult males. *J Sports Med.* 19:323–326.

121. Tanaka, K., and T. Nakanishi. 1996. Obesity as a risk factor for various diseases: necessity of lifestyle changes for healthy aging. *Appl Human Sci.* 15(4):139–148.

122. Tcheng, T. K., and C. Tipton. 1973. Iowa wrestling study: anthropometric measurements and the prediction of a "minimal" body weight for high school wrestlers. *Med Sci Sports.* 5(1):1–10.

123. Thorland, W. G., G. O. Johnson, T. G. Fagot, G. D. Tharp, and R. W. Hammer. 1981. Body composition and somatotype characteristics of Junior Olympic athletes. *Med Sci Sports Exerc.* 13(5):332–338.

124. Thorland, W. G., C. M. Tipton, T. G. Lohman, R. W. Bowers, T. J. Housh, G. O. Johnson, J. M. Kelly, R. A. Opplinger, and T. K. Tcheng. 1991. Midwest wrestling study: prediction of minimal weight for high school wrestlers. *Med Sci Sports Exerc.* 23(9):1102–1110.

125. Timson, T. R., and G. L. Etheridge. 1980. Hydrostatic weighing at residual volume and functional residual capacity. *J Appl Physiol Respir Environ Exerc Physiol.* 49(1):157–159.

126. Tipton, C. M. (ed.). 1974. The influence of exercise on the morphology and metabolism of the isolated fat cell. *Fed Proc.* 33(8):1947–1968.

127. Tipton, C. M., and Tcheng, T. K. 1970. Iowa wrestling study. *JAMA.* 214(7):1269–1274.

128. Toriola, A. L. 1984. Influence of 12-week jogging on body fat and serum lipids. *Br J Sports Med.* 18(1):13–17.

129. Tremblay, A., and B. Buemann. 1995. Exercise-training, macronutrient balance and body weight control. *Int J Obes Relat Metab Disord.* 19(2):79–86.

130. Vaccaro, P., and M. Clinton. 1981. The effects of aerobic dance conditioning on the body composition and maximal oxygen uptake of college women. *J Sports Med.* 21:291–294.

131. Van der Kooy, K., and J. C. Seidell. 1993. Techniques for the measurement of visceral fat: a practical guide. *Int J Obes Relat Metab Disord.* 17(4):187–196.

132. Vogel, J. A., and K. E. Friedl. 1992. Body fat assessment in women. Special considerations. *Sports Med.* 13(4):245–269.

133. Wardle, J. 1995. The assessment of obesity: theoretical background and practical advice. *Behav Res Ther.* 33(1):107–117.

134. Watson, A. W. S. 1979. A three-year study of the effects of exercise on active young men. *Eur J Appl Physiol.* 40:107–115.

135. Watson, A. W. S., and D. J. O'Donovan. 1977. The effects of five weeks of controlled interval training on youths of diverse pre-training condition. *J Sports Med.* 17:139–146.

136. Webster, S., R. Rutt, and A. Weltman. 1990. Physiological effects of a weight loss regimen practiced by college wrestlers. *Med Sci Sports Exerc.* 22(2):229–234.

137. Weltman, A., and V. Katch. 1981. Comparison of hydrostatic weighing at residual volume and total lung capacity. *Med Sci Sports Exerc.* 13(3):210–213.

138. White, J., J. L. Mayhew, and F. C. Piper. 1980. Prediction of body composition in college football players. *J Sports Med.* 20:317–324.

139. Wilmore, J. 1969. The use of actual, predicted and constant residual volumes in the assessment of body composition by underwater weighing. *Med Sci Sports.* 1(2):87–90.

140. Wilmore, J. H. 1983. Body composition in sport and exercise: directions for future research. *Med Sci Sports Exerc.* 15(1):21–31.

141. Wilmore, J. H., and A. R. Behnke. 1969. An anthropometric estimation of body density and lean body weight in young men. *J Appl Physiol.* 27(1):25–31.

142. ———. 1970. An anthropometric estimation of body density and lean body weight in young women. *Am J Clin Nutr.* 23:267–274.

143. Wilmore, J. H., C. H. Brown, and J. A. Davis. 1977. Body physique and composition of the female distance runner. *Ann NY Acad Sci.* 301:764–776.

144. Wilmore, J. H., P. A. Vodak, R. B. Parr, R. N. Girandola, and J. E. Billing. 1980. Further simplification of a method for determination of residual lung volume. *Med Sci Sports Exerc.* 12:216–218.

145. Wood, P. D. 1993. Impact of experimental manipulation of energy intake and expenditure on body composition. *Crit Rev Food Sci Nutr.* 33(4–5):369–373.

146. Worsley, A., W. Coonan, D. Leitch, and D. Crawford. 1984. Slim and obese children's perceptions of physical activities. *Int J Obesity.* 8:201–211.

147. Yarasheski, K. E. 1994. Growth hormone effects on metabolism, body composition, muscle mass, and strength. *Exerc Sport Sci Rev.* 22:285–312.

148. Zahorska-Markiewicz, B. 1980. Thermic effect of food and exercise in obesity. *Eur J Appl Physiol.* 44:321–325.

Selected Readings

Bjorntorp, P. 1996. The regulation of adipose tissue distribution in humans. *Int J Obes Relat Metab Disord.* 20:291–302.

Going, S., D. Williams, and T. Lohman. 1995. Aging and body composition: biological changes and methodological issues. *Exerc Sport Sci Rev.* 23:411–458.

Goran, M. I. 1995. Variation in total energy expenditure in humans. *Obes Res.* (3 suppl.)1:59–66.

Muls, E., K. Kempen, G. Vansant, and W. Saris. 1995. Is weight cycling detrimental to health? A review of the literature in humans. *Int J Obes Relat Metab Disord.* 19 Suppl 3:S46–50.

Stefanick, M. L. 1993. Exercise and weight control. *Exerc Sport Sci Rev.* 21:363–396.

Wang, Z. M., S. Heshka, R. N. Jr Pierson, and S. B. Heymsfield. 1995. *Am J Clin Nutr.* 61:457–465.

Wilmore, J. H. 1996. Increasing physical activity: alterations in body mass and composition. *Am J Clin Nutr.* 63(3 suppl.):456S–460S.

section

6

Humoral Responses and Performance Aids

The activity of all cells takes place within a fluid environment. This environment, referred to as the *milieu interieur* by the French physiologist, Claude Bernard, must be precisely regulated with respect to particle content, temperature, and hydrogen ion concentration. Exercise, as well as environmental factors, tends to temporarily unbalance or disrupt the homeostatic mechanisms that, at rest, normally maintain a constant internal environment. For example, we have previously studied how particles such as ions and nutrients move into and out of cells, how oxygen and carbon dioxide diffusion relates to their partial pressures, and how disruptions may be implicated in causing impending fatigue during exercise as well as cellular adaptations to training.

In this section we will study how the endocrine system, through its release of hormones into the blood (e.g., humoral factors), aids in the overall homeostatic regulation of the internal environment, again under resting and exercise conditions (chapter 17); and we will study what influence, if any, drugs and so-called ergogenic aids have on these and other regulatory mechanisms during exercise and athletic performance (chapter 18). The potential for overlap of content here is real and apparent because many drugs and ergogenic aids are analogs of endogenous hormones. We marvel at the profound changes in cellular function that can be brought about by minute changes in the circulating concentrations of drugs and hormones. Unfortunately, sometimes with deleterious effects!

The following chapters are contained in this section:

17

Exercise and the Endocrine System

As mentioned in the introduction to this section, the internal environment in which all cells function must be precisely regulated with respect to content, temperature, and hydrogen ion concentration. Such a task is indeed difficult, requiring many homeostatic mechanisms, some of which have already been mentioned. However, there are two major control systems around which all homeostatic mechanisms function: (1) *the nervous system,* some functions of which have already been presented in other parts of this text; and (2) *the endocrine system,* a system that, by way of chemical substances called *hormones,* controls specific cellular functions and responses. This chapter describes the hormonal or endocrine system with respect to maintenance of homeostasis during both resting and exercising conditions. We will also explore the impact of training on circulating blood levels of selected hormones.

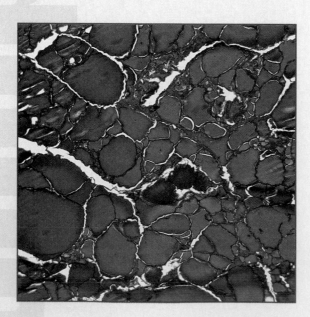

Characteristics of Hormone Action

Hormonal Responses to Exercise and Training

Summary

The major concepts to be learned from this chapter are as follows:

- A hormone is a chemical substance secreted into the body fluids by an endocrine gland and has a specific effect on the activities of other organs.
- An endocrine gland is ductless and secretes a hormone directly into the blood or lymph.
- Many hormones operate through cyclic AMP which is viewed as a "second messanger" and amplifier.
- The predominant hormonal control system is the negative feedback mechanism. In this mechanism, the secretion of the hormone is turned off or decreased due to the end result of the response caused by that hormone.
- The numerous hormones can be learned by organizing them according to glandular source, target tissues, and primary actions.
- Exercise and exercise training have an effect on blood levels of most hormones.
- Combinations of hormones are currently being studied in an effort to better identify their responses to acute and chronic exercise.

Characteristics of Hormone Action

A **hormone** can be defined as a discrete chemical substance that is secreted into the body fluids by an endocrine gland and that has a specific effect on the activities of other cells, tissues, and organs.[27] The cell, tissue, or organ on which a hormone has an effect is called the **target cell, target tissue,** and **target organ,** respectively.

The **endocrine glands** are ductless and are composed of epithelial cells in which hormones are manufactured or stored. Because the hormone is secreted directly into the blood or lymph, the endocrine glands are referred to as *glands of internal secretion.*

As just mentioned, hormones cause a specific effect on the activities of target organs. This effect, which may require minutes or hours to occur, is brought about mainly by increasing or decreasing an ongoing cellular process rather than by initiating a new one. For example, hormones may:[23] (1) activate enzyme systems, (2) alter cell membrane permeability, (3) cause muscular contraction or relaxation, (4) stimulate protein synthesis, or (5) cause cellular secretion.

Three general characteristics of hormone action that need to be discussed are (1) specificity of hormone action, (2) physiological mechanisms of hormone action, and (3) control of hormone secretion.

Specificity of Hormone Action

Although some hormones have an effect on all tissues of the body, most have an effect only on a specific target organ. This specificity is accomplished by the presence of a specific **hormone receptor** located within the cell membrane of the target organ. As shown in figure 17.1, the receptor is specific to and can react with only one hormone. It is analogous to a lock and key; only a specific key (hormone) will fit the lock (receptor), thus opening the way for a given action. Hormones may be so specific that they affect only a specific part of an organ or tissue. For example, antidiuretic hormone (ADH) affects cells of the collecting tubules in the kidney but not those of the ascending limb of the loop of Henle.

It is thought that hormones that cause an effect on all the tissues of the body also work by the receptor mechanism. However, in this case, the receptor is more general and widespread so that all the cells have them. Examples are the receptors for thyroxin and growth hormone.

Mechanisms of Hormone Action

Physiologically, how does a hormone cause an effect on a cell? There are many different physiological mechanisms of hormonal action. However, the most common mechanism of action of the majority of hormones is the **cyclic AMP**

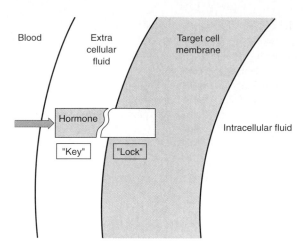

Figure 17.1

Specificity of hormone action is accomplished by the presence of a specific hormone receptor ("lock") located within the cell membrane of the target organ. The receptor is specific to and can react only with one hormone ("key").

mechanism. AMP is an abbreviation for adenosine monophosphate, a compound similar to ATP. Because it is involved in the mechanism of action of so many hormones, it is often referred to as a *messenger for hormone mediation.*

The cyclic AMP mechanism is shown schematically in figure 17.2. A hormone, on reaching the cell via the blood, interacts with its specific receptor located within the cell membrane. This interaction activates an enzyme called *adenyl cyclase,* which is also located within the cell membrane. In turn, the activated adenyl cyclase causes cyclic AMP to be formed from ATP, which is located inside the cell in the cytoplasm. Once cyclic AMP is formed, one or more of the physiological responses mentioned before can occur (figure 17.2). The response ceases when cyclic AMP is destroyed. The particular response that occurs depends on the type of cell itself. For example, thyroid cells stimulated by cyclic AMP form thyroid hormone, whereas epithelial cells of the renal tubules are affected by cyclic AMP by increasing their permeability to water. Also, several hormones may cause the same response in a given cell. Fat cells, for instance, can be stimulated through the cyclic AMP mechanism to break down triglycerides by the hormones epinephrine, norepinephrine, adrenocorticotropic hormone, and glucagon.

It is thought that cyclic AMP is not the only type of intracellular hormone mediator. Other such substances might include: (1) *prostaglandins,* a series of lipid compounds present in most cells throughout the body, and (2) a compound called *cyclic guanosine monophosphate,* which is similar to cyclic AMP. In addition, the intracellular hormone mediator mechanism is not the only mechanism whereby hormones can elicit a cellular effect. For example, insulin causes a direct effect on the permeability of cell

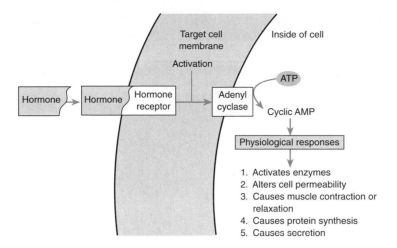

Figure 17.2

The cyclic AMP mechanism of hormone action. A hormone, on reaching the cell via the blood, interacts with its specific receptor located within the cell membrane. This interaction activates an enzyme called adenyl cyclase, which is also located within the membrane. The activated adenyl cyclase causes cyclic AMP to be formed from ATP, which is located inside the cell. Once cyclic AMP is formed, physiological responses can occur.

membranes to glucose, whereas the catecholamine hormones cause a direct effect on membrane permeability to various ions.

Control of Hormone Secretion

Because hormones have a precise effect on cellular function, their secretion must also be precisely controlled. How is this accomplished? Again, several control systems exist. One of these is the nervous system. However, the predominant hormonal control system is the **negative feedback mechanism.** This mechanism was mentioned earlier in the control of the cardiorespiratory system (chapter 9) and in body temperature regulation (chapter 19). In this control mechanism, the secretion of the hormone is turned off or decreased as a result of the response caused by that hormone.

An example of this is illustrated in figure 17.3. An increase in blood glucose concentration stimulates the pancreas to secrete the hormone insulin. Insulin causes an increase in cellular glucose uptake, which decreases the blood glucose concentration. This decrease in blood glucose "feeds back" to the pancreas, having a "negative" (decreased) effect on the secretion of insulin (hence, the term *negative feedback*). In other words, the end result of the action of insulin (decreased blood glucose) causes its secretion to be turned off or reduced.

Although this is a relatively simple example, some hormones are controlled by a more complex version of the negative feedback mechanism. For instance, the secretion of thyroxin from the thyroid gland is stimulated by another hormone called thyroid-stimulating hormone, or TSH, from the anterior pituitary gland. The negative feedback in this case is provided by the level of thyroxin in the blood. When it is high, secretion of TSH is reduced; when it is low, TSH

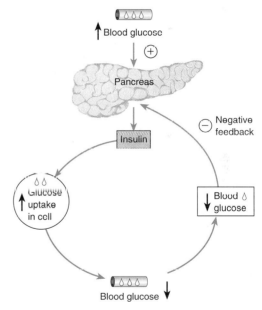

Figure 17.3

An example of negative feedback control of hormone secretion. An increase in blood glucose concentration stimulates the pancreas to secrete the hormone insulin. Insulin causes an increase in cellular glucose uptake which decreases the blood glucose concentration. This decrease in blood glucose "feeds back" to the pancreas, having a negative (decreased) effect on the secretion of insulin.

secretion is increased. In still other feedback systems, several endocrine glands and their hormones might be involved.

As mentioned previously, the nervous system is also involved in the control of hormone secretion. For example, epinephrine and norepinephrine from the adrenal medulla are secreted in direct response to stimulation by the sympathetic nervous system. The release of antidiuretic hormone

(ADH) from the posterior pituitary gland is also under control from the brain. Actually, the control of hormone secretion by the nervous system is not surprising. These two systems must, and do, work together to bring about the precise regulation necessary for maintenance of homeostatic function.

Circulating Concentrations of Hormones

Numerous factors other than hormone production or secretion rate can influence the circulating concentration (referred to as level[s]) of any given hormone. Arena et al.[3] succinctly state this in their review of the effects of intensive physical exercise on the reproductive hormones and menstrual cycle of female athletes. The endocrine equilibrium that regulates bodily functions can be affected by physical, psychological, and environmental factors. That is to say, blood levels of hormones depend on a balance between production, metabolism, binding, compartmentalization, and clearance rates.

Intensive physical exercise may affect this balance via different mechanisms, such as stress associated with competition, dieting, reduction of body fat, body weight, hydration status and a host of environmental factors. Couple all this with the fact that circulating levels of hormones are very small and in some cases require special assay procedures to even detect their presence. Since resting levels are so small it requires very little added hormone to increase existing values by several fold. For these reasons, it is risky, and sometimes outright dangerous, to indiscriminately take supplemental hormones in an effort to improve one's athletic performance. Look for more on this in the next chapter on drugs and ergogenic aids.

The Hormones and Their Glands

Table 17.1 contains a list of hormones, their origin or endocrine gland, their stimulating factors, their target organs, and a brief description of their actions. The following features in the table should be noted.

The Pituitary Gland, or Hypophysis

The pituitary gland, also called the **hypophysis,** releases many hormones. The pituitary gland is an extremely small gland located at the base of the brain and is connected to the **hypothalamus** (figure 17.4). Physiologically, it has two distinctive lobes, each of which secretes specific hormones.

1. The **posterior lobe,** also referred to as the **neurohypophysis** (because of its direct connection with the hypothalamus of the brain), is responsible for the secretion of **antidiuretic hormone (ADH),** or vasopressin, which functions mainly to promote water reabsorption from the collecting tubules of the kidney.

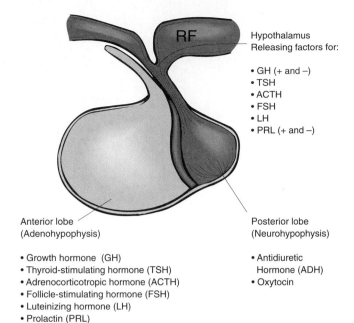

Hypothalamus
Releasing factors for:

• GH (+ and –)
• TSH
• ACTH
• FSH
• LH
• PRL (+ and –)

Anterior lobe
(Adenohypophysis)

Posterior lobe
(Neurohypophysis)

• Growth hormone (GH)
• Thyroid-stimulating hormone (TSH)
• Adrenocorticotropic hormone (ACTH)
• Follicle-stimulating hormone (FSH)
• Luteinizing hormone (LH)
• Prolactin (PRL)
• Endorphins

• Antidiuretic
  Hormone (ADH)
• Oxytocin

Figure 17.4

The pituitary gland (hypophysis) has two distinct lobes, each of which secretes specific hormones—the posterior lobe, also referred to as the neurohypophysis, and the anterior lobe, also called the adenohypophysis. Note the close proximity of the hypothalamus, which produces releasing factors and "hormones," which regulate the release of the majority of hormones from the adenohypophysis. The pituitary gland is sometimes called the "master gland" because of its control over the secretion of hormones by various endocrine glands located throughout the body.

The other hormone secreted from the neurohypophysis is **oxytocin.** Its main functions are stimulation of milk ejection and contraction of the pregnant uterus.

2. The **anterior lobe,** also called the **adenohypophysis,** secretes the following hormones: (a) **growth hormone (GH),** or somatotropin (STH), which stimulates growth and development; (b) **thyroid-stimulating hormone (TSH),** which stimulates production and release of the thyroid hormones; (c) **adrenocorticotropic hormone (ACTH),** or corticotropin, which stimulates the production and release of the glucocorticoid hormones from the adrenal cortex; (d) **follicle-stimulating hormone (FSH),** which promotes growth of the ovarian follicle in the female and spermatogenesis in the male; (e) **luteinizing hormone (LH),** or lutropin, which stimulates ovulation, formation of the corpus luteum, and hormone secretion in the female, and stimulates secretion of interstitial cells in the male; (f) **prolactin (PRL),** which stimulates secretion of milk after pregnancy; and (g) **endorphins,** which are related to relief of pain and production of euphoria.

17.1

A summary of major endocrine glands, hormones secreted, target cells or organs, and the primary actions of the hormones

Endocrine gland	Hormone(s)	Target cells or organ	Primary action
Hypothalamus	Releasing hormones	Anterior pituitary	Production of releasing factors or substances that regulate the production of hormones from the anterior pituitary
Anterior pituitary	Growth hormone (GH)	All body cells	Growth promotion and increase in size of all tissues until full maturation; stimulates protein synthesis; increases fat mobilization and use as a fuel source; but decreases carbohydrate utilization
	Thyroid-stimulating hormone (TSH)	Thyroid gland	Stimulates thyroxin (T4) and triiodothyronine (T3) produced and released by the thyroid gland
	Adrenocorticotropin (ACTH)	Adrenal cortex	Regulates the rate of secretion of hormones from the adrenal cortex (outer portion)
	Follicle-stimulating hormone (FSH)	Ovaries or testes	Starts growth of follicles in ovaries and stimulates secretion of estrogen from the ovaries; promotes sperm development in testes
	Luteinizing hormone (LH)	Ovaries or testes	Promotion of estrogen and progesterone secretion by the ovaries; causes the follicle to rupture and release ovum; promotes testosterone secretion by the testes
	Prolactin (PRL)	Breasts	Stimulation of breast tissue development and secretion of milk
Posterior pituitary	Antidiuretic hormone (ADH)	Kidneys	Reduction in the quantity of water excreted as urine; constriction of blood vessels with some elevation of blood pressure
	Oxytocin	Uterus and breasts	Stimulates uterine muscles to contract; supports milk secretion by the breasts

Note: Table information based on references 8, 33, and 78.

17.1
(Cont'd.)

Endocrine gland	Hormone(s)	Target cells or organ	Primary action
Thyroid	Thyroxine and triiodothyronine	All body cells	Increases the rate of metabolic heat production by cells; speeds heart rate and increases myocardial contractility
	Calcitonin	Bones	Inhibits calcium ion (Ca^{++}) release into the blood from bone
Parathyroid	Parathyroid hormone	Bones, intestines, kidneys	Increases calcium ion (Ca^{++}) concentration in extracellular fluids through its combined actions on bones, intestines, and kidneys
Adrenal cortex	Glucocorticoids (cortisol)	Most body cells	Anti-inflammatory action; also partial regulation of metabolism of carbohydrates, fats, and proteins; stress response syndrome
	Mineralocorticoids (aldosterone)	Kidneys	Increases sodium (Na^+) retention and potassium (K^+) excretion via the kidneys
	Androgens and estrogens	Testes, ovaries, breasts	Supports the development of the male and female secondary sex characteristics
Adrenal medulla	Epinephrine	Most body cells	Increases heart rate, myocardial contractility, skeletal muscle blood flow and oxygen consumption; also glycogen mobilization
	Norepinephrine	Most body cells	Constriction of arterioles and venules resulting in an elevation of blood pressure

As may be seen, the pituitary gland is a very important endocrine gland and because of its many hormones, it is sometimes referred to as the "master" gland. This title might be challenged from the perspective of the hypothalamus. After all, it produces the releasing factors that stimulate or inhibit the release of all hormones produced by the adenohypophysis, except for the endorphins. For the most part, tagging **releasing factor** onto the hormone name or abbreviation describes these hypothalamic substances—for example, GH, TSH, ACTH, FSH, LH, and PRL releasing factors. Note, however, that growth hormone and prolactin also have hypothalamic factors that inhibit their release. These are appropriately named *growth hormone release inhibiting hormone* (GHRIH), or **somatostatin,** and *prolactin inhibiting factor* (PIF), or **prolactostatin.** The presence of hypothalamic releasing and inhibiting factors is shown with positive and negative signs in figure 17.4. Once again, this is a perfect example of the tightly coupled workings of the

table 17.1
(Cont'd.)

Endocrine gland	Hormone(s)	Target cells or organ	Primary action
Pancreas	Insulin	All body cells	Decreases blood glucose by lowering circulating levels; increases the utilization of glucose and the synthesis of fat
	Glucagon	All body cells	Increases blood glucose by stimulating its release from the liver; stimulates the breakdown of protein and fat
	Somatostatin	Islets of Langerhans and G-I tract	Inhibits the secretion of both insulin and glucagon
Kidneys	Renin	Adrenal cortex	Assists in blood pressure regulation via aldosterone-angiotensin mechanism
	Erythropoietin	Bone marrow	Increased production of erythrocytes
Gonads **Ovaries**	Estrogen	Sex organs, adipose tissue	Promotes development of female sex organs and characteristics; provides increased storage of fat; assists in menstrual cycle regulation
	Progesterone	Sex organs	Assists in menstrual cycle regulation
Testes	Testosterone	Sex organs, muscle tissue	Promotes development of male sex organs and secondary sex characteristics including growth of testes, scrotum and penis, facial hair and deepening of voice; promotes protein synthesis and muscle growth

neural and endocrine systems as they function jointly to regulate and control physiological functions throughout the organism.

The Adrenal Glands

The adrenal glands, as their name implies, sit on top of the kidneys. Physiologically, the adrenal gland is really two separate endocrine glands: the *adrenal medulla,* or inner portion of the gland, and the *adrenal cortex,* or outer portion.

1. The **adrenal medulla** is similar to and under the direct influence of the sympathetic nervous system. Its hormones are also similar to the nervous system in that they secrete **epinephrine** and **norepinephrine.**[*] These two hormones are referred to as **catecholamines.** The catecholamines are the type of

---

[*]Norepinephrine is the neurotransmitter released from sympathetic postganglionic fibers of the autonomic nervous system.

table

17.2

Comparison of epinephrine and norepinephrine in humans

Parameter	Epinephrine	Norepinephrine
Heart		
Heart rate	+ +	+
Force of contraction	+ + +	+
Cardiac output	+ + +	+
Vascular effects		
Mean arterial pressure	+	+ + +
Systolic pressure	+ +	+ + +
Diastolic pressure	+, 0, −	+ +
Total peripheral resistance	−	+ +
Metabolic effects		
Hyperglycemia	+ + +	0, +
Heat production	+ +	0, +
Blood lactic acid (result of glucose utilization)	+ + +	0, +
Fatty acid mobilization	+ + +	0
Central nervous system stimulation	+ + +	+ + +

+ = increase; 0 = no change; − = decrease.

From Barbara R. Landau, *Essential Human Anatomy and Physiology.* Copyright © 1976 Scott, Foresman & Company. Reprinted by permission of the author.

hormones referred to earlier that have effects on all the tissues of the body. A comparison of the physiological effects of epinephrine and norepinephrine in the human is given in table 17.2.

2. The **adrenal cortex** secretes some forty hormones that belong to the class of compounds known as **steroids.** They are divided into the following three groups on the basis of their major actions.

a. The **mineralocorticoids** primarily affect electrolyte metabolism. The most important mineralocorticoid is **aldosterone,** which functions to increase the reabsorption of sodium from the distal tubules of the kidney. This, in turn, causes the reabsorption of chloride and water.

b. The **glucocorticoids,** although named because of their effects on glucose metabolism, also have an effect on protein and fat metabolism. The most important glucocorticoid is **cortisol.** The glucocorticoids (principally cortisol) promote the increased synthesis of glucose (gluconeogenesis) from amino acids, depress liver lipogenesis, and mobilize fat from adipose tissues. Two other effects of cortisol are maintenance of vascular reactivity (without cortisol, the blood vessels are unable to respond to circulating catecholamines) and inhibition of the inflammatory reaction, the normal response of tissues to injury. Because of this latter action, glucocorticoids are often administered in massive pharmacological doses as anti-inflammatory agents.

c. The **androgens** cause development of male secondary sex characteristics. Androgens are primarily secreted by the testes in males, but production by the adrenals occurs in both sexes. The most important androgen is *testosterone.* The female counterpart to the androgens are the **estrogens.** The effects of oral ingestion of androgens by some athletes for the sole purpose of improving athletic performance are discussed in the next chapter (p. 496).

The Pancreas

The two major hormones secreted by the **pancreas** are **insulin** and **glucagon.** Both of these hormones are secreted by the cells of the *islets of Langerhans,* insulin from the beta cells and glucagon from the alpha cells. Insulin is *hypoglycemic* (i.e., it lowers the blood glucose levels). It does this by increasing the rate of glucose transport through the membranes of most cells in the body. The mechanisms of this process are discussed in Appendix B. Aside from its effects on cellular glucose uptake, insulin increases fat deposition in the adipocytes (fat cells). A lack of insulin results in *diabetes mellitus.*

Glucagon has effects that are the opposite of insulin. Therefore, secretion of glucagon causes increased blood glucose levels. Glucagon has two major effects on carbohydrate or glucose metabolism: (1) *glycogenolysis,* or the breakdown of glycogen; and (2) increased *gluconeogenesis,* or the synthesis of glucose from molecules that are not themselves carbohydrates, such as protein.

The Thyroid Gland

The **thyroid gland** is located on the upper part of the trachea just below the larynx (voice box). Its principal hormones are **thyroxin** and **triiodothyronine,** although it also secretes a hormone called **calcitonin.** Both thyroxin and triiodothyronine require small amounts of iodine (1 mg per week) for their formation. To prevent iodine deficiency, common table salt is iodized. The release of thyroxin and triiodothyronine is controlled by the thyroid-stimulating hormone (TSH) secreted from the adenohypophysis.

The major action of the thyroid hormones is a general increase in the metabolic rate. Some specific functions associated with this increased metabolism are (1) an increased protein synthesis making the thyroid hormones necessary for normal growth and development in the young, (2) an increased quantity of intracellular enzymes, (3) an increased size and number of mitochondria, (4) an increased cellular uptake of glucose and enhanced glycolysis and gluconeogenesis, and (5) an increased mobilization and oxidation of fatty acids.

Calcitonin causes a decrease in the blood calcium level. This hormone works in conjunction with the parathyroid hormone, which is discussed next.

The Parathyroid Glands

The **parathyroid glands** are tiny glands embedded in the dorsal surface of the thyroid gland. **Parathyroid hormone (PTH)** is the hormone they secrete. This hormone, together with calcitonin, regulates the calcium equilibrium in the body. PTH causes more calcium to be absorbed from the digestive tract; therefore, less calcium is lost through the feces and urine. This, along with its action of removing calcium from the bone, causes an increase in the blood calcium level. Calcitonin acts in the opposite way from PTH; in other words, it causes a decrease in blood calcium levels by preventing the removal of calcium from the bone.

The Ovaries and the Testes

As endocrine glands, the **ovaries** (female) and the **testes** (male) produce the sex hormones, **androgens** in the male and **estrogens (estradiol)** and **progesterone** in the female. In males, the most important androgen is **testosterone.** You may recall that the production and release of the sex hormones are under the control of luteinizing hormone (LH) from the adenohypophysis. The androgens promote secondary sex characteristics and are recognized as promoting protein anabolism (synthesis) and reducing protein catabolism (breakdown). As will be pointed out in the next chapter, excessive dosages of anabolic steroids cause harmful side effects.

Estrogens from the ovaries have actions in the female comparable to those of androgens in the male. They are responsible for the development and function of the uterus, uterine tubes, and vagina and promote the secondary sex characteristics of the female. The estrogens and progesterone work, along with FSH and LH, to regulate the menstrual cycles of women. In addition, as mentioned in chapter 14, estrogens are thought to provide protection against atherosclerosis and thus, coronary heart disease.

Progesterone is secreted in large quantities only after ovulation. It promotes further development of the uterus and mammary glands.

Other Production Sites

A few substances with hormone-like qualities are produced by various tissues of the body other than the endocrine glands. For example, under hypoxic conditions, the kidney synthesizes **erythropoietin,** which in turn stimulates bone marrow to increase production of red blood cells. Because erythropoietin is produced at one location and is carried via the blood to a second location where it exerts its biological effect, it meets most of the definitional qualifications for a hormone. Likewise, **prostaglandins** are produced by a variety of body tissues including the blood vessels, skeletal muscles, and the heart. Prostaglandins vary in their makeup and actions but primarily influence blood flow regulation through their ability to produce vasodilation. Finally, the **somatomedins** are a class of substances produced by the liver and several other tissues. These substances stimulate the growth of muscle and cartilage through stimulation of various phases of protein synthesis. The somatomedins themselves are comprised of amino acid chains that are produced as a result of increased growth hormone release from the adenohypophysis. Consequently, they are often viewed as factors that support growth hormone action rather than as hormones in their own right.

Hormonal Responses to Exercise and Training

Exercise and training cause blood levels of some of the hormones previously mentioned to either increase or decrease in comparison to resting values. The increases or decreases often directly reflect adjustments in the rate of hormone secretion by an endocrine gland. You should be aware, however, that changes in blood levels also may reflect changes in metabolic turnover rates or clearance rates and hemoconcentration effects. For example, an increase in the circulating plasma concentration (level) of a given hormone during exercise might be due to an increased rate of secretion, a reduced turnover or clearance of the hormone, a reduction in plasma volume due to water losses in sweat, or a combination of one or more of these factors. Some other factors that might affect blood levels of hormones are

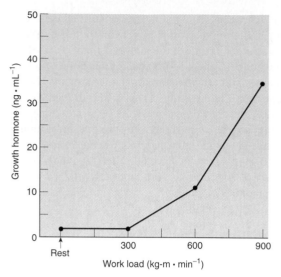

Figure 17.5

Response of growth hormone (GH) to bicycle exercise. With light loads, blood levels of GH do not increase. However, with higher loads, GH increases substantially.

(Based on data from Sutton and Lazarus.[65])

training status and psychological state,[34] as well as the intensity of the work load[90] and hypoxia.[39] Current research techniques allow rather precise explanations for observed changes in circulating hormone levels.

Although the physiological significance of many of these changes is not presently known, the fact that they even respond to exercise is in itself significant. The following is a brief review of the effects of exercise and training on hormonal responses. Excellent in-depth reviews of this topic have been written by Métivier[54] and by Terjung[76] and more recently by others.[19,20,33]

Growth Hormone (GH)

Growth hormone (GH) secreted from the adenohypophysis increases in the blood during exercise, being more pronounced the greater the exercise intensity.[25,31,32,46] There is some evidence that the increases may be due to increases in body temperature rather than the effects of the exercise per se.[9] An example of the response of growth hormone is shown in figure 17.5. In this study,[74] exercise was performed for 20 minutes on a bicycle ergometer. Notice that with light exercise loads (e.g., 300 kg-m · min^{-1}), there was no increase in the concentration of growth hormone in the blood. However, at a work load of 900 kg-m · min^{-1}, the peak increase in growth hormone was about thirty-five times the resting value. Although not shown in the figure, growth hormone does not immediately increase during exercise, but rather gradually increases with time. This finding refutes the idea that an increased release of growth hormone during exercise plays a significant role in fatty acid mobilization and metabolism.

The response of growth hormone to exercise appears to be related to the fitness level of the individual.[32,67,75] This is demonstrable in two ways: (1) there is a lesser increase in growth hormone during exercise of the same intensity in the trained individual than in the untrained and (2) the decrease in growth hormone following exhaustive exercise is faster in the trained than in the untrained individual. Although the significance of these differences between trained and untrained individuals is not known exactly, it has been suggested that chronic physical training establishes a difference in the control processes of growth hormone.[77]

An excellent review of the effects of exercise and training on the response of growth hormone has been written by Shephard and Sidney.[71]

Thyroid and Parathyroid Hormones

The intensity and duration of exercise apparently has considerable influence over whether circulating levels of thyroid hormones will be altered during activity. For example, swimming 0.18 to 0.9 kilometers or pedalling a bicycle ergometer for 90 minutes at a moderate intensity had no effect on thyroid hormone concentrations that could not be explained by hemoconcentration effects.[65] Likewise, neither prolonged submaximal or short-term maximal exercise produced any consistent pattern of change in circulating levels of thyroid hormones.[68] Serum concentrations of thyroid hormones also were unaffected by prolonged submaximal exercise in the form of a 9-hour, 37-kilometer march.[79]

The thyroid hormones, thyroxin and triiodothyronine, are increased during prolonged strenuous exercise,[66] as is shown in figure 17.6. Blood levels of thyroid-stimulating hormone (TSH) are also shown in the figure. In this study, the exercise consisted of a 70-kilometer (43.4 miles) cross-country ski race, which required between 5 and 7½ hours to complete. The most interesting change is not the fact that both thyroxin and triiodothyronine increased during the race, but that they were actually below their pre-race levels for several days after the race. This, coupled with postrace elevations of TSH, reflects obvious deviations in the ordinary balance between secretion, distribution, and removal of the individual hormones.

There is considerable conflict concerning TSH changes with exercise. There is evidence that at low submaximal work loads, TSH does not change either during exercise or within the subsequent 24 hours.[78] These findings have been confirmed for bicycle ergometry exercise at 15, 30, and 40% of maximal work capacity.[25] Other studies indicate a continuous rise in TSH levels during and up to 15 minutes after prolonged submaximal exercise but a decrease during maximal exercise.[68] Nevertheless, the most probable physiological explanation for observed changes in thyroid hormones with heavy exercise is as follows:[66]

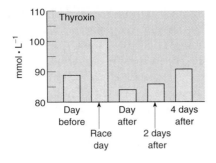

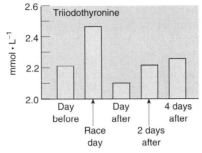

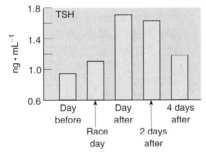

Figure 17.6

Thyroxin, triiodothyronine, and thyroid-stimulating hormone (TSH) before, during, and after a 70-kilometer (43.4 miles) cross-country ski race. The most interesting change is not the fact that both thyroxin and triiodothyronine increased during prolonged strenuous exercise, but that they were actually below their pre-race levels for several days after the race.

(Based on data from Refsum and Strömme.[66])

1. The prolonged and marked rise in blood levels of TSH is most probably due to a persistent peripheral deficit in thyroid hormone caused by exercise. This stimulates TSH release from the adenohypophysis.
2. The increase in thyroxin and triiodothyronine at the end of exercise may be due to an early TSH-induced release of these hormones, whereas the subsequent decrease of thyroxin and triiodothyronine following exercise may be due to an inability of the thyroid gland to meet the enhanced cellular demands for these hormones. This results in the marked rise in TSH observed in the first few days following exercise (figure 17.6).

Incidentally, another interesting finding concerning the response of the thyroid hormones to exercise is that they are similar in magnitude to those found in many hyperthyroid patients.[77] However, the hormonal levels in response to exercise are not accompanied by any clinical signs of hyperthyroidism. Signs of hyperthyroidism include increased basal metabolic rate, intolerance to heat, increased sweating, weight loss, diarrhea, weakness, fatigue, nervousness, and insomnia.

Little is known concerning the responses of parathyroid hormone and calcitonin to exercise or physical training. One study of six normal men before, during, and after maximal treadmill exercise (Bruce protocol) indicated no change in PTH levels.[84]

Antidiuretic Hormone (ADH) and Aldosterone

Antidiuretic hormone (ADH) is a hormone released from the neurohypophysis. Aldosterone is a mineralocorticoid released from the adrenal cortex. Both of these hormones are involved in the regulation and control of electrolytes, water metabolism, and fluid volume. During exercise, considerable water and sodium can be lost, particularly during prolonged exercise in the heat. The hormonal control mechanism for maintenance of fluid (plasma) volume during exercise is as follows:

1. Exercise causes the release of antidiuretic hormone (ADH) from the posterior pituitary (neurohypophysis) and the release of renin, an enzyme that breaks down protein, from specialized cells located in the kidney. The stimuli for these changes are (a) an increased sympathetic nervous system activity, (b) sodium loss, (c) a decreased plasma volume, and (d) an increased plasma osmolarity.*
2. ADH causes water retention by acting on the collecting tubules of the kidney. Renin acts on a plasma protein called angiotensin I to form angiotensin II. Angiotensin II stimulates the adrenal cortex to release aldosterone. Aldosterone increases the reabsorption of sodium from the distal tubules of the kidney. This in turn causes the passive reabsorption of water. Thus both water and sodium are conserved, an antidiuretic (emphasis on anti) effect.

Because of this mechanism, it is not surprising to find that aldosterone, renin, angiotensin II, and ADH all increase substantially during exercise.[10,13,14,41,45] Similar levels of blood ADH were found for trained and untrained subjects who performed maximal treadmill exercise, so there may not be a clear training effect for this hormone.[21]

---

*Osmolarity refers to the number of osmotically active particles in a solution. Osmosis is defined in Appendix B.

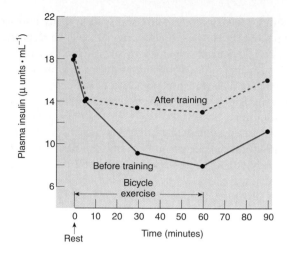

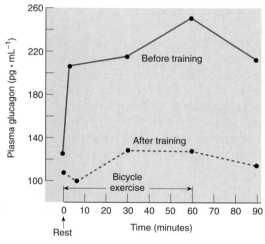

Figure 17.7

Changes in insulin and glucagon during and following 60 minutes of bicycle exercise before and after 10 weeks of physical training. Blood insulin levels decreased whereas glucagon levels increased during the exercise. Both responses are blunted by physical training.

(Based on data from Gyntelberg et al.[28])

Insulin and Glucagon

As mentioned previously, insulin causes an increase in cellular uptake of glucose resulting in a lowered blood glucose level. In addition to this function, insulin also inhibits glucose release from the liver and fatty acid release from adipose tissue. Glucagon, on the other hand, causes just the opposite effects (i.e., glucose mobilization from the liver through glycogenolysis and gluconeogenesis) and fatty acid mobilization from the adipocytes (fat cells). During exercise, in which both glucose and fatty acids are needed as metabolic fuels, glucagon has been shown to increase and insulin to decrease.[2,23,28,89]

An example of these changes before and after exercise training is presented in figure 17.7. The exercise bout in this case consisted of 60 minutes of submaximal bicycle

exercise at an intensity that required 60% of the subjects' max $\dot{V}O_2$. The training program consisted of running and cycling 40 minutes per day, four times per week for 10 weeks. As shown in the figure, blood insulin levels decreased, whereas glucagon levels increased during the exercise. Although this was generally true both before and after training, the most pronounced changes occurred before training. The lesser response of insulin and glucagon following the training program can be explained by a decreased catecholamine (epinephrine and norepinephrine) response to submaximal exercise that also results from physical training, as will be discussed next. Both the glucagon and insulin responses are thought to be mediated in large part by the release of the catecholamines.[28]

Before we leave this area, you should be aware of some special relationships that are known to exist between blood glucose levels during exercise and circulating levels of insulin and glucagon. These relationships have been summarized in detail by Terjung.[76] Decreased insulin levels during exercise do not mean that glucose uptake by muscle cells is reduced. In fact, it is enhanced. It appears that a small amount of insulin is adequate and necessary to "permit" this exercise-related increase in glucose uptake. This increase in insulin "sensitivity," where less or the same amount is able to do the job, is present for at least 48 hours after 1 hour of moderate exercise.[56]

The increased glucose clearance must be matched, however, by an equivalent or greater glucose supply in order to avoid the condition called **hypoglycemia.** This is where glucagon comes into the picture. Glucose output by the liver is influenced by appropriate changes in both insulin and glucagon. The mechanism that controls glucagon release is not clearly known but appears to be related to glucose demand in a manner that is not necessarily reflected in changes in blood glucose levels. Once again, sympathetic neural influences have been implicated because it is known that the catecholamines stimulate glucagon release in rats and that running causes increases in glucagon, catecholamines, and cyclic AMP in human subjects.[58,59] Decreases in insulin levels during exercise, however, appear to be related directly to diminished insulin secretion rates.

The Catecholamines: Epinephrine and Norepinephrine

As pointed out earlier, the catecholamines secreted by the adrenal medulla are physiologically related closely to the actions of the sympathetic nervous system. Therefore, because the sympathetic system is activated under "fight or flight" conditions, an elevated blood concentration of catecholamines would be expected during bouts of exercise. This, in fact, is the case.[11,13,23,29,35,58,62,64,89] The increase in these hormones is related to the work intensity—the greater the intensity, the greater the increase. This rule holds true with some limitations. The increases are similar during

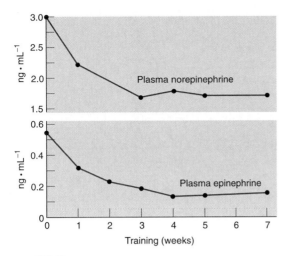

Figure 17.8

Blood levels of catecholamines (epinephrine and norepinephrine) decrease during submaximal exercise with exercise training.

(Based on data from Winder et al.[89])

submaximal exercise for both male and female subjects.[18] Brief repetitive maximal exercise such as all-out 6-second sprints caused greater blood epinephrine levels (18 × resting levels) in males; norepinephrine levels were similar.[7] There does appear to be a lower limit of submaximal exercise that must be exceeded. For example, mild to moderate treadmill exercise did not produce any significant increase in venous plasma epinephrine levels in normal male subjects.[85] At the other end of the exercise intensity-duration continuum, incremental treadmill tests leading to exhaustion produced a cumulative effect that led to a disproportionally large increase in catecholamines.[48]

The increases in plasma epinephrine and norepinephrine during both progressive and continuous exercise are highly correlated with plasma cyclic AMP concentrations.[61] In these studies, plasma catecholamines were significantly elevated by the time subjects reached 80% of max $\dot{V}O_2$ in the progressive experiments and after exercising continuously for 10 minutes at 80% of max $\dot{V}O_2$. The fact that the increases in cyclic AMP levels always followed increases in catecholamine levels further implicates the central role of the sympathetic nervous system in mediating a variety of perceived and real stresses during exercise.[61] There is some evidence that, although exercise induces a response of the sympathetic nervous system, psychological stress induces primarily an adrenal response.[12]

In addition, as mentioned above, the increased blood levels of catecholamines during submaximal exercise are not as great following exercise training.[63,89] This is shown in figure 17.8. Note the large magnitude of the drop (e.g., norepinephrine dropped 50% and epinephrine 70%) and the rapid onset of the response. After just 1 week of training, there was a 40% decrease in epinephrine and a 25% de-

crease in norepinephrine. Another reported effect of training is that plasma catecholamine levels at the time of exhaustion are higher in trained athletes than they are in sedentary subjects.[40] These higher levels in athletes could not be explained by differences in catecholamine clearance and were assumed to be due to increased rates of secretion as the athletes endured the exercise tests for much longer periods of time.

The increased levels of catecholamines are obviously important contributors to exercise performance. For example, as pointed out in table 17.2, epinephrine and norepinephrine have a variety of positive effects on the cardiovascular and metabolic systems with respect to aiding exercise performance. On the other hand, the decrease in catecholamine response seen during exercise following training also appears to be in the direction of "bettering" performance. Such lower levels of these hormones, for instance, would imply a lesser overall "stress" on all systems performing. Furthermore, the lower exercise heart rate that is also a result of physical training can be explained, at least in part, by this decreased catecholamine response (p. 320).

The Sex Hormones

Studies dealing with the responses of the sex hormones (androgens in the male and estrogens in the female) are not numerous. Nevertheless, it has been demonstrated that both androgens (testosterone) and estrogens (estradiol) are increased with exercise.[24,36,38,73] A review of gonadal secretory variations and control mechanisms during exercise has been written by Métivier.[55] He reports that blood testosterone levels increased in both young and old men following an acute work bout on a motor-driven treadmill. These findings are consistent with reports of increased androgen levels in highly trained athletes in response to maximal but not to submaximal exercise.[73] They also are consistent with reports that plasma testosterone responses to bicycle ergometer tests are more closely related to work intensity than they are to work duration or total work output.[35] Blood testosterone levels are known to increase with a variety of heavy resistance exercise protocols.[42] One report sounded a note of caution in that increases in peripheral venous plasma testosterone concentrations, which were proportional to exercise intensity, could nearly all be accounted for through decreases in plasma volume.[88]

All of these studies were conducted using male subjects, as might be expected. Women, however, have only approximately one-tenth to one-half as much circulating testosterone as males, and it is therefore possible to study exercise-induced changes. For example, 30 minutes of running at each subject's own pace caused a significant elevation of plasma testosterone in six women recreational runners.[70] A comparison of serum testosterone and androstenedione responses to weight lifting in men and women has also been made.[87] The ovaries and adrenals are the main source of androstenedione and testosterone production in women, whereas the testes and adrenals serve this function in men. At rest, testosterone levels were ten times higher in men, whereas androstenedione levels were 43% higher in women. Immediately after 30 minutes of weight lifting, testosterone levels increased in men but not women and were restored to resting levels within 30 minutes. On the other hand, androstenedione responses were similar in men and women in that levels decreased below pre-exercise levels at the 2-hour time point in recovery. Such studies ultimately should prove useful in better understanding gender-specific responses to different types of exercise and training.

An example of the responses to exercise of the blood levels of the ovarian hormones, estradiol (the most important estrogen), progesterone, follicle-stimulating hormone (FSH), and luteinizing hormone (LH) (the last two from the adenohypophysis) is shown in figure 17.9. Both estradiol and progesterone increase more or less linearly with exercise (figure 17.9A). Follicle-stimulating hormone also increases with exercise, but the response is not large in magnitude nor does it appear to be related to the exercise intensity. The blood concentration of LH does not appear to be affected by exercise (figure 17.9B). These responses were measured during the luteal phase of the menstrual cycle (6 to 9 days after ovulation). The hormonal responses during the follicular phase of the cycle (6 to 9 days after the beginning of menstruation) were somewhat different. Estradiol was the only hormone to increase with exercise during the follicular phase.

Additional studies have verified the findings shown in figure 17.9 and have provided some new insights regarding the effects of exercise on the sex hormones. Many of these studies have been reviewed and summarized by Shangold.[70] In one of these studies, ten young women performed 30 minutes of intense cycle ergometer exercise.[5] This resulted in a significant increase in progesterone and estradiol levels but produced no change in FSH or LH levels. The same response patterns have been reported for testosterone, FSH, and LH for male subjects.[25] After 8 to 11 weeks of training, the women in the first study[5] displayed marked irregularities in their menstrual cycles, which made it impossible to retest in the same cycle phase. Yet, when subjects were tested with the same absolute work loads used before training, no changes in serum progesterone, estradiol, or LH were observed. Training apparently suppressed the release of these sex hormones or altered some aspect of clearance so circulating levels remained unchanged.

LH also has been studied in young male sprinters and long-distance runners.[43] No changes in LH levels were found after maximal short-term running or after moderate (90 minutes, 4.3 min/km) or intense (45 minutes, 3.3 min/km) long-term running. One-half hour after the long-term runs, LH dropped to about half of the pre-run levels. Plasma testosterone was significantly decreased after the intense long-term run and remained depressed for up to 3 hours after the end of exercise. It was concluded that changes

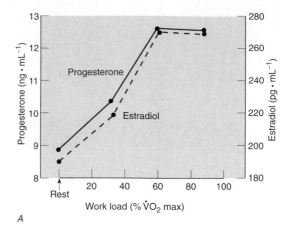

A

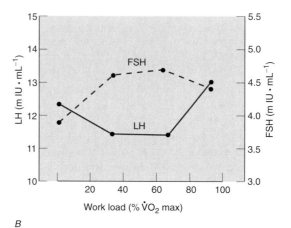

B

Figure 17.9

Responses to exercise of the ovarian hormones during the luteal phase of the menstrual cycle (6 to 9 days after ovulation). As shown in *A*, both estradiol (estrogen) and progesterone increase linearly with exercise. In *B*, follicle-stimulating hormone (FSH) also increases with exercise, but the response is not large in magnitude nor does it appear to be related to the exercise intensity. The blood concentration of luteinizing hormone (LH) does not appear to be affected by exercise.

(Based on data from Jurkowski et al.[36])

in testosterone and LH levels depend more on the intensity of exercise than on its duration. These findings also verify earlier reports[25] that some exercise-induced changes in sex hormone levels may not be apparent until after the cessation of activity.

It was mentioned above that the menstrual cycles of females became irregular with rigorous physical training. The irregular periods can, in fact, lead to a stoppage of menses altogether, which is called **amenorrhea.** This means that the ovaries would reduce their production of estrogenic steroids. Such reductions in female athletes have raised considerable concern because of known relationships between estrogen deficiency and **osteoporosis.** Osteoporosis is a condition of the bones where they become thin and brittle due to loss of mineral content and are therefore more susceptible to fractures. This condition is especially common in postmenopausal women.

Although there is evidence that amenorrhea may only predispose female athletes to a reduced bone mineral content when combined with excessive body thinness[49], and that female marathon runners maintain their bone mass longer than do sedentary women of similar age and body size,[6] the concerns persist with good reason. For example, a comparison of amenorrheic elite distance runners to those with regular menses (called **eumenorrheic**) disclosed a diminished bone mineral density in the lumbar spines of the amenorrheic group and a higher incidence of running-related fractures. It was concluded that, although intense exercise may reduce the impact of amenorrhea on bone mass (because amenorrheic runners who trained more intensely had denser bones than amenorrheic runners who trained less intensely), amenorrheic runners as a group remain at elevated risk for exercise-related fractures. In terms of our discussion of exercise effects on sex hormones, the amenorrhea of women athletes has been related to a decrease in resting gonadotropin levels, namely LH and FSH. The decreases in LH and FSH are believed to be related to an alteration in hypothalamic control as a result of rigorous training.[19] Recall here that LH and FSH both are under regulatory control of hypothalamic releasing factors (see figure 17.4). The consequence of this is that resting estradiol levels of amenorrheic athletes are only one-fourth to one-third of eumenorrheic athletes.[19,52]

The changes in the blood concentration of the male and female sex hormones during exercise are not well understood with respect to their roles in performance. Aside from the relationship of testosterone to muscular strength little significance can be attached to these hormonal responses. Further research will be needed to clarify this problem.

The Glucocorticoids (Cortisol) and Adrenocorticotropic Hormone (ACTH)

The responses to exercise of the adrenal cortex hormone, cortisol, are inconsistent and varied.[62,63] For example, with light or moderate exercise, there may be no change or a small decrease in blood levels of cortisol. However, if the exercise is prolonged to exhaustion, an increase in cortisol may be seen.[16,25,58] In addition, physical training does not appear to alter the responses of cortisol to exercise. The changes in cortisol secretion with exercise are presumably stimulated by an increased release of adrenocorticotropic hormone (ACTH) from the adenohypophysis. Venous plasma levels of ACTH have been reported to increase to two and five times above resting levels, respectively, following 20 minutes of running at 80% of max $\dot{V}O_2$ and a progressive run to exhaustion.[16]

An increased secretion of cortisol is a general response to stress. Therefore, in mild or light exercise where the stress may be low, no change in cortisol can be detected. On the other hand, during exhaustive exercise, stress is maximal, and cortisol would be expected to increase. One way in which cortisol might benefit exercise performance would be its gluconeogenic effect on the liver. Gluconeogenesis, you will recall, involves the formation of glucose from noncarbohydrate sources (e.g., protein) and would, therefore, make more glucose available as a metabolic fuel.

Prostaglandins and Endorphins

Exercise and training research related to these hormone-like substances, which are produced by a variety of tissues in the body, is rather limited. Many of the experiments involve electrical stimulation of muscles in anesthetized dogs and center on the role of prostaglandins in mediating blood flow changes. Although prostaglandins are released during direct muscle stimulation,[91] there is no clear evidence that these locally synthesized products are important to the maintenance of blood flow during exercise.[4] At this point, it is likely most appropriate to conclude that the prostaglandins may have some influence over resting blood flow because of their known ability to produce vasodilation.

Shangold's[70] review indicates that the opioid peptides, which would include beta-endorphin, are increased in the blood during exercise and that this response is facilitated by training. Interpretation of these observations are made difficult for two reasons. First, these substances are produced by so many different tissues in the body that it is impossible to know where the endorphins that are showing up in the blood are coming from (i.e., what is the source of production?). If the source is uncertain, then it is difficult to place any physiological or functional significance on the increased levels that are induced by exercise. Second, many of the endorphins are produced in regions of the brain or central nervous system (e.g., hypothalamus, pituitary gland, spinal cord) and may never leave these regions to show up in the peripheral circulation. There is recent evidence, however, that the exercise-induced activation of the endogenous opioid system may serve to regulate the secretion of several hormones during and after exercise.[17] Because the list of hormones that might be regulated includes epinephrine, the endorphins might eventually be implicated in a variety of exercise- and training-related matters.

A summary of the effects of exercise and training on hormonal changes is presented in table 17.3.

Hormonal Response Combinations

Researchers are beginning to look more at hormone responses to exercise in terms of systems and clusters,[69] such as the hypothalamic-pituitary-adrenal axis, the

17.3

Summary of changes in blood hormone levels during exercise and training

Hormone	Exercise changes	Training changes	Significance
Hypothalamic release hormones	Some likely increase with increased intensity	Unknown but by association a dampened effect is likely	Close neural tie-in to movement/stress
Growth hormone	Increases with increasing exercise intensities	Lesser response in trained subjects	Increase in fatty acid mobilization and gluconeogenesis
Thyroid stimulating hormone	Increases with increasing exercise intensities	Unknown	Unknown
Adrenocorticotropin	Increases with increasing exercise intensities	Unknown	Increases availability of glucocorticoids
Thyroxine	Little or no change	Increase of thyroxin turn-over without toxic effects	Unknown
Calcitonin and parathyroid hormone	Unclear	Unknown	Important for normal bone development and bone health
Glucocorticoids (cortisol)	Increases with increasing exercise intensities	Increases less for the same work rate, may increase more with exhaustion	Increased glycogen deposition, liver gluconeogenesis, lipolysis and anti-inflammatory effect

*Antidiuretic hormone (ADH) and renin are believed to respond in a similar manner.
Note: Table information based on references 8, 33, 78.

reninangiotensin-aldosteroneaxis,[15,50]and the anabolic/catbolic steroid hormones.[1] For example, endurance athletes show a greater activation of the pituitary-adrenocortical system in response to two hours of stationary cycling at 60% of max$\dot{V}O_2$ max than do untrained subjects.[83] Additionally, the interactions of pituitary, adrenal and testicular function have been investigated by Vasankari, et al.[81] In this study a long-lasting somatostatin analog was injected to study the possible endocrine effects of exercise-induced GH secretion. A surprise finding was a direct increase in secretion of testosterone by the testes. All of this speaks to the complex interactions of the endocrine system rather than it being simply a collection of independent glands releasing their own specific hormones.

The comparative effect of running and meditation on mood and the release of three hormones from the hypothalamic-pituitary-adrenocortical (HPA) axis has been studied.[30] Similar increases in corticotropin-releasing hormone (CRH) and elevations of mood occurred after both activities. Researchers concluded that positive *affect* is associated with plasma CRH immunoreactivity but that physical exercise is not an essential requirement for CRH release. That is to say, equal benefits might be obtained through meditation.

There also are studies of the fuel substrate regulatory and counterregulatory hormones that work to regulate blood levels of carbohydrates and lipids.[22,57] Blood glucose levels are tightly controlled during moderate-intensity exercise with glucose release from the liver controlled by glucagon and insulin. During high-intensity exercise this control is lost, and blood glucose levels increase—primarily because of a disproportionate increase in catecholamine release for a given increment in work intensity.[86] Such a disproportionate catecholamine increase has been shown at maximal intensity for subjects performing supine-graded exercise as part of a study of heart hemodynamics.[37] Also

table 17.3 (Cont'd.)

Hormone	Exercise changes	Training changes	Significance
Mineralocorticoids* (aldosterone)	Increases with increasing rates of performing work	May increase less for the same absolute work rate	Maintenance of plasma volume
Epinephrine	Little change with short periods of light work, increases with intensity and duration	Increases less for the same absolute work rate	Increases blood glucose, muscle blood flow, heart rate and contractility
Norepinephrine	Relative marked increase with increases in work rate; unsure of adrenal vs. sympathetic source	Increases less for the same absolute work rate	Blood pressure control, heart rate, and contractility
Insulin	Decreases with increasing rates of performing work	Decreases less after training	Reduces the stimulus to utilize blood glucose
Glucagon	Increases with exercise duration but decreases from an elevated level with high intensity/short duration activity	Increases less following training	Increases blood glucose by glycogenolysis and gluconeogenesis
Erythropoietin	Unknown, but postulated to increase with exercise	Unknown	Increased production of RBCs
Estrogen and progesterone	Increases with higher rates of performing work	Unknown	Unknown
Testosterone	Increases with higher rates of performing work	Unknown	Unknown

there is a known "blunting" or response reduction in the circulating level of several hormones involved in blood glucose regulation as a result of training. The greatest impact is seen in the initial 10 days of endurance-exercise training.[53]

The following is intended to provide additional insights into the breadth of research in the general area of exercise, training, and hormones. For example, no differences in male-versus-female subjects were found during performance of endurance exercise for such regulatory hormones as epinephrine, norepinephrine, growth hormone, insulin, or cortisol.[22] Another example is the finding that glucagon-to-insulin ratios, but not cortisol levels, were lower in subjects who drank a high-concentration carbohydrate solution during prolonged intermittent exercise.[57] Once again, the effects of exercise on these counterregulatory hormones would not be so well known if they were simply studied in isolation.

The effects of various components of overall exercise stress on hormone concentrations have also been studied. It has been suggested that endocrine response thresholds exist for both exercise intensity and duration.[82] This implies that the endocrine system would respond when the exercise intensity is "high enough" but that it also would respond to lower intensity exercise that lasts "long enough." Intense interval exercise in the form of treadmill running to exhaustion produced large post-exercise increases in testosterone (38%) and growth hormone (2000%) in trained male athletes.[26] In an extreme application of combined intensity and duration, Lehmann et al.[47] have attempted to induce an overtraining syndrome in middle- and long-distance runners by doubling their training volume over a period of three weeks. The runners performed poorly and displayed a 50% reduction in nocturnal catecholamine excretion, whereas numerous other hormones remained unchanged. The reduction might indicate a decrease in sympathetic neural activity as a result of chronic exhaustion and prove to be an important marker for overtraining.

The effects of resistance training on selected hormone concentrations have produced some equally interesting results. The concentration of blood testosterone rises steadily during the night after subjects perform heavy resistance exercises to exhaustion, whereas human growth hormone (GH) and cortisol are elevated for less than one hour.[51] Serum growth hormone concentration increases about 18-fold above resting measures in older men (mean age of 60 years) after a single session of resistive training.[60] These increases were found even after 16 weeks of progressive training, which also had no effect on resting growth hormone concentrations. It is possible that the increase in serum growth hormone that accompanies each workout session could have a significant anabolic effect and promote muscle growth. An interesting question has been raised by Tiidus[80] as to whether estrogen can protect human females from muscle damage due to exercise. The suggested mechanism would rest with the known antioxidant and membrane stabilizing properties of estrogens. These properties have been shown to provide protection from exercise-induced muscle damage in female, but not male rats. All of these studies point to the potential for important outcomes and applications of exercise-hormone research.

Summary

The intent of this chapter was to describe the hormonal or endocrine system with respect to maintenance of homeostasis during both resting and exercising conditions.

A hormone is a chemical substance secreted into the body fluids by an endocrine gland and has a specific effect on the activities of other organs (target organs). An endocrine gland is ductless and secretes a hormone directly into the blood or lymph. The actions of hormones on target organs include: (1) activation of enzyme systems, (2) alterations of cell membrane permeability, (3) muscular contraction or relaxation, (4) protein synthesis, or (5) cellular secretion. These actions are brought about through a mechanism referred to as the cyclic AMP mechanism.

Some hormones have an effect only on a specific target organ. This specificity is accomplished by the presence of a specific hormone receptor located within the cell membrane of the target organ. The receptor is specific to, and can only react with, one hormone.

The predominant hormonal control system is the negative feedback mechanism. In this mechanism, the secretion of the hormone is turned off or decreased due to the end result of the response caused by that hormone. The nervous system is also involved in the control of hormone secretion, primarily through the functions of the hypothalamus and the sympathetic branch of the autonomic nervous system.

The hormones and their endocrine glands include the following:

1. *The Pituitary Gland.* Antidiuretic hormone (ADH) and oxytocin (from the posterior lobe), growth hormone (GH), thyroid-stimulating hormone (TSH), adrenocorticotropic hormone (ACTH), follicle-stimulating hormone (FSH), luteinizing hormone (LH), prolactin (PRL), and endorphins (from anterior lobe).
2. *The Adrenal Glands.* The catecholamines, epinephrine and norepinephrine (adrenal medulla), mineralocorticoids, glucocorticoids, and androgens (adrenal cortex).
3. *Pancreas.* Insulin and glucagon.
4. *The Thyroid Gland.* Thyroxin (T_4), triiodothyronine (T_3), and calcitonin.
5. *The Parathyroid Glands.* Parathyroid hormone (PTH).
6. *The Ovaries and Testes.* Estrogen and progesterone in females and testosterone in males.

Blood levels of hormones known to increase with exercise include: (1) growth hormone, (2) catecholamines, (3) ACTH, (4) glucocorticoids, (5) mineralocorticoids, (6) glucagon, (7) testosterone, (8) estrogen, (9) progesterone, (10) TSH, (11) thyroxin, and (12) triiodothyronine. Blood levels of LH and FSH do not change with exercise, whereas insulin decreases with exercise.

The effects of training on hormone levels with exercise are quite variable. A pattern toward lesser responses (releases) after training exists for several hormones. Exceptions are insulin, which decreases less after training, and endorphins, which increase more after training. Some current topics in sports medicine that are based in endocrinology include:

1. Altering growth and muscle mass by abusing GH and anabolic steroids;
2. Amenorrhea in women athletes, predisposing them to osteoporosis caused by estrogen deficiency; and
3. Anti-depressive effects of exercise via the release of immunoreactive opioid peptides, including beta-endorphin.

Questions

1. Define the terms *hormone* and *endocrine gland*.
2. Explain the mechanism of specificity of hormone action.
3. Describe the mechanisms of hormone action.
4. How is hormone secretion controlled?
5. Construct a table listing the endocrine glands and their hormones.
6. Why is the pituitary gland called the "master" gland?
7. Construct a table listing the hormonal responses to exercise. Where possible, describe the significance of such changes.

8. Outline the effects of training on hormone release during and following exercise (i.e., which ones increase, decrease, stay the same?).

9. Why are prostaglandins and endorphins considered "hormone-like" substances?

10. Describe several diseases or sports-related concerns that have an endocrinological basis.

References

1. Adlercreutz, H., M. Harkonen, K. Kuoppasalmi, H. Naveri, I. Huhtaniemi, H. Tikkanen, K. Remes, A. Dessypris, and J. Karvonen. 1986. Effect of training on plasma anabolic and catabolic steroid hormones and their response during physical exercise. *Int J Sports Med.* 7:27–28.

2. Ahlborg, G., and P. Felig. 1976. Influence of glucose ingestion on fuel-hormone response during prolonged exercise. *J Appl Physiol.* 41(5):683–688.

3. Arena, B., N. Maffulli, F. Maffulli, and M. A. Morleo. 1995. Reproductive hormones and menstrual changes with exercise in female athletes. *Sports Med.* 19(4):278–87.

4. Beaty, O., III, and D. E. Donald. 1979. Contribution of prostaglandins to muscle blood flow in anesthetized dogs at rest, during exercise, and following inflow occlusion. *Circ Res.* 44:67–75.

5. Bonen, A., W. Y. Ling, K. P. MacIntyre, R. Neil, J. C. McGrail, and A. N. Belcastro. 1979. Effects of exercise on the serum concentrations of FSH, LH, progesterone, and estradiol. *Europ J Appl Physiol.* 42:15–23.

6. Brewer, V., B. M. Meyer, M. S. Keele, S. J. Upton, and R. D. Hagan. 1983. Role of exercise in prevention of involutional bone loss. *Med Sci Sports Exerc.* 15(6):445–449.

7. Brooks, S., M. Nevill, L. Meleagros, H. Lakomy, G. Hall, S. Bloom, and C. Williams. 1990. The hormonal responses to repetitive brief maximal exercise in humans. *Eur J Appl Physiol.* 60:144–148.

8. Bunt, J. 1986. Hormonal alterations due to exercise. *Sports Med.* 3:331–345.

9. Christensen, S. E., O. L. Jorgensen, N. Moller, and H. Orskov. 1984. Characterization of growth hormone release in response to external heating: comparison to exercise induced release. *Acta Endrocrinol.* 107:295–301.

10. Convertino, V. A., P. J. Brock, L. C. Keil, E. M. Bernauer, and J. E. Greenleaf. 1980. Exercise training—induced hypervolemia: role of plasma albumin, renin, and vasopressin. *J Appl Physiol.* 48(4):665–669.

11. Cousineau, D., R. J. Ferguson, J. deChamplain, P. Gauthier, P. Côté, and M. Bourassa. 1977. Catecholamines in coronary sinus during exercise in man before and after training. *J Appl Physiol.* 43(5):801–806.

12. Dimsdale, J. E., and J. Moss. 1980. Plasma catecholamines in stress and exercise. *JAMA.* 243(4):340–342.

13. Fagard, R., A. Amery, T. Reybrouck, P. Lijnen, E. Moerman, M. Bogaert, and A. De-Schaepdryver. 1977. Effects of angiotensin antagonism on hemodynamics, renin, and catecholamines during exercise. *J Appl Physiol.* 43(3):440–444.

14. Fagard, R., P. Lijnen, and A. Amery. 1985. Effects of angiotensin II on arterial pressure, renin and aldosterone during exercise. *Eur J Appl Physiol.* 54:254–261.

15. Fallo, F. 1993. Renin-angiotensin-aldosterone system and physical exercise. *J Sports Med Phys Fitness.* 33(3):306–312.

16. Farrell, P. A., T. L. Garthwaite, and A. B. Gustafson. 1983. Plasma adrenocorticotropin and cortisol responses to submaximal and exhaustive exercise. *J Appl Physiol.* 55(5):1441–1444.

17. Farrell, P. A., A. Gustafson, T. Garthwaite, R. Kalkhoff, A. Cowley, Jr., and W. Morgan. 1986. Influence of endogenous opioids on the response of selected hormones to exercise in humans. *J Appl Physiol.* 61:1051–1057.

18. Favier, R., J. M. Pequignot, D. Desplanches, M. H. Mayet, J. R. Lacour, L. Peyrin, and R. Flandrois. 1983. Catecholamines and metabolic responses to submaximal exercise in untrained men and women. *Eur J Appl Physiol.* 50:393–404.

19. Fisher, E. C., M. E. Nelson, W. R. Frontera, R. N. Turksoy, and W. J. Evans. 1986. Bone mineral content and levels of gonadotropins and estrogens in amenorrheic running women. *J Clin Endocrinol Metab.* 62:1232–1236.

20. Francesconi, R. 1988. Endocrinological responses to exercise in stressful environments. *Exercise and Sports Science Reviews.* 16:255–284.

21. Freund, B., J. Claybaugh, M. Dice, and G. Hashiro. 1987. Hormonal and vascular fluid responses to maximal exercise in trained and untrained males. *J Appl Physiol.* 63:669–675.

22. Friedman, B., and W. Kindermann. 1989. Energy metabolism and regulatory hormones in women and men during endurance exercise. *Eur J Appl Physiol.* 59:1–9.

23. Galbo, H., J. J. Holst, N. J. Christensen, and J. Hilsted. 1976. Glucagon and plasma catecholamines during beta-receptor blockade in exercising man. *J Appl Physiol.* 40(6):855–863.

24. Galbo, H., L. Hummer, I. B. Petersen, N. J. Christensen, and N. Bie. 1977. Thyroid and testicular hormone responses to graded and prolonged exercise in man. *Eur J Appl Physiol.* 36:101–106.

25. Gawel, M. J., D. M. Park, J. Alaghband-Zadeh, and F. C. Rose. 1979. Exercise and hormonal secretion. *Postgrad Med J.* 55:373–376.

26. Gray, A. B., R. D. Telford, and M. J. Weidemann. 1993. Endocrine response to intense interval exercise. *Eur J Appl Physiol.* 66(4):366–371.

27. Guyton, A. C. 1996. *Textbook of Medical Physiology,* 9th ed. Philadelphia: W. B. Saunders.

28. Gyntelberg, F., M. J. Rennie, R. C. Hickson, and J. O. Holloszy. 1977. Effect of training on the response of plasma glucagon to exercise. *J Appl Physiol.* 43(2):302–305.

29. Hagberg, J. M., R. C. Hickson, J. A. McLane, A. A. Ehsani, and W. W. Winder. 1979. Disappearance of norepinephrine from the circulation following strenuous exercise. *J Appl Physiol.* 47(6):1311–1314.

30. Harte, J. L., G. H. Eifert, and R. Smith. 1995. The effects of running and meditation on beta-endorphin, corticotropin-releasing hormone and cortisol in plasma, and on mood. *Biol Psychol.* 40(3):251–265.

31. Hartley, L. H. 1975. Growth hormone and catecholamine response to exercise in relation to physical training. *Med Sci Sports.* 7(1):34–36.

32. Hartley, L. H., J. W. Mason, R. P. Hogan, L. G. Jones, T. A. Kotchen, E. H. Mongey, F. E. Wherry, L. L. Pennington, and P. T. Ricketts. 1972. Multiple hormonal responses to graded exercise in relation to physical training. *J Appl Physiol.* 33(5):602–606.

33. Howlett, T. 1987. Hormonal responses to exercise and training: a short review. *Clin Endocrin.* 26:723–742.

34. Hyyppa, M., S. Aunola, and V. Kuusela. 1986. Psychoendocrine responses to bicycle exercise in healthy men in good physical condition. *Int J Sports Med.* 1:89–93.

35. Jezová, D., M. Vigaš, P. Tatár, R. Kvetňanský, K., Nazar, H. Kaciuba-Uścilko, and S. Kozlowski. 1985. Plasma testosterone and catecholamine responses to physical exercise of different intensities in men. *Eur J Appl Physiol.* 54:62–66.

36. Jurkowski, J. E., N. L. Jones, W. C. Walker, E. V. Younglai, and J. R. Sutton. 1978. Ovarian hormonal responses to exercise. *J Appl Physiol.* 44(1):109–114.

37. Kanstrup, I. L., J. Marving, N. Gadsboll, H. Lonborg-Jensen, and P. F. Hoilund-Carlsen. 1995. Left ventricle haemodynamics and

vaso-active hormones during graded supine exercise in healthy male subjects. *Eur J Appl Physiol.* 72(1–2):86–94.

38. Keizer, H. A., J. Poortman, and G. S. J. Bunnik. 1980. Influence of physical exercise on sex-hormone metabolism. *J Appl Physiol.* 48(5):765–769.

39. Kjaer, M., J. Bangsbo, G. Lortie, and H. Galbo. 1988. Hormonal response to exercise in humans: influence of hypoxia and physical training. *Am J Physiol.* 254:R197–R203.

40. Kjaer, M., N. J. Christensen, B. Sonne, E A. Richter, and H. Galbo. 1985. Effect of exercise on epinephrine turnover in trained and untrained male subjects. *J Appl Physiol.* 59(4):1061–1067.

41. Kosunen, K. J., and A. J. Pakarinen. 1976. Plasma renin, angiotensin II, and plasma and urinary aldosterone in running exercise. *J Appl Physiol.* 41(1):26–29.

42. Kraemer, W., L. Marchitelli, S. Gordon, E. Harman, J. Dziados, R. Mello, P. Frykman, D. McCurry, and S. Fleck. 1990. Hormonal and growth factor responses to heavy resistance exercise protocols. *J Appl Physiol.* 69:1442–1450.

43. Kuoppasalmi, K., H. Näveri, M. Härkönen, and H. Adlercreutz. 1980. Plasma cortisol, androstenedione, testosterone and luteinizing hormone in running exercise of different intensities. *Scand J Clin Invest.* 40:403–409.

44. Landau, B. R. 1976. *Essential Human Anatomy and Physiology.* Glenview, IL: Scott, Foresman.

45. Landgraf, R., R. Häcker, and H. Buhl. 1982. Plasma vasopressin and oxytocin in response to exercise and during a day-night cycle in man. *Endokrinologie.* 79(2):281–291.

46. Lassarre, C., F. Girard, J. Durand, and J. Raynand. 1974. Kinetics of human growth hormone during submaximal exercise. *J Appl Physiol.* 37(6):826–830.

47. Lehmann, M., U. Gastmann, K. G. Petersen, N. Bachl, A. Seidel, A. N. Khalaf, S. Fischer, and J. Keul. 1992. Training-overtraining: performance, and hormone levels, after a defined increase in training volume versus intensity in experienced middle- and long-distance runners. *Br J Sports Med.* 26(4):233–242.

48. Lehmann, M., P. Schmid, and J. Keul. 1985. Plasma catecholamine and blood lactate cumulation during incremental exhaustive exercise. *Int J Sports Med.* 6:78–81.

49. Linnell, S. L., J. M. Stager, P. W. Blue, N. Oyster, and D. Robertshaw. 1984. Bone mineral content and menstrual regularity in female runners. *Med Sci Sports Exerc.* 16(4):343–384.

50. Luger, A., P. Deuster, P. Gold, D. Loriaux, and G. Chrousos. 1988. Hormonal responses to the stress of exercise. *Adv Exp Med Biol.* 245:273–280.

51. McMurray, R. G., T. K. Eubank, and A. C. Hackney. 1995. Nocturnal hormonal responses to resistance exercise. *Eur J Appl Physiol.* 72(1–2):121–126.

52. Marcus, R., C. Cann, P. Madvig, J. Minkoff, M. Goddard, M. Bayer, M. Martin, L. Gaudiani, W. Haskell, and H. Genant. 1985. Menstrual function and bone mass in elite women distance runners. *Anns Intern Med.* 102(2):158–163.

53. Mendenhall, L. A., S. C. Swanson, D. L. Habash, and A. R. Coggan. 1994. Ten days of exercise training reduces glucose production and utilization during moderate-intensity exercise. *Am J Physiol.* 266:E136–E143.

54. Métivier, G. 1975. The effects of long lasting physical exercise and training on hormonal regulation. In Howald, H., and J. R. Poortmans (eds.), *Metabolic Adaptation to Prolonged Physical Exercise.* Basel, Switzerland: Birkhäuser Verlag, pp. 276–292.

55. Métivier, G. 1985. Pituitary and gonadal secretory variations and control mechanism during physical exercise. *J Sports Med.* 25:18–26.

56. Mikines, K. 1988. Effect of physical exercise on sensitivity and responsiveness to insulin in humans. *Am J Physiol.* 254:E248–E259.

57. Mitchell, J., D. Costill, J. Houmard, M. Flynn, W. Fink, and J. Beltz. 1990. Influence of carbohydrate ingestion on

counterregulatory hormones during prolonged exercise. *Int J Sports Med.* 11:33–36.

58. Näveri, H. 1985. Blood hormone and metabolite levels during graded cycle ergometer exercise. *Scand J Clin Invest.* 45:599–603.

59. Näveri, H., K. Kuoppasalmi, and M. Härkonen. 1985. Plasma glucagon and catecholamines during exhaustive short-term exercise. *Eur J Appl Physiol.* 53:308–311.

60. Nicklas, B. J., A. J. Ryan, M. M. Treuth, S. M. Harman, M. R. Blackman, B. F. Hurley, and M. A. Rogers. 1995. Testosterone, growth hormone and IGF-I responses to acute and chronic resistive exercise in men aged 55–70 years. *Int J Sports Med.* 16(7):445–450.

61. Painter, P. C., E. T. Howley, and J. N. Liles. 1982. Change in plasma cAMP and catecholamines in men subjected to the same relative amount of physical work stress. *Aviat Space Environ Med.* 53(7):683–686.

62. Peguignot, J. M., L. Peyrin, and G. Pirès. 1980. Catecholamine-fuel interrelationships during exercise in fasting men. *J Appl Physiol.* 48(1):109–113.

63. Péronnet, F., J. Cléroux, H. Perrault, D. Cousineau, J. deChamplain, and R. Nadeau. 1981. Plasma norepinephrine response to exercise before and after training in humans. *J Appl Physiol.* 51(4):812–815.

64. Péronnet, F., J. Cléroux, H. Perrault, G. Thibault, D. Cousineau, J. deChamplain, J. C. Guilland, and J. Klepping. 1985. Plasma norepinephrine, epinephrine and dopamine β-hydroxylase activity during exercise in man. *Med Sci Sports Exerc.* 17(6):683–688.

65. Premachandra, B. N., W. W. Winder, R. Hickson, S. Lang, and J. O. Holloszy. 1981. Circulating reverse triiodothyronine in humans during exercise. *Eur J Appl Physiol.* 47:281–288.

66. Refsum, H. E., and S. B. Strömme. 1979. Serum thyroxine, triiodothyronine, and thyroid-stimulating hormone after prolonged heavy exercise. *Scand J Clin Invest.* 39:455–459.

67. Rennie, M. J., and R. H. Johnson. 1974. Alterations of metabolic and hormonal responses to exercise by physical training. *Eur J Appl Physiol.* 33:215–226.

68. Schmid, P., W. Wolf, E. Pilger, G. Schwaberger, H. Pessenhofer, H. Pristautz, and G. Leb. 1982 TSH, T_3, rT_3 and fT_4 in maximal and submaximal physical exercise. *Eur J Appl Physiol.* 48:31–39.

69. Schürmeyer, T., K. Jung, and E. Nieschlag. 1984. The effect of an 1100 km run on testicular, adrenal and thyroid hormones. *Intern. J Andro.* 7:276–282.

70. Shangold, M. M. 1984. Exercise and the adult female: hormonal and endocrine effects. *Exer Sports Sci Rev.* 12:53–79.

71. Shephard, R. J., and K. H. Sidney. 1975. Effects of physical exercise on plasma growth hormone and cortisol levels in human subjects. In Wilmore, J. H., and J. F. Keogh (eds.), *Exercise and Sport Sciences Reviews,* vol. 3. New York: Academic Press, pp. 1–30.

72. Sundsfjord, J. A., S. B. Stromme, and A. Aakvaag. 1975. Plasma aldosterone, plasma renin activity and cortisol during exercise. In Howald, H., and J. R. Poortmans (eds.), *Metabolic Adaptation to Prolonged Exercise.* Basel, Switzerland: Birkhäuser Verlag, pp. 308–314.

73. Sutton, J. R., M. J. Coleman, J. Casey, and L. Lazarus. 1973. Androgen responses during physical exercise. *Br Med J.* 1:520–522.

74. Sutton, J. R., and L. Lazarus. 1976. Growth hormone in exercise: comparison of physiological and pharmacological stimuli. *J Appl Physiol.* 41(4):523–527.

75. Sutton, J. R., J. D. Young, L. Lazarus, J. B. Hickie, and J. Maksvytis. 1969. The hormonal response to physical exercise. *Aust Ann Med.* 18:84–90.

76. Terjung, R. L. 1979. Endocrine response to exercise. *Exer Sports Sci Rev.* 7:153–180.

77. Terjung, R. L. 1979. Endocrine systems. In Strauss, R. H. (ed.),

Sports Medicine and Physiology. Philadelphia: W. B. Saunders, pp. 147–165.

78. Terjung, R. L., and C. M. Tipton. 1971. Plasma thyroxine and thyroid-stimulating hormone level during submaximal exercise in humans. *Am J Physiol.* 220:1840–1845.

79. Theilade, P., J. M. Hansen, L. Skovsted, and J. P. Kampmann. 1979. Effect of exercise on thyroid parameters and on metabolic clearance rate of antipyrine in man. *Acta Endocrinol.* 92:271–276.

80. Tiidus, P. M. 1995. Can estrogens diminish exercise induced muscle damage? *Can J Appl Physiol.* 20(1):26–38.

81. Vasankari, T., U. Kujala, S. Taimela, A. Torma, K. Irjala, and I. Huhtaniemi. 1995. Effects of a long acting somatostatin analog on pituitary, adrenal, and testicular function during rest and acute exercise: unexpected stimulation of testosterone secretion. *J Clin Endocrinol Metab.* 80(11):3298–3303.

82. Viru, A. 1992. Plasma hormones and physical exercise. *Int J Sports Med.* 13(3):201–209.

83. Viru, A., K. Karelson, and T. Smirnova. 1992. Stability and variability in hormonal responses to prolonged exercise. *Int J Sports Med.* 13(3):230–235.

84. Vora, Nila, M., S. C. Kukreja, P. A. J. York, E. N. Bowser, G. K. Hargis, and G. A. Williams. 1983. Effect of exercise on serum calcium and parathyroid hormone. *J Clin Endocrinol Metab.* 57:1067–1069.

85. Warren, J. B., N. Dalton, C. Turner, T. J. H. Clark, and P. A. Toseland. 1984. Adrenaline secretion during exercise. *Clin Sci.* 66:87–90.

86. Wasserman, D. H. 1995. Regulation of glucose fluxes during exercise in the postabsorptive state. *Annual Rev Physiol.* 57:191–218.

87. Weiss, L. W., K. J. Cureton, and F. N. Thompson. 1983. Comparison of serum testosterone and androstenedione responses to weight lifting in men and women. *Eur J Appl Physiol.* 50:413–419.

88. Wilkerson, J. E., S. M. Horvath, and B. Gutin. 1980. Plasma testosterone during treadmill exercise. *J Appl Physiol.* 49(2):249–253.

89. Winder, W. W., J. M. Hagberg, R. C. Hickson, A. A. Ehsani, and J. A. McLane. 1978. Time course of sympatho-adrenal adaptation to endurance exercise training in man. *J Appl Physiol.* 45(3):370–374.

90. Winder, W. W., R. C. Hickson, J. M. Hagberg, A. A. Ehsani, and J. A. McLane. 1979. Training-induced changes in hormonal and metabolic responses to submaximal exercise. *J Appl Physiol.* 46(4):766–771.

91. Young, E. W., and H. V. Sparks. 1980. Prostaglandins and exercise hyperemia of dog skeletal muscle. *Am J Physiol.* 238:H190–H195.

Selected Readings

American College of Sports Medicine. 1975. Symposium on hormonal responses in exercise. *Med Sci Sports.* 7(1):1–36.

Arena, B., N. Maffulli, F. Maffulli, and M. A. Morleo. 1995. Reproductive hormones and menstrual changes with exercise in female athletes. *Sports Med.* 19:278–287.

Fellmann, N. 1992. Hormonal and plasma volume alterations following endurance exercise. A brief review. *Sports Med.* 13:37–49.

Tremblay, M. S., S. Y. Chu, and R. Murcika. 1995. Methodological and statistical considerations for exercise-related hormone evaluations. *Sports Med.* 20:90–108.

Wasserman, D. H. 1995. Regulation of glucose fluxes during exercise in the postabsorptive state. *Annu Rev Physiol.* 57:191–218.

18 Drugs and Ergogenic Aids

Almost all athletic and medical associations, including the American College of Sports Medicine, the International Olympic Committee (IOC), the United States Olympic Committee (USOC), and the American Medical Association are strongly against the use of drugs in sports. Athletes identified as using them are banned from competition. Joining such organizations in raising their voices against drug use are coaches, trainers, team physicians, physical educators, and the athletes themselves. Unfortunately, there is also widespread clandestine support of the use of certain illegal pharmacologic agents among other coaches, trainers, physicians, and athletes. The practice not only is contrary to the moral code underlying all athletics but also is potentially injurious to the health of the athlete. This chapter discusses the effects of drugs and so-called ergogenic aids on physiological responses and on physical performance.

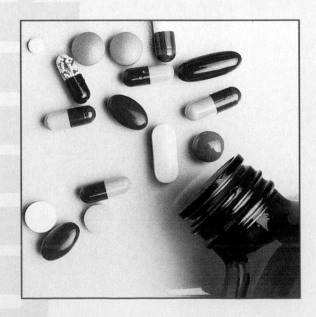

Ergogenic Aids (EA) Defined

Problems in Research Design

Nutrition Aids

Pharmacological Agents

Physiological Agents

Classification of "Contemporary" Ergogenic Aids

Sports and Drug Testing

Summary

The major concepts to be learned from this chapter are as follows:

- An ergogenic aid is anything that improves or is thought to improve physical performance.
- The lack of objective and consistent information regarding the effects of drugs and ergogenic aids is in part attributable to individual physiological and psychological variations among people.
- A placebo is an inert substance with the identical physical characteristics of a real drug.
- By far, the majority of studies dealing with the effects of drugs and other so-called ergogenic aids show little if any positive influence on exercise performance.
- Numerous "contemporary" ergogenic aids are being studied to determine their mechanism of action, effectiveness index, and inherent level of risk to users and abusers.
- The taking of drugs or other so-called ergogenic aids for the sole purpose of improving exercise performance may be dangerous to health and is illegal in sports competition.

Doping is the administration of or the use by a competing athlete of any substance foreign to the body or of any physiological substance taken in abnormal quantity or taken by an abnormal route of entry into the body, with the sole intention of increasing in an artificial and unfair manner his/her performance in competition. When necessity demands medical treatment with any substance which because of its nature, dosage, or application is able to boost the athlete's performance in competition in an artificial and unfair manner, this is to be regarded as doping.

U.S.O.C. Drug Control Program Protocol[100]

Ergogenic Aids (EA) Defined

An **ergogenic aid,** simply defined, is any substance, process, or procedure that may, or is perceived to, enhance performance through improved strength, speed, response time, or the endurance of the athlete. Another area of interest in ergogenic aids is to hasten recovery. The nature of the action of any supposed ergogenic aid may be elicited through the following: (1) directly act on muscle fiber; (2) counteract fatigue products; (3) improve fuel supply needed for muscular contraction; (4) affect the heart and circulatory system; (5) affect the respiratory center; (6) delay the onset of fatigue or the perception of fatigue; and (7) counteract the inhibitory effects of the central nervous system on muscular contraction and other functions.

Frequently, ergogenic aids are thought of only as pharmacologic agents that may be consumed to give the athlete an advantage. Pharmacological agents constitute only one of several classes of ergogenic aids. Others include nutritional (carbohydrates, proteins, vitamins, minerals, water, and electrolytes); physiological (oxygen, blood boosting, conditioning, and recovery procedures); psychological (hypnosis, suggestion, and rehearsal); and mechanical (improved body mechanics, clothing, equipment, and skill training) components.[111] In its broadest sense, one could call anything that can be related to an improvement in work or performance an ergogenic aid. Obviously, some ergogenic aids are clearly acceptable as adjuncts to improved performance and safety. Such things as training and conditioning, use of water, improved equipment, carbohydrate loading, vitamin (questionable effects) and iron supplements, warm-up techniques, rehearsal strategies, and cool-down techniques are within the spirit of competition.

The use of anabolic steroids, amphetamines, and other pharmacological agents are clearly outside the bounds of the spirit of competition and have been declared illegal by national and international sports governing bodies and denounced by medical societies and sports medicine groups. In this chapter, we will present information on selected nutritional, physiological, and pharmacological agents that have been of interest for some time. Keep in mind that psy-chological and mechanical components as defined here can also play a very important role in athletic performance. The reader is referred to Williams' *Ergogenic Aids in Sports* for information in these two areas.[111]

In the later portion of the chapter our emphasis will shift to what we have chosen to call "contemporary" ergogenic aids. While some of the earlier ones have remained of interest, we have chosen to emphasize the "new kids on the block" that currently are being used, abused, and much researched. This should give readers a sense of history and also make you aware of what is happening at the present time in this most dynamic and rapidly changing area.

Ergogenic aids affect people differently, as might be expected. For some, studies show a positive influence on work performance and for others, no effect whatsoever. What might prove effective with the athlete may prove inconsequential to the nonathlete and vice versa. Certain ergogenic aids may influence a person's endurance performance but may have little or no effect on activities requiring short bursts of strength and power. Look for these differences as you, like others, attempt to identify and consolidate the scientific evidence about whether ergogenic aids make any "real" or "significant" difference in performance. If they don't, they aren't true aids!

Problems in Research Design

Unquestionably, the lack of objective and consistent information regarding the effects of ergogenic aids is in part attributable to (1) considerable individual physiological and psychological variations among people and (2) difficulties in developing foolproof research protocols.

For example, a company wished to learn the effects of lighting in an industrial plant on the performance of the workers. As the illumination increased, so did work production. But when the researchers decreased illumination, production did not decrease! Apparently, the results were a consequence of the workers realizing that they were in an experiment (and consequently developed an *esprit de corp*) and not solely because of increased illumination.

Studies testing the efficacy of new drugs use placebos to deal with possible psychological contaminants. For example, if we tell you that a certain pill will help you to run faster (suggestion), you might run faster simply because of what we have said. Who knows whether it was the pill or the suggestion? A **placebo** is an inert substance with the identical physical characteristics of the real drug without any of its chemical qualities. In experiments the placebo is randomly administered to half the subjects and the actual drug is administered to the other half. Neither the investigator nor the subjects know which is which. Frequently, such a design is referred to as a **double-blind study.** Although this design appears to be foolproof, some subjects in the placebo group still improve, confusing the final results of the study. In other cases, subjects taking the drug experience noticeable changes

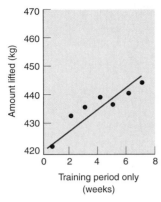
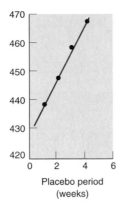

Figure 18.1

The amount of weight that could be lifted each week during a weight-training program is shown on the left. On the right is the amount of weight that could be lifted each week during a placebo period. The placebo period consisted also of a weight-training program, but in addition, the subjects were given placebo pills daily and told that the pills contained 10 mg of Dianabol, an oral anabolic steroid. Notice the greater increase in the amount of weight lifted weekly (indicated by the steepness of the line) when the subjects thought they were taking steroid pills.

(Based on data from Ariel and Saville.[5])

in their body (e.g., skin complexion, acne) or feelings (e.g., aggressiveness) and as a result, "unblind" the study.

The ability to experimentally isolate the true effect of any drug or ergogenic aid is extremely difficult and in many cases nearly impossible. This has been scientifically demonstrated,[5] as shown in figure 18.1. The amount of weight that could be lifted each week during a weight-training program is shown on the left. On the right is the amount of weight that could be lifted each week during a placebo period. The placebo period consisted also of a weight-training program, but in addition, the subjects were given placebo pills daily with the information that they contained 10 mg of Dianabol, an oral anabolic steroid. Notice the much greater gain in the amount of weight lifted weekly (as indicated by the steepness of the line) when the subjects thought they were taking steroid pills. This very nicely points out the psychological effects that some drugs have on physical performance.

We should be alerted to the fact that just because one study shows positive results, it might not necessarily be true or apply to all individuals. Early studies are often criticized because of research design weaknesses. However, they served a very useful purpose, namely, in giving other researchers a base on which to design more "air-tight" studies.

Prime interest in ergogenic aids deals mostly with the effects of drugs on athletic performance and of steroids on increasing muscle size and strength. Those interested in a thorough and current overview of the effects of drugs and ergogenic aids should consult the excellent series of review papers listed at the end of the chapter under selected readings. Other outstanding resources are *Ergogenic Aids in Sport,* edited by Melvin H. Williams[111], and the review articles by E. C. Percy[75] and Smith and Perry.[91]

Nutrition Aids

There are a variety of nutrition supplements (figure 18.2) and manipulations that may or may not be beneficial to the athlete. Among these are the manipulation of carbohydrate stores for endurance events, water and electrolytes, and vitamin and mineral supplements.

Carbohydrates

As discussed in chapter 2, carbohydrates and fatty acids are the primary sources of fuel for muscular contraction. For activities where work intensity exceeds 70% to 90% of the aerobic capacity of the athlete, muscle glycogen stores and utilization are critical. Both absolute and relative muscle glycogen depletion are related to the intensity of the work (chapter 2, figure 2.18).

A process called **glycogen-loading** (carbohydrate-loading) may be incorporated to elevate muscle glycogen stores above their normal resting levels prior to endurance competition (chapter 15). This procedure involves several days of preparation including 4 to 6 days of tapering aerobic training while maintaining a normal carbohydrate intake (approximately 50% of total calories) for the first three days. During the last 3 days, the athlete increases carbohydrate intake to 70% of the total caloric intake.[88] This will result in significant increases in glycogen storage and is not as severe a regimen as has been described by others.[7]

Generally, carbohydrate loading is applicable in athletic events where the athlete is continuously in motion for more than an hour at a time. This practice may also have applicability for events with an anaerobic component (1500 m) to the extent that lowered levels of muscle glycogen can have adverse effects on lactate production (anaerobic power).[87] Under circumstances where multiple events are run or swum in a single day, carbohydrate loading is appropriate.[87] For these purposes, simply increasing the dietary intake of carbohydrates for 48 to 72 hours prior to competition is adequate.

The practice of ingesting glucose 30 to 45 minutes before competition, once felt to be harmful,[15,25,41] is no longer frowned upon given an athlete has eaten a small meal within the past several hours and undertakes adequate warm-up. Fructose ingestion appears to blunt the shift in blood glucose versus glucose ingestion.[53] One final point: With the storage of 1 gram of glycogen about 2.7 grams of water will be taken into storage. Thus, with a storage of 500 gm of glycogen an additional storage of about 1.4 kg (3 lb) of water will occur. So the athlete should not be surprised to have a precompetition weight gain. This can be an advantage or disadvantage depending on the event.

Water and Electrolytes

The importance of water ingestion and maintenance of electrolyte levels was discussed in chapter 15. Water loss in amounts as low as 2% to 3% of body weight can impair

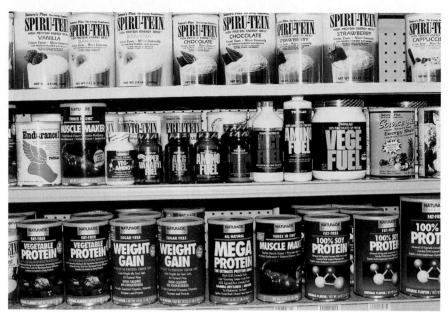

Figure 18.2
Typical display of the wide variety of so called "ergogenic aids" often found in contemporary fitness and health food stores.

performance through disruption of circulatory and thermoregulatory functions.[56,64] The diet normally contains sufficient electrolytes to compensate for any acute losses experienced through activity. Exception is noted where very high sweat rates over a period of days may occur.[72] A concerted effort will be needed to ensure added electrolyte intake, especially as it relates to potassium.

Vitamins and Minerals

In spite of widespread usage, there appears to be little compelling evidence for supplemental intake of various vitamins and minerals, with the exception of iron[6,54] and possibly vitamin C.[12] Most vitamins, when taken in excess, are merely excreted in the urine.[55] There is no justification for the consumption of megadoses of vitamins. As discussed in chapter 15, none of the known vitamins, when taken in excess of their recommended daily allowance, produces an ergogenic effect.

One consideration for recommending vitamin supplementation to athletes relates to those who restrict caloric intake to "make weight" (wrestlers, boxers, or jockeys, among others) or to keep body weight to a minimum for cosmetic and other reasons (gymnasts, dancers, and figure skaters, among others). Because vitamin intake is closely related to caloric intake, it would not be inappropriate to take a multivitamin/mineral supplement on a regular basis for those who restrict caloric intake.[12]

Iron

In many instances there is a legitimate concern for iron deficiency among athletes and the general population. Iron is an important component in hemoglobin of the red blood cell.

Although iron deficiency is more prevalent among women, it can also occur in men. The monitoring of iron intake, along with a clinical evaluation, is recommended for those who may be showing signs of an iron deficiency anemia, such as early fatigue while on training runs or loss of aerobic power. Daily iron needs for males and females are about 10 mg and 15 mg, respectively.[6,54]

Pharmacological Agents

The practice of using various pharmacological agents and drugs has raised the most controversy and presents more ethical, legal, and clinical questions than any other area. The indiscriminate use of pharmacological agents also poses the greatest threat to the health and welfare of the athlete.[33] Most of the contemporary controversy centers on the use of anabolic/androgenic steroids, human growth hormone, and blood boosting abuses. Other substances of concern include amphetamines and, to a lesser degree, bicarbonates and caffeine.

Anabolic-Androgenic Steroids

Starting in the 1950s, the use and abuse of **anabolic-androgenic steroids** to enhance performance has grown. Used mostly, in the beginning, by performers in the weight events in track and field, and in body building, the use has spread across a wide variety of sports among both males and females. The anabolic-androgenic steroids are derivatives of the male sex hormone, testosterone, secreted by the testes. Testosterone causes the particular physical characteristics of the male body. With production accelerating between the ages of 11 and 13 in males, testosterone quickens the onset of puberty and is continually produced throughout life.

Secretion of testosterone causes descent of the testes into the scrotum and enlargement of the testes, penis, and scrotum. It also affects the secondary male characteristics including (1) distribution of hair, (2) voice, (3) growth and development of bones, and (4) development of musculature following puberty.

The drug trade names, with generic names for a few of the synthetic testosterone preparations include: Adroyd (Oxymetholone), Dianabol (methandrostenolone), Deca-Durabolin (Nandrolone), Maxibolin (Ethylestrenol), Nilevar (Norethandrolone), and Winstrol (Stanozolol).[118] These drugs are chemically structured to emphasize the anabolic (protein-building) attributes of testosterone while minimizing the androgenic (producing masculine characteristics) properties. Recognizing the problems we mentioned earlier in designing scientific studies to probe the effects of drugs on performance and development, many studies have been completed with equivocal results.[19,40,42,47,60,81,95,106]

It appears that steroids increase strength and muscle mass for some but not for others. Perhaps the real issue is that of side effects. Physicians are most concerned with the effects of these drugs on the liver. Under no circumstances should persons with histories of liver ailment involve themselves with steroid experimentation. Women taking steroids have developed acne and exhibited positive symptoms on liver function tests.

The American College of Sports Medicine conducted a comprehensive survey of the world literature and carefully analyzed the claims made for and against the efficacy of anabolic-androgenic steroids in improving human physical performance.[3] The following is its position statement:

1. Anabolic-androgenic steroids in the presence of an adequate diet can contribute to increases in body weight, often in the lean mass compartment.
2. The gains in muscular strength achieved through high-intensity exercise and proper diet can occur by the increased use of anabolic-androgenic steroids in some individuals.
3. Anabolic-androgenic steroids do not increase aerobic power or capacity for muscular exercise.
4. Anabolic-androgenic steroids have been associated with adverse effects on the liver, cardiovascular system, reproductive system, and psychological status in therapeutic trials and in limited research on athletes. Until further research is completed, the potential hazards of the use of the anabolic-androgenic steroids in athletes must include those found in therapeutic trials.
5. The use of anabolic-androgenic steroids by athletes is contrary to the rules and ethical principles of athletic competition as set forth by many of the sports

governing bodies. The American College of Sports Medicine supports these ethical principles and deplores the use of anabolic-androgenic steroids by athletes.

There are reports in which weight lifters, consuming a variety of steroids, showed a consistent pattern of low to very low blood levels of HDL-C (high-density lipoprotein cholesterol).[23,27,63,76,81] HDL-C levels below about 35 mg · 100 mL^{-1} of blood are associated with high risk for premature coronary artery disease.[23] The mean value for HDL-C for all the studies was 21 mg · 100 mL^{-1} for the "users" and 49 for the nonusers. This is, perhaps, one of the most harmful and earliest manifestations of ongoing consumption of large doses of steroids. A summary of the results of these studies appears in table 18.1. In one study where both female and male steroid users were included, the patterns were similar, regardless of gender.[23] In another, weight-lifter users and nonusers were compared with non-weight-lifter nonuser controls.[97] In two of the studies where subjects stopped taking the steroids for a period of time, HDL-C levels rebounded to normal values within three to six weeks.[27,73] Thus, it is possible to reverse the low HDL-C levels but the ominous question remains: What is the effect on the possible development of coronary artery disease while HDL-C levels are depressed? This question is particularly pertinent for those athletes who continue usage over several years.

The prolonged use of oral anabolic-androgenic steroids (C_{17}-alkylated derivatives of testosterone) has resulted in liver disorders in some persons. Some of these disorders are apparently reversible with the cessation of drug usage, but others are not. The administration of anabolic-androgenic steroids to men may result in a decrease in testicular size and function and a decrease in sperm production. Although these effects appear to be reversible when small doses of steroids are used for short periods of time, the reversibility of the effects of large doses over extended periods of time is unclear.

Strauss and colleagues reported the results of a survey of ten female weight lifters who were using a variety of steroids, both injectable and oral, over a prolonged period of time.[96] Table 18.2 shows the responses by the participants to a questionnaire. Questions were asked to determine if the respondents had noticed changes in any of the items included in the list in table 18.2. The responses were subjective in nature and, as such, do not represent a scientifically controlled research design. The results are insightful nonetheless.

Serious and continuing efforts should be made to educate male and female athletes, coaches, physical educators, physicians, trainers, and the general public regarding the inconsistent effects of anabolic-androgenic steroids on improvement of human physical performance and the potential dangers of taking certain forms of these substances, especially in large doses, for prolonged periods.

table 18.1

Summary of studies examining the effects of anabolic steroids on HDL-C levels in weight lifters.*

Reference	Gender	Weight lifter user		Weight lifter nonuser		Non-weight-lifter nonuser	
		Total cholesterol	HDL-C	Total cholesterol	HDL-C	Total cholesterol	HDL-C
17	M	291	24	183	52		
60	M	183	26	176	50		
84	M		35		54		54
20	M	218	17	204	45	210	46
(OFF)†			(43)				
70	M	223	16			210	50
(OFF)†		(200)	(52)				
Mean		229	21	188	49	210	48
17	F	216	31			183	52

*Values are in mg · 100 mL^{-1} of blood.

†OFF following a reference means that the subjects in the study stopped consuming the anabolic steroid.

Growth Hormone

Over the years, athletes desiring weight gain have combined the use of illegal anabolic-androgenic steroids with growth hormones.[68] Biosynthetic human growth hormone (rGH) can be obtained relatively easily, whereas formerly it could be obtained only from the pituitary glands of cadavers.[73] One study reported reduction in fat weight and increases in fat-free weight in eight well-trained men on a resistance training program.[29] Although there are no other laboratory-controlled studies available to examine the effects of rGH on athletes (and there likely will not be any), certain athletes are blindly using this substance hoping for short-term gains and ignoring possible long-term side effects. The potential side effects are as ominous as those for anabolic steroids.

Amphetamines

It generally is reported that amphetamines are the most popular drugs for "increasing" athletic performance among those inclined toward usage. **Amphetamine** (Benzedrine being a popular brand) is a synthetically structured drug closely related to epinephrine. Like epinephrine, it produces stimulation of the central nervous system, resulting in increased alertness in motor and physical activity, decreased fatigue, and sometimes insomnia. Most often there is a rise in blood pressure with increased heart rate and perhaps some cardiac irregularities such as extrasystoles (extra beats) and **paroxysmal tachycardia** (sudden rapid heart rate). Also, there is a moderate rise in metabolism, which may be accompanied by some loss in weight. Excessive dosages result in hyper-excitability and insomnia followed by depression. This may be accompanied by abdominal cramps, hematuria (discharge of blood into the urine), collapse, convulsions, and coma.

Characteristically, amphetamines affect people differently. For this reason, small doses are administered initially to ascertain individual reactions. Certainly, amphetamines are contraindicated for easily excitable people and for those with high blood pressure.

Scientific investigations of the effects of amphetamines on endurance performance have not always produced consistent findings.[46,65,83,115] Most studies, though, have shown no significant influence of amphetamines on endurance performance. In one well-designed study,[115] it was shown that variant dosages of amphetamines do not affect heart rate or maximal endurance capacity during submaximal exercise. Although maximal heart rate was found to be significantly increased, such an effect does not appear to be related to endurance capacity. Another study[90] showed that ephedrine, a medication similar in action to amphetamines, has no effect on several measures of physical work capacity. Incidentally, in the 1972 Olympic Games, an American swimmer, Rick DeMont, was denied an earned gold medal because he was taking ephedrine for his asthmatic condition (it was prescribed).

Chandler and Blair examined amphetamines and athletic success, including strength, power, speed, anaerobic and aerobic capacity, and heart rate.[20] The results were mixed with one of two strength components unaffected. Also, leg power, speed, and aerobic capacity were unaffected. Acceleration, anaerobic capacity, time to exhaustion on the treadmill, preexercise heart rate, and maximal heart rate were all increased with drug (amphetamine) use.

table 18.2

Results of a survey of ten female weight lifters who were users of both injectable and oral anabolic-androgenic steroids.*

Questions†	Increased	Decreased	No change
1. Increased facial hair	9		1
2. Clitoris enlargement	8		2
3. Libido	6	1	3
4. Breast size		5	5
5. Menstruation (2 hysterectomized)		7 (or stopped)	1
6. Aggressiveness	8		2
7. Acne	6		4
8. Body hair	5		5
9. Scalp hair loss	2		8
10. Appetite	8		2
11. Body fat	8		2

*From Strauss et al.[96]

†The questions were designed to acquire respondents' perceptions of the effects of the steroids on the items listed.

We remind the reader again that, regardless of any real or perceived benefits, amphetamines are classified as controlled substances (Class II drugs) and are, without equivocation, banned for athletic competition, even when they are prescribed for clinically justifiable reasons.

Alkaline (Bicarbonate) Ingestion

In chapter 2, we pointed out that during anaerobic exercise, blood and muscle pH decrease, whereas lactic acid concentrations increase. Both of these factors (decreased pH and increased lactic acid concentration) have been implicated in the muscular fatigue process (p. 159).

Working from these facts, early researchers reasoned that increasing the body's alkali reserve (buffering system) prior to heavy exercise might significantly retard the decrease in pH, thus delaying fatigue and increasing exercise performance. Their reasoning was correct in that Dr. D. B. Dill and colleagues of the Harvard Fatigue Laboratories showed that runners in an alkaline state could run 13% longer on a treadmill before fatiguing.[32]

The preceding results were substantiated in two later studies, both of which used the same dosage of sodium bicarbonate of 300 mg · kg^{-1} of body weight as the alkalinizing agent.[62,108] In the first study, exercise to exhaustion was increased from 4.5 minutes to 7.3 minutes with bicarbonate loading. When ammonium chloride was ingested (making the blood more acidic) endurance time deteriorated to 2.6 minutes.[51] In the second study, running time in an 800-m run was improved by almost 3 seconds (from 2:05.8 to 2:02.9). Because of high pH values and HCO$_3^-$ in the urine, this form of doping would be relatively easy to detect.[108]

Caffeine

The many people who feel that a cup of coffee helps them "get going" in the morning may well have a scientifically valid point. However, the ergogenic effect of caffeine has remained controversial.[24] A review of the literature on the ergogenic effects of caffeine on psychomotor performance, muscular strength, and endurance performance shows that there is an abundance of disagreement. Addressing only the issue of endurance performance, one group of studies supports the ergogenic effect of improving endurance time and/or total work output,[11,26,38,39,59,70,84] whereas others have shown no improvement in endurance performance.[14,18,77,85]

Some rationale for the divergence of results may be found in the variety of experimental designs used in the cited references. Other factors relate to the caffeine tolerance of various individuals,[80] chronic users versus nonusers, level of fitness (as it relates to fatty acid metabolism), and variable responsiveness by Type I or Type II muscle fibers.

Caffeine is found in coffee, tea, various soft drinks, cocoa, chocolate, and some over-the-counter drugs. The average consumption in the United States is about 200 mg per day, which is equivalent to about two cups of coffee. The International Olympic Committee has set a standard of greater than 12 mcg · mL^{-1} in the urine as doping. This is the equivalent of six to eight cups of coffee consumed in one sitting and then being tested within two to three hours following consumption.[101]

If an ergogenic effect of caffeine does exist, it is probably related to caffeine's role in aiding the mobilization of free fatty acids. You should recall that fatty acids are the usable form of fat as a fuel for the aerobic system. Thus caffeine may have a glycogen-sparing effect in that it enables more fat to be used as a fuel, with less usage of glycogen. As previously mentioned, glycogen-sparing reduces muscle fatigue (p. 317).

Pangamic Acid (Vitamin B-15)

Of considerable interest has been a chemical compound called *pangamic acid* or *vitamin B-15*. According to the Federal Drug Administration, there is no scientific evidence to suggest that pangamic acid is a vitamin. It further states that pangamic acid is not only an illegal drug but is possibly dangerous. Nevertheless, coaches and athletes around the world have claimed that chronic ingestion of pangamic acid improves physical and athletic performance.

Two studies, utilizing treadmill performance, are cited.[45,48] In the first study, submaximal treadmill running at 70% of aerobic capacity showed no beneficial effects.[45] The second study, using much more elaborate procedures, failed to show any significant effect of pangamic acid on maximal performance.[48]

Physiological Agents

Of the physiological methods for improving performance, the two most often cited are blood doping and the use of supplemental oxygen. A third, very ominous, method, which is another form of blood doping, is the use of EPO (erythropoietin) to stimulate the increase in red blood cell concentration. Blood doping is, again, an illegal procedure, and supplemental oxygen has little practical benefit.

Blood Doping

Before proceeding with a description of **blood doping,** we will describe the position of the USOC relevant to this phenomenon.

> The practice of blood doping . . . is considered a form of doping by the United States Olympic Committee, and is therefore prohibited. Blood doping is the intravenous (I.V.) injection of blood (whole, packed red blood cells, or blood substitute) into an athlete's body, whether that blood be the athletes' own blood, or that of another person for the purpose of enhancing performance. . . . Any evidence confirming . . . that the practice of blood doping . . . was administered to an athlete will be cause for punitive action, comparable to that for using a banned substance, relative to anyone implicated by that evidence. . . .[100]

Further, the American College of Sports Medicine position stand concerning blood doping clearly condemns the practice for sport while recognizing the scientific and medical value of infusion of autologous red blood cell (RBC).[2]

As with other banned practices, blood doping is considered to be unethical and, consequently, unjustifiable in sport.

Blood doping, the removal and subsequent reinfusion of blood, is done to temporarily increase blood volume and, most importantly, raise the number of RBC. As was discussed in chapter 8, RBC contain hemoglobin. Thus overloading the blood with hemoglobin would increase the oxygen-carrying capacity of the blood and lead to an increased endurance performance.

Scientific studies of blood doping and endurance performance have produced conflicting results. Several studies have shown that blood doping increases endurance performance between 13% and 39% (measured by a treadmill run to exhaustion) and maximal oxygen consumption between 5% and 31% in both nonathletic subjects and highly trained endurance athletes.[10,16,17,35,36,43,78,79] An equal number of studies (mostly from earlier literature), however, have found no effects of blood doping on endurance performance, maximal oxygen consumption, heart rate responses during exercise, or perceived exertion.*[30,74,103,110,113,114]

An examination of research design differences clarifies much of the conflicting evidence. Two critical factors become apparent: (1) when between 800 and 1200 mL of blood, or its equivalent, is reinfused (as opposed to 450 to 500 mL), aerobic capacity and endurance increase and (2) when five to six weeks elapse before reinfusion, "positive" results also are seen.[109]

In practice, two sources of blood are available, autologous (reinfusion of one's own blood) and homologous (infusion from a donor).[50] By law, blood that is refrigerated cannot be stored for more than 21 days before usage. On the other hand, frozen supplies may be used after much longer periods of time.

Blood doping should not be recommended at any level of endurance competition. However, perhaps even more convincingly, blood doping should not be attempted because of the methodology involved (i.e., blood withdrawal and reinfusion). Some possible complications resulting from blood doping are:[2,31] (1) blood incompatibilities, (2) viral disease transmission, (3) septicemia (a morbid blood infection), (4) air embolism, and (5) thrombosis (blood clot).

Another technique for boosting RBC became apparent in the late 1980s. **Erythropoietin (EPO),** a hormone produced by the kidneys, stimulates the production of RBC under conditions of hypoxia (chronic low oxygen tension in the blood) and anemia. Human EPO can now be produced outside the human body with a recombinant DNA technique and is identified as rEPO. As in so many other situations, the artificial production of an agent designed for clinical usage has been brought into the athletic world; in this case, for endurance athletes.[28] rEPO is capable of stimulating levels of red blood cell production that reach toxic, life-

---

*Perceived exertion is a measure of how difficult the subjects believe the exercise is that they are performing (see chapter 14).

threatening levels. With hematocrit (chapter 8) levels above 55%, blood clots more readily form, increasing the danger for a stroke or coronary thrombosis. The endurance athlete who has infused rEPO and participates in an event where dehydration is probable magnifies the danger.

Oxygen

Studies have been conducted regarding the ergogenic effects of breathing oxygen (1) prior to exercise, (2) during exercise, and (3) during recovery from exercise.

O₂ Breathing prior to Exercise

There is some evidence that breathing oxygen immediately prior to exercise has some beneficial effects on performance, provided that the exercise is performed while holding the breath.[64,116] Studies in which oxygen was breathed prior to a non-breath-holding type of exercise show very little if any effect on performance.[37,71,86]

O₂ Breathing during Exercise

There is a rather large body of information indicating that breathing oxygen-enriched air (33% to 100% oxygen) has a beneficial effect on exercise performance.[1,8,51,58,71,117] During maximal work, these benefits include a greater endurance capacity, and during submaximal work, lower heart rate, lower blood lactic acid accumulation, and lower minute ventilation have been observed. The mechanism responsible for this change is the increased partial pressure of oxygen, which facilitates the transport of dissolved oxygen in plasma (physical solution) increasing diffusion across the alveolar-capillary and tissue-capillary membranes (chapter 8). As an ergogenic aid for improving athletic performance, breathing oxygen during exercise is not useful simply because it is not practical.

O₂ Breathing during Recovery

We are certain you have seen oxygen being administered to professional athletes during time-outs or rest breaks. Although there is not a great deal of research on this practice, any beneficial effects, either on the recovery process itself or on performance of a subsequent work bout, are inconsequential.[13,37,51,62] Although there may be a psychological effect, there is no physiological basis for use of oxygen during recovery.

Classification of "Contemporary" Ergogenic Aids

Table 18.3 contains a list of 29 so called ergogenic aids that currently are being researched for their mechanism of action and whether or not they are truly "ergogenic" by the definition given previously. Note that they have been placed

---

table 18.3

Classification of "contemporary" ergogenic aids

Nutritional (food and drink)

Amino acids[67]
Antioxidant vitamins[102]
Branched-chain amino acids (BCAAs)[69]
Ginseng[9]
High fat diet[89]
Minerals[22]
    Boron[49]
    Calcium[98]
    Chromium[52]
    Iron[44]
    Zinc[54]

Pharmacologic (drugs and hormones)

Anabolic-androgenic steroids (AAS)[91]
Epoetin (rEPO)[92]
Erythropoietin (EPO)[34]
Growth hormone (GH)[119]
Peptide hormones and analogues[66]

Physiological (natural and loading)

Bicarbonate loading[57]
Blood doping[4]
Carnitine[104]
Choline[112]
Creatine[82]
Phosphate loading[99]

Psychological (CNS stimulants and sympathomimetics)

Amphetamines[105]
Beta 2-agonists (Clenbuterol)[93]
Caffeine[94]
Cocaine[107]
Ephedrine[92]
Phenylpropanolamine[92]
Pseudoephedrine[92]

---

in four categories. This placement is arbitrary because many of them could reasonably fall under more than one heading. Note also the parenthetical descriptions for each category. These also are arbitrary and forced, but they do allow discussion of a wide variety of food, drug, natural, and stimulant substances in some organized fashion. Each of the substances is followed by a current reference that should provide a quick starting point for a more thorough search of the recent literature (perhaps a term paper topic).

Additional important information about each contemporary ergogenic aid is found in table 18.4. This represents our effort to consolidate a large amount of information into

18.4

table

Proposed mechanisms, most likely application, arbitrary index of effectiveness, and risks/regulations notation for contemporary ergogenic aids

Ergogenic aid	Proposed mechanism	Most likely application	Index of effectiveness	Risks/ regulations
Amino acids	Enhanced protein synthesis	Muscle & other tissue building	Not beneficial if adequate dietary protein	Little/FDA as a food
Antioxidant vitamins	Reduce damage by free radicals	Less tissue destruction & enhanced repair	Too little data to index effectiveness	Little/FDA as OTC drug
Branched chain amino acids	Provide more energy to muscle	Prolong endurance exercise	Not beneficial if adequate nutrition	Little/FDA as a food
Ginseng	Unclear; "restorative" tonic	Offset fatigue; psychological support	Unwarranted claims	Little/FDA as a food
High-fat diets	Raise plasma FFA; spare muscle glycogen	Enhance endurance performance	Probably beneficial	Much health risk/no regulation
Minerals	Supplement inadequate intake	Restricting food to maintain body weight	Probably beneficial if deficient	Little/no regulation
Boron	Increase testosterone level/effect	Improve strength and muscle mass	Unwarranted claims	Little/no regulation
Calcium	Increase bone mineral density	Offset risk of developing osteoporosis	Clearly beneficial if ammenorheic	Little/no regulation
Chromium	Unclear; gain strength and LBM	Supplement weight training program	Unwarranted claims	Little/no regulation
Iron	Offset iron deficiency anemia	Improve endurance performance	Not beneficial unless truly anemic	Little/no regulation
Zinc	Essential to protein synthesis	Offset loss in sweat and urine	Not beneficial unless truly deficient	Moderate/no regulation
Anabolic-androgenic steroids	Reverse corticosteroid catabolic effects	Weight training for strength & muscle mass	Clearly beneficial if negative nitrogen balance	Much/IOC, USOC, and NCAA
Epoetin and Erythropoietin	Increase RBC production; O_2 transport	Enhanced endurance performance	Probably beneficial	Moderate/IOC, USOC, and NCAA

FDA = U.S. Food and Drug Administration
IOC = International Olympic Committee
USOC = United States Olympic Committee
NCAA = National Collegiate Athletic Association

RBC = Red blood cell
LBM = Lean body mass
FA = Fatty acid

CNS = Central nervous system
SNS = Sympathetic nervous system

18.4
(Cont'd.)

Ergogenic aid	Proposed mechanism	Most likely application	Index of effectiveness	Risks/ regulations
Growth hormone	Counteract insulin; spare AA for anabolism	Increase LBM and "sculpted" appearance	Unwarranted claims	Much risk of acromegaly/ IOC, USOC
Peptide hormones & analogues	Increase levels & release of several hormones	Anabolic & O_2 transport effects specific to hormone	Too little data to index effectiveness	Moderate & specific/ IOC
Bicarbonate loading	Buffer effects of lactic- acidosis	High intensity performance lasting 1–7 min	Probably beneficial	Little/no regulation
Blood doping	Increase hematocrit & O_2 transport	Submaximal & maximal endurance exercise	Clearly beneficial	Moderate/IOC, USOC
Carnitine	Increase transport of long chain FA into mitochondria	Endurance exercise, more FA oxidation, spare muscle glycogen	Probably beneficial	Little/no regulation
Choline	Ensure adequate quantities of acetylcholine	Widespread since relates to possible site of fatigue	Too little data to index effectiveness	Little/no regulation
Creatine	Enhance body stores of creatine phosphate	Short duration, high-intensity efforts, 1–3 min	Probably beneficial	Little/no regulation
Phosphate loading	Unclear; delay fatigue by buffering	Wide if fatigue related; moreso for endurance exercise	Probably beneficial	Little/no regulation
Amphetamines	Indirect SNS & excess CNS stimulation	Widespread; masks body's symptoms of fatigue	Clearly beneficial	Much risk of dependence/ IOC, USOC
Beta2 agonists	Bronchodilator, dilate skin, muscle, blood vessels	Increase endurance performance; increase LBM, decrease body fat	Probably beneficial to breathing only	Little/IOC, USOC
Caffeine	CNS stimulant; increase lipolysis, glycogen sparing	Prolonged endurance exercise; possibly short intense (5 min.) exercise	Probably beneficial to endurance exercise	Little/IOC, USOC and NCAA
Cocaine	Blocks catecholamine uptake; increases SNS & CNS activity	Widespread; masks body's symptoms of fatigue	Unwarranted claims	Much/IOC, USOC, and NCAA
Ephedrine	Sympathomimetic; CNS stimulation, bronchodilator	Prolong endurance; some fatigue masking	Probably beneficial	Moderate/IOC, USOC, and NCAA

one useful presentation. Review this table carefully to get an overall impression of several important aspects of each ergogenic aid. First review the headings that are used in the table. The "ergogenic aid" listing is the same as for table 18.3, except that epoetin and erythropoietin are combined (blood doping), and ephedrine is used to also represent phenylpropanolamine and pseudoephedrine. These combinings are logical since the actions of the substances are nearly identical. Next note the heading for the "proposed mechanism" of the substance. This provides a very short description of how the ergogenic aid "might" work. Not all of the mechanisms are understood at the same level, and some are still regarded as unclear. Under the heading of "most likely application," a short description is given for the specific type of activity, aspect of body composition, or physiological response where the proposed ergogenic aid would reasonably exert its greatest effect. In some cases the effects are singular and narrow, and in other cases they are multiple and widespread. For example, brochodilation would be relatively specific, whereas masking fatigue would be quite general.

The final two categories of "index of effectiveness" and "risks/regulations" are even more judgmental and the reader is alerted to the rather arbitrary decisions that are made in the process. For example, "clearly beneficial" is meant to indicate that the research literature is generally supportive that the ergogenic aid is truly effective. "Probably beneficial" is used to indicate that there is less certainty but that there is at least equivocal data to support both a true effect and no effect. "Not beneficial" means that there is little support and that the ergogenic aid may only be effective in the presence of another condition, such as an inadequate diet or actual deficiency of a nutrient. The effectiveness index of "unwarranted claims" is used to indicate that research has been done but that there is a general lack of support to the claims made for the ergogenic aid—that is to say, it is highly unlikely that the proposed substance is truly an ergogenic aid. The final index used is "too little data to index effectiveness"; this is an important index that does not lend support at this time but leaves the door open for further investigation.

The terms used to describe the level of risk related to using a specific ergogenic aid are "little," "moderate," and "much." Caution must be used here, since even a "little" risk may be more than one should be willing to take. This holds especially true for substances that are relatively safe to take in small amounts for a brief period of time but that become exponentially more harmful when the dosage is increased or prolonged. Likewise, a substance that puts the user at "little" risk may really be more harmful if and when all the side effects are known or considered. The "moderate" risk index is used with substances that have well known and documented side effects that place the user at elevated risk. For example, the risks of infection or clotting with blood doping. The use of "much" as a risk index means that use of the substance is outright dangerous to the immediate

or long-term health of the user. Recall here that the user of amphetamines and cocaine have caused the deaths of some outstanding athletes and that human growth hormone abuse can cause irreversible acromegaly (abnormal bone growth).[61]

Finally, note the "regulations" indication of whether the substance is not regulated at all, is listed in some category by the FDA, or is banned by the IOC, USOC, or NCAA. Those interested in the moral and ethical issues that surround the use of contemporary ergogenic aids are directed to the excellent article by Williams.[112]

Sports and Drug Testing

Prior to the 1984 Olympic Games in Los Angeles, the application of sanctions against athletes detected with various drugs in their systems was inconsistent and uneven. There are a variety of reasons for this. One reason was that drug-testing protocols were not reliable. With the development of newer methods of drug detection and equipment using gas chromatography/mass spectrometry, the detection of minute levels of foreign substances in the bodies of athletes has been made possible.

The United States Olympic Committee formally established its own drug-testing program during a meeting at the 1983 Pan-American Games in Caracas.[21] The USOC uses a laboratory at the University of California at Los Angeles that is certified by the International Olympic Committee. The USOC Drug Control Program protocol defines the drug-testing program and details of the procedures including human rights and "chain of custody" expectations.[100] All athletes who are selected for the U.S. Olympic Team at the Olympic Trials will be tested. If the Olympic Trials occur more than 60 days prior to the Olympic Games, athletes will be retested prior to departing for the games. National governing bodies of the various sports may request formal testing during sanctioned competition.

The International Rowing Federation has initiated random drug testing among its members to be conducted at any time. If an athlete tests positive, then he or she is banned for life from rowing as a competitor, coach, and official.*

The National Collegiate Athletic Association, in its 1986 annual meeting, approved a drug-testing program for athletes participating in its various championships, including football bowl games. Several athletes have been barred from national championship contests as a consequence of this program. With the USOC and the NCAA drug-testing programs, a new environment for the conduct of sporting events is evolving that should provide more equitable competition for all athletes.

---

*Personal communication with Frederick C. Hagerman, Chair of the I.O.C. Medical Committee for the 1992 Olympic Games.

Summary

An ergogenic aid is anything that improves, or is thought to improve, physical performance. Ergogenic aids may be classified as nutritional, pharmacological, physiological, psychological, or mechanical.

The lack of objective and consistent information regarding the effects of drugs and ergogenic aids is in part attributable to individual physiological and psychological variations among people. To deal with possible psychological effects, a placebo is used in the research design.

Nutritional aids in the form of carbohydrate loading can enhance endurance performance by providing larger initial glycogen stores in muscle, thus delaying the onset of fatigue. The intake of supplemental vitamins generally has no benefit for the athlete and is harmless, except in some instances where megadoses of vitamins might be ingested. Maintaining water and electrolyte balance is essential to optimal performance.

Anabolic-androgenic steroids can be effective in increasing body mass and strength; however, the potential dangers and risks of taking steroids are well documented. There are inherent dangers for both male and female users of this class of drugs. Human growth hormone has been used alone and in combination with steroids. This represents a further heightening of risk to the health of an individual. The intake of steroids and growth hormone for the sole purpose of improving physique and athletic performance is not justifiable and is both illegal and ill-advised.

The American College of Sports Medicine, the United States Olympic Committee, the International Olympic Committee, and other sports-governing bodies have all taken strong stands against the use of the various pharmacological substances. Steroids, human growth hormone, and amphetamines represent the largest classes of banned substances.

Among physiological agents, blood doping represents a major concern. Because of both ethical and clinical reasons, any form of blood doping is not recommended. The practice is illegal in national and international competition. The introduction of recombinant erythropoietin represents an ominous new source of concern for the welfare of athletes. Oxygen can have short-term benefits if breathed prior to breath-holding activities. Otherwise, supplemental oxygen is ineffective.

The ingestion of alkaline salts (sodium bicarbonate) appears to increase endurance during heavy, short-term exercise. Caffeine has shown equivocal results related to the amount of endurance performance before fatigue.

There are ongoing research efforts to evaluate the proposal mechanism of action for many contemporary ergogenic aids. These efforts include the arbitrary indexing of the effectiveness, inherent risks, and source of any regulatory sanctions related to the use of each substance or practice.

Drug testing in sports has become a highly sophisticated and reliable procedure. The use of gas chromatography/mass spectrometry has made the detection of doping substances, even in very minute levels, in urine samples easily detectable.

Questions

1. Define an ergogenic aid.
2. What are some of the problems associated with obtaining consistent and objective information on the effects of ergogenic aids?
3. How do anabolic-androgenic steroids affect performance?
4. What are the physiological effects of amphetamines?
5. What is blood doping, and does it improve athletic performance?
6. What is the role of erythropoietin in blood doping?
7. Explain the effects of bicarbonate, oxygen, and caffeine on athletic performance.
8. Outline the proposed mechanism of action for three different "muscle building" ergogenic aids. How are they different?
9. List three so-called ergogenic aids that are not beneficial unless a true deficiency or undesirable bodily condition exists.
10. Identify four contemporary ergogenic aids that are "probably" effective and, at the same time, expose the user to "little" risk. Would you use them?
11. Choose the three contemporary ergogenic aids that you believe present the greatest short- or long-term risk to the user, i.e. clearly the riskiest to use although they may be of "clear" or "probable" effectiveness. Would you use these? Why or why not?
12. If you knew for sure that substance "X" was a "true ergogenic aid," but could not be detected by any means, would you advocate its use by recreational athletes? How about elite athletes?

References

1. Allen, P. D., and K. B. Pandolf. 1977. Perceived exertion associated with breathing hyperoxic mixtures during submaximal work. *Med Sci Sports.* 9(2):122–127.
2. American College of Sports Medicine. 1987. ACSM position stand on blood doping as an ergogenic aid. *Med Sci Sports Exerc.* 19(5):540–543.
3. American College of Sports Medicine. 1984. ACSM position stand on the use of anabolic-androgenic steroids in sports. *Med Sci Sports Exerc.* 19(5):534–539.
4. American College of Sports Medicine. 1996. ACSM position stand on the use of blood doping as an ergogenic aid. *Med Sci Sports Exerc.* 28:i–viii.
5. Ariel, G. N., and W. Saville. 1972. Anabolic steroids: the physiological effects of placebos. *Med Sci Sports.* 4(2):124–126.
6. Aronson, V. 1986. Vitamins and minerals as ergogenic aids. *Physician Sportsmed.* 14(3):209–212.
7. Åstrand, P. O., and Rodahl, K. 1986. *Textbook of Work Physiology,* 3rd ed. New York: McGraw-Hill.

8. Bannister, R., and D. Cunningham. 1954. The effects on the respiration and performance during exercise of adding oxygen to the inspired air. *J Physiol Lond.* 125:118–137.

9. Bahrke, M. S., and W. P. Morgan. 1994. Evaluation of the ergogenic properties of ginseng. *Sports Med.* 18:229–248.

10. Belko, A. 1987. Vitamins and minerals—an update. *Med Sci Sports Exerc.* 19(5):S191–S196.

11. Bell, R. D., R. T. Card, M. A. Johnson, T. A. Cunningham, and F. Baker. 1977. Blood doping and athletic performance. *Aust J Sports Med.* 8(2):133–139.

12. Berglund, B., and P. Hemmingsson. 1982. Effects of caffeine ingestion on exercise performance at low and high altitudes in cross-country skiers. *Int J Sports Med.* 3:234–236.

13. Bjorgum, R. K., and B. J. Sharkey. 1966. Inhalation of oxygen as an aid to recovery after exertion. *Res Q.* 37:462–467.

14. Bond, V., R. Adams, R. Balkissoon, J. McRae, and R. J. Tearny. 1987. Effects of caffeine on cardiorespiratory function and glucose metabolism during rest and graded exercise. *J Sports Med Phys Fit.* 20:135–137.

15. Bonen, J., S. A. Malcolm, R. D. Kilgour, K. P. MacIntyre, and A. N. Belcastro. 1981. Glucose ingestion before and during intense exercise. *J Appl Physiol.* 50:766–771.

16. Buick, F. J., N. Gledhill, A. B. Froese, L. Spriet, and E. C. Meyers. 1978. Double blind study of blood boosting in highly trained runners. *Med Sci Sports.* 10(1):49.

17. ———. 1980. Effect of induced erythrocythemia on aerobic work capacity. *J Appl Physiol.* 48:636–642.

18. Butts, N. K., and D. Crowell. 1985. Effect of caffeine ingestion on cardiorespiratory endurance in men and women. *Res Q.* 56:301–305.

19. Casner, S., R. Early, and B. Carlson. 1971. Anabolic steroid effects on body composition in normal young men. *J Sports Med Phys Fit.* 11:98–103.

20. Chandler, J. V., and S. N. Blair. 1980. The effect of amphetamine on selected physiological components related to athletic success. *Med Sci Sports Exerc.* 12(1):65–69.

21. Clarke, K. S. 1984. Sports medicine and drug control programs of the U.S. Olympic Committee. *J Allergy Clin Immunol.* 73:740–744.

22. Clarkson, P. M. 1991. Minerals: exercise performance and supplementation in athletes. *J Sports Sci.* 9:91–116.

23. Cohen, J. C., W. M. Faber, A. J. Spinnler, and T. D. Noakes. 1986. Altered serum lipoprotein profiles in male and female power lifters ingesting anabolic steroids. *Physician Sportsmed.* 14(6):131–136.

24. Costill, D. L. 1978. Performance secrets. *Runners World.* 13(7):50–55.

25. Costill, D. L., E. Coyle, G. Dalsky, W. Evans, W. Fink, and D. Hoopes. 1977. Effects of elevated plasma FFA and insulin on muscle glycogen usage during exercise. *J Appl Physiol.* 43:695–699.

26. Costill, D. L., G. P. Dalsky, and W. J. Fink. 1978. Effects of caffeine ingestion on metabolism and exercise performance. *Med Sci Sports.* 10(3):155–158.

27. Costill, D. L., D. R. Pearson, and W. J. Fink. 1984. Anabolic steroid use among athletes: changes in HDL-C levels. *Phys Sports Med.* 12(6):112–117.

28. Cowart, V. 1989. Erythropoietin: a dangerous new form of blood doping. *Phys Sportsmed.* 17(8):114–118.

29. Crist, D. M., G. T. Peake, P. A. Egan, and D. L. Waters. 1988. Body composition response to exogenous GH during training in highly conditioned adults. *J Appl Physiol.* 54:366–370.

30. Cunningham, K. G. 1978. The effect of transfusional polycythemia on aerobic work capacity. *J Sports Med.* 18:353–358.

31. Desbleds, M., J. P. Rapp, P. Dumas, and P. Jolis. 1979. Risk of blood transfusion doping in athletes. *Med Sport (Paris).* 53(4):191–194.

32. Dill, D. B., H. T. Edwards, and J. H. Talbott. 1932. Alkalosis and the capacity for work. *J Biol Chem.* 97:58–59.

33. Eichner, E. R. 1993. Ergolytic drugs in medicine and sports. *Am J Med.* 94(2):205–211.

34. Ekblom, B., and B. Berglund. 1991. Effect of erythropoietin administration on maximal aerobic power. *Scand J Med Sci Sports.* 1:88–93.

35. Ekblom, B., A. Goldbard, and B. Gullbring. 1973. Response to exercise after blood loss and reinfusion. *J Appl Physiol.* 33(2):175–180.

36. Ekblom, B., G. Wilson, and P. O. Åstrand. 1976. Central circulation during exercise after venesection and reinfusion of red blood cells. *J Appl Physiol.* 40:379–383.

37. Elbel, E., D. Ormond, and D. Close. 1961. Some effects of breathing O_2 before and after exercise. *J Appl Physiol.* 16:48–52.

38. Erickson, M. A., R. J. Schwartzkopf, and R. D. McKenzie. 1987. Effects of caffeine, fructose, and glucose ingestion on muscle glycogen utilization during exercise. *Med Sci Sports Exerc.* 19:579–583.

39. Essig, D., D. L. Costill, and P. J. Van Handel. 1980. Effects of caffeine ingestion on utilization of muscle glycogen and lipid during leg ergometer cycling. *Int J Sports Med.* 1:86–90.

40. Fahey, T. D., and C. H. Brown. 1973. The effects of anabolic steroids on the strength, body composition and endurance of college males when accompanied by a weight training program. *Med Sci Sports.* 5(4):272–276.

41. Foster, C., D. L. Costill, and W. J. Fink. 1979. Effects of preexercise feedings on endurance performance. *Med Sci Sports.* 11(1):1–5.

42. Fowler, W. H., G. W. Garner, and G. H. Egstrom. 1965. Effect of an anabolic steroid on physical performance of young men. *J Appl Physiol.* 20:1038–1040.

43. Frye, A., and R. Ruhling. 1977. RBC infusion, exercise, hemoconcentration, and VO_2. *Med Sci Sports.* 9(1):69.

44. Galloway, R., J. McGuire. 1994. Determinants of compliance with iron supplementation: supplies, side effects, or psychology? *Soc Sci Med.* 39(3):381–390.

45. Girandola, R. N., R. A. Wiswell, and R. Bulbulian. 1980. Effects of pangamic acid (B-15) ingestion on metabolic response to exercise. *Med Sci Sports Exerc.* 12(2):98.

46. Golding, L. A., and R. J. Barnard. 1963. The effects of d-amphetamine sulfate on physical performance. *J Sports Med Phys Fit.* 3:221–224.

47. Golding, L., J. Freydinger, and S. Fishel. 1974. Weight, size and strength—unchanged with steroids. *Phys Sportsmed.* 2:39–43.

48. Gray, M. E., and L. W. Titlow. 1983. Effect of pangamic acid on maximal treadmill performance. *Med Sci Sports Exerc.* 14(6):277–280.

49. Green, N. R., A. A. Ferrando. 1994. Plasma boron and the effects of boron supplementation in males. *Environ Health Perspect.* (102 suppl.)7:73–77.

50. Guyton, A. C. 1996. *Textbook of Medical Physiology,* 9th ed. Philadelphia: W.B. Saunders.

51. Hagerman, F. C., R. W. Bowers, E. L. Fox, and W. Ersing. 1968. The effects of breathing 100 percent oxygen during rest, heavy work, and recovery. *Res Q.* 39(4):965–974.

52. Hallmark, M. A., T. H. Reynolds, C. A. DeSouza, C. O. Dotson, R. A. Anderson, and M. A. Rogers. 1996. Effects of chromium and resistive training on muscle strength and body composition. *Med Sci Sports Exerc.* 28(1):139–144.

53. Hargreaves, M. W., D. L. Costill, A. Katz, and W. J. Fink. 1985. Effects of fructose on muscle glycogen usage during exercise. *Med Sci Sports Exerc.* 17(3):360–363.

54. Haymes, E. M. 1983. Proteins, vitamins, and iron. In Williams, M. H. (ed.), *Ergogenic Aids in Sports.* Champaign, IL: Human Kinetics Publishers.

55. Haymes, E. M. 1991. Vitamin and mineral supplementation to athletes. *Int J Sport Nutr.* 1(2):146–169.

56. Herbert, W. G. 1983. Water and electrolytes. In Williams, M. H. (ed.), *Ergogenic Aids in Sports.* Champaign, IL: Human Kinetics Publishers.

57. Horswill, C. A. 1995. Effects of bicarbonate, citrate, and phosphate loading on performance. *Int J Sport Nutr.* 5:S111–S119.

58. Hughes, R., M. Clode, R. Edwards, T. Goodwin, and N. Jones. 1968. Effect of inspired O_2 on cardiopulmonary and metabolic responses to exercise in man. *J Appl Physiol.* 24(3):336–347.

59. Ivy, J. L., D. L. Costill, W. J. Fink, and R. W. Lower. 1979. Influence of caffeine and carbohydrate feedings on endurance performance. *Med Sci Sports.* 11(1):6–11.

60. Johnson, L., G. Fisher, L. J. Silvester, and C. Hofheins. 1972. Anabolic steroid: effects on strength, body weight, oxygen uptake and spermatogenesis upon mature males. *Med Sci Sports.* 4(1):43–45.

61. Jonas, A. P., R. T. Sickles, and J. A. Lombardo. 1992. Substance abuse. *Clin Sports Med.* 11(2):379–401.

62. Jones, N. L., J. R. Sutton, R. Taylor, and C. J. Toews. 1977. Effect of pH on cardiorespiratory and metabolic responses to exercise. *J Appl Physiol.* 43(6):959–964.

63. Kantor, M. A., A. Bianchini, D. Bernier, S. P. Sady, and P. D. Thompson. 1985. Androgens reduce HDL-cholesterol and increase hepatic triglyceride lipase activity. *Med Sci Sports Exerc.* 17(4):462–465.

64. Karpovich, P. 1959. The effect of oxygen inhalation on swimming performance. *Res Q.* 5(2):24.

65. ———. 1959. Effect of amphetamine sulphate on athletic performance. *JAMA.* 170:558–561.

66. Kicman, A. T., and D. A. Cowan. 1992. Peptide hormones and sport: misuse and detection. *Br Med Bull.* 48(3):496–517.

67. Kreider, R. B., V. Miriel, and E. Bertun. 1993. Amino acid supplementation and exercise performance. Analysis of the proposed ergogenic value. *Sports Med.* 16(3):190–209.

68. Lombardo, J. A., R. C. Hickson, and D. R. Lamb. 1991. Anabolic/androgenic steroids and growth hormone. In Lamb, D. R., and M. H. Williams (eds.), *Perspectives in Exercise Science, vol. 4: Ergogenics.* Dubuque, IA: Brown & Benchmark, pp. 249–284.

69. MacLean, D. A., T. E. Graham, and B. Saltin. 1994. Branched-chain amino acids augment ammonia metabolism while attenuating protein breakdown during exercise. *Am J Physiol.* 267: E1010–1022.

70. McNaughton, L. 1987. Two levels of caffeine ingestion on blood lactate and free fatty acid responses during incremental exercise. *Res Q Exerc Sport.* 58:255–259.

71. Miller, A. 1952. Influence of oxygen administration on the cardiovascular function during exercise and recovery. *J Appl Physiol.* 5:165–168.

72. Murphy, R. J. 1963. The problem of environmental heat in athletics. *Ohio State Med J.* 59:799.

73. Murray, T. H. 1986. Human growth hormone in sports—no. *Phys Sportsmed.* 14(5):29.

74. Pate, R. R., J. McFarland, J. Van Wyk, and A. Okocha. 1979. Effects of blood reinfusion on endurance exercise performance in female distance runners. *Med Sci Sports.* 11(1):97.

75. Percy, E. C. 1978. Ergogenic aids in athletics. *Med Sci Sports.* 10(4):298–303.

76. Peterson, G. E., and T. D. Fahey. 1984. HDL-C in five elite athletes using anabolic-androgenic steroids. *Phys Sportsmed.* 12(6):120–130.

77. Powers, S. K., S. Dodd, J. Woodyard, and M. Magnum. 1986. Caffeine alters ventilatory and gas exchange kinetics during exercise. *Med Sci Sports Exerc.* 18:101–106.

78. Robertson, D., D. Wade, R. Workman, R. L. Woosley, and J. A. Oates. 1981. Tolerance to the humoral and hemodynamic effects of caffeine in man. *J Clin Invest.* 67:1111–1117.

79. Robertson, R., R. Gilcher, K. Metz, H. Bahnson, T. Allison, G. Skrinar, A. Abbott, and R. Becker. 1978. Effect of red blood cell reinfusion on physical working capacity and perceived exertion at normal and reduced oxygen pressure. *Med Sci Sports.* 10(1):49.

80. Robertson, R., R. Gilcher, K. Metz, C. Casperson, A. Abbott, T. Allison, G. Skrinar, K. Werner, S. Zelicoff, and J. Drause. 1979.

81. Rogozkin, V. 1979. Metabolic effects of anabolic steroids on skeletal muscle. *Med Sci Sports.* 11(2):160–163.

82. Rossiter, H. B., E. R. Cannell, and P. M. Jakeman. 1996. The effect of oral creatine supplementation on the 1000-m performance of competitive rowers. *J Sports Sci.* 14(2):175–179.

83. Ryan, A. J. 1959. Use of amphetamines in athletics. *JAMA.* 170:562.

84. Sasaki, H., J. Maeda, S. Usui, and T. Ishiko. 1987. Effects of sucrose and caffeine ingestion on performance of prolonged strenuous running. *Int J Sports Med.* 8:261–265.

85. Sasaki, H., I. Takaoka, and T. Ishiko. 1987. Effects of sucrose and caffeine ingestion on running performance and biochemical responses to endurance running. *Int J Sports Med.* 8:203–207.

86. Sharkey, B. 1961. *The Effect of Preliminary Oxygen Inhalation on Performance in Swimming.* Master's thesis: West Chester State College, West Chester, PA.

87. Sherman, W. M. 1983. Carbohydrates, muscle glycogen, and muscle glycogen supercompensation. In Williams, M. H. (ed.), *Ergogenic Aids in Sports.* Champaign, IL: Human Kinetics Publishers.

88. Sherman, W. M., D. L. Costill, W. J. Fink, and J. M. Miller. 1981. The effect of exercise and diet manipulation on muscle glycogen and its subsequent utilization during performance. *Int J Sports Med.* 2:114–118.

89. Sherman, W. M., and N. Leenders. 1995. Fat loading: the next magic bullet? *Int J Sport Nutr.* (5 suppl.):S1–S12.

90. Sidney, K. H., and N. M. Lefcoe. 1977. The effect of ephedrine on the physiological and psychological responses to submaximal and maximal exercise in man. *Med Sci Sports* 9(2):95–99.

91. Smith, D. A., and P. J. Perry. 1992. The efficacy of ergogenic agents in athletic competition. Part I: androgenic-anabolic steroids. *Ann Pharmacother.* 26:520–528.

92. Smith, D. A., and P. J. Perry. 1992. The efficacy of ergogenic agents in athletic competition. Part II: other performance-enhancing agents. *Ann Pharmacother.* 26:653–659.

93. Spann, C., and M. E. Winter. 1995. Effect of clenbuterol on athletic performance. *Ann Pharmacother.* 29(1):75–77.

94. Spriet, L. L. 1995. Caffeine and performance. *Int J Sport Nutr.* (5 suppl.):S84–99.

95. Stone, M. H., and H. Lipner. 1978. Responses to intensive training and methandrostenelone administration. I. Contractile and performance variables. *Pflugers Arch.* 375(2):141–146.

96. Strauss, R. H., M. T. Liggett, and R. R. Lanese. 1985. Anabolic steroid use and perceived effects in ten weight trained women athletes. *JAMA.* 253:2871–2873.

97. Strauss, R. H., J. E. Wright, G. A. M. Finerman, and D. H. Catlin. 1983. Side effects of anabolic steroids in weight-trained men. *Phys Sportsmed.* 11(12):87–95.

98. Teegarden, D., and C. M. Weaver. 1994. Calcium supplementation increases bone density in adolescent girls. *Nutr Rev.* 52(5):171–173.

99. Tremblay, M. S., S. D. Galloway, and J. R. Sexsmith. 1994. Ergogenic effects on phosphate loading: physiological fact or methodological fiction? *Can J Appl Physiol.* 19:1–11.

100. United States Olympic Committee. 1986. *Drug control program protocol.* Colorado Springs, CO: U.S. Olympic House.

101. United States Olympic Committee. 1989. *Drug free: U.S. Olympic committee drug education handbook—1989–92.* Colorado Springs, CO.

102. Van der Hagen, A. M., D. P. Yolton, M. S. Kaminski, and R. L. Yolton. 1993. Free radicals and antioxidant supplementation: a review of their roles in age-related macular degeneration. *J Am Optom Assoc.* 64(12):871–878.

103. Videman, T., and T. Rytomaa. 1977. Effect of blood removal and autoinfusion on heart rate response to a submaximal workload. *J Sports Med.* 17:387–390.

Central circulation and work capacity after red blood cell reinfusion under normoxia and hypoxia in women. *Med Sci Sports.* 11(1):98.

104. Vulkovich, M., D. Costill, and W. Fink. 1994. L-carnitine supplementation: effect on muscle carnitine content and glycogen utilization during exercise. *Med Sci Sports Exerc.* 26:1122–1129.

105. Wadler, G. I., and B. Hainline. 1989. Amphetamine. In *Drugs and the Athlete.* Philadelphia: F. A. Davis.

106. Ward, P. 1973. The effect of an anabolic steroid on strength and lean body mass. *Med Sci Sports.* 5(4):277–282.

107. Welder, A. A., and R. B. Melchert. 1993. Cardiotoxic effects of cocaine and anabolic-androgenic steroids in the athlete. *J Pharmacol Toxicol Methods.* 29(2):61–68.

108. Wilkes, D., N. Gledhill, and R. Smyth. 1983. Effects of acute induced metabolic alkalosis on 800-m racing time. *Med Sci Sports Exerc.* 15(4):277–280.

109. Williams, M. H. 1983. Blood doping. In M. H. Williams (ed.), *Ergogenic Aids in Sports.* Champaign, IL: Human Kinetics Publishers.

110. Williams, M. H. 1975. Blood doping—does it really help athletes? *Phys Sportsmed.* Jan:52.

111. Williams, M. H. (ed.), 1983. *Ergogenic Aids in Sports.* Champaign, IL: Human Kinetics Publishers.

112. Williams, M. H. 1994. The use of nutritional ergogenic aids in sports: is it an ethical issue? *Int J Sport Nutr.* 4(2):120–131.

113. Williams, M. H., H. Goodwin, R. Perkins, and J. Bocrie. 1973. Effect of blood reinjection upon endurance capacity and heart rate. *Med Sci Sports.* 5(3):181–185.

114. Williams, M. H., M. Lindhiem, and R. Schuster. 1978. The effect of blood-infusion upon endurance capacity and ratings of perceived exertion. *Med Sci Sports.* 10(2):113–118.

115. Williams, M. H., and J. Thompson. 1973. Effect of variant dosages of amphetamine upon endurance. *Res Q.* 44(4):417–422.

116. Wilmore, J. 1972. Oxygen. In Morgan, W. (ed.), *Ergogenic Aids and Muscular Performance.* New York: Academic Press, pp. 321–342.

117. Wilson, G. D., and H. G. Welch. 1975. Effects of hyperoxic gas mixtures on exercise tolerance in man. *Med Sci Sports* 7(1):48–52.

118. Wright, J. E., and V. S. Cowart, 1990. Steroids. Carmel, IN: Benchmark Press (Brown & Benchmark).

119. Yarasheski, K. E., J. J. Zachweija, T. J. Angelopoulos, and D. M. Bier. 1993. Short-term growth hormone treatment does not increase muscle protein synthesis in experienced weight lifters. *J Appl Physiol.* 74:3073–3076.

Selected Readings

Clarkson, P. M. 1996. Nutrition for improved sports performance. Current issues on ergogenic aids. *Sports Med.* 21:393–401.

Greenhaff, P. L. 1995. Creatine and its application as an ergogenic aid. *Int J Sport Nutr.* 5:S100–110.

Kanter, M. M., and M. H. Williams. 1995. Antioxidants, carnitine, and choline as putative ergogenic aids. *Int J Sport Nutr.* 5:S120–131.

Kreider, R. B., V. Miriel, and E. Bertun. 1993. Amino acid supplementation and exercise performance. Analysis of the proposed ergogenic value. *Sports Med.* 16:190–209.

Sawka, M. N., M. J. Joyner, D. S. Miles, R. J. Robertson, L. L. Spriet, and A. J. Young. 1996. American College of Sports Medicine. Position Stand. The use of blood doping as an ergogenic aid. *Med Sci Sports Exerc.* 28:i–viii.

Smith, D. A., and P. J. Perry. 1992. The efficacy of ergogenic agents in athletic competition. Part II: Other performance-enhancing agents. *Ann Pharmacother.* 26:653–709.

Spriet, L. L. 1991. Blood doping and oxygen transport. In Lamb, D. R., and M. H. Williams (eds.), *Perspectives in Exercise Science, Vol. 4: Ergogenics.* Dubuque, IA: Brown & Benchmark, pp. 213–248.

Thein, L. A., J. M. Thein, and G. L. Landry. 1995. Ergogenic aids. *Phys Ther.* 75:426–439.

Williams, M. H. 1994. The use of nutritional ergogenic aids in sports: is it an ethical issue? *Int J Sport Nutr.* 4:120–131.

section 7

The Environment

If you had knowledge of how, physiologically, an athlete—such as a triathlete—can die from heat stroke, you would never knowingly contribute to such a tragedy. As a matter of fact, you, being informed, could now help influence teachers, coaches, and athletic trainers about preventing such hazards. If everyone were informed about proper clothing, fluid needs, what situations to avoid, and warning signs and symptoms, there could be literally no heat-related deaths in physical education, road races, and expeditions. Similarly, sport scuba diving and exercise at high altitude can be potentially dangerous if the performer does not have a thorough understanding of the effects that go along with rapid changes to higher (scuba) or lower (altitude) barometric pressures. The information contained in this section will help you better appreciate the important problems that confront clinicians, coaches, and trainers charged with working in these different environments.

Chapter 19 thoroughly explores the body's acute (short-term) and chronic (long-term) adaptations to different thermal environments (hot and cold). Chapter 20 completes this section with coverage of the physiological adjustments to different barometric pressures: hyperbaric (scuba), hypobaric (altitude), and microgravity (space).

Traveling to, living, and working under water, in highlands, and in space has allowed us to learn much about man's ability to tolerate environmental stresses as well as the physiologic changes that occur in response. Remember, the physiologic strain placed on the body while exercising in all of the above conditions can be harmful, and in rare cases, life threatening—making your knowledge in these areas that much more important.

The following chapters are contained in this section:

19

Temperature Regulation: Exercise in the Heat and Cold

One of the principles of environmental physiology is the familiar one of homeostasis.[26] When challenged with different ambient temperatures (heat or cold), the body strives to maintain internal temperature in a narrow range. Add to this the myriad of physiological adjustments that occur with exercise, students should begin to appreciate the complexity with which the body functions during exercise in various environmental conditions. In some cases the adjustments with exercise produce heat to keep us warm in a cold environment. On the other hand, the same exercise related heat production risks *overheating* the human "machine" in a hot environment.

What are the risks of overheating the body? Well, the *Annual Survey of Football Injury Research*[56] reports that a total of 89 football fatalities were attributable to heat stroke between 1931 and 1995 (figure

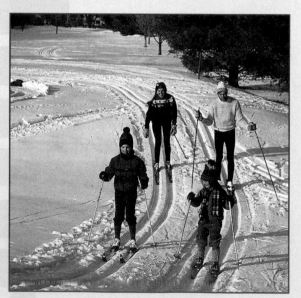

19.1). The deaths of these young men were tragic, for all were preventable. However, heat-related illnesses are not unique to football alone. Why do they happen? Lack of knowledge, misinformation, and not paying attention to the known "warning signs" on the part of the coaches and exercise enthusiasts all likely contribute. It is our intention to ensure that you do not contribute toward such accidents, and that you educate others toward improved safety and first-aid treatment.

Heat Balance

Temperature Regulation

Exercise in the Heat

Exercise in the Cold

Other Factors That Influence Thermoregulation

Summary

The major concepts to be learned from this chapter are as follows:

- Body heat balance is achieved when heat loss equals heat production (gain).
- The body loses heat through convection, conduction, radiation, and evaporation of sweat. Heat is gained by the body mainly through metabolism, but it may also be gained from the environment through radiation, convection, and conduction.
- The major function of the thermoregulatory system is to maintain a relatively constant internal body temperature (37° C) at rest as well as during exercise.
- The seriousness of overexposure to heat while exercising is exemplified not only by a decrease in work performance, but also by a predisposition to serious heat illnesses and even death.
- Heat illnesses during exercise can be significantly reduced through (a) adequate water (and electrolyte) replacement, (b) acclimatization to heat, and (c) awareness of the limitations imposed by the combination of exercise, clothing, and environmental heat.
- Exercise in the cold does not usually present a serious hazard; however, prolonged exposure can.
- After adjustments for fitness level, body composition, and body surface area have been made, few differences remain between males and females relative to heat or cold tolerance. What differences do exist relate to sweating function and menstrual cycle phase.

Heat Balance

Throughout the day, and across all types of activity levels (rest to running) and environments, the body constantly regulates itself to maintain a safe, constant body temperature. Therefore, one's body temperature represents a careful balance between heat production and heat loss. Recall that energy production within the body results in heat being liberated. To maintain a constant internal temperature, this heat must be dissipated. If not, it will be stored by the body and cause body temperature to increase.

As you sit and read this book, your body temperature remains near 98.6° F (37° C*). Such heat balance, as shown schematically in figure 19.2, is ultimately dependent on your ability to offset heat *gained* from both metabolism and the environment with heat *loss.*

$$heat\ balance = heat\ gain - heat\ loss$$

Heat Exchange

The exchange of heat with your surrounding environment occurs through several important mechanisms. The body gains or loses heat through *convection, conduction, radiation,* and *evaporation* (figure 19.3).

Convection

Convection is defined as the transfer of heat from one place to another by the motion of a heated substance. For example, an electric fan blowing over the surface of the skin removes air warmed by the body and replaces it with cooler air. In this case, although the skin is not moving, the air blowing across the skin is. Also, holding your arm out the window of a moving car produces the same result. As long as cooler air blows across the surface of the body, heat can be lost. *Also, the amount of heat loss due to convection is directly related to the speed and temperature of the air flow over the surface of the body.* The individual who is running (i.e., moving) can lose heat by convection just as one can lose heat by standing in a breeze. The faster velocities achieved during cycling make this method a particularly effective means of heat transfer. Convection also occurs within the body when blood flow carries heat from the muscles to the core and then to the skin.

Conduction

Conduction is the transfer of heat between two objects of different temperatures that are in direct contact with each other. The direction of heat flow is always from the warmer to the cooler object. When we touch a piece of ice, for example, heat is conducted from the surface of the hand to the

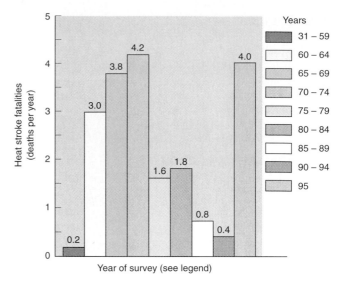

Figure 19.1

The rate of heat stroke fatalities in high school and college football from 1931 to 1995 in 5-year increments (except for 1931 to 1959 and 1995).

(Data from Mueller and Schindler.[56])

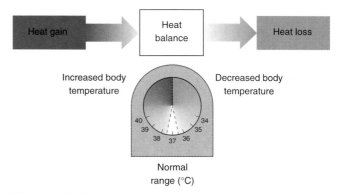

Figure 19.2

Heat balance. When heat gain and heat loss are equal, the amount of heat stored does not change, and therefore body temperature remains constant. When heat gain is greater than heat loss, body temperature will increase, and when heat loss exceeds heat gain, body temperature will decrease.

ice, whereas when we touch a hot stove, heat is transferred from the stove to the hand (ouch!). Conduction is directly related to the temperature difference between the two surfaces in contact with one another. The greater the temperature difference between two objects the greater the heat loss from the hotter to the colder object.

Radiation

Radiation accounts for about 60% of the heat loss from an undressed person resting quietly in a room at 70° F. The principle of radiation is based on the fact that molecules within a body are constantly vibrating and, as a consequence,

---

*° F = (1.8 × ° C) + 32, and ° C = (° F − 32) × 0.56.

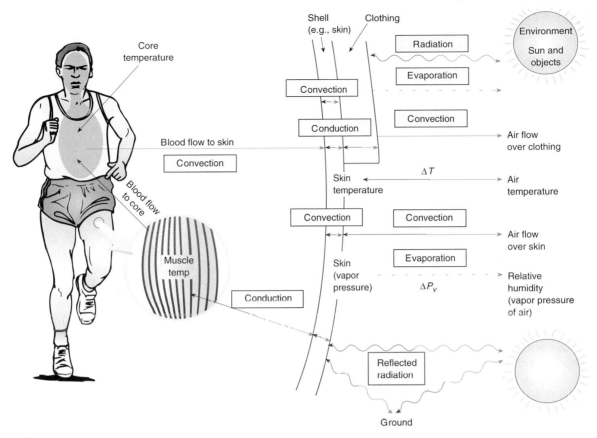

Figure 19.3

Avenues of heat transfer are depicted in the rectangles. Heat production increases dramatically in the muscle with exercise. Internally, conduction and convection are important in the transfer of heat both from muscle to core to shell to skin and from muscle to shell to skin. Externally, during heavy exercise, evaporation accounts for practically all of the heat transfer. Other external mechanisms important at rest include radiation, convection, and conduction. Important factors include ΔT (temperature difference between the skin and the air) and ΔP_v (vapor pressure difference between skin and air).

heat in the form of electromagnetic waves operating in the infrared range is continuously being given off. Figure 19.3 shows the variations in radiant heat across the body surface area. **Radiation,** then, is the transfer of heat between objects through electromagnetic wave activity. For example, when we are seated in the classroom we are radiating heat to the walls of the room. At the same time heat is being radiated from the walls to us! We *gain* heat through radiation when surrounding objects are warmer than our bodies; we *lose* heat through radiation when our body temperature is warmer than surrounding objects. A person seated in a dry sauna with the temperature set at 120° F would obviously gain more heat from the radiating light bulbs and heating elements than he or she could lose through radiation.

With this in mind, whether you are on the athletic field or running trail, a considerable amount of heat can be gained from the sun through radiation. This is especially true when (1) there is little or no cloud cover and (2) when the time of day is between 12:00 noon and 4:00 P.M. Because of the position of the sun during this period, the radiation from the sun is more concentrated.

Evaporation

The primary mechanism of heat loss during exercise is through the evaporation of sweat from the surface of the skin. Even while resting, *insensible perspiration* occurs, which rids the body of any excessive heat being produced. Insensible perspiration is the small amount of extracellular fluid that continually diffuses through the skin and the respiratory surfaces and evaporates unnoticed. Because it evaporates rapidly, we do not notice the moisture, hence the term *insensible.*

Evaporation is the term applied when a liquid is changed to a vapor or a gas. Energy is required for this change and it is obtained from the immediate surroundings. This extraction of energy results in cooling. When we work hard and sweat profusely, our bodies will be cooled only if the sweat evaporates from the surface of the skin—that is, if it changes from a liquid into a vapor on the surface of the skin. If the sweat cannot evaporate and merely drips from the body, no cooling of the body can take place. For every mL of sweat evaporated, the body can lose approximately 0.580 kcal of heat (or, 1L of sweat evaporated = 580 kcal).

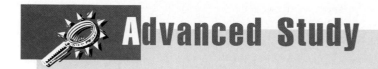

Advanced Study

Sweat

The formation and secretion of sweat is called hidropoesis (hidro = sweat; poesis = formation). Sweat is a weak solution of sodium chloride in water, along with urea and small quantities of potassium ion, other electrolytes, and lactic acid. The sweat glands, which number over 2.5 million in a person living in a temperate climate, are controlled or regulated by the sympathetic nervous system. Stimulation of the anterior hypothalamus—preoptic area—of the brain by an increased temperature (heat) in the blood circulating through this area leads to sweating. Nerve impulses from the hypothalamus travel down nerves found in the spinal cord and then through the sympathetic outflow to the skin. These nerves then innervate the sweat glands through the release of acetylcholine. The sweat glands can also be stimulated by the epinephrine and norepinephrine (adrenaline and noradrenaline) that is circulating in the blood. During exercise the latter method is important because these hormones are released in greater amounts by the adrenal medulla during exercise, thus increasing sweat production and facilitating heat loss.

The sweat gland itself is a tubular structure consisting of two parts:

1. A deep (subdermal) coiled portion that secretes the sweat (precursor secretion) and
2. A duct portion that passes through the dermal and epidermal layers of the skin and terminates in a pore.

The composition of the precursor secretion is, except for proteins, quite similar to that of plasma. The concentrations of sodium and chloride are about 140 $meq \cdot L^{-1}$ and 104 $meq \cdot L^{-1}$, respectively. However, as the precursor secretion flows through the duct portion of the gland toward the pore, its chemical composition is modified as most of the sodium and chloride are reabsorbed. The extent of this reabsorption varies depending on the sweat rate. When sweat rate is low the precursor fluid passes through the duct slowly, allowing for almost all of the sodium and chloride to be reabsorbed and dropping the concentration of these two ions to as low as 5 $meq \cdot L^{-1}$ each. In fact, much of the water is also reabsorbed because of the low osmotic pressure of the precursor fluid. This leaves the resulting sweat with higher concentrations of urea, lactic acid, and potassium.

On the other hand, when the sweat glands receive strong stimulation from the sympathetic nervous system, the duct portion may absorb only 50% of the sodium and chloride. Additionally, both the higher osmotic pressure of sweat and its higher flow rate cause less water to be reabsorbed and as a result, the other constituents (urea, potassium, and lactic acid) of sweat are only moderately elevated when compared to plasma.[10,39]

To carry out the sweating process, there are two kinds of sweat glands in the body. *Eccrine* sweat glands, which are the most numerous, secrete a dilute, watery sweat that is involved in thermal regulation. These glands are widely distributed over the body surface, being more heavily concentrated on the palms of the hands, soles of the feet, the neck, and the trunk. The *apocrine* sweat glands secrete a "thicker" sweat that is not used for thermal regulation. Rather, this kind of sweat is secreted in response to emotional stress. Apocrine sweat glands are found principally in the pubic and axillary (underarm) areas.

Heat Production (Gain)

The unit of heat energy most commonly used is the calorie, which we previously defined as the heat required to raise the temperature of 1 gram of water 1° C (chapter 4). The kilocalorie (kcal), as the name implies, is the amount of heat required to raise the temperature of 1 kg of water 1° C. The *specific heat of water* (the heat required to change the temperature of a unit mass of water one degree) is therefore 1 kcal per kg of water per degree centigrade (1 kcal $\cdot$ kg^{-1} $\cdot$ ° C^{-1}). The overall or combined specific heat of the body's tissues (bone, muscle, and so on) is 0.83 kcal $\cdot$ kg^{-1} $\cdot$ ° C^{-1}. Therefore, a person weighing 70 kg (154 pounds) must "store" 58 kcal of heat (0.83 × 70) to increase the body temperature 1° C.

Also recall from chapter 4 that the amount of heat or energy produced during metabolism is dependent on the food being oxidized. For the above person weighing 70 kg, resting $\dot{V}O_2$ would be between 250 and 300 mL $\cdot$ min^{-1} (or 0.25 to 0.3 L $\cdot$ min^{-1}). The caloric equivalent of one liter of oxygen ranges between 4.69 and 5.05 kcal, depending on the food being metabolized (see table 4.3). A person resting quietly usually oxidizes about 66% fat and 33% carbohydrate

(R = 0.82), which means that for each liter of oxygen consumed, 4.83 kcal of heat will be produced. Therefore, the heat production of a resting person via metabolism would be about 1.45 kcal $\cdot$ min^{-1} (0.3 L of O_2 × 4.83 kcal $\cdot$ L^{-1}), or 87 kcal $\cdot$ h^{-1}. If all of this heat was stored and none lost, body temperature would increase approximately 1.5° C $\cdot$ hr^{-1}. This increase was calculated as follows:

$$\frac{\text{Resting energy expenditure}}{\text{Body weight} \times \text{the specific heat of the body}} =$$

$$\frac{87 \text{ kcal} \cdot \text{h}^{-1}}{70 \text{ kg} \times 0.83 \text{ kcal} \cdot \text{kg}^{-1} \cdot {}^{\circ}\text{C}^{-1}} = 1.5° \text{ C} \cdot \text{hr}^{-1}$$

The net result would increase body temperature from 37.0° C (normal) to 38.5° C (or 98.6° F to 101.3° F). This increase usually does not occur at rest because, under most environmental conditions, the 87 kcal $\cdot$ h^{-1} of heat produced can be easily dissipated through convection, conduction, radiation, and evaporation. However, on an extremely hot day the *potential* rise in body temperature of a runner, whose heat production may be 10 to 15 times that of rest, is staggering.

For example, let us assume that an athlete consumes, on average, 2 liters of oxygen per minute doing an activity for 1 hour. At the end of this hour the VO$_2$ would equal 120 liters (60 min × 2 L $\cdot$ min^{-1}). Assuming again that R = 0.82 (or 4.83 kcal $\cdot$ L^{-1} of O_2), the total heat energy produced would equal 580 kcal $\cdot$ h^{-1} (120 L $\cdot$ min^{-1} × 4.83 kcal $\cdot$ L^{-1}). If all of this heat were stored and none lost, what would the increase in body temperature be if the person weighed 80 kg (remember, the specific heat of body tissue is 0.83 kcal $\cdot$ kg$^{-1} \cdot$ °C^{-1})?

$$\frac{580 \text{ kcal} \cdot \text{h}^{-1}}{80 \text{ kg} \times 0.83 \text{ kcal} \cdot \text{kg}^{-1} \cdot {}^{\circ}\text{C}^{-1}} = 8.7° \text{ C} \cdot \text{hr}^{-1}$$

Left unchecked, the above increase in body temperature would likely result in heat stroke and death. This example should make us keenly aware of the extreme importance and unique ability of our body to thermoregulate and maintain heat balance during activity.

In addition to metabolism, heat can also be gained by the body from the environment through radiation, convection, and conduction (figure 19.3). This occurs when the air and/or the objects surrounding the body are warmer than the body itself.

Assessment of Body Temperature

Body temperature directly reflects the amount of heat gained by metabolism and/or the environment. Since the temperature of the body tends to vary across different tissues, an average temperature (mean body temperature) can be determined by obtaining *internal* or **core temperature** and a *weighted average of skin* temperature. Several techniques can be employed to measure the body's core temperature including rectal, tympanic (i.e., ear), and/or

esophageal methods. While researchers rightfully debate which method is most accurate, rectal temperature remains in widespread use.

Since skin temperature can vary depending on the air temperature and the evaporation of sweat, an average temperature may be obtained by placing thermal sensors (thermistors) on the skin across different areas of the body. The mean skin temperature may be calculated using the following equation[78]:

$$T_{skin} = (0.1 \times T_{arms}) + (0.6 \times T_{trunk}) + (0.2 \times T_{legs}) + (0.1 \times T_{head})$$

Notice that the thermal sensor for each body part is multiplied by a constant. These constants represent the corresponding percentage of the total skin area for that region of the body. Given the temperatures for various areas of the body listed below, compute T_{skin}.

$$T_{arms} = 35.1° \text{ C} \qquad T_{trunk} = 36.5° \text{ C}$$

$$T_{legs} = 37.1° \text{ C} \qquad T_{head} = 36.4° \text{ C}$$

Did your answer for $T_{skin} = 36.5°$ C?

Once core temperature and mean skin temperature have been determined we can calculate mean body temperature by using the following formula:

$$T_{mean} = (0.4 \times T_{skin}) + (0.6 \times T_{core})$$

Notice that skin and core temperature account for 40% and 60% of mean body temperature, respectively.

Mechanisms of Heat Exchange

When discussing the interaction of conduction, convection, radiation, and evaporation, it is best to do so using the core-shell model of heat production and transfer. The *core* of the body may be described as the *deep body* tissues of the thoracic cavity (heart and lungs), head (brain), and neck. Core temperature, often represented by rectal temperature, is maintained within a very narrow range of 2° to 3° C. The *shell* represents the *outer body* tissues at and below the surface of the skin. Temperatures at this level may vary over a range of 11° C or more, depending on the thermal stress. While the vital organs of the body can be considered as the core compartment, there is no clear anatomical landmark that separates the core from the shell.

Figure 19.3 depicts the effects of the various components of the heat exchange system on the core-shell model. Key points to remember are:

1. Heat flows down the *temperature gradient* from muscle (where the heat is produced) → to the core → to the skin via convection;
2. Some heat is conducted directly to the surface of the skin from both muscle and the core; and
3. The transfer of heat from the skin to the environment depends on (a) the temperature gradient between the

skin and the air for both convection and radiation and (b) the rate of evaporation, which is greatly dependent on the difference in vapor pressure between the skin and the environment.[60,93]

The rate of convective transfer of heat from *muscle to core to skin* is also dependent on blood flow. When blood vessels, such as those within the skin, are *less* constricted, more blood flow is directed to the skin, and heat transfer takes place rather rapidly. If the temperature gradient between the skin and the environment is maintained, heat loss is facilitated (figure 19.3). Also, the temperature gradient between the shell and the core must remain at least 2° F to maintain heat loss; otherwise, the shell acts as an insulating layer.

Increased sweating makes the skin wet, which raises its vapor pressure. When the relative humidity (RH) is low (e.g., 10% to 20%), the vapor pressure in the environmental air is also low. Consequently, a vapor pressure gradient is established and evaporative heat loss is enhanced. In contrast, if RH is high (e.g., 80% to 90%), meaning the environmental air is more saturated with water, then *the difference* between the skin vapor pressure and the environmental vapor pressure is low, and heat cannot be dissipated effectively. Literally, the water on the skin has no place to evaporate to when environmental air is already holding as much water as it can (RH = 100%). These latter conditions, especially during exercise, exaggerate heat storage within the body, as sweat literally drips off the skin!

Temperature Regulation

The function of the *thermoregulatory system* is to maintain a relatively constant internal (core) body temperature. At rest and during exercise the system strives to keep the temperature at 37° C, which, for our purposes, is called the *reference temperature.*

The thermoregulatory system of the body (figure 19.4) uses the following components to carry out its function:

1. A *thermal regulatory center* located in the central nervous system that coordinates incoming sensory information with outgoing regulatory action;
2. *Thermal receptors* or *sensors,* which are sensitive to thermal stimuli (heat and cold) and provide input to the coordinating center located in the central nervous system; and
3. *Thermal effectors* or *organs,* which are directed by the coordinating center to produce regulatory or corrective changes.

The Thermal Regulatory Center

The thermal regulatory center is located in a subcortical area of the brain called the **hypothalamus.** The role of this center is somewhat analogous to that of a thermostat in a room. The temperature of the room (internal body temperature) is measured by a thermometer (receptor organs or sensors) and compared with a set point (T_{set}, 37° C). If the measured temperature deviates from T_{set}, the thermostat (hypothalamic center) automatically relays information to the heating or cooling systems (thermal effectors), which correct the room (body) temperature to the T_{set} value. The return to T_{set} then automatically shuts off the effector system.

Thermal Receptors

The human body has at least three major thermal receptor areas: these are located in the *anterior hypothalamus* (central receptors), the *skin* (peripheral receptors), and the *spinal cord/abdominal viscera/great veins* (deep body receptors).

In the anterior hypothalamus there are a large number of heat and cold sensitive neurons, all of which are sensitive to small temperature fluctuations (0.2 to 0.5° F) within the arterial blood perfusing them. The ratio of heat-sensitive to cold-sensitive neurons is 3 to 1. As you might expect, the heat-sensitive neurons increase their firing rate as the temperature of the blood passing through that area is increased. Conversely, the cold-sensitive neurons increase their firing rate as the temperature of blood passing through the anterior hypothalamus falls.

Thermal changes on the skin, brought about by fluctuations in environmental temperature, are "evaluated" by at least three types of sensory receptors: cold receptors, warmth receptors, and pain receptors. Along with cold or warmth receptors, the pain receptors respond to "freezing cold" or "burning hot".

The cold and warmth receptors are located just underneath the surface of the skin, each serving an area that is approximately 1 mm in diameter. Throughout different areas of the body there are 3 to 10 times more cold than warmth receptors. As a result, these receptors (and the deep body receptors) mainly concern themselves with detecting cold rather than warmth. To date, the exact nature of the warmth fiber has not been identified. It is thought to consist mainly of free nerve endings. On the other hand the cold-sensitive nerve ending has been identified as a small myelinated nerve ending that extends into the bottom of the basal epidermal cells of the skin.

Both the central receptors located in the hypothalamus and the other receptors are neurally connected to a regulatory or control center in the posterior part of the hypothalamus. Sensory input to this area triggers *involuntary* reflexes that will help eliminate or conserve heat as needed. In addition, skin receptors and other sensory systems (e.g., vision) provide information to the cerebral cortex. These cortical connections provide us with a means for *voluntary* or behavioral regulation, such as seeking shaded or sunny areas, initiating or avoiding physical exercise, removing or adding clothing, and stretching out or curling up in warm or cool environments, respectively.

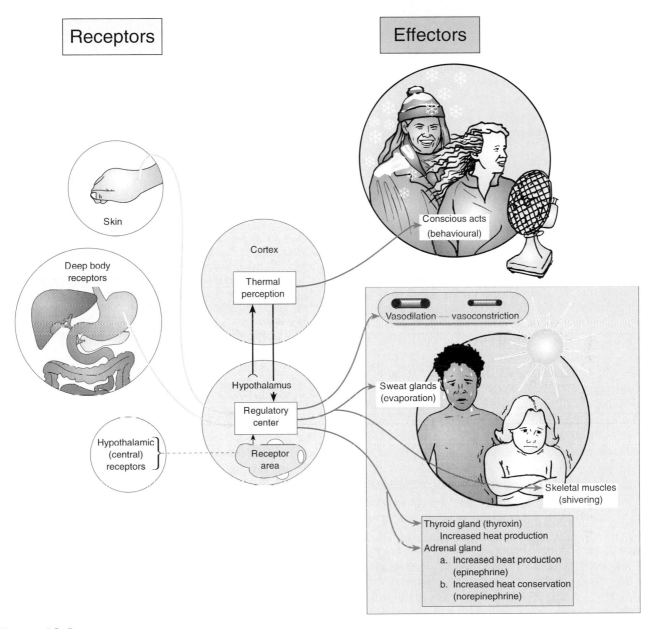

Figure 19.4

A summary of the thermoregulatory system. The internal body temperature is measured by receptor organs (yellow) and compared to a set point (37° C). If the temperature deviates from the set point, the hypothalamic center automatically relays information to the effector organs (green), which correct the temperature to the set point value through the mechanisms shown on the right. The return to the set point value then automatically shuts off the effector system. The cortical connections provide us with a means for voluntary regulation of body temperature.

The central and peripheral receptors are usually coordinated to provide accurate information to the hypothalamus. However, there are instances when the input can be misleading. For example, after prolonged exercise events that evoke excessive sweating (and evaporation), the skin may feel cool even though core temperature is still elevated (hyperthermic). Because of this the signal supplied by the peripheral receptors to the hypothalamus may give the sensation that you are cold—even though internal temperature is high. This is why thermal wraps are provided to partici-

pants following prolonged endurance events such as a marathon. Doing so warms the surface of the skin and provides the appropriate signal to the temperature regulatory center.

One final point about the temperature regulatory center. Earlier we said that the internal body temperature is compared with T_{set}—usually 37° C or 98.6° F. As a result of this comparison, adjustments are made by the body that lead to heat loss or heat conservation. T_{set}, however, can be changed, and this is thought to be an important role of the peripheral receptors. For example, when the skin is warmed, T_{set} is reduced. In effect, this causes sweating, cutaneous vasodilation, and body cooling to occur sooner. The opposite is true when the skin is exposed to cold—that is, T_{set} is increased so that responses that lead to heat conservation or heat production occur sooner.

Thermal Effectors

The thermal effector organs are the *skeletal muscles,* the *smooth muscles encircling the arterioles* that supply blood to the skin, the eccrine *sweat glands,* and certain *endocrine glands.* These are the sites that carry out actions to help correct (restore) core temperature. For example, in a warm or hot environment, the arterioles supplying blood to the skin dilate (cutaneous vasodilation), and sweating occurs to facilitate heat loss. On the other hand, in a cold environment, the skeletal muscles contribute to shivering, which increases metabolic heat production. The mechanism of shivering occurs when body temperature falls (as sensed in the hypothalamus) just below a critical level. In this example, motor neurons are stimulated to increase muscle tone throughout the body, to the extent that shivering is noticed. During maximal shivering body heat production can rise 4 to 5 times above normal. At the same time cutaneous vasoconstriction occurs, which contributes further to heat conservation.

The importance of vasomotor control (by dilation and constriction) of the arterioles supplying blood to the skin stems from the fact that heat from the body core must first be transported, by circulatory conduction and convection, to the surface before it can be lost to the environment by conduction, convection, radiation, and evaporation. With cutaneous vasoconstriction, blood flow to the skin is decreased and, hence, so is the transfer of heat from the body core (heat conservation). The opposite is true for cutaneous vasodilation; where increased blood flow to the skin allows for increased dissipation of deep body heat to the environment.

The endocrine glands involved in temperature regulation contribute to both short-term and long-term heat production. During cold exposure, increased levels of *epinephrine* and *norepinephrine* arise from the adrenal medulla and cause increased heat production by increasing the metabolic rate of the cell. The extent of this *chemical* or *nonshivering thermogenesis* is directly related to the amount of *brown fat* that exists in the animal's tissues. In adult humans very, very little brown fat is present; therefore, heat production via this method of chemical thermogenesis is limited to a 10% to 15% increase. In newborn infants (neonates), however, some brown fat is present, which contributes to the maintenance of normal body temperature. Over several weeks of exposure to cold, metabolic heat production is also increased because of increased output of *thyroxine* from the thyroid gland. Thyroxine increases the rate of cellular metabolism, representing another form of chemical thermogenesis.

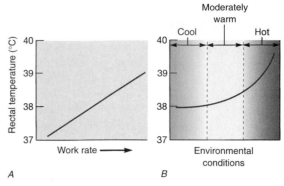

A

B

Figure 19.5

A. Relationship between rectal temperature and work rate in a cool environment. Although environmental conditions remain constant as the work rate increases, the rectal temperature increases proportionately. *B.* At a constant work rate, the rise in rectal temperature is the same in a cool to moderately warm environment, but it rises disproportionately in a hot environment because of the added resistance to heat loss.

Exercise in the Heat

Elevations in environmental temperature reduce the thermal gradient between the environment and the skin surface and between the skin surface and the body core. All of this opposes heat loss by the body. We have seen that body heat can actually be gained, when the temperature of the environment is greater than the temperature of the skin. By the same token, increased humidity represents a barrier to heat loss via the evaporative mechanism. As discussed earlier, it does so by decreasing the vapor pressure gradient between the moisture in the air and the moisture (sweat) on our skin. During prolonged exercise in a hot environment, these barriers to heat loss can lead to an excessive increase in rectal temperature and severely limit one's ability to perform work in the heat. During intense, *short-term* work, when heat production may well exceed the heat-dissipating capacity made possible through physical means (evaporation, conduction), physical exhaustion usually occurs before rectal temperature can reach a limiting or dangerous level.

In a cold or cool environment, activities that can be maintained for an hour or even more are seldom limited by an excessive increase in internal or rectal temperature. Under these conditions nearly all the metabolic heat produced can be easily dissipated by the circulatory and sudomotor (sweating) adjustments referred to previously. In fact, when exercising in cold to moderately warm environments the elevation of rectal temperature during exercise, although proportional to the intensity of work (and therefore to metabolic rate), is independent of environmental temperatures (figure 19.5).

table 19.1

Effects of environmental heat loads on sweat rate and heart rate responses during 15 minutes of moderate work*

Dry bulb temperature (° C)	Wet bulb temperature (° C)†	Relative humidity (%)	Sweat rate (L · hr⁻¹)	Heart rate (beats · min⁻¹)
22	14.7	45	0.4	150
35	26.0	50	1.0	155
35	33.4	90	1.6	165

*Based on data from Fox et al.[28]
†See text (p. 526) for definition of wet bulb temperature.

Circulatory System and Sweating Mechanism

Internal body heat produced during exercise, mainly by the liver and skeletal muscles, is carried by the blood (e.g., convection) to the surface (via cutaneous vasodilation), where conduction, convection, radiation, and particularly evaporation take place (review figure 19.3). The cooled blood then returns to the warmer core and the cycle is repeated. Typical body temperature changes that occur during exercise in a comfortable environment (room temperature) are shown in figure 19.6. Internal or rectal temperature increases to a new level soon after starting to exercise and remains at this new level until recovery. At the same time, skin temperature decreases slightly, mostly due to increased convective and evaporative cooling. The net result of these changes is an *increase* in the *thermal gradient* between the skin and the core.

On the other hand, hot/humid environments reduce thermal and vapor pressure gradients and, as a result, greatly increase the demands placed on the circulatory system and sweating mechanism. This is evidenced by greater increases in heart rate and sweating during exercise in hot as compared to cool environments (table 19.1). More blood must be circulated and more sweat secreted by the sweat glands to lose any given quantity of heat. Please note that in hot, dry environments, where temperature is high and relative humidity low, heat stress is reduced because the evaporation of sweat is more efficient. The major circulatory demands while working in the heat are:

1. A large blood flow through the working muscles to provide for the increased exchange of O_2 and CO_2 (and to carry away the increased heat produced in the muscles);
2. As previously indicated, the large increase in skin blood flow to (a) move "warm blood" from the core to the shell where it is "cooled" and to (b) supply the sweat glands with water.

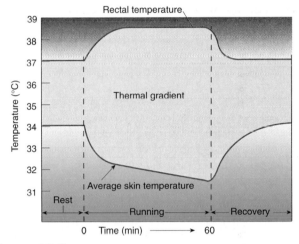

Figure 19.6

Rectal and skin temperatures during and following 60 minutes of running at 6 miles per hour. During exercise, rectal temperature increases while skin temperature decreases, thus increasing the thermal gradient between skin and core.

To accomplish these tasks, there is "competition" for cardiac output. Adequate blood flow to the muscles and skin is usually not a problem during light to moderate exercise in the heat. However, with more intense exercise the muscles "win out" at the expense of skin blood flow, which can impair the body's ability to dissipate heat. When this occurs, core temperature will rise and threaten thermal injury. This scenario can be worsened by a progressive dehydration (water loss) that can occur during exercise.

Cardiovascular Drift

As mentioned previously, during moderate intensity exercise in a warm environment blood is distributed to both the active skeletal muscles and the skin. In fact, there is a slight "pooling" of blood at the cutaneous level that facilitates

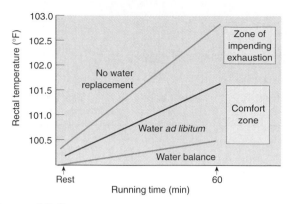

Figure 19.7

Schematic representation of progressive water loss during one hour of exercise in a hot and moderately humid environment. When water consumption equals sweat loss (water balance), rectal temperature is lowest, compared with no replacement and water *ad libitum*.

Source: Data from G. Pitts, et al., "Work in the Heat as Affected by Intake of Water, Salt, and Glucose" in Journal of Applied Physiology, 1944, 142:253–259, American Physiological Society, Bethesda, MD.

heat transfer. All of this leads to less blood being returned to the heart, which leads to a decrease in left ventricular end-diastolic volume, a reduced stroke volume and, if left uncompensated, a reduced cardiac output. However, to maintain cardiac output during exercise, the drop in stroke volume is compensated for by an increase in heart rate. This phenomenon, referred to as *cardiovascular drift*, explains why higher heart rates are observed when exercising at the same intensity in a hot versus a cool climate (table 19.1).

Dehydration

The high sweat rates (0.5 to $2.0 \text{ L} \cdot \text{h}^{-1}$) that are needed to adequately cool the body via evaporation during exercise in the heat can lead to excessive losses of water, salt, and other electrolytes. When this occurs, work performance and tolerance to heat are greatly reduced, and hyperthermia (excessive internal body temperature) and the risk of a serious heat disorder are imminent.[15,19,38,73,81,83,93] As little as a 1% to 3% decrease in body weight caused by **dehydration** can impair physiologic and performance responses.[4,59,84] Armstrong and colleagues[6] showed that a diuretic induced dehydration approximating 2% resulted in an approximate 7% increase in 1,500 m and 10,000 m run times.

The most serious consequence of profuse sweating is loss of body water. This leads to a decrease in blood volume[49,82] and, if severe enough, to a decrease in sweating rate and evaporative cooling. Figure 19.7 shows the effects of progressive water deficiency on rectal temperature while exercising in the heat.

It cannot be emphasized enough that adequate fluid replacement, equal to what was lost in sweat, is essential

for preventing dehydration and thermal injury. Fluids should be administered before, during, and after prolonged work bouts in the heat. Adequate hydration by voluntary intake (thirst mechanism) alone takes several days. Therefore, during day-to-day heat exposure it is necessary to "enforce" the consumption of liquids (water), even though there may be no apparent thirst. A more detailed description of fluid replacement and the composition/role of commercially prepared drinks is covered later in this chapter and in chapter 15.

Exercise Metabolism

In addition to the effects exercising in the heat can have on the circulatory system, blood volume, and sweat rate, it can influence cellular metabolism as well. For example, exercising in the heat can lead to a greater reliance on anaerobic glycolysis for energy production. Also, a decrease in muscle glycogen utilization and a reciprocal increase in blood lactate concentration have been reported.[23,24,25] It appears that the consequences of trying to maintain the same work rate in a warmer versus a cooler environment leads to an increased energy requirement, secondary to increases in sweat production and respiration.

Thermal Injury

The consequences of overexposure to heat while exercising is exemplified not only by a decrease in work performance but also by an increased risk for one of several types of heat illness.[46] These disorders are listed below and graphically depicted in figure 19.8:

1. heat cramps
2. heat syncope
3. heat exhaustion (two types)
   a. water depletion
   b. salt depletion
4. heat stroke

1. *Heat Cramps.* **Heat cramps** are characterized by muscle spasms or twitching in the arms, legs, and possibly, the abdomen. Such a disorder occurs more frequently in the unacclimatized individual.

2. *Heat Syncope.* Heat syncope is characterized by a general weakness and fatigue, hypotension (low blood pressure), occasionally blurred vision, pallor (paleness), syncope (brief loss of consciousness), and elevated skin and core temperature. Heat syncope usually occurs in the unacclimatized person.

3. *Heat Exhaustion—Water Depletion.* Water-depletion **heat exhaustion** is characterized by reduced sweating, although there is a large weight loss, dry tongue and mouth ("cotton mouth"), thirst, elevated skin and core temperature, weakness, and loss of

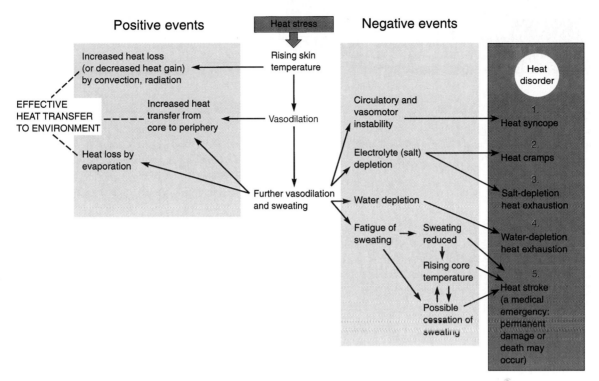

Figure 19.8

When an athlete is exposed to a heat stress during exercise, a number of events occur including elevated skin temperature, vasodilation, and sweating. Generally, these are positive and facilitate effective heat transfer to the environment, which helps to minimize a rise in core temperature (extreme left). Prolonged exercise in extreme conditions, however, can lead to a variety of heat disorders (extreme right).

(From Licht[50] and Nash.[64])

coordination. Another sign is that the urine is very concentrated, almost an orange color. Water-depletion heat exhaustion can occur in an acclimatized individual.

4. *Heat Exhaustion—Salt Depletion.* Salt-depletion **heat exhaustion** is characterized by headache, dizziness, fatigue, nausea, possible vomiting and diarrhea, syncope, and muscle cramps. Salt-depletion heat exhaustion is insidious, in that it usually takes 3 to 5 days to develop. It can occur in an acclimatized individual.

5. *Heat Stroke.* **Heat stroke** *is a life-threatening, medical emergency.* The sweating mechanism has become fatigued, although some sweating may still be occurring. Additionally, both skin and core temperatures are elevated (core temperature may well exceed 105° F or 40.5° C) and there is muscle flaccidity, involuntary limb movement, seizures and coma, vomiting, diarrhea, tachycardia (rapid) or shallow heart beat, and possibly death. The individual may be irrational and hallucinating if not in a coma. Heat stroke may occur to any individual under the proper conditions. The appearance of any one of these features should be taken seriously and emergency procedures begun immediately.

Immediate corrective action for the first four disorders includes rest, removing excess clothing, moving the subject to a cooler environment, and ensuring fluid and/or electrolyte replacement. Corrective action and care for heat stroke entails contacting emergency assistance and aggressive attempts to lower skin and core temperature through ice packs and/or spraying or submersing the subject in cold (12° C) water. In the hospital setting intravenous fluids and medications are also given and a rectal thermometer is used to assess core temperature, which may reach 110° F (43.3° C). When temperature is lowered to 102° F (38.9° C), the subject is moved to a bed and covered. Overexposure to the cold bath can cause body temperature to fall dangerously low.

In the field it is the responsibility of a coach or trainer to recognize the symptoms of heat stroke and act accordingly. The athlete with heat stroke should never be left alone to "rest." If an emergency should occur, a prearranged, rehearsed plan of care should be available. This includes access to a telephone.

The most frequent common denominators for the above conditions are (1) heat exposure, (2) physical activity, (3) loss of water and electrolytes, and (4) heat storage (usually reflected by a high core temperature; hyperthermia).

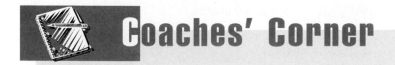

Coaches' Corner

Exercise in the Heat

Highlights of the ACSM position stands on "The Prevention of Thermal Injuries During Distance Running"[3] and "Exercise and Fluid Replacement"[2] are featured below.

Race Organization

1. To minimize the effects of solar radiation, races should be organized to avoid the hottest summer months and the hottest part of the day. As there are great regional variations in environmental conditions, the local weather history will be most helpful in scheduling an event to avoid unacceptable times. Organizers should be cautious of unseasonably hot days in the early spring, as entrants will almost certainly not be heat acclimatized.

2. The environmental heat stress prediction for the day should be obtained from the meteorological service. It can be measured as wet bulb globe temperature (WBGT) (see page 426). If the WBGT is above 31° C (88° F), consideration should be given to rescheduling or delaying the race until safer conditions prevail. If below 28° C, participants should simply be alerted to the degree of heat stress.

3. An adequate supply of water should be available before the race and every 2 to 3 km during the race. Competitors should be encouraged to consume 500 mL two hours before exercise. During exercise, participants should start drinking early and at regular intervals to replace the water lost through sweating, or should consume the maximal amount that can be tolerated. Fluids should be served in containers that allow adequate volumes to be ingested with ease and with minimal interruption of exercise.

4. Race officials should be educated as to the warning signs of a competitor's impending collapse. Each official should be identifiable and warn runners to stop if they appear to be in distress.

Competitor Education

Recognizing that all athletes are not well versed in the hazards of thermal stress, the ACSM suggests distributing guidelines before the race, providing publicity in the press, and holding clinics and seminars. Persons particularly prone to heat illness include the obese, the unfit, the dehydrated, those unacclimatized, those with a previous history of heat stroke, and anyone who exercises while ill. Children are more susceptible than adults. Specific points include the following:

1. Adequate levels of pre-event training, especially in the heat, will improve fitness and promote heat acclimatization. Participants should do as much training as possible at the time of day at which the race will be held.

2. Fluid consumption before and during the race is indicated, particularly in longer runs (e.g., marathon).

3. Illness prior to and at the time of the event precludes participation.

4. Participants should be advised of the early symptoms of heat injury. These include clumsiness, stumbling, excessive sweating (and also cessation of sweating), headache, nausea, dizziness, apathy, and any gradual impairment of consciousness.

However, the single most important factor, from a clinical standpoint, is loss of body water. Inattention to heat cramps, heat syncope, and heat exhaustion can lead to heat stroke. Even in persons who do recover from heat stroke, there may be some permanent damage to the central nervous system (thermoregulatory center in the hypothalamus). As a result of this damage, the body loses some of its ability to regulate body temperature. This leads to decreased heat conductance from the body's core to the skin, explaining why people who have survived heat stroke are more prone to heat disorders in the future.[85]

Normally, most people will voluntarily stop working and seek shelter from the heat when heat cramps, syncope, or exhaustion sets in. However, highly competitive athletes are more vulnerable to heat disorders, in general, and heat stroke, in particular. Reasons for this include: (1) athletes are often highly competitive (motivated) and, therefore, more likely to overextend themselves; (2) they have a sense of immortality; (3) they sometimes are required to wear heavy protective equipment, which impedes heat dissipation by reducing the surface area for evaporation; and (4) incomprehensible as it may seem, coaches may deny the athlete water during prolonged contests or practice sessions—which further lowers the athlete's resistance to heat tolerance. These factors, either singularly or combined, apply to both the "comfortable" environment and the hot environment. For example, rectal temperatures equal to or greater than 40° C (104° F) are not uncommon, even in athletes who compete at environmental temperatures as low as 5° to 16° C (41° to 61° F).

The seriousness of heat illnesses in sports may be best illustrated by the frequency of heat stroke deaths among high school and college football players, which was briefly discussed earlier (see figure 19.1). Please note the tragic number of deaths for 1995 alone: 4 deaths! Apparently, coaches, trainers, and the athletes themselves continue to be uninformed or disrespectful of the risks associated with exercising in thermal environments that pose a potential for heat stroke. Continued education; a stronger, more widespread message; and improved compliance to set guidelines are all needed.

Heat illnesses, however, are not confined to football alone. Any sport or physical activity is potentially hazardous for heat illness. This includes both wrestling, where athletes often lose large quantities of water to "make weight," and outdoor track-and-field events.[14,40,41] Although more common in professional, intercollegiate, or interscholastic athletics, heat-related disorders can also develop in the leisure exerciser. This problem is evident if one observes the frequency of heat stroke events reported in novice and competitive athletes participating in community "fun runs" and triathlons.[40,41] Literally millions of people are now participating in these activities, and given the fact that many of the events are held during the hotter months, the potential for heat illness is clear.[92] Concerned about the hot weather conditions under which distance races and fun runs are sometimes held, the American College of Sports Medicine (ACSM) issued a position stand on "The Prevention of Thermal Injuries During Distance Running."[3] The position stand is *divided into four sections* dealing with (1) the medical director, (2) race organization, (3) medical support, and (4) competitor education.

Acclimatization to Heat and Physical Conditioning

Tolerance of, and the ability to work comfortably in, the heat are improved through *heat acclimatization*.[7,15,54,96,97] The process of heat acclimatization leads to improved circulatory, sweating, metabolic, and symptomatic responses (table 19.2). As a result, heat dissipation is facilitated and changes in rectal temperature are minimized. Acclimatization can be accomplished by using a 5- to 10-day progressive exercise program performed in the heat. Simply sitting (at the beach) or resting in a hot environment produces little, if any, heat acclimatization for exercise. Athletes or leisure exercisers who plan to acclimatize to the heat should do their training during the warmer periods of the day. However, exercise intensity and exercise duration for the first few days of acclimatization should be reduced to below 70% $\dot{V}O_2$ max and <20 min, respectively. In addition,

table 19.2

19.2

Physiological adjustments while working in the heat following acclimatization

Physiological mechanism	Physiological adjustments
Circulatory system	
Pulse rate	↓
Skin blood flow	
Time to onset	↓
Skin blood flow (dry heat)	↑
Skin blood flow (humid heat)	↔
Blood volume	↑
Blood pressure	↔
Sweating mechanism	
Sweat rate	
Time to onset	↓
Sweat volume	↑
Evaporation	↑
Salt loss in sweat	↓
Metabolic	
Muscle glycogen utilization	↓
Blood lactate	↓
Oxygen consumption	↔
Subjective symptoms	
Nausea	↓
General discomfort	↓

↑ = increase; ↓ = decrease; ↔ = no change

individuals should consume as much fluids as possible and pay attention to the signs and symptoms of heat injury.

The relationship between physical conditioning and heat acclimatization has been extensively studied and is worthy of further comment.[21,35,45,62,70,71,75,76,79,86,87,99] Exercise training conducted indoors or outdoors during the winter months promotes some degree of heat acclimatization, even though the person had not been exposed to environmental heat since the preceding summer.[33,75,76] In fact, estimates are that exercise training produces at least 50% to 65% of the total physiological adjustment resulting from heat acclimatization.[33,70] An example of this is shown in figure 19.9. As can be seen, when subjects were neither trained nor acclimatized, the sweating response does not start until a relatively high internal body temperature is reached (37.7° C). On the other hand, when the subjects are exercise-trained, the onset of sweating occurs at a lower internal temperature (37.5° C)—and at the lowest temperature (37.2° C) when the subjects are both trained and acclimatized to the heat. Furthermore, the rate of increase of sweating (as evidenced by the steepness of the slopes of the lines)

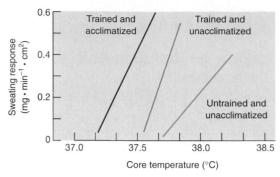

Figure 19.9

In untrained and unacclimatized subjects, the sweating response starts at a relatively high body temperature (37.7° C). When subjects are trained, the onset of sweating occurs at a lower temperature (37.5° C), and when subjects are both trained and acclimatized sweating begins at an even lower body temperature (37.2° C). Furthermore, not only is the onset of sweating faster under these latter conditions, but its rate of increase is also greater (as evidenced by the steepness of the slopes of the lines).

(Based on data from Nadel.[61])

improves with training—and is improved even more with training and acclimatization (figure 19.9). Yamazaki et al.[98] have shown that in response to *intermittent exercise* (somewhat more representative of typical activities of daily living and some sports), exercise-trained individuals demonstrate a more prompt sweating response and are able to better maintain a constant body temperature than are untrained individuals.

The faster onset and greater rate of sweating experienced as a result of exercise training reduces skin temperature (increases the thermal gradient between core and skin temperatures) and greatly enhances body cooling. Also, the marked elevation in metabolic rate and, therefore, in heat production during training, can cause rectal temperatures to approach 40° C at the end of a strenuous workout. Such elevations in rectal temperatures likely serve as a stimulus for the circulatory and sweating adjustments that occur in the acclimatized individual.

Exercise training also promotes an expansion in blood volume. In fact, as little as three days of training (two hours per day) has been shown to increase plasma volume by 20% and increase total blood volume by 12%.[37] Although these changes are not as extensive as what occurs in individuals who train in the heat, a greater blood volume does serve to reduce the circulatory strain that can occur when an unacclimatized person exercises in the heat.

Fluid Replacement

Water and electrolyte replacement before, during, and following work in the heat is essential.[18] It is not unusual for an athlete to lose 5 to 10 pounds (mostly water loss—i.e., sweat) during a heavy practice session or during a game.

Such large weight losses can occur even when water is available. To prevent progressive dehydration over several days, coaches and trainers should be sure the athletes are weighed before and after each practice session.

The unrestricted availability of water is a must at all times during scheduled practices, workouts, and games. The "superhydrated" athlete suffers no impairment of performance or efficiency.[11,38] However, large amounts of water should not be consumed at any one time during exercise because the athlete may feel uncomfortable under these conditions. The best procedure is to schedule frequent water breaks as well as to encourage the drinking of water *ad libitum.*

For athletic teams the consumption of water can be facilitated by maintaining several water stations strategically located around the practice field or along the training route. Ice-water buckets, pressurized garden-spray containers, and thermos jugs are containers that can be properly located and easily maintained.[57]

During competition and training in hot and/or humid weather, coaches, trainers, athletes, and exercise enthusiasts should follow the "drinking" guidelines outlined in table 19.3. Under most circumstances plain water is the best and the most available drink. There are, however, many sport drinks meant to replace not only lost water but carbohydrates and electrolytes as well. Of these drinks, those that provide hydration without "staying in the stomach" are best. Drinks associated with a slowed gastric emptying can increase gastric irritability, impair rehydration, and decrease performance. A cooler drink (15° to 21° C or 59° to 70° F) that is hypotonic and has a concentration of sugar below 4% to 8% is usually a good place to start. However, replacement drinks containing sugar, even in the correct concentration, are usually only helpful in events or activities lasting 1 hour or longer. Please note that we encourage the consumption of a cool drink. Contrary to a previously popular belief, cold drinks do not cause stomach cramps and, in fact, are related to increased palatability. Such cramps are likely more related to the volume of liquid consumed (too much in too short a period of time), rather than to the temperature of the drink.[2]

One final comment relative to the consumption of sport drinks during competition. Given differences among athletes relative to their gastrointestinal tolerance to a specific solution, it makes good sense that the beverage first be tested over several training sessions before it is used in competition. More information on fluid replacement and sport drinks can be found in chapter 15.

Water Loss vs. Fat Loss

The loss of body water does not play any role in the loss of body fat. Thus, deliberately causing excessive water loss through fluid deprivation or sweating for the purpose of losing weight is unnecessary and, in fact, quite hazardous. For example, among wrestlers the practice of exercising in

19.3

Guidelines for fluid intake and exercise[2]

Content of drink

The drink should be:
- hypotonic (few solid particles per unit of water)
- plain water is the most important
- for events greater than 1 hour, a drink low in sugar (4–8 grams per 100 mL) may be helpful
- cool (15° to 22° C or 59° to 70° F)
- palatable

Amount to be ingested before competition

Consume adequate fluids in the 24 hour period before an event.
Drink 500 mL (17 ounces) of water (or a drink low in sugar) 2 hours before start of the event.

Amount to be ingested during competition

During event, drink 100–200 mL (3–6.5 ounces) every 10 to 15 min (approximately 600 to 1200 mL $\cdot$ hr^{-1}).

Postevent diet and fluid intake

Following practice or an event, consume water beyond that indicated by thirst. Consume a balanced diet, including complex carbohydrates, vitamins, and minerals (sodium, potassium).

Value of drinks

Water and low sugar drinks are of value during competition and during long practice sessions under warm conditions in both team and individual sports.

---

sweatsuits and rubber jackets (often done in warm environments) to "make weight" can impair physiologic and academic performance; impact normal growth and development; and, though rare, lead to heat illness, pulmonary emboli, pancreatitis, and reduced immune function.[4] The athlete or performer may think he is "melting off" pounds, but this has nothing to do with real weight loss. Moreover, water weight that is lost using these unsafe practices is almost entirely replaced within 24 hours. Real weight loss involves the true loss of body fat, which occurs when there is a *sustained* negative calorie balance: daily caloric intake (calories available in food) is less than daily caloric output (energy expended during activity, see chapter 16).

Electrolyte Replacement

Sweat is hypotonic (the amount of solid particles is lower in sweat than in plasma) and, therefore, is very low in sodium and, to an even lesser extent, potassium. Unless the individual has consumed excessive quantities of fluid during exercise or has maintained a high sweat rate over an extended period of time, such as an ultra-endurance event conducted over several days,[66] the risk of the body's serum sodium level becoming abnormally low (hyponatremia, <130 mmol $\cdot$ L^{-1}) is negligible. During these situations the prevalence of hyponatremia can approach 10% of "collapsed participants."[66] The consumption of supplementary salt tablets represents an unnecessary practice for most athletes, provided adequate nutrition is maintained. The average individual consumes 7 to 15 g of sodium daily, which is far more than what is lost in the sweat and needed for bodily function. Potassium losses can be restored through the diet as well. For instance, one 8 oz. glass of orange juice has enough potassium to replace that lost in one liter of sweat.

Clothing

Heat disorders can also occur when the clothing worn by the athlete prevents or limits the ability of the body to dissipate the heat generated by the exercising muscles. Several examples of this include: the wearing of protective equipment needed to participate in an activity, wearing too much clothing, and the use of certain fabrics that trap excess heat against the body. Consider the following study where nine men ran on a treadmill for 30 minutes at 9.6 km $\cdot$ hr^{-1} (6 mph). Each subject completed three separate test conditions: the first wearing shorts only, the second in a full

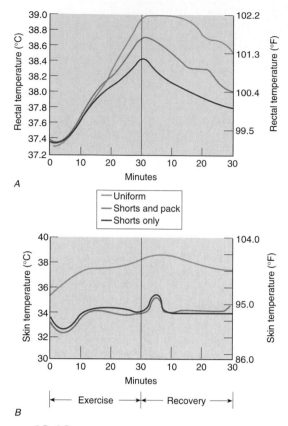

Figure 19.10

The effects of wearing a football uniform on rectal and skin temperatures during 30 minutes of running at 6 miles per hour. *A.* The uniform retards heat loss, causing rectal temperature to climb during exercise and remain elevated during recovery. *B.* Skin temperatures while wearing the uniform also rise considerably owing to reduction in evaporative cooling. Environmental conditions were 78° F and 35% relative humidity.

Source: Data from D. K. Mathews, et al., "Physiological Responses During Exercise and Recovery in a Football Uniform" in Journal of Applied Physiology, *1969, 26:611–615, American Physiological Society, Bethesda, MD.*

football uniform, and the third in shorts plus a backpack weighing the same as the uniform (13 pounds). The temperature of the room for all runs was 23.9° C (78° F), with a relative humidity of 35%—a normal, comfortable situation.

As shown in figure 19.10*A*, the increase in rectal temperature while wearing the uniform was 1.5 times greater (average, 39.0° C) than when shorts only were worn.[52] Also, the weight of the uniform alone, as shown by the increase in rectal temperature while carrying the pack, also represents an important factor that contributes to thermal stress. Finally, the heat-loss barrier imposed by the uniform led to an excessively high skin temperature in those areas covered by both pads and clothing (figure 19.10*B*). In fact, the full football uniform covers 50% of the body. The uniform prevented the evaporation of sweat and greatly impaired body cooling. In addition to this, the researchers observed (1) an

almost twofold increase in loss of body water because of profuse sweating and (2) a significantly higher heart rate or circulatory strain.

Perhaps even more startling was the slow return of rectal temperature during recovery when the full uniform was worn versus the other two test conditions. This is an extremely important point to remember. For example, a 16-year-old boy reported to his first football practice on a hot day and was required to wear a complete uniform. After a period of time, he felt ill. The coach then placed him in the shade, did not remove his uniform and left him unattended for about 2 hours. Later, the boy was found unconscious and was taken to the hospital, where he died of heat stroke. Although the likelihood of wearing a full uniform the first day of football is less today than it was years ago,* the lessons learned from this tragedy are quite clear.

In the above text the football uniform was used as an example of how clothing can affect evaporative cooling and lead to heat illnesses. Similar problems can also arise if one is inappropriately dressed, regardless of the type of physical activity. The following clothing recommendations should be considered (to aid in heat dissipation) when weather conditions warrant:

1. Wear short sleeve, netted jerseys that are loose fitting and light in color. Use short versus long socks.
2. Minimize the taping of exposed skin surfaces.
3. Whenever feasible, remove protective equipment (arm pads, gloves, helmets). During rest periods, remove as much clothing as feasible to expose skin surface (e.g., raise jersey to expose abdominal area).
4. On a hot, humid day exercising without a shirt is not recommended because direct and reflected radiation from the sun to the skin can facilitate heat gain. Instead, use light-colored cotton fabric; this will allow for heat exchange and limit heat absorption from solar radiation.

Assessing Environmental Heat Stress

As we have learned, the actual environmental stress imposed on the body is more than just ambient temperature. Factors such as humidity and radiant heat from our surroundings also play a big role in our ability to dissipate heat. The most accurate means for measuring environmental heat stress is the **wet bulb globe temperature (WBGT).** The WBGT index was developed by the armed forces for use in determining stress on unconditioned trainees participating in physical activity while wearing army fatigues. It takes into account temperature (dry bulb), relative humid-

---

*Most state high school and collegiate governing bodies now require several days of conditioning in shorts and T-shirts prior to wearing full gear.

ity (wet bulb), and radiation (globe). The wet bulb globe temperature can be assessed indoors or outdoors and consists of:

1. Ordinary air temperature (as measured with a dry bulb thermometer),
2. Temperature as affected by wind and humidity (measured with a wet bulb thermometer), and
3. Temperature as affected by radiant heat from the sun (measured with a black globe thermometer—temperature measured inside a copper globe painted flat black).

Figure 19.11 shows the combination of thermometers used to take the WBGT. If used outside, the device is placed in the open, away from trees, buildings, or other objects that cast shadows or influence air movement. To compute WBGT, the following formula are used:[1]

Outdoor WBGT (° F) = (0.7 × WB) + (0.2 × G) + (0.1 × DB)

Indoor WBGT = (0.7 × WB) + (0.3 × G)

Where:

WB = wet bulb temperature
G = black globe temperature (radiant energy)
DB = dry bulb temperature

If, for example, the wet bulb temperature is 75° F, the black globe temperature is 110° F, and the dry bulb temperature is 85° F, then

Outdoor WBGT = (0.7 × 75) + (0.2 × 110) + (0.1 × 85)
    WBGT = 83° F
Indoor WBGT = (0.7 × 75) + (0.3 × 110)
    WBGT = 86° F

Both the National Institute for Occupational Safety and Health[65] and the ACSM[3] have developed criteria to help categorize the heat stress imposed by different environments (table 19.4). The highest warning level is for a WBGT index of 23° to 28° C (73° to 82° F). If the WBGT index is ≥31° C (88° F), it is advisable not to participate.[94] For team practices, exercise programs, and individual exercise prescriptions, warning systems such as the one shown in table 19.4 should be used by coaches, leaders, trainers, and individual exercisers—as an alert about the potential risk of thermal stress. Please note that these precautions mostly apply to tennis, track and field, soccer, field hockey, training workouts, and other activities where heavy protective clothing is not a problem.

The outdoor WBGT computed in the above example (83° F) falls just above the red/high risk level. This raises the question of what to do when the WBGT is below the "consider cancelling" value of 88° F but above the red level of 82° F. And, what should be done if protective clothing is involved, such as helmets or padding? Clearly, attempts

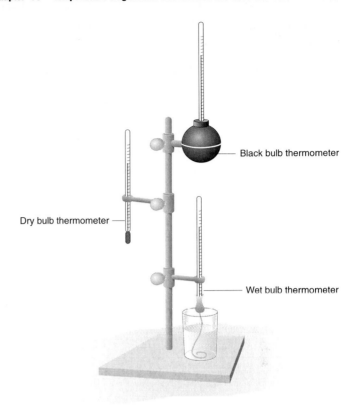

Figure 19.11

An instrument that simultaneously measures solar radiation (black bulb or globe thermometer), air temperature (dry bulb thermometer), and relative humidity computed via the wet bulb thermometer in conjunction with the dry bulb thermometer. A combination of the three temperatures recorded is used in computing the wet bulb globe temperature (WBGT) index.

should be made to improve conditions, such as through the use of fans (if indoors), altering time of day, removing clothing (shorts and helmets, no pads), decreasing intensity level, including more frequent rest periods, and seeking shade whenever possible.[1]

In lieu of the preferred WBGT method of measuring thermal stress, a simpler approach called the wet bulb temperature (WBT) can be used. The WBT is obtained by first wetting a wick wrapped around the bulb of a thermometer and then determining the effect of evaporation of moisture on the thermometer's temperature reading. The thermometer used in this technique is called a wet bulb thermometer. Along with a regular or **dry bulb thermometer,** it is contained in an instrument called a *sling psychrometer.*

The actual measurement of the WBT involves dipping the wick of the wet bulb thermometer in water and spinning the entire instrument (called slinging) for 1½ minutes. The water in the wick will lower the temperature reading based on the amount of water vapor (relative humidity) in the environment. The lower the relative humidity, the lower the temperature reading will be on the wet bulb

table

19.4

ACSM flag warning system for alerting participants to the potential risk of various thermal conditions*

Flag/status	WBGT Index	Comment
1. Red/High risk	23 to 28° C (73 to 82° F)	This signal would indicate that all participants should be aware that heat injury is possible, particularly among persons sensitive to heat or humidity.
2. Amber/Moderate risk	18 to 23° C (65 to 73° F)	It should be remembered that the air temperature, possibly humidity, and almost certainly the radiant heat will increase during the course of the race if conducted in the morning or early afternoon.
3. Green/Low risk	Below 18° C (65° F)	This is no guarantee that heat illness will not occur but indicates only that risk is low.
4. White/Low risk	Below 10° C (50° F)	Low risk for hyperthermia but possible risk for hypothermia.

*From the American College of Sports Medicine Position Stand[3] and the National Institute for Occupational Safety and Health.[65]
This system is based on the WBGT index, which takes into account temperature, radiation, and relative humidity. If WBGT index is >31° C (88° F), it is advisable to reschedule the practice or event.

thermometer. On the other hand, when the air is completely saturated with water vapor (near 100% humidity), the temperature for the wet bulb thermometer will equal the temperature of the dry bulb thermometer, since the water in the wick has no place to go. The action of spinning the instrument reflects the effect of wind on evaporation. Guidelines have been established regarding exercise levels or practice schedules per the WBT (table 19.5).[58] Guidelines such as this are just that: guidelines! A final decision as to what extent exercise habits or plans should be modified are also based on age, gender, body composition, prior acclimatization, fitness level, and health status (college student versus heart patient).

Exercise in the Cold

Activities in the cold can be classified under two general headings: (1) sporting events and (2) wilderness experiences. Each presents its own unique interaction between the environment and the participant. Winter sporting events such as alpine and nordic skiing, snow-shoeing, or snow-boarding and year around activities (running) rarely present serious problems. This is because: (1) exposure time in the cold is usually limited, (2) access to shelter is readily available, (3) adequate protective clothing for heat conservation can be worn or is available, and (4) muscular exercise generates large increases in heat production.

On the other hand, wilderness experiences such as hiking, backpacking, mountain climbing, ice fishing, scuba diving, and ski-touring in isolated areas can increase the risk of cold injury, overexposure, and, in rare instances, death.

Physiological Responses during Exercise in the Cold

In the resting individual, a number of acute and chronic physiological and behavioral responses can be witnessed in response to cold exposure. These include:

1. Peripheral vasoconstriction, which shunts blood away from the surface of the skin to the core. The vasoconstriction of the smooth muscles in arterioles reduces blood flow to the shell to conserve heat in the body's core.
2. Chemical or nonshivering thermogenesis (see page 518), which involves stimulation of the thyroid gland and the adrenal medulla—the latter of which leads to release of epinephrine and norepinephrine. The end effect is an increased metabolic rate meant to increase/maintain core temperature.
3. Shivering, which involves uncontrolled, synchronous muscular contraction, can elevate heat production up to 4 to 5 times resting levels—but the response is generally less than this.

19.5

Guidelines for exercise or conducting practice on persons wearing heavy, protective clothing in a hot and/or humid environment based on wet bulb temperature

Wet bulb temperature	Precaution
Less than 60° F	None necessary
61° to 66° F	Observe all athletes and team members for signs of heat illness, particularly those who lose considerable weight
67° to 72° F	Water must be available for *ad libitum* consumption
73° to 77° F	In addition to the above, alter practice schedule to provide rest period every 30 minutes
78° F or higher	Practice postponed or modified so intensity of effort is reduced (e.g., shorts only instead of full uniform; skill drills emphasized instead of speed or endurance drills)

Modified from Murphy and Ashe.[58]

Behavioral responses include: (1) wearing appropriate attire, (2) avoiding the cold by remaining indoors, and (3) altering exercise intensity to generate more heat production. In other words, we try to avoid the cold whenever we can! However, in the event that we plan to or must exercise or work in the cold, a good understanding of the physiological responses that occur during exercise is warranted.

Oxygen Consumption

Is the energy cost ($\dot{V}O_2$) of performing in the cold different than under normal conditions? At submaximal work loads (less than 50% to 60% of maximum), the energy or oxygen cost of a particular work task is greater by 11% to 45%.[8,17,44,77,91] This increase is mostly due to the peripheral vasoconstriction (and possibly muscle shivering) that occurs. However, as exercise intensity exceeds 50% to 60% of max $\dot{V}O_2$, there appears to be no difference between working in the cold and in normal temperatures. Eventually, the heat production from, and demand for blood flow to, the metabolically active skeletal muscles warms the periphery and overrides the cold-induced vasoconstriction mentioned above.

The above-mentioned increase in $\dot{V}O_2$ during submaximal exercise pertains to exercise initiated in the cold when core temperature was normal. Berg and coworkers conducted a unique experiment where they first cooled the core temperature (immersion in a cold bath) of their subjects before asking them to perform submaximal exercise.[8] With core temperature starting at 34° C, they observed that $\dot{V}O_2$ at a standardized work load was 30% higher when compared to exercising in the cold after starting at normal core temperature. An application from this information

would include advising athletes who are about to perform in the cold to stay as warm as possible until the competition begins.

Maximal Work Capacity

When subjects have a normal core temperature, the effects of cold weather on maximal aerobic capacity ($\dot{V}O_2$) are negligible.[53] However, when core temperature is again lowered by submersion in cold water and then followed by a standard maximal test, the results are quite different.[9] In this study subjects showed a decrease in maximal $\dot{V}O_2$ that was related to the decrease in core temperature. That is, the lower the core temperature, the greater the measured decrease in $\dot{V}O_2$ max. In fact, there was a 5% to 6% decrease in aerobic capacity for each 1° C decrease in core temperature. The take home message here is don't allow hypothermia to occur.

Muscular Function

In activities where individuals are adequately insulated against the cold, muscular strength, muscle endurance, and exercise performance are unaffected. However, if there is insufficient insulation against the cold, both the ability to develop muscle force and the ability to perform coordinated movement are impaired. Oksa and colleagues[68] asked their subjects to perform fast overhead throws using different weighted balls following 60 minutes of exposure in warm and cold environments. Cooling decreased velocity of the thrown ball, skin temperature, and muscle temperature (triceps brachii). These changes were associated with a 30% to 42% increase in the time to achieve the maximal level of

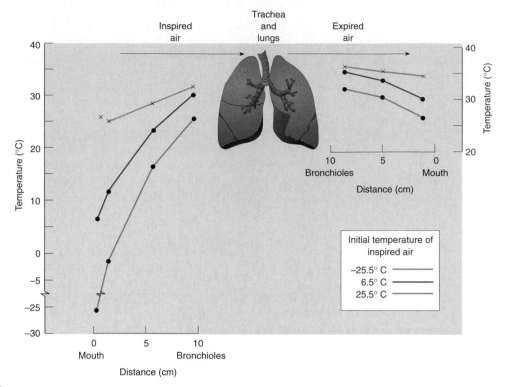

Figure 19.12

Air is rapidly warmed as it enters the nasal passage. Regardless of the temperature of inspired air from −25° C to 25° C, by the time the air reached 9 cm into the nasal passage it had been warmed to at least 25° C. The left side of the figure represents inspired air and its pattern of warming. The right side of the figure shows expired air cooling slightly but remaining at higher temperatures at each measurement site. This illustrates, in part, the "conditioning" of inspired air.

Source: Data from P. Webb, "Air Temperature in Respiratory Tracts of Resting Subjects in the Cold" in Journal of Applied Physiology, *1951, 4(11):378–382, American Physiological Society, Bethesda, MD.*

muscle activity. Also, the activity of the antagonist muscle (deltoid) was increased, which influenced coordination of movement. Clearly, recruitment of motor units are affected as a result of muscle cooling.

Metabolic Responses

The cold-induced vasoconstriction, which shunts blood away from the skin and subcutaneous tissue, can also impact energy substrate utilization. For example, exposure to a cold environment diverts blood away from subcutaneous tissues and, as a result, the mobilization of free-fatty acids from adipocytes (fat cells) is impaired. Thus, even though exposure to cold increases levels of epinephrine and norepinephrine (which are known to increase free-fatty acid mobilization), free-fatty acid levels are not as high as one might expect.[25] Because of this, muscle glycogen is utilized at a higher rate in cold than in warm conditions.[100]

Cold Exposure and the Respiratory Tract

Anyone who has exercised in the cold has likely experienced varying levels of throat irritation. Over the years, a myth has persisted that this irritation and/or the cold weather itself represents a sign, or contributes to, the freezing of lung tissue. However, the evidence concerning this issue suggests otherwise. The danger of lung tissue freezing under weather conditions experienced in any athletic setting is very, very remote (figure 19.12).[16,42]

In general, inhaled air is "conditioned" in the upper respiratory passageways (oral/nasal passages, trachea, bronchus), which involves both temperature elevation to within 2% or 3% of body temperature and increasing the moisture content to also within 2% to 3% of full saturation. In fact, a number of studies have been performed where cool to cold air was introduced into the respiratory system, and all of them indicated that air is adequately warmed and moistened by the time it reaches the bronchi.[42,55,95]

Now that we have established that lung tissue does not freeze, what, then, is the reason for throat irritation during prolonged exercise in the cold? We mentioned earlier that air is "conditioned" as it enters the respiratory passages. Conditioning occurs when both heat and moisture are rapidly added to the incoming air. The heat and moisture come from the mucosal linings of the trachea. Because there is a *loss* of moisture from mucosal tissue, the tissue becomes dryer and, thus, irritated. The use of a breathable

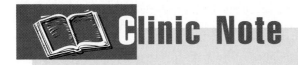

Clinic Note

Cold-Induced Angina

It is well established that some heart patients with angina (chest pain resulting from myocardial ischemia) often report that their symptoms are more easily provoked or are more severe when exposed to the cold, particularly on a windy day. The physiologic mechanism responsible for this cold-weather-induced problem remains uncertain. Some clinicians have speculated that the cold-induced angina results from an increase in heart rate or blood pressure, while others state that it is caused by vasoconstriction of the coronary arteries.

Confounding the issue is the fact that not all heart patients with angina experience an increase in angina when exposed to cold. Marchant and co-workers[51] identified seven patients with angina who did not experience an increase in symptoms when exposed to the cold (cold-tolerant) and seven patients who did (cold-intolerant). All of their patients underwent exercise testing in both cold (6° C) and warm (25° C) environments. The severity of angina in the cold-tolerant patients was similar in both the cold and warm exercise environments. However, the cold-intolerant patients experienced an increase in the severity or duration of

their angina when exposed to the cold versus the warm environment. According to their research, exposure to cold caused an increase in blood pressure among all 14 patients. However, in cold-tolerant patients this increase in blood pressure was associated with a more normal increase in heart rate during exercise. In cold-intolerant patients the increase in blood pressure was associated with an exaggerated heart rate response to cold, thus increasing the oxygen demand of the heart even further.

Taking this discussion one step further, imagine the increased stress placed on the heart of any cardiac patient who finds himself having to perform combined arm and leg activity in the cold. For example, snow shoveling, even in normal persons, can be quite strenuous and lead to near maximal increases in heart rate, blood pressure, and myocardial oxygen consumption.[29] Given all of this, you should now appreciate why patients with heart problems are often asked to avoid shoveling snow or, if they must do so, to proceed at a much slower pace and with adequate rest periods.

---

face mask provides a barrier between the environmental air and the respiratory passages, which helps moisten and warm the inhaled air before it enters the trachea, reducing irritability.

Heat Loss from the Head

Another common belief is that 50% or more of the body's heat loss occurs through the head (which occupies approximately 7% to 9% of total body surface area). Is this myth true? Studies have shown that the rate of heat loss from the head is inversely related to the environmental temperature.[30] In other words, the lower the environmental temperature, the greater the heat loss from the head. At rest, the rate of heat loss from the head accounts for approximately 30% to 35% (not 50%) of total heat loss.[30,67] With modest exercise, this value decreases to about 20% of the heat produced.[67] A simple solution of wearing a cap can significantly reduce heat loss through the head. By the same token, the individual who is exercising in the cold and becomes too warm can remove the cap to enhance heat loss.

An equation for approximating heat loss from the head area is as follows:[30]

$$H = 284.8 - (7.55)(T)$$

Where:

$$H = \text{heat loss rate in kcal} \cdot \text{m}^{-2} \cdot \text{hr}^{-1}$$
$$T = \text{air temperature in } °C$$
$$284.8 = \text{a constant}$$

Factors That Influence Heat Loss in the Cold

There are a number of factors that can influence the body's ability to maintain a constant core temperature when exposed to a cold environment. These are outlined in the following discussion.

Body Surface Area and Body Composition

The size and shape of the body affect the amount of heat required to maintain a constant internal temperature. When the ratio of body surface area to body mass is considered, a smaller person is required to produce more heat to maintain body temperature than is a larger person. With respect to subcutaneous fat, which serves as an important and natural insulation layer in humans, thermal conductivity is relatively low. This is because subcutaneous fat is not well vascularized. As a result, persons with a low percentage of body fat are more prone to shivering than are persons who are overfat.

Acclimation and Acclimatization

More than 20 years ago (1977) Buskirk[13] defined **acclimation** as a physiological change that reduces the strain of experimentally induced stressful changes in specific climatic factors. Acclimation may be observed under controlled *acute* exposure either in laboratory chambers or in the environment. Acclimation to cold includes both heat conserving (peripheral vasoconstriction) and heat producing (nonshivering or chemical thermogenesis, shivering, and/or increased physical activity) mechanisms. **Acclimatization,** on the other hand, represents chronic physiological changes occurring within the individual that allows him or her to better adjust to changes in the natural environment.

Have you ever wondered why your hands or cheeks sometimes suddenly appear flushed when you are exposed to the cold? As discussed previously, the initial vasomotor response to cold exposure is peripheral vasoconstriction, which diverts blood flow from the skin to the core. If, however, skin temperature reaches about 3° to 4° C, peripheral vasodilation suddenly occurs. The body *acclimates* and the skin becomes reddened and a feeling of warmth prevails. This is the body's attempt to warm the skin surface, which is, indeed, quite successful. Local skin temperature will rise 11° or 12° C for a period of time, before vasoconstriction reoccurs. Continued exposure results in a periodic fluctuation between vasodilation and vasoconstriction.

Consider these questions: does the athlete *acclimate* to the cold? And does the athlete *acclimatize* to the cold? The answer to the first question is "yes, just like everyone else." However, the answer to the second question is "probably yes." The reason for the indefinite answer to the second question has to do with the nature of our Western culture, with its modern conveniences of well-heated homes, air conditioning, and proper clothing. We actually live in a microclimate that is generally quite comfortable. Therefore, the process of acclimatization is difficult to ascertain. Intuitively, one could say that some acclimatization occurs among athletes who exercise through seasonal climatic changes. However, there is little evidence to suggest that cold acclimatization influences thermoregulatory responses during exercise.[100]

Water Immersion

The physiological burden of exposure to cold water has generated a significant amount of interest by researchers. In general, heat transfer is 4 to 5 times greater in water than in air. The accelerated heat transfer is predominantly due to thermal *conduction,* which is 26 times greater in water than in air.

Individuals are capable of maintaining a constant core temperature in water temperatures of 32° C (90° F). However, below this, the risk of hypothermia (low core temperature) increases exponentially according to both the decline in water temperature and exposure time. For an athlete (e.g., triathlete, swimmer) who is exercising in the water, the above suggests that water temperature and the length of time one is exposed to the water be monitored.

Windchill

The most immediate threat to an individual exposed to the cold is the influence of wind on the rate of surface skin cooling. The term *windchill* dates back to the work of Siple[88] and Siple and Passel[89] and represents another name for the dry, convective cooling power of the atmosphere. Heat loss from the body in such a manner is expressed in kilocalories per square meter of body surface area per hour ($kcal \cdot m^{-2} \cdot hr^{-1}$).

The wind chill index (table 19.6) demonstrates the cooling effects of the wind. As the wind velocity increases for a given ambient temperature, its cooling effect on bare skin is accelerated. For instance, when the ambient temperature is 40° F and accompanied by a 40 mph wind, it feels like 10° F. In addition, the wind chill index is color-coded to emphasize the impact of different cold wind exposures on health risk.

Health Risks of Cold Exposure

Exposure to the cold and wind can lead to two conditions: (1) freezing of human flesh (frostbite) and (2) hypothermia (lowering of body temperature). Of the two we will first discuss frostbite, because it can progress more rapidly than hypothermia and, in extreme conditions, it can occur in less than one minute.

Frostbite

Frostbite occurs when skin temperature reaches between −2° C and −6° C (28.4° F to 21.2° F). For a variety of reasons, including vasomotor activity and metabolism, an environmental temperature lower than −29° C (−20° F) is required to freeze exposed areas such as ear lobes, fingers, and facial skin. The two key factors that contribute to frostbite, and to hypothermia for that matter, are the rate of heat loss from the skin and the length of time one is exposed to the elements.

Siple and Passel[89] developed the following formula for calculating heat loss:

$$K_0 = [\sqrt{100V} + 10.5 - V] [33 - T]$$

19.6

The wind chill index

Wind velocity (mph)	Ambient temperature (°F)										
	50	**40**	**30**	**20**	**10**	**0**	**−10**	**−20**	**−30**	**−40**	**−50**
	(Equivalent temperature [°F])										
5	48	37	27	16	6	−5	−15	−26	−36	−47	−57
10	40	28	16	4	−9	−24	−33	−46	−58	−70	−83
15	36	22	9	−5	−18	−32	−45	−58	−72	−85	−99
20	32	18	4	−10	−25	−39	−53	−67	−82	−96	−110
25	30	16	0	−15	−29	−44	−59	−74	−88	−104	−118
30	28	13	−2	−18	−33	−48	−63	−79	−94	−109	−125
35	27	11	−4	−20	−35	−51	−67	−82	−98	−113	−129
40	26	10	−6	−21	−37	−53	−69	−85	−100	−115	−132
	Minimal risk				Increased risk				Great risk		

Where:

K_0 = heat loss in $kcal \cdot m^{-2} \cdot hr^{-1}$
V = wind velocity in $meters \cdot sec^{-1}$
T = environmental temperature in $°C$
10.5 = a constant
33 = the assumed normal skin temperature in $°C$
(Note: 1 mph = 0.447 $meters \cdot sec^{-1}$)

At a temperature of 0° F, a wind speed of only 10 mph can *threaten* a person with frostbite. An athlete who is very active and generating body heat is able to tolerate lower temperatures and higher winds before experiencing frostbite. In fact, it is not uncommon for runners who are adequately clothed to train when the temperature is −20° F. Other factors moderating the onset of frostbite include: (1) the radiant effect of the sun, (2) the amount of insulating clothing, (3) whether or not the clothing is wet and, if so, how much, and (4) relative humidity.

Consider the following—a runner is exercising at a 7:30 mile pace (8 mph), in an environment with wind velocity at 12 mph and a temperature of 15° F (−9.5° C). When running with the wind, the effective wind velocity is 4 mph (12 mph − 8 mph) (1.8 m · s⁻¹). Using the Siple and Passel[89] formula for computing heat loss, we compute it to be approximately 937 $kcal \cdot m^{-2} \cdot hr^{-1}$. This rate is generally well tolerated by properly clothed runners. However, when the runner turns into the wind, the effective wind velocity becomes 20 mph (12 mph + 8 mph). The calculated rate of heat loss now becomes 1335 $kcal \cdot m^{-2} \cdot hr^{-1}$, which represents a value consistent with frostbite. Factors that are "protective" to the runner in this scenario include a relatively high metabolic rate (7:30 per mile pace) and proper clothing.

Hypothermia

Prolonged exposure to cold or bitterly cold conditions can lead to hypothermia. **Hypothermia** is diagnosed when core temperature has fallen to 95° F (35° C). Ironically, some runners experience hypothermia in conditions that others would judge to be quite comfortable. For example, take the 1985 Boston marathon. Weather conditions that day were described as being warm (76° F), sunny, and humid. During that event 250 persons were treated for hyperthermia; however, 75 other persons were treated for hypothermia. How can hypothermia occur under these conditions? For starters, those affected usually represented the slower runners, meaning that their rate of heat production was not as high as the front runners. Also, they had become dehydrated, with reduced total blood volume. Add to this increased heat loss due to increases in evaporation, convection, and conduction, and to sudden cooling by being sprayed with cold water—all of which represent likely possibilities during a race of this nature. Fluid replacement by intravenous route and ingestion of water generally alleviated the hypothermia within 30 minutes to 1 hour.

Training in the Cold

The primary concern of the individual exercising in the cold is to maintain a comfortable microclimate and body temperature. As a result, what the individual wears becomes an important matter. Additionally, the type of activity and its related level of heat production can affect what the athlete or the leisure exerciser wears. For example, under the same climatic conditions a downhill skier should use more insulation than a runner.

In 1941 Gagge, Burton, and Bazett[32] introduced the concept of a standardized insulating unit, called the "clo." One clo is the amount of insulating material required to keep a person comfortable—equivalent to sitting in a room at 70° F, with a relative humidity less than 50% and with an air movement of 20 feet per minute. When exercising in a cold environment, and heat production increases and the clothing becomes wet, the clo value of the insulating clothing is dramatically altered. Wearing several pieces of lightweight clothing in layers represents a sensible approach to addressing this problem. Materials such as polypropylene that "wick" moisture away from the surface of the skin to the outer layers of the garment are also recommended. Removing moisture away from the skin surface reduces heat loss resulting from conduction. If the individual heats up too much, a layer may then be removed to prevent overheating. Also, although an activity (especially one greater than 6 METs) may be sufficient to maintain body temperature in the cold, it does little for exposed body areas such as the nose, ears, and fingers that remain susceptible to cold injury. Therefore, the individual should wear some sort of protective covering such as mittens, a cap, or a face mask.

Other Factors That Influence Thermoregulation

Before concluding our chapter on thermoregulation, it is necessary that we discuss two other factors that affect heat balance.

Age

Older adults appear to be less tolerant of the heat than younger individuals. Additionally, they may not achieve the same degree of acclimatization as their younger counterparts. The above is due, in part, to (1) a reduced sweat gland function,[47] (2) a reduced skin blood flow,[48] and (3) a lower thirst mechanism creating a lag in fluid intake.[69] Consequently, older adults are more susceptible to heat injury.[5] To what extent, if any, exercise training offsets this age-related decline in heat tolerance is not known. Well-trained older athletes seem to tolerate heat in a manner that is similar to that of fitness-matched younger athletes.[80] However, given the limited research in this area, specific conclusions cannot be drawn. Considering the above, for the inactive or occasionally active older person who finds herself involved in heavy work or vigorous exercise in a hot environment, it would be prudent to take the necessary steps to reduce heat injury. Such actions might include more frequent rests in a cooler environment and consuming fluids beyond thirst.

Aging (and not simply a reduced $\dot{V}O_2$) also appears to diminish one's ability to maintain core temperature at rest and during moderate exercise in the cold.[22] Potential reasons for the poorer cold tolerance in older versus younger persons may be a lower metabolic heat production and/or an increase in thermal conductance.

Gender Differences

Do males and females tolerate hot and cold environments differently? Well, factors related to aerobic power (max $\dot{V}O_2$), relative energy expenditure during work, subcutaneous fat thickness, and body surface area to body mass ratio make it difficult to answer this question directly. In fact, earlier studies that reported a greater tolerance to heat in males than in females did not control for many of these variables.[20,63,72]

For example, we have already shown that exercise training is associated with improved heat tolerance. Consequently, the higher aerobic capacity generally observed in males than in females may account for some of the observed differences in heat tolerance. The early studies, which identified heat tolerance differences between gender, asked the females to work at the same absolute work rate as males. Again, given the generally lower peak aerobic power that is found in females than males, the absolute work rates the females were asked to perform at represented a higher relative work intensity of maximum for them as compared to the males. More recent studies controlled for the intensity of effort, by making it relative to one's own peak aerobic power (e.g., 70% of peak), and found similar thermoregulatory responses.[21,27,34,90,96]

Skinfold thickness may also account for some of the reported gender differences in thermoregulatory response. Remember that a person's ability to dissipate heat is inversely related to their amount of subcutaneous fat, because fat acts as an insulator. Since females generally have greater amounts of body fat than males, it seems obvious their ability to dissipate heat will be impeded when exercising in a hot environment. However, when males and females are matched for skinfold thickness, there are no apparent differences in skin or core temperature.[43]

Thermoregulatory differences between gender can also be explained by the differences in body surface area to body mass ratio that occur between females and males. In an extremely hot environment the larger surface area to mass ratio that is present in females is related to greater heat gain. Therefore, females may be at a disadvantage in these climates. In contrast, in moderately warm temperatures, having their larger surface area to mass ratio allows for improved heat dissipation, since more body surface area is exposed to the environment. When differences in body surface area to body mass are controlled, gender-related differences relative to tolerating heat are markedly narrowed, if not abolished.

There is one clear gender-related difference that impacts thermoregulation. Specifically, males have a higher overall sweat rate and a higher sweat rate per gland than females during light to moderate exercise.[12,31] This is despite

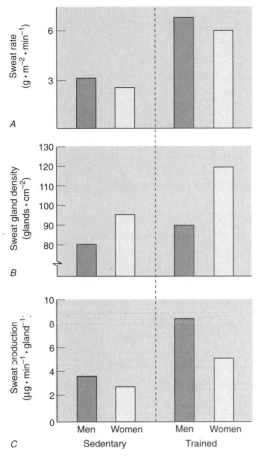

Figure 19.13

Differences in sweat rate, sweat gland density, and sweat production per gland between males and females. Notice that the differences remain, and in some instances, become greater with training.[12]

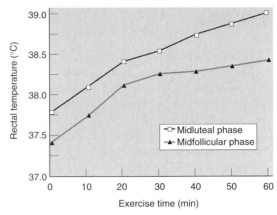

Figure 19.14

Rectal temperature during 60 minutes of cycle exercise performed at a room temperature of 22° C and 60% relative humidity in midfollicular and midluteal phases. Note the absence of a plateau in core temperature during the midfollicular condition.[74]

the fact that females have more sweat glands per unit of skin area (figure 19.13).[12] Frye and Kamon observed that males had an approximate 35% greater average sweat rate than females following three hours of light exercise (30% of maximum) in a hot, dry environment.[31] This difference in sweat rate between males and females is narrowed with training and acclimatization, but average sweat rate remains higher in males.[12,31] Interestingly, females showed a lowering of sweat rate response when exposed to humid heat versus dry heat. This response was not observed in males.[31] The ability of females to suppress the sweating response once the skin is moist, in an environment where heat loss due to evaporation is impaired, may protect them from dehydration during exercise. This may be a particularly important mechanism that also helps protect the cardiovascular system in females, since they generally have smaller blood volumes and, therefore, may not tolerate plasma losses as well.

Finally, evidence exists that indicates that the thermoregulatory response in premenopausal females varies through the menstrual cycle.[90] The temperature set point in

the hypothalamus is increased, on average, 0.47° C during the luteal (post-ovulatory) phase versus the follicular phase.[90] This means that sweating and vasodilation occur at a higher core temperature during the luteal phase of the cycle. Pivarnik and associates showed that during 60 minutes of cycling at 65% of peak $\dot{V}O_2$, core temperature was greater, and never plateaued, during the midluteal versus midfollicular phase of the cycle (figure 19.14).[74] The difference in core temperature between the luteal and follicular phases increased from 0.3° C at rest to 0.6° C at the end of exercise. Skin blood flow also tends to be greater during the luteal phase, suggesting that heat transfer to the skin surface (thermal gradient) is influenced by menstrual cycle phase.

As you might have guessed, females also respond differently than males when exposed to cold environments. Although the increased body fat in females does provide insulation against the cold, both their larger body surface area to body mass ratio and smaller muscle mass (i.e., lower heat production) facilitate body cooling. This faster cooling rate observed in females than males occurs when they are exposed to either cold air or cold water. These differences occur not only at rest but also when exercising in a cold environment.[90] Graham[36] observed a decrease in core temperature in females following two hours of exercise in the cold. In contrast, core temperature was maintained in males.

The higher hypothalamic temperature threshold observed in females during the luteal phase of their menstrual cycle also impacts cold exposure. Specifically, heat production through muscular activity are initiated at a higher core temperature during the luteal phase as compared to the follicular phase of the menstrual cycle.[90] What remains unclear is whether or not the higher hypothalamic temperature threshold during the luteal phase results in altered responses while exercising in the cold.

Summary

Heat balance is obtained when the same amount of heat is lost as is produced or gained. Heat is lost from the body through convection, conduction, radiation, and evaporation. Convection is defined as the transfer of heat from one place to another by the motion of a heated substance (e.g., air). Conduction is heat exchange between two objects of different temperatures that are in direct contact with each other. Radiation involves the transfer of heat between objects through electromagnetic waves. Heat loss through evaporation is the result of changing a liquid (e.g., sweat) to a vapor. Heat is gained by the body mainly through metabolism, but the body can also gain heat from the environment through radiation, convection, and conduction.

The function of the thermoregulatory system is to maintain a relatively constant internal body temperature both at rest and during exercise. The basic components of the thermoregulatory system are (1) the thermal regulatory (coordinating) center located in the hypothalamus, which receives information from the receptors and initiates outgoing regulatory actions via the effector organs; (2) thermal receptors located in the hypothalamus (central receptors) of the brain and in the skin (peripheral receptors); and (3) thermal effectors or organs such as the skeletal muscles, the smooth muscles of the arterioles, the sweat glands, and the endocrine glands.

The principal means by which the body loses heat during exercise or exposure to heat are (1) circulatory adjustments of increased blood flow to the skin resulting from cutaneous vasodilation and (2) evaporative cooling resulting from increased secretion of sweat. Internal body heat produced mainly by the liver and skeletal muscles is carried by the blood (circulatory convection) to the surface, where conduction, convection, radiation, and, particularly, evaporation take place. The cooled blood then returns to the warmer core, and the cycle is repeated.

The seriousness of overexposure to heat during exercise is exemplified not only by a decrease in work performance, but also by a predisposition to heat illness. These disorders are categorized in order of ascending severity as (1) heat cramps, (2) heat syncope, (3) water-depletion heat exhaustion, (4) salt-depletion heat exhaustion, and (5) heat stroke. The most frequent common denominators for all these illnesses are (1) heat exposure, (2) loss of water, and (3) heat storage, usually reflected by high internal body temperature. However, the single most important factor, from a clinical standpoint, is loss of body water. Also, inattention to heat cramps, heat syncope, and heat exhaustion can lead to heat stroke and, finally, to death.

Heat disorders in athletics can be significantly reduced through (1) acclimatization to heat and improving aerobic fitness; (2) adequate fluid replacement; and (3) awareness of the limitations imposed by exercising in environmental heat.

Individuals respond to the cold through both physiological and behavioral means. Physiological responses include peripheral vasoconstriction, nonshivering (chemical) thermogenesis, and shivering. Behavioral responses include wearing appropriate attire, avoiding the cold, and altering physical activity levels. Lung tissue is not normally in danger of freezing because air is conditioned (warmed and moistened) by the bronchiole mucosa. The exposed head can be a significant source of heat loss during exercise. However, it probably does not exceed 30% of total heat loss during exercise. The energy cost ($\dot{V}O_2$) of submaximal work is elevated due to shivering while the person exercises. Maximal $\dot{V}O_2$ is not affected unless the core temperature is reduced.

Windchill is an important concept because it provides a means by which heat loss from the body can be calculated. Wind velocity and temperature are the key factors in calculating windchill. Two consequences of exposure to the cold are frostbite and hypothermia. Human flesh freezes when its temperature reaches between $-2°$ and $-6°$ C. Hypothermia can occur under conditions that can be characterized as mild. Factors important to cold tolerance include body surface area to body mass ratio, body composition, water immersion, acclimation, and physical conditioning. With proper clothing, an athlete can train successfully in cold environments.

Older individuals do not tolerate environmental extremes as well as younger individuals. A lower heat tolerance is probably a result of a decrease in thermal effector responses or a lag in the thirst mechanism, either of which may contribute to heat injury. Limited information is available regarding the physiological responses of older individuals exercising in environmental extremes.

Factors related to aerobic capacity, relative energy expenditure during work, subcutaneous fat thickness, and body surface area to body mass ratio are primary determinants to gender differences observed in hot or cold environments. Once accounted for, some narrow differences still exist between males and females relative to their responses to different environmental conditions. These differences appear due to gender-specific differences in sweat rate and the menstrual cycle phase.

Questions

1. Describe the manner by which the body loses heat.
2. Compare and contrast convection versus conduction.
3. Why is evaporation impaired in a hot, humid environment?
4. Describe in detail how the body may gain heat.
5. Explain the function of the thermoregulatory system

relative to a constant temperature. Identify the function of the hypothalamus, thermal receptors, and thermal effectors.

6. Explain the principal means by which heat is lost during exercise or exposure to heat.

7. Explain how water depletion during exercise can lead to serious heat disorders.

8. How would you regulate salt and water replacement as a consequence of exercising in the heat? List "fluid replacement" guidelines for athletes.

9. What effect does excessive sweating have on plasma volume and cardiovascular function? Explain cardiovascular drift.

10. What instruments are available to assess environmental heat stress? Include in your response wet bulb temperature and wet bulb globe temperature.

11. What procedures would you follow to protect the athlete against heat illness during stressful environmental conditions?

12. What are the emergency procedures for a heat stroke casualty?

13. Describe the effects of cold exposure on the energy cost of exercise during submaximal and maximal effort.

14. Does cold exposure affect energy metabolism or muscle function? If yes, explain your answer.

15. Can the lungs freeze during exercise in the cold? Explain your answer.

16. What is windchill, and why is it important to understand?

17. Briefly describe the two health risks associated with cold exposure.

18. How might cold exposure affect heart patients who experience angina (chest pain caused by lack of oxygen to their heart muscle)?

19. Compare and contrast how males versus females respond to heat stress; include such factors as fitness level, skinfolds thickness, sweat rate, and number of sweat glands per unit of skin area.

References

1. American College of Sports Medicine. 1995. *Guidelines for Exercise Testing and Prescription,* 5th ed. Baltimore: Williams & Wilkins. pp. 288–296.

2. American College of Sports Medicine Position Stand. 1996. Exercise and fluid replacement. *Med Sci Sports Exerc.* 28(1):i–vii.

3. American College of Sports Medicine Position Stand. 1984. The prevention of thermal injuries during distance running. *Med Sci Sports Exerc.* 16:ii.

4. American College of Sports Medicine Position Stand. 1996. Weight loss in wrestlers. *Med Sci Sports Exerc.* 28(2):ix–xii.

5. Applegate, W. B., J. W. Runyan, L. Brasfeld, M. L. Williams, C. Konigsberg, and C. Fauche. 1981. Analysis of the 1980 heat wave in Memphis. *J Am Geriatrics Society.* 29:337–342.

6. Armstrong, L. E., D. L. Costill, and W. J. Fink. 1985. Influence of diuretic-induced dehydration on competitive running performance. *Med Sci Sports Exerc.* 17(4):456–461.

7. Bass, D., C. Kleeman, M. Quinn, A. Henschel, and A. Hegnauer. 1955. Mechanisms of acclimatization to heat in man. *Medicine.* 34:323–380.

8. Bergh, U. 1980. Human power at subnormal body temperature. *Acta Physiol Scand.* (Suppl. 478):1–39.

9. Bergh, U., and B. Ekblom. 1979. Physical performance and peak power at different body temperatures. *J Appl Physiol.* 45(5):885–889.

10. *Best and Taylor's Physiologic Basis of Medical Practice,* 1985. West, J. B. (ed.). 11th ed. Baltimore: Williams and Wilkins, pp. 1229–1231.

11. Blyth, C., and J. Burt. 1961. Effects of water balance on ability to perform at high ambient temperatures. *Res Q.* 32:301–307.

12. Buono, M. J., and N. T. Sjoholm. 1988. Effect of physical training on peripheral sweat production. *J Appl Physiol.* 65(2):811–814.

13. Buskirk, E. R. 1977. Temperature regulation with exercise. In Hutton, R. S. (ed.), *Exercise and Sport Sciences Reviews,* vol. 5. Santa Barbara: Journal Publishing Affiliates.

14. Buskirk, E., and D. Bass. 1974. Climate and exercise. In Johnson, W., and E. Buskirk (eds.), *Science and Medicine of Exercise and Sports,* 2d ed. New York: Harper and Brothers, pp. 190–205.

15. Buskirk, E., P. Iampietro, and D. Bass. 1958. Work performance and dehydration, effects of physical condition and heat acclimatization. *J Appl Physiol.* 12:189–194.

16. Claremont, A. D. 1976. Taking winter in stride. *Phys Sports Med.* 4:65–68.

17. Claremont, A. D., F. Nagle, W. D. Redden, and G. A. Brooks. 1975. Comparison of metabolic, temperature, heart rate and ventilatory responses to exercise at extreme ambient temperatures (0° and 35° C). *Med Sci Sports Exerc.* 7(2):150–153.

18. Costill, D. L. 1977. Fluids for athletic performance: why and what you should drink during prolonged exercise. In *The New Runners Diet.* Moutain View, CA: World Publications.

19. Craig, E., and E. Cummings. 1966. Dehydration and muscular work. *J Appl Physiol.* 21:670–674.

20. Cunningham, D. J., J. A. J. Stolwijk, and C. B. Wenger. 1978. Comparative thermoregulatory responses of resting men and women. *J Appl Physiol.* 45(6): 908–915.

21. Drinkwater, B. L., J. E. Denton, I. C. Kupprat, T. S. Talag, and S. M. Horvath. 1976. Aerobic power as a factor in women's response to work in hot environments. *J Appl Physiol.* 41.815–821.

22. Falk, B., O. Bar-or, J. Smolander, and G. Frost. 1994. Response to rest and exercise in the cold: effects of age and aerobic fitness. *J Appl Physiol.* 76(1):72–84.

23. Febbraio, M., R. Snow, M. Hargreaves, C. G. Stathis, I. Martin, and M. Carey. 1994. Muscle metabolism during exercise and heat stress in trained men: effect of acclimation. *J Appl Physiol.* 76(2):589–597.

24. Febbraio, M., R. Snow, C. G. Stathis, M. Hargreaves and M. Carey. 1994. Effect of heat stress on muscle energy metabolism during exercise. *J Appl Physiol.* 77(6):2827–2831.

25. Fink, W., D. L. Costill, P. Van Handel, and L. Getchell. 1975. Leg muscle metabolism during exercise in the heat and cold. *Eur J Appl Physiol.* 34:183–190.

26. Folk, G. E. 1974. *Textbook of Environmental Physiology,* 2d ed. Philadelphia: Lea & Febiger, pp. 393–394.

27. Fortney, S. M., and L. C. Senay. 1979. Effect of training and heat acclimation on exercise responses of sedentary females. *J Appl Physiol.* 47(5):978–984.

28. Fox, E. L., H. S. Weiss, R. L. Bartels, and E. P. Hiatt. 1966. Thermal responses of man during rest and exercise in a helium oxygen environment. *Arch Environ Health.* 13:23–28.

29. Franklin, B. A., P. Hogan, K. Bonzheim, D. Bakalyar, E. Terrien, S. Gordon, and G. C. Timmis. 1995. Cardiac demands of heavy snow shoveling. *JAMA.* 273:880–882.

30. Froese, G., and A. C. Burton. 1957. Heat loss from the human head. *J Appl Physiol.* 10:235–241.

31. Frye, A. J., and E. Kamon. 1981. Responses to dry heat of men and women with similar aerobic capacities. *J Appl Physiol Respirat Environ Exercise Physiol.* 50(1):65–70.

32. Gagge, A. P., A. C. Burton, and H. C. Bazett. 1941. A practical system of units for the description of the heat exchange of man with his environment. *Science.* 94(2445):428–430.

33. Gisolfi, C. V. 1973. Work-heat tolerance derived from interval training. *J Appl Physiol.* 35:349–354.

34. Gisolfi, C. V., and J. S. Cohen. 1979. Relationships among training, heat acclimation, and heat tolerance in men and women: the controversy revisited. *Med Sci Sports.* 11(1):56–59.

35. Gisolfi, C. V., N. C. Wilson, and B. Claxton. 1977. Work-heat tolerance of distance runners. *Ann NY Acad Sci.* 301:139–150.

36. Graham, T. E. 1983. Alcohol ingestion and the sex difference on the thermal responces to mild exercise in a cold environment. *Human Biology.* 55:463–476.

37. Green, H. J., L. L. Jones, and D. C. Painter. 1990. Effects of short-term training on cardiac function during prolonged exercise. *Med Sci Sports Exerc.* 22(4):488–493.

38. Greenleaf, J., and B. Castle. 1971. Exercise temperature regulation in man during hypohydration and hyperhydration. *J Appl Physiol.* 30:847–853.

39. Guyton, A. C., and J. E. Hall. 1996. *Textbook of Medical Physiology,* 9th ed. Philadelphia: W. B. Saunders Co., pp. 914–915.

40. Hanson, P. G. 1979. Heat injury in runners. *Phys Sports Med.* 7(6):91–96.

41. Hanson, P. G., and S. W. Zimmerman. 1979. Exertional heatstroke in novice runners. *JAMA.* 242(2):154–157.

42. Hartung, G. H., L. G. Myhre, and S. A. Nunneley. 1980. Physiological effects of cold air inhalation during exercise. *Aviat Space Environ Med.* 51:591–597.

43. Haymes, E. M., and C. L. Wells. 1986. *Environment and Human Performance.* Champaign, IL: Human Kinetics Publishers.

44. Hellström, B., K. Berg, and V. Lorentzen. 1970. Human peripheral re-warming following exercise in the cold. *J Appl Physiol.* 29:191–199.

45. Henane, R., R. Flandrois, and J. P. Charbonnier. 1977. Increase in sweating sensitivity by endurance conditioning in man. *J Appl Physiol.* 43:822–828.

46. Hubbard, R. W. 1979. Effects of exercise in the heat on predisposition to heatstroke. *Med Sci Sports.* 11(1):66–71.

47. Kenny, W. L., and R. K. Anderson. 1988. Response of older and younger women in dry and humid heat without fluid replacement. *Med Sci Sports Exerc.* 20:155–160.

48. Kenny, W. L., C. G. Tankersley, D. L. Newswanger, D. E. Hyde, S. M. Puhl. 1990. Age and hypohydration independently influence the peripheral vascular response to heat stress. *J Appl Physiol.* 68:1902–1908.

49. Kozlowski, S., and B. Saltin. 1964. Effects of sweat loss on body fluids. *J Appl Physiol.* 19:1119–1124.

50. Licht, S. (ed.). 1964. *Medical Climatology.* New Haven: Elizabeth Licht.

51. Marchant, B., G. Donaldson, K. Mridha, M. Scarborough, and A. D. Timmis. 1994. Mechanisms of cold intolerance in patients with angina. *J Am Coll Cardiol.* 23:630–636.

52. Mathews, D. K., E. L. Fox, and D. Tanzi. 1969. Physiological responses during exercise and recovery in a football uniform. *J Appl Physiol.* 26:611–615.

53. Matsui, H., K. Shimaoka, M. Miyamura, and K. Kobayashi. 1978. Seasonal variation of aerobic work capacity in ambient and constant temperature. In Folinsbee, L. J., et al. (eds.), *Environmental Stress: Individual Human Adaptations.* New York: Academic Press, pp. 279–292.

54. Mitchell, D., L. C. Senay, C. H. Wyndham, A. J. van Rensburg, G. G. Rogers, and N. B. Strydom. 1976. Acclimatization in a hot, humid environment: energy exchange body temperature, and sweating. *J Appl Physiol.* 40:768–778.

55. Moritz, A. R., and J. R. Weisiger. 1945. Effects of cold air on the air passages and lungs. *Arch Int Med.* 75:233–240.

56. Mueller, F. O., and R. D. Schindler. 1996. *Annual Survey of Football Injury Research 1931–1995.* Overland Park, KS: National Collegiate Athletic Association; Waco, TX: American Football Coaches Association; Kansas City, MO: The National Federation of State High School Associations.

57. Murphy, R. J. 1963. The problem of environmental heat in athletics. *Ohio State Med J.* 59(8).

58. Murphy, R. J., and W. Ashe. 1965. Prevention of heat illness in football players. *JAMA.* 194:650–654.

59. Murray, R. 1995. Fluid needs in hot and cold environments. *Int J Sports Nutrition.* 5(suppl):S62–S72.

60. Nadel, E. R. 1979. Control of sweating rate while exercising in the heat. *Med Sci Sports Exerc.* 11(1):31–35.

61. Nadel, E. R. 1978. Temperature regulation during exercise. In Houdus, Y., and J. D. Guieu (eds.), *New Trends in Thermal Physiology.* Paris: Masson, pp. 143–153.

62. Nadel, E. R., K. B. Pandolf, M. F. Roberts, and J. A. J. Stolwijk. 1974. Mechanisms of thermal acclimation to exercise and heat. *J Appl Physiol.* 37:515–520.

63. Nadel, E. R., M. F. Roberts, and C. B. Wenger. 1978. Thermoregulatory adaptations to heat and exercise: comparative responses of men and women. In Folinsbee, L. J., et al. (eds.), *Environmental Stress: Individual Human Adaptations.* New York: Academic Press, pp. 29–38.

64. Nash, H. L. 1985. Treating thermal injury: disagreement heats up. *Phys Sports Med.* 13(7):134–144.

65. National Institute for Occupational Safety and Health: Criteria for a recommended standard . . . occupational exposure to hot environments. 1986. (DHHS, NIOSH Publ. No. 86-113). U.S. Department of Health and Human Services, Washington, D.C.

66. Noakes, T. D., R. J. Norman, R. H. Buck, J. Godlonton, K. Stevenson, and D. Pittaway. 1990. The incidence of hyponatremia during prolonged ultraendurance exercise. *Med Sci Sports Exerc.* 22(2):165–170.

67. Nunneley, S. A., S. J. Troutman, and P. Webb. 1971. Head cooling in work and heat stress. *Aerospace Med.* 42:64–68.

68. Oksa, J., H. Rintamaki, T. Makinen, J. Hassi, and H. Rusko. 1995. Cooling-induced changes in muscular performance and EMG activity of agonist and antagonist muscles. *Aviat Space Environ Med.* 66(1):26–31.

69. O'Neil, P. A., E. B. Faragher, L. Davies, R. Wears, K. McClean, D. Fairweather. 1990. Reduced survival with increasing plasma osmolality in elderly continuing care patients. *Age Aging.* 19:68–71.

70. Pandolf, K. B. 1979. Effects of physical training and cardiorespiratory physical fitness on exercise-heat tolerance: recent observations. *Med Sci Sports.* 11(1):60–65.

71. Pandolf, K. B., R. L. Burse, and R. F. Goldman. 1977. Role of physical fitness in heat acclimatization, decay and reinduction. *Ergonomics.* 20:399–408.

72. Paolone, A. M., C. L. Weils, and G. T. Kelly. 1978. Sexual variations in thermoregulation during heat stress. *Aviat Space Environ Med.* 49:715–719.

73. Pitts, G., R. Johnson, and F. Consolazio. 1944. Work in the heat as affected by intake of water, salt and glucose. *Am J Physiol.* 142:253–259.

74. Pivarnik, J. M., C. J. Marichal, T. Spillman, and J. R. Morrow. 1992. Menstrual cycle phase affects temperature regulation during endurance exercise. *J Appl Physiol.* 72(2):543–548.

75. Piwonka, R., and S. Robinson. 1967. Acclimatization of highly trained men to work in severe heat. *J Appl Physiol.* 22:9–12.

76. Piwonka, R., S. Robinson, V. Gay, and R. Manalis. 1965. Preacclimatization of men to heat by training. *J Appl Physiol.* 20:379–383.

77. Pugh, L. G. C. 1967. Cold stress and muscular exercise, with special reference to accidental hypothermia. *Br Med J.* 2:333–337.

78. Ramanathan, L. N. 1964. A new weighing system for mean surface temperature of the human body. *J Appl Physiol.* 19(3)531.

79. Roberts, M. F., C. B. Wenger, J. A. J. Stolwijk, and E. R. Nadel.

1977. Skin blood flow and sweating changes following exercise training and heat acclimation. *J Appl Physiol.* 43:133–137.

80. Robinson, S. 1967. Training acclimatization and heat tolerance. *Can Med Assoc J.* 96:795–800.

81. Saltin, B. 1964. Aerobic and anaerobic work capacity after dehydration. *J Appl Physiol.* 19:1114–1118.

82. Saltin, B. 1964. Aerobic work capacity and circulation at exercise in man. *Acta Physiol Scand.* 62 (Suppl. 230):1–52.

83. Saltin, B. 1964. Circulatory response to submaximal and maximal exercise after thermal dehydration. *J Appl Physiol.* 19:1125–1132.

84. Sawka, M. N., R. P. Francesconi, A. J. Young, and K. B. Pandolf. 1984. Influence of hydration level and body fluids on exercise performance in the heat. *JAMA.* 252:1165–1169.

85. Shapiro, Y., A. Magazanik, R. Vdassin, G. M. Ben-Baruch, E. Shvartz, and Y. Shoenfeld. 1979. Heat intolerance in former heatstroke patients. *Ann Intern Med.* 90(6):913–916.

86. Shvartz, E., A. Bhattacharya, S. J. Sperindle, P. J. Brock, D. Sciaraffa, and W. J. Van Beaumont. 1979. Sweating responses during heat acclimation and moderate conditioning. *J Appl Physiol.* 46(4):675–680.

87. Shvartz, E., Y. Shapiro, A. Magazanik, A. Meroz, H. Birnfeld, A. Mechtinger, and S. Shibolet. 1977. Heat acclimation, physical fitness, and responses to exercise in a temperate and hot environment. *J Appl Physiol.* 43:678–683.

88. Siple, P. A. 1939. *Adaptation of the Explorer to the Climate of Antarctica.* Doctoral dissertation: Clark University, Worcester, MA.

89. Siple, P. A., and C. F. Passel. 1945. Measurement of dry atmospheric cooling in subfreezing temperatures. *Proc Am Philosophical Soc.* 89:177–199.

90. Stephenson, L. A., and M. A. Kolka. 1993. Thermoregulation in Women. In Holloszy, J. O. (ed.) *Exercise and Sport Science Reviews.* Baltimore: Williams & Wilkins, pp. 231–262.

91. Strømme, S., K. Lange-Andersen, and R. W. Elsner. 1963. Metabolic and thermal responses to muscular exertion in the cold. *J Appl Physiol.* 18(4):756–763.

92. Sutton, J. R. 1991. Heat illness. In Strauss, R. H. (ed.), *Sports Medicine.* Philadelphia: W. B. Saunders, pp. 345–358.

93. Taylor, H., A. Henschel, O. Mickelson, and A. Keys. 1943. The effect of sodium chloride intake on the work performance of man during exposure to dry heat and experimental heat exhaustion. *Am J Physiol.* 140:439.

94. Vogel, J. A., P. B. Rock, B. H. Jones, and G. Havenith. 1993. Environmental considerations in exercise testing and training. In: American College of Sports Medicine, *Resource Manual for Guidelines for Exercise Testing and Prescription,* 2d ed. Philadelphia: Lea & Febiger, pp. 129–147.

95. Webb, P. 1951. Air temperature in respiratory tracts of resting subjects in the cold. *J Appl Physiol.* 4(11):378–382.

96. Wells, C. L. 1980. Responses of physically active and acclimatized men and women to exercise in a desert environment. *Med Sci Sports Exerc.* 12(1):9–13.

97. Wyndham, C. H., G. G. Rogers, L. C. Senay, and D. Mitchell. 1976. Acclimatization in a hot, humid environment: cardiovascular adjustments. *J Appl Physiol.* 40:779–785.

98. Yamazaki, F., N. Nobuharu, R. Sone, and H. Ikegami. 1996. Response of sweating and body temperature to sinusoidal exercise in physically trained men. *J Appl Physiol.* 80(2):491–495.

99. Yoshida, T., S. Nakai, A. Yorimoto, T. Kanabata, and T. Morimoto. 1995. Effect of aerobic capacity on sweat rate and fluid intake during outdoor exercise in the heat. *Eur J Appl Physiol.* 71(2–3):235–239.

100. Young, A. J. 1990. Energy substrate utilization during exercise in extreme environments. In: Pandolf, K. B. and Holloszy, J. O. (eds.) *Exercise and Sport Science Reviews.* Baltimore: Williams & Wilkins, pp. 66–117.

Selected Readings

Benzinger, R. 1969. Heat regulation: homeostasis of central temperature in man. *Physiol Rev.* 49:671–759.

Consolazio, C. F., R. E. Johnson, and L. J. Pecora. 1963. *Physiological Measurements of Metabolic Function in Man.* New York: McGraw-Hill.

Gisolfi, C. V. (ed.). 1979. Symposium on the thermal effects of exercise in the heat. *Med Sci Sports.* 11(1):30–71.

McMurray, R. G., and S. M. Horvath. 1979. Thermoregulation in swimmers and runners. *J Appl Physiol.* 46(6):1086–1092.

Noakes, T. D. 1993. Fluid replacement during exercise. In: Holloszy, J. O. (ed.), *Exercise and Sport Science Reviews.* Baltimore: Williams and Wilkins, pp. 297–330.

Nunneley, S. 1978. Physiological responses of women to thermal stress: a review. *Med Sci Sports.* 10(4):250–255.

Paton, B. C. 1991. Cold injuries. In: Strauss, R. H. (ed.), *Sports Medicine,* 2d ed. Philadelphia: WB Saunders, pp. 359–388.

Patterson, M., D. Warlters, A. Nigel, and S. Taylor. 1994. Attenuation of the cutaneous blood flow response during combined exercise and heat stress. *Eur J Appl Physiol.* 69(4):367–369.

20

Performance Underwater, at High Altitude, and during and after Microgravity

The principal focus of this chapter will be exercise performance under a variety of environmental conditions, including hyperbaria (scuba), hypobaria (altitude) and microgravity (space). Humans are exploring new environments, "climbing higher," "going deeper," and challenging new frontiers in space. It is important for you to understand the physiological effects of a variety of environmental stresses on human performance.

Scuba (self-contained underwater breathing apparatus) diving, in addition to being fun, offers a wonderful opportunity to learn a great deal about physiology in a very interesting and exciting manner. The physiology of just one dive could actually fill a textbook, and the importance of this information is dramatically illustrated by the fact that if the knowledge is not applied, a single dive could be fatal.

Focusing on altitude considerations, it is not unusual in this jet age for athletic teams to be suddenly whisked to competition in cities that are at greater altitudes than the place where the athletes trained. The day of competition will be too late to wonder about the effects of low pressure on performance and the

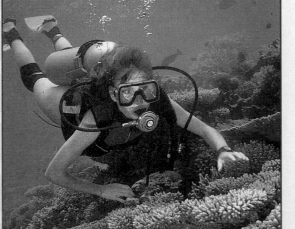

advisability of administering oxygen to your team; one must plan in advance.

Humans are inhabiting space for longer and longer periods of time. It will be important to understand the role of exercise in monitoring and sustaining physiological function in space and upon return to a gravitational environment. This has relevance to extended deconditioning on earth, caused by bedrest, inactivity, and aging.

The purpose of this chapter is to provide the knowledge that will allow you to serve as a knowledgeable reference source for those who wish to learn about performance while scuba diving, at altitude, and in a microgravity environment.

Effects of Changes in Pressure and Temperature on Gas Volumes

Physical and Physiological Principles of Scuba

Performance at Altitude

Performance during and after Microgravity Exposure

Summary

The major concepts to be learned from this chapter are as follows:

- When the pressure on a given volume of gas is increased, the volume decreases (Boyle's Law).
- When the temperature of a given volume of gas is increased, the volume increases (Charles's Law).
- The partial pressures of gases in a mixture remain constant and act independently of each other (Dalton's Law).
- The amount of gas a fluid will absorb under pressure varies in direct proportion to the partial pressure of the gas (Henry's Law).
- Scuba (self-contained underwater breathing apparatus) diving is an excellent sport and can be performed without accident, provided that physiological concepts are understood and applied.
- At altitudes over 5000 feet (1524 meters), the ability to perform endurance activities is decreased due to hypoxia—i.e., the lowered partial pressure of oxygen in the air.
- Endurance performance at altitude may sometimes be improved with continued stay at altitude due to the acclimatization process.
- Acclimatization to altitude involves: (1) increasing pulmonary ventilation, (2) increasing red blood cell and hemoglobin concentrations, (3) eliminating bicarbonate in the urine, and (4) tissue changes.
- Training at altitude might enhance endurance performance at sea level but only in unconditioned, nonathletic individuals.
- For the highly trained athlete, the training intensity required for maintenance of peak performances cannot be achieved at altitude.
- Performance during microgravity exposure is altered in several ways: maximal oxygen consumption decreases (with simulated microgravity) proportional to the length of exposure.
- During extended periods of microgravity, heart rate is higher during submaximal exercise.
- Muscle size and strength decrease with long-term exposure to microgravity.
- Exercise has the potential to be an effective countermeasure for long-term microgravity exposure.

Effects of Changes in Pressure and Temperature on Gas Volumes

Comprehension of the physiological factors associated with physical performance below the sea and at altitude requires knowledge of the gas laws. Familiarity with these laws will help us to make valid judgments regarding how the individual may be physiologically affected, whether skiing in Squaw Valley (altitude of 6000 or more feet) or donning scuba gear and searching the ocean floors.

Effects of Pressure Changes on Gas Volume

It is quite interesting to note that when you increase the pressure on a given volume of gas, the volume diminishes. Whereas, when you increase the pressure on a given volume of water, the volume remains just about the same. If, for example, a given amount of gas is subjected to twice the pressure, the volume will be *reduced* by one-half. By the same token, if the pressure should be diminished by one-half, the volume will *double*. Water volume is not affected by pressure changes, whereas gas volumes are significantly altered. You will realize shortly that these are important considerations for us to be aware of, particularly in scuba diving. The gas law that relates pressure and volume of a gas is called **Boyle's law.** A more comprehensive treatment of the gas laws appears in appendix C.

Effects of Temperature Changes on Gas Volume

Gas volume is affected not only by pressure but also by temperature. Heating a gas causes it to expand. As a matter of fact, if you hold pressure on the gas constant and raise the temperature from 0° C to 100° C, the volume increases almost 37%. However, temperature change has an insignificant effect on the volume of water, just as does pressure change. The gas law that relates temperature and volume of a gas is called **Charles's law.**

Weight of Air and Water

Air has weight and at sea level exerts 14.7 pounds of pressure per square inch (psi). This 14.7 psi is equal to a **barometric pressure** of 760 millimeters of mercury (mmHg) and is also referred to as one atmosphere of pressure. As we ascend in altitude, the amount of air above us decreases and, as a result, the pressure diminishes. For example, at 5000 feet the pressure is reduced to 12.2 psi; at 10,000, 10.1 psi;

and at 15,000, 8.3 psi. At 60,500 feet, only 1 psi of pressure is exerted by air.

On the other hand, as we descend below the surface of the sea, we have in addition to the 14.7 psi of pressure exerted by the atmosphere, the weight of the water above us. Sea water, because of the salt content, weighs 64 pounds per cubic foot, whereas fresh water weighs 62.4 pounds per cubic foot. The density* of water (i.e., its weight per cubic foot) remains constant as one descends to the ocean depths because, as was mentioned earlier, water is essentially noncompressible. Because of this factor, the weight of water is proportional to the depth. That is, at 33 feet under the surface the weight of water alone will be equal to one atmosphere, or 14.7 psi of pressure. Why is this so?

If the weight of sea water equals 64 pounds per cubic foot, and a diver descends to 33 feet, what is the pressure (or weight of the water) on the diver at this depth in terms of pounds per square inch?

33 feet × 64 pounds per cubic feet
= 2112 pounds per square foot†
1 square foot (12 inch × 12 inch)
= or 144 square inches

Converting pounds per square foot to pounds per square inch:

$$\frac{2112 \text{ pounds per square foot}}{144 \text{ square inches per square foot}} = 14.7 \text{ psi}$$

Therefore, at a depth of 33 feet, the water would cause a pressure on the diver of 14.7 psi. The total pressure on the diver, or what is referred to as the absolute pressure, will be equal to 29.4 psi because to the weight of the water must be added the weight of the atmosphere (14.7 psi + 14.7 psi = 29.4 psi). Figure 20.1 depicts the increased pressure as one descends to 99 feet.

Effects of Pressure and Concentration on Gas Absorption

The absorption of gases by the body during scuba diving is governed by two laws. These same laws apply at sea level and in higher altitude conditions. **Dalton's Law** states that the partial pressure of gases in a mixture remains constant and will act independently of each other. The compressed air used in diving tanks is a mixture of gases just as is room air. The main constituents are nitrogen 79%, oxygen 20.94%, carbon dioxide 0.03%, and other inert gases in very small concentrations. The concentrations or fractions of the constituent gases are not changed even though the gases are compressed in the tank. The gas molecules are compressed

---

*Density equals the mass per unit volume.
†One square foot represents the bottom surface area of the column of water which is 33 feet high.

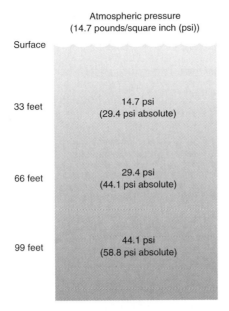

Atmospheric pressure
(14.7 pounds/square inch (psi))

Surface

33 feet   14.7 psi
                (29.4 psi absolute)

66 feet   29.4 psi
                (44.1 psi absolute)

99 feet   44.1 psi
                (58.8 psi absolute)

Figure 20.1

Depth and pressure relationships. As the diver descends from the surface of the water at sea level to a depth of 99 feet, the absolute pressure increases from 14.7 psi to 58.8 psi.

together, but there remains the same fraction of molecules per given volume. Keep in mind that these compressed gases are inhaled through a regulator valve, so it "feels" like breathing on the surface.

The partial pressure, which is the critical consideration to absorption, of any gas can be calculated by simply multiplying the decimal fraction of the gas by the pressure to which it is exposed. For example, the ambient barometric pressure of approximately 760 mmHg or 14.7 psi (1 atmosphere) is used at sea level. This would yield partial pressures for nitrogen $.79 \times 760 = 600$ mmHg, for oxygen $.2094 \times 760 = 159$ mmHg, and for carbon dioxide $.0003 \times 760 = 0.23$ mmHg. As you have learned, the pressure below the water surface is greater so an appropriate number of whole and fractional atmospheres would be used for pressure depending on the depth of the dive. Remember a depth of 33 feet is equivalent to one more atmosphere for a total of two, one above sea level and one below. The pressure used in calculating the partial pressures would be $2 \times 760 = 1520$ mmHg, so the partial pressures would double: $.79 \times 1520 = 1200$ mmHg for N_2, $.2094 \times 1520 = 318$ mmHg for O_2, and $.0003 \times 1520 = 0.46$ for CO_2. Simply put, the *partial pressures of gases in a mixture increase in proportion to the depth of the dive*. For practice, calculate the oxygen partial pressure of compressed air at a depth of 16.5 feet. Did you get 239 mmHg? [$.2094 \times (760 \text{ mmHg} \times 1.5 \text{ atmospheres})$]. Great!

The second important law is **Henry's Law**, which states that the amount of gas a fluid will absorb under pressure varies in direct proportion to the partial pressure of the

gas. At sea level, blood absorbs a gas at one atmosphere, at two atmospheres it will absorb twice as much of this gas proportional to its partial pressure. We now more clearly see the importance of the partial pressure calculation. The amount of a gas that is absorbed by the blood and other tissue fluids is directly proportional to the partial pressure, which is directly proportional to the ambient pressure as governed by the depth of the dive. The reverse is also true. Champagne is bottled under pressure, so on removal of the cork, carbon dioxide previously in solution produces bubbles when the pressure is reduced. Likewise, gases in tissues may "bubble out" if a diver ascends too rapidly. This is called the bends, which we will discuss later in the chapter.

Physical and Physiological Principles of Scuba

We have learned that: (1) gas volume is affected by both pressure and temperature; (2) air has weight, and the greater the altitude, the less it weighs; (3) water is noncompressible (at 5000 feet below the surface a cubic foot of water weighs the same as at the surface); (4) at 33 feet below the surface of the sea, the water pressure is equivalent to one atmosphere; (5) the absorption of any gas by body fluids is proportional to its partial pressure; and (6) gases, once absorbed into tissue fluids, will form bubbles if pressure is too quickly released. Remember that the body contains air cavities, the most important being the lungs; and that the body (with the exception of air cavities) is essentially water and therefore noncompressible. These considerations are important to understand diving medicine[13,33] and some attendant hazards.[5]

Air Embolus

The term **embolus** comes from a Greek word meaning "plug"; it is used in physiology to refer to any material that enters the bloodstream and obstructs a blood vessel. We may consider the alveoli of the lungs as millions of small balloons. Let us suppose that, at a depth of 33 feet, a diver inhales a volume of air from his or her tank, holds the breath, and then proceeds to the surface. If the diver should be foolish enough to do this, the lungs would rupture and death would result. This is true because, as we have learned, gas volume is affected by pressure; the volume of gas the diver inhaled at a depth of 33 feet would double by the time he or she reached the surface, causing the alveoli to rupture. See figure 20.2.

Even under five feet of water, if a volume of air is breathed from the scuba tank and the breath is held while surfacing, overdistension of the lungs will occur. This in turn can cause rupture of the alveoli and perhaps pulmonary hemorrhage. The more severe rupture results in shattering

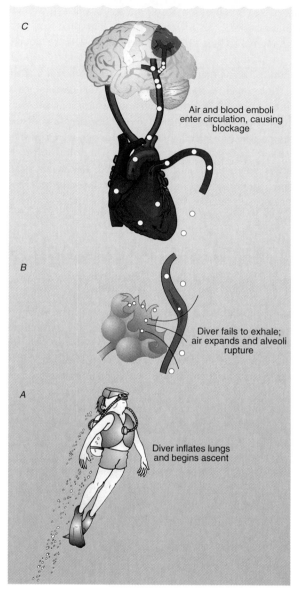

Figure 20.2
Formation of emboli as a diver ascends without exhaling.

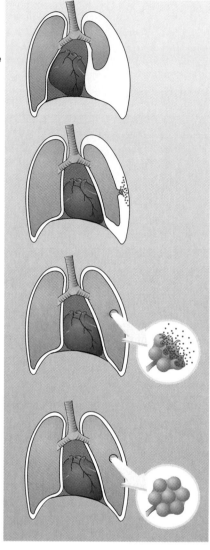

Figure 20.3
Spontaneous pneumothorax, caused by diver's failure to exhale during ascent.

of lung tissue, capillaries, and veins, and free air may be forced into the capillaries, forming emboli. The emboli may then enter the mainstream of the circulatory system, and the bubbles of air may find their way into the arteries of the heart and brain. As a consequence, circulatory blockage by the emboli and even death may occur. Probably the single most important consideration when giving scuba instruction is that *a diver must exhale as he or she surfaces. NEVER HOLD YOUR BREATH!*

Spontaneous Pneumothorax

Following rupture of lung tissue (alveoli), an accumulation of air or gas in the pleural cavity (intrathoracic space) may occur. This is referred to as a **pneumothorax.** As the diver con-

tinues to ascend, the pressure decreases, and the air that is in the pleural cavity, as a consequence of the lung rupture, will continue to expand, causing the ruptured lung to collapse (figure 20.3). In addition, the increasing volume of air will cause the collapsed lung and the heart to be pushed toward the opposite side of the chest. As a consequence, the diver may go into shock, and if the pneumothorax is sufficiently severe, death may result. Treatment requires surgical intervention with a syringe and needle to remove the air pocket.

Nitrogen Narcosis

Nitrogen narcosis is dependent primarily on the depth of the dive and secondarily on the length of time at that depth. Nitrogen narcosis affects the central nervous system: first

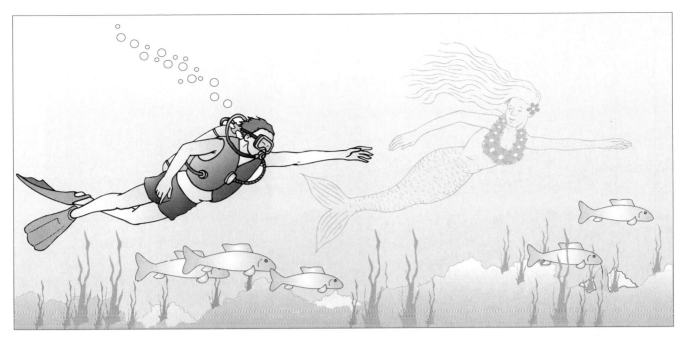

Figure 20.4

Nitrogen narcosis. Nitrogen has a narcotic effect on the nervous system similar to that of alcohol. Prolonged stay at depth may produce a euphoric condition such as is illustrated by the diver chasing the mermaid.

there is a sense of dizziness, then a slowing of mental processes, euphoria, and a fixation of ideas (figure 20.4).

The exact cause of these symptoms is difficult to explain. However, it is felt that because nitrogen is quite soluble in fatty tissue, the deeper the dive (i.e., exceeding 100 feet), the more nitrogen is forced into solution within the body. Its effects on the central nervous system are similar to those of alcohol. As a consequence, the "martini rule" has been formulated: 100 feet has the same effect as one martini on an empty stomach; 200 feet, two to three martinis; 300 feet, four martinis; and 400 feet, "tee many martoonis!"

One must recognize that the effects are quite individualistic and some people may be affected at moderate depths (50 feet or less)—the severity of the symptoms is unique to the individual. The U.S. Navy suggests the maximum depth for scuba should be set at 200 feet, with a practical limiting depth of 130 feet.[40]

The Bends

Nitrogen is inert—that is, this gas does not take part in respiratory exchange. The amount inhaled is equal to the amount exhaled.[20] As a diver descends, the pressure about the diver increases; this increased pressure will force nitrogen into solution within the blood. The deeper the dive, the greater the length of time for the dive, and the greater the exercise intensity, the more nitrogen will go into solution. The same principle prevails in carbonation of soft drinks.

The carbon dioxide (CO_2) is forced into the liquid under high pressure and the bottle is capped. When the cap is removed, the CO_2 escapes into the air in the form of bubbles because of the decreased pressure. Very rapid ascent by a diver to regions of lower pressure is similar to removal of the cap from the soda bottle in that the dissolved gas (nitrogen) is liberated in the form of bubbles. These nitrogen bubbles (gas emboli) may cause the **bends** (i.e., circulatory blockage and tissue damage) (figure 20.5). Exercise hastens the onset of the bends in that it is analogous to shaking a bottle of soda, causing a rapid and large release of gas bubbles. Pain is usually felt at the joints or ligaments and tendons first, within 24 hours following exposure; indeed, 85% of those suffering from the bends will have symptoms within four to six hours. Other symptoms besides pain in the legs or arms include dizziness, paralysis, shortness of breath, fatigue, and collapse with unconsciousness.

There is only one way in which the bends may be successfully treated and that is by recompression. The individual is placed into a chamber into which air is pumped, elevating the pressure and hence forcing the nitrogen bubbles back into solution. The diver then undergoes slow decompression, which allows the nitrogen to gradually come from solution (without the formation of bubbles) and be exhaled. This recompression process may require two to three hours to complete.[31]

Those responsible for the welfare of divers should be aware of the location of the nearest recompression chamber. The prevention of the bends requires a thorough knowledge of the recommended ascent patterns for divers from various

Surface

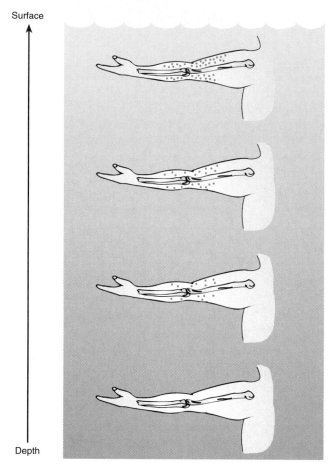

Depth

Figure 20.5

Bends. Increased pressure forces nitrogen into solution. Decreased pressure releases this nitrogen from solution into the blood and causes formation of gas bubbles in the tissues.

depths who had been submerged for various durations. These data can be found in the United States Navy Diving Manual.[40]

Oxygen Poisoning

The breathing of 100% oxygen, and the depth and duration of the dive are factors in the production of **oxygen poisoning** (figure 20.6). As was mentioned earlier, increasing the pressure of a gas over a liquid will cause more of the gas to go into solution. If oxygen is forced into solution, the tissues would first use the oxygen in solution as it is more readily available than is the oxygen carried by the red cell. At the same time, if the red blood cells are adequately loaded with oxygen, carbon dioxide, which is continually being formed, cannot be removed. Remember that the red blood cell carries oxygen from the alveoli to the cells and transports CO_2 from the cells to the alveoli. Because the red blood cell cannot dispose of the oxygen, it cannot as readily take on the CO_2, causing a buildup of CO_2 in body tissues. Excess CO_2 and O_2 in the tissues disturbs cerebral blood flow, resulting in the following symptoms of oxygen

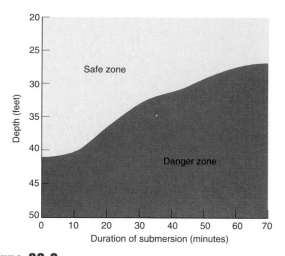

Figure 20.6

Oxygen poisoning is dependent on duration of submersion and depth of dive.

poisoning: tingling of fingers and toes, visual disturbance, acoustic hallucinations, sensations of abnormality, confusion, muscle twitching, unpleasant respiratory sensations, nausea, vertigo, lip twitching, and convulsions.

There is no place in amateur diving for the use of pure oxygen. One might ask why pure oxygen is ever used. Consider the Navy's UDT (Underwater Demolition Team) being given a project to destroy an enemy vessel. If you were the person on watch and observed bubbles coming toward your ship, what might you surmise? Quite obviously someone is "up to no good!" Navy divers must use a closed breathing system so that bubbles of expired air do not come to the surface, revealing their presence. The unit works by employing a chemical to absorb the CO_2 produced, and returning, hopefully, only oxygen and nitrogen to the tank. Unfortunately, a good chemical for ridding the expired air of all CO_2 has not as yet been perfected. The result is a possible buildup of CO_2, which may cause the diver to eventually lose consciousness.

Energetics of Swimming with Scuba

Swimming with scuba requires a greater energy utilization than swimming in water or moving in air. When swimming, the fluid medium provides a greater resistance to movement, and thus the $\dot{V}O_2$ is higher at a given swimming velocity. Scuba further increases the energy requirements primarily as a result of the extra drag caused by the scuba tank and the altered body position during swimming with scuba. In addition, swimming underwater requires the use of more leg kick because the arms are unable to provide significant forward propulsion.[29] Highly skilled swimmers have a significantly lower energy cost of swimming.[15a] While no studies have examined the energy cost of scuba between skilled and unskilled divers, one would predict that the skilled divers would be more efficient.

Because the legs are so important to movement in water, fins are used to enhance propulsion. In a recent study by Pendergast et al.,[29] divers preferred a large rigid fin over a small flexible fin. It is interesting to note that this type of fin was preferred although it had the higher energy cost.

In summary, Pendergast et al.[29] make the following recommendations to recreational divers:

1. Divers should maintain neutral buoyancy and maintain a horizontal position in the water to decrease the energy cost of swimming with scuba.
2. Divers should determine a balance between kicking frequency and kicking depth that will minimize drag and maximize efficiency.
3. Consider your swimming speed when selecting additional gear. Additional gear, like dry suits and double tanks, increases the energy cost of swimming only slightly at lower speeds, but at higher speeds the increase in energy cost can be significant.
4. Use a medium-sized, flexible fin to provide adequate propulsive force but not at a high energy cost.

Performance at Altitude

Acute Effects of Altitude

As we ascend above sea level, the barometric pressure (P_B) decreases as the weight of the atmosphere becomes less. The *percentage* of oxygen in the air remains 20.93, but the number of oxygen molecules per unit volume decreases. This means that, when at altitude, to receive the same number of molecules in a breath of air that we receive at sea level, we must breathe more air. The main reason for lessened performance at altitude is a consequence of the lowered oxygen partial pressure (PO_2). This lowered PO_2 results in **hypoxia,** which is lack of adequate oxygen. Some of the important physiological adjustments to acute altitude exposure are listed below.

1. *Increased pulmonary ventilation (hyperventilation).* This response is immediate (within a few hours) upon arrival at altitude, being more pronounced during the first few days, then stabilizing after about a week at altitude. The most important result of hyperventilation is an increased alveolar PO_2. This ensures a greater saturation of hemoglobin (Hgb) with oxygen (see figure 8.11, p. 205). Also, you may remember that with hyperventilation, excessive amounts of CO_2 are "blown off," thus decreasing both the alveolar PCO_2 and the H^+ concentration (increased pH) in the alveolus and blood.
2. *Increased resting and submaximal cardiac output.* The acute increase in cardiac output observed at altitude is a result of an increase in heart rate. The higher the altitude, the greater the heart rate. There is no change in stroke volume[12] in that the contractile function of the heart is maintained.[35]

3. *Elevation of pulmonary vascular resistance.* This results in higher blood pressures in the pulmonary circulation (pulmonary hypertension). In severe cases, it can lead to altitude sickness (pulmonary edema) and other physiological problems.

These major physiological changes are immediate and greatly aid in delivering oxygen to the tissues when oxygen is hard to come by (i.e., under hypoxic conditions). It is important to point out that some individuals become very sick when they go to altitude. The symptoms of mountain sickness may include pulmonary edema, nausea, vomiting, headache, rapid pulse, and anorexia (loss of appetite).[21,23]

A word of warning: severe cases of mountain sickness cause symptoms not unlike pneumonia—fever and congestion of the lungs (pulmonary edema)—even at an altitude of 10,000 feet. In more than one instance the diagnosis has been that these people were suffering from pneumonia; they were given antibiotics and left at altitude. As a result, the patients have died. Emergency treatment of severe mountain sickness consists of administering oxygen or removal to lower altitude or both. Services of a physician should be obtained at once.

Conditioned versus Nonconditioned Persons

Studies have shown that on first arriving at altitude, conditioned subjects have no greater advantage over their non-conditioned contemporaries beyond what they would have at sea level.[6] Fit persons will be able to perform more work, just as they can at sea level, than the unfit, but at a diminished output. They will not acclimatize any more rapidly, nor will they be any more immune to the discomforts of mountain sickness.[7] As a matter of fact, in one set of altitude studies[6,7] the most highly trained person became so ill at 3,800 meters that he had to be removed to a lower altitude, where he stayed for 2 days. He then returned to 3,800 meters for another two weeks, during which time he was a little better off, but not much.

Acute Effects of Altitude on Exercise Performance

At altitudes of over 5000 feet (1524 meters), the ability to perform physical work is affected—the higher the altitude, the more severe the effects. This is illustrated by the data shown in Figure 20.7. In the past, studies have established that there is a reduction in endurance capacity as measured by maximal oxygen consumption of 3% to 3.5% for every 300 meters ascended above 1500 meters.[10] Cymerman et al.[14] related the maximum oxygen consumption to the partial pressure of oxygen in the inspired air (figure 20.8). In one study, it has been proposed that impairment may begin as one ascends from sea level to moderate altitudes below

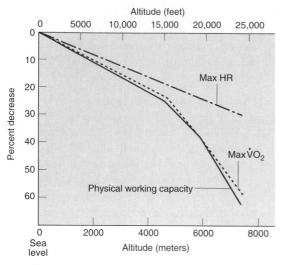

Figure 20.7

At altitudes of about 3000 feet (914 meters), small decrements in maximal oxygen consumption can be observed. At 5000 feet (1524 meters) and above, the decrement in max $\dot{V}O_2$ is 3 to 3.5% for every 1000 feet ascended. Physical working capacity and max $\dot{V}O_2$ are reduced by 60% or more at extremely high altitudes.

(Based on data from Squires and Buskirk[34] and Pugh.[30])

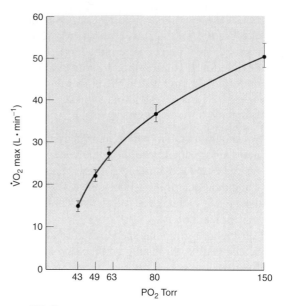

Figure 20.8

Plot showing a reduction of relative $\dot{V}O_2$ max with lower partial pressures of inspired oxygen as would be breathed at higher altitudes.[14]

1500 meters. The concept of a threshold for aerobic impairment may be misleading.[34] In figure 20.7, work performance and max $\dot{V}O_2$ are reduced by 60% or more at extremely high altitudes (i.e., at around 7600 meters).[20,43] Although such reductions in physical performance are quite large as they stand, these values were obtained on acclimatized and very fit mountain climbers. Acclimatization, as we will discuss later, refers to certain physiological adjustments that are brought about through continued exposure to altitude and which significantly improve performance. In unacclimatized subjects, the $\dot{V}O_2$ max decreases about the same as the acclimatized subject.[41]

Although more than 15 million people live at an altitude higher than 10,000 feet (3000 meters), most athletic competition in the United States takes place in areas located below this altitude. This means that because the effects of altitudes below 1500 meters are not great, from a practical standpoint, we need to be concerned mainly with the effects on athletic competition of altitudes between 1500 and 4500 meters. A review of the effects of hypoxia on human performance has been provided by Welch.[42]

Before discussing these results, we should point out that altitude mainly affects endurance or aerobic activities rather than sprint or anaerobic events. This makes sense because as has already been emphasized, hypoxia significantly reduces oxygen availability. The hypoxia may be reflected in a lower $\dot{V}O_2$ max and a lesser oxygen supply to the heart.[43,25] In shorter duration activities, especially those that are not dependent on aerobic metabolism, altitude is thought to have less of an effect. Interestingly, low levels of lactate

have been reported following exhaustive exercise at altitude.[17] This subsequently has been referred to by many investigators as the "lactate paradox." Studies have proposed that a reduced level of lactate in blood and muscles may serve a protective effect by minimizing reductions in the acidity (pH) of the muscle cell.[10]

The Oxygen Dissociation Curve and Altitude

What factors limit performance at altitude? You will recall from chapter 8 (p. 205) our discussion on the oxyhemoglobin dissociation curve. Briefly, the alveolar partial pressure of oxygen provides the pressure for the diffusion of oxygen into the alveolar capillaries as blood passes through the lungs. As we ascend to altitude, barometric pressure decreases and, as a consequence, so does the partial pressure of oxygen in the alveoli. This phenomenon is presented in table 20.1. As air enters the alveoli, we must subtract the partial pressure of water (47 mmHg at a temperature of 37°C). Assuming an alveolar oxygen concentration of 14.75%, we can see the effect on the partial pressure of oxygen in the lungs (P_AO_2).

At sea level, arterial blood is approximately 96% to 98% saturated with oxygen. At the conclusion of exhaustive exercise, the arterial saturation is still well maintained. As one ascends to altitude, arterial saturation at rest is lower. However, more importantly, the level of saturation of arterial blood following exhaustive work is diminished. This is

20.1
table

Effect of increasing altitude on the partial pressure of oxygen in the lungs (P$_A$O$_2$)

Altitude	Barometric pressure (mm Hg)	P$_B$ – 47 (mm Hg)	Alveolar oxygen fraction	P$_A$O$_2$ (mm Hg)
Sea level	760	713	.1475	105.0
5000 feet	638	591	.1475	87.0
7200 feet	586	539	.1475	79.5
10,000 feet	530	483	.1475	71.2

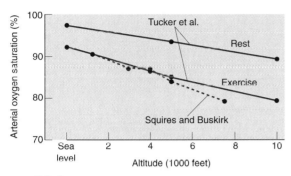

Figure 20.9

Changes in arterial oxygen saturation (SaO$_2$) with different altitudes. Resting and postexercise data from Tucker et al.[39] and postexercise data from Squires and Buskirk.[34]

illustrated in figure 20.9, where the difference between rest and exercise arterial oxygen saturation was 5.1%, 9.4%, and 10.8% at sea level, 1500 meters, and 3000 meters, respectively.[39] Also shown in Figure 20.9 are the postexercise data from another study involving different altitudes.[34] Note the remarkable agreement between the two studies for the level of arterial oxygen saturation following exercise.[34,39] One may conclude from these data not only that the resting arterial saturation for oxygen is lowered at altitude but also that saturation is progressively less complete during more intense work at higher altitude.

Acclimation to Altitude Exposure

It is widely accepted that hypoxia stimulates a number of acclimatization mechanisms, depending on altitude and duration of stay. The important physiological changes that take place during acclimatization to altitude include:[24]

1. *Increased number of red blood cells and hemoglobin concentration.* This is rapid during the first few weeks at altitude, with the increase becoming more gradual thereafter. The function of this response is to increase the oxygen content of the arterial blood.

2. *Elimination of bicarbonate (HCO$_3^-$) in the urine.* This adjustment requires several days. Although this mechanism per se does not enhance oxygen availability, its main function is to maintain blood pH at near normal values. Remember, with hyperventilation and loss of CO$_2$, the blood pH tends to increase; elimination of bicarbonate is offsetting, causing a decrease in pH.

3. *Tissue level changes.* These changes include (a) increased muscle and tissue capillarization, (b) increased myoglobin concentration, (c) increased mitochondrial density, and (d) enzyme changes that enhance the oxidative capacity. Unlike the previously mentioned acclimatization processes, these cellular changes take more time. In fact, they are most developed in long-time residents of high-altitude regions.

When the person returns from a 3- to 4-week sojourn at altitude, he or she will lose these changes brought about by acclimatization within a period of about two to four weeks.

Acclimatization and Exercise Performance at Altitude

The longer you remain at altitude, the better your performance becomes, but it never quite reaches the values that are obtained at sea level. As mentioned, the improved performance during a stay at altitude is brought about through **acclimatization.** The number of weeks to acclimatize depends on the altitude—i.e., for 2700 meters, about 7 to 10 days; for 3600 meters, 15 to 21 days; and for 4600 meters, 21 to 25 days. These are only approximations; a great deal depends on the individual. As a matter of fact, a few people will never acclimatize and will continue to suffer **mountain** (or **altitude) sickness**[21,23] while at altitude. This happens even with people who were born and raised at altitude. Suddenly, for unknown reasons, they lose their acclimatization and suffer from mountain sickness.

table

20.2

Average physical and physiological characteristics of high-school athletes

	Athletes native to 3100 meters	Athletes native to 300 meters
Age	17 years	17 years
Height	176 cm	175 cm
Weight	68 kg	66 kg
Max $\dot{V}O_2$ (low altitude)	66 ml·kg^{-1}·min^{-1}	66 ml·kg^{-1}·min^{-1}

From Robert F. Grover, et al., "Muscular Exercise in Young Men Native to 3,100 m Altitude." in *Journal of Applied Physiology*, 1967, 22(3):555–64. Copyright © 1967 American Physiological Society. Reprinted by

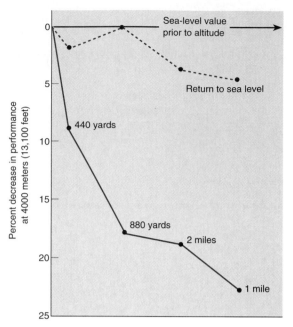

Figure 20.10

Decreases in running performances at 13,000 feet (4000 meters). The decreases in performance are most pronounced in the longer events where the oxygen system is the predominant energy pathway. Notice that the performances did not exceed their prealtitude values on returning to sea level.

(Based on data from Buskirk et al.[9])

Several studies on the effect of altitude on athletic performance have been conducted involving both high school and college athletes. The results provide important information regarding the effects of training and acclimatization on competitive athletic performances. This section will focus on the effects of altitude on endurance or aerobic activities rather than on sprint or anaerobic events, because, as already mentioned, hypoxia significantly reduces oxygen availability, and thus performance, in endurance events.

The Lexington-Leadville Study[22]

The primary purpose of this very interesting study with high-school athletes was to determine whether lifelong acclimatization to altitude would give the native an advantage over the newcomer in regard to track performance. Two groups of athletes were studied:

1. Five members of the track team of Lafayette High School, Lexington, Kentucky (altitude, 300 meters or 1000 feet); and
2. Five athletes from Lake County High School, Leadville, Colorado (altitude, 3100 meters or 10,200 feet).

The Leadville students had to be selected from other sports (skiing, basketball, or football) as the high school had no organized track team. They did, however, have four months of training prior to a track meet with the Kentucky high school track team. Table 20.2 contains the physical and physiological characteristics of these young athletes. The interesting thing to note is the high maximum oxygen consumption values these young men obtained while running on a treadmill. The data may be compared with those appearing in table 4.8, page 89.

The experiment consisted of having two track meets between the teams, one in Leadville and the other in Lexington. In Leadville, the competition was held on the twentieth day of residence at altitude for the Kentucky team. Table 20.3 contains the running times for the track events at both altitudes. The Kentucky team (who incidentally were the Kentucky State Champions in 1964) was superior and won the competition at both low and high altitudes. These track times show that hypoxia as a consequence of altitude affects the long-term resident just as it does the newcomer during strenuous activity. The athlete or team that is highly successful in competition at sea level should be equally successful at altitude.

The faster times obtained by the Kentucky team in the 220- and 440-yard sprints at altitude may be due in part to the lessened atmospheric density at 3100 meters (about one-third less dense than that at sea level). At any rate, these results clearly indicate that anaerobic events are not adversely affected by moderate altitude.

The Pennsylvania State University Study[9]

A study of equal interest was conducted by E. Buskirk and others of Pennsylvania State University. They took several members of Penn State's track team to Nunoa, Peru, which is at an altitude of 13,000 feet (4000 meters). Figure 20.10 shows the average decreases in running performance

20.3 table

Running times for track events at 300 and 3100 meters*

| Running Distances | | Lexington team Altitude (meters) | | Leadville team Altitude (meters) | |
		300	3100	300	3100
Yards	Meters	Time (min:sec)		Time (min:sec)	
220	201	0:24.0	0:22.4	0:25.7	0:27.0
440	402	0:54.0	0.51.0	1:03.5	0:52.5
880	804	2:10.0	2:11.5	2:24.7	2:30.0
1760	1608	4:49.0	5:10.9	5:23.5	5:35.0

From Robert F. Grover, et al., "Muscular Exercise in Young Men Native to 3,100 m Altitude." in *Journal of Applied Physiology,* 1967, 22(3):555–64. Copyright © 1967 American Physiological Society. Reprinted by permission.

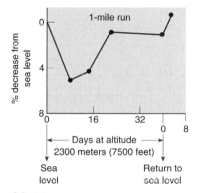
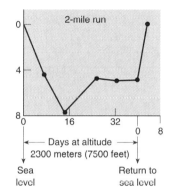
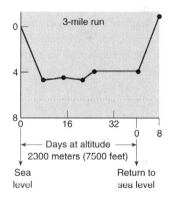

Figure 20.11

Decreases in running performances at 7500 feet (2300 meters). These results indicate that even at moderate altitude, physical performance, particularly if it relies heavily on the aerobic system, will be impaired and will not always improve with acclimatization.

(Based on data from Faulkner et al.[19])

experienced by the runners. The running times were obtained after 40 to 57 days at altitude, that is, after acclimatization had occurred. As was the case with the high-school runners, the decreases in performance were most pronounced in the longer events, where the oxygen system is the predominant energy pathway.

Following three weeks of residence at altitude, the runners began participating in soccer with the Indian natives. After five weeks of residence the track runners were as good as the natives, with four of the runners eventually playing on the winning team! During a track meet held at 13,000 feet, the runners won over the best times for the Indians by one minute in the one-mile event and by two minutes in the two-mile event. These results again point out that altitude effects the working capacity of the native in much the same manner as it does the newcomer to altitude.

It is of further interest to note from figure 20.1 that upon return to sea level the athletes' performances were not improved as a result of training at altitude. As a matter of fact, performances in the one-mile and two-mile events were slower the third and fifteenth days after return from altitude.

The Michigan-Penn State Study[18]

In another study by Dr. Buskirk and associates, twelve athletes, some of whom were top-rated middle-distance runners, were studied at various altitudes over a five- to six-week period. The results of their time trials at an altitude of 7500 feet (2300 meters) are shown in figure 20.11. Three points are worth noting: First, all performances were not quite as good as at sea level. Second, the decrease in performance was related, once again, to the duration of the event; the longer the race, the greater the oxygen needed and the poorer the performance. Third, the two- and three-mile performances were not improved with acclimatization as was the performance in the mile run. Also of interest is that the maximal aerobic power did not improve with acclimatization.

These results indicate that even at moderate altitude (7500 feet), physical performance, particularly if it relies heavily on the aerobic system, will be impaired and will not always improve with acclimatization.

The California-Colorado Study[1]

In this study, twelve middle-distance runners, each having recently completed a competitive track season, were divided into two groups. One group trained for three weeks at sea level (Davis, California) running 19.3 km (12 miles) per day. The other group trained with an identical training program at an altitude of 2300 meters or 7500 feet (Colorado Springs, Colorado). The two groups then exchanged sites and followed similar training programs for an additional three weeks. Periodically, the runners ran two-mile competitive time trials and had their maximal aerobic powers (max $\dot{V}O_2$) determined on a motor-driven treadmill. The results are shown in figure 20.12. Three features are observable: (1) both the max $\dot{V}O_2$ and two-mile performance were significantly decreased at days 1 and 3 of altitude; (2) only a slight (2%) improvement in max $\dot{V}O_2$ and the two-mile performance was made after 18 to 20 days of acclimatization to altitude; and (3) performances equaled but did not exceed their pre-altitude values on returning to sea level. The authors concluded that there is no potentiating effect of hard endurance training at 2300 meters over equivalently severe sea-level training on sea-level max $\dot{V}O_2$ or on two-mile performances in already well-conditioned middle-distance runners.[1]

The Ohio State Studies[6,7,8]

Twenty-five young college men were studied at Columbus, Ohio (altitude, 750 feet or 230 meters) and at the Barcroft Research Station, White Mountain, California (altitude, 12,470 feet or 3800 meters). The following conclusions were reached:

1. The physical fitness of healthy individuals, measured at sea level, is not a sufficient index of their ability to perform hard physical work at high terrestrial altitudes.
2. Physical fitness appears to bear no relationship to the occurrence of symptoms of acute altitude sickness. The extremely fit person is as likely to become ill as is the sedentary person.
3. Ability to perform hard physical work at high altitudes improves markedly during three weeks of continuous residence at such altitudes. It does not, however, approach sea-level work capacity during this period of time.

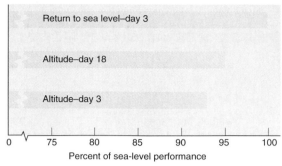

2-mile run

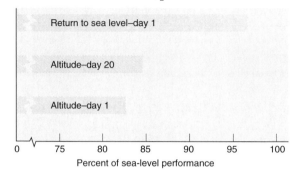

Max $\dot{V}O_2$

Figure 20.12

Performance in the two-mile run and maximal aerobic power (max $\dot{V}O_2$) during exposure to an altitude of 7500 feet (2300 meters). Note that (1) both max $\dot{V}O_2$ and two-mile performances were significantly decreased at days 1 or 3 of altitude; (2) only a slight (2%) improvement in max $\dot{V}O_2$ and the two-mile run was made after 18 to 20 days of acclimatization; and (3) performances equaled but did not exceed their prealtitude values on returning to sea level.

(Based on data from Adams et al.[1])

4. Some subjects, regardless of physical condition, do not tolerate altitude well and may be expected to become ineffective or ill.
5. All healthy individuals, other than those with a predisposition to altitude sickness, can work steadily for one-half hour or more at a level that is roughly half their sea-level capacity at 12,500 feet immediately after arrival.
6. Only a minority will be able to sustain one-half hour of work at two-thirds of their sea-level work capacity even after eight days at altitude.

Training and Altitude

When Mexico City (elevation, 7400 feet or 2250 meters) was named as the site for the 1968 Olympic games, coaches immediately asked: How can we train our athletes to best withstand any effects of altitude on their performance? Should they train only at altitude? If so, at what altitude and

table 20.4

Time trials in running before, during, and after training at an altitude of 7500 feet (2300 meters)*

Event	Time at sea level (min:sec)	Time at altitude (min:sec)			Time on return to sea level (min:sec)	
		Day 3	**Day 14**	**Day 21**	**Day 1**	**Day 21**
880-yard run	2:41	2:48	2:38	2:37	2:32	2:32
1-mile run	6:07	6:30	—	6:15	5:49	5:38
2-mile run	13:08	13:45	13:09	—	12:22	11:57

*Based on data from Faulkner, Daniels, and Balke.[18]

for how long? Should they train intermittently at altitude and at sea level? Because the answers to these questions were not available, a great deal of research was initiated.

From a theoretical viewpoint, training at altitude could produce more rapid and even greater physiological changes than could training at sea level only. The reason for this is that altitude hypoxia is a stress that produces physiological changes (acclimatization) similar to those caused by physical training. For example, total blood volume, hemoglobin, red blood cell count, mitochondrial concentration, and muscle enzyme changes have all been shown to be enhanced in both types of stress. To a certain extent, this idea has been supported experimentally. For example, in several well-controlled studies using nonathletes[3,32] greater increases in maximal aerobic power and endurance time were seen when the training sessions were conducted at altitude (7400 to 11,300 feet) rather than at sea level. In addition, we have shown that some effects of eight weeks of interval training can be maintained for an additional 12 weeks by use of two three-hour exposures to a simulated altitude of 15,000 feet (4572 meters). During the exposures, the subjects did not perform any exercise, but merely rested.[4] Other studies[2,18] have shown improved performances at sea level after training at altitude and at simulated altitude.[37] Some of the results are given in table 20.4. However, in these studies, it was not determined whether the increased sea-level performances were due to altitude exposure per se or to the fact that the subjects eventually increased their fitness level during the conditioning at altitude. In other words, it is possible that their performances would have been improved with further training even at sea level.

Figures 20.10, 20.11, and 20.12 show that in studies involving highly trained athletes, performance on return from altitude was not much different from prior performance at sea level; if anything, some were poorer. This would indicate that for the highly trained athlete, training at and acclimatization to altitude does not improve perfor-

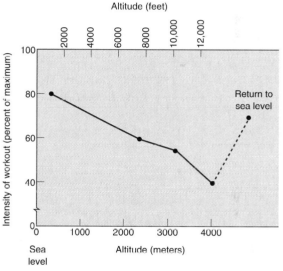

Figure 20.13

Intensity of training workouts for six collegiate runners at various altitudes. Even though their coach was present at all workouts, it is clear that altitude greatly reduced their training efforts.

(Based on data from Kollias and Buskirk.[26])

mance. Also, as already pointed out, maximal aerobic power and performance of these athletes do not always improve with altitude acclimatization. One of the major reasons for this might be that the training programs required for these athletes cannot be sustained at altitude at an intensity and duration commensurate with that at sea level.[26] This can be seen from figure 20.13, which gives the intensity of the training workouts for six collegiate runners at various altitudes. Although their coach was present at all workouts, it is clear that altitude greatly reduced their training efforts.

It remains to be seen whether training at altitude significantly improves athletic performance upon returning to sea level. More recently studies have attempted to provide appropriate experimental designs to answer this question.[27,36] However, even in these studies, methodological problems preclude one from saying that altitude training is beneficial. In addition to answering that basic question, more studies need to address the duration of the activity, timing of return to sea level, and other relevant questions. If you wish to train your athletes at altitude for whatever reason, the following guidelines may prove to be helpful:[15]

1. Adequate training facilities and training atmospheres must be available.
2. The bulk of time spent at altitude should be at moderate altitude (6500 to 7500 feet).
3. Short exposure to higher altitude should be included regularly during the general training period at moderate elevation.
4. Steady altitude exposures should be limited to periods of two to four weeks, with intermittent sea-level or lower elevation trips scheduled to insure maintenance of muscular power and normal competitive rhythm and intensity of effort.
5. Training at altitude should emphasize maintenance of muscular power yet be geared to include normal or near normal overall amounts of work.
6. Important sea-level efforts should be scheduled about two weeks after leaving altitude.

Performance during and after Microgravity Exposure

At present, human space travel is a very costly endeavor and restricted to only a few select individuals. However, with the planned space station, a possible trip to Mars, and a permanent habitation facility either in space or on the moon, more humans will be spending longer periods of time in microgravity environments.

Several problems have been noted with the limited data collected on the long term effects of microgravity. Three major problems have emerged: bone demineralization, muscle atrophy, and cardiovascular deconditioning. Bone demineralization occurs primarily as a result of lack of stress on bone tissue and a greater resorption rate of existing bone tissue. Loss of bone has been noted in several of the longer Russian flights.[11] Muscle atrophy and a concomitant loss of strength has been reported after both Russian and U.S. space flights. It appears as if the degree of muscle atrophy is dependent on the time exposed to microgravity. Cardiovascular deconditioning is a catch-all term for the overall changes in the cardiovascular system with exposure to microgravity. Three major results of

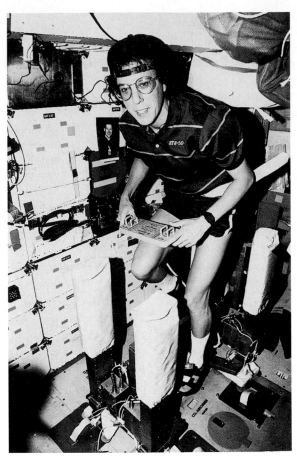

Figure 20.14
Astronaut exercising on a stepping ergometer during space travel.

cardiovascular deconditioning have been documented: a loss of $\dot{V}O_2$ max, alterations in orthostatic tolerance, and an increase in exercise heart rate secondary to loss of fluid volume.

Orthostatic tolerance describes the inability to maintain blood pressure with changes in posture—i.e., moving from the supine to the erect posture. Many of these same changes have been documented with the aging process. Knowledge of the efficacy of exercise in remediating these changes will have important spinoffs in aging research.

Given these changes, it is readily apparent that the exercise responses will be affected both during microgravity exposure and upon return to the earth. You would think that many studies would have been performed in space; however, few studies have looked at the changes in exercise performance during space flight because of the difficulty in controlling on-board activities. While few controlled studies have taken place in space (figure 20.14), a number of studies have used simulated microgravity to look at the effects of microgravity on exercise performance. One way to simulate microgravity is bedrest. When you are in bed for long periods of time, your body is not exposed to the normal gravity loads that we are subjected to when we are mobile. Therefore, bones and muscles are subjected to less stress and as a result they experience the previously mentioned effects. A specialized form of bed rest is head-down tilt bedrest. In this simulation, the subjects head is positioned at 6 degrees below the feet. In this position, fluid shifts from the feet to the head, thus simulating the fluid shifts that occur in space. Another technique used to simulate microgravity is head-out water immersion. For obvious reasons, this technique is limited to the study of the short-term effects of microgravity.

Exercise Performance during Microgravity

One consistent finding with exposure to simulated microgravity (bedrest) is a decrease in $\dot{V}O_2$ max proportional to the length of the bedrest (figure 20.15). Because of the methodological difficulties in performing a maximal oxygen consumption test in space, reductions in $\dot{V}O_2$ max have not been well documented in true microgravity conditions. In spite of these problems, measurements of $\dot{V}O_2$ max were performed during the Skylab mission. Surprisingly, in that study $\dot{V}O_2$ max actually increased (figure 20.16).[28] How is this possible? Exercise was an important part of the daily operations in Skylab. The crew members may have increased their $\dot{V}O_2$ max because they trained more in space than they did on the earth. It is important to note that it is probably difficult to get a true $\dot{V}O_2$ max in microgravity, thus what was actually being measured was the peak $\dot{V}O_2$.

If maximal responses are altered, at least during simulated microgravity, what are the effects of microgravity on submaximal exercise responses? Submaximal responses seem to be dependent on the length of exposure. In Skylab experiments, heart rates in response to a standardized work rate (approximately 75% of $\dot{V}O_2$ max) were not different in flight compared to preflight measurements.[28] Skylab missions were 28, 59, and 84 days long. In one of the Russian Salyut missions, one that lasted 140 days, different responses were observed. Heart rates during the mission were higher than heart rates obtained at the same work rate before the mission.[44] They also report a decrease in stroke volume in flight. This is likely a consequence of a decrease in cardiac filling caused by a decrease in blood volume and not a reduction in the contractile function of the heart.

Muscle atrophy is a common finding with prolonged microgravity. In a recent study, muscle biopsies were taken on astronauts before and after 5 to 11 days of space flight.[16] These results are summarized in table 20.5. Overall, there was a reduction in fiber cross-sectional area in both fiber types; however, the authors note that there was a great deal of variability between subjects. When they looked at the physical activities of the astronauts involved in the study, they noticed that the degree of atrophy of fiber types might be related to the amount of physical activity performed in flight.

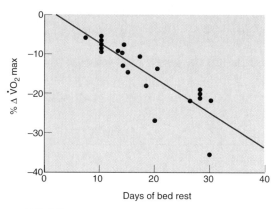

Figure 20.15
Plot showing that decreases in $\dot{V}O_2$ max are proportional to the length of exposure to simulated microgravity (days of bed rest).[11]

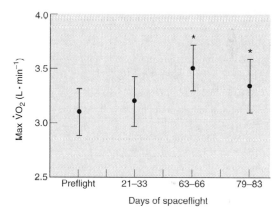

Figure 20.16
Plot showing a significant improvement (see) in absolute $\dot{V}O_2$ max during the latter phases of a Skylab mission.[28]

These anatomical changes have been reflected in functional changes in muscle. Muscle strength has been shown to decrease in the Skylab missions.[38] Strength loss was greater in the legs than in the arms, probably due to lack of postural stress on the legs. This will be an important factor to consider when designing exercise programs for astronauts.

Exercise Performance after Exposure to Microgravity

Upon return to a gravitational environment, it is generally agreed that work performance is affected in many ways. It has been suggested that $\dot{V}O_2$ max decreases upon return to Earth. While $\dot{V}O_2$ max measurements have been made postflight, they all have been confounded by the use of countermeasures designed to minimize the physical changes that accompany exposure to microgravity. Many bed rest studies have demonstrated reductions in $\dot{V}O_2$ max. For example,

20.5

Muscle fiber size and enzymatic properties before and after spaceflight*

	Type I fibers			Type II fibers		
	Preflight	**Postflight**	**%Δ**	**Preflight**	**Postflight**	**%Δ**
% Fiber type	44 ± 11	37 ± 9	−16	56 ± 10	61 ± 7	+11
Fiber CSA (μm^2)	5472 ± 1789	4655 ± 1475	−15	5517 ± 2479	4279 ± 1680	−22
ATPase activity	383 ± 73	376 ± 73	− 2	471 ± 79	513 ± 84	+ 9
SDH activity	232 ± 65	203 ± 66	−13	184 ± 55	158 ± 48	−14
GPD activity	5.9 ± 4.7	10.6 ± 11.4	+80	25.0 ± 7.9	23.0 ± 12.9	− 8

*Values are means ± standard deviations; size is expressed as cross-sectional area (CSA). For type analyses, the total number of fibers was 1,875 fibers. All enzyme measures (ATPase = myofibrillar adenosinetriphosphate; SDH = succinate dehydrogenase; GPD = α-glycerophosphate dehydrogenase) were made on a total of 714 fibers. From V. R. Edgerton, et al., "Human Fiber Size and Enzymatic Properties After 5 and 11 Days of Spaceflight" in *Journal of Applied Physiology*, 78:1733–1739, 1995. Copyright © 1995 American Physiological Association, Bethesda, MD. Reprinted by permission.

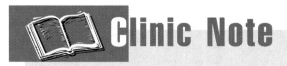

Clinic Note

Aging in Space

Many similarities exist between aging and exposure to microgravity. It is well documented that bone mass, muscle mass, and muscle force production all decline with age. Somewhere in the middle of the third decade of life, formation of new bone fails to keep up with bone resorption and there is a reduction of bone mass. Some of the loss of bone is a direct result of disuse in older adults. In a study by Krolner and Toft (1983), subjects lost 1% of their bone per week during one month of bed rest. Similar findings from space flights have been reported (Leblanc and Schneider, 1991). Maximum grip strength of elderly males (mean age = 79) was one-half that of younger individuals (mean age = 25 yr) (Burke et al., 1953). This is a result of significant reductions in muscle mass in the elderly (Larsson et al., 1978).

As exercise has been proposed as a means of minimizing changes in physical function with microgravity, so has it been proposed to improve physical function in older adults. Many of the results from simulated microgravity experiments could have a direct bearing on physical function in older adults. Many of the same exercise programs proposed for astronauts in space could benefit older adults.

combined results from five studies demonstrated a reduction in $\dot{V}O_2$ max of 5.2% to 9.7%.[11]

One would predict that muscle cross-sectional area, and thus muscle strength, would decline given the lack of gravity in space. While these adaptations would not have negative consequences in space, upon return to earth, function would be significantly impaired. Numerous studies have documented decreases in cross-sectional area and strength with both simulated and true microgravity.[12] Interestingly, in many of the Russian flights where exercise is an integral part of the daily routine, muscle strength declines are minimal. The Russians have used a wide variety of exercise devices to maintain strength. The most unique of these is a suit called the penguin suit. Springs connected to the appendages provide a continuous load to the arms and legs. Cosmonauts wear the suit for up to eight hours a day in an attempt to maintain a resistive stress on the muscles of the torso and appendages.

Exercise as a Countermeasure

For humans to work and live in microgravity environments, many of the negative adaptations that occur will need to be offset by countermeasures specifically designed to maintain human function. To this point, many countermeasures have been proposed, including: simulated gravity on the spacecraft, salt intake and fluid loading to restore plasma volume, and exercise.

At this point you would probably agree that the potential for exercise as a countermeasure for microgravity is limitless. Many studies are now focused on determining the ideal exercise to minimize changes in bone mineralization, muscle atrophy, and cardiovascular deconditioning. The types of exercise being considered include aerobic and high-resistance exercise (both concentric and eccentric). Several recent studies have suggested that eccentric exercise has a great deal of potential as an exercise countermeasure especially since there are relatively few eccentric types of contractions performed while living/working in a microgravity environment.[11] It has been well documented on Earth that eccentric exercise can improve muscle function. Consideration must be given to the potential for muscle tearing and other injuries with this type of exercise when recommending it for use as an in-flight countermeasure.

Summary

Four laws govern the manner in which gas volumes, partial pressures, and absorption of gases by liquids (blood) are influenced. These are Boyle's pressure/volume Law, Charles's temperature/gas volume Law, Dalton's partial pressure Law, and Henry's liquid absorption Law. An understanding of these laws allows for an understanding of many differences in physiological responses and risks associated with hyperbaric (scuba) and hypobaric (high altitude) environments.

Scuba is an excellent sport and can be performed safely, provided that the physiological concepts are understood and applied. Make sure that you select the gear (wet/dry suit, fins, type of tank) that best suits your specific needs. Do not hold your breath when ascending!

At altitudes over 5000 feet (1524 meters), the ability to perform physical work is decreased due to hypoxia (lowered PO_2). However, physical performance at moderate altitude may sometimes be improved with continued stay at altitude due to the acclimatization process. This involves (1) increased red blood cell and hemoglobin concentrations, (2) elimination of bicarbonate (HCO_3^-) in the urine, and (3) in those chronically exposed to altitude, tissue level changes. Increased physical fitness alone does not acclimatize the individual to altitude.

Altitude mainly affects endurance or aerobic activities rather than sprint or anaerobic events. This is because the major problem is hypoxia, which significantly reduces oxygen availability. While anaerobic performance is not significantly influenced, the lactate response is blunted at altitude.

Training at altitude might enhance performance at sea level but well controlled studies have not been performed to document any improvement. For the highly trained athlete, the training intensity required for maintenance of peak performance cannot be achieved at altitude.

Exposure to simulated and true microgravity results in decreases in muscle cross-sectional area and strength; in simulated microgravity, to decreases in $\dot{V}O_2$ max. Exercise is a viable countermeasure for the physical changes that occur during microgravity exposure. The type and duration of exercise that will be most effective in maintaining function still needs to be determined.

Questions

1. For a mixture of gases, how is the partial pressure calculated?
2. Why is knowing the partial pressure of a gas in a mixture so important to determining its absorption by body fluids?
3. What happens to gases in liquids when the pressure that put them there is released very quickly?
4. Discuss the effects of increasing and decreasing the pressure, while holding temperature constant, on (a) a given volume of water, and (b) a given volume of gas.
5. At 33 feet below the surface of the sea, the weight of water above the diver will be equal to 1 additional atmosphere. Why is this true?
6. Describe how a diver may suffer an air embolism.
7. What is spontaneous pneumothorax, and how is it treated?
8. What is the effect of nitrogen narcosis on a diver?
9. How may one avoid developing the bends during a dive?
10. What are the physiological principles underlying oxygen poisoning while diving?
11. What is the importance of the eustachian tube for one who descends below the surface of the sea or ascends to altitude?
12. Define acclimatization to altitude and discuss the physiology involved.
13. How is performance affected at altitude?
14. How does training at altitude affect performance at altitude and at sea level?
15. What are three problems related to bone and muscle tissue that are known to occur with prolonged exposure to microgravity?
16. Similarly, three major problems of cardiovascular deconditioning have been documented with prolonged exposure to microgravity. What are they?
17. What are the overall effects on maximal exercise performance from exposure to simulated microgravity (bedrest)? What are the effects on submaximal exercise responses?
18. When muscles atrophy as a result of spaceflight, is most of the size reduction in Type I or Type II muscle fibers?
19. Generally speaking, what is the effect of spaceflight on $\dot{V}O_2$ max measures made after return to earth? What has confounded these measures?

20. What countermeasures have been advocated to offset the negative adaptations that occur when humans work and live in microgravity environments?

21. What types of exercise are being considered important as countermeasures? Have all the details on this matter been worked out? Why/why not?

References

1. Adams, W. C., E. M. Bernauer, D. B. Dill, and J. B. Bomar. 1975. Effects of equivalent sea-level and altitude training on $\dot{V}O_2$ max and running performance. *J Appl Physiol.* 39(2):262–266.

2. Balke, B., F. Nagle, and J. Daniels. 1965. Altitude and maximum performance in work and sports activity. *JAMA.* 194:646–649.

3. Banister, E. W., and W. Woo. 1978. Effects of simulated altitude training on aerobic and anaerobic power. *Eur J Appl Physiol.* 38:55–69.

4. Bason, R., E. Fox, C. Billings, J. Klinzing, K. Ragg, and E. Chaloupka. 1973. Maintenance of physical training effects by intermittent exposure to hypoxia. *Aerospace Med.* 44(10):1097–1100.

5. Becker, G. 1983. Recurrent alternobaric facial paralysis resulting from scuba diving. *Laryngoscope.* 93:596–598.

6. Billings, C., R. Bason, D. Mathews, and E. Fox. 1971. Cost of submaximal and maximal work during chronic exposure at 3,800 m. *J Appl Physiol.* 30(3):406–408.

7. Billings, C., R. Brashear, D. Mathews, and R. Bason. 1969. Medical observations during twenty days at 3800 meters. *Arch Environ Health.* 18:987–995.

8. Billings, C., D. Mathews, R. Bartels, E. Fox, R. Bason, and D. Tanzi. 1968 (June). *The Effects of Physical Conditioning and Partial Acclimatization to Hypoxia on Work Tolerance at High Altitudes.* Columbus, OH: Ohio State University Research Foundation Report RF 2002–2004.

9. Buskirk, E., J. Kollias, R. Akers, E. Prokop, and E. Picon-Reátegui. 1967. Maximal performance at altitude and on return from altitude in conditioned runners. *J Appl Physiol.* 23(2):259–266.

10. Buskirk, E., J. Kollias, E. Picon-Reátegui, R. Akers, E. Prokop, and P. Baker. 1967. Physiology and performance of track athletes at various altitudes in the United States and Peru. In Goddard, R. (ed.), *The International Symposium on the Effects of Altitude on Physical Performance.* Chicago: The Athletic Institute.

11. Convertino, V. A. 1996. Exercise and adaptation to microgravity environments. In Fregley, M. J., and C. M. Blatteis. (eds), *Handbook of Physiology, section 4: Environmental Physiology.* New York: Oxford University Press, pp. 815–843.

12. Convertino, V. A. 1990. Physiological Adaptations to Weightlessness: Effects on Exercise and Work Performance. In J. Holloszy (ed.), *Exercise and Sport Science Reviews.* Baltimore: Williams and Wilkins, pp. 119–166.

13. Crook, R. 1977. Basic medical implications of scuba diving. *J Otolaryngology.* 6:519–523.

14. Cymerman, A., J. T. Reeves, J. R. Sutton, P. B. Rock, B. M. Groves, M. K. Malconian, P. M. Young, P. D. Wagner, and C. S. Houston. 1989. Operation Everest II: maximal oxygen uptake at extreme altitude. *J Appl Physiol.* 66:2446–2453.

15. Daniels, J. 1972. Effects of altitude on athletic accomplishment. *Mod Med.* June 26:73–76.

15a. DiPrampero, P. E., D. R. Pendergast, D. R. Wilson, and D. W. Rennie. 1974. Energetics of swimming in man. *J Appl Physiol.* 37:1–5.

16. Edgerton, V. R., M. Y. Zhou, Y. Ohira, H. Klitgaard, B. Jiang, B. Bell, B. Harris, B. Saltin, P. D. Gollnick, R. R. Roy, M. K. Day, and M. Greenhisen. 1995. Human fiber size and enzymatic

    properties after 5 and 11 days of spaceflight. *J Appl Physiol.* 78:1733–1739.

17. Edwards, H. T. 1936. Lactic acid in rest and work at high altitude. *Am J Physiol.* 116:367–375.

18. Faulkner, J., J. Daniels, and B. Balke. 1967. Effects of training at moderate altitude on physical performance capacity. *J Appl Physiol.* 23(1):85–89.

19. Faulkner, J., J. Kollias, C. Favour, E. Buskirk, and B. Balke. 1968. Maximum aerobic capacity and running performance at altitude. *J Appl Physiol.* 24(5):685–691.

20. Fox, E., and R. Bowers. 1973. Steady-state equality of respiratory gaseous N_2 in resting man. *J Appl Physiol.* 35:143–144.

21. Green, I. D., and R. F. Fletcher (eds.). 1979. Acute mountain sickness. *Postgrad Med J.* 55(645):441–515.

22. Grover, R., J. Reeves, E. Grover, and J. Leathers. 1967. Muscular exercise in young men native to 3,100 m altitude. *J Appl Physiol.* 22(3):555–564.

23. Houston, C. S. 1976. High altitude illness: disease with protein manifestations. *JAMA.* 236(19):2193–2195.

24. Hurtado, A. 1964. Acclimatization to high altitudes. In W. Weihe (ed.), *The Physiological Effects of High Altitude.* New York: Macmillan, pp. 1–17.

25. Kaijser, L., J. Grubbstrom, and B. Berglund. 1990. Coronary circulation in acute hypoxia. *Clin Physiol.* 10:259–263.

26. Kollias, J., and E. Buskirk. 1974. Exercise and altitude. In Johnson, W., and E. Buskirk (eds.), *Science and Medicine of Exercise and Sports,* 2d ed. New York: Harper and Row, pp. 211–227.

27. Levine, B. D., and J. Stray-Gunderson. 1992. A practical approach to altitude training: where to live and train for optimal performance enhancement. *Int J Sp Med.* 13:S209–S212.

28. Michel, E. L., J. A. Rummel, C. F. Sawin, M. C. Buderer, and J. D. Lem. 1977. Results of Skylab medical experiment M171— metabolic activity. In R. S. Johnston and L. F. Dietlein (eds.), *Biomedical Results from Skylab: NASA SP-37,* pp. 372–387.

29. Pendergast, D. R., M. Tedesco, D. M. Nawrocki, and N. M. Fisher. 1996. Energetics of underwater swimming with scuba. *Med Sci Sports Exerc.* 28(5):573–580.

30. Pugh, L. 1964. Muscular exercise at great altitudes. In W. Weihe (ed.), *The Physiological Effects of High Altitude.* New York: Macmillan, pp. 209–210.

31. Radermacher, P., B. Santak, C. Muth, J. Wenzel, L. Vogt, M. Hahm, and K. Falke. 1990. Nitrogen partial pressures in man after decompression from simulated scuba dives. *Scand J Clin Lab Invest.* (50 suppl.) 203:217–221.

32. Roskamm, H., F. Landry, L. Samek, M. Schlager, H. Weidemann, and H. Reindell. 1969. Effects of a standardized ergometer training program at three different altitudes. *J Appl Physiol.* 27(6):840–847.

33. Segadal, K., A. Gulsvik, and G. Nicolaysen. 1990. Respiratory changes with deep diving. *Eur Respir J.* 3:101–108.

34. Squires, R. W., and E. R. Buskirk. 1982. Aerobic capacity during acute exposure to simulated altitude, 914 to 2286 meters. *Med Sci Sports Exerc.* 14(1): 36–40.

35. Suarez, J. M., J. K. Alexander, and C. S. Houston. 1987. Enhanced left ventricular systolic performance at high altitude during Operation Everest II. *Am J Cardiol.* 60:137–142.

36. Terrados, N., E. Jansson, C. Sylven, and L. Kaijser. 1990. Is hypoxia a stimulus for synthesis of oxidative enzymes and myoglobin? *J Appl Physiol.* 68:2369–2372.

37. Terrados, N., J. Melichna, C. Sylven, E. Jansson, and L. Kaijser. 1988. Effects of training at simulated altitude on performance and muscle metabolic capacity in competitive road cyclists. *Eur J Appl Physiol.* 57:203–209.

38. Thornton, W. E., and J. A. Rummel. 1977. Muscular deconditioning and its prevention in spaceflight. In R. S. Johnston and L. F. Dietlein (eds.), *Biomedical Results from Skylab: NASA SP-37,* pp. 191–197.

39. Tucker, A., J. M. Stager, and L. Cordain. 1984. Arterial O_2 saturation and maximum O_2 consumption in moderate-altitude runners exposed to sea level and 3,050 m. *JAMA.* 252(20):2867–2871.

40. *U. S. Navy Diving Manual.* 1970. Washington, D.C.: Department of Navy.

41. Ward, M. P., J. S. Milledge, and J. B. West. *High Altitude Medicine and Physiology.* London: Chapman and Hall Medical, 1995.

42. Welch, H. 1987. Effects of hypoxia and hyperoxia on human performance. *Exercise and Sport Sciences Reviews.* 15:191–221.

43. West, J. 1990. Limiting factors for exercise at extreme altitudes. *Clin Physiol.* 10:265–272.

44. Yegorov, A. D., O. G. Itsekhovsky, A. P. Polyakova, V. F. Turchanimova, I. V. Alferova, V. G. Savelyeva, M. V. Domracheva, T. V. Batenchuk-Tusko, V. G. Doroshev, and Y. A. Kobzev. 1981. Results of studies of hemodynamics and phase structure of the cardiac cycle during functional test with graded exercise during 140 days aboard the Salyut-6 station. *Kosm Biol Aviakosm Med.* 15(3):18–22.

Selected Readings

American Medical Association. 1974. Standards for cardiopulmonary resuscitation (CPR) and emergency cardiac care (ECC). Supplement to *JAMA.*

Bentz, R. L. 1979. Development of the Navy Mark 14 Underwater Breathing Apparatus. *Nav Eng J.* 91(2):91–98.

Crosbie, W. A., J. W. Reed, and M. C. Clarke. 1979. Functional characteristics of the large lungs found in commercial divers. *J Appl Physiol.* 46(4):639–645.

Davies, C. T. M., and A. J. Sargeant. 1974. Effects of hypoxic training on normoxic maximal aerobic power output. *Eur J Appl Physiol.* 33:227–236.

Fox, E. L. 1979. *Sports Physiology.* Philadelphia: W. B. Saunders, pp. 185–188.

Goddard, R. (ed.). 1967. *The International Symposium on the Effects of Altitude on Physical Performance.* Chicago: The Athletic Institute.

Heath, D., and D. R. Williams. 1979. The lung at high altitude. *Invest Cell Pathol.* 2(3):147–156.

Hegnauer, A. (ed.). 1969. *Biomedicine Problems of High Terrestrial Elevations.* Natick, MA: U. S. Army Research Institute of Environmental Medicines.

Humpeler, E., K. Inama, and P. Deetjen. 1979. Improvement of tissue oxygenation during a 20 days-stay at moderate altitude in connection with mild exercise. *Klin Wochenschr.* 57(6):267–272.

Hurtado, A. 1964. Animals in high altitudes: resident man. In *Handbook of Physiology, Section H, Adaptation to the Environment.* Washington, D.C.: American Physiological Society.

Luce, J. M. 1979. Respiratory adaptations and maladaptation to altitude. *Physician Sportsmed.* 7(6):54–59, 62–65, 68–69.

Maher, J. T., L. G. Jones, and L. H. Hartley. 1974. Effects of high-altitude exposure on submaximal endurance capacity of men. *J Appl Physiol.* 37(6):895–898.

Margaria, R. (ed.). 1967. *Exercise at Altitude.* New York: Excerpta Medica Foundation.

Miles, S. 1962. *Underwater Medicine.* Philadelphia: J. B. Lippincott.

Pugh, L. 1967. Athletes at altitude. *J Physiol.* 192:619–646.

Rattner, B. A., S. P. Gruenau, and P. D. Altland. 1979. Cross-adaptive effects of cold, hypoxia, or physical training on decompression sickness in mice. *J Appl Physiol.* 47(2):412–417.

Strauss, R. H. (ed.). 1976. *Diving Medicine.* New York: Grune & Stratton.

Weihe, W. (ed.). 1964. *The Physiological Effects of High Altitude.* New York: Macmillan.

Appendices

Appendix A

Symbols, Abbreviations, and Norms

Selected Symbols and Abbreviations

ADP	=	adenosine diphosphate
ATP	=	adenosine triphosphate
$a - vO_2diff$	=	arterial-mixed venous oxygen difference
$°C$	=	degrees Celsius (centigrade)
CA	=	carbonic anhydrase
Ca^{++}	=	calcium ion
CO_2	=	carbon dioxide
d	=	distance
db	=	dry bulb (temperature)
e^-	=	electron
F	=	force
FA or FFA	=	fatty acid or free fatty acid
FFB	=	fat-free body
F_x	=	fractional (decimal) concentration of a gas
g	=	black globe temperature
H	=	hydrogen atom
H^+	=	hydrogen ion
Hgb	=	hemoglobin
$HgbO_2$	=	oxyhemoglobin
HCO_3^-	=	bicarbonate ion
Hg	=	mercury
HR	=	heart rate
H_2CO_3	=	carbonic acid
H_2O	=	water
kcal	=	kilocalorie
$kcal \cdot min^{-1}$	=	kilocalories per minute
kg	=	kilogram
L	=	liter
LBW	=	lean body weight
m	=	meter
max $\dot{V}O_2$	=	maximal volume of oxygen that can be consumed per minute during exercise (expressed in $L \cdot min^{-1}$ or $mL \cdot kg^{-1} \cdot min^{-1}$)
meq	=	milliequivalent

MET	=	metabolic equivalent: ≈ 3.5 ml of O_2 consumed per kg of body weight per minute ($mL \cdot kg^{-1} \cdot min^{-1}$)
min	=	minute
mL	=	milliliter
mm	=	millimeter
mmol	=	millimole
Na^+	=	sodium ion
O_2	=	oxygen
P	=	power
P_B	=	barometric pressure
PC (or CP)	=	phosphocreatine of creatine phosphate
P_{CO_2}	=	partial pressure or carbon dioxide
Pi	=	inorganic phosphate
P_{mean}	=	mean arterial pressure
P_{N_2}	=	partial pressure of nitrogen
P_{O_2}	=	partial pressure of oxygen
P_X	=	partial pressure of gas "X"
$\dot{Q}$	=	cardiac output in liters per minute ($L \cdot min^{-1}$)
RM	=	repetition maximum
s	=	second
SV	=	stroke volume
t	=	time
T_sP_r	=	total systemic peripheral resistance
$\dot{V}$	=	volume per minute
$\dot{V}_E$	=	minute ventilation, or amount of air expired ($L \cdot min^{-1}$)
$\dot{V}O_2$	=	volume of oxygen consumed per minute ($L \cdot min^{-1}$ or $mL \cdot kg^{-1} \cdot min^{-1}$)
V_T	=	tidal volume
WB	=	wet bulb
WBGT	=	wet bulb globe temperature
WBT	=	wet bulb temperature

Symbols and Abbreviations Used by Pulmonary Physiologists*†

Before 1950, each pulmonary physiologist had developed a jargon of his or her own. In 1950 a group of American pulmonary physiologists, as a way to lessen confusion, agreed to use a standard set of symbols and abbreviations. The symbols below are used in equations in this book and in most original articles published since 1950; they cannot be applied to earlier articles.

Special Symbols

– Dash above any symbol indicates a *mean value*.
· Dot above any symbol indicates a *time derivative*.

For Gases

Primary Symbols (large capital letters)

V = gas volume
$\dot{V}$ = gas volume per unit time
P_x = gas pressure (gas "X")
$\bar{P}$ = mean gas pressure
F = fractional concentration in dry gas phase
f = respiratory frequency (breaths per unit time)
D = diffusing capacity

R = respiratory exchange ratio

Examples

V_A = volume of alveolar gas
$\dot{V}O_2$ = O_2 consumption per minute
$P_{A_{O_2}}$ = alveolar O_2 pressure
$\bar{P}_{C_{O_2}}$ = mean capillary O_2 pressure
$F_{I_{O_2}}$ = fractional concentration of O_2 in inspired gas

D_{O_2} = diffusing capacity for O_2 (ml O_2 per minute per mm Hg)
R = $\dot{V}_{CO_2}/\dot{V}_{O_2}$

Secondary Symbols (small capital letters)

I = inspired gas
E = expired gas
A = alveolar gas
T = tidal gas
D = dead space gas
B = barometric
STPD = 0° C, 760 mm Hg, dry
BTPS = body temperature and pressure saturated with water vapor
ATPS = ambient temperature and pressure saturated with water vapor

Examples

$F_{I_{CO_2}}$ = fractional concentration of CO_2 in inspired gas
$\dot{V}_E$ = volume of expired gas (L · min^{-1})
$\dot{V}_A$ = alveolar ventilation per minute
V_T = tidal volume
V_D = volume of dead space gas
P_B = barometric pressure

For Blood

Primary Symbols (large capital letters)

Q = volume of blood
$\dot{Q}$ = volume of blood flow per unit time

C = concentration of gas in blood
S = percent saturation of Hgb with O_2 or CO

Examples

Qc = volume of blood in pulmonary capillaries
$\dot{Q}$c = blood flow through pulmonary capillaries per minute

Ca_{O_2} = ml O_2 in 100 ml arterial blood
$S\bar{v}_{O_2}$ = saturation of Hgb with O_2 in mixed venous blood

---

*From Comroe, J. H., et al. 1962. *The Lung*, 2d ed. Chicago: Year Book Medical Publishers, Inc., 1962. (Based on report in *Fed Proc.* 9:602–605.)
†Bartels, H. B., et al. 1973. Glossary on respiration and gas exchange. *J Appl Physiol.* 34:549–558.

Secondary Symbols (small letters)

a = arterial blood
v = venous blood
c = capillary blood

Examples

Pa_{CO_2} = partial pressure of CO_2 in arterial blood
$P\bar{v}_{O_2}$ = partial pressure of O_2 in mixed venous blood
Pc_{CO_2} = partial pressure of CO_2 in pulmonary capillary
blood

For Lung Volumes

VC	= vital capacity	= maximal volume that can be expired after maximal inspiration
IC	= inspiratory capacity	= maximal volume that can be inspired from resting expiratory level
IRV	= inspiratory reserve volume	= maximal volume that can be inspired from end-tidal inspiration
ERV	= expiratory reserve volume	= maximal volume that can be expired from resting expiratory level
FRC	= functional residual capacity	= volume of gas in lungs at resting expiratory level
RV	= residual volume	= volume of gas in lungs at end of maximal expiration
TLC	= total lung capacity	= volume of gas in lungs at end of maximal inspiration

Typical Values for Pulmonary Function Tests

These are values for a healthy, resting, recumbent 70 kg adult (1.7 square meters of surface area), breathing air at sea level, unless other conditions are specified. They are presented merely to give approximate figures. These values may change with position, age, size, gender, and altitude; variability occurs among members of a homogeneous group under standard conditions.

Lung Volume (BTPS)

Inspiratory capacity, mL	3600
Expiratory reserve volume, mL	1200
Vital capacity, mL	4800
Residual volume (RV), mL	1200
Functional residual capacity, mL	2400
Thoracic gas volume, mL	2400
Total lung capacity (TLC), mL	6000
RV/TLC × 100, percent	20

Ventilation (BTPS)

Tidal volume, mL	500
Frequency, respirations per minute	12
Minute volume, mL · min^{-1}	6000
Respiratory dead space, mL	150
Alveolar ventilation, mL · min^{-1}	4200

Alveolar Ventilation/Pulmonary Capillary Blood Flow

$\dot{V}_A$ (L · min^{-1}) / blood flow (L · min^{-1})	0.8
Physiologic shunt / cardiac output × 100, percent	<7
Physiologic dead space / tidal volume × 100, percent	<30

Pulmonary Circulation

Pulmonary capillary blood flow, mL · min^{-1} 5400
Pulmonary artery pressure, mm Hg .... 25 / 8
Pulmonary capillary blood volume, mL 90
Pulmonary "capillary" pressure (wedge), mm Hg 8

Alveolar Gas

Oxygen partial pressure, mm Hg 104
CO_2 partial pressure, mm Hg 40

Diffusion and Gas Exchange

O_2 consumption (STPD), resting, mL · min^{-1} 240
CO_2 output (STPD), resting, mL · min^{-1} 192
Respiratory exchange ratio, R (CO_2 output / O_2 uptake) 0.8
Diffusing capacity, O_2 (STPD) resting, mL O_2 · min^{-1} · mm Hg^{-1} .... >15
Maximal diffusing capacity, O_2 (STPD), exercise, mL O_2 · min^{-1} · mm Hg^{-1} 60

Arterial Blood

O_2 saturation (saturation of Hgb with O_2), percent 97.1
PO_2 (partial pressure of O_2), mm Hg 98
PCO_2 (partial pressure of CO_2), mm Hg 40
Alveolar-arterial PO_2 difference, mm Hg 9
O_2 saturation (breathing 100% O_2), percent 100
PO_2 (breathing 100% O_2), mm Hg 640
pH 7.4

Mechanics of Breathing

Maximal voluntary ventilation (BTPS), L · min^{-1} 170
Forced expiratory volume, percent in 1 second 83
                                percent in 3 seconds 97
Maximal expiratory flow rate (for 1 liter) (ATPS), L · min^{-1} .... >400
Maximal inspiratory flow rate (for 1 liter) (ATPS), L · min^{-1} .... >300
Compliance of lungs and thoracic cage, L · cm H_2O^{-1} 0.1
Compliance of lungs, L · cm H_2O^{-1} 0.2
Airway resistance, cm H_2O · L^{-1} · s^{-1} 1.6
Pulmonary resistance, cm H_2O · L^{-1} · s^{-1} 1.9
Work of quiet breathing, kg-m · min^{-1} 0.5
Maximal work of breathing, kg-m · breath^{-1} 10
Maximal inspiratory and expiratory pressures, mm Hg 60–100

The Cell

Life is maintained at the cellular level and is dependent primarily on the movement of food, electrolytes, gases, and waste products into and out of the cell. When this delicate equilibrium is interrupted, serious consequences prevail, and death may occur if the situation is not remedied immediately. Comprehending the principles of cellular exchange is extremely important if trainers, clinicians, physical educators, and coaches are to be knowledgeable about their professions. For example, the principles of cellular exchange play an important part in respiration, gas exchange, metabolism, and thermoregulation.

The interior of the cell is composed of organic and inorganic materials dissolved in H_2O; these substances are constantly involved in a myriad of chemical reactions to produce energy, and hence maintain life. Outside of every cell is the **interstitial fluid,** whose composition is quite similar to the interior of the cell. Food and gases move from the blood through the interstitial fluid and into the cell, while waste materials produced in the cell move through the interstitial fluid and into the blood. Forces are constantly at work to maintain this dynamic equilibrium. Diffusion, facilitated diffusion, osmosis, electrical potential, and active transport are the forces that allow this delicate balance between the inside and the outside of the cell to be maintained.

Diffusion

Because of its kinetic energy, each molecule is in constant vibration, and as a result, those contained within a given volume are constantly colliding with one another. This vibrating and colliding results in a mixing of the molecules throughout the system. This randomness of movement, or **diffusion,** is an excellent mixing device and is the most important means by which particles move into and out of the cell. *In diffusion, particles always move from a region of higher concentration to one of lower concentration.* For example, oxygen (O_2) moves from the capillary to the interstitial fluid and from the interstitial fluid into the cell. By the same token, carbon dioxide (CO_2) moves from the cell through the interstitial fluid and into the capillaries. There

are by far a greater number of O_2 molecules in the blood moving about in random fashion, which is why more diffuse from the blood toward the cell. By the same token, CO_2 is produced in the cell, and the random motion of these molecules will result in their greater diffusion out of the cell through the interstitial fluid and into the capillaries. When the concentration of molecules is greater on one side of a membrane than on the other, a *diffusion gradient* exists. One might say that the O_2 has a "downhill grade" toward the cell, whereas CO_2 has a "downhill grade" toward the capillary. Figure B.1 diagrammatically portrays this phenomenon.

Facilitated Diffusion

Each cell is surrounded by a membrane that is very thin—only two molecules thick. The cell membrane is made up of two classes of molecules: lipids (fats) and protein, and is called a lipid matrix (figure B.2). As we have just seen, in ordinary or free diffusion, carbon dioxide, oxygen, and some other compounds (e.g., fatty acids and alcohol) move easily across the cell membrane. To accomplish this they must (1) pass through the pores of the outer membrane, (2) dissolve into the matrix, (3) diffuse to the inner membrane, and (4) finally pass through the inner membrane wall and into the interior of the cell.

Glucose, however, because of its larger molecular weight, cannot diffuse through the pores of the cell membrane. Consequently, it must find some other means of diffusing through to the inner membrane wall. This is accomplished with the help of a carrier protein. Figure B.2 shows how it works. The carrier protein (let's call it X) binds with glucose at the outer membrane of the matrix, forming a compound we can call glucose-X. Through a change in the conformation of the carrier protein, glucose-X transports glucose to the inner membrane of the lipid matrix, where the carrier protein breaks away—allowing glucose to pass through to the inside of the cell. The carrier protein is ready to once again transport glucose to the inside of the cell. This process is called **facilitated diffusion** because the carrier protein facilitates the transport of glucose into the cell.

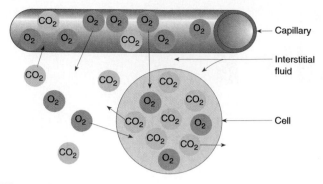

Figure B.1

Diffusion between cell and capillary. Because of a higher concentration of CO_2 in the cell, more CO_2 moves toward the capillary; on the other hand, a greater concentration of O_2 in the capillary causes more O_2 to move toward and into the cell by diffusion. Water, CO_2, and O_2 pass freely into and out of the cell.

Osmosis

Small molecules and other particles, such as CO_2 and O_2, pass into and out of the cell membrane through pores, with ease, as was discussed previously. However, certain molecules are too large to find passage through the pores of the cell membrane and, as a result, too little or too much water moves into or out of the cell causing it to swell or shrink. The reason for this may be explained in the following manner. Consider a cell with only water on the inside and outside. As water molecules pass easily into and out of the cell through diffusion, there will be an equal number of molecules on either side of the cell membrane; a diffusion gradient does not exist. Now suppose there were a number of large nondiffusible particles (too large to get through the pores) on the outside of the membrane, which reduces the concentration of water on that side of the membrane. This means that as the number of moles of dissolved particles in a solution increases, the mole fraction of water decreases (i.e., pure water becomes less pure). Water will then flow down its concentration gradient from the high water concentration side (in the above example, from inside of the cell) to the lower water concentration side (outside of the cell)—which, by the way, is the definition of **osmosis.** Osmosis is a special case of diffusion that occurs when you have: (1) a semipermeable membrane, and (2) a liquid containing more particles on one side of the membrane.

Osmosis can be demonstrated using a U-tube with a semipermeable membrane that separates pure water from a solution of sodium chloride (NaCl). The relatively large sodium (Na^+) and chloride (Cl^-) ions find it difficult to move through the membrane. As a result of the presence of these particles on one side of the membrane, the concentration of water is lowered. Water will then diffuse, as it normally does, from the high-water concentration (water only) side of the semi-permeable membrane to lower water con-

centration side. It will continue to do so until the pressure on the side of the membrane containing Na^+ and Cl^- produces a force tending to drive molecules out of its compartment that is equal to the force tending to drive molecules into the compartment. This force is called **osmotic pressure** and works against the tendency of water to diffuse into a compartment of higher concentration of ions.

Figure B.3 depicts two U-tubes with a semipermeable membrane separating the solutions. In figure B.3, the solutions (A_1 and A_2) on either side of the membrane contain an *equal* number of Na^+ and Cl^-. The membrane is not permeable to these ions; however, water will pass through from one side to the other in equal amounts. As a result, the solutions are said to be **isotonic** to each other. Also in figure B.3, side B_1 contains fewer Na^+ and Cl^- than side B_2. Gradually more water molecules will diffuse to B_2. Solution B_2 is said to be **hypertonic** to side B_1. Conversely, B_1 is said to be **hypotonic** to side B_2.

A practical application of this principle can be observed using red blood cells in three different saline solutions: (1) a solution isotonic to the internal mixture of the cell, (2) a solution hypertonic to the internal mixture of the cell, and (3) a solution hypotonic to the internal mixture of the cell. Can you deduce what would happen to the cell in each of the three conditions? Figure B.4 contains three test tubes with the aforementioned solutions. Observe what has happened in each instance to the red blood cell.

Electrical Forces

The capacity for producing electrical effects is called **electrical potential.** When certain compounds, such as NaCl, are placed in water, they ionize—that is, the sodium breaks away from the chlorine, resulting in a positively charged sodium ion (cation), or Na^+, and a negatively charged chloride ion (anion), or Cl^-. Like charges repel, and unlike charges attract. An important difference between the intracellular fluid and the interstitial fluid is the concentration of ions. Sodium, calcium, and chloride concentrations are many times greater outside the cell; on the other hand, potassium, magnesium, and phosphate concentrations are greater inside the cell. As a result of the distribution of these ions, the fluid inside of the cell has a negative charge (between -75 and -95 millivolts) when expressed relative to the fluid outside the cell.

This negative *electrochemical force* on the inside of the cell tends to attract the positively charged cations into the cell and to drive the negatively charged anions out of the cell. For example, K^+ would tend to diffuse from the cell because of its high concentration, but the influence of the internal negative charge would cause the K^+ to remain within the cell. These two forces (diffusion gradient and electrochemical force) are *almost* equal but are sufficiently unequal to favor the movement of K^+ outside the cell. The opposite is true for Cl^-. Chloride ions have a high interstitial

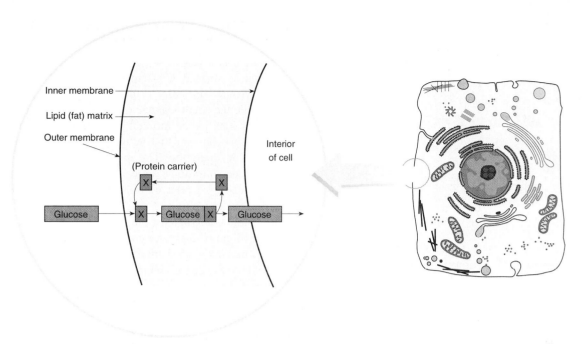

Figure B.2

The membrane of a cell is composed of a lipid (fat) matrix. Relative to facilitated diffusion, a carrier protein (X) combines with glucose just inside the outer membrane of the matrix, forming a compound called glucose-X. The glucose diffuses across to the inner membrane of the matrix. The carrier then breaks away, and glucose passes into the cell.

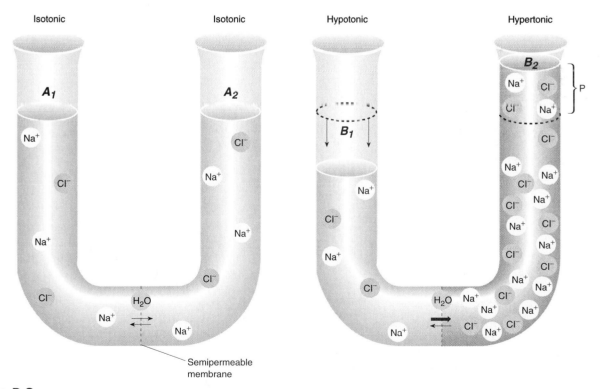

Figure B.3

U-tubes with semipermeable membranes separating the solutions. Solutions A_1 and A_2 contain an equal number of Na^+ and Cl^- ions. Water will pass in both directions through the semipermeable membrane in equal amounts; the solutions are isotonic to each other. Solution B_1 contains fewer Na^+ and Cl^- ions than solution B_2. More water molecules will therefore diffuse to solution B_2. This will continue until solutions on both sides of the membrane are of equal concentrations, or osmotic pressure (P) overcomes further movement.

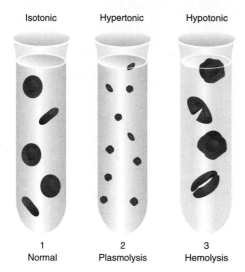

Isotonic   Hypertonic   Hypotonic

1   2   3
Normal   Plasmolysis   Hemolysis

Figure B.4

Three test tubes containing isotonic, hypertonic, and hypotonic solutions. In test tube 1, the solution is isotonic, and therefore the cells retain their normal size and shape. In tube 2, the solution is hypertonic to the interior of the cells, causing them to lose water and shrink (plasmolysis). In tube 3, the solution is hypotonic, causing the cells to "take on" water and swell or even burst (hemolysis).

concentration, which would cause diffusion into the cell, but the electric forces are sufficient to keep the Cl^- from entering the cell. In other words, the chloride ions inside the cell are in electrochemical equilibrium with those on the outside.

Active Transport

Sodium is a large ion because it attracts water molecules about its surface. Consequently, although it is a cation, it experiences difficulty in penetrating the pores of the cell. Despite the small leakage of sodium into the cell, the number of ions inside the cell remains small, which suggests that a mechanism that actively removes sodium from the cell is in operation. The movement of substances against their concentration gradients by the expenditure of metabolic energy is referred to as **active transport.** Remember, when sodium moves from the inside to the outside of the cell, it is going against the concentration gradient ("uphill," for sodium is in greater concentration outside the cell). It is also moving against the electrochemical force, because the inside of the cell is electrically negative, and unlike charges attract. Exactly how this comes about is unknown, but we observe that as sodium leaves the cell, K^+ enters. This phenomenon, which is referred to as the **sodium-potassium pump,** maintains an equilibrated movement of Na^+ and K^+ against the diffusion gradient and the electrochemical forces.

Diffusion, both free and facilitated, osmosis (hydraulic pressure), electrochemical potential, and active transport are the forces that move materials into and out of the cell. This is a dynamic process going on continuously. The time factor for a given particle to diffuse from the capillary to the cell and vice versa is measured in microseconds at the cellular level. Upsetting this equilibrium, as mentioned earlier, can result in serious physiological consequences.

Appendix C

The Gas Laws

Gas volume is dependent on temperature and pressure. For example, a given number of gas molecules occupies a greater volume at a higher temperature and lower pressure than at a lower temperature and higher pressure. By the same token, an unequal number of gas molecules could occupy the same volume, but only at different temperature or pressures. In other words, two gas volumes of one liter each could contain an unequal number of gas molecules only if the temperature or pressure of the two volumes were different. On the other hand, whenever the temperature and pressure of two equal volumes of gases are the same, the two volumes will always contain the same number of molecules. Because of a change or difference in temperature or pressure from day-to-day or from one laboratory to another, respiratory gas volumes must be corrected to a reference temperature and pressure so that valid comparisons can be made.

ATPS Conditions

The conditions of temperature and pressure at the precise time a respiratory gas volume is measured are abbreviated **ATPS**. This abbreviation means ambient temperature and pressure, saturated with water vapor. Ambient temperature refers to the temperature of the gas in the device measuring volume (i.e., spirometer) and ambient pressure refers to the environment or barometric pressure at the time of the measurement. The volume is also assumed to be saturated with water vapor at spirometer temperature because a water-sealed wet spirometer is often the instrument used for making the measurement (chapter 7). In other words the gas is collected over water and is assumed to be saturated with water vapor. It is this volume, under various ATPS conditions, which must be corrected to a reference temperature and pressure before any comparisons can be made.

STPD Conditions

There are two reference conditions of temperature and pressure with which you will be concerned. The first of these is standard temperature and pressure, dry, abbreviated **STPD**.

Standard temperature is $0°$ C and standard pressure is 760 mm Hg. "Dry" means that the volume occupied by molecules of water vapor has been adjusted for (i.e., the gas volume at STPD is that volume occupied by all gas molecules except those of water vapor). The number of gas molecules and the volume they occupy under STPD conditions is constant and independent of the particular gas involved. In other words, one mole of any gas (e.g., 32 grams of oxygen) at STPD contains 6.02×10^{23} molecules and occupies 22.4 liters. Therefore, a volume of gas under STPD conditions represents the number of gas molecules present. Corrections of gas volumes from ATPS to STPD are made whenever we need to know the *amount* or number of gas molecules (e.g., when calculating the amount of oxygen consumed and the amount of carbon dioxide produced). Such corrections always result in a reduction of volume for several reasons: (1) ambient (spirometer) temperature is higher than $0°$ C, for example, from $20°$ to $25°$ C; (2) ambient pressure in most parts of the country is below 760 mm Hg; and (3) the gas is "dried."

BTPS Conditions

The other reference point for making gas volume corrections is body temperature and pressure, saturated with water vapor, abbreviated **BTPS**. Body temperature is $37°$ C and body pressure is the same as ambient pressure. Corrections of gas volumes from ATPS (or from STPD, for that matter) to BTPS are made when we are interested in knowing the *volume* of air that is ventilated by the lungs versus the number of gas molecules present. When air at room temperature (e.g., $22°$ C) is inspired, its volume will expand in the lungs as a result of: (1) the increase in temperature (from $22°$ to $37°$ C) and (2) the addition of water vapor molecules because of the increase in temperature. Corrections to BTPS are necessary, therefore, for all respiratory gas measurements dealing with volume (e.g., vital capacity, tidal volume, minute volume, and maximal breathing capacity).

Calculation of Volume Corrections

Calculations of gas volume corrections for differences in temperature, pressure, and water vapor are based on several gas laws irrespective of the specific correction to be made. Remember that correction from ATPS to STPD is made when we are concerned with the amount or number of gas molecules present, such as in calculating oxygen consumption and carbon dioxide production; on the other hand, correction to BTPS is made when we are concerned with the volume occupied by the gas molecules, such as in determining lung volumes.

Temperature Correction

Gas volume is directly related to temperature, so that increasing or decreasing the temperature of a gas (at constant pressure) causes a proportional increase or decrease, respectively, in volume. This is known as *Charles's law*. It states that the change in temperature as determined by the ratio of the initial temperature (T_1) to that of the final or corrected temperature (T_2) is equal to the change in volume or to the ratio of the initial volume (V_1) to that of the final or corrected volume (V_2). In mathematical form:

$$\frac{T_1}{T_2} = \frac{V_1}{V_2} \qquad (1)$$

The units for temperature in this case are those of either the Absolute (A) or the Kelvin (K) scale, in other words, $273°$ K $= 0°$ C; $°$ K $= 273° + °$ C (e.g., $22°$ C $= 273° + 22° = 295°$ K).

Rearranging equation (1) to solve for V_2:

$$V_2 = \frac{V_1 \times T_2}{T_1} \qquad (2)$$

In correcting a gas volume to standard temperature ($0°$ C):

V_1 = volume ATPS (V_{ATPS})
V_2 = volume corrected to standard temperature (V_{ST})
T_1 = absolute gas meter temperature ($273°$ K $+$ T$°$ C)
T_2 = absolute standard temperature ($273°$ K)

and

$$V_{ST} = V_{ATPS} \frac{273°}{273° + T} \qquad (3)$$

In correcting to body temperature (BT) or $37°$ C, then:

V_2 = volume corrected to body temperature (V_{BT})
T_2 = absolute body temperature
$\quad = 273°$ K $+ 37°$ C $= 310°$

and

$$V_{BT} = V_{ATPS} \frac{310°}{273° + T} \qquad (4)$$

Pressure and Water Vapor Corrections

Gas volume is inversely related to pressure, so that increasing or decreasing the pressure of a gas (at constant temperature) causes a proportional decrease or increase, respectively, in volume. This is known as *Boyle's law*. It states that the change in pressure is determined by the ratio of the initial pressure (P_1) to the final or corrected pressure (P_2) is equal to the volume change or the ratio of the final or corrected volume (V_2) to the initial volume (V_1). In other words:

$$\frac{P_1}{P_2} = \frac{V_2}{V_1} \qquad (5)$$

Again, rearranging to solve for V_2:

$$V_2 = V_1 \left(\frac{P_1}{P_2} \right) \qquad (6)$$

Pressure is measured in millimeters of mercury (mm Hg).

Correction for water vapor is made along with the correction for pressure even though water vapor pressure is dependent only on temperature. (See Table C.1 for the vapor pressure of water at selected temperatures.) When the gas volume is to be "dried," as in STPD, the vapor pressure of water at ambient temperature T_1 (P_{H_2O}) is subtracted from the ambient or initial pressure (P_1) as follows:

$$V_2 = V_1 \left(\frac{P_1 - P_{H_2O}}{P_2} \right) \qquad (7)$$

For example, correcting to standard pressure (760 mm Hg, dry or SPD), we would have:

$$V_{SPD} = V_{ATPS} \left(\frac{P_1 - P_{H_2O}}{760} \right) \qquad (8)$$

When the gas volume is to be saturated, as in BTPS, P_{H_2O} is subtracted from P_1 as previously, but in addition the vapor pressure of water at T_2 or body temperature (P_{H_2O}') is subtracted from P_2 or body pressure. In other words:

$$V_2 = V_1 \left(\frac{P_1 - P_{H_2O}}{P_2 - P_{H_2O}'} \right) \qquad (9)$$

The reason why this procedure accounts for the increase in volume due to the addition of water vapor molecules when the temperature is increased to body temperature is because

C.1

Water vapor pressure (P_{H_2O}) at selected gas collection (ambient) temperatures*

Ambient temperature (°C)	P_{H_2O} (mm Hg)	Ambient temperature (°C)	P_{H_2O} (mm Hg)
18	15.5	28	28.3
19	16.5	29	30.0
20	17.5	30	31.8
21	18.7	31	33.7
22	19.8	32	35.7
23	21.1	33	37.7
24	22.4	34	39.9
25	23.8	35	42.2
26	25.2	36	44.6
27	26.7	37	47.1

*For computer programming purposes, the following equation may be used: $P_{H_2O} = 13.955 - 0.6584T + 0.0419T^2$, where T = ambient temperature

body pressure (P_2) obviously must equal ambient pressure (P_1), therefore no correction for pressure per se is necessary in going from ATPS to BTPS; in other words, $\frac{P_1}{P_2} = 1$. When P_{H_2O} and P_{H_2O}' are subtracted from P_1 and P_2, respectively, the resulting ratio, which is greater than 1, is proportional to the increase in volume due to the addition of water vapor molecules.

When correcting to body pressure, saturated with water vapor (BPS):

$$V_{BPS} = V_{ATPS}\left(\frac{P_1 - P_{H_2O}}{P_2 - 47 \text{ mm Hg}}\right) \qquad (10)$$

The 47 mm Hg pressure is the vapor pressure of water at body temperature.

Combined Correction Factors

We can now combine the temperature, pressure, and water vapor corrections into one equation for STPD and one equation for BTPS. Correcting from ATPS to STPD, we would combine equation (3) for temperature and equation (8) for pressure and water vapor as follows:

$$V_{STPD} = V_{ATPS}\left(\frac{273°}{273° + T}\right)\left(\frac{P_1 - P_{H_2O}}{760}\right) \qquad (11)$$

Correcting from ATPS to BTPS we would combine equations (4) and (10) for temperature and water vapor pressure, respectively:

$$V_{BTPS} = V_{ATPS}\left(\frac{310°}{273° + T}\right)\left(\frac{P_1 - P_{H_2O}}{P_2 - 47}\right) \qquad (12)$$

Problems

Suppose you have collected in a spirometer 100 L of expired gas. At the time you measured the gas volume, ambient temperature in the spirometer was 22° C, ambient pressure was 747 mm Hg, and P_{H_2O} at 22° C is equal to 19.8 mm Hg.

1. Correct the volume from ATPS to STPD.
2. Correct the volume from ATPS to BTPS.
3. Correct the volume from STPD to BTPS.

Solutions

1. Using equation (11) and substituting, we have:

$$V_{STPD} = 100 \text{ L}\left(\frac{273°}{295°}\right)\left(\frac{727.2 \text{ mm}}{760 \text{ mm}}\right)$$
$$= 100 \,(0.925)(0.957)$$
$$= 100 \,(0.885)$$
$$= \mathbf{88.5 \text{ L}}$$

2. Using equation (12) and substituting, we have:

$$V_{BTPS} = 100 \text{ L}\left(\frac{310°}{295°}\right)\left(\frac{727.2 \text{ mm}}{700 \text{ mm}}\right)$$
$$= 100 \,(1.051)(1.039)$$
$$= 100 \,(1.092)$$
$$= \mathbf{109.2 \text{ L}}$$

3. You can also use equation (12) for this solution but remember that the gas volume to be corrected is under conditions of STPD and not ATPS. Therefore, in equation (12):

    a. V$_{STPD}$ replaces V$_{ATPS}$.
    b. 273° + T now represents standard temperature, or 273° K + 0° C.

c. P$_1$ represents standard pressure, or 760 mm Hg, and P$_{H_2O}$ at 0° C is negligible. Therefore,

$$V_{BTPS} = 88.5 \text{ L} \left(\frac{310°}{273°}\right)\left(\frac{760 \text{ mm}}{700 \text{ mm}}\right)$$
$$= 88.5 \,(1.136)(1.086)$$
$$= 88.5 \,(1.233)$$
$$= \mathbf{109.2 \text{ L}}$$

Appendix D

Calculation of Oxygen Consumption and Carbon Dioxide Production

Oxygen Consumption

The amount of oxygen consumed per minute ($\dot{V}_{O_2}$) is equal to the difference between the amount of oxygen inspired ($\dot{V}_{I_{O_2}}$) and the amount of oxygen expired ($\dot{V}_{E_{O_2}}$) or:

$$\dot{V}_{O_2}(\text{STPD}) = \dot{V}_{I_{O_2}}(\text{STPD}) - \dot{V}_{E_{O_2}}(\text{STPD}) \qquad (13)$$

To use equation (13), the following variables must be measured:

1. $\dot{V}_E$ the volume of air exhaled per minute.
2. $F_{E_{O_2}}$ the fractional concentration of oxygen in exhaled air.
3. $F_{I_{O_2}}$ the fractional concentration of oxygen in inspired air.*
4. $F_{E_{CO_2}}$ the fractional concentration of carbon dioxide in expired air.
5. $F_{I_{CO_2}}$ the fractional concentration of carbon dioxide in inspired air.

An *amount* is defined as a volume times a concentration. The volume in this case, as you will recall, is a volume that has been corrected to STPD. All volumes referred to from here on are STPD. In a 100 L volume of gas containing 20% oxygen ($F_{O_2} = 0.2$) and 80% nitrogen ($F_{N_2} = 0.8$), the *amount* of oxygen is equal to 20 liters (100 L $\times$ 0.2) and the amount of nitrogen is equal to 80 liters (100 L $\times$ 0.8). As a result, the amount of oxygen inspired per minute according to equation (13) is equal to:

$$\dot{V}_{I_{O_2}} = (\dot{V}_I)(F_{I_{O_2}}) \qquad (14)$$

The same is true for the amount of oxygen expired; that is:

$$\dot{V}_{E_{O_2}} = (\dot{V}_E)(F_{E_{O_2}}) \qquad (15)$$

Substituting equations (14) and (15) into equation (13), we have:

$$\dot{V}_{O_2} = (\dot{V}_I)(F_{I_{O_2}}) - (\dot{V}_E)(F_{E_{O_2}}) \qquad (16)$$

Because $F_{I_{O_2}}$, $\dot{V}_E$, and $F_{E_{O_2}}$ are either known or measured directly, only $\dot{V}_I$ and $\dot{V}_{O_2}$ are unknown. Therefore, we must measure or calculate $\dot{V}_I$ to solve equation (16) for $\dot{V}_{O_2}$.

You may first think that $\dot{V}_I$ equals $\dot{V}_E$ (i.e., that the volume we inspire is the same as that which we expire). This is true if, and only if, the amount of CO_2 given off is equal to the amount of oxygen consumed. In other words, $\dot{V}_I = \dot{V}_E$ only when $\dot{V}_{CO_2} = \dot{V}_{O_2}$ or when R = 1. When more O_2 is consumed than CO_2 given off, $\dot{V}_E$ is less than $\dot{V}_I$. The opposite is true (i.e., $\dot{V}_E$ is greater than $\dot{V}_I$, when $\dot{V}_{CO_2}$ is greater than $\dot{V}_{O_2}$).

Rather than *measuring* $\dot{V}_I$ directly, there is a simpler method by which we can calculate it accurately. The calculation for determining $\dot{V}_I$, referred to as the Haldane transformation,[2] is based on the fact that the *amount* of nitrogen we inspire is equal to that which we expire:

$$(\dot{V}_I)(F_{I_{N_2}}) = (\dot{V}_E)(F_{E_{N_2}}) \qquad (17)$$

Solving for $\dot{V}_I$, we have:

$$\dot{V}_I = (\dot{V}_E)\left(\frac{F_{E_{N_2}}}{F_{I_{N_2}}}\right) \qquad (18)$$

Where:

$F_{I_{N_2}}$ = fractional concentration of nitrogen in inspired air
$F_{E_{N_2}}$ = fractional concentration of nitrogen in expired air

The factor $\left(\dfrac{F_{E_{N_2}}}{F_{I_{N_2}}}\right)$ is referred to as the *Nitrogen factor* and is designated N_F.

The above relationship holds true because nitrogen is neither consumed nor produced by the body; it is physiologically inert and, therefore, the amounts inspired and expired over time are essentially equal.†

---

*If fresh air (i.e., outside air) is inspired, then $F_{I_{O_2}}$, and $F_{I_{CO_2}}$, and $F_{I_{N_2}}$, will be 0.2093, 0.0004, and 0.7903 respectively.

†The concept of equality of respiratory gaseous nitrogen in man has been challenged, mainly by one laboratory,[1,3,4,5] and with it, the accuracy of calculating oxygen consumption by the Haldane transformation.[2] However, subsequent studies from a number of different laboratories,[6,7,8,9,10] have shown that nitrogen differences are small and inconsistent and do not significantly affect oxygen consumption values calculated by assuming nitrogen equality.

Because the sum of the fractional concentrations of oxygen, carbon dioxide, and nitrogen* equals 1.0 (for both inspired and expired gas volumes), we can calculate $F_{I_{N_2}}$ and $F_{E_{N_2}}$ from the following:

$$1 = F_{I_{O_2}} + F_{I_{CO_2}} + F_{I_{N_2}} \qquad (19)$$

or

$$F_{I_{N_2}} = 1 - (F_{I_{O_2}} + F_{I_{CO_2}}) \qquad (20)$$

and

$$1 = F_{E_{O_2}} + F_{E_{CO_2}} + F_{E_{N_2}} \qquad (21)$$

or

$$F_{E_{N_2}} = 1 - (F_{E_{O_2}} + F_{E_{CO_2}}) \qquad (22)$$

Therefore, substituting equations (20) and (22) in equation (18), we have:

$$\dot{V}_I = (\dot{V}_E) \frac{[1 - (F_{E_{O_2}} + F_{E_{CO_2}})]}{[1 - (F_{I_{O_2}} + F_{I_{CO_2}})]} \qquad (23)$$

or

$$\dot{V}_I = (\dot{V}_E)(N_F) \qquad (24)$$

Now we have the means to finally calculate oxygen consumption. Referring to equation (16), we can make appropriate measurements and calculations and solve for $\dot{V}_{O_2}$ ($F_{E_{O_2}}$ and $\dot{V}_E$ are measured, $\dot{V}_I$ is calculated using the nitrogen factor, and $F_{I_{O_2}}$ is assumed to be 0.2093, unless otherwise indicated).

$$\dot{V}_{O_2} = (\dot{V}_I)(F_{I_{O_2}}) - (\dot{V}_E)(F_{E_{O_2}})$$

"True" Oxygen

If the concentrations of gases in inspired air are as follows (usually the case),

$$F_{I_{O_2}} = .2093 \qquad F_{E_{O_2}} = 0.0004 \qquad F_{E_{N_2}} = .7903$$

then equation (16), with substitutions, may be rearranged to the following:

$$\dot{V}_{O_2} = (\dot{V}_E) \left[\frac{1 - (F_{E_{O_2}} + F_{E_{CO_2}})}{0.7903} \right](.2093) - (\dot{V}_E)(F_{E_{O_2}}) \qquad (25)$$

or

$$\dot{V}_{O_2} = (\dot{V}_E)[(F_{E_{N_2}})(0.265) - F_{E_{O_2}}] \qquad (26)$$

The factor $[(F_{E_{N_2}})(0.265) - F_{E_{O_2}}]$ is called "true" oxygen.

---

*These relationships are based on the fact that oxygen, carbon dioxide, and nitrogen are the only gases, for all practical purposes, in inspired and expired air. The small concentrations of rare gases, such as argon and helium, which are also physiologically inert, are included in the nitrogen fraction.

Carbon Dioxide Production

Calculation of CO_2 production per minute is based on the same general process as with the calculation of oxygen consumption. The basic question is:

$$\dot{V}_{CO_2} = \dot{V}_{E_{CO_2}} - \dot{V}_{I_{CO_2}} \qquad (27)$$

or

$$\dot{V}_{CO_2} = (\dot{V}_E)(F_{E_{CO_2}}) - (\dot{V}_I)(F_{I_{CO_2}}) \qquad (28)$$

If $\dot{V}_{O_2}$ is calculated first, as is generally the case, then all the factors to the right of equation (28) are known and $\dot{V}_{CO_2}$ can be determined in a short time.

"True" Carbon Dioxide

If we take equation (28) and substitute $\dot{V}_E$ times the nitrogen factor for $\dot{V}_I$ and 0.0004 for the $F_{I_{CO_2}}$, we will see the following:

$$\dot{V}_{CO_2} = (\dot{V}_E)(F_{E_{CO_2}}) -$$
$$(\dot{V}_E)\left[\frac{1 - (F_{E_{O_2}} + F_{E_{CO_2}})}{0.7903} \right](0.0004) \qquad (29)$$

$$\dot{V}_{CO_2} = (\dot{V}_E)(F_{E_{CO_2}} - [(1 - [F_{E_{O_2}} + F_{E_{CO_2}}])(0.0005)]) \qquad (30)$$

or

$$\dot{V}_{CO_2} = (\dot{V}_E)[F_{E_{CO_2}} - (F_{E_{N_2}})(0.0005)] \qquad (31)$$

Along the same line of reasoning as with oxygen, the factor $(F_{E_{N_2}})(0.0005)$ could be called "true" carbon dioxide.

Because the factor $(F_{E_{N_2}})(0.0005)$ results in a very small value for the volume of inspired CO_2 it may be neglected and equation (31) may be written:

$$\dot{V}_{CO_2} = (\dot{V}_E)(F_{E_{CO_2}}) \qquad (32)$$

Respiratory Exchange Ratio (R)

In Chapter 4, the importance of the R-value is discussed. The equation is presented here, again, to place it in the context of the metabolic calculations we have just described.

$$R = \frac{\dot{V}_{CO_2}}{\dot{V}_{O_2}} \qquad (33)$$

Problems

Suppose you have made a 5-minute collection of expired air from a resting subject breathing fresh air with the following results:

$\dot{V}_{E(ATPS)} = 35$ L in 5 minutes $P_B = 745$ mm Hg

$F_{E_{O_2}} = 0.1640$ $T = 24°$ C

$F_{E_{CO_2}} = 0.0420$ $P_{H_2O} = 22.4$ mm Hg at 24° C

$F_{I_{O_2}} = 0.2093$ $P_{H_2O} = 47$ mm Hg at 37° C

$F_{I_{CO_2}} = 0.0004$

1. What is the subject's $\dot{V}_{O_2}$?
2. What is the subject's $\dot{V}_{CO_2}$?
3. What is the subject's R-value?
4. What is the subject's $\dot{V}_{E(BTPS)}$?

Solutions

1. To calculate $\dot{V}_{O_2}$, the first thing we should do is place the $\dot{V}_E$ on a per-minute basis by dividing 35 L by 5 minutes and then convert $\dot{V}_{E(ATPS)}$ to $\dot{V}_{E(STPD)}$ by use of the STPD correction factor. From equation (11):

$$\dot{V}_{E(STPD)} = (7.0 \text{ L} \cdot \text{min}^{-1})\left(\frac{273}{273 + 24}\right)\left(\frac{745 - 22.4}{760}\right)$$
$$= (7)(0.919)(0.951)$$
$$= (7)(0.874)$$
$$= \mathbf{6.116 \text{ L} \cdot \text{min}^{-1}}$$

Then, find $\dot{V}_I$ by using the nitrogen factor (equation 23):

$$\dot{V}_{I(STPD)} = (\dot{V}_E)\frac{[1 - (F_{E_{O_2}} + F_{E_{CO_2}})]}{[1 - (F_{I_{O_2}} + F_{I_{CO_2}})]}$$
$$= (6.116 \text{ L} \cdot \text{min}^{-1})\left(\frac{0.7940}{0.7903}\right)$$
$$= (6.116)(1.005)$$
$$= \mathbf{6.147 \text{ L} \cdot \text{min}^{-1}}$$

Using equation (16) and substituting, we have:

$$\dot{V}_{O_2} = (6.147 \text{ L} \cdot \text{min}^{-1})(0.2093) -$$
$$(6.116 \text{ L} \cdot \text{min}^{-1})(.1640)$$
$$= 1.287 \text{ L} \cdot \text{min}^{-1} - 1.003 \text{ L} \cdot \text{min}^{-1}$$
$$= \mathbf{0.284 \text{ L} \cdot \text{min}^{-1}}$$

2. For CO_2 production, equation (28) is appropriate:

$$\dot{V}_{CO_2} = (6.116 \text{ L} \cdot \text{min}^{-1})(0.0420) -$$
$$(6.147 \text{ L} \cdot \text{min}^{-1})(.0004)$$
$$= 0.257 \text{ L} \cdot \text{min}^{-1} - 0.002 \text{ L} \cdot \text{min}^{-1}$$
$$= \mathbf{0.255 \text{ L} \cdot \text{min}^{-1}}$$

(Note how small the quantity for inspired CO_2 is. In most instances this can be ignored, but for precision, it should be included.)

3. The R-value (equation 33) is then:

$$R = \frac{0.255}{0.284} = \mathbf{0.90}$$

4. To calculate $\dot{V}_{E(BTPS)}$, we would apply equation (12) from Appendix C:

$$\dot{V}_{E(BTPS)} = (7 \text{ L} \cdot \text{min}^{-1})\left(\frac{310}{273 + 24}\right)\left[\frac{(745 - 22.4)}{(745 - 47)}\right]$$
$$= (7)(1.044)(1.035)$$
$$= (7)(1.081)$$
$$= \mathbf{7.567 \text{ L} \cdot \text{min}^{-1}}$$

References

1. Cissik, J., and R. Johnson. 1972. Myth of nitrogen equality in respiration: its history and implications. *Aerospace Med.* 43:755–758.
2. Cissik, J., and R. Johnson. 1972. Regression analysis for steady state N_2 inequality in O_2 consumption calculations. *Aerospace Med.* 43:589–591.
3. Cissik, J., R. Johnson, and B. Hertig. 1972. Production of gaseous nitrogen during human steady state exercise. *Physiologist.* 15:108.
4. Cissik, J., R. Johnson, and D. Rokosch. 1972. Production of gaseous nitrogen in human steady-state conditions. *J Appl Physiol.* 32:155–159.
5. Dudka, L., H. Inglis, R. Johnson, J. Pechinski, and S. Plowman. 1971. Inequality of inspired and expired gaseous nitrogen in man. *Nature.* 232:265–267.
6. Fox, E. L., and R. Bowers. 1973. Steady-state equality of respiratory gaseous N_2 in resting man. *J Appl Physiol.* 35(1):143–144.
7. Herron, J., H. Saltzman, B. Hills, and J. Kylstra. 1973. Differences between inspired and expired volumes of nitrogen in man. *J Appl Physiol.* 35(4):546–551.
8. Luft, U., L. Myhre, and J. Loeppky. 1973. Validity of Haldane calculation for estimating respiratory gas exchange. *J Appl Physiol.* 34(6):864–865.
9. Wagner, J., S. Horvath, T. Dahms, and S. Reed. 1973. Validation of open-circuit method for the determination of oxygen consumption. *J Appl Physiol.* 34(6):859–863.
10. Wilmore, J., and D. Costill. 1973. Adequacy of the Haldane transformation in the computation of exercise V_{O_2} in man. *J Appl Physiol.* 35(1):84–89.

Selected Readings

Consolazio, C., R. Johnson, and L. Pecora. 1963. *Physiological Measurements of Metabolic Functions in Man.* New York: McGraw-Hill.

Holly, R. G. 1993. Fundamentals of cardiorespiratory exercise testing. In *ACSM's Resource Manual for Guidelines for Exercise Testing and Prescription* (2d ed.). Philadelphia: Lea & Febiger, pp. 247–257.

Appendix E

Nomogram for Calculating Body Surface Area, Conversion Table for Body Mass in Pounds to Kilograms, and Nomogram for Calculating Body Mass Index from Inches and Pounds

Body Surface Area

The nomogram for calculating body surface area in square meters (m^2) from height, measured either in centimeters (cm) or feet (ft) and inches (in) and from body weight, measured either in kilograms (kg) or pounds (lb), is given in figure E.1. The nomogram is used by placing one end of a straightedge on the body height and the other end on the body weight. Where the straightedge intersects the middle scale is the body surface area.

As an example, consider the following:

Weight	= 154 lb or 70 kg
Height	= 5 ft 9 in or 175 cm
Surface area	= **1.84 m²**

Conversion of Body Weight from Pounds to Kilograms

The conversion of body weight from pounds to kilograms is presented in table E.1. To use the table, find the appropriate body weight in pounds and read the equivalent body weight in kilograms from the table. For example, a body weight of 173 pounds is equal to **78.5 kg.**

Nomogram for Calculating Body Mass Index from Inches and Pounds

One method used to define obesity is to calculate body mass index (BMI). This is a person's weight in kilograms divided by height in meters squared. For example, an 86 kg person who is 1.91 m tall has a body mass index of: $86 \div (1.91^2) =$ **24 kg · m⁻².** Figure E.2 provides a nomogram for determining body mass index using pounds for weight and inches for height.

Health risks for males and females begin when body mass index exceeds ~ 25. A body mass index above 30 is often used as the cutoff for obesity and is associated with an even greater risk for health problems, such as diabetes, heart disease, certain cancers, and diseases of the digestive tract.

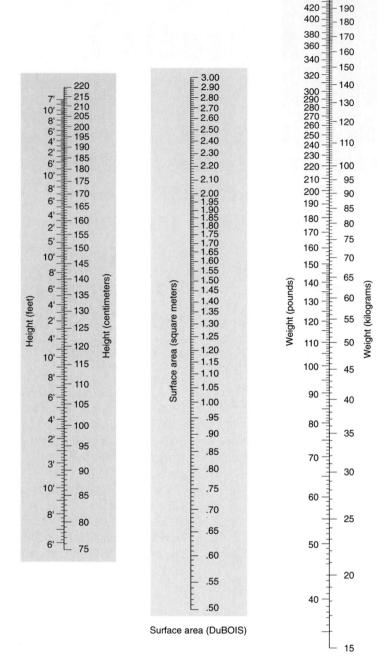

Figure E.1

Nomogram for computing surface area.

Source: Data from W. M. Boothby and R. B. Sandiford, 1920.

E.1

table

Conversion of pounds to kilograms

Pounds*	0	1	2	3	4	5	6	7	8	9
100	45.4	45.9	46.3	46.8	47.2	47.7	48.1	48.6	49.0	49.5
110	49.9	50.4	50.8	51.3	51.7	52.2	52.7	53.1	53.6	54.0
120	54.5	54.9	55.4	55.8	56.3	56.7	57.2	57.6	58.1	58.6
130	59.0	59.5	59.9	60.4	60.8	61.3	61.7	62.2	62.6	63.1
140	63.6	64.0	64.5	64.9	65.4	65.8	66.3	66.7	67.2	67.6
150	68.1	68.6	69.0	69.5	69.9	70.4	70.8	71.3	71.7	72.2
160	72.6	73.1	73.5	74.0	74.4	74.9	75.4	75.8	76.3	76.7
170	77.2	77.6	78.1	**78.5**	79.0	79.4	79.9	80.3	80.8	81.3
180	81.7	82.2	82.6	83.1	83.5	84.0	84.4	84.9	85.3	85.8
190	86.3	86.7	87.2	87.6	88.1	88.5	89.0	89.4	89.9	90.3
200	90.8	91.2	91.7	92.2	92.6	93.1	93.5	94.0	94.4	94.9
210	95.3	95.8	96.2	96.7	97.1	97.6	98.1	98.5	99.0	99.4
220	99.9	100.3	100.8	101.2	101.7	102.1	102.6	103.0	103.5	104.0
230	104.4	104.9	105.3	105.8	106.2	106.7	107.1	107.6	108.0	108.5
240	109.0	109.4	109.9	110.3	110.8	111.2	111.7	112.1	112.6	113.0

*1 pound = 0.454 kg; 1 kg = 2.205 pounds

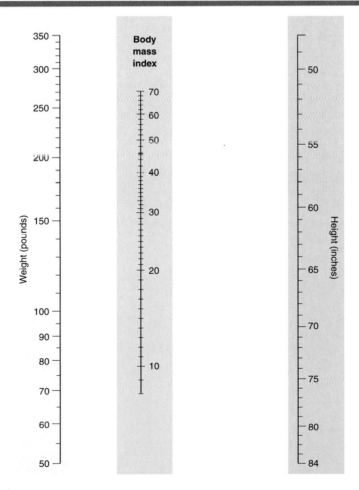

Figure E.2

To determine body mass index using this nomogram, make a mark next to the person's weight (without clothes) along the left-hand scale, then make another mark next to their height (without shoes) on the right-hand scale. The point at which a line connecting these two points crosses the scale in the middle is their body mass index.

Appendix F

Tests of Anaerobic and Aerobic Power

Anaerobic Power Tests

The ability to develop considerable power is a prime factor in athletic success. Power (kg-m · min^{-1}) is performance of work (force in kg × distance in meters) expressed per unit of time (min). The development of maximal or peak power is related to muscular strength and especially to the amount and rate of utilization of the ATP-PC system. Several tests have been developed over the years to assess and reflect one's ability to employ the ATP-PC system during very short-duration tasks. Two of these tests are discussed below, while a third—the Wingate anaerobic test—is described in detail in chapter 4 (p. 85) because of its widespread use in assessing anaerobic characteristics. Another advantage of the longer-duration (30-sec) Wingate test is that in addition to evaluating anaerobic power (ATP-PC system), it assesses anaerobic capacity (i.e., glycolysis) as well.

Sargent's Jump Test

Measuring the difference between how high a person can reach while standing and the height to which he or she can jump and touch (similar to basketball tipoff) has erroneously been used as a power test of the legs. Although the Sargent jump test may categorize the ability of an athlete to jump vertically one time, if body weight and the speed in performing the jump are not included as part of the measurement, one cannot regard it as a true index of muscle power. Certainly, a 56.3-kg (124-pound) female who jumps vertically 0.46 m (1.5 feet) produces less power than the 60.0-kg (132-pound) female who also jumps 0.46 m. Additionally, the brief nature of the test—one single jump—likely does not maximally tax the ATP-PC system.

Margaria-Kalamen Power Test

R. Margaria[4] suggested an excellent test of power, which has been modified by J. Kalamen (figure F.1).[3] The modification results in greater power output than in Margaria's original

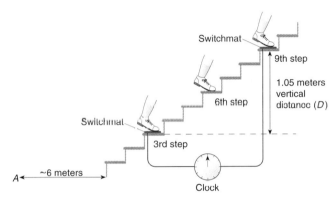

Figure F.1

Margaria-Kalamen power test. Subject starts at point A and runs as rapidly as possible up the flight of stairs, taking them three at a time. The time it takes to traverse the distance between stair 3 and stair 9 is recorded to a hundredth of a second. The power generated is a product of the subject's weight and the vertical distance (D), divided by the time. An example appears in the text.

test. The subject stands ~ 6 m in front of a staircase. At his pleasure he runs up the stairs as rapidly as possible, taking three at a time. An electronic switchmat is placed on the third and ninth stair. (An average stair is about 17.4 cm high.) A clock starts as the person steps on the first switchmat (on the third step) and stops as he steps on the second (on the ninth step). Time is recorded to a hundredth of a second. It is best to administer the test several times, recording the best score. Power output is computed using the formula:

$$P = \frac{W \times D}{t}$$

Where:

P = power
W = weight of person
D = vertical height between third and ninth steps
t = elapsed time from third to ninth steps

Therefore, for a 75-kg athlete who covers 1.05 m in 0.49 seconds, power is:

$$P = \frac{75 \times 1.05}{0.49} = 161 \text{ kg-m} \cdot \text{sec}^{-1}$$

Kalamen,[3] using 23 nonathletic males, obtained a mean power output of 168.5 kg-m · sec^{-1}. Some standards based on these data, plus those of Margaria et al.,[4] are listed in table F.1. When evaluating seven sprinters from the Ohio State University track team, a mean power output of 200 kg-m · sec^{-1} was obtained. Furthermore, power outputs between 240 and 271 kg-m · sec^{-1} have been reported for professional football players (backs).[2] The greater power outputs of these trained athletes support the validity of this test.

Tests of Maximal Aerobic Power

The measurement of aerobic power is ordinarily accomplished through the determination of oxygen consumption ($\dot{V}O_2$). Maximal oxygen consumption ($\dot{V}O_2$ max) is dependent on age, gender, body size, and exercise training habits. Typical values for $\dot{V}O_2$ max among males and females are given in chapter 4 (page 89). Chapter 4 also discusses many protocols and methods for directly measuring and for estimating $\dot{V}O_2$.

Direct Methods for Assessing Aerobic Power

Deciding the correct treadmill speed/elevation to start a test aimed at directly measuring $\dot{V}O_2$ can be simplified by choosing one of the protocols shown in chapter 4 (tables 4.6 and 4.7; page 87). Alternately, the *Saltin-Åstrand Method*[5] can help determine where to set the initial work load. In this technique the subject first performs a 5-minute submaximal bicycle ergometer ride, where heart rate and oxygen consumption are measured during the last minute. These data are then used to predict the subject's max $\dot{V}O_2$. Using a nomogram (figure F.2), this is done by connecting, with a straightedge, the point on the $\dot{V}O_2$ scale with the corresponding point on the pulse (heart) rate scale. The predicted max $\dot{V}O_2$ is read from the middle scale. Then, from table F.2, the predicted max $\dot{V}O_2$ is used to determine the appropriate *starting* speed and inclination of the treadmill so that the running test will last between 6–10 minutes.

For example, suppose a male subject's predicted max $\dot{V}O_2$ were 45 mL · kg^{-1} · min^{-1}. Based on table F.2, the starting speed and inclination of the treadmill would be 12.5 km per hour (7.8 miles per hour) and 5.2% grade, respectively. After three minutes at this level, the treadmill is then elevated 2.7% every 3 minutes until the subject is exhausted. Consecutive 1-minute gas collections using the Douglas bag method or an automated metabolic cart are

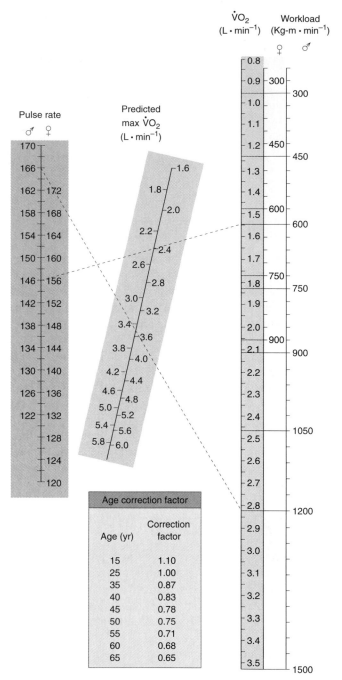

Age correction factor

Age (yr)	Correction factor
15	1.10
25	1.00
35	0.87
40	0.83
45	0.78
50	0.75
55	0.71
60	0.68
65	0.65

Figure F.2

This nomogram calculates aerobic work capacity from submaximal pulse rate, and either $\dot{V}O_2$ (cycling, running, or walking) or workload during cycling. Using a straightedge, the point on the $\dot{V}O_2$ scale shall be connected with the corresponding point on the pulse rate scale and the predicted maximal O_2 uptake read on the middle scale. A female subject reaches a heart rate of 156 at a $\dot{V}O_2$ of 1.54 L · min^{-1}; predicted max $\dot{V}O_2$ = 2.4 L · min^{-1}. A male subject reaches a heart rate of 166 while cycling at a work load of 1200 kg-m · min^{-1}; predicted max $\dot{V}O_2$ = 3.5 L · m^{-1} (exemplified by dotted lines). To convert L · min^{-1} to mL · kg^{-1} · min^{-1}, multiply by 1000 and divide by subject's body weight in kg.

Source: Data from I. Åstrand, "Aerobic Work Capacity in Men and Women with Special Reference to Age," in Acta Physiologica Scandinavica, *49 Supplement 169, 1–92, 1960, Scandinavian Physiological Society, Stockholm, Sweden.*

F.1

Classifications for anaerobic power based on the Margaria-Kalamen test (ATP-PC system)*

| | **Males** | | | | |
| | **Age Groups (yr)** | | | | |
Classification	**15–20**	**21–30**	**31–40**	**41–50**	**Over 50**
Poor	Under 113†	Under 106†	Under 85†	Under 65†	Under 50†
Fair	113–149	106–139	84–111	65–84	50–65
Average	150–187	140–175	112–140	85–105	66–82
Good	188–224	176–210	144–168	106–125	83–98
Excellent	Over 224	Over 210	Over 168	Over 125	Over 98
	Females				
	Age Groups (yr)				
Classification	**15–20**	**21–30**	**31–40**	**41–50**	**Over 50**
Poor	Under 92†	Under 85†	Under 65†	Under 50†	Under 38†
Fair	92–120	85–111	65–84	50–65	38–48
Average	121–151	112–140	85–105	66–82	49–61
Good	152–182	141–168	106–125	83–98	62–75
Excellent	Over 182	Over 168	Over 125	Over 98	Over 75

*Based on data from Kalamen,[3] and Margaria, et al.[4]
†kg-m · sec^{-1}

F.2

Starting work load used for the Saltin-Åstrand maximal aerobic power test

| **Predicted max $\dot{V}_{O_2}$, (mL · kg^{-1} · min^{-1})** | **Males** | | | **Females** | | |
| | **Speed** | | **Grade** | **Speed** | | **Grade** |
	(mi · hr^{-1})	**(km · hr^{-1})**	**(%)**	**(mi · hr^{-1})**	**(km · hr^{-1})**	**(%)**
below 40	6.2	10.0	5.2	6.2	10.0	2.7
40–54	7.8	12.5	5.2	6.2	10.0	5.2
55–75	9.3	15.0	5.2	7.8	12.5	5.2
above 75	10.9	17.5	5.2			

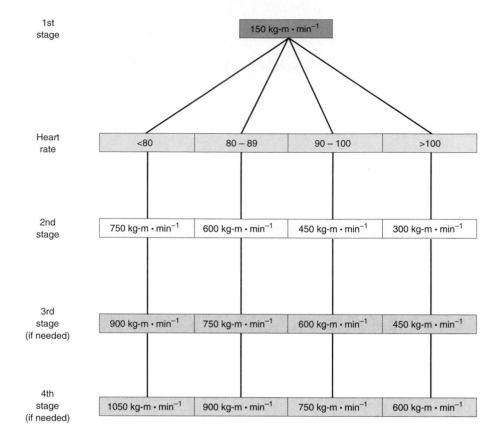

Figure F.3

Set the first workload at 150 kg-m · min⁻¹. Based on heart rate toward the end of the third minute of exercise, the 2nd workload is set as shown above. Similarly, 3rd and 4th workloads are set if needed. Two consecutive heart rates must be obtained in the 110 to 150 beats · min⁻¹ range. Workloads are based on a pedal speed of 50 rpm.

also performed. Prior to the test, the subject warms up for 10 minutes at a work load that is ~50% of his or her predetermined starting load.

Indirect Methods for Assessing Aerobic Power

As you may have concluded from the preceding descriptions, direct assessment of max $\dot{V}O_2$ is limited in that the test is difficult, exhausting, and may require somewhat costly equipment for measuring $\dot{V}O_2$. For this reason, several methods for predicting max $\dot{V}O_2$ from submaximal exercise data have been developed. Following are two such methods, both of which involve a cycle ergometer.

Åstrand-Ryhming Nomogram[1]

The Åstrand-Ryhming nomogram, shown in figure F.2, was developed for prediction of max $\dot{V}O_2$ from submaximal data. It involves a single-stage test lasting six minutes that

is based on the idea that heart rate during submaximal cycling or walking increases linearly (in a straight line) with $\dot{V}O_2$.

Here is how to use the nomogram:

1. Using a cycle ergometer, a work rate is selected that will elicit a heart rate of between 125 and 170 beats · min⁻¹. Typical work rates might be 300 or 600 kg-m · min⁻¹ for an unconditioned male and 300 or 450 kg-m · min⁻¹ for an unconditioned female. In all cases, one-minute determinations of heart rate are made during the fifth and sixth minutes of work, and an average value for the two is computed.

2. The heart rate and work rate are then applied to the nomogram shown in figure F.2 to predict the max $\dot{V}O_2$. Using a straightedge, the point on the workload (kg-m · min⁻¹) scale is connected with the corresponding point on the pulse (heart) rate scale. The predicted max $\dot{V}O_2$ is read from the middle scale.

3. If the subject is older than 25 years, an appropriate age correction factor (given as an insert in figure F.2)

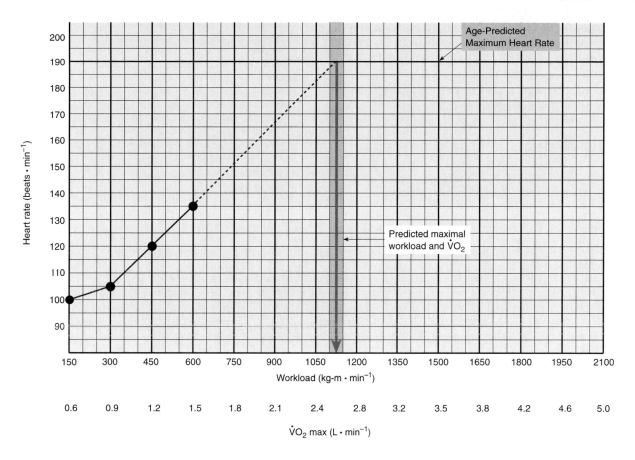

Figure F.4

Estimated $\dot{V}O_2$ max using the YMCA protocol in a 30-year-old male. Two rates between 110 and 150 beats $\cdot$ min^{-1} were obtained during exercise and used to extrapolate to a line set at age-predicted maximum heart rate (220 $-$ 30 = 190 beats $\cdot$ min^{-1}). A vertical line is dropped to X-axis and estimates a peak workload of 1125 kg-m $\cdot$ min^{-1}, which is equivalent to a $\dot{V}O_2$ max of approximately 2.6 L $\cdot$ min^{-1}.

must be applied to the predicted max $\dot{V}O_2$. For example, for a 45-year-old female with a predicted max $\dot{V}O_2$ of 2.4 L $\cdot$ min^{-1}, her age-corrected max $\dot{V}O_2$ would be 2.4 $\times$ 0.78 = 1.87 L $\cdot$ min^{-1}.

Whenever any variable is predicted rather than measured, the question most often asked is, How accurate is it? In the case of the Åstrand-Ryhming nomogram (figure F.2), the standard deviation from the measured max $\dot{V}O_2$ is $\pm$ 15%. As an example of what this means, for every 1000 persons whose max $\dot{V}O_2$ is predicted to be 3.0 L $\cdot$ min^{-1}, 25 of them will have actual max $\dot{V}O_2$ values less than 2.1 L $\cdot$ min^{-1}, and 25 will be greater than 3.9 L $\cdot$ min^{-1}. This clearly points out that such predictions are at best only rough approximations of the true aerobic power. Precise values can be determined only by direct methods.

YMCA (Young Men's Christian Association) Physical Working Capacity Test[6]

The YMCA protocol uses two to four, 3-minute stages of continuous exercise to produce two consecutive heart rates that fall between 110 to 150 beats $\cdot$ min^{-1}. Having two heart rates in this range is needed to predict $\dot{V}O_2$ max. Heart rates are measured during the final 15 to 30 seconds of each three-minute stage. The algorithm for guiding work rate at each three-minute stage is given in figure F.3. The two heart rates measured between 110 and 150 beats $\cdot$ min^{-1} are plotted on a graph (figure F.4) and used to extrapolate a line that intersects another line drawn at age-predicted maximum heart rate. From this point a vertical line is drawn to intersect with the X-axis, resulting in an estimate of $\dot{V}O_2$ max. Again, keep in mind that an estimated $\dot{V}O_2$ max works well for broadly categorizing an individual's level of aerobic fitness; however, directly measured values are more accurate and must be used when assessing response to an intervention or for research purposes.

References

1. Åstrand, P., and I. Ryhming. 1954. A nomogram for calculation of aerobic capacity (physical fitness) from pulse rate during submaximal work. *J Appl Physiol.* 7:218–221.

2. Fox, E., and D. Mathews. 1974. *Interval Training: Conditioning for Sports and General Fitness.* Philadelphia: W. B. Saunders.

3. Kalamen, J. 1968. *Measurement of Maximum Muscular Power in Man.* Doctoral dissertation: The Ohio State University, Columbus, OH.

4. Margaria, R., I. Aghemo, and E. Rovelli. 1966. Measurement of muscular power (anaerobic) in man. *J Appl Physiol.* 21:1662–1664.

5. Saltin, B., and P. Åstrand. 1967. Maximal oxygen uptake in athletes. *J Appl Physiol.* 23:353–358.

6. Golding, L. A., C. R. Myers, and W. E. Sinning. 1989. *Y's Way to Physical Fitness,* 3d ed. Champaign, Human Kinetics, p. 89–124.

Appendix G

Measuring Efficiency

In chapter 4 a variety of devices called *ergometers* were described which are available to study the energetics of physical activity. Care must be taken to ensure that, regardless of the type of equipment, such equipment remains calibrated. Doing so will allow the tester to be sure that the work rate he/she wants to impose on the person being tested is, in fact, the work rate that is being put out. You may also remember from chapter 4 that work output is used in our equation for measuring efficiency:

$$\% \text{ Efficiency} = \frac{\text{useful work output (kcal)}}{\text{work input (kcal)}} \times 100$$

Recall that work, power, or energy units can be used when computing efficiency, as long as the units in both the numerator and denominator are the same. The steps involved with measuring efficiency using two common ergometers are given below. The same principles can be applied to other devices as well.

Measuring Efficiency on a Cycle Ergometer

Figure G.1 depicts a mechanically braked cycle ergometer. A belt that runs around the rim of a flywheel can be adjusted to provide tension using an adjustable dial.* By increasing tension on the wheel, more friction, and thus greater resistance, is provided. The cycle gearing and wheel circumference have been designed so that one complete turn of the pedals moves a point on the rim 6 meters (the rim is 1.6 meters in circumference). Using a metronome set at 100 counts per minute (50 rpm) a scale is provided that is graduated in *kiloponds (kp)*. One kp is the force acting on the mass of 1 kg at the normal acceleration of gravity. The braking power, in kp, multiplied by the distance pedaled in meters yields work in *kilopond-meters (kp-m)*. If the distance "traveled" is related to time, then power can be expressed as kp-m $\cdot$ min^{-1}. Power can also be expressed as watts, kg-m $\cdot$ min^{-1}, or joules $\cdot$ sec^{-1}.

The relationship among the various work units *at 50 rpm* is 1 kp = 300 kp-m = 300 kg-m.* From table 4.2 (page 76) we see that the work units can be converted to power units of kilocalories (kcal) or kilojoules (kJ).[†]
1 kcal = 426.78 kg-m $\cdot$ min^{-1} = 4.186 kJ $\cdot$ min^{-1}.

There are other cycle ergometers available for laboratories and personal usage that are electronically braked and compensate for variations in pedal frequency. That is, if the subject pedals at a faster rate, the resistance is lowered so that total work output is held constant. Nonetheless, the mechanically braked cycle described previously represents a less expensive, reliable research ergometer.

In the following example, a subject exercises for 10 minutes on a cycle ergometer at a resistance of 3 kp. The task is to determine efficiency for the 10 minutes.

1. *Work Output.* To determine work output, we need to know the resistance (3 kp), the total time (10 min), the pedaling rate (50 rpm), and the distance the rim of the flywheel travels (6 meters per revolution).

   a. Determine the work performed.

   W = F $\times$ D
   W = (3 kp) $\times$ (50 rpm $\times$ 10 min $\times$ 6 m per revolution)
   W = (3 kp) $\times$ (3000 m)
   W = 9000 kp-m
   = 9000 kg-m[‡]

   b. Convert to kilocalories.

   1 kcal = 426.78 kg-m, therefore
   Total kcal = 9000 kg-m $\div$ 426.78 kg-m $\cdot$ kcal^{-1}
   = 21.09 kcal

2. *Work Input.* To determine work input, we need to know the R-value (respiratory exchange ratio, see chapter 4), to determine the caloric equivalent of a liter of O_2. Recall that R can only be determined under steady-state conditions, thus the work must be submaximal.

---

*Note that this relationship changes with changes in pedal frequency.

[†]Joule is the international unit for work. 1 kp = 9.80665 Newtons (N). A Newton-meter is expressed in joules.
[‡]Remember, for our purposes 1 kp-m = 1 kg-m.

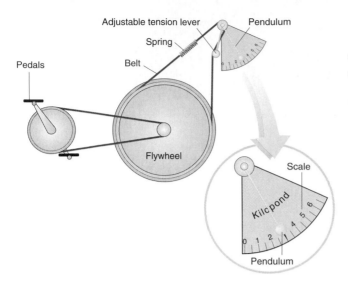

Figure G.1

Components of a mechanically braked cycle ergometer. A weighted flywheel has a belt around its circumference. The belt is connected with a small spring on one end and has an adjustable tension lever on the other end. A pendulum balance indicates the resistance in kiloponds. The inset shows the pendulum at a resistance of 3 kiloponds.

G.1

Angles of incline and corresponding percent grade*

θ (degrees)	sine θ	Tangent θ	Percent Grade
1	0.0175	0.0175	1.75
2	0.0349	0.0349	3.49
3	0.0523	0.0523	5.23
4	0.0698	0.0698	6.98
5	**0.0872**	0.0872	8.72
6	0.1045	0.1051	10.51
7	0.1219	0.1228	12.28
8	0.1392	0.1405	14.05
9	0.1564	0.1584	15.84
10	0.1736	0.1763	17.63
15	0.2588	0.2680	26.80
20	0.3420	0.3640	36.40

*Note that sine and tangent are equal for the first 5 degrees, but as the angle increases, the difference between sine and tangent increases.

Given:

R = 0.85 (from table 4.4; 1 L of O_2 = 4.865 kcal)
$\dot{V}O_2$ = 2.0 L · min^{-1}
Exercise time = 10 minutes

c. Determine total oxygen consumed.

Total VO_2 = (2.0 L · min^{-1}) × (10 min)
= **20 L of O_2**

d. Total kcal consumed = (20 L of O_2) ×
(4.865 kcal · L^{-1})
= **97.3 kcal**

3. *Efficiency.*

e. Efficiency = $\dfrac{21.09 \text{ kcal}}{97.30 \text{ kcal}}$ × 100 = **21.7%**

Measuring Efficiency on a Treadmill

If a subject were walking or running horizontally on the treadmill, he or she would not be performing "useful" work, and therefore efficiency could not be computed. Sometimes this is difficult for a student to resolve because we know it requires *energy* to walk or run—but according to the physicist, we are not doing any *work*. Recall that work is moving an object through a distance. The subject walking along a horizontal is raising and lowering the center of gravity the same distance; therefore, one cancels the other. All the energy expended by the subject is lost as heat without performing any useful work. The same is true if you hold a 2.2 kg weight in front of you at arm's length; because you are not moving the weight, no useful work is being performed, even though you are expending energy.

To determine efficiency using a treadmill, the device must be positioned so the subject walks up a grade; in other words, the horizontal angle of the treadmill must be greater than 0 degrees. Usually the slope or incline of the treadmill is reported as percent grade rather than in degrees. Percent grade may be defined as units (meters) of vertical rise per 100 horizontal units (meters) of run. It may also be determined by multiplying the tangent of the angle times 100, as shown in table G.1. Determining work output and work input while walking or running on an elevated treadmill is more involved and is accomplished in the following manner.

1. *Work Output.* Work output is equal to the weight of the subject times the vertical distance he or she would have been raised in walking or running up the incline of the treadmill; in other words, work equals force (weight of subject) times distance. Measuring the weight of the subject poses no problem (e.g., 73 kg); however, computing vertical distance is somewhat more involved. Referring to figure G.2, the measurements and computations are made in the following manner:

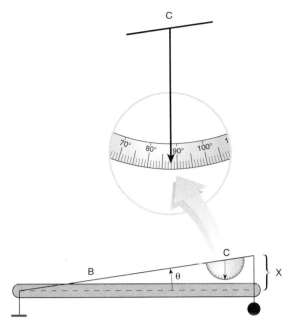

Figure G.2

Determination of work output using inclined treadmill. Angle theta (θ) is determined by use of inclinometer at point C. The reading of 88 degrees at point C on the treadmill is equivalent to 2 degrees at angle θ (180 degrees − [90 degrees + 88 degrees] = 2 degrees). The vertical distance the subject would travel, X, is computed as outlined in the text.

The vertical distance (X) = Sine of angle theta (θ) × B,
$$X = \text{Sine } \theta \times B$$

where,

B = the distance traveled along the incline

For example, assume angle θ is 5 degrees. The angle may be measured with an inclinometer at point C (figure G.2). Sine θ of 5 degrees (from table G.1) equals 0.0872. The value of B (distance traveled) is calculated by knowing the speed of the treadmill belt and the duration of exercise. For example, the distance traveled while walking on the incline at 4.8 km · hr^{-1} for 30 minutes (0.5 hour) is 2.4 km, or:

$$B = 4.8 \text{ km} \cdot \text{hr}^{-1} \times 0.5 \text{ hr} = 2.4 \text{ km};$$

Therefore,

$$X = \text{Sine } \theta \times B$$
$$= 0.0872 \times 2.4 \text{ km} = \mathbf{0.2093 \text{ km}}$$

Changing vertical distance (X) to meters:

$$X = 0.2093 \text{ km} \times 1000 \text{ m} \cdot \text{km}^{-1} = \mathbf{209.3 \text{ meters}}$$

Therefore, work output (W) becomes:

W = 73 kg (weight of subject) × 209.3 meters
W = **15,278 kg-m** of work accomplished during 30 minutes

For calculating efficiency, the work output may also be expressed in power units (work per unit of time). For power calculation, convert work output to work output per unit of time, or:

$$\text{Power} = \frac{15,278 \text{ kg-m}}{30 \text{ minutes}} = \mathbf{509 \text{ kg-m} \cdot \text{min}^{-1}}$$

2. *Work Input.* Work input (i.e., energy expenditure) during steady-state submaximal exercise (aerobic) can be expressed in terms of net $\dot{V}O_2$ per unit of time. Assuming the net $\dot{V}O_2$ for the subject while walking is 1.2 L · min^{-1}, we must convert this measurement to identical units expressed as power output—that is, it must be expressed in kg-m · min^{-1}. The first consideration is to convert L of O_2 per minute to kcal · min^{-1}. This is done by using R and then referring to table 4.4 to obtain the proper caloric equivalent.

Given:

$$R = 0.82; 1 \text{ L of } O_2 = 4.83 \text{ kcal}$$

Therefore,

1.2 L of O_2 per min × 4.83 kcal · L^{-1} = **5.8 kcal · min^{-1}**
1 kcal · min^{-1} = 426.8 kg-m · min^{-1} (table 4.2)

Therefore,

5.8 kcal · min^{-1} × 426.8 kg-m · kcal^{-1} =
2475 kg-m · min^{-1}

3. *Efficiency.*

$$\text{Efficiency} = \frac{509 \text{ kg-m} \cdot \text{min}^{-1}}{2475 \text{ kg-m} \cdot \text{min}^{-1}} \times 100 = \mathbf{20.6\%}$$

Appendix H

Six Key Equations to Remember

Calculation of Important Variables in Cardiorespiratory Physiology—Including $\dot{V}O_2$ max Using the Fick Equation

In chapters 4 and 7 through 12, a great deal of attention was given to the measurement of oxygen consumption ($\dot{V}O_2$) and various other variables often used in exercise physiology. This section provides a detailed review of the six basic equations you need to understand and be able to compute given the necessary data. At the time of examination, professors often expect you to memorize these equations; therefore, we suggest you practice them until they become second nature. The six basic equations and their associated units are:

1. $\dot{V}_E$ (L · min^{-1}) = $V_T \times$ f
2. $\dot{Q}$ (L · min^{-1}) = heart rate $\times$ stroke volume
3. P_{mean} (mm Hg) = diastolic blood pressure $\div \frac{1}{3}$ pulse pressure
4. T_sP_r (mm Hg · L^{-1} · min^{-1}) = $P_{mean} \times \dot{Q}$
5. a $\overline{v}O_2$ diff (mL · L^{-1}) = arterial O_2 concentration − mixed venous O_2 concentration
6. $\dot{V}O_2$ (L · min^{-1}) = $\dot{Q} \times$ a − $\overline{v}O_2$ diff

By the way, on rearranging these equations you should be able to solve for unknowns elsewhere in the equation. For example, given $\dot{V}_E$ and V_T, compute f. To accomplish this you need to rearrange the equation so that the unknown variable is isolated on one side of the equation, with the other variables located on the other side of the equation (e.g., f = $\frac{\dot{V}_E}{V_T}$).

When moving variables across the equal sign they must change sign (+, −) or change position (above or below) the present or implied division line. Practice this if you are rusty!

Finally, when working through this material, keep several overall issues in mind. First, consider the importance we place on a high level of human performance and health, and how five major bodily systems must be inte-

grated to achieve a high $\dot{V}O_2$ max. Can you think of what these systems are before going ahead? More importantly, can you now see why a compromised function of one or more of these systems would show up as a reduced $\dot{V}O_2$ max?

Second, given the above and while working through these equations, try to understand why measured $\dot{V}O_2$ max is considered by most exercise scientists as the single best overall indicator of a person's cardiorespiratory fitness or aerobic capacity. Third, also reflect on the way (increase, decrease, no change) that factors such as age, gender, body size, type of test (cycle vs. treadmill), amount of active muscle mass involved, mechanical efficiency, body composition, level of training, training type (resistance vs. Fartlek), and motivation may have on an individual's $\dot{V}O_2$ max.

For the following information, the "example" person is a 50-year-old, sedentary male who weighs 80 kg. A contrast will often be made between resting and maximal exercise responses. Additionally, assume that this person possesses no blood disorders. Specifically, the blood's O_2-carrying capacity is not compromised in that hematocrit, hemoglobin, and red blood cell counts are all normal. And there is no anemia, polycythemia, or iron deficiency.

Lungs

Our interest here is in calculating the volume of air taken into the lungs per unit time. We assume that there is no compromised lung tissue that would reduce diffusion capacity or the subject's ability to exhale effectively, such as cystic fibrosis, emphysema, or other forms of obstructive lung disease. Minute ventilation ($\dot{V}_E$) equals tidal volume (V_T, L · breath^{-1}) times frequency of breathing (f, breaths · min^{-1}).

$$\dot{V}_E = V_T \times f$$
$$\dot{V}_E(rest) = 0.5 \text{ L} \cdot breath^{-1} \times 12 \text{ breaths} \cdot min^{-1}$$
$$= \mathbf{6 \text{ L} \cdot min^{-1}}$$
$$\dot{V}_E(max) = 3 \text{ L} \cdot breath^{-1} \times 40 \text{ breaths} \cdot min^{-1}$$
$$= \mathbf{120 \text{ L} \cdot min^{-1}}$$

a. Note that $\dot{V}_E$ increased 20 times
b. Calculate $\dot{V}_E$ if V_T = 2 L · breath^{-1} and f = 30 breaths · min^{-1}

c. Note that the equation can be rearranged to solve for

$$V_T = \frac{\dot{V}_E}{f} \text{ and } f = \frac{\dot{V}_E}{V_T}. \text{ Try this!}$$

Heart

A similar calculation to determine the volume of blood pumped from the heart per unit of time (minute) is defined as cardiac output ($\dot{Q}$), where heart rate (HR) is in beats · min^{-1}, and volume pumped with each beat or stroke volume (SV) is in mL · beat^{-1}. Once again, we assume that there is no compromise to cardiac function, such as valvular defects, post-infarct scar tissue, or progressive heart failure.

$$\dot{Q} = HR \times SV$$
$$\dot{Q} \text{ (rest)} = 70 \text{ beats} \cdot \text{min}^{-1} \times 70 \text{ mL} \cdot \text{beat}^{-1}$$
$$= 4900 \text{ mL} \cdot \text{min}^{-1}$$
$$= \textbf{4.9 L} \cdot \textbf{min}^{-1}$$
$$\dot{Q} \text{ (max)} = 170 \text{ beats} \cdot \text{min}^{-1} \times 110 \text{ mL} \cdot \text{beat}^{-1}$$
$$= 18700 \text{ mL} \cdot \text{min}^{-1}$$
$$= \textbf{18.7 L} \cdot \textbf{min}^{-1}$$

a. Note that $\dot{Q}$ increased 3.8 times (only!)
b. Calculate $\dot{Q}$ if HR = 130 beats · min^{-1} and SV = 90 mL · beat^{-1}
c. Note that the equation can be rearranged to solve for

$$SV = \frac{\dot{Q}}{HR} \text{ and } HR = \frac{\dot{Q}}{SV}. \text{ Try this!}$$

Circulation

The primary consideration with the function of this system is what happens to systolic (SBP) and diastolic (DBP) blood pressure and total systemic peripheral resistance (T_sP_r), since blood flow is altered by the relationship that flow is directly proportional to pressure and inversely proportional to resistance—i.e., Flow $= \frac{\text{Pressure}}{\text{Resistance}}$. Note that this proportionality equation can be rearranged to indicate the following relationships: Pressure = Flow × Resistance and Resistance $= \frac{\text{Pressure}}{\text{Flow}}$. Try this later!

We assume that there are no regions of compromised blood flow from atherosclerotic plaque formation, or occlusion or narrowing of blood vessels caused by other diseases. The units for SBP and DBP are millimeters of mercury (mm Hg) while the units for T_sP_r are mm Hg over L · min^{-1} which will be shown later.

SBP (rest)	= 125 mm Hg
DBP (rest)	= 75 mm Hg
Pulse pressure (PP)	= SBP − DBP
	= 125 mmHg − 75 mm Hg
	= **50 mm Hg**
Mean BP or P_{mean} (rest)	= DBP + ⅓ PP
	= 75 mm Hg + 17 mm Hg
	= **92 mm Hg**

SBP (max)	= 200 mm Hg
DBP (max)	= 80 mm Hg
PP (max)	= SBP − DBP
	= 200 mm Hg − 80 mm Hg
	= **120 mm Hg**
P_{mean} (max)	= DBP + ⅓ PP
	= 80 mm Hg + 40 mm Hg
	= **120 mm Hg**

a. Note that P_{mean} increased 1.3 times
b. Calculate P_{mean} if SBP = 165 and DBP = 75
c. What explanation is there for adding ⅓ of pulse pressure onto DBP to yield the P_{mean}? Why not just calculate the arithmetic average?

Total systemic peripheral resistance reflects the partial closing of some vascular fields (shunting effect) and the opening of many others (capillaries). The equation is an application of $T_sP_r = \frac{P_{mean}}{\dot{Q}}$ and reflects the resistance encountered by the heart's output (remember units are L · min^{-1} so it's an expression of flow rate), when blood is squeezed out into the elastic aorta and into the closed vascular system. The P_{mean} calculated above is used in this calculation. The final units of mm Hg over L · min^{-1} may seem strange at first glance but they make sense. It is appropriate to write these units on a single line as mm Hg · L^{-1} · min^{-1}.

$$T_sP_r = \frac{P_{mean}}{\dot{Q}}$$

$$T_sP_r \text{ (rest)} = \frac{92 \text{ mm Hg}}{4.9 \text{ L} \cdot \text{min}^{-1}} = \frac{18.7 \text{ mm Hg}}{\text{L} \cdot \text{min}^{-1}}$$

$$= \textbf{18.7 mm Hg} \cdot \textbf{L}^{-1} \cdot \textbf{min}^{-1}$$

$$T_sP_r \text{ (max)} = \frac{120 \text{ mm Hg}}{18.7 \text{ L} \cdot \text{min}^{-1}} = \frac{6.4 \text{mm Hg}}{\text{L} \cdot \text{min}^{-1}}$$

$$= \textbf{6.4 mm Hg} \cdot \textbf{L}^{-1} \cdot \textbf{min}^{-1}$$

a. Note that T_sP_r decreased to ⅓ of resting value. Why?
b. Note that it is only coincidental that T_sP_r at rest and $\dot{Q}$ at maximal exercise have the same numerical value of 18.7. The units are different!
c. Calculate T_sP_r if P_{mean} = 105 mm Hg and $\dot{Q}$ = 11.7 L · min^{-1}

d. Note that the equation can be rearranged to solve for

$$P_{mean} = T_sP_r \times \dot{Q} \text{ and } \dot{Q} = \frac{P_{mean}}{T_sP_r}$$

e. With a combined increase in blood pressures (especially SBP because DBP didn't change much) and a decrease in T_sP_r, what happens to blood flow to working muscles during strenuous exercise?

Muscles

The major concern with the skeletal muscle system is the capability of this tissue to take up oxygen (often influenced by mitochondrial adaptations that occur because of training vs. a sedentary existence). This capability is reflected through differences in the amounts of oxygen carried to the muscles in contrast to the amounts carried away from the muscles. The amounts are expressed as concentrations of oxygen in arterial (a) and mixed venous ($\bar{v}$) blood. The calculation is called "av O_2 difference" and is shown as $a - \bar{v}O_2$ diff. The concentrations are in units of mL $O_2 \cdot$ 100 mL^{-1} of blood which is called volumes percent (vol %). It is best to convert these units to mL $O_2 \cdot L^{-1}$ of blood for subsequent calculations.

aO_2 (rest)	= 20 mL $O_2 \cdot$ 100 mL^{-1} blood
	= 20 vol %
	= 200 mL $O_2 \cdot L^{-1}$ blood
$\bar{v}O_2$ (rest)	= 16 mL $O_2 \cdot$ 100 mL^{-1} blood
	= 16 vol %
	= 160 mL $O_2 \cdot L^{-1}$ blood
$a-\bar{v}O_2$ diff (rest)	= (200 − 160) mL $O_2 \cdot L^{-1}$ blood
	= **40 mL $O_2 \cdot L^{-1}$ blood**
aO_2 (max)	= 200 mL $O_2 \cdot L^{-1}$ blood
	(Note that it is unchanged!)
$\bar{v}O_2$ (max)	= 40 mL $O_2 \cdot L^{-1}$ blood
	(Note that it is much lower!)
$a-\bar{v}O_2$ diff (max)	= (200 − 40) mL $O_2 \cdot L^{-1}$ blood
	= **160 mL $O_2 \cdot L^{-1}$ blood**

a. Note that $a-\bar{v}O_2$ diff increased 4 times with maximal exercise

b. Calculate $a-\bar{v}O_2$ diff if aO_2 = 20 vol % and $\bar{v}O_2$ = 10 vol % (conversions first, please!)

c. Do you see that a larger $a-\bar{v}O_2$ diff means more blood-borne O_2 is extracted by muscle?

Oxygen Consumption

This calculation brings together some of the others, i.e., the amount of oxygen consumed during a given period of exercise (say a minute) is related to both the amount of oxygen delivered in the blood ($\dot{Q}$) and the amount of oxygen extracted from the blood ($a-\bar{v}O_2$ diff). The basic equation is an application of the Fick principle: $\dot{V}O_2 = \dot{Q} \cdot a-\bar{v}O_2$ diff. Remember that the units for $\dot{Q}$ are $L \cdot min^{-1}$ and for $a-\bar{v}O_2$ diff, use mL $O_2 \cdot L^{-1}$ so the liters cancel and you are left with mL $O_2 \cdot min^{-1}$. This is converted to the customary units for oxygen uptake of $L \cdot min^{-1}$ by dividing by 1000.

$\dot{V}O_2$	$= \dot{Q} \cdot a-\bar{v}O_2$ diff
$\dot{V}O_2$ (rest)	= 4.9 L $\cdot min^{-1} \times$ 40 mL $O_2 \cdot L^{-1}$
	= 196 mL $\cdot min^{-1}$
	= **.196 L $\cdot$ min^{-1}**
$\dot{V}O_2$ (max)	= 18.7 L $\cdot min^{-1} \times$ 160 mL $O_2 \cdot L^{-1}$
	= 2992 mL $\cdot min^{-1}$
	= **2.99 L $\cdot$ min^{-1}**

a. Note that the O_2 uptake increased 15 times. Is this as high as it can go?

b. Express $\dot{V}O_2$ max relative to body weight (80 kg), i.e., in units of mL $\cdot kg^{-1} \cdot min^{-1}$ (do you get 37.4 with the decimal in the correct place?).

c. Calculate $\dot{V}O_2$ if $\dot{Q}$ = 11.7 L $\cdot min^{-1}$ and $a-\bar{v}O_2$ diff is 100 mL $O_2 \cdot L^{-1}$ blood

d. Note that the equation can be rearranged to solve for

$$\dot{Q} = \frac{\dot{V}O_2}{a-\bar{v}O_2} \text{ diff and } a-\bar{v}O_2 \text{ diff} = \frac{\dot{V}O_2}{\dot{Q}} \text{ try this!}$$

glossary

A

A Band   That area located in the center of the sarcomere containing both actin and myosin.

Acceleration Sprint   A training method in which running speed is gradually increased from jogging to striding and finally to sprinting.

Acclimation   Short-term or acute changes that occur in the body to lessen the physiological strain that develops in response to changes in climatic factors.

Acclimatization   Pertaining to certain physiological adjustments brought about through continued exposure to a different climate, for example, changes in altitude and heat.

Accommodating Resistance   A feature unique to isokinetic testing or training apparatus where a counterforce is provided so that the speed of contraction is controlled.

Acetylcholine (ACh)   A chemical substance involved in several important physiological functions such as transmission of an impulse from one nerve fiber to another across a synapse.

Acid   A chemical compound that gives up hydrogen ions (H^+) in solution.

Acidosis   A condition of reduced alkali reserve (bicarbonate) of the blood and other body fluids; usually, but not always, associated with an increase in H-ion concentration and a fall below normal in pH.

Actin   A protein involved in muscular contraction.

Action Potential   The electrical activity developed in a muscle or nerve cell during activity or depolarization.

Active Transport   The movement of substances or materials against their concentration gradients by the expenditure of metabolic energy.

Actomyosin   A protein complex formed from actin and myosin when myosin cross-bridges form a chemical bond with selected sites on actin filaments.

Acute Muscular Soreness   Pain that occurs during or immediately after performance of relatively high-intensity exercise; associated with inadequate blood flow.

Adenine   An aromatic base that when linked to ribose forms adenosine, the molecular foundation for ATP, ADP, and AMP.

Definitions followed by an asterisk (*) are from the Publications Advisory Committee, IOC Medical Commission, and personal communication with H. G. Knuttgen.

Adenohypophysis   The anterior lobe of the pituitary gland; *aden* means "in relationship to a gland," in this case the hypophysis (pituitary); secretes six major hormones.

Adenosine   The molecular foundation for ATP, ADP, and AMP, comprised of a five-carbon sugar (ribose) linked to an aromatic base (adenine).

Adenosine Diphosphate (ADP)   A complex chemical compound which, when combined with inorganic phosphate (Pi), forms ATP.

Adenosine Triphosphate (ATP)   A complex chemical compound formed with the energy released from food and stored in all cells, particularly muscles. Only from the energy released by the breakdown of this compound can the cell perform work.

Adipocyte   A fat cell; a cell that stores fat.

Adipose Tissue   Fat tissue.

Adrenal Cortex   Outer portion of the adrenal gland; secretes some forty different hormones known as steroids, which can be categorized as mineralocorticoids, glucocorticoids, and androgens.

Adrenal Medulla   Inner portion of the adrenal gland; often viewed as a direct extension of the sympathetic nervous system; secretes epinephrine and norepinephrine.

Adrenocorticotropic Hormone (ACTH; or Corticotropin)   A hormone secreted by the anterior lobe of the pituitary gland that stimulates the production and release of the glucocorticoid hormones from the adrenal cortex.

Aerobic   In the presence of oxygen.

Aerobic Glycolysis   See *Glycolysis.*

Aerobic Power   Maximal rate at which an individual can consume oxygen during the performance of all-out, exhaustive exercise; "best" index of cardiorespiratory fitness.

Aerobic System   Term used to denote the entire series of biochemical reactions and pathways whereby ATP can be synthesized from food-fuels but only in the presence of oxygen. Includes aerobic glycolysis, Krebs Cycle, and ETS.

Aerotitis   Inflammation or disease of the ear.

Afferent Nerve   A neuron that conveys sensory impulses from a receptor to the central nervous system.

Alactacid Oxygen Debt   That portion of the recovery oxygen used to resynthesize and restore ATP + PC in muscle following exercise. The rapid recovery phase.

Aldosterone   A mineralocorticoid.

Alkali Reserve   The amount of bicarbonate (base) available in the body for buffering.

Alkaline   Pertaining to a base.

Alkalosis   Excessive base (bicarbonate ions) in the extracellular fluids.

All-or-None Law   A stimulated muscle or nerve fiber contracts or propagates a nerve impulse either completely or not at all; in other words, once stimulated, it causes a maximal response.

Alpha-Gamma Coactivation   Firing of both alpha and gamma motoneurons to the same muscle at nearly the same time to produce desired voluntary contractions.

Alpha Motor Neuron   A type of efferent nerve cell that innervates extrafusal muscle fibers.

Alveolar-Capillary Membrane   The thin layer of tissue dividing the alveoli and the pulmonary capillaries where gaseous exchange occurs.

Alveolar Ventilation   The portion of inspired air that reaches the alveoli.

Alveoli (plural); Alveolus (singular)   Tiny terminal air sacs in the lungs where gaseous exchange between the blood and the pulmonary capillaries occurs.

Ambient   Pertaining to the surrounding environment.

Amenorrhea   Stoppage of menstrual cycles; not uncommon in female athletes practicing rigorous endurance training or severely restricting their body weight; often preceded by irregular menses.

Amino Acid Deamination   Metabolic process where the nitrogen containing amino radical (NH_2) is removed from the amino acid molecule.

Amino Acids   The basic structural unit of proteins having an amino radical component (NH_2) that contains nitrogen and a carboxyl group (COOH).

Amphetamine   A synthetically structured drug closely related to epinephrine; it produces stimulation of the central nervous system.

Anabolic   Protein building.

Anabolic-Androgenic Steroid   A compound that promotes tissue-building and male-like bodily characteristics; it is conducive to the constructive (building up) process of metabolism.

Anaerobic   In the absence of oxygen.

Anaerobic Glycolysis   The incomplete chemical breakdown of carbohydrate. The anaerobic reactions in this breakdown release energy for the manufacture of ATP as they produce lactic acid (anaerobic glycolysis is known as the lactic acid system).

Anaerobic Power   The development of maximal or peak power during exertion; measured as work (force in kg $\times$ distance in meters) expressed per unit of time (min).

Anaerobic Threshold   That intensity of work load or oxygen consumption at which anaerobic metabolism is accelerated.

Anatomical Dead Space (V_D)   That volume of fresh air that remains in the respiratory passages (nose, mouth, pharynx, larynx, trachea, bronchi, and bronchioles) and does not participate in gaseous exchange.

Androgen   Any substance that possesses masculinizing (male-like) properties.

Anemia   A lack of sufficient red blood cells or hemoglobin.

Aneurysm   Blood-filled pouches that balloon out from a weak spot in the arterial wall.

Annulospiral Nerve   Sensory (afferent) nerve from central region of muscle spindle; sends impulses to CNS with whole muscle stretch or intrafusal fiber shortening.

Anorexia Nervosa   A clinical disorder of eating associated with loss of appetite, distorted body image, and an intense fear of fatness or weight gain.

Anterior Lobe   The portion of the pituitary gland located furthest from the spinal cord (anterior position); also called the adenohypophysis.

Anthropometry   The measurement of the size and proportions of the human body.

Antidiuretic Hormone (ADH; also called Vasopressin)   A hormone secreted by the posterior lobe of the pituitary gland that functions mainly to promote water reabsorption from the collecting tubules of the kidney.

Antioxidants   Substances that provide electrons that reduce free radicals associated with other molecules.

Apnea (Apneic)   Cessation of breathing.

Aqueous   Pertaining to water.

Arterial Mixed Venous Oxygen Difference (a-$\bar{v}O_2$ diff)   The difference between the oxygen content of arterial and mixed venous blood.

Artery   A vessel carrying blood away from the heart.

Atherosclerosis   A disease of the arteries in which lipid (fat) material and cholesterol accumulate on the inside walls of the arteries.

ATP   See *Adenosine Triphosphate*.

ATPase   An enzyme that facilitates the breakdown of ATP.

ATP-PC System   An anaerobic energy system in which ATP is manufactured when phosphocreatine (PC) is broken down. This system represents the most rapidly available source of ATP for use by muscle. Activities performed at maximum intensity for a period of 10 seconds or less derive energy (ATP) from this system.

ATPS   Ambient temperature, pressure, saturated (see appendix C).

Atrioventricular Node (A-V Node)   A specialized area of tissue located in the right atrium of the heart from which the electrical impulse initiated by the sino-atrial node spreads throughout the heart.

Atrophy   A reduction in the cross-sectional area of muscle, muscle fibers, or other tissues due to injury, disuse, disease, immobilization, or similar factors.

Autonomic Nervous System   A self-controlled system that helps to control activities such as those involving movement and secretion by the visceral organs, urinary output, body temperature, heart rate, adrenal secretion, and blood pressure.

Axon   A nerve fiber.

B

Barometric (Atmospheric) Pressure (P_B)   The force per unit area exerted by the earth's atmosphere. At sea level, it is 14.7 pounds per square inch or 760 mm of mercury (mm Hg).

Baroreceptors   Receptors predominantly located in the walls of the carotid arteries and the aortic arch that are sensitive to transluminal (across the wall) stretch; when activated, they increase the afferent firing rate to the cardiorespiratory center of the medulla.

Basal Ganglia   Subcortical portion of brain that, along with the thalamus, provides an information loop back to the premotor cortex to assist in the selection and initiation of chosen movements.

Bends (Decompression Sickness)   A condition induced by the evolution of nitrogen bubbles resulting from rapid decompression (gas emboli) and which may cause circulatory blockage and tissue damage.

Beta-Oxidation   The series of reactions by which fat is broken down from long carbon chains to two carbon units in preparation for entry into the Krebs Cycle.

Bicarbonate Ion (HCO_3^-)   A by-product of the dissociation (ionizing) of carbonic acid.

Bioenergetics   The study of energy transformations in living organisms.

Biopsy   The removal and examination of tissue from the living body.

Black Globe Thermometer   An ordinary thermometer placed in a black globe. The black bulb temperature measures radiant energy or solar radiation and is one of three temperatures used to compute the WBGT index.

Blood Doping   The removal and subsequent reinfusion of blood, undertaken to temporarily increase oxygen-carrying red blood cells.

Blood Glucose   Simple form of sugar (carbohydrate) circulating in blood; levels are regulated mainly through the glycogen stored in the liver.

Blood Pressure   The force per unit area exerted by the blood against the inside walls of an artery; the driving force that moves blood through the circulatory system.

Body Mass Index (BMI)   A much-used indication of the "size" of an individual in relationship to his or her height; ratio of wt:ht squared using units of kilograms and meters.

Boyle's Law   The volume occupied by a gas (at constant temperature) is reduced or expanded in direct proportion to the pressure placed around it; very important to underwater diving.

Bradycardia   A heart rate less than 60 beats per minute.

BTPS   Body temperature, pressure, saturated (see appendix C).

Buffer   Any substance in a fluid that lessens the change in hydrogen ion (H^+) concentration which otherwise would occur by adding acids or bases.

C

Calcitonin   A hormone secreted by the thyroid gland that causes a decrease in the blood calcium level. It is thought that calcitonin may also be secreted from the parathyroid glands.

Calorie (cal)   A unit of work or energy equal to the amount of heat required to raise the temperature of one gram of water 1° C.

Calorimeter   Measures heat production from oxidized food stuffs (bomb-type) or heat production from the human body (live-in type).

c-AMP Amplification   Impact of a hormone on a membrane causing cyclic AMP to form on the inside surface; has effect of multiplying the hormone effect.

Capillary   A fine network of small vessels located between arteries and veins where exchanges between tissue and blood occur.

Carbamino Compounds   The end product obtained from the chemical combination of plasma proteins and/or hemoglobin (Hgb) and carbon dioxide (CO_2).

Carbaminohemoglobin   A carbamino compound formed in the red blood cells when CO_2 reacts with Hgb.

Carbohydrate   Any of a group of chemical compounds, including sugars, starches, and cellulose; contains carbon, hydrogen, and oxygen only.

Carbonic Anhydrase   An enzyme that speeds up the reaction of carbon dioxide (CO_2) with water (H_2O).

Cardiac Cycle   Contraction (systole) and relaxation (diastole) of the heart.

Cardiac Output ($\dot{Q}$)   The amount of blood pumped by the heart in one minute; the product of the stroke volume and the heart rate.

Cardiorespiratory Endurance   The ability of the lungs and heart to take in and transport adequate amounts of oxygen to the working muscles, allowing activities that involve large muscle masses (e.g., running, swimming, bicycling) to be performed over long periods of time.

Cardiovascular Drift   A compensatory increase in heart rate that usually occurs during prolonged endurance exercise in response to a decrease in stroke volume; cardiac output is maintained as a result.

Catecholamines   Epinephrine and norepinephrine.

Cell Body   See *Soma*.

Central Command   Neurons originating in the motor cortex that influence the cardiorespiratory (ventilation and cardiovascular) center of the medulla on their way to initiate a skeletal muscle action.

Central Nervous System   The spinal cord and brain.

Central Neural Fatigue   Decrease in muscle force attributable to a decline in motoneuronal output.

Cerebellum   That division or part of the brain concerned with coordination of movements.

Cerebral Cortex   That portion of the brain responsible for mental functions, movements, visceral functions, perception, and behavioral reactions, and for the association and integration of these functions.

Cerebral Thrombosis   A blood clot in the brain.

Charles's Law   The volume occupied by a gas (at constant pressure) is reduced or expanded in direct proportion to its temperature.

Chemical Transmitter Substance   Stored in vesicles within the synaptic knobs of axons; released with the arrival of an impulse into the synaptic cleft or gap.

Cholesterol   A fatlike compound found in animal tissues that contributes to the development of atherosclerosis.

Cholinesterase   A chemical that deactivates or breaks down acetylcholine.

Chronotropic   Rate of myocardial contractions (beats $\cdot$ min^{-1}).

Cisterns   The terminal ends of the longitudinal tubules of the sarcoplasmic reticulum which store Ca^{++}; also called outer cisterns, outer vesicles, and terminal cisternae.

Concentric Contraction*   Muscle action in which the ends of the muscle are drawn closer.

Conditioning   Augmentation of the energy capacity of muscle through a physical exercise program. Conditioning is not primarily concerned with the skill of performance, as would be the case in training.

Conduction   The transfer of heat between objects of different temperatures in direct contact with each other.

Continuous Work   Exercises performed to completion without relief periods.

Convection   The transfer of heat from one place to another by the motion of a heated substance—e.g., air or water.

Core Temperature   Temperature of deep body tissues such as head, thorax, and digestive system.

Cori Cycle   A process where lactic acid from muscle metabolism diffuses into the blood and is carried to the liver for conversion to glucose where it can be used, stored, or released into the blood.

Coronary Heart Disease   Narrowing (atherosclerosis) of a coronary artery, causing ischemic symptoms, spasms, and infarctions.

Cortisol   A glucocorticoid.

Coupled Reactions   Two series of chemical reactions, one of which releases energy (heat) for use by the other.

Creatine Kinase (CK)   Enzyme that catalyzes (speeds) the breakdown of phosphocreatine to reform ATP in the presence of ADP (i.e., PC + ADP $\overset{CK}{\rightarrow}$ ATP + C).

Cristae   A series of inward membrane folds and convolutions within mitochondria that contain the enzyme systems required for aerobic metabolism.

Cross-Bridges   Extensions of myosin.

Cross-Innervate   A surgical procedure in experimental animals where the nerve fibers to Type I and Type II muscle fibers are crossed over and reattached.

Cross-Training or **Transfer of Training**   A theory that developing one region of the body will result in improvement of other regions; also used to describe potential benefits of combined running, biking, swimming, and/or weight training.

Cryogenic   Pertaining to the production of low temperatures.

Cyclic AMP Mechanism   The most common mechanism for the action of hormones on their target cells; hormones arrive at receptors and activate adenyl cyclase to speed cyclic AMP formation from ATP resulting in numerous specific actions.

Cytochromes   Co-enzyme carriers containing iron (Fe^{++} and Fe^{+++} forms) that pass on hydrogens and their associated electrons in the electron transport system.

Cytoplasm   Cell fluid that makes up the inside of cells; in muscle cells it is called sarcoplasm.

Dalton's Law   The partial pressures of gases in a mixture remain constant and will act independently of each other.

Dehydration   The condition that results from excessive loss of body water.

Delayed Muscular Soreness   Pain and stiffness that occurs 1 to 2 days after the performance of exercise that is of a type or intensity uncommon to the performer.

Delayed Onset Muscular Soreness (DOMS)   See *Delayed Muscular Soreness*.

Dendrites   Short extensions from the body of a nerve cell.

Density   The mass per unit volume of an object.

Depolarization   A positive change (spike) away from the resting membrane potential of neural or muscle cells; loss of semipermeability and in-rushing of Na^+.

Detraining   Changes in body structure or function caused by reduction or cessation of regular physical training.

Diaphragmatic Pleura   See *Pleura*.

Diastole   The resting phase of the cardiac cycle.

Diastolic Blood Pressure (DBP)   The lowest pressure existing in the arteries.

Diastolic Volume   The amount of blood that fills the ventricle during diastole.

Diffusion   The random movement of molecules due to their kinetic energy.

Disaccharides   Double sugars such as sucrose and maltose; carbohydrates where two molecular ring structures are bonded.

Dopamine   An excitatory neurotransmitter chemical.

Double-Blind Study   An experimental protocol in which neither the investigators nor the subjects know which group is receiving a placebo and which group the real drug or treatment.

Douglas Bag   A rubber-lined, canvas bag used for collection of expired gas. Rubber meterologic balloons now are used.

Drug   A chemical substance given with the intention of preventing or curing disease or otherwise enhancing the physical or mental welfare of humans or animals.

Dry Bulb Thermometer   A common thermometer used to record temperature of the air.

Dynamic Contraction   See *Concentric Contraction.*

Dynamic Flexibility   The opposition or resistance of a joint to motion; forces opposing movement rather than the range of movement itself, which is static flexibility.

Dysmenorrhea   Painful menstruation.

Dyspnea   Labored breathing.

E

Eccentric Contraction*   Muscle action in which a force external to the muscle overcomes the muscle force and the ends of the muscle are drawn further apart.

Ectomorphy   A body type component characterized by linearity, fragility, and delicacy of body.

Efferent Nerve   A neuron that conveys impulses away from the central nervous system to an organ of response such as skeletal muscle.

Efficiency   The ratio of work output to work input expressed as a percentage.

Electrical Potential   The capacity for producing electrical effects, such as an electric current, between two bodies (e.g., between the inside and outside of a cell).

Electrocardiogram (ECG)   A recording of the electrical activity of the heart.

Electrolyte   A substance that ionizes in solution, such as salt (NaCl), and is capable of conducting an electrical current.

Electron   A negatively charged particle.

Electron Micrographs   Photographs of tissues as magnified thousands of times in an electron microscope.

Electron Transport System (ETS)   A series of chemical reactions occurring in mitochondria, in which electrons and hydrogen ions combine with oxygen to form water, and ATP is resynthesized. Also referred to as the *respiratory chain.*

Embolus (singular); Emboli (plural)   A clot or other plug transported by the blood and forced into a small vessel, thus obstructing circulation.

Endocrine Gland   An organ or gland that produces an internal secretion (hormone).

Endomorphy   A body type component characterized by roundness and softness of the body.

Endomysium   A connective tissue surrounding a muscle fiber or cell.

Endorphins   One of several substances in the general category of endogenous opioid peptides that may provide mood-altering, pain-reduction, and relaxing benefits; implicated in phenomena known as "runner's high" and "exercise addiction."

Endurance*   The time limit of a person's ability to maintain either an isometric force or a power level involving combinations of concentric and/or eccentric muscle actions.

Energy*   The capability of producing force, performing work, or generating heat (SI unit: joule).

Energy Capacity   The maximal amount of energy that can be liberated by a metabolic system; independent of time but using all available stores of fuel substrate.

Energy Continuum   A conceptual model whereby the energy required for mostly anaerobic, mixed, and mostly aerobic activities is provided via a greater or lesser use of the same metabolic pathways.

Energy Nutrients   Sources of usable energy from food; carbohydrates, fats, and proteins.

Energy State Regulation   A mechanism of control over cellular metabolism that is tightly linked to the ongoing use of energy and the rate of ADP production.

Energy System   One of three metabolic systems involving a series of chemical reactions resulting in the formation of waste products and the manufacture of ATP.

Engram   A memorized motor pattern stored in the brain; a permanent trace left by a stimulus in the tissue protoplasm.

Enzyme   A protein compound that speeds up a chemical reaction.

Epimysium   A connective tissue surrounding the entire muscle.

Epinephrine   A hormone secreted by the medulla of the adrenal gland that has effects on the heart, the blood vessels, metabolism, and the central nervous system.

Ergogenic Aid   Any factor that improves work performance.

Ergometer   An apparatus or device, such as a treadmill or stationary cycle, used for measuring the physiological effects of exercise.

Erythropoietin   A hormone, naturally produced by the kidney, which stimulates the formation of red blood cells within bone marrow.

Essential Hypertension   Abnormally high blood pressure in humans that has no known cause and therefore no known cure; most common type of high blood pressure.

Essential Nutrients   Nutrients that cannot be manufactured by the body or are manufactured at a pace that is slower than the body's needs (e.g., linoleic acid).

Estradiol   A hormone of the estrogen category; the primary form produced by the human ovaries; produces female secondary sex characteristics and causes estrus in animals.

Estrogen   A general category of female sex hormones; the principal one produced by the human ovary is estradiol.

Eumenorrheic   The presence of regular menstrual cycles.

Evaporation   The loss of heat resulting from changing a liquid to a vapor.

Excitation   A response to a stimulus.

Excitatory Postsynaptic Potential (EPSP)   A transient increase in electrical potential (depolarization) from its resting membrane potential in a postsynaptic neuron.

Exercise*   Any and all activity involving the generation of force by the activated muscle(s). Exercise can be quantified mechanically as force, torque, work, power, or velocity of progression.

Exercise Intensity*   A specific level of muscular activity that can be quantified in terms of power (energy expenditure or work performed per unit of time), the opposing force (e.g., by free weight stack), isometric force sustained, or velocity of progression.

Exercise Physiology   Scientific study of how the body, from a functional standpoint, responds, adjusts, and adapts to acute exercise and chronic training.

Exercise Pressor Reflex   An afferent feedback mechanism to the cardiorespiratory areas of the medulla that originates in the skeletal muscles, mainly via mechanoreceptors and metaboreceptors.

Exercise-Recovery   The performance of light exercise during recovery from exercise.

Expiratory Reserve Volume (ERV)   Maximal volume of air expired from end-expiration.

Extracellular   Outside the cell.

Extrafusal Fiber   A typical or normal muscle cell or fiber.

F

Facilitated Diffusion   Diffusion that takes place with the help of a carrier substance.

Fartlek Training (Speed Play)   An informal interval-training-type method for endurance performance that involves alternating a fast and a slow training pace over natural terrain. Neither the work nor relief intervals are precisely timed. It is the forerunner of the interval training system.

Fasciculus (singular); Fasciculi (plural)   A group or bundle of skeletal muscle fibers held together by a connective tissue called the perimysium.

Fast Component (of recovery)   The initial, rapid decline in oxygen consumption at the start of recovery from exercise, usually lasting 3 to 4 minutes (reported in liters); formerly alactacid oxygen debt.

Fast-Twitch (FT) Fiber   A muscle fiber characterized by fast contraction time, high anaerobic capacity, and low aerobic capacity, all making the fiber suited for high-power output activities. Also known as Type II fiber.

Fat   A compound containing glycerol and fatty acids.

Fatigue   A state of discomfort and decreased efficiency resulting from prolonged or excessive exertion.

Fat-Soluble Vitamins   A category of vitamins that are fat soluble and consequently are stored in the body in the liver and fatty tissues; need not be supplied each day but excessive accumulations can cause toxic effects; vitamins A, D, E, and K.

Fatty Acid (Free Fatty Acid)   The usable form of degraded triglycerides.

Fiber:Nerve Ratio (F:N)   The number of muscle fibers in a motor unit in relationship to the motor neuron axon that is innervating it.

Fibrillation   Irregularity in force and rhythm of the heart, or quivering of the muscle fibers, causing inefficient emptying.

Fibrinolysis   The dissolving of a blood clot.

Flaccid   Lacking muscular tonus.

Flavin Adenine Dinucleotide   An acceptor and carrier of hydrogens from the Krebs cycle to the electron transport system.

Flexibility   See *Static Flexibility* or *Dynamic Flexibility*.

Flexometer   An instrument used for measuring the range of motion about a joint (static flexibility).

Follicle-Stimulating Hormone (FSH)   A hormone secreted by the anterior lobe of the pituitary gland that promotes growth of the ovarian follicle in the female and spermatogenesis in the male.

Foot-Pound (ft-lb)   A work unit; that is, application of a one-pound force through a distance of one foot.

Force*   That which changes or tends to change the state of rest or motion in matter (SI unit: Newton). A muscle generates force in a muscle action.

Frank-Starling Mechanism   A change in cardiac performance (i.e., stroke work) as a function of preload or stretch of the cardiac muscle prior to contraction.

Free Weight*   An object of known mass, not attached to a supporting or guiding structure, which is used for physical conditioning and competitive lifting.

Fulcrum   The axis of rotation of a lever.

Functional Residual Capacity (FRC)   Volume of air in the lungs at resting expiratory level.

Fusimotor Neurons   The nerve cells of the CNS whose thin axons innervate the intrafusal fibers of the muscle spindles; also called *gamma motor neurons*.

G

Gamma-Aminobutyric Acid (GABA)   An inhibitory neurotransmitter substance.

Gamma Motor Neuron   A type of efferent nerve cell that innervates the ends of an intrafusal muscle fiber.

Gamma System (Gamma Loop)   The contraction of a muscle as a result of stretching the muscle spindle by way of stimulation of the gamma motor neurons.

Glucagon   A hormone secreted by the alpha cells of the pancreas that causes increased blood glucose levels.

Glucocorticoids   A class of hormones secreted by the cortex of the adrenal gland that promote the increased synthesis of glucose from amino acids (gluconeogenesis), depress liver lipogenesis (formation of fat), mobilize fat in adipose tissues, maintain vascular reactivity, and inhibit the inflammatory reaction.

Gluconeogenesis   The manufacturing of carbohydrates from noncarbohydrate sources such as fat and protein.

Glucose   A sugar.

Glucose-Alanine Cycle   Glucose made in the liver from pyruvic acid that is carried there in the form of alanine; the alanine being originally formed in muscle by combining $-NH_2$ radicals from metabolized amino acids with pyruvate.

Glycine   A simple amino acid, thought to be the main inhibitory transmitter in the spinal cord.

Glycogen   A polymer of glucose; the form in which glucose (sugar) is stored in the body, mainly in muscles and the liver.

Glycogen-Loading (supercompensation)   A diet or exercise-diet procedure that elevates muscle glycogen stores to concentrations two to three times normal.

Glycogen Sparing   The diminished utilization of glycogen that results when other fuels are available (and are used) for activity. If, for instance, fat is used to a greater extent than usual, glycogen is "spared"; glycogen will thus be available longer before ultimately being depleted.

Glycogenesis   The manufacture of glycogen from glucose.

Glycogenolysis   The breakdown of glycogen to glucose.

Glycolysis   The incomplete chemical breakdown of glycogen. In aerobic glycolysis, the end product is pyruvic acid; in anaerobic glycolysis (lactic acid system), the end product is lactic acid.

Golgi Tendon Organ   A proprioceptor located within a muscular tendon, which ultimately inhibits muscle contraction.

Gradation   The ability of muscles to produce forces of varying strength; from very light to maximal force or tension.

Growth Hormone [GH; also called Somatotropin (STH)]   A hormone secreted by the anterior lobe of the pituitary gland that stimulates growth and development.

H-Zone   The area in the center of the A band where the cross-bridges are absent.

Half-Reaction Time   Method of estimating speed at which a chemical or physiological reaction or change occurs (e.g., in 30 seconds one half of fast oxygen recovery component is completed).

HDL Cholesterol   That portion of total plasma cholesterol that is transported or carried by high-density lipoproteins, higher levels of which carry an inverse relationship to the development of atherosclerosis.

Heart Attack   The blocking of blood flow to a portion of the heart muscle. Also *myocardial infarction.*

Heart Rate Reserve   The difference between the resting heart rate and the maximal heart rate.

Heat   A form of energy.

Heat Cramps   Painful muscular contractions caused by prolonged exposure to environmental heat.

Heat Exhaustion   A condition of fatigue caused by prolonged exposure to environmental heat. May be associated with headache, nausea, and vomiting.

Heat Stroke   A disorder caused by overexposure to heat and characterized by high body (rectal) temperature, hot, dry skin (usually flushed), and unconsciousness. It can be fatal.

Hematuria   Discharge of blood into the urine.

Hemoconcentration   Concentration of the blood.

Hemodilution   Dilution of the blood.

Hemodynamics   The study of the physical laws governing blood flow.

Hemoglobin (Hgb)   A complex molecule found in red blood cells, which contains iron (heme) and protein (globin) and is capable of combining with oxygen.

Hemolysis   The rupture of a cell, such as the red blood cell.

Henry's Law   The amount of gas that a fluid will absorb under pressure varies in direct proportion to the partial pressure of the gas.

High-Energy Phosphogens   Includes ATP, ADP, and CP—all of which contain one or two high-energy phosphate bonds that can be split to liberate usable energy.

Hormone   A discrete chemical substance secreted into the body fluids by an endocrine gland; has a specific effect on the activities of other cells, tissues, and organs.

Hormone Receptor   A region of the membranes of target cells that is specific to and can react with only one hormone; analogous to a lock and key mechanism.

Humidity   Pertaining to the moisture in the air.

Hydraulic Pressure   The force per unit area resulting from a vertical column of water of a certain height.

Hypercapnia   Presence of an abnormally large amount of CO_2 in the circulating blood; increased partial pressure of CO_2 resulting in extra stimulation of respiratory area.

Hypernatremia   Increased sodium concentration in the blood.

Hyperplasia   An increase in the number of cells in a tissue or organ.

Hyperpolarization   An overshoot of the repolarization process so that the cell membrane potential goes below the normal resting level.

Hypertension   High blood pressure.

Hyperthermia   Increased body temperature.

Hypertonic   Pertaining to a solution having a greater tension or osmotic pressure than the one with which it is being compared.

Hypertrophy   An increase in the size of a cell or organ.

Hyperventilation   Excessive ventilation of the lungs caused by increased depth and frequency of breathing and usually resulting in elimination of carbon dioxide.

Hypervolemia   An increased blood volume.

Hypoglycemia   Lower than normal blood sugar level due to inadequate supply or regulation; may be the result of excessive blood insulin.

Hypophysis   Another name for the pituitary gland; made up of the anterior lobe, called the adenohypophysis, and the posterior lobe, called the neurohypophysis.

Hypotension   Abnormally low blood pressure.

Hypothalamus   That portion of the brain that exerts control over visceral activities, water balance, body temperature, and sleep.

Hypothermia   An abnormally low (less than 35° C) body temperature.

Hypotonic   Pertaining to a solution having a lesser tension or osmotic pressure than the one with which it is being compared.

Hypoxia   Lack of adequate oxygen due to a reduced oxygen partial pressure.

I

I Band   That area of a myofibril containing actin and bisected by a Z line.

Immune System   A highly integrated system of bodily functions responsible for detecting the presence of and maintaining resistance to disease.

Inert   Having no action.

Inhibitory Postsynaptic Potential (IPSP)   A transient decrease in electrical potential (hyperpolarization) in a postsynaptic neuron from its resting membrane potential.

Inorganic Phosphate (Pi)   Simple form of phosphorus not in association with carbon, which would make it organic. A by-product of ATP when it is split to ADP and Pi and used in resynthesizing ATP in the process of oxidative-phosphorylation.

Inotropic   Force of myocardial contraction; a shift in the Frank-Starling curve to the right or to the left.

Inspiratory Capacity (IC)   Maximal volume of air inspired from resting expiratory level.

Inspiratory Reserve Volume (IRV)   Maximal volume of air inspired from end-inspiration.

Insulin   A hormone secreted by the beta cells of the pancreas that causes increased cellular uptake of glucose.

Intermittent Work   Exercises performed with alternate periods of relief, as opposed to continuous work.

Interneuron (Internuncial Neuron)   A nerve cell located between afferent (sensory) and efferent (motor) nerve cells. It acts as a "go-between" between incoming and outgoing impulses.

Interstitial   Pertaining to the area or space between cells.

Interstitial Fluid   The fluid between the cells.

Interval Sprinting   A method of training whereby an athlete might alternately sprint 50 m and jog 60 m for distances of 4 to 5 km.

Interval Training   A system of physical conditioning in which the body is subjected to short but regularly repeated periods of work stress interspersed with adequate periods of relief.

Intrafusal Fibers   Muscle cells (fibers) that house the muscle spindles.

Intramuscular Glycogen   Complex carbohydrate stored within muscle cells; the glucose subunits are used as a ready source of energy for muscle metabolism.

Ion   An electrically charged particle.

Iron   A mineral found in the heme groups of red blood cells and in the cytochromes of the mitochondrion; very important to O_2 transport, metabolism, and energy levels.

Ischemia   Local and temporary deficiency of blood and oxygen, chiefly caused by narrowing of a blood vessel.

Isoforms   Proteins that have the same basic make-up but also slight modifications that alter their function (e.g., in muscle both heavy- and light-chain myosin exist).

Isokinetic Contraction   Contraction in which the tension developed by the muscle while shortening at constant speed is theoretically maximal over the full range of motion.

Isometric Contraction*   Muscle action in which the ends of the muscle are prevented from drawing closer together, with no change in length.

Isotonic   Pertaining to solutions having the same tension or osmotic pressure.

Isotonic Contraction   Contraction in which the muscle shortens with varying tension while lifting a constant load. Also referred to as a *dynamic* or *concentric contraction.*

J

Joint Receptors   A group of sense organs located in joints concerned with kinesthesis.

K

Kilocalorie (kcal)   A unit of work or energy equal to the amount of heat required to raise the temperature of one kilogram of water 1° C.

Kilogram-Meters (kg-m)   A unit of work.

Kilojoules (kJ)   A unit of energy.

Kinesiology   Scientific study of human movement. Includes such aspects of study as exercise physiology, motor learning/control, and biomechanics.

Kinesthesis   Awareness of body position.

Krebs Cycle   A series of chemical reactions occurring in mitochondria, in which carbon dioxide is produced and hydrogen ions and electrons are removed from carbon atoms (oxidation). Also referred to as the *tricarboxylic acid cycle* (TCA), or *citric acid cycle.*

L

Lactacid Oxygen Debt   That portion of the recovery oxygen used to remove accumulated lactic acid from the blood following exercise. The slow recovery phase.

Lactate Threshold   The point during exercise where a nonlinear increase in blood lactate occurs.

Lactic Acid (Lactate)   A fatiguing metabolite produced during anaerobic glycolysis; resulting from the incomplete breakdown of glucose (sugar).

Lactic Acid System (LA System)   An anaerobic energy system in which ATP is manufactured when glucose (sugar) is broken down to lactic acid. High-intensity efforts requiring 1 to 3 minutes before energy (ATP) is primarily drawn from this system. More commonly referred to as *anaerobic glycolysis.*

LDL Cholesterol   That portion of total plasma cholesterol that is transported or carried by low-density lipoproteins, higher levels of which carry a direct relationship to the development of atherosclerosis.

Lean Body Mass (Weight)   The body weight minus the weight of the body fat.

Lever   A rigid bar (such as a bone) that is free to rotate about a fixed point or axis called a fulcrum (such as a joint).

Linear   Pertaining to a straight line.

Lipid   A term used when discussing fats in the body.

Longitudinal Fiber Splitting   Development of new muscle fibers from existing ones as a result of intense chronic "weight training"; shown only in experimental animals.

Longitudinal Tubules   Portions of the sarcoplasmic reticulum that run parallel to the muscle myofibrils and terminate in the outer vesicles.

Luteinizing Hormone (LH) or **Interstitial Cell-Stimulating Hormone (ICSH)**   A hormone secreted by the anterior lobe of the pituitary gland that stimulates ovulation, formation of the corpus luteum, and hormone secretion in the female; and stimulates secretion by interstitial cells in the male.

M

Mass***   The quantity of matter of an object that is reflected in its inertia (SI unit: kilogram).

Maximal Aerobic Power   See *Maximal Oxygen Consumption*.

Maximal Oxygen Consumption (max $\dot{V}O_2$)   The maximal rate at which oxygen can be consumed per minute; the power or capacity of the aerobic or oxygen system.

Maximum Voluntary Contraction (MVC)   The greatest force output that an individual can generate from a muscle group through only volitional control.

Mechanoreceptors   Peripheral nerve endings primarily activated by shape changes in the contracting skeletal muscle.

Medulla Oblongata   That portion or area of the brain continuous above with the pons and below with the spinal cord and containing the cardiorespiratory control area.

Membrane   A thin layer of tissue that covers a surface or divides a space or organ.

Menarche   The onset of menstruation.

Menses   The monthly flow of blood from the genital tract of women.

Menstruation   The process or an instance of discharging the menses.

Mesomorphy   A body type component characterized by a square body with hard, rugged, and prominent musculature.

MET (Metabolic Equivalent)   The amount of oxygen required per minute under resting, sitting conditions. It is approximately 3.5 mL of oxygen consumed per kilogram of body weight per minute (mL · kg^{-1} · min^{-1}).

Metabolic System   A system of biochemical reactions that cause the formation of waste products (metabolites) and the manufacture of ATP; for example, the ATP-PC, anaerobic glycolysis, and oxygen systems.

Metabolism   The sum total of the chemical changes or reactions occurring in the body.

Metabolite   Any substance produced by a metabolic reaction.

Metaboreceptors   Peripheral nerve endings primarily activated by metabolic changes (e.g., pH) in and around contracting skeletal muscle.

Microgravity   A gravitational field that is experienced in orbital space flight; very much less than at sea level but not entirely "weightless."

Millimole   One thousandth of a mole.

Mineralocorticoids   A class of hormones secreted by the cortex of the adrenal gland, that function to increase the reabsorption of sodium from the distal tubules of the kidney. The most important mineralocorticoid is aldosterone.

Minerals   Inorganic compounds found in the body that are important to proper bodily function; calcium, magnesium, phosphorus, potassium, sodium, iron, iodine, and chlorine are common examples.

Minute Ventilation   The amount of air inspired ($\dot{V}_I$) or expired ($\dot{V}_E$) in one minute; usually it refers to the expired amount.

Mitochondrion (singular); Mitochondria (plural)   A subcellular structure found in all cells in which the reactions of the Krebs Cycle and electron transport system take place.

Mole   The gram-molecular weight or gram-formula weight of a substance. For example, one mole of glucose. $C_6H_{12}O_6$ weighs $(6 \times 12) + (12 \times 1) + (6 \times 16) = 72 + 12 + 96 = 180$ grams, where the atomic weight of carbon (C) = 12; hydrogen (H) = 1; and oxygen (O) = 16.

Moment (Moment Arm)   The perpendicular distance from the line of action of the force to the point of rotation.

Monosaccharides   Simple sugars such as glucose, fructose, and galactose; carbohydrates comprised of only one molecular ring structure and formula $C_6H_{12}O_6$.

Motor Endplate   The neuromuscular or myoneural junction.

Motor Engrams   Memorized motor patterns that are stored in the motor area of the brain.

Motor Fiber   See *Efferent Nerve*.

Motor Neuron (Motoneuron)   A nerve cell, which when stimulated, affects muscular contraction. Most motoneurons innervate skeletal muscle.

Motor Unit   An individual alpha motor nerve and all the muscle fibers it innervates.

Mountain (or Altitude) Sickness   Failure to acclimatize after going to a higher altitude, resulting in symptoms similar to pneumonia and/or flu-like illnesses.

Multiple Motor Unit Summation   The varying of the number of motor units contracting within a muscle at any given time.

Muscle Bundle   A fasciculus.

Muscle Spindle   A proprioceptor (stretch receptor) surrounded by intrafusal muscle fibers.

Muscle Spindle Reflex   Discharge of impulses from muscle spindles due to stretch, which results in CNS reflex maintenance of active muscle tonus in the same muscles.

Muscular Endurance   The ability of a muscle or muscle group to perform repeated contractions against a light load for an extended period of time.

Muscular Strength   The force or tension that a muscle or group of muscles can exert against a resistance in one maximal effort.

Muscular Tonus (Tone)   Resiliency and resistance to stretch in a relaxed, resting muscle.

Myelin Sheath   A structure composed mainly of lipid (fat) and protein that surrounds some nerve fibers (axons).

Myelinated Nerve Fiber   A nerve fiber containing a myelin sheath.

Myofibril   That part of a muscle fiber containing two protein filaments, myosin and actin.

Myofilaments   Contractile proteins (actin and myosin) located within muscle myofibrils.

Myogenic Factors   Substances found within muscle fibers that regulate the properties specific to the fiber type, such as contractile speed and power production during contraction.

Myoglobin   An oxygen-binding pigment similar to hemoglobin that gives the red muscle fiber its color. It acts as an oxygen store and aids in the diffusion of oxygen.

Myokinase (MK)   Enzyme found in muscle cells that catalyzes (speeds) the reformation of ATP in the presence of ADP (i.e., ADP + ADP $\xrightarrow{MK}$ ATP + AMP).

Myosin   A protein involved in muscular contraction.

Myosin-ATPase (m-ATPase)   Myofibrillar adenosine triphosphatase; an enzyme found in myosin that catalyzes ATP degradation to ADP and Pi; a marker for muscle fiber contraction speed.

N

Necrosis   Death of a cell or group of cells in contact with living tissue.

Negative Energy Balance   A condition in which less energy (food) is taken in than is given off; body weight decreases as a result.

Negative Feedback Mechanism   A system of regulatory control where a change from normal is detected and an adjustment is effected until normal levels are reestablished.

Negative Work   Force times distance applied in the same direction as the pull of gravity; assisted by gravity.

Nerve Cell   See *Neuron*.

Nerve Conduction Velocity   The speed of travel of nerve impulses along nerve axons or fibers; faster for large fibers and faster still for medullated (insulated) ones.

Nerve Impulse   An electrical disturbance at the point of stimulation of a nerve that is self-propagated along the entire length of the axon.

Net Oxygen Cost   The amount of oxygen, above resting values, required to perform a given amount of work. Also referred to as *net cost of exercise*.

Neurohypophysis   The posterior lobe of the pituitary gland; so called because of its direct connection with the hypothalamus of the brain; secretes ADH and oxytocin.

Neuromuscular (Myoneural) Junction   The union of a muscle and its nerve. Also referred to as the *motor endplate*.

Neuron   A nerve cell consisting of a cell body (soma), with its nucleus and cytoplasm, dendrites and axon.

Nicotinamide Adenine Dinucleotide   An acceptor and carrier of hydrogen from various reaction sites in the cytosol and Krebs Cycle to the electron transport system.

Nitrogen Balance   A monitor of daily protein balance; a positive nitrogen balance means that nitrogen intake from protein is equal to or slightly greater than nitrogen loss.

Nitrogen Narcosis (Raptures of the Deep)   A condition affecting the central nervous system (much as does alcohol) due to the forcing (by pressure) of nitrogen into solution within the body; symptoms include dizziness, slowing of mental processes, euphoria, and fixation of ideas.

Nodes of Ranvier   Those areas on a medullated nerve that are devoid of a myelin sheath.

Nomogram   A graph enabling one to determine by aid of a straightedge the value of a dependent variable when the values of two independent variables are known.

Nonmyelinated Nerve Fiber   A nerve fiber entirely devoid of a myelin sheath.

Norepinephrine   A hormone secreted by the medulla of the adrenal gland that has effects on the heart, the blood vessels, metabolism, and the central nervous system. Also, the major neurotransmitter substance released at the ends of the sympathetic postganglionic fibers of the autonomic nervous system.

O

Obesity   An excessive accumulation and storage of fatty tissue; greater than 20% above ideal body weight for size, age, and gender; also, a BMI over 30.

One Repetition Maximum (1 RM)   The largest amount of weight that can be lifted only once without a substantial period of rest and recovery.

Osmosis   The diffusion through a semipermeable membrane of a solvent such as water from a lower to a more concentrated solution.

Osmotic Pressure   The force per unit area needed to stop osmosis.

Osteoporosis   Condition of the bones where they become very thin and brittle due to loss of mineral content; bones are susceptible to deformation and fracture.

Outer Vesicles   The terminal ends of the longitudinal tubules of the sarcoplasmic reticulum which store Ca^{++}; also called outer cisterns and terminal cisternae.

Ovaries   Reproductive glands of the female that contain the ova or germ cells; production site of estrogen (estradiol) and progesterone; lesser amounts of testosterone and androstenedione (male hormones).

Overload Principle   Progressively increasing the volume of exercise during workouts over the course of the training program as fitness capacity improves.

Overtraining   Imbalance between high volume and/or high intensity training and adequate recovery, resulting in disturbances in physical performance, biologic function, and mood state.

Oxidation   The removal of electrons.

Oxidation-reduction   Biochemical reactions where hydrogens (and/or electrons) are removed from a molecule (oxidation). When hydrogens are added to a molecule it is called reduction. Combining oxygen with hydrogen involves both oxidation and reduction.

Oxidative Phosphorylation   Process within the electron transport system of the mitochondrion that couples the liberation of energy from hydrogens to the synthesis of ATP and the formation of metabolic H_2O.

Oxidative State Regulation   A mechanism of control of cellular metabolism that is closely linked to the relative availability of oxygen and subsequent activation of the electron transport system enzyme, cytochrome oxidase.

Oxygen Consumption   The amount or rate at which oxygen can be consumed per minute.

Oxygen Debt   The amount of oxygen consumed during recovery from exercise, above that ordinarily consumed at rest in the same time period. There is a rapid component (alactacid) and a slow component (lactacid).

Oxygen Deficit   The time period during exercise in which the level of oxygen consumption is below that necessary to supply all the ATP required for the exercise; the time period during which an oxygen debt is contracted.

Oxygen Poisoning (Toxicity)   A condition caused by breathing oxygen under high pressure. Symptoms include tingling of fingers and toes, visual disturbances, auditory hallucinations, confusion, muscle and lip twitching, nausea, vertigo, and convulsions.

Oxygen System   An aerobic energy system in which ATP is manufactured when food (principally sugar and fat) is broken down. This system produces ATP most abundantly and is the prime energy source during long-lasting (endurance) activities.

Oxygen Transport System ($\dot{V}O_2$)   Composed of the stroke volume (SV), the heart rate (HR), and the arterial-mixed venous oxygen difference (a-$\bar{v}O_2$ diff.). Mathematically, it is defined as $\dot{V}O_2 = SV \times HR \times$ a-$\bar{v}O_2$ diff.

Oxyhemoglobin ($HgbO_2$) · Hemoglobin chemically combined with oxygen.

Oxyhemoglobin ($HgbO_2$) Dissociation Curve   The graph of the relationship between the amount of oxygen combined with hemoglobin and the partial pressure of oxygen.

Oxytocin   A hormone secreted by the posterior lobe of the pituitary gland that stimulates milk ejection and contraction of the pregnant uterus.

P

Pancreas   Endocrine gland responsible for the synthesis and secretion of two hormones important to blood glucose regulation; insulin from its beta cells and glucagon from its alpha cells.

Parasympathetic   Pertaining to the craniosacral portion of the autonomic nervous system.

Parathyroid Gland   Tiny endocrine glands imbedded in the dorsal surface of the thyroid gland; secretes parathyroid hormone (PTH), which increases Ca^{++} absorption.

Parathyroid Hormone (PTH)   A hormone secreted by the parathyroid gland that causes an increase in the blood calcium levels; also called parathormone.

Parietal Pleura   See *Pleura*.

Paroxysmal Tachycardia   A sudden onset of rapid heart rate; from paroxysmal meaning sharp or sudden and tachycardia meaning an increased heart rate, usually faster than 100 beats · min^{-1}.

Partial Pressure   The pressure exerted by a single gas in a gas mixture or in a liquid.

Passive (resting) Recovery   A period following exercise when no cool-down movement or less intense activity is practiced, i.e., the subject remains sedentary during recovery from exercise.

PC   See *Phosphocreatine*.

Perimysium   A connective tissue surrounding a fasciculus or muscle bundle.

Periodization   The structured, sequential development of athletic skill or the physiologic capacity brought about by organizing training regimens into blocks of time (macrocycles, mesocycles).

Periosteum   A fibrous membrane surrounding bone.

Peritoneum   The thin membrane that secretes serous fluid and lines the walls of the abdominal cavity and encloses the viscera.

Peritonitis   Inflammation of the peritoneum.

pH   The power of the hydrogen ion; the negative logarithm of the hydrogen ion concentration.

Phenotypic Properties   Characteristics of a muscle fiber specific to its classification type, such as contraction speed and rate of fatigue.

Phosphagen   A group of compounds; collectively refers to ATP and PC.

Phosphagen System   See *ATP-PC System*.

Phosphocreatine (PC)   A chemical compound stored in muscle, which when broken down aids in manufacturing ATP.

Phospholipids   A class of waxy compounds characterized by phosphoric acid as a hydrolysis product along with a long chain carbon compound such as a fatty acid or sphingol.

Photosynthesis   The process whereby green plants manufacture their own food from carbon dioxide, water, and energy from the sun.

Placebo   An inert substance having the identical physical characteristics of a real drug.

Plasma   The liquid portion of the blood.

Plasmolysis   The shrinking of a cell such as the red blood cell.

Pleura (singular); Pleurae (plural)   A thin membrane that secretes serous fluid and lines the thoracic wall (parietal pleura), the diaphragm (diaphragmatic pleura), and the lungs (visceral pleura).

Pleural Cavity   The potential space between the parietal and visceral pleura.

Plyometrics   A method of strength and power training that involves an eccentric loading of muscles and tendons followed by a quickly timed concentric contraction.

Pneumothorax   The entrance of air into the pleural cavity.

Polycythemia   An increased production of red blood cells.

Polysaccharides   Complex sugars such as glycogen and starch; carbohydrates where numerous glucose molecules are attached to one another in chainlike structures.

Polyunsaturated Fatty Acid   A long chain of carbon atoms bonded to hydrogen atoms, which includes two or more double bonds between carbon atoms in place of hydrogen atoms.

Ponderal Index   Body height divided by the cube root of body weight.

Positive Energy Balance   A condition in which more energy (food) is taken in than is given off; body weight increases as a result.

Positive Work   Force times distance applied in opposition to the pull of gravity.

Posterior Lobe   The portion of the pituitary gland located closest to the spinal cord (posterior position); also called the *neurohypophysis.*

Postsynaptic Neuron   A nerve cell located distal to a synapse.

Power*   The rate of performing work; the product of force and velocity. The rate of transformation of metabolic potential energy to work or heat (SI unit; watt).

Preload   Stretch placed on the cardiac muscle fiber(s) just prior to contraction.

Premotor Area   The area of the brain just forward of the primary motor cortex.

Pressure   Force per unit area.

Primary Motor Cortex   That area of the brain (cortex) containing groups of motor neurons other than Betz cells.

Progesterone   A hormone secreted by the ovary that promotes further development of the uterus and mammary glands.

Progressive-Resistance Exercise (PRE)   Comprehensive term to cover a wide variety of muscular strength or endurance training practices where progressive overload is emphasized.

Prolactin or **Lactogenic Hormone (LTH)**   A hormone secreted by the anterior lobe of the pituitary gland that stimulates secretion of milk after pregnancy.

Prolactostatin   A substance produced by the hypothalamus that on release can inhibit the secretion of prolactin from the adenohypophysis; also called prolactin inhibiting factor (PIF).

Proprioceptive Neuromuscular Facilitation (PNF)   A method for improving joint flexibility by contracting against opposition, then relaxing and stretching further.

Proprioceptor   Sensory organs found in muscles, joints, and tendons, which give information concerning movement and position of the body (kinethesis).

Prostaglandins   A class of hormones found in nearly all cellular membranes; have a fatty acid as their molecular base; may regulate resting blood flow through vasodilation; numerous other effects suggested.

Protein   A compound containing amino acids.

Protein Expression   The end result of multiple sources of control that results in the synthesis of specific structural or enzymatic proteins.

Proton   A positively charged particle.

Protoplasm   Living matter, the substance of which animal and vegetable tissues are formed.

Psychrometer   An instrument used for measuring the relative humidity.

Pulmonary Circuit   The flow of arterial blood from the heart to the pulmonary (lung) capillaries and of venous blood from the pulmonary capillaries back to the heart.

Pyramidal (Corticospinal) Tract   The area in which impulses from the motor area of the cortex are sent down to the anterior motoneurons of the spinal cord.

Pyruvic Acid   A three-carbon by-product resulting from the metabolism of glucose within the cytoplasm of the cell; enters Krebs Cycle for further breakdown (oxygen available) or is converted to lactic acid (oxygen lacking).

Q_{10} Effect   An increase in the speed of cellular metabolic reactions as a result of an increase in body temperature. The 10 is from culture studies indicating that reaction speeds double with a 10 degree (C) increase in temperature.

Radiation   The transfer of heat between objects through electromagnetic waves.

Rate-Limiting Enzymes   A few enzymes that serve as "gate-keepers"—i.e., they control the rate at which glycolytic and mitochondrial metabolic reactions are allowed to proceed.

Rate-Pressure Product   The product of heart rate and systolic blood pressure, which provides a noninvasive estimate of myocardial oxygen consumption.

Receptor   A sense organ that receives stimuli.

Reciprocal Inhibition   Basic reflex that causes antagonist muscle group to relax while agonist group is undergoing concentric contraction.

Recovery Oxygen   Net amount of oxygen consumed during recovery from exercise; oxygen consumed in excess of the amount consumed at rest over the same time period (reported in liters).

Reflex   An automatic response induced by stimulation of a receptor.

Relative Humidity   Ratio of water vapor in the atmosphere to the amount of water vapor required to saturate the atmosphere at the same temperature.

Releasing Factor   A group of specific substances produced by the hypothalamus that can stimulate or inhibit the release of all hormones produced by the adenohypophysis with the exception of the endorphins.

Relief Interval   In an interval-training program, the time between work intervals as well as between sets.

Repetition Maximum (RM)   The maximal load that a muscle group can lift over a given number of repetitions before fatiguing. For example, a 10 RM load is the maximal load that can be lifted over ten repetitions.

Repetitions   In an interval-training program, the number of work intervals within one set. For example, six 220 m runs would constitute one set of six repetitions.

Repolarization   A negative change back toward the resting membrane potential (reverse spike) of neural or muscle cells; semi-permeability restored, K^+ pumped out.

Residual Volume (RV)   Volume of air remaining in the lungs at end of maximal expiration.

Respiration   A cellular process where food substrates are broken down to CO_2 and H_2O in the presence of O_2 to liberate chemical energy.

Respiratory Exchange Ratio (R)   The ratio of the amount of carbon dioxide produced by the body to the amount of oxygen consumed ($\dot{V}CO_2/\dot{V}O_2$).

Rest-Recovery   Resting during recovery from exercise.

Rest-Relief   In an interval-training program, a type of relief interval involving moderate moving about, such as walking and flexing of arms and legs.

Resting Membrane Potential   The electrical difference between the inside and outside of the cell (i.e., across the cell membrane) at rest.

Ribose   A five-carbon sugar molecule that when linked to adenine forms adenosine, the molecular foundation for ATP, ADP, and AMP.

Risk Factor   A condition, trait, or habit that is associated with an increased risk or danger of developing a specific health problem in the future.

S

Saline   A 0.9% salt solution that is isotonic to the blood.

Saltatory Conduction   The propagation of a nerve impulse from one node of Ranvier to another along a medullated fiber.

Sarcolemma   The muscle cell membrane.

Sarcomere   The distance between two Z lines; the smallest contractile unit of skeletal muscle.

Sarcopenia   Aging associated muscle wasting that results in lower basal metabolic rate, weakness, reduced activity levels, decreased bone density, and lowered caloric needs.

Sarcoplasm   Muscle protoplasm.

Sarcoplasmic Reticulum   A network of tubules and vesicles surrounding the myofibril.

Saturated Fatty Acids   A fatty acid where all carbon atoms of the chain structure are filled with hydrogen atoms (i.e., there is no double bonding); often found in animal fats, eggs, and dairy products.

Second Wind   A phenomenon characterized by a sudden transition from an ill-defined feeling of distress or fatigue during the early portion of prolonged exercise to a more comfortable, less stressful feeling later in the exercise.

Semipermeable Membrane   A membrane permeable to some but not all particles or substances.

Sensory Fiber   See *Afferent Nerve.*

Sensory Neuron   A nerve cell that conveys impulses from a receptor to the central nervous system. Examples of sensory neurons are those excited by sound, pain, light, and taste.

Serotonin   An excitatory neurotransmitter chemical.

Serous Fluid   A watery fluid secreted by the pleurae.

Set   In an interval training program, a group of work and relief intervals.

Sinoatrial Node (S-A Node)   A specialized area of tissue located in the right atrium of the heart, which originates the electrical impulse to initiate the heartbeat.

Size Principle   Recruitment of motor units within muscle on the basis of the size of their motoneurons; small ones recruited first, then intermediate, then large ones.

Sliding Filament Theory   A proposed mechanism for muscle action where shortening and elongation are the result of actin protein filaments sliding inward and outward over myosin protein filaments.

Slow Component (of recovery)   The slow decline in oxygen consumption during recovery (reported in liters) lasting up to 60 minutes or more; follows the initial fast component; formerly lactacid oxygen debt.

Slow-Twitch (ST) Fiber   A muscle fiber characterized by slow contraction time, low anaerobic capacity, and high aerobic capacity, all making the fiber suited for low-power output activities. Also known as *Type I fiber.*

Sodium-Potassium Pump   A cellular phenomenon requiring ATP energy to remove Na^+ from and move K^+ into the cell interior against their diffusion gradients and electrochemical forces.

Soma   The cell body of a neuron.

Somatic   Pertaining to the body.

Somatomedins   A class of substances produced by the liver and several other tissues as a result of growth hormone influence; comprised of amino acid chains; stimulate the growth of muscle and cartilage by turning on phases of protein synthesis.

Somatostatin   A substance produced by the hypothalamus that on release can inhibit the secretion of growth hormone from the adenohypophysis; also called *growth hormone release inhibiting hormone (GHRIH).*

Somatotype   The body type or physical classification of the human body.

Spatial Summation   An increase in responsiveness of a nerve resulting from the additive effect of numerous nearby stimuli.

Specific Gravity   The ratio of the density of an object to the density of water.

Specific Heat   The heat required to change the temperature of a unit mass of a substance by one degree.

Specificity of Training   Principle underlying construction of a training program for a specific activity or skill and the primary energy system(s) involved during performance. For example, a training program for sprinters would consist of repeated bouts of sprints in order to develop both sprinting performance and the ATP-PC system.

Spirometer   A device used to collect, store, and measure either inspired or expired gas volume.

Sports Medicine   Umbrella term that refers to all aspects of sport and exercise science, especially as used in the U.S.; examples are kinesiology, cardiac rehabilitation, adult fitness, and athletic medicine.

Sprint Training   A type of training system employing repeated sprints at maximal speed.

Squeeze   Extravasation of blood into the conjunctivae of the eyes while descending underwater as a result of inadequate equilibration of pressures inside and outside of the diving mask; exhale into mask to equilibrate.

Static Contraction   See *Isometric Contraction.*

Static Flexibility   The range of motion about a joint; usually measured with a goniometer or flexometer as the arc in degrees at the end when there is no joint motion.

Steady State   Pertaining to the time period during which a physiological function (such as $\dot{V}O_2$) remains at a constant (steady) value.

Steroid   A general class of hormones including derivatives of the male sex hormone, testosterone, which has masculinizing properties.

Stimulus (singular); Stimuli (plural)   An agent, act, or influence that modifies the activity of a receptor or irritable tissue.

STPD   Standard temperature, pressure, dry (see appendix C).

Strength*   The maximal force or torque a muscle or muscle group can generate at a specific or determined velocity.

Stretch Reflex   Contraction of muscles to produce movement or tension due to muscle spindle stretch via a sharp tap on tendon or pull of gravity on skeleton.

Stroke   Interference with the blood supply to the brain causing necrosis; due to embolus, thrombus, or burst vessel; due to cerebral artery atherosclerosis or aneurysm.

Stroke Volume (SV)   The amount of blood pumped by the left ventricle per beat of the heart.

Sudomotor   Pertaining to activation of the sweat glands.

Supplemental Motor Area (SMA)   Medial portion of cortical area 6, which is called the sports skills area; sends axons to directly innervate distal motor units.

Sympathetic   Pertaining to the thoracolumbar portion of the autonomic nervous system.

Synapse   The connection or junction of one neuron to another.

Synaptic Cleft   The gap or space between presynaptic and postsynaptic neurons.

Synaptic Knobs   Expanded regions on the ends of axon that store a chemical transmitter substance (neurotransmitter) for release across the synaptic cleft.

Systemic Circuit   The flow of arterial blood from the heart to the body tissues (such as the muscles) and of the venous blood from the tissues back to the heart.

Systole   The contractile or emptying phase of the cardiac cycle.

Systolic Blood Pressure (SBP)   The highest pressure existing in the arteries; the result of ventricular systole.

T

T-System and **T-Tubules**   Invaginations of the sarcolemma that function as part of the sarcoplasmic reticulum; also called *transverse tubules.*

Tachycardia   A heart rate greater than 100 and less than 250 beats per minute.

Tapering   The concept of decreasing training duration by ~ 80% to 90% some five days to three weeks before athletic competition, which may or may not be accompanied by an associated increase in training intensity.

Target Cell (also **Target Tissue**)   The specific cells or tissues on which hormones exert their biological effect; see also target organ; tropic used as a suffix with a hormone identifies the target organ (e.g., somatotropic hormone).

Target Heart Rate (THR)   A predetermined heart rate to be obtained during exercise.

Target Organ   The organ on which a hormone has an effect.

Telemetry   Transmission of physiological measurements via radio waves. Requires a sensor and transmitter worn by the subject and a distant receiver/recorder to obtain and record the signals, e.g., HR and ECG measurement on a track runner or swimmer.

Temperature   The degree of sensible heat or cold.

Temporal Summation   An increase in responsiveness of a nerve, resulting from the additive effect of frequently occurring stimuli.

Tension   Force applied to a structure that does not move; in muscle, the static or isometric tension developed with the recycling of ATP at cross-bridge sites.

Testes   Reproductive glands of the male that produce the germ cells (spermatozoa); production site of androgens (testosterone and androstenedione).

Testosterone   The male sex hormone secreted by the testicles; it possesses masculinizing properties.

Tetanus   The maintenance of tension of a motor unit at a high level as long as the stimuli continue or until fatigue sets in.

Thalamus Subcortical portion of the brain that, along with the basal ganglia, provides an information loop back to the premotor cortex to assist in the selection and initiation of chosen movements.

Thermodynamics The science of the transformation of heat and energy.

Threshold for Excitation The minimal electrical level at which a neuron will transmit or conduct an impulse.

Thrombus A blood clot that remains at the point of its formation.

Thyroid Gland Endocrine gland located on the upper part of the trachea just below the larynx (voice box); major hormones secreted are thyroxin and triiodothyronine (raises metabolism of all cells) and calcitonin (inhibits Ca^{++} removal from bone).

Thyroid-Stimulating Hormone (TSH) A hormone secreted from the anterior lobe of the pituitary gland that stimulates production and release of the thyroid hormones, thyroxin and triiodothyronine.

Thyroxin A hormone secreted by the thyroid gland that causes an increase in metabolic rate.

Tidal Volume Volume of air inspired or expired per breath.

Tissue-Capillary Membrane The thin layer of tissue dividing the capillaries and an organ (such as skeletal muscle); site at which gaseous exchange occurs.

Tonic Neck Reflexes Assists young children under the age of 4 to 6 months to correct losses in balance; elicited by rotational movements of the head.

Torque* The effectiveness of a force to overcome the rotational inertia of an object. The product of force and the perpendicular distance from the line of action of the force to the axis of rotation (SI unit; netwon-meter).

Total Lung Capacity (TLC) Volume of air in the lungs at the end of maximal inspiration.

Training An exercise program to develop an individual for a particular event. Increasing skill of performance and energy capacities are of equal consideration.

Training Distance In an interval training program, the distance of the work interval; for example, running 200 m.

Training Duration The length of the training program.

Training Effect Temporary or extended changes in body structure or function caused by repeated bouts of exercise.

Training Frequency The number of times per week for the training workout.

Training Time The rate at which the work is to be accomplished during a work interval in an interval training program.

Transverse Tubules Function to connect outer vesicles of the sarcoplasmic reticulum to one another; run at right angles or transversely to myofibrils of muscle.

Triglycerides The storage form of fatty acids.

Triiodothyronine A hormone secreted by the thyroid gland that causes an increase in metabolic rate.

Trophic Pertaining to nutrition or nourishment.

Tropomyosin A protein involved in muscular contraction.

Troponin A protein involved in muscular contraction.

Twitch A brief period of contraction followed by relaxation in the response of a motor unit to a stimulus (nerve impulse).

Type I Muscle Fiber Commonly used classification for muscle fibers that display characteristics of slow twitch, nonfatigue, and mostly oxidative metabolism.

Type II$_A$ Muscle Fiber Commonly used classification for muscle fibers that display characteristics of fast twitch, medium fatigue, and combined oxidative and glycolytic metabolism.

Type II$_B$ Muscle Fiber Commonly used classification for muscle fibers that display characteristics of fast twitch, rapid fatigue, and mostly glycolytic metabolism.

Type II$_C$ Muscle Fiber Commonly used classification for muscle fibers that display characteristics of fast twitch but cannot be further classified; predominant early fetal type but very few present after maturity.

U

Unsaturated Fatty Acids A fatty acid where all the carbon atoms of the chain structure are not filled with hydrogen atoms (i.e., there is double bonding); found mostly in vegetable oils.

V

Valsalva Maneuver Making an expiratory effort with the glottis closed.

Vasoconstriction A decrease in the diameter of a blood vessel (usually an arteriole) resulting in a reduction of blood flow to the area supplied by the vessel.

Vasodilation An increase in the diameter of a blood vessel (usually an arteriole) resulting in an increased blood flow to the area supplied by the vessel.

Vasomotor Pertaining to vasoconstriction and vasodilation.

Vegan People who eat no animal products.

Vein A vessel carrying blood toward the heart.

Venoconstriction A decrease in the diameter of a vein.

Venous return Amount of blood returned to the right heart via the systemic venous system.

Ventilatory Efficiency The amount of ventilation required per liter of oxygen consumed (i.e., $\dot{V}_E/\dot{V}_{O_2}$).

Viscera (plural); Viscus (singular) The internal organs of the body.

Visceral Pertaining to the viscera.

Visceral Pleura See *Pleura*.

Vital Capacity (VC) Maximal volume of air forcefully expired after maximal inspiration.

Vitamin An organic material in the presence of which important chemical (metabolic) reactions occur.

W

Water-Soluble Vitamins   A category of vitamins that are water soluble and consequently are not stored in the body and must be constantly supplied in the diet; examples are vitamin C and B-complex vitamins.

Watt   A unit of power.

Wave Summation   Increase in force due to an additive effect caused by rapid stimulation of a single motor unit.

WBGT (Wet Bulb Globe Temperature) Index   An index calculated from dry bulb, wet bulb, and black bulb temperatures. It indicates the combined severity of the environmental heat conditions.

Weight*   The force exerted by gravity on an object (SI unit: newton; traditional unit: kilogram of weight). (Note: mass = weight $\cdot$ acceleration due to gravity^{-1}).

Wet Bulb Thermometer   An ordinary thermometer with a wetted wick wrapped around the bulb. The wet bulb's temperature is related to the amount of moisture in the air. When the wet bulb and dry bulb temperatures are equal, the air is completely saturated with water and the relative humidity is equal to 100%.

Work*   Force expressed through a displacement but with no limitation on time (SI unit: joule). (Note: 1 newton $\times$ 1 meter = 1 joule.)

Work Interval   That portion of an interval-training program consisting of the work effort.

Work-Relief   In an interval-training program, a type of relief interval involving light or mild exercise such as rapid walking or jogging.

Work-Relief Ratio   In an interval-training program, a ratio relating the duration of the work interval to the duration of the relief interval. As an example, a work-relief ratio of 1:1 means that the durations of the work and relief intervals are equal.

Z

Z Line   A protein band that defines the distance of one sarcomere in the myofibril.

Credits

LINE ART AND TEXT CREDITS

Figure 1.1   Reprinted with permission of the American College of Sports Medicine, *ACSM's Membership Directory,* May 1995–April 1996. © American College of Sports Medicine 1993.

Figure 7.14   From Arthur C. Guyton, *Textbook of Medical Physiology,* 6th ed. Copyright © 1981 W. B. Saunders Company, Philadelphia, Pennsylvania. Reprinted by permission.

Figure 7.15   From Arthur C. Guyton, *Textbook of Medical Physiology,* 6th ed. Copyright © 1981 W. B. Saunders Company, Philadelphia, Pennsylvania. Reprinted by permission.

Figure 13.2   From A. M. Gordon, et al., "Variation in Isometric Tension with Sarcomere Length in Vertebrate Muscle Fibers," in *Journal of Physiology* (London), 1966, 184:170–192. Copyright © 1966 The Physiology Society, London. Reprinted by permission.

Figure 17.2   From Arthur C. Guyton, *Textbook of Medical Physiology,* 6th ed. Copyright © 1981 W. B. Saunders Company, Philadelphia, Pennsylvania. Reprinted by permission.

List 1–5   From American College of Sports Medicine, 1984. "ACSM position stand on the use of anabolic-androgenic steroids in sports." In *Medicine Science in Sports Exercise,* 1984, 19(5):534–539. Copyright © 1984 Williams & Wilkins, Baltimore, MD. Reprinted by permission.

Appx Figure F.1   From B. Saltin and P. Åstrand, "Maximal Oxygen Uptake in Athletes." In *Journal of Applied Physiology,* 1967, 23:353–358. Copyright © 1967 American Physiological Society, Bethesda, MD. Reprinted by permission.

PHOTO CREDITS

Chapter 1 Opener: Planet Art; **Chapter 2 Opener:** Health and Medicine; **Chapter 3 Opener:** © Marc Romanelli/Image Bank; **Chapter 4 Opener:** Courtesy Henry Ford Health Systems; **Figure 4.14:** Photo courtesy of Polar Electro Inc.; **Chapter 5 Opener:** © Ed Reschke; **Chapter 6 Opener:** © Ed Reschke; **Figure 6.14:** Photo courtesy Steven Keteyian; **Chapter 7 Opener:** Photo courtesy Steven Keteyian; **Chapter 8 Opener:** © David M. Phillips/Science Source/Photo Researchers, Inc.; **Chapter 10 Opener:** © Garry Gay/Image Bank; **Chapter 11 Opener:** © Bill Bachman/Photo Researchers, Inc.; **Chapter 12 Opener:** Source: © Gerhart Gsheidle/Peter Arnold, Inc.; **Chapter 13 Opener:** Source: © Bachmann/Photo Researchers, Inc.; **Chapter 14 Opener:** Tony Stone Images/Bruce Ayers; **Chapter 15 Opener:** © Explorer/Photo Researchers, Inc.; **Chapter 16 Opener:** Source: Philippe Plailly/Eurelios/Science Photo Library/Photo Researchers, Inc.; **Figure 16.1:** Source: Dr. Ray Clark & Mervyn Goff/Science Photo Library/Photo Researchers, Inc.; **Figures 16.2a,b:** Source: R. B. Mazess, Lunar Radiation Corporation, Madison, WI; **Figure 16.4:** Source: Prof. P. Motta/Dept. of Anatomy/University "LA SAPIENZA," Rome/Science Photo Library/Photo Researchers, Inc.; **Figure 16.9:** Source: © Manny Millan/Sports Illustrated; **Figure 16.10:** Source: © Tony Freeman/PhotoEdit; **Chapter 17 Opener:** Source: John Burbridge/Science Photo Library/Photo Researchers, Inc.; **Chapter 18 Opener:** Source: Lou Jones/The Image Bank; **Figure 18.2:** Source: Courtesy of Mark Perkins; **Chapter 19 Opener:** © Hanson Carroll/Peter Arnold, Inc. **Chapter 20 Opener:** Source: © Tony Stone Images/Chris Harvey; **Figure 20.14:** Source: NASA

Index